DENTAL HYGIENE
Applications to Clinical Practice

Rachel Kearney Henry, RDH, MS
Assistant Professor
Dental Hygiene Graduate Program Director
Ohio State College of Dentistry, Division of Dental Hygiene

Maria Perno Goldie, RDH, BA, MS
Past President, International Federation of Dental Hygienists
Past President, American Dental Hygienists' Association
Owner, Seminars for Women's Health and Sex-Based Medicine
Editorial Director, RDH eVillage Focus
Cofounder, International Dental Hygiene Educator's Forum

F.A. Davis Company • Philadelphia

F. A. Davis Company
1915 Arch Street
Philadelphia, PA 19103
www.fadavis.com

Printed in the United States of America

Last digit indicates print number: 10 9 8 7 6 5 4 3 2 1

Publisher: Quincy McDonald
Developmental Editor: Patricia Gillivan
Director of Content Development: George Lang
Art and Design Manager: Carolyn O'Brien

As new scientific information becomes available through basic and clinical research, recommended treatments and drug therapies undergo changes. The author(s) and publisher have done everything possible to make this book accurate, up to date, and in accord with accepted standards at the time of publication. The author(s), editors, and publisher are not responsible for errors or omissions or for consequences from application of the book, and make no warranty, expressed or implied, in regard to the contents of the book. Any practice described in this book should be applied by the reader in accordance with professional standards of care used in regard to the unique circumstances that may apply in each situation. The reader is advised always to check product information (package inserts) for changes and new information regarding dose and contraindications before administering any drug. Caution is especially urged when using new or infrequently ordered drugs.

Library of Congress Cataloging-in-Publication Data

Names: Henry, Rachel Kearney, author. | Goldie, Maria Perno, author.
Title: Dental hygiene : applications to clinical practice / Rachel Kearney
  Henry, Maria Perno Goldie.
Description: Philadelphia : F.A. Davis Company, [2016] | Includes
  bibliographical references and index.
Identifiers: LCCN 2015047564 | ISBN 9780803625686
Subjects: | MESH: Dental Care | Oral Hygiene
Classification: LCC RK60.5 | NLM WU 29 | DDC 617.6/01--dc23 LC record
available at http://lccn.loc.gov/2015047564

I am dedicating this book to all of my current, former, and future students. Because you have decided to pursue a career in dental hygiene, I am able to do what I truly love, teach. I hope that your experiences during school carry with you for a lifetime, especially the love of learning. There is always something to learn, no matter how many degrees you attain or how long you have been practicing.

I would also like to thank those people who have given me the opportunity to learn more, try new things, and take risks. I would not be where I am without the opportunities I was given at The Ohio State University and all of the people there who supported, encouraged, and made those opportunities possible.

Finally, to my daughter, Harper, as a parent I am always trying to be an example for you without limiting your possibilities and potential. May this book be one example of hard work, creativity, and determination that you can look up to.

—R.C.K.

My parents, Rose and Raymond Perno (both now deceased),
for always inspiring me to strive for more...
My husband George, for his support
Rachel Kearny Henry, my co-editor,
for working diligently these last few years to get this text published...
To my many mentors who have set examples for excellence...
And to all others who have contributed to the production of this textbook.

—M.P.G.

Preface

The profession of dental hygiene has evolved in its 100-plus years of existence and continues to evolve. Expectations of dental hygienists continue to increase. In addition to performing oral prophylaxis and scaling and root planing, individuals entering and working in this field must be able to think critically, use evidence-based practices, and advocate for their patients. Although much of this book focuses on the process of care and clinical skills, being a dental hygienist involves more than just clinical care. Dental hygienists must demonstrate professionalism, advocate for patients and the profession, and develop leadership skills.

ORGANIZATION

This book is organized following the process of care assessment, diagnosis, planning, implementation, evaluation, and documentation. The process of care is bookended by a chapter overview of the profession of dental hygiene and information on skill sets and foundational knowledge important in the practice of dental hygiene and by a chapter on lifelong learning in the profession.

Each chapter begins with a statement of relevance to clinical practice. As the book's title implies, the focus of each chapter is to relate the content to scenarios, skills, and situations that dental hygiene clinicians face daily. Each chapter has strong relevance to the clinical practice of a dental hygienist. Information and topics were carefully chosen to be beneficial and relatable to the practice of dental hygiene.

FEATURES

- *Application to Clinical Practice:* This feature is included in most chapters and highlights the application of knowledge to clinical practice, translating didactic knowledge to practical experiences.
- *Advancing Technologies:* Because dental hygiene is a technology-rich field, it would be difficult to cover all technology used in the profession of dental hygiene.

This feature highlights new and emerging technologies used in practice.
- *Evidence-Based Practice:* A chapter in the book is devoted to evidence-based practice, but this feature also appears throughout the entire book, highlighting cases in which evidence-based practice can be applied.
- *Spotlight on Public Health:* With the high demand for oral health services in such venues as long-term care facilities, nursing homes, and other settings influenced by the change in demographics, this feature presents information on the access-to-care issue, as well as highlighting what dental hygienists are doing to improve access to care.
- *Teamwork:* Teamwork and interdisciplinary collaboration are essential to successful oral health care. The Teamwork feature addresses opportunities for alliances with other oral health professionals, other health professionals, and the community.
- *Professionalism:* Professionalism can encompass a wide range of issues, including ethics, appearance, professional organization involvement, and attitude. This feature focuses on what it means to be a professional and how this applies to the career of dental hygiene.
- *Procedures:* Procedures are written in a step-by-step format with rationales to help students understand how and why a step should be performed.
- *Case Study and Review:* A case study with associated questions is presented at the end of each chapter to give students an opportunity to apply chapter content to clinical situations.
- *Active Learning:* Each student has his or her own learning style, whether it is visual, auditory, read/write, or kinesthetic. These exercises address different types of learners to create a strong learning environment and to help students develop critical thinking skills.

SUPPORT MATERIALS

DentalCareDecisions.com: Dental Care Decisions combines a fully searchable eBook with a wide variety of multisensory applications that build student recognition of key equipment and anatomical features, develop critical retention of important dental procedures, build students' ability to communicate with clients and colleagues, test students' content knowledge on applicable material, and push students to make critical clinical and administrative decisions based on realistic simulated audio scenarios. The students' progress, time spent, and performance in Dental Care Decisions is captured by the system and provided to the student and his or her instructor. In addition, a collaborative work environment is provided through small-group functionality and a group discussion board. Access to Dental Care Decisions is provided through the use of an access code that is provided for free in each new copy of the text. Codes may also be purchased at DentalCareDecisions.com and through access cards sold in the student's bookstore.

Student Workbook: Additional practice activities and study support are provided by a separate for-sale workbook available with the text. Written to provide specific support for the text, the workbook provides the perfect portable support tool to study for examinations or for the National Board Dental Hygiene Examination.

Instructor Resources: Instructional support is provided to adopters through the protected instructor area for the text at davisplus.fadavis.com. Support materials include a full test bank, lecture PowerPoint, *Instructor's Guide*, image resource library with all of the images from the text, and resource packs that provide easy transfer of the instructor materials to the most popular learning management systems.

TO THE STUDENT

As you read this book, keep in mind that you are becoming a professional. With the knowledge and skill you gain from reading this book and completing your program, and the education provided to you by your faculty, you are taking on a responsibility. This responsibility is one of advocacy, education, quality care, and community. Being a dental hygienist is a demanding and rewarding career. We sincerely hope that the profession of dental hygiene will give you as much as it has given to us.

Contributors

Brooke Agado, RDH, BS
Idaho State University
Pocatello, ID
Chapter 38, Respiratory

Cynthia C. Amyot, MSDH, EdD
University of Missouri
Kansas City, MO
Chapter 2, Legal and Ethical Considerations

Deb Astroth, RDH, BS
Examiner for the Central Regional Dental Testing
Service, Inc
*Chapter 18, Dental Hygiene Diagnosis, Treatment Plan,
Documentation, and Case Presentation*

Susan Badanjak, RDH, ADH
OralChroma Breathomics/Halitomics Educator
Montreal, Canada
Chapter 6, Evidence-Based Care

Shirley Beaver, RDH, PhD
Fox College Dental Hygiene Program
University of Illinois at Chicago College of Dentistry
Chicago, IL
Chapter 4, Health Education and Promotion

Kathryn Bell, RDH, MS
Pacific University
Eugene, OR
Chapter 43, Immune System

Lisa Bilich, RDH, BS, MEd
Eastern Washington University
Cheney, WA
Chapter 35, Maintenance

Ann Brunick, RDH, MS
University of South Dakota
Vermillion, SD
Chapter 32, Nitrous Oxide/Oxygen Sedation

Lillian Caperila, RDH, MEd
Premier Dental Products Company
Chapter 28, Management of Dentin Hypersensitivity

Michele Carr, RDH, MA
Ohio State University
Columbus, OH
Chapter 25, Power Scaling

Christine Charles, RDH, BS
Retired, Johnson & Johnson
Chapter 14, Indices

Aubreé Chismark, MSDH, RDH
West Coast University
Anaheim, CA
Chapter 29, Polishing

Ugo Covani, MD, DDS
University of Pisa
Istituto Stomatologico Toscano
Lido di Camaiore, Italy
*Chapter 27, Nonsurgical and Surgical Periodontal
Therapy*

Ann-Marie C. DePalma, CDA, RDH, MEd, FADIA,
FAADH
Patterson Dental
Chapter 52, Practice Management

Catherine Draper, RDH, MS
Foothill College
Los Altos Hills, CA
Chapter 23, Prostheses and Appliances

Bernadette Alvear Fa, DDS
University of the Pacific
San Francisco, CA
Chapter 36, Introduction to Special Needs

Deborah Finnegan, RDH
Middlesex Community College
Lowell, MA
Chapter 6, Evidence-Based Care

Jackie Foskett, RDH, BA, CH
Healing Hypnotherapy
Chapter 31, Dental Fear and Anxiety Management

Jacques Freudenthal, RDH, MHE
Idaho State University
Pocatello, ID
Chapter 21, Cariology and Caries Management

Danielle Furgeson, RDH, EFDA
Clinical Assistant Professor, University of Michigan
Ann Arbor, MI
Chapter 40, Mental Health

Nicole Giesey, RDH, BSDH, MSPTE
Youngstown State University
Youngstown, OH
Chapter 30, Esthetics

Maria Perno Goldie, RDH, BA, MS
Chapter 1, Dental Hygiene as a Profession
Chapter 5, Immunology and the Oral Systemic Link
Chapter 47, Men's and Women's Health Issues

Shawneen M. Gonzalez, DDS, MS
Oregon Health & Science University
Portland, OR
Chapter 15, Radiology

Sara Gordon, DDS, MSc
University of Washington
Seattle, WA
Chapter 10, Extraoral and Intraoral Examination

Gwen Grosso, RDH, MS
University of New Haven
New Haven, CT
Chapter 33, Local Anesthesia

JoAnn R. Gurenlian, RDH, PhD
Idaho State University
Pocatello, ID
Chapter 8, Comprehensive Medical and Oral Health History
Chapter 18, Dental Hygiene Diagnosis, Treatment Plan, Documentation, and Case Presentation

Ellen R. Guritzky, AAS, RDH, BS, MSJ
Crosstex, A Cantel Medical Company
Little Falls, NJ
Chapter 28, Management of Dentin Hypersensitivity

Ann L. Hague, PhD, MS, RD, LD, RDH, CLT
The RiteBite
Lewis Center, OH
Chapter 16, Dietary Assessment and Nutritional Counseling

Lisa Handa, BS, RDHAP, MS
Miles of Smiles, Inc.
Chapter 46, Pediatric Patient

R. Donald Hoffman, DMD, MEd, PhD
University of Pittsburgh
Pittsburgh, PA
Chapter 37, Cardiovascular Disease

Janet Jaccarino, CDA, RDH, MA
School of Health Related Professions
Rutgers, the State University of New Jersey
Wayne, NJ
Chapter 39, Sensory Disability: Vision and Hearing Impairment

Carol A. Jahn, RDH, MS
Water Pik, Inc.
Chapter 19, Devices

Kris Johnson, RDHAP, BA, MSDH(c)
Aptos, CA
Chapter 54, Lifelong Learning

Tara Johnson, RDH, PhD
Idaho State University
Pocatello, ID
Chapter 45, Cancer

Mark G. Kacerik, RDH, MS
University of New Haven
New Haven, CT
Chapter 51, Dental and Medical Emergencies

Juli Kagan, RDH, MEd
Nova Southeastern University
Fort Lauderdale, FL
Chapter 24, Ergonomics

Diane P. Kandray, RDH, MEd
Youngstown State University
Youngstown, OH
Chapter 12, Hard Tissue Examination

Rachel C. Kearney, RDH, MS
Ohio State College of Dentistry
Columbus, OH
Chapter 9, Assessment Instruments
Chapter 22, Sealants

Noel Kelsch, RDHAP
Chapter 50, Alternative Practice Settings

Ashlynn Le, RDH, MA
West Coast University
Anaheim, CA
Chapter 26, Instrumentation Principles and Techniques

Susan Long, RDH, EdD
University of Arkansas for Medical Sciences
Little Rock, AR
Chapter 11, The Periodontal Examination

Deborah Lyle, RDH, BS, MS
Water Pik, Inc.
Chapter 17, Risk Assessment

Stacy McCauley, RDH, MS
Inspired Hygiene
Chapter 3, Communication Skills

L. Teal Mercer, RDH, MPH
University of New Haven
West Haven, CT
Chapter 33, Local Anesthesia

Anne H. Missig, RDH, MA, BA
Chapter 41, Neurological Impairments

Amy Molnar, RDH, MDH
The Ohio State University
Columbus, OH
Chapter 46, Pediatric Patient

Kay Murphy, CDA, RDH, MS
City College of San Francisco
San Francisco, CA
Chapter 48, The Elderly

Christine N. Nathe, RDH, MS
The University of New Mexico
Albuquerque, NM
Chapter 53, Career Development

Kristina Okolisan-Mulligan, RDH, BS
University of Detroit Mercy
Detroit, MI
Chapter 10, Extraoral and Intraoral Examination

Jonathan B. Owens, RDH, MS
Howard University
Washington, DC
Chapter 54, Lifelong Learning

Ruthie Palich, RDH, BSAS, MHHS
Youngstown State University
Youngstown, OH
Chapter 30, Esthetics

Jennifer Pieren, RDH, MS
Youngstown State University
Youngstown, OH
Chapter 20, Dentifrices and Mouthrinses

Renee G. Prajer, RDH, MS
University of New Haven
New Haven, CT
Chapter 51, Dental and Medical Emergencies

Angelina E. Riccelli, BS, MS, RDH
University of Pittsburgh
Pittsburgh, PA
Chapter 37, Cardiovascular Disease

Massimilliano Ricci, DDS, PhD
Oral Surgeon, Private Practice
Istituto Stomatologico Toscano
Tuscany, Italy
Chapter 27, Nonsurgical and Surgical Periodontal Therapy

Sandra Roggow, RDH, BA
Director of Communications
fiteBac Skin Care, LLC
Chapter 42, Endocrine System

Jessica Salisbury, RDH, MSA
The Ohio State University
Columbus, OH
Chapter 5, Immunology and the Oral Systemic Link

Kathi R. Shepherd, RDH, MS
University of Detroit Mercy
Detroit, MI
Chapter 10, Extraoral and Intraoral Examination

Suzanne Smith, RDH, MEd
Youngstown State University
Youngstown, OH
Chapter 7, Exposure and Infection Control

Silvia A. Stefan, RDH, MHHS
Youngstown State University
Youngstown, OH
Chapter 13, Biofilm, Calculus, and Stain

Paul Subar, DDS, EdD
University of the Pacific
San Francisco, CA
Chapter 36, Introduction to Special Needs

Mechee Thomas, RDH, BSAS, MSPTE
Youngstown State University
Youngstown, OH
Chapter 30, Esthetics

Maureen Vendemia, RDH, MEd
Professor Emeritus
Youngstown State University
Youngstown, OH
Chapter 7, Exposure and Infection Control

Janet Weber, RDH, MEd
University of Maryland
College Park, MD
Chapter 44, Hematological Considerations

Ann O'Kelley Wetmore, RDH, BSDH, MSDH
Eastern Washington University
Cheney, WA
Chapter 34, Evaluation

Kristin Wolf, BA, RDH, MSHS
Retired from Cuyahoga Community College
Cleveland, OH
Chapter 49, Physical Impairment

Allen Wong, DDS, EdD
University of the Pacific
San Francisco, CA
Chapter 36, Introduction to Special Needs

Douglas A. Young, DDS, MBA, MS, EdD
University of the Pacific
San Francisco, CA
Chapter 36, Introduction to Special Needs

Reviewers

Crystal Adams, RDH, BS
Dental Hygiene
Catawba Valley Community College
Taylorsville, NC

Susan Alexander, MEd, RDH
Dental Hygiene
Weber State University
Ogden, UT

Joanna Allaire, RDH, MDH
Periodontics and Dental Hygiene
The University of Texas School of Dentistry
Houston, TX

Jordan Rae Anderson, RDH, BS, MDH
Dental Hygiene
University of Louisiana at Monroe
Monroe, LA

Lynn D. Austin, RDH, MPH (ABD)
Allied Health
Western Kentucky University
Bowling Green, KY

Deborah Blythe Bauman, BSDH, MS
Dental Hygiene
Old Dominion University
Norfolk, VA

Josette Beach, RDH, MS
Dental Sciences
Portland Community College
Portland, OR

Christine French Beatty, RDH, PhD
Dental Hygiene Program
Texas Woman's University
Denton, TX

Sandra N. Beebe, RDH, PhD
Dental Hygiene/Health Care Management
Southern Illinois University Carbondale
Carbondale, IL

Stephanie Bossenberger, RDH, MS
Dental Hygiene
Weber State University
Ogden, UT

Denise Bowers, RDH, PhD
Dental Hygiene
James A. Rhodes State College
Lima, OH

Constance Clark, MEd, RDH
Allied Health
Columbus State Community College
Columbus, OH

Dawn E. Conley, RDH, MEd
Dental
Camden County College
Blackwood, NJ

Shelly M. Costley, RDH, MEd
Dental Hygiene
Weber State University
Ogden, UT

Ann E. Curtis, RD, RDH, MS, CAS
Dental Health
University of Maine at Augusta
Bangor, ME

Tammy Deese, RDH
Dental Hygiene/Health Science
Darton State College
Albany, GA

Alice S. Derouen, RDH, MEd
Dental Sciences
Horry Georgetown Technical College
Conway, SC

Lisa M. Duddy, DHSc, MHSc, RDH
Dental Hygiene
New York University
New York, NY

Melissa Efurd, RDH, EdD
Dental Hygiene
University of Arkansas for Medical Sciences
Little Rock, AR

Michelle M. Florencki, RDH, MEd
Dental Hygiene Program
Cuyahoga Community College
Cleveland, OH

Jacquelyn L. Fried, RDH, BA, MS
Health Promotion and Policy
University of Maryland Dental School
Baltimore, MD

Josephine Galliano, MEd, RDH
Dental Hygiene
Chabot College
Hayward, CA

Jane Gauthier, RDH, MEd, CHES
Dental Hygiene
Quinsigamond Community College
Worcester, MA

Theresa Grady, RDH, MEd
Math, Science and Health Careers
Community College of Philadelphia
Philadelphia, PA

Patricia D. Guenther, RDH, MA
Allied Health & Human Service
Lansing Community College
Lansing, MI

Christine A. Halvorson, CDA, RDH, BS
Allied Dental Programs
Asheville-Buncombe Technical Community College
Asheville, NC

Stephanie Harrison, RDH, BS, MA
Dental Hygiene
Community College of Denver
Denver, CO

Linda Hecker, CDA, RDH, BS, MA
Dental Hygiene
Burlington County College
Pemberton, NJ

Harold Henson, RDH, MEd, PhD
Associate Professor
Interim Director, Dental Hygiene Program; Director
for the Center for Teaching and Learning
The University of Texas at Houston School
of Dentistry
Houston, TX

Janet L. Hillis, RDH, MA
Dental Hygiene
Iowa Western affiliated with Creighton University
School of Dentistry
Council Bluffs, IA

Kathleen Hodges, RDH, MS
Department of Dental Hygiene, Office of Medical
and Oral Health
Idaho State University
Pocatello, ID

Kim T. Isringhausen, BSDH, RDH, MPH
Dental Hygiene
Virginia Commonwealth University School
of Dentistry
Richmond, VA

Laura Joseph, RDH, BS, MS, EdD
Dental Hygiene
Farmingdale State College of New York
Farmingdale, NY

Tobin Korsch, RDH, BSDH, MS
Dental Hygiene
NWCCD–Sheridan College
Sheridan, WY

Demetra Logothetis, RDH, MS
Dental Hygiene
University of New Mexico
Albuquerque, NM

Frances McConaughy, RDH MS
Dental Hygiene
Weber State University
Ogden, UT

Jacquelyne L. Mack, RDH, MS, MPA
Dental
Florida State College at Jacksonville
Jacksonville, FL

Paula Malcomson, BA, BEd
Dental Programs
Fanshawe College
London, Ontario, Canada

Robin Blatt Matloff, RDH, BSDH, JD
Dental Hygiene
Mount Ida College
Newton, MA

Bernice A. Mills, RDH, MS
Dental Hygiene
University of New England
Portland, ME

Tammy Morgan-Schubert, RDH
Health Sciences—Dental
Cambrian College
Sudbury, Ontario, Canada

Jo Ann Allen Nyquist, BSDH, MA, EDS
Dental
Wayne County Community College District
Detroit, MI

Mary S. Pelletier, CRDH, MEd
Dental Hygiene
Indian River State College
Fort Pierce, FL

Pamela P. Quinn, RDH, BSE, MSEd
Dental Hygiene
SUNY Canton
Rome, NY

Amanda Richardson, RDH, BS, MDH
Dental Hygiene
University of Louisiana at Monroe
Monroe, LA

Leah Rising, RDH, MS
Associate Professor, Dental Hygiene and Dental
Assisting Programs
Gulf Coast Community College
Panama City, FL

Laurel L. Risom, RDH, BS, MPH
Dental Hygiene
University of Bridgeport
East Lyme, CT

Shawna Rohner, RDH, BS, MS
School of Dental Health Science
Pacific University
Hillsboro, OR

Michelle M. Singley, RDH, EDM
Dental Hygiene
Lewis and Clark Community College
Godfrey, IL

Margaret J. Six, RDH, MSDH
Dental Hygiene
West Liberty University
West Liberty, WV

Rebecca M. Smith, RDH, BHSA, MPH, EdD
Dental Hygiene
Miami Dade College
Miami, FL

C. Kelly Turner, BA (Kin), RDH
Health Sciences: Dental
Fanshawe College of Applied Arts and Technology
London, Ontario, Canada

Cynthia P. Wampler, RDH, MS
Dental Programs
Florida State College at Jacksonville
Jacksonville, FL

Cheryl Westphal, RDH, MS
Dental Hygiene
New York University
New York, NY

Rosalyn Word, RDH, MPA
Dental Hygiene
Tennessee State University
Nashville, TN

Mary Yeomans, BLS, BS, RDH
Program Coordinator Dental Hygiene
Cambrian College of Applied Arts and Technology
Sudbury, Ontario, Canada

Debbie Zuern, RDH, BS, MEd
Dental Hygiene
Darton College
Albany, GA

Acknowledgments

Many people helped us turn this vision into reality, including:

- The contributors, who shared their expertise and remained committed and patient throughout the process
- Quincy McDonald, Publisher, who supported and guided us
- Pat Gillivan, Developmental Editor, whose editorial skills helped shape the text
- F. A. Davis editorial and production teams, who helped with this publication
- The Ohio State University Dental School, for allowing us to use their laboratory for the textbook photo shoot
- Jason Torres, photographer, for his creativity and skills in taking many of the photos for this textbook

Contents
at a Glance

PART I INTRODUCTION TO DENTAL HYGIENE

Chapter 1 Dental Hygiene as a Profession, 2
Chapter 2 Legal and Ethical Considerations, 8
Chapter 3 Communication Skills, 24

PART II THE DENTAL HYGIENIST'S ROLE IN THE DELIVERY OF HEALTH CARE

Chapter 4 Health Education and Promotion, 40
Chapter 5 Immunology and the Oral Systemic Link, 54
Chapter 6 Evidence-Based Care, 70

PART III INFECTION CONTROL

Chapter 7 Exposure and Infection Control, 84

PART IV ASSESSMENT

Chapter 8 Comprehensive Medical and Oral Health History, 120
Chapter 9 Assessment Instruments, 154
Chapter 10 Extraoral and Intraoral Examination, 166
Chapter 11 The Periodontal Examination, 190
Chapter 12 Hard Tissue Examination, 216
Chapter 13 Biofilm, Calculus, and Stain, 230
Chapter 14 Indices, 240
Chapter 15 Radiology, 254
Chapter 16 Dietary Assessment and Nutritional Counseling, 270
Chapter 17 Risk Assessment, 290

PART V DIAGNOSIS AND PLANNING

Chapter 18 Dental Hygiene Diagnosis, Treatment Plan, Documentation, and Case Presentation, 304

PART VI TREATMENT

Preventative Treatment
Chapter 19 Devices, 318
Chapter 20 Dentifrices and Mouthrinses, 334
Chapter 21 Cariology and Caries Management, 344
Chapter 22 Sealants, 364
Chapter 23 Prostheses and Appliances, 374
Therapeutic Treatment
Chapter 24 Ergonomics, 394
Chapter 25 Power Scaling, 408
Chapter 26 Instrumentation Principles and Techniques, 416
Chapter 27 Nonsurgical and Surgical Periodontal Therapy, 432
Chapter 28 Management of Dentin Hypersensitivity, 448
Chapter 29 Polishing, 460
Chapter 30 Esthetics, 474

PART VII ANXIETY AND PAIN MANAGEMENT

Chapter 31 Dental Fear and Anxiety Management, 490
Chapter 32 Nitrous Oxide/Oxygen Sedation, 512
Chapter 33 Local Anesthesia, 526

PART VIII EVALUATION

Chapter 34 Evaluation,   548
Chapter 35 Maintenance,   566

PART IX CARING FOR PATIENTS WITH SPECIAL NEEDS

Chapter 36 Introduction to Special Needs,   580
Chapter 37 Cardiovascular Disease,   590
Chapter 38 Respiratory,   610
Chapter 39 Sensory Disability: Vision and Hearing Impairment,   620
Chapter 40 Mental Health,   634
Chapter 41 Neurological Impairments,   646
Chapter 42 Endocrine System,   662
Chapter 43 Immune System,   672
Chapter 44 Hematological Considerations,   690
Chapter 45 Cancer,   706
Chapter 46 Pediatric Patient,   722

Chapter 47 Men's and Women's Health Issues,   736
Chapter 48 The Elderly,   750
Chapter 49 Physical Impairment,   772
Chapter 50 Alternative Practice Settings,   790

PART X EMERGENCY MANAGEMENT

Chapter 51 Dental and Medical Emergencies,   802

PART XI FUTURE VISION

Chapter 52 Practice Management,   820
Chapter 53 Career Development,   834
Chapter 54 Lifelong Learning,   842
Glossary,   854
Photo and Illustration Credits for Part Openers and Chapter Openers,   876
Index,   878

Contents

PART I INTRODUCTION TO DENTAL HYGIENE

Chapter 1 Dental Hygiene as a Profession,   2
Relevance to Clinical Practice,   3
Dental Hygiene,   3
History of the Dental Hygiene Profession,   4
Scope of Practice of Dental Hygienists,   4
  Standards of Practice and the Process of Care,   4
Roles of a Dental Hygienist,   4
  Clinician,   4
  Corporate,   4
  Public Health,   5
  Researcher,   5
  Educator,   5
  Administrator,   5
  Advocate,   5
Professional Organizations,   5
The Future of Dental Hygiene,   5
Case Study,   6
Case Study Exercises,   6
Review Questions,   6
Active Learning,   7
References,   7
Chapter 2 Legal and Ethical Considerations,   8
Relevance to Clinical Practice,   9
Law and Ethics,   9
Law and the Practice of Dental Hygiene,   10
  Licensure,   10
  State Dental Boards,   10
  Criminal and Civil Law,   11
  Managing Risk,   12
Ethical Principles and Core Values,   12
  Autonomy,   12
  Beneficence,   15
  Nonmaleficence,   15
  Justice,   15
  Veracity,   16
  Confidentiality,   16
  Societal Trust,   18
Ethical Decision-Making Model,   18

Case Study,   20
Case Study Exercises,   20
Review Questions,   20
Active Learning,   21
References,   21
Chapter 3 Communication Skills,   24
Relevance to Clinical Practice,   25
What Is Communication?,   25
  Definition,   25
  Types of Communication,   25
Why Do We Have Communication Breakdowns?,   27
Dialoguing with the Patient,   28
Motivational Interviewing: Strategies to Elicit Real
  Change,   30
  The Spirit of Motivational Interviewing: Three Pillars,   31
Creating Value for the Dental Hygiene Appointment
  Through Communication,   32
Practicing Dental Hygiene in a Multicultural
  Society,   33
Case Study,   36
Case Study Exercises,   36
Review Questions,   37
Active Learning,   37
References,   38

**PART II THE DENTAL HYGIENIST'S ROLE IN
THE DELIVERY OF HEALTH CARE**

Chapter 4 Health Education and Promotion,   40
Relevance to Clinical Practice,   41
Health and Wellness,   41
Health Promotion,   42
U.S. Health-Care System,   42
  Health Disparities,   42
  Healthy People 2020,   42
Behavioral Change Models,   44
  Maslow's Hierarchy of Needs,   44
  Learning Ladder,   44
  Locus of Control,   44

Theory of Reasoned Action/Planned Behavior,   45
Social Learning and Social Cognitive Theories,   45
Health-Promotion Models,   45
Health Belief Model,   45
Transtheoretical/Stages of Change Model,   46
Dental Hygiene Process of Care,   46
Assessment,   46
Dental Hygiene Diagnosis,   47
Planning,   47
Implementation,   47
Evaluation,   47
Documentation,   47
Prevention and Promotion for Specific
Populations,   47
Infants and Children (Birth to 12 Years),   47
Adolescents (13–18 Years),   47
Elderly,   48
Smoking Cessation,   48
Five A's of Tobacco Cessation,   48
Ask. Advise. Refer.,   48
Smoking Cessation for Adolescents,   49
Changing Habits,   49
Case Study,   50
Case Study Exercises,   50
Review Questions,   51
Active Learning,   51
References,   51

**Chapter 5 Immunology and the Oral Systemic
Link,   54**
Relevance to Clinical Practice,   55
Immune System,   55
Innate and Acquired Immunity,   56
Complement Cascade,   56
Research,   57
Pathogenesis of Periodontal Diseases, Chronic
Inflammation, and Risk Assessment,   57
Oral–Systemic Connections,   60
Cardiovascular Diseases,   60
Diabetes,   61
Respiratory Infections,   63
Pregnancy,   64
Improving Outcomes,   64
Case Study,   65
Case Study Exercises,   65
Review Questions,   65
Active Learning,   66
References,   66

Chapter 6 Evidence-Based Care,   70
Relevance to Clinical Practice,   71
What Is Evidence-Based Care in Dental Hygiene
Practice?,   72
The Evidence-Based Process,   72

Good Clinical Question Framework,   72
Scenario A,   72
PICO Question,   72
Scenario B,   72
Levels of Evidence,   73
Meta-analysis,   73
Systematic Review,   73
Randomized Controlled Trial,   74
Cohort Study,   74
Case–Control Study,   74
Case Series and Case Report,   74
Literature Review,   74
In Vitro and Animal Studies,   74
Literature Search,   74
Peer-Reviewed Articles,   75
Resources,   75
Evidence Evaluation,   75
Evidence Evaluation Example,   76
Evidence Application,   76
Outcome Evaluation,   76
Parts of a Scientific Paper,   76
Title,   76
Abstract,   76
Introduction,   76
Materials/Methods,   76
Results,   76
Discussion/Conclusion,   76
Conflicts of Interest,   76
Acknowledgments,   77
References,   77
Introduction to Writing a Scientific Paper,   77
Formulate the Idea and Conduct Research,   77
Write the First Draft,   77
*Editing: Choosing Precise Words and Using Proper
Grammar,*   77
Continuity, Sentence Length, and Flow,   77
Plagiarism,   78
Case Study,   78
Case Study Exercises,   78
Review Questions,   79
Active Learning,   79
References,   80

PART III INFECTION CONTROL

Chapter 7 Exposure and Infection Control,   84
Relevance to Clinical Practice,   85
Transmissible Diseases,   85
HIV/AIDS,   86
Hepatitis,   86
Hepatitis A,   87
Hepatitis B,   88

Hepatitis C,   88

Hepatitis D,   88

Hepatitis E,   88

Human Herpesviruses 1 to 8,   89

Human Herpesviruses 1 and 2,   89

Human Herpesvirus 3,   89

Human Herpesvirus 4,   90

Human Herpesvirus 5,   90

Human Herpesviruses 6 and 7,   90

Human Herpesvirus 8,   90

Tuberculosis,   90

Other Diseases and Conditions,   91

Resources and References for Infection Control,   93

Engineering and Work Practice Controls,   94

Personal Protective Equipment,   95

Protective Clothing,   95

Protective Eyewear,   95

Masks,   96

Face Shields,   96

Gloves,   96

Infection Control in the Patient Care Area,   99

*Clinical Contact Surfaces and Housekeeping
   Surfaces,*   100

Cleaning and Disinfection,   100

Surface Barriers,   100

Dental Radiograph Equipment and the Darkroom,   100

Dental Unit Water Lines,   102

Evacuation Systems,   102

Dental Laboratory,   102

Environmental Protection,   103

Instrument Processing,   103

Area,   103

Transportation,   103

Cleaning and Decontamination,   104

*Preparation, Packaging, and Sterilization
   Monitoring,*   104

Sterilization   105

Chemical Disinfectants,   106

Disposal of Waste and Sharps,   108

Preventive Steps,   109

Patient,   109

Dental Health-Care Personnel,   109

Health Maintenance,   109

Hair,   109

Jewelry,   110

Hand Care: Fingernails and Skin,   110

Hand Lotions,   110

*Selection, Storage, and Dispensing of Hand Hygiene
   Products,*   110

Hand Hygiene Methods,   111

Exposure Control Plans,   112

Record-Keeping and Documentation,   112

Case Study,   114

Case Study Exercises,   114

Review Questions,   114

Active Learning,   115

References,   115

PART IV ASSESSMENT

**Chapter 8 Comprehensive Medical and Oral
   Health History,   120**

Relevance to Clinical Practice,   121

Role and Importance of the Patient History,   121

Patient Interview,   121

Types of Record Forms,   122

History-Taking Preparation,   122

Focus of Health Histories,   123

Samples of Health Histories,   123

Elements of the Health History,   127

Biographical Data,   127

Chief Complaint,   129

General Health,   130

Oral History,   130

Personal Psychosocial History,   138

Medication History,   139

Vital Signs,   140

Decision-Making,   147

Premedication,   148

Updating the Health History,   150

Case Study,   151

Case Study Exercises,   151

Review Questions,   151

Active Learning,   152

References,   152

Chapter 9 Assessment Instruments,   154

Relevance to Clinical Practice,   155

What Are Assessment Instruments?,   155

Mouth Mirror,   155

Purpose,   155

Design,   156

Types,   156

Grasp,   157

Retraction,   157

Clear Vision,   157

Explorer,   157

Purpose,   157

Design,   158

Types,   158

Grasp,   158

Activation and Technique,   158

Periodontal and Furcation Probes,   160

Purpose,   160

Types and Design,   161

Grasp,   161
Activation and Technique,   161
Summary,   163
Case Study,   163
Case Study Exercises,   163
Review Questions,   163
Active Learning,   164
References,   164

Chapter 10 Extraoral and Intraoral Examination,   166
Relevance to Clinical Practice,   168
Objectives of the Extraoral and Intraoral Examination,   168
Common Oral Pathology,   168
Common Variations From Normal,   168
Common Reactive Lesions,   170
Oral Cancer,   172
How and Why Does Oral Cancer Arise?,   172
What Is the Appearance of Oral Cancer?,   173
How Is Oral Cancer Diagnosed?,   174
What Is the Treatment and Prognosis of Dysplasia and of Oral Cancer?,   175
Extraoral and Intraoral Examination,   176
Diagnostic Aids,   182
Use of Imaging for Screening,   182
Vital Tissue Staining and Other Visualization Adjuncts,   184
Biopsy Techniques,   185
Types of Biopsies,   185
Submitting a Biopsy,   186
Generating a Pathology Report,   187
Case Study,   187
Case Study Exercises,   187
Review Questions,   188
Active Learning,   188
References,   188

Chapter 11 The Periodontal Examination,   190
Relevance to Clinical Practice,   191
Introduction to Periodontal Anatomy,   191
Gingiva,   191
Cementum,   193
Periodontal Ligament,   193
Alveolar Bone,   193
Periodontal Examination,   194
Periodontal Risk Assessment,   194
Periodontal Screening Examination,   195
Comprehensive Periodontal Assessment,   195
Procedure,   196
Radiographic Evaluation of the Periodontium,   204
Adjunctive Techniques,   205
Microbiological Testing,   205

Biochemical Assays of Gingival Crevicular Fluid,   205
Subgingival Temperature,   205
Genetic Tests,   206
Classification of Periodontal Diseases,   206
Charting Examination Findings,   208
Case Study,   212
Case Study Exercises,   212
Review Questions,   213
Active Learning,   213
References,   213

Chapter 12 Hard Tissue Examination,   216
Relevance to Clinical Practice,   217
Dental Charts,   217
Tooth Numbering Systems,   217
Universal,   217
Palmer Notation,   217
International Standards Organization,   217
Charting Dental Conditions,   219
Classification of Dental Caries,   221
Identifying Noncarious Lesions,   223
Abfraction,   223
Abrasion,   223
Attrition,   223
Decalcification,   223
Erosion,   224
Hypoplasia,   224
Hypocalcification (Hypomineralization),   224
Analysis of Occlusion,   224
Class I,   224
Class II,   224
Class III,   225
Malrelations of Teeth,   225
Anterior Crossbite,   225
Posterior Crossbite,   225
Edge-to-Edge Bite,   225
End-to-End Bite,   226
Open Bite,   226
Underjet,   226
Overbite,   226
Overjet,   227
Measuring Overbite and Overjet,   227
Malposition of Individual Teeth,   227
Occlusal Considerations,   227
Pulp Testing,   227
New Technology for Identification of Dental Caries,   227
Case Study,   228
Case Study Exercises,   228
Review Questions,   229
Active Learning,   229
References,   229

Chapter 13 Biofilm, Calculus, and Stain,   230
   Relevance to Clinical Practice,   231
   Soft Deposits,   231
      Acquired Pellicle,   231
      Biofilm,   231
      Materia Alba,   232
      Food Debris,   232
   Oral Malodor,   232
   Hard Deposits,   233
      Calculus Formation,   233
      Calculus Location,   233
      Forms of Calculus,   233
      Calculus Detection,   233
      Calculus Removal,   235
   The Body's Response to Biofilm and Calculus,   235
   Staining and Tooth Discoloration,   235
      Intrinsic Stains,   235
      Extrinsic Stains,   236
   Case Study,   236
   Case Study Exercises,   236
   Review Questions,   237
   Active Learning,   237
   References,   237
Chapter 14 Indices,   240
   Relevance to Clinical Practice,   241
   What Are Indices?,   241
   Types of Clinical Indices,   242
      Dental Caries Indices,   243
      Indices That Measure Oral Hygiene Status (Plaque Biofilm, Debris, and Calculus),   244
      Indices That Measure Gingival and Periodontal Health Status,   247
      Indices Contribute to Oral Disease Risk Assessment,   249
   Case Study,   250
   Case Study Exercises,   250
   Review Questions,   250
   Active Learning,   251
   References,   251
Chapter 15 Radiology,   254
   Relevance to Clinical Practice,   255
   ALARA,   255
   What Are X-rays?,   255
      Definition,   255
      History,   256
   Radiographic Terms,   256
      Definition,   256
      Relative Radiopacities/Radiolucencies,   258
      Normal Radiographic Appearances,   258
   Dental Imaging Systems,   259
      Types,   259
      Analog Film,   261
      Computed Radiography,   262
      Digital Radiography,   262

   Ionizing Radiation Protection Guidelines,   263
      Terminology,   263
      Effects on Biological Matter,   263
      Background Radiation Dose,   263
      Lead Apron and Thyroid Collar,   263
      Collimation,   264
      Radiation Exposure to the Operator,   264
      Prescription of Radiographs,   264
   Radiation Safety,   266
   Case Study,   266
   Case Study Exercises,   266
   Review Questions,   267
   Active Learning,   267
   References,   268
Chapter 16 Dietary Assessment and Nutritional Counseling,   270
   Relevance to Clinical Practice,   271
   Impact of Dietary Risk Factors on Oral Health,   271
      Oral Manifestations Associated With Nutrient Imbalance,   271
      Malnutrition and Periodontitis,   272
      Malnutrition and Oral Tissue Development,   272
      Fluid Imbalance and Xerostomia,   272
      Fermentable Carbohydrates and Dental Caries,   273
      Protective Foods and Beverages and Dental Caries,   273
      Dietary Pattern and Dental Caries,   273
      Consistency of Foods and Dental Caries,   273
      Dental Erosion,   273
   Impact of Dental/Oral Health on Diet,   273
   Dietary Assessment Procedures,   274
      Dietary Assessment Tools,   275
      Effective Communication Skills,   275
      Twelve Steps to Dietary Assessment,   277
   Interdisciplinary Care,   283
   Summary,   285
   Case Study,   286
   Case Study Exercises,   286
   Review Questions,   287
   Active Learning,   287
   References,   288
Chapter 17 Risk Assessment,   290
   Relevance to Clinical Practice,   291
   Oral Risk Assessment,   291
      Definitions,   291
      Modifiable Risk Factors,   292
      Nonmodifiable Risk Factors,   297
   Systematic Approach to Risk Assessment,   298
   Case Study,   299
   Case Study Exercises,   299
   Review Questions,   300
   Active Learning,   300
   References,   300

PART V DIAGNOSIS AND PLANNING

Chapter 18 Dental Hygiene Diagnosis, Treatment Plan, Documentation, and Case Presentation,   304
Relevance to Clinical Practice,   305
Dental Hygiene Diagnosis,   305
  Historical Perspective,   305
  Current Clinical Practice Standards,   305
  Definition,   305
  Purpose,   306
  Diagnostic Terminology,   306
Formulating the Dental Hygiene Diagnosis,   307
  Case Examples,   308
Treatment Plan,   308
  Treatment Options,   310
  Risk and Benefits of Treatment,   310
  Financial Implications,   310
  Case Examples,   310
Case Presentation,   312
Consent,   313
Documentation,   313
Case Study,   314
Case Study Exercises,   315
Review Questions,   315
Active Learning,   316
References,   316

PART VI TREATMENT

Chapter 19 Devices,   318
Relevance to Clinical Practice,   319
Toothbrushes,   319
  Manual Toothbrushes,   319
  Power Toothbrushes,   319
  The Scientific Evidence,   320
  Brush Selection and Usage,   321
Mechanical Interdental Cleaning,   322
  Dental Floss,   324
  Interdental Brushes,   325
  Wood Sticks,   326
  Floss Holders, Automated Flossers, and Toothpicks,   327
Pulsating Oral Irrigation,   327
  The Scientific Evidence,   328
Patient Education,   330
Case Study,   331
Case Study Exercises,   331
Review Questions,   331
Active Learning,   332
References,   332

Chapter 20 Dentifrices and Mouthrinses,   334
Relevance to Clinical Practice,   335
Regulation and Classification of Dentifrices and Mouthrinses,   335
Dentifrice,   335
  Inactive Ingredients in Dentifrices and Indications for Use,   335
  Active Ingredients in Dentifrices and Indications for Use,   336
Mouthrinses,   336
  Inactive Ingredients in Mouthrinses and Indications for Use,   336
  Active Ingredients in Mouthrinses and Indications for Use,   337
  Discussion,   338
Prescription Products,   338
Adverse Reactions and Special Considerations,   338
American Dental Association Seal of Acceptance,   339
Case Study,   340
Case Study Exercises,   340
Review Questions,   341
Active Learning,   341
References,   342

Chapter 21 Cariology and Caries Management,   344
Relevance to Clinical Practice,   345
Definitions and Terminology,   345
Cause of the Infection,   346
  Multifactorial Disease,   346
  Demineralization/Remineralization Process,   347
Preventive and Therapeutic Therapies,   348
  Fluoride Pastes, Gels, Foams, and Varnishes,   348
  Chlorhexidine Mouthrinses and Varnish,   349
  Additional Measures,   349
Classification of Carious Lesions,   350
  G.V. Black's Classification,   350
  Classification Systems by Caries Type,   350
Caries Detection Methods,   352
  Visual Inspection,   352
  Tactile Detection,   352
  Radiographic Detection,   352
  Emerging Technologies,   352
Caries Management,   353
  Dental Hygienist's Role in Caries Management,   353
  Risk Assessment,   354
Case Study,   359
Case Study Exercises,   359
Review Questions,   359
Active Learning,   360
References,   361

Chapter 22 Sealants,   364
Relevance to Clinical Practice,   365
What Are Sealants?,   365
  Definition,   365
  Composition,   365
  How Sealants Work,   366
Indications for Sealants,   366
  Risk Assessment,   366
  Tooth Anatomy,   366
  Contraindications,   366
Sealant Placement,   367
Retention and Replacement,   371
Discussion Issues,   371
  Bisphenol A and Estrogenicity,   371
  Sealants and Incipient Caries,   371
Case Study,   372
Case Study Exercises,   372
Review Questions,   372
Active Learning,   373
References,   373

Chapter 23 Prostheses and Appliances,   374
Relevance to Clinical Practice,   375
What Are Oral Appliances and Prostheses?,   375
Oral Appliances,   375
  Dental Hygiene Considerations,   376
  Patient Education,   378
  Why Replace Missing Teeth?,   378
  Understanding the Options for Tooth Replacement,   378
Oral Prostheses,   379
  Fixed Partial Denture,   379
  Types of Fixed Partial Dentures,   379
  Dental Hygiene Care Considerations,   379
  Patient Education,   379
  Removable Partial Dentures,   380
  Complete Dentures,   380
  Dental Hygiene Care Considerations,   380
  Professional Prosthesis and Appliance Care,   381
Complications Associated With Dental Prostheses and Appliances,   383
  Patient Education,   384
Dental Implants,   384
  From an Unpredictable Art to Standard of Care,   384
  Types of Dental Implants,   385
  Parts of an Endosteal Implant,   385
  Implant Restorations,   386
  Implant Prosthesis Retention Options,   386
  Implant–Bone–Soft Tissue Interfaces,   386
  Peri-implant Disease,   387
  Dental Hygiene Considerations,   387
  Discussion Issues,   390
Summary,   390
Case Study,   391
Case Study Exercises,   391

Review Questions,   391
Active Learning,   392
References,   392

Chapter 24 Ergonomics,   394
Relevance to Clinical Practice,   395
Ergonomics,   395
Common Dental Musculoskeletal Disorders,   395
  Prevention,   396
Low-Back Pain,   396
Anterior Version Pelvic Position,   396
Operator Stool,   397
  Chair Options,   398
Taking a Stand,   399
Posture,   399
  Loupes and Lighting,   400
Hand Instruments,   400
  Selecting Instruments,   400
Automated Instruments (Handpieces),   401
  Additional Tips to Improve Posture,   401
  Fitness Outside the Operatory,   401
Operatory and Office Exercises,   401
  Navel In and Up,   401
  Hands,   401
  Neck Stretches,   402
  Shoulder Stretches,   402
  Upper Body Stretches,   403
  Legs,   404
Summary,   405
Case Study,   405
Case Study Exercises,   405
Review Questions,   405
Active Learning,   406
References,   406

Chapter 25 Power Scaling,   408
Relevance to Clinical Practice,   409
What Are Power Scaling Devices?,   409
Types of Power Scaling Devices,   409
  Mechanism of Action,   409
  Frequency,   409
  Amplitude,   410
  Lavage,   410
  Advantages of Power Scaling Devices,   410
  Disadvantages of Power Scaling Devices,   410
  Indications for Use,   410
  Contraindications,   410
  Tip Types,   411
  Specialty Tips,   411
  Tip Designs,   411
Care and Maintenance of Equipment,   413
Microultrasonic Instruments,   413
Case Study,   414
Case Study Exercises,   414
Review Questions,   415

Active Learning,   415
References,   415
Chapter 26 Instrumentation Principles and Techniques,   416
Relevance to Clinical Practice,   417
Instrument Design,   418
    Handle,   418
    Shank,   418
    Working End Design,   419
Instrument Identification,   419
    Working End Identification,   420
    Instrument Classification,   420
Instrument Activation,   420
    Grasp,   420
    Adaptation,   420
    Angulation,   421
    Activation,   421
    Instrumentation Strokes,   421
    Using the Anterior Sickle,   423
    Using the Posterior Sickle,   423
    Calculus Removal Stroke with Universal Curet,   424
    Using the Universal Curet for the Anterior Region,   425
    Using the Universal Curet for the Posterior Region,   425
Types of Instruments,   425
    Gracey Curets,   425
    Hoes,   426
    Files,   426
Instrument Sharpening,   428
    Differentiating a Sharpened Instrument From a Dull One,   428
    Sharpening Stones,   428
    Principles of Sharpening,   428
Sharpening Curets,   428
    Gracey Curets,   428
    Universal Curets,   429
    Sickles,   429
Case Study,   429
Case Study Exercises,   429
Review Questions,   430
Active Learning,   430
References,   430
Chapter 27 Nonsurgical and Surgical Periodontal Therapy,   432
Relevance to Clinical Practice,   433
Oral–Systemic Link,   433
Nonsurgical Therapy,   433
    Local Drug Delivery,   435
    Systemic Antibiotics,   437
    Lasers,   437
    Perioscopy,   438
    Indications and Contraindications for Use of the Perioscope,   438

Using the Perioscopy System,   439
Periodontal Surgery: An Overview,   440
Periodontal Healing: What Is the Key?,   440
What Is the Correct Approach in Periodontology?,   440
What Are the Indications to a Surgical Approach?,   441
What Is the Aim of a Surgical Approach?,   441
Types of Periodontal Surgery,   441
    Gingivectomy,   441
    Flap Procedures,   441
    Replaced Flap,   441
    Repositioned Flap,   442
    Regenerative Periodontal Surgery,   442
    Complications of Periodontal Surgery,   442
    Sutures and Periodontal Dressings,   442
Dental Hygiene Considerations,   444
Periodontal Maintenance,   445
Case Study,   445
Case Study Exercises,   445
Review Questions,   445
Active Learning,   446
References,   446
Chapter 28 Management of Dentin Hypersensitivity,   448
Relevance to Clinical Practice,   449
Definition of Dentin Hypersensitivity,   449
    Dental Structures,   449
Causative and Predisposing Factors,   450
Prevalence of Dentin Hypersensitivity,   450
Dental Hygiene Diagnosis of Dentin Hypersensitivity,   452
Management of Dentin Hypersensitivity,   452
    Treatment Options,   453
    Delivery Modes,   454
    Treatment and Patient Education Plan,   454
Home-Applied Treatment Options,   455
Professional Treatment Options,   456
    Potassium Nitrate,   456
    Potassium Oxalates,   456
    Calcium Compounds,   456
    Adhesives and Resins,   456
    Miscellaneous Procedures,   456
    Laser Therapy,   456
    Restorative or Periodontal Plastic Procedures,   457
Case Study,   457
Case Study Exercises,   457
Review Questions,   458
Active Learning,   458
References,   458
Chapter 29 Polishing,   460
Relevance to Clinical Practice,   461
Stains,   461
    Extrinsic Stains,   461
    Intrinsic Stains,   461

Polishing,   461
  Selective Polishing,   461
  Abrasive Agents,   461
  Finishing Strips,   462
  Mohs Hardness Value,   462
  Therapeutic Polishing,   462
  Polishing Restorations,   463
  Manual Polishing,   463
  Power Polishing,   465
  Air Polishing,   468
  Air-Polishing Powders,   468
Case Study,   470
Case Study Exercises,   470
Review Questions,   470
Active Learning,   471
References,   471

Chapter 30 Esthetics,   474
Relevance to Clinical Practice,   475
What Are Esthetic Restorations?,   475
Indirect Esthetic Restorations,   476
  Inlay and Onlay,   476
  Crown,   476
  Materials,   476
  Traditional Crowning Process,   476
  Computer-Aided Design/Computer-Aided Manufacturing
    Restorations,   477
  Advantages and Disadvantages of Computer-Aided
    Design/Computer-Aided Manufacturing,   477
  Porcelain Veneer,   477
Direct Esthetic Restorations,   478
  Composites,   478
  Glass Ionomer,   478
  Dental Hygiene Considerations for Esthetic
    Restorations,   479
  Patient Education for Esthetic Restorations,   479
Tooth Whitening,   480
  External Methods,   480
  Internal,   481
Indications and Contraindications for Whitening,   482
Side Effects of Whitening,   482
Whitening Outcomes on Various Types of Enamel
  Conditions,   483
  Tobacco Use,   483
  Tetracycline Stains,   483
  Dental Fluorosis,   483
  Hypocalcification,   483
  Combination Therapy,   484
Patient Education for Post-Whitening Care,   484
Professionalism and Esthetic Dentistry,   484
  Ethical and Safety Considerations,   484
  Presenting a Treatment Plan,   484
Case Study,   485

Case Study Exercises,   485
Review Questions,   486
Active Learning,   486
References,   486

PART VII ANXIETY AND PAIN MANAGEMENT

**Chapter 31 Dental Fear and Anxiety
  Management,   490**
Relevance to Clinical Practice,   491
Definitions,   491
The Effects of Dental Anxiety,   492
  Onset and Etiology of Dental Fear and Anxiety,   492
Stress Response: The Sympathetic and
  Parasympathetic Nervous Systems in
  Action,   494
Management Program,   495
  Components of a Dental Fear and Anxiety Management
    Program,   495
  Cognitive and Behavioral Management,   499
  Pain Control Management,   505
Consideration and Management of the Anxious
  Child,   506
Summary,   506
Case Study,   507
Case Study Exercises,   508
Review Questions,   508
Active Learning,   509
References,   509

**Chapter 32 Nitrous Oxide/Oxygen
  Sedation,   512**
Relevance to Clinical Practice,   513
Introduction,   513
Indications,   514
Contraindications,   514
Gas Properties,   515
Respiratory Physiology,   515
Armamentarium,   516
Sedation Expectations,   518
  Ethical and Legal Responsibilities,   519
Preoperative Assessment,   519
Informed Consent,   519
Minimizing Trace Gas,   521
Recommendations for Best Practices,   522
Summary,   522
Case Study,   522
Case Study Exercises,   522
Review Questions,   523
Active Learning,   523
References,   523

Chapter 33 Local Anesthesia, 526
Relevance to Clinical Practice, 527
Local Anesthesia, 527
Nerve Conduction, 527
Amide and Ester Agents, 530
Pharmacokinetics, 530
Dosage, 531
Topical Anesthesia, 533
Injection Techniques, 538
Posterior Superior Alveolar Nerve Block, 538
Infiltration for Posterior Superior Alveolar, Middle
Superior Alveolar, and Anterior Superior Alveolar
Blocks, 538
Infraorbital Nerve Block, 539
Greater Palatine Block, 539
Nasopalatine Nerve Block, 540
Inferior Alveolar Nerve Block, 540
Gow-Gates, 541
Buccal Nerve Block, 541
Mental/Incisive (M/I) Nerve Block, 541
Adverse Systemic Reactions, 542
Medical Conditions, 542
Malignant Hyperthermia, 542
Methemoglobinemia, 542
Adverse Local Reactions, 542
Hematoma, 542
Paresthesia, 542
Trismus, 544
Needle Breakage, 545
Epithelial Desquamation, 545
Postinjection Lesions, 545
Case Study, 545
Case Study Exercises, 545
Review Questions, 545
Active Learning, 546
References, 546

PART VIII EVALUATION

Chapter 34 Evaluation, 548
Relevance to Clinical Practice, 549
What Is Evaluation?, 549
Taxonomy of Evaluation, 549
Evaluation Tools, 549
Evidence-Based Decision-Making, 554
Evaluation of Assessment Data, 554
Evaluation of Diagnosis, 555
Oral Pathology, 555
Evaluation of Plan, 556
Evaluation of Implementation, 556
Evaluation of Care, 556
Qualitative Evaluation, 557

Quantitative Evaluation of Treatment Outcomes
and Prognosis, 557
Referrals, 558
Professionalism and Quality Assurance, 561
Summary, 561
Case Study, 562
Case Study Exercises, 562
Review Questions, 563
Active Learning, 563
References, 563
Chapter 35 Maintenance, 566
Relevance to Clinical Practice, 567
What Is Oral Health?, 567
Definition, 567
Oral Health Versus Systemic Health, 567
Criteria for Determining a Maintenance
Care Plan, 567
Assessment, 567
Medical and Dental History, 567
Intraoral and Extraoral Examination, 568
Radiographs and Dental Charting, 568
Oral Risk Assessment, 568
Periodontal Charting, 570
Evaluation of Deposits, 570
Homecare, 571
Dental Hygiene Diagnosis, 571
Dental Hygiene Treatment Plan, 571
Informed Consent, 571
Maintenance Therapies, 572
Debridement, 572
Polishing, 573
Special Care for the Implant, 573
Locally Delivered Antimicrobials, 574
Continuing Care Intervals, 574
Evaluation, 575
Documentation, 575
Case Study, 575
Case Study Exercises, 575
Review Questions, 576
Active Learning, 576
References, 576

**PART IX CARING FOR PATIENTS WITH SPECIAL
NEEDS**

Chapter 36 Introduction to Special Needs, 580
Relevance to Clinical Practice, 581
Defining Special Needs, 581
Changing Terminology, 581
History, 582
Specific Categories, 582
Management of Patients, 583

Understanding Best Practices,　586
　　Behavioral Management,　586
　　Medical Management,　586
　　Dental Implications,　587
　　Dental Management,　587
Summary,　588
Case Study,　588
Case Study Exercises,　588
Review Questions,　588
Active Learning,　589
References,　589

Chapter 37 Cardiovascular Disease,　590
Relevance to Clinical Practice,　591
Cardiovascular Disease,　592
　　Physiology of the Heart,　592
　　Association Between Oral and Systemic Health,　593
Disease Processes,　596
　　Arrhythmias,　596
　　Bradycardia,　596
　　Tachycardia,　596
　　Heart Block,　597
Atherosclerosis,　597
　　Risk Factors,　598
Hypertension,　598
　　Risk Factors,　599
　　Treatment of Hypertension,　599
Infective Endocarditis,　600
　　Types of Endocarditis,　600
Rheumatic Heart Disease,　600
Ischemic Heart Disease,　601
　　Angina Pectoris,　601
　　Myocardial Infarction or Acute Myocardial Infarction,　602
　　Chronic Ischemic Heart Disease,　602
　　Sudden Cardiac Death,　602
Heart Failure,　603
Congenital Heart Disease,　603
　　Common Forms of Congenital Heart Disease,　603
Valvular Heart Disease,　604
Anticoagulant Therapy,　605
Post–Cardiovascular Surgery,　605
Summary,　606
Case Study,　606
Case Study Exercises,　606
Review Questions,　606
Active Learning,　607
References,　607

Chapter 38 Respiratory,　610
Relevance to Clinical Practice,　611
Overview of the Respiratory System,　611
Oral–Respiratory Disease Link,　611
Respiratory Disease,　612
Acute Respiratory Infections,　613

Asthma,　614
　　Etiology and Classification,　614
　　Signs and Symptoms,　615
　　Dental Hygiene Considerations,　615
Chronic Obstructive Pulmonary Disease (COPD),　615
　　Signs and Symptoms,　616
　　Dental Hygiene Considerations,　617
Cystic Fibrosis,　617
　　Dental Hygiene Considerations,　617
Tuberculosis (TB),　617
　　Symptoms, Diagnosis, and Treatment,　617
　　Dental Hygiene Considerations,　618
Case Study,　618
Case Study Exercises,　618
Review Questions,　618
Active Learning,　619
References,　619

Chapter 39 Sensory Disability: Vision and Hearing Impairment,　620
Relevance to Clinical Practice,　621
Vision Impairment,　622
　　Causes,　622
　　Oral Clinical Findings,　622
　　Patient Factors,　622
　　Communication,　624
　　Guiding and Seating the Patient,　625
　　Dental Hygiene Considerations,　626
　　Oral Self-Care Instruction,　626
Hearing Impairment,　627
　　Causes and Types of Hearing Loss,　627
　　Patient Factors,　628
　　Communication,　628
　　Dental Hygiene Considerations,　630
　　Oral Factors, Self-Care, and Prevention,　630
The Deaf-Blind Patient,　630
Summary,　631
Case Study,　631
Case Study Exercises,　631
Review Questions,　632
Active Learning,　632
References,　632
Resources,　633

Chapter 40 Mental Health,　634
Relevance to Clinical Practice,　635
What Are Mental Disorders?,　635
　　Definition,　635
　　Categories,　635
　　Pervasive Developmental Disorders,　635
　　Mood Disorders and Bipolar Disorder,　636
　　Schizophrenia,　637
　　Eating Disorders,　638
　　Substance Dependence and Abuse,　639

Summary,   641
Case Study,   643
Case Study Exercises,   643
Review Questions,   643
Active Learning,   644
References,   644

Chapter 41 Neurological Impairments,   646
Relevance to Clinical Practice,   647
What Are Neurological Impairments?,   647
  Definition,   647
  Categories,   647
Common Neurological Impairments,   647
  Amyotrophic Lateral Sclerosis,   649
  Bell Palsy,   650
  Cerebral Palsy,   651
  Huntington Disease,   652
  Myasthenia Gravis,   653
  Parkinson Disease,   654
  Stroke,   656
Critical-Thinking Process,   658
Case Study,   659
Case Study Exercises,   659
Review Questions,   660
Active Learning,   660
References,   660

Chapter 42 Endocrine System,   662
Relevance to Clinical Practice,   663
Endocrine System,   663
  Pituitary Gland, Pineal Gland, and Hypothalamus,   663
  Thyroid Gland and Parathyroid Glands,   664
  Adrenal Gland,   664
  Pancreas—Islets of Langerhans,   665
  Gonads,   665
Diabetes Mellitus,   665
  Dental Hygiene Considerations,   666
Disease Processes of the Pituitary Gland,   667
  Cushing Syndrome,   667
  Acromegaly,   667
  Thyroid Disorder,   668
  Cancer of the Thyroid,   668
  Diseases of the Adrenal Gland,   669
  Dental Hygiene Considerations and Precautions,   669
Case Study,   669
Case Study Exercises,   669
Review Questions,   669
Active Learning,   670
References,   670

Chapter 43 Immune System,   672
Relevance to Clinical Practice,   673
Basic Concepts of Immunity,   673
  Self Versus Nonself and Immunological Memory,   673
  Innate and Adaptive Immune Systems,   674
  Cells of the Immune Response,   674

  Chemokines and Cytokines,   674
  Autoimmune Diseases,   674
  Immunodeficiency Diseases,   674
Disease That Affect Overall and Oral Health,   675
  Sjögren Syndrome,   675
  Myasthenia Gravis,   676
  Scleroderma,   677
  Multiple Sclerosis,   679
  Rheumatoid Arthritis,   680
  Systemic Lupus Erythematosus,   681
  Adrenal Insufficiency,   681
  Fibromyalgia,   682
  HIV/AIDS,   683
  Lichen Planus,   684
  Erythema Multiforme,   685
Treating Patients With Transplants,   686
  Dental Hygiene Considerations,   686
Case Study,   687
Case Study Exercises,   687
Review Questions,   688
Active Learning,   688
References,   688

Chapter 44 Hematological Considerations,   690
Relevance to Clinical Practice,   691
Clot Formation,   691
Clotting Determination,   692
  Bleeding Time,   692
  International Normalized Ratio,   692
  Prothrombin Time,   693
  Partial Thromboplastin Time,   693
  Thrombocytopenia,   693
Blood-Thinning Drugs,   693
  Acetylsalicyclic Acid (Aspirin),   693
  Clopidogrel (Plavix),   694
  Coumadin (Warfarin),   695
  Other "Blood-Thinning" Medications,   696
  Antibiotics,   696
  Statins,   696
  Herbal Medications,   697
Bleeding Disorders,   697
  Von Willebrand Disease,   697
  Hemophilia,   698
Red Blood Cell Disorders,   698
  Anemia,   698
  Iron Deficiency,   699
  B_{12} Deficiency,   699
  Pernicious Anemia,   699
  Celiac Sprue,   700
  Sickle Cell Anemia,   700
  Aplastic Anemia,   700
  Polycythemia,   701
White Blood Cell Disorders,   701
  Leukemia,   701
  Hodgkin Disease,   701

Occupational Exposure Recommendations,   702
  Hepatitis,   702
HIV/AIDS,   703
Summary,   703
Case Study,   703
Case Study Exercises,   703
Review Questions,   704
Active Learning,   704
References,   705

Chapter 45 Cancer,   706
Relevance to Clinical Practice,   707
What Is Cancer?,   707
  Staging,   707
  Grading,   707
Cancer Incidence, Risk Factors, and Most Common Types,   708
Chemotherapy-Associated Complications,   709
Cancer Therapy and Acute Oral Complications,   709
  Mucositis,   710
Oral Cancer as a Subset of Head and Neck Cancers,   712
  Demographics,   714
Oral Cancer Therapies and Oral Complications,   715
  Long-Term Oral Complications,   716
Treatment-Planning Strategies,   718
  Before Cancer Therapy or After Diagnosis of Oral Cancer,   718
  During Cancer Therapy,   718
  After Cancer Therapy or With a History of Oral Cancer,   718
Summary,   718
Case Study,   719
Case Study Exercises,   719
Review Questions,   719
Active Learning,   720
References,   720

Chapter 46 Pediatric Patient,   722
Relevance to Clinical Practice,   723
Evolution and Goals of Pediatric Dentistry,   723
  A Paradigm Shift: Surgical Model Versus Medical Model,   723
Public Health Rationale on Pediatric Oral Health,   723
Unique Aspects of Pediatric Dentistry,   723
  The Dental Home,   724
  Anticipatory Guidance,   724
  Role of the Dental Hygienist,   724
  Physical, Emotional, and Mental Development,   725
The Developing Dentition,   725
  Primary Dentition,   725

  Mixed Dentition,   726
  Permanent Dentition,   726
Oral Health Considerations for Pediatric Patients,   726
  Dental Caries,   726
  Non-nutritive Habits,   727
  Malocclusion,   727
  Dental Trauma,   727
Behavior Guidance Techniques,   728
  Communicative Management,   728
  Physical Techniques,   729
The Dental Appointment,   729
  Before Dental Hygiene Care,   729
  During Dental Hygiene Care,   730
  After Dental Hygiene Care,   732
Case Study,   733
Case Study Exercises,   733
Review Questions,   733
Active Learning,   734
References,   734

Chapter 47 Men's and Women's Health Issues,   736
Relevance to Clinical Practice,   737
Sex Versus Gender,   737
Life Cycles,   738
  Puberty,   738
  Childbearing Years,   739
  Preconception,   739
  Pregnancy,   740
  Epulis Gravidarum,   741
  Postpartum,   742
  Menopause and After Menopause,   742
  Biphosphonate-Related Osteonecrosis of the Jaw,   743
  Osteoradionecrosis,   743
Domestic Violence,   744
  Dental Hygiene Considerations,   744
Men's Health,   744
  Diseases of the Prostate,   744
Dental Decay and the Sexes,   745
Case Study,   746
Case Study Exercises,   746
Review Questions,   746
Active Learning,   747
References,   747
Resources,   749

Chapter 48 The Elderly,   750
Relevance to Clinical Practice,   751
Demographics of Aging,   751
  Chronic Conditions,   751
  Physical and Cognitive Disabilities,   751
  Homebound and Institutionalized Adults,   751
What Is Aging?,   753

Physiological Aging, 754
  Cardiovascular System, 754
  Respiratory System, 754
  Gastrointestinal System, 755
  Urinary System, 755
  Endocrine System, 755
  Brain and Nervous System, 755
  Immune System, 755
  Musculoskeletal System, 756
  Sensory System, 756
  Integumentary System, 756
Common Pathophysiological Diseases of the
  Elderly, 757
  Alzheimer Disease, 757
Other Common Systemic Diseases in the
  Elderly, 760
  Arthritis, 761
  Chronic Obstructive Pulmonary Disease, 762
  Diabetes, 762
  Cardiovascular Disease, 763
  Osteoporosis, 763
  Parkinson Disease, 763
  Stroke, 763
Normal and Pathological Oral Changes in the
  Elderly, 764
  Lips, 765
  Oral Mucosa, 765
  Tongue, 765
  Salivary Glands, 765
Common Pathological Oral Conditions, 765
  Xerostomia, 765
  Oral Candidiasis, 765
  Angular Cheilitis, 765
  Oral Cancer, 766
  Dentition, 767
  Periodontal Structures, 767
  Periodontal Diseases, 767
Case Study, 768
Case Study Exercises, 768
Review Questions, 768
Active Learning, 769
References, 769

Chapter 49 Physical Impairment, 772
Relevance to Clinical Practice, 773
Physical Impairment, 773
  Definition, 773
  Prevalence, 773
  Historical Perspective, 773
Barriers to Health-Care Access, 773
  Financial Barriers, 773
  Architectural Barriers, 775
  Transportation Barriers, 775
  Attitudinal Barriers, 775
  Other Barriers to Care, 775

Etiology, 776
Classification of Impairments, 776
Disability Etiquette, 776
  Communication, 776
  Wheelchair Etiquette, 777
  Physical Contact, 777
  Other Considerations, 777
The Dental Hygiene Appointment, 777
  Oral Hygiene Instructions, 780
  Teaching the Patient, 780
  Modifying Recommendations, 781
  Teaching the Caregiver, 781
Conditions, 784
  Inherited and Genetic Conditions, 784
  Congenital Conditions, 785
  Developmental and Acquired Conditions, 786
Case Study, 788
Case Study Exercises, 788
Review Questions, 788
Active Learning, 789
References, 789

Chapter 50 Alternative Practice Settings, 790
Relevance to Clinical Practice, 791
Access to Care, 791
Alternative Practice, 791
Alternative Practice Settings, 791
  Mobile Dental Clinics, 791
  Portable Units, 792
  Simplified Portable Units, 792
  Independent Practice Hygienist Karine Strickland,
    RDHAP 792
  Freestanding Building, 793
  Shelby Kahl, Owner and Operator of a Freestanding
    Clinic 793
  Backpack, 794
  Flying Hygienists, 794
  Kelly Nance, Flying Hygienist 794
Beyond the Dental Office: Venues and Services, 795
  Skilled Nursing Facilities and Intermediate
    Care Facilities, 796
  Hospitals, 796
  Schools, 797
  Private Homes, 797
  Street Outreach, 797
  Institutions and Prisons, 798
  Workplace, 798
Administration of Care, 798
  Charting, 798
  Allowable Duties, Venues, and Supervision, 798
  Dental Hygiene Practice Act, Level of Supervision,
    and Scope of Duties, 799
  Restorative, 799
Case Study, 799
Case Study Exercises, 799

Review Questions,   799
Active Learning,   800
References,   800

PART X EMERGENCY MANAGEMENT

Chapter 51 Dental and Medical
    Emergencies,   802
Relevance to Clinical Practice,   803
Emergency Prevention,   803
    Medical History Assessment,   803
    Physical Observation,   804
    Psychological Assessment,   804
    Medical Consultation,   804
    Oral Trauma Prevention,   805
Emergency Preparation and Organization,   805
    Training,   805
    Emergency Contacts,   806
    Action Plan,   806
    Equipment,   806
    Documentation,   808
Medical and Dental Emergency Management,   808
Case Study,   815
Case Study Exercises,   816
Review Questions,   816
Active Learning,   817
References,   817

PART XI FUTURE VISION

Chapter 52 Practice Management,   820
Relevance to Clinical Practice,   821
Leadership,   821
    Trust and the Drama Triangle,   822
    Vision, Mission, and Goals,   822
Communication,   823
    Communication Barriers,   823
    Components of Communication,   823
Business of Dentistry and Dental Hygiene,   824
    Production and Collection Goals,   824
    Patient Financial Options,   825
    The Dental Hygienist's Role in Accounts Receivable,   825
    Current Dental Terminology and Periodontal
        Diseases,   826
    Reaching Hygiene Goals,   827
    Team Communication,   828
    Routing Slips,   828
    Other Meetings,   828
    Patient Scheduling,   828
    The Appointment Book,   829
    Scheduling,   829

    Communication to Avoid Cancellations and
        No-Shows,   829
    Hygiene/Dentist Discussion,   830
    Hygiene Retention,   830
    Professionalism and Appearance,   831
    Habits of Effective Offices,   831
Case Study,   832
Case Study Exercises,   832
Review Questions,   832
Active Learning,   833
References,   833
Resources,   833

Chapter 53 Career Development,   834
Relevance to Clinical Practice,   835
Employment Opportunities,   835
Finding a Position,   836
Resume Writing,   838
Interviewing,   838
Career Development,   838
Summary,   840
Case Study,   840
Case Study Exercises,   840
Review Questions,   840
Active Learning,   841
References,   841

Chapter 54 Lifelong Learning,   842
Relevance to Clinical Practice,   843
What Is Lifelong Learning?,   843
Adult Versus Child Learners,   843
Critical Thinking,   844
Evidence-Based Practice,   844
Advanced Education,   846
    Degree-Completion Programs,   846
    Master's Degree Programs,   846
    Doctoral Degrees,   846
    Direct Access,   847
    Alternative Practice Models,   847
Continuing Education,   847
    The Standards for Clinical Dental Hygiene Care,   848
    State Requirements,   848
    Professional Organizations,   848
    Delivery of Continuing Education,   849
Case Study,   850
Case Study Exercises,   850
Review Questions,   850
Active Learning,   851
References,   851
Glossary,   854
Photo and Illustration Credits for Part Openers
    and Chapter Openers,   876
Index,   878

Part I

Introduction to Dental Hygiene

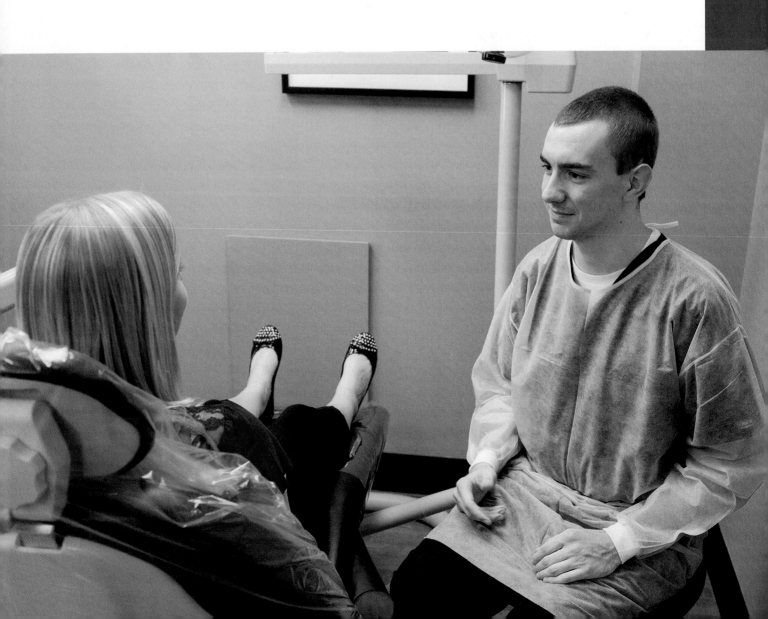

Chapter 1 | Dental Hygiene as a Profession

Maria Perno Goldie RDH, BA, MS

KEY TERMS

American Dental Hygienists' Association (ADHA)

dental hygiene process of care

dental hygiene treatment plan

dental hygienist

International Federation of Dental Hygienists (IFDH)

National Dental Hygienists' Association (NDHA)

public health

registered dental hygienist

scope of practice

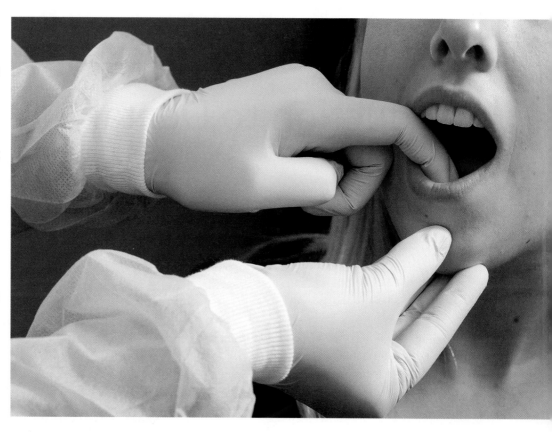

LEARNING OBJECTIVES

After reading this chapter, the student should be able to:

1.1 Define the term *dental hygienist.*
1.2 Describe the history and evolution of dental hygiene practice.
1.3 Describe the roles of the dental hygienist.
1.4 List and explain the dental hygiene process of care.
1.5 Summarize the standards of care for dental hygiene.
1.6 Explain the importance of dental hygiene professional organizations.

KEY CONCEPTS

• A registered dental hygienist (RDH) is a licensed oral health-care professional who specializes in preventive oral health.
• Evidence-based decision-making is the foundation of dental hygiene education, practice, and research.
• The American Dental Hygienists' Association (ADHA) is the professional organization that represents dental hygienists in the United States.
• Dental hygienists are graduates of accredited dental hygiene education programs in colleges and universities, and they must take a written

national board examination and a clinical examination before they are licensed to practice.
* The profession of dental hygiene must embrace change, focus on growth and development, and plan for its future, as well as the future oral health needs of the public.

RELEVANCE TO CLINICAL PRACTICE

Entering into a career in dental hygiene is more than just taking a new job. Dental hygiene is a rewarding profession and career choice. **Dental hygienists** are essential members of the dental team and interdisciplinary health-care teams. The profession of dental hygiene began as a **public health** profession and has since evolved into a discipline that continues to grow. The potential for dental hygienists who are clinically trained and have expanded their education is great.

The profession of dental hygiene is more than 100 years old. It is essential that dental hygienists be aware of the profession's history and are part of its future.

DENTAL HYGIENE

The practice of dental hygiene was developed to deliver oral health education and preventive oral health care to children. It has matured and transformed to a profession that provides oral health services to a broad spectrum of the community.

A discipline is knowledge or a concentration in one academic field of study or profession. In each discipline, practitioners are identified by the science that is the foundation of practice. Although dental hygiene has some features of a discipline, such as a focus on disease prevention and oral health promotion, the body of knowledge based on research by dental hygienists is relatively scarce, and frequently not connected to theoretical or conceptual frameworks. A conceptual framework is a system of concepts, assumptions, expectations, beliefs, and theories that supports and informs the research in a particular discipline.[1]

Dental hygiene could improve its contribution to the public by evolving as a professional discipline. Building the dental hygiene body of knowledge as a foundation for practice would lead to the profession's designation as a professional discipline. The field needs dental hygiene scientists who systematically research questions related to substantive areas of the dental hygiene discipline. Dental hygiene scholars who are research scientists and are dedicated to examining how their science relates to the dental hygiene's mission, values, and effects on humanity are also needed.

Three conceptual models have been proposed for the profession of dental hygiene. Conceptual models can provide a shared language and framework for the discipline to define the process of care. The oral health-related quality of life,[2] patient self-care commitment,[3] and the human needs models[4] have been proposed. The oral health-related quality of life model is composed of six primary domains. As a cohesive model, it may serve as a foundation for assessing, planning, implementing, and evaluating outcomes to dental hygiene care. The patient self-care commitment model is composed of five domains. This model proposes that the relationships among the five domains, and the interaction between the patient and the dental hygienist, can enable patients to make decisions that will improve their own health through commitment and adherence. The human needs conceptual model provides a formal structure for recognizing and understanding the distinctive needs of the patient that can be met through dental hygiene care.

A dental hygienist is a licensed, preventative oral health professional who provides a variety of oral health services to patients. Dental hygienists are graduates of accredited dental hygiene education programs in colleges and universities. The credential RDH stands for **registered dental hygienist.** In Indiana, the designation is LDH, licensed dental hygienist. Each state defines its licensure requirements; all states except Alabama require graduation from an accredited dental hygiene program and passing a national written examination and a regional clinical examination. Dental hygienists work in a variety of settings including private dental offices, schools, public health clinics, hospitals, managed care organizations, correctional institutions, nursing homes, and corporate businesses.

HISTORY OF THE DENTAL HYGIENE PROFESSION

The preventative dental hygiene movement began in 1910 in Cleveland, Ohio, where the Oral Hygiene Committee of the National Dental Association began a publicly funded program for oral hygiene education and dental prophylaxis for children in schools.[5] Although this movement was one of the first to focus on oral hygiene and prophylaxis, it was not until a few years later that dental hygienists were charged with this duty. In 1913, Dr. Alfred C. Fones coined the term *dental hygienist* and began the first dental hygiene education program in Bridgeport, Connecticut. Dr. Fones envisioned dental hygienists as specialists in the science of health and the prevention of oral disease. In particular, Dr. Fones taught dental hygienists to remove plaque biofilm and calculus deposits from the teeth. The first graduating class of dental hygienists worked in schools and later in hospitals. Irene Newman, who worked as Dr. Fones' assistant and graduated from the Fones School of Dental Hygiene, became the first licensed dental hygienist in the United States in 1917. By 1936, 30 states were licensing dental hygienists.[6] The profession of dental hygiene began with a strong public health focus. As time evolved the focus shifted to a private practice model. As the profession continues to evolve it is likely that the profession will again shift to delivering dental hygiene care in public health settings.

SCOPE OF PRACTICE OF DENTAL HYGIENISTS

Each state has its own rules and regulations concerning the treatment and **scope of practice** that dental hygienists can provide. Dental hygienists perform a variety of preventative, educational, and therapeutic services.

Standards of Practice and the Process of Care

Dental hygiene is defined as the science and practice of the recognition, treatment, and prevention of oral diseases.[7] The **American Dental Hygienists' Association (ADHA)** published *Standards for Clinical Dental Hygiene Practice* to provide an evidence-based framework for dental hygiene practice. The document includes six standards that follow the **dental hygiene process of care:** assessment, diagnosis, planning, implementation, evaluation, and documentation. The purpose of the dental hygiene process of care is to provide a framework where the individualized needs of the patient can be met, and to identify the causes of a condition that can be treated or prevented by the dental hygienist. Assessment is the collection, analysis, and documentation of the health status of the patient. Dental hygiene assessments may include patient history, clinical evaluation, and risk

assessment. Diagnosis is identifying an existing or potential oral health problem that a dental hygienist can treat. A dental hygiene diagnosis is made using the assessment data that have been collected and professional critical-thinking and decision-making skills. Planning is identifying recommended treatment and outcomes related to the established assessments and diagnosis. This is often called a **dental hygiene treatment plan.** Implementation is the delivery of dental hygiene treatment as established in the treatment plan. Evaluation is the process of reviewing the outcomes of the treatment that was delivered. The final step is documentation. Documentation is recording a complete and accurate record of data, treatment plan, treatment implemented, evaluation, and recommendations.[8] Specific techniques for all steps in the process of care are outlined in this book.

ROLES OF A DENTAL HYGIENIST

Traditionally, dental hygienists have been viewed in a clinical role, but dental hygienists have opportunities to serve in many professional roles (Fig. 1-1).

Clinician

The role as a clinician is the basis of the dental hygiene profession. Dental hygienists in a clinical role use the dental hygiene process of care to prevent and treat oral diseases in collaboration with other health professionals. Clinical employment settings may include private dental practices, community clinics, hospitals, prison facilities, nursing homes, and schools.

Corporate

Corporations in the oral health industry employ dental hygienists. They may be part of the sale of oral health products, development of products, or the marketing

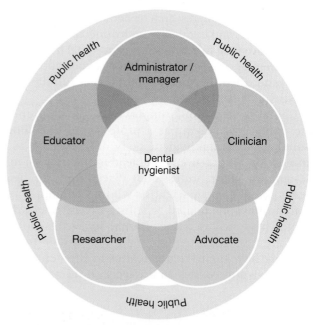

Figure 1-1. Professional roles of the dental hygienist.

of oral health products. Corporate positions may include sales representatives, researchers, or corporate educators and administrators.

Public Health

Federal or state government or nonprofit organizations often fund public health programs. Dental hygienists may provide clinical or administrative services in public health settings. Some examples of public health employment are in Indian Health Services, Head Start programs, school sealant programs, and community clinics.

Researcher

Dental hygienists can play a role in research in several different settings. Dental hygienists' clinical expertise and knowledge of research methods make them a valuable member of a research team. Research is commonly conducted in colleges and universities, corporations, governmental agencies, and nonprofit organizations.

Educator

More than 300 accredited dental hygiene programs in the United States are in need of qualified educators to contribute to the education of future dental hygienists. Full-time educators must have a bachelor's or higher degree, and part-time faculty must have a bachelor's degree or be enrolled in a bachelor's degree program.[9] Outside of a college or university setting, corporations also employ educators to provide continuing education to dental hygienists. Educators may be clinical instructors, lecturers, professors, program directors, or corporate educators.

Administrator

Administrative roles for dental hygienists may overlap with other roles listed in this chapter. Administrators apply organizational management skills, manage resources, and implement and evaluate programs. Examples of administrative positions include clinical director, program director, executive director, and corporate director.

Advocate

Dental hygienists are advocates in conjunction with many other professional roles. Dental hygienists may advocate for their patients, for their profession, and for policy that supports improving the oral health of the public. Dental hygienists may find themselves in many of these roles throughout their careers, and many times the roles of a professional dental hygienist complement each other in one employment setting. It is important to keep in mind that dental hygienists have the potential to expand beyond a traditional clinical role.

PROFESSIONAL ORGANIZATIONS

When entering a profession, there is often an organized group of professionals who make up the professional organization. Professional organizations represent those who are in the profession and the organization's goals. The largest professional organization representing dental hygienists in the United States is the ADHA. The ADHA was founded in 1923 and is headquartered in Chicago. The core ideology of the ADHA is to "lead the transformation of the dental hygiene profession to improve the public's oral and overall health."[7] The ADHA offers resources for dental hygienists related to evidence-based clinical recommendations, education, advocacy, and representation. The ADHA also offers dental hygienists opportunities for professional development and leadership opportunities within the profession.[10] Membership in the ADHA is not mandatory, but is recommended. In 1932, the **National Dental Hygienists' Association (NDHA)** was founded to provide a professional foundation for minority dental hygienists. The NDHA's mission includes increasing the number of minority dental hygienists, assisting in the access to oral care for underserved communities, and promoting the highest educational and ethical standards for dental hygienists.[11] Dental hygiene professional organizations extend beyond the United States. The **International Federation of Dental Hygienists (IFDH)** is composed of representatives from dental hygiene professional organizations in 25 countries. The IFDH was established in 1986 and serves to unite dental hygiene associations from around the world with the common cause of promoting dental health.[12] Professional organizations are essential in maintaining dental hygiene as a profession and improving the oral health of the public.

THE FUTURE OF DENTAL HYGIENE

The landscape of the United States and the world is changing, and the way health care is delivered is also changing. This includes the way dental hygiene care is and will be delivered. One challenge that the profession must address is eliminating the barriers to receiving dental care. To address barriers to access, predominantly in underserved and vulnerable populations, states are considering increasing the oral health-care workforce. This will include dental hygienists, who typically perform preventive oral health services. To increase access to basic oral health care, some states are positioning dental hygienists outside of traditional dental offices or private practices. States also have explored changing supervision or reimbursement rules for existing dental hygienists, as well as creating new professional certifications for advanced practice dental hygienists.[13] An expanded scope of practice for dental hygienists has proved safe and effective, as shown by outcomes of pilot programs.[14] As the profession continues to evolve, dental hygienists will participate in improving oral health care globally. The profession of dental hygiene is essential to improving the health of the public.

Case Study

Beth has been a dental hygienist for 17 years. One of the Beth's patients, Andrea, is seriously considering dental hygiene as a career and will begin taking her prerequisite course work in the fall. Beth has talked with Andrea about her career and what being a dental hygienist requires. Andrea has many questions and is very enthusiastic about becoming a dental hygienist.

Case Study Exercises

1. When Andrea asks Beth about how many examinations she needed to take to become a dental hygienist, Beth should outline which of the following?
   A. Dental hygienists take a written national board examination and a clinical examination before they are licensed to practice.
   B. Dental hygienists take a written national board examination only.
   C. Dental hygienists only need to graduate from an accredited dental hygiene program to become licensed to practice.
   D. Dental hygienists do not require any examinations to be licensed.

2. Andrea knows a dental hygienist who works at the state health department. This hygienist is working within what professional role of the dental hygienist?
   A. Corporate
   B. Public health
   C. Researcher
   D. Educator
   E. Advocate

3. Beth discusses with Andrea how she cares for patients. Which part of the process of care includes patient history, clinical evaluation, and risk assessment?
   A. Diagnosis
   B. Planning
   C. Implementation
   D. Assessment
   E. Evaluation

4. What future opportunities in dental hygiene should Beth highlight for Andrea?
   A. Future solutions to allow more access to dental care
   B. Expanded practice locations and settings
   C. Global improvement of oral health care
   D. A public health–focused future of the profession
   E. All of the above

Review Questions

1. A dental hygienist is a licensed, preventative oral health professional. Dental hygienists are licensed by the individual states.
   A. Both statements are true.
   B. Both statements are false.
   C. The first statement is true, the second is false.
   D. The first statement is false, the second is true.

2. The first licensed dental hygienists worked in a private practice setting. Public health settings were the first area where dental hygienists were utilized.
   A. Both statements are true.
   B. Both statements are false.
   C. The first statement is true, the second is false.
   D. The first statement is false, the second is true.

3. Dental hygienists perform a variety of preventive, educational, and therapeutic services. Which of the following is NOT a service typically provided by a dental hygienist?
   A. Conducting oral health-care assessments that include the review of patients' health history, dental charting, oral cancer screening, and evaluation of gum disease/health
   B. Filing teeth for tooth movement procedures, such as Invisalign

   C. Exposing, processing, and interpreting dental radiographs, standard or digital
   D. Removing deposit such as plaque and calculus from above and below the gumline using hand or ultrasonic instruments
   E. Appling cavity-preventive agents such as fluorides and sealants to the teeth

4. The dental hygiene process of care is a framework where the individualized needs of the patient can be met. _____ is the one item that goes across all facets of the dental hygiene process of care.
   A. Assessment
   B. Diagnosis
   C. Planning
   D. Implementation
   E. Documentation

5. Order the dental hygiene process of care.
   _2_ A. Diagnosis
   _6_ B. Documentation
   _1_ C. Assessment
   _3_ D. Planning
   _5_ E. Evaluation
   _4_ F. Implementation

Active Learning

1. Diagram the process of care and give examples of procedures completed within each area.
2. Research and identify dental hygienists working each professional role. Interview one dental hygienist and discover his or her career path in achieving that role.
3. Create a promotional video encouraging dental hygienists to become members of one of the professional associations. ▪

REFERENCES

1. Cobban SJ, Edgington EM, Compton SM. An argument for dental hygiene to develop as a discipline. *Int J Dent Hyg.* 2007;5(1):13-21.
2. Williams KB, Gadbury-Amyot CC, Bray KK, Manne D, Collins P. Oral health-related quality of life: a model for dental hygiene. *J Dent Hyg.* 1998;72(2):19-26.
3. Calley KH, Rogo E, Miller DL, Hess G, Eisenhauer L. A proposed client self-care commitment model. *J Dent Hyg.* 2000;74(1):24-35.
4. Darby ML, Walsh MM. Application of the human needs conceptual model to dental hygiene practice. *J Dent Hyg.* 2000;74(3):230-237.
5. Picard A. Making the American mouth: dentists and public health in the twentieth century. New Brunswick (NJ): Rutgers University Press; 2009. p. 226. http://www.loc.gov/catdir/toc/ecip0825/2008035426.html
6. American Dental Hygienists' Association. 100 years of dental hygiene. http://www.adha.org/timeline. Updated 2012. Accessed July 11, 2014.
7. American Dental Hygienists' Association. *American Dental Hygienists' Association Policy Manual.* http://www.adha.org/resources-docs/7614_Policy_Manual.pdf. Updated 2013. Accessed July 11, 2014.
8. American Dental Hygienists' Association. *Standards for Clinical Dental Hygiene Practice.* http://www.adha.org/resources-docs/7261_Standards_Clinical_Practice.pdf. Updated 2008. Accessed July 11, 2014.
9. American Dental Association. Accreditation standards for dental hygiene education programs. http://www.ada.org/~/media/CODA/Files/dh.ashx. Updated January 1, 2013. Accessed August 27, 2014.
10. American Dental Hygienists' Association. American Dental Hygienists' Association mission and history. http://www.adha.org/mission-history. Updated 2014. Accessed July 11, 2014.
11. National Dental Hygienists' Association Website. http://www.ndhaonline.org. Updated 2013. Accessed July 11, 2014.
12. International Federation of Dental Hygienists Website. http://www.ifdh.org/about.html. Updated 2014. Accessed July 11, 2014.
13. Rhea M, Bettles C; American Dental Hygienists' Association. Dental hygiene at the crossroads of change. http://www.adha.org/resources-docs/7117_ADHA_Environmental_Scan.pdf. Updated 2011. Accessed July 11, 2014.
14. National Governors' Association. The role of dental hygienists in providing access to oral health care. NGA Paper 2014. http://www.nga.org/files/live/sites/NGA/files/pdf/2014/1401DentalHealthCare.pdf.

Chapter 2 | Legal and Ethical Considerations

Cynthia C. Amyot, MSDH, EdD

KEY TERMS

autonomy
beneficence
confidentiality
civil law
criminal law
ethical decision-making
fiduciary
justice
nonmaleficence
societal trust
veracity

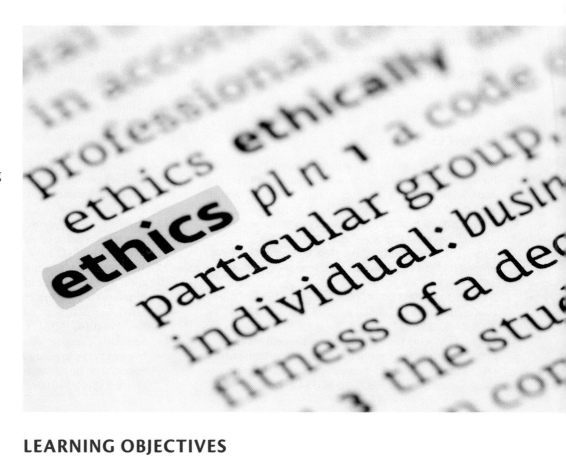

LEARNING OBJECTIVES

After reading this chapter, the student should be able to:

2.1 Compare and contrast law and ethics as they interface within the practice of dental hygiene.

2.2 Explain how the practice of dental hygiene is defined through statutory law and how a thorough understanding of the law is necessary.

2.3 Distinguish between criminal and civil law as they pertain to the practice of dental hygiene and strategies that assist in risk management.

2.4 Analyze how the ethical principle and core value of autonomy factors into both patient and provider autonomy.

2.5 Identify ways in which informed consent comes into play when discussing the issue of autonomy in health care.

2.6 Explore how dental hygiene professional organizations around the world address the issue of beneficence in their ethical codes and values, and discuss common themes.

2.7 Provide a rationale for how current access to health-care issues and beneficence interface, and develop strategies for addressing these issues.

2.8 Debate how nonmaleficence can lead to conflict when trying to balance good against harm for the same patient.

2.9 Explore the issue of justice through the eyes of legislators and policy makers who must grapple with issues of allocation of limited resources.

2.10 Define what is meant by a fiduciary relationship between patient and provider, and, in the context of the ethical principle and core value of veracity, discuss the idea of shared decision-making.

2.11 Evaluate the impact of the Health Insurance Portability and Accountability Act (HIPAA) on the ethical principle and core value of confidentiality.

2.12 Assess the factors that combine to create trust—for example, reciprocity, moral obligation, and trustworthiness—in the context of the practice of dentistry and dental hygiene, and compare with other health professions.

2.13 Use an ethical decision-making model when presented with an ethical dilemma to assist with critically thinking and problem-solving through an appropriate course of action.

KEY CONCEPTS

- The public trusts that the hygienist, as a licensed health-care provider, will practice legally and ethically.
- To practice legally and ethically, the dental hygienist must have a full understanding of ethical principles and core values and a full understanding of the law that will serve to guide decision-making.
- Use of an ethical decision-making model that incorporates professional codes of ethics, standards of care, and the law is key to critically thinking and problem-solving when faced with an ethical dilemma.

RELEVANCE TO CLINICAL PRACTICE

Martin Luther King said, "Intelligence is not enough . . . intelligence plus character—that is the true goal of education." Why discuss legal and ethical considerations in a dental hygiene textbook? In addition to developing clinical expertise, it is critical that dental hygiene students understand what it means legally to be a licensed practitioner and how ethics factors into the life and work of a health-care professional.

As in any health-care profession, legal and ethical issues arise in dentistry and dental hygiene. This chapter is devoted to introductory legal and ethical principles and their application to clinical practice. The **ethical decision-making** model is presented as a way to resolve ethical dilemmas. The American, Canadian, and International Dental Hygiene codes of ethics are all presented.

LAW AND ETHICS

Law and ethics are not the same. Laws are rules created by a society to arbitrate its citizens' relationships with each other. Ethics are moral principles that guide law creation and individual behavior. The judiciary, legislature, and public officials create and enforce laws for the general public. State boards of dentistry or dental hygiene promulgate laws related to dental hygiene practice. Whereas laws carry with them a punishment for violations, ethics do not. Ethics and ethical behavior originate from an individual's or group's moral values.

Experts agree that knowledge of the relevant law is one of the key elements in truly understanding the field of ethics.[1] For example, suppose that you are a dental hygienist infected with HIV. You discovered that you were infected at an early stage of the virus and immediately started a multidrug treatment regimen (highly active antiretroviral therapy [HAART]). You are aware that studies show the average life expectancy of an HIV-infected individual is 32 years from the time of infection if treatment is started when the CD4 count is less than $350/\mu L$.[2] You are further aware that the chance of transmitting HIV to your patients is extremely low.[3] In addition, you know that individuals with HIV/AIDS are covered under the Americans with Disabilities Act and, therefore, are not required to report their status.[4] The law would state that as an HIV-infected oral health-care worker you do not legally have to disclose your HIV status and, therefore, can continue to work as long as you are not putting the patient at risk for exposure.[5] In contrast, the ethical principle of **nonmaleficence,** which states "do no harm," makes you wonder whether you should reveal your HIV status to patients, thereby allowing them the autonomy to decide whether they wish to seek care from you. Resources available to assist in the decision-making process include: professional codes of ethics from the American Dental Hygienists' Association (ADHA),[6] the Canadian Dental Hygienists' Association (CDHA),[7] and the International Federation of Dental Hygienists (IFDH);[8] dental hygiene practice acts; professional standards of care;[9] and applicable laws. Knowledge of the Americans with Disabilities Act is critical to this decision-making process.[10]

As licensed professionals it is incumbent upon dental hygienists to thoroughly understand the laws that pertain to the practice of dental hygiene in the states, provinces, or countries where they are practicing. Ignorance of the law is not an acceptable defense in a court of law.

LAW AND THE PRACTICE OF DENTAL HYGIENE

Licensure

The purpose of licensure is to ensure the safety and well-being of the public to whom the professional provides services, in this case, dental hygiene care. The licensure process for dental hygienists in the United States consists of the successful completion of the National Board Dental Hygiene Examination, a passing score on a clinical licensure examination, and completion of a jurisprudence examination on the laws of the particular state(s) where one is seeking licensure to practice dental hygiene. Individual states have differing requirements for licensure to practice, and not all states offer reciprocity of licensure (recognition of the validity of licenses granted by other states). This system of licensure is possible because the U.S. Constitution reserves many rights to the states, and regulation of occupational licenses is deemed to be a state's right. This constitutional law was observed as early as 1898 when a U.S. Supreme Court decision authorized states to set their own requirements for licensure of physicians.[11] This

decision still serves today as the basis for supporting state over federal regulations in health-care licensure, including dental hygiene. Therefore, when obtaining licensure, it is necessary to review the state practice acts for the state or states where one plans to practice.

In the United States, dental practice acts and licensure are regulated within the individual states' legislative branch of government (the other two branches are executive and judicial). Dental hygiene practice acts are statutory law. Statutory law is written law set down by a legislature to regulate the conduct of individuals, businesses, among others. For dental hygiene, statutory laws outline such areas as the allowable scope of practice, requirements necessary to obtain a dental hygiene license, and dental supervision requirements. Statutory law can only be changed by the state legislature.

When state lawmakers enact legislation, such as dental hygiene practice acts, the details of implementation are often left to state agencies.[12] A mechanism commonly used to implement legislation is rulemaking. A rule is a statement of general applicability that interprets and implements law or defines the practice and procedure requirements of an agency of a state government. In other words, rulemaking is lawmaking in areas that the legislature has decided are too specific or detailed to be handled by legislation. For example, state legislators, who may have little or no expertise related to the practice of dentistry and dental hygiene, delegate their lawmaking power to an agency (such as a state dental board) by passing a law granting rulemaking authority to the agency. The agency then adopts and enforces rules. In dentistry and dental hygiene, state agencies are generally appointed by the governor.

State Dental Boards

State dental boards (executive branch) are responsible to the legislature to regulate the practice of dentistry and dental hygiene in their respective states. This is called *self-regulation* and is unique to professions whereby the public exhibits an increased level of trust that professionals will exercise due diligence to ensure quality of care. Some of the functions carried out by the state dental boards can be found in Box 2-1.

The rulemaking process is ongoing, and state dental boards may promulgate (put into effect) rules at any time, provided they follow the provision of the law or statute. A rule can be changed by the board or by a person petitioning the board to promulgate, amend, or repeal a rule. It is in the best interests of dental hygiene professionals to work toward legislative changes in the practice act passed by state legislators that result in statutory law, rather than a rule or regulation, which may be changed by a dental board and may not be representative of the profession. An example would be a rule that is created by a dental board to allow dental hygienists to administer local anesthesia. If this is not in the form of a statutory law, the rule can be changed at any time by the dental board.

> ### Box 2-1. *Examples of State Dental Board Functions*
>
> State dental boards may:
> - Determine the qualifications of applicants for licensure to practice.
> - Issue licenses to those persons who meet the standards of professional competences set forth in the state.
> - Maintain high standards of professional competence and ethical conduct among members of the profession through the requirement of continuing education for licensure.
> - Enforce dental law to ensure the protection of the public. ■

State legislative processes generally include two legislative bodies: the Senate and the House of Representatives. It is necessary for a concept (bill) to become a law to make any statutory changes. Both houses (Senate and House of Representatives) must pass a bill after it has spent time in specific committees, which may amend, or make changes, to each respective bill. It is not unusual for a bill to "die" in committee only to have its most vital ideas added to a different bill. This process functions as a political compromise between legislators. If both houses fail to pass a bill, the bill will not become a law. If both houses pass the bill, it is necessary for the governor to sign it into law, or if the governor vetoes the bill, both houses have the ability to override the veto by a two-thirds majority vote.

Canada has differing regulation and licensure requirements across provinces for the practice of dental hygiene; however, dental hygienists in Canada operate in a more autonomous manner than dental hygienists in the United States. For example, although many dental hygienists in the United States are regulated under state dental boards that often include minimal representation of dental hygienists, Canadian dental hygienists enjoy self-regulation with regulatory agencies completely separate from dentistry. These regulatory bodies are referred to as "Colleges of Dental Hygienists" such as the College of Dental Hygienists of Manitoba, the College of Registered Dental Hygienists of Alberta, and so on across the provinces.[13]

Regardless of the regulating process, dental hygienists must be aware of the laws that pertain to the practice of dental hygiene where they practice. Most licensing bodies now have practice acts posted on their websites for easy and ready access. Likewise, professional organizations are increasingly providing information via the Web that can serve as resources in decision-making. For example, the ADHA Governmental Affairs section (available online at http://www.adha.org/governmental_affairs/practice_issues.htm) provides information about permitted services and supervision levels by state, continuing education requirements for licensure renewal, and so on.

Criminal and Civil Law

There are two types of statutory law: criminal and civil. A violation of **criminal law** is considered a crime against society as outlined by statutory law, and the state (government) may institute criminal proceedings in a court of law. Because statutory law requires that dental hygienists be licensed to practice, an example of a criminal law violation in dental hygiene would be providing dental hygiene treatment without a license. A prosecutor with intent to punish an offender has the burden of providing proof of the offense "beyond a reasonable doubt." A conviction of guilt requires a unanimous decision by a jury. In criminal law the consequences for the offender are great and can involve a fine (payment with either money or community service), a prison sentence, or in some states, the death penalty. Considering the magnitude of the potential consequences, the requirement for "beyond a reasonable doubt" when determining the outcome of a case becomes evident.

A **civil** offense is a wrongful act against a person that violates his or her person (body), privacy, or property or contractual rights. **Civil law** is made up of two categories: tort law and contract law. Tort law is described as a civil wrong that results from a breach of legal duty that exists by virtue of society's expectations of performance.[14] There can be intentional tort and unintentional tort (negligence). Examples of intentional torts include assault and battery, misrepresentation, defamation, and breach of confidentiality, where the intention is clearly to harm someone. Unintentional torts, or negligence, occur in instances where the dental hygienist's actions or inactions result in harm to the patient even though there was never the intent to inflict harm. An example of an unintentional tort could be failing to perform periodontal probing, a standard of care, which results in undiagnosed periodontal disease. The standard of care or standard of practice refers to the concept that reasonable persons of ordinary prudence with comparable education, skill, and training, under similar circumstances, would perform the same function.[14] Thus, a dental hygiene professional who fails to perform periodontal probing would be at fault because it is a function that any well-educated dental hygienist would have performed in a comparable situation.

Standards tend to be higher for health-care professionals because of their advanced skills and knowledge, and because of the impact on patient health and well-being. Standards of care are determined through evidence-based education, professional organizations such as the ADHA, which publishes standards such as *Standards for Clinical Dental Hygiene Practice*,[9] and other health-care organizations such as the Centers for Disease Control and Prevention or the American Academy of Periodontology. Professional negligence that results in harm to the patient, such as in the example of the dental hygienist not performing periodontal probing, is considered malpractice. Strategies for avoiding malpractice include a philosophy of lifelong learning, the practice of good communication skills that involves listening and seeking to understand the other person's point of view, as well as an understanding of the limits of one's abilities and scope of practice.

The second category of civil law is contract law, which includes both implied and expressed contracts. An example of an implied contract is when a patient calls the dental office to schedule an appointment; making the appointment (i.e., the agreement to give and receive care) implies that the patient will show up at the scheduled time and that the provider will extend care. Expressed contracts involve oral or written agreements. Treatment plans that have been discussed, agreed on, and signed are an example of an expressed contract. This example of contract law, treatment/care plans, involves informed consent, which is discussed more fully in this chapter under the ethical principle of **autonomy.**

In civil law, a crime is committed against an individual; therefore, the initiator of legal action is the individual. The outcome can include such things as nominal, compensatory, or punitive damages. In civil cases, there must be a majority vote by a jury (>50%). Civil cases are most often the result of lawsuits that are brought against dentists and dental hygienists, and arise from three of the most common actions relating to health care: (a) failure to obtain informed consent, (b) professional malpractice, and (c) breach of contract.

Managing Risk

Avoiding lawsuits and managing one's risk is best accomplished by thoroughly understanding the law and good documentation practices. It is generally accepted that the following elements make for good documentation: date, reasons for the visit, radiographs and other diagnostic tools (as applicable), examination and findings, treatment rendered, patient instructions, prescriptions (as applicable), laboratory results (as applicable), patient perception whether satisfaction or dissatisfaction, evaluation of outcome, referral (as applicable), and recare/recall.[15] As a licensed professional it is critical that dental hygienists obtain professional liability insurance before they begin practicing. Should a dental hygienist be named in a lawsuit, professional liability insurance may provide coverage and protection of the hygienist's personal and professional assets. Many hygienists mistakenly believe that they are covered under their dentist employer's liability insurance. The principle that an employer may generally be held liable for the wrongful acts of an employee if the employee was acting within the scope of his or her employment is known as respondeat superior or "let the master answer."[14] However, the employer's policy represents the dental hygienist only if the dentist is named in the lawsuit. Should the employer and dental hygienists be named in the suit and the employer's name is later dropped, the insurance policy of the employer may not cover the dental hygienist.[16] Most policies cost a minimal amount and offer necessary coverage in the event of a lawsuit.

In addition to a thorough understanding of the law, it is also incumbent upon the dental hygienist to understand the ethical principles and core values of the profession of dental hygiene. A hallmark of a professional is the use of these principles and values to guide decision-making, and particularly in the health sciences they provide guidance for decision-making when it comes to patient care.

ETHICAL PRINCIPLES AND CORE VALUES

The health professions have historically been guided by the Hippocratic Oath, which is believed to have been written by Hippocrates in the late fifth century BC.[17] Hippocrates is often thought of as the father of Western medicine, and even today centuries later doctors still take the oath, thereby swearing to practice medicine ethically. Many of the statements in the modern version of the oath apply to the practice of dental hygiene (Box 2-2). The statement "I will prevent disease whenever I can, for prevention is preferable to cure" is particularly relevant to the practice of dental hygiene, which was founded on the concept of prevention.

Society expects that the healing professions are guided by ethical principles and core values, and in response the ADHA, the CDHA, and the IFDH have developed codes of ethics intended to guide the practice of dental hygiene (Box 2-3). Central to these three codes of ethics are principle core values. Values can be defined as those things that are important to or valued by an individual or organization, or both, and as such should be the basis for the behavior of the individual and members of the organization. These core values are outlined in Table 2-1.

Autonomy

Autonomy is the ethical principle and core value of self-determination. The ability to be self-governing and self-directing is central to autonomy. An autonomous individual freely chooses his or her thoughts, actions, and behavior relevant to his or her needs and independent from the will of others. Autonomy arises from the Kantian principle of respect for persons. Immanuel Kant was an 18th-century German philosopher who believed that every human being is a rational person and, therefore, one's self-respect and respect for the value of rationality would not allow oneself to be treated as a means to an end (i.e., used for purposes not beneficial to oneself).

In health care, autonomy comes into play as individuals are permitted to make decisions about their health. The health-care provider has a duty to provide a patient with all the pertinent and unbiased information a patient would need to make a decision about treatment options (informed consent). There are times when what the professional believes is best for the

Box 2-2. *Modern Version of the Hippocratic Oath*

"I swear to fulfill, to the best of my ability and judgment, this covenant:

I will respect the hard-won scientific gains of those physicians in whose steps I walk, and gladly share knowledge as is mine with those who are to follow.

I will apply, for the benefit of the sick, all measures [that] are required, avoiding those twin traps of overtreatment and therapeutic nihilism.

I will remember that there is art to medicine as well as science, and that warmth, sympathy, and understanding may outweigh the surgeon's knife or the chemist's drug.

I will not be ashamed to say "I know not," nor will I fail to call in my colleagues when the skills of another are needed for a patient's recovery.

I will respect the privacy of my patient, for their problems are not disclosed to me that the world may know. Most especially must I tread with care in matters of life and death. If it is given to me to save a life, all thanks. But it may also be within my power to take a life; this awesome responsibility must be faced with great humbleness and awareness of my own frailty. Above all, I must not play at God.

I will remember that I do not treat a fever chart, a cancerous growth, but a sick human being, whose illness may affect the person's family and economic stability. My responsibility includes these related problems, if I am to care adequately for the sick.

I will prevent disease whenever I can, for prevention is preferable to cure.

I will remember that I remain a member of society, with special obligations to all my fellow human beings, those sound of mind and body as well as the infirm.

If I do not violate this oath, may I enjoy life and art, respected while I live and remembered with affection thereafter. May I always act so as to preserve the finest traditions of my calling and may I long experience the joy of healing those who seek my help." ■

Written in 1964 by Louis Lasagna, Academic Dean of the School of Medicine at Tufts University, and used in many medical schools today.
The Hippocratic Oath: Modern Version. Doctors' Diaries. WGBH Educational Foundation. Retrieved September 11, 2010. http://www.pbs.org/wgbh/nova/body/hippocratic-oath-today.html.

---

patient is not what the patient selects to do. When there is a conflict between the professional's recommendations and the patient's desires, two scenarios may develop. First, if the patient selects from treatment options that are consistent with the standards of care, the professional may ethically act on the patient's choice. However, if the professional believes that the treatment option the patient is requesting is not consistent with standards of care, the professional can exercise his or her autonomy and refuse to render treatment. In the example in Table 2-1, if the patient requests a simple prophylaxis even though assessment of the patient's condition clearly indicates periodontal disease, the dental hygienist would exercise his or her autonomy by refusing to treat the patient, because a prophylaxis is not considered the standard of care for active periodontal disease.

Box 2-3. *Dental Hygiene Codes of Ethic*

American Dental Hygienists' Association Code of Ethics for Dental Hygienists: http://www.adha.org/resources-docs/7611_Bylaws_and_Code_of_Ethics.pdf.
Canadian Dental Hygienists' Association Code of Ethics: http://www.cdha.ca/pdfs/Profession/Resources/CDHA_Code_of_Ethics_public.pdf.
International Federation of Dental Hygienists Code of Ethics: http://www.ifdh.org/dt/ifdh_Code_of_Ethics.pdf. ■

Professional guidelines are available to assist the dental health professional in the decision-making process. For example, the position paper "Guidelines for Periodontal Therapy" by the American Academy of Periodontology clarifies for both patients and providers what is considered a standard of care. It provides treatment procedures for individuals diagnosed with periodontal disease that go beyond basic therapy (prophylaxis), which has been shown to not be effective in arresting the disease process.[18]

Informed Consent

The concept of informed consent has taken on new meaning in today's health-care environment. The basis for obtaining informed consent is the principle of respect for autonomy. In the past, patients and practitioners considered decision-making the responsibility of the professional. This form of provider care was termed *paternalistic*, where the health-care provider rarely or never consulted the patient regarding treatment choices and the patient was willing to abdicate responsibility for decision-making to the professional. In current health-care practice, decision-making is a process that involves both the patient and the practitioner. Shared decision-making has become a critical aspect of informed consent. Because informed consent is based on the patient exercising autonomy in decision-making, the practitioner (in this case, the dental hygienist) has the responsibility to provide the patient with all relevant information needed to make a decision, and the patient has the responsibility to consider all relevant

Table 2-1. *Core Values Identified in the American Dental Hygienists' Association, Canadian Dental Hygienists' Association, and International Federation of Dental Hygienists Codes of Ethics*

Core Value	Example
Autonomy—self-determination of the patient	A patient presents with active periodontal disease. In consultation with the dentist the dental hygienist presents a treatment plan to the patient that includes four quadrants of scaling and root planing. The patient has the right to accept or refuse the treatment recommendations.
Beneficence—taking actions that serve the best interests of the patient	A patient presents with a small chip on the incisal edge of a central incisor. Two approaches to care would be a small composite (tooth-colored) restoration or a porcelain veneer. The patient has been out of work for the past 6 months and currently does not have any medical or dental coverage. Considering all of the unique circumstances of this patient, it could be argued that the small composite would be in the best interest of the patient at this point in time.
Nonmaleficence—do no harm	A patient who recently read in a magazine that amalgam fillings are toxic wants the dentist to take out all of her amalgam fillings and replace them with composite resins. The patient has amalgam fillings in 12 of her posterior teeth and only 1 of the 12 fillings is defective. You cannot justify removing 11 perfectly sound fillings.
Justice—the fair treatment of individuals; equitable allocation of health-care dollars and resources	A dental hygienist who graduated 3 years ago has returned to his hometown in rural Kansas after working in a major metropolitan area. Despite the fact that there are no practicing dentists in his county or any of the surrounding counties, he is hoping to find a sponsoring dentist to support his practice of dental hygiene using his newly acquired Extended Care Permit (ECP)—legislation that allows the dental hygienist to provide dental hygiene care without the presence of a dentist. The decay rate in this county and the surrounding counties is much higher than the national average. He hopes to approach the schools to set up an ECP practice to treat those children who are unserved or underserved.
Veracity—to tell the truth	Economic times have been harsh and dentistry has not been immune to the effects of the bad economy. Dr. Smith's practice has experienced a severe downturn in overall production and income. To cut costs, she has decided to lay off her dental hygienist who has worked for her for the past 15 years. In place of the hygienist, Dr. Smith has hired a scaling assistant. According to the practice acts, the scaling assistant is not to work below the gumline. A patient presents with periodontal disease and 4- to 5-mm pocketing. Dr. Smith has presented a treatment plan that includes scaling and root planing. The patient has a niece who is a dental hygienist in another state and she asks Dr. Smith if the dental hygienist will be performing the scaling procedures. To follow the principle of veracity, Dr. Smith would be required to inform the patient that a scaling assistant will be performing the procedure above the gumline and that Dr. Smith will provide scaling and root planing below the gumline.
Confidentiality—personal and/or medical information given to a health-care provider will not be disclosed to others unless the patient has given informed consent	A patient presents to the practice and discloses during the health history that she is HIV-positive. You live in a small town and as luck would have it your patient is dating a family friend. You are very concerned about the safety of your friend but at the same time you are held accountable to the core value of confidentiality.
Societal trust—promotion of a mutual trust between the profession and the larger public (similar to societal trust is the principle of accountability covered in the Canadian Dental Hygienists' Association Code of Ethics)	You have witnessed one of your colleagues using illicit drugs in the dental office. Dentistry is a self-regulated profession, which means that the public trusts that dental professionals will regulate the conduct of colleagues and discipline those practitioners who operate outside the values and ethics established by the profession's codes of ethics. Out of concern for the patients and the core value of societal trust, you have placed a call to the state dental board to report your colleague's actions.

information provided when deciding how to proceed (Box 2-4). When a patient understands the relevant information and freely consents to proposed treatment or procedures, the patient has provided an informed consent. The patient also has the right to make an informed refusal. Respecting the autonomy of patients as self-determining agents is to recognize their right to make their own choices and determine their own destiny. As shown in the preceding example, in an environment of informed consent and shared decision-making, the health-care provider can also exercise autonomy and refuse to treat when it would be against the practitioner's best judgment given his or her knowledge and expertise on best practices and standards of care.

Beneficence

Beneficence is the ethical principle and core value that pertains to "doing good." It is incumbent upon health-care providers to use their knowledge and skills to benefit the patient. Founded in the Hippocratic tradition (see Box 2-2), and included in the ADHA, CDHA, and IFDH codes of ethics (see Box 2-3), dental hygienists profess their primary role in promoting the well-being of individuals and the public by engaging in health promotion/disease prevention activities. In fact, dental hygiene as a profession in the United States started out in the public health sector providing oral health-care services to children in schools.[19] However, over the years dental hygienists have migrated from the public health setting to primarily a private practice fee-for-service delivery model. Now, the pendulum may be swinging back the other way. Recent initiatives such as the U.S. Surgeon General Report on Oral Health (2000) and subsequent National Call to Action (2003), the Canadian Oral Health Strategy (2005), and other international oral health documents have brought awareness to the lack of public access to oral health-care services.[20–22] These documents collectively identify inequities and disparities in oral health care along with barriers to achieving optimal oral health for all citizens. As a result, dental hygienists are increasingly becoming more involved in the public health arena providing services to unserved and underserved populations. Both the National Call to Action and the Canadian Oral Health

Strategy reports promote legislative changes for increasing access to oral health-care services, with dental hygienists figured prominently into these changes. Opportunities to further engage in health-promotion and disease-prevention strategies as outlined in dental hygiene codes of ethics around the world will hopefully become more of a reality in the years ahead.

Nonmaleficence

Considered the founding principle of all health professions, nonmaleficence is the ethical principle and core value that a health-care provider's first obligation is to do no harm, or physical injury. As with beneficence, this principle is also founded in the Hippocratic Oath. Patients are in a vulnerable position when seeking health care. It should be expected that no additional harm will result. Standard of care comes into play with nonmaleficence in that health-care providers act ethically when they apply all the measures that prevent harm. To distinguish beneficence from nonmaleficence, Beauchamp and Childress[23] use the following classification:

Beneficence
1. One ought to prevent harm.
2. One ought to remove harm.
3. One ought to do or promote good.

Nonmaleficence
1. One ought _not_ to inflict harm.

Note that all of the statements of beneficence involve positive action toward preventing or removing harm, and promoting good. In contrast, the nonmaleficence statement is stated in the negative, to refrain from inflicting harm. Although ideally the dental hygienist would be able to avoid harm, it is not always possible. For example, when the dental hygienist performs scaling and root planing on a patient with periodontal disease, the result is loss of attachment level, which can lead to exposed roots and increased root sensitivity.[24,25] This is not avoidable when performing this procedure and yet is considered the standard of care for patients diagnosed with periodontal disease. In this instance, causing a degree of harm will lead to a greater good, which is to bring the disease process under control. This example demonstrates that it is not always possible for the health-care provider to avoid harm and promote good. In this case, the "harm" is the side effect of a positive treatment. It is comparable with a drug that is given to treat a condition but may have a positive, neutral, or negative side effect.

Justice

Justice is the ethical principle and core value concerned with providing individuals or groups what is owed, due, or deserved. Justice is defined as *fairness,* or described as the principle of *equality.* In health care, this might include such things as equal access to health-care resources and patients' rights. In dentistry, justice is most often discussed in terms of public policy issues and has been referred to as distributive justice. All societies

> ### Box 2-4. *Generally Accepted Elements of Informed Consent*
>
> - Patient competence: confirmation of patient competency
> - Understanding: understandable language used
> - Disclosure: the nature of the condition
> - Proposed treatment: including the inherent and potential hazards of the proposed treatment, the alternatives to that treatment, if any, and the results likely if the patient remains untreated ■

grapple with the issue of resource distribution. Distributive justice is concerned with the allocation of resources in large social systems. Legislators and policy makers grapple with the issues of allocation. An example of this is the legislative actions in the state of Minnesota. On May 13, 2009, Minnesota Governor Tim Pawlenty signed into law Senate Bill 2083 establishing the basic and advanced dental therapist. The legislation was enacted in response to a lack of access to oral health-care services for the citizens of Minnesota. Expanding the scope of education and practice for dental hygienists (advanced dental therapist) is an effort to address the issue of access for unserved and underserved populations in the state by increasing the number of dental hygiene practitioners able to provide direct oral health-care services, both preventive and restorative.[12] As discussed previously, the practice of dental hygiene has largely been rendered in private practice fee-for-service settings in North America, and national data have clearly illustrated that this model of delivery is not reaching large segments of the population. Being able to distribute oral health-care services in the public health/safety net arena through the use of practitioners such as the basic and advanced dental therapists in Minnesota has the potential to have a positive impact on the oral health of all citizens.

Veracity

Veracity is the ethical principle and core value related to honesty. The ADHA, CDHA, and IFDH codes of ethics unequivocally state that dental hygienists accept their obligation to tell the truth and seek truth and honesty in all relationships. Veracity binds both the health practitioner and the patient in an association of truth. The patient must tell the truth in order that appropriate care can be provided; likewise, the practitioner must disclose factual information so the patient can exercise personal autonomy. The nature of the relationship between provider and patient is defined as a **fiduciary** relationship. A fiduciary relationship is any relationship between persons in which one person acts for another in a position of trust.[14] Fiduciary obligation acknowledges that there are always inequalities in knowledge and power in patient encounters with health providers and that these inequalities require health providers to act in the best interests of the patient (fiduciary obligation) and to honor the trust placed in them by patients and society as a whole. The example in Table 2-1 related to veracity illustrates patients' expectation that they will be provided services that meet the standard of care and that they must rely on the honesty of the health providers to be truthful at all times. It is highly unlikely that the average dental patient will be aware of legislative rules and regulations for dentistry, and in this example, of the rules and regulations involving a scaling assistant in the state of Kansas. It is therefore incumbent upon practitioners to inform patients about the practitioners providing their treatment, including their qualifications.

Confidentiality

Confidentiality is the ethical principle and core value that in health care deals with nondisclosure of personal information about the patient, which could potentially cause harm. In the provider–patient relationship, patients should expect that when they disclose personal information it will remain confidential. Therefore, it is not surprising that the ADHA, CDHA, and IFDH codes of ethics cover the issue of patient confidentiality.

The issue of confidentiality of private health information became a matter of law in the United States in 1996 when Congress enacted the Health Insurance Portability and Accountability Act (HIPAA) to ensure "portability" of health insurance as individuals changed employment or insurance coverage, or both. The final HIPAA Privacy Rule took effect on April 14, 2003.[26] HIPAA protected health information (PHI) includes individually identifiable health information transmitted or maintained in any form or medium, which is held by a covered entity (CE) or its business associate, and:

1. Identifies the individual or offers a reasonable basis for identification
2. Is created or received by a CE or an employer
3. Relates to a past, present, or future physical or mental condition, provision of health care, or payment for health care

CEs under HIPAA include:

1. Health-care providers who transmit any health information in electronic form in connection with a transaction covered by the rule—for example, billing
2. Health plans that assume the risk of paying for medical/dental treatments—for example, an HMO
3. Health-care clearinghouses, which are public or private entities that standardize health information received from another entity, for example, a billing service that processes or facilitates the processing of data from one format into a standardized billing for a receiving entity

Table 2-2 outlines the basic tenets of the Privacy Rule. The Privacy Rule preempts state laws that are less stringent or contrary to the rule, but does not preempt more stringent state privacy laws. The Privacy Rule specifies that health information is determined to be Individually Identifiable Health Information on the basis of 18 identifiers, which are outlined in Table 2-3. As a health-care provider it is critical that one has a thorough understanding of HIPAA and the dental hygienist's role in ensuring that the patient's privacy is protected.

Under HIPAA, individuals have the right to access their PHI; to request amendment of their PHI; to receive an accounting or record of certain disclosures of their PHI within a period of 6 years before their request; effective April 14, 2003, the right to request restrictions on uses and disclosures of their PHI; the right

Table 2-2. *Seven Principles of the Privacy Rule*

1	Quality and Availability of Care: Nothing in the Privacy Rule should interfere with the delivery of quality health care or threaten the financial stability of health-care organizations.
2	Notice: A patient has the right to know what information is maintained about him or her and how that information may be used or disclosed.
3	Minimum Necessary: The workforce of health-care organizations should access and use only the minimum necessary information about patients to accomplish their assigned duties.
4	Onward Transfer: Patients have an ownership interest in their protected health information and a right to control subsequent uses and disclosures of this information. They also have the right to request an accounting of all such disclosures.
5	Data Security/Privacy/Integrity: Those who store, process, transmit, or use protected health information have an obligation to reasonably protect its confidentiality and to prevent unauthorized alterations.
6	Access: Patients have a right to inspect their confidential information to ensure its accuracy and completeness, and to request that erroneous information be corrected.
7	Enforcement: Patients have a right to redress of privacy violations. Health-care organizations must reasonably prevent and detect the abuse of their patient information, mitigate further loss, and sanction offenders.

Table 2-3. *Eighteen Potential Identifiers for Protected Health Information (26)*

1	Names
2	All geographic subdivisions smaller than a State, including street address, city, county, precinct, zip code, and their equivalent geocodes, except for the initial three digits of the zip code if, according to the current publicly available data from the Bureau of Census a. The geographic unit formed by combining all zip codes with the same three initial digits contains more than 20,000 people; and b. The initial three digits of a zip code for all such geographic units containing 20,000 or fewer people is changed to 000
3	Elements of dates (except year) for dates directly related to an individual, including birth date, admission date, discharge date, date of death; and all ages over 89 and all elements of dates (including year) indicative of such age, except that such ages and elements may be aggregated into a single category of age 90 or older
4	Telephone numbers
5	Fax numbers
6	Electronic mail addresses
7	Social security numbers
8	Medical record numbers
9	Health plan beneficiary numbers
10	Account numbers
11	Certificate/license numbers
12	Vehicle identifiers and serial numbers
13	Device identifiers and serial numbers
14	Web Universal Resource Locators (URLs)
15	Internet Protocol (IP) address numbers
16	Biometric identifiers, including fingerprints and voice prints
17	Full-face photographic images and any comparable images
18	Any other unique identifying number, characteristic, or code, except as permitted

to request receipt of communication of their PHI by alternative means or location (e.g., at home or at work, by mail or telephone only); and the right to revoke their authorization for the use or disclosure of their PHI for other than treatment, payment, or health-care operations.[27]

Instances of permitted use and disclosure of PHI without authorization by the individual include:

- For the purpose of treatment, payment, or health-care operations
- Where disclosure is required by law
- For public health activities
- For victims of abuse, neglect, or domestic violence
- For health-care oversight activities
- For judicial and administrative proceedings in response to a court order
- For law enforcement purposes (pursuant to a court order) or to disclose the death of an individual under suspicious circumstances
- To a coroner or medical examiner regarding decedents, or to a funeral director, consistent with applicable laws
- For research after de-identification
- For research through a limited dataset
- For research pursuant to a waiver of authorization issued by a Privacy Board or Institutional Review Board (IRB)

In those instances where researchers wish to obtain authorization from patients for use of PHI, required elements must be included in the authorization. To learn more about the required elements, refer to the Privacy Rule.

In addition to the Privacy Rule, the Department of Health and Human Services released the final HIPAA Security Rule in the *Federal Register* on February 20, 2003. The Security Rule became effective for enforcement on April 25, 2005. The final HIPAA Security Rule applies only to PHI that is transmitted in electronic form at the CE or business associate. It is important to be knowledgeable about this rule in the current environment of technology and paperless patient records. Electronic devices covered under HIPAA include memory devices in computers (hard drives) and any removable or transportable digital memory medium, such as magnetic tape or disk, optical disk or digital memory card, and devices used to exchange information already in electronic form. This includes the Internet, extranet, leased lines, dial-up lines, private networks, and the physical movement of removable or transportable electronic storage devices. A CE has some flexibility in implementing these specifications. It has the option of determining alternative security measures that are reasonable and appropriate with its available resources for protecting PHI. The language used in the rule is:

- *Required*—standards that are essential for compliance
- *Addressable*—one of many options that by itself is not essential

The CE performs a risk assessment that takes into account such things as the size, complexity, and capabilities of the CE; the CE's technical infrastructure, hardware, and software capabilities; cost of implanting security measures; and probability and criticality of potential risks to electronic PHI. If the CEs determine during the risk assessment that the set specifications are not reasonable and appropriate to implement, they must: (a) document why it would not be reasonable and appropriate to implement the specification, and (b) implement an equivalent alternative measure.

Confidentiality is a critical principle, so critical that since 2003 the government has deemed it necessary to pass legislation to safeguard and protect the confidentiality of patients.

Societal Trust

Trust is a core value that is incorporated into all three of the dental hygiene codes of ethics (ADHA, CDHA, and IFDH). In alignment with veracity, this core value seeks to ensure that the professions of dentistry and dental hygiene remain trustworthy in the eyes of the public. Welch and colleagues[28] define **social trust** as follows:

> Social trust is the mutually shared expectation, often expressed as confidence, that people will manifest sensible and, when needed, reciprocally beneficial behavior in their interactions with others.

The authors explain that participants in these relationships can confidently have recourse to such relationships to fulfill various needs. Therefore, a patient–provider relationship of trust allows the patient to have confidence in the practitioner recommendations, and the practitioner is rewarded by the patient seeking his or her counsel and treatment. Researchers have determined a variety of factors that combine to create trust, including reciprocity, moral obligation, trustworthiness, social relations, cooperation, and familiarity. Further research suggests that social trust has beneficial effects on individuals, communities, the workplace, institutions, and even nations. Trust makes people healthier, happier, and more hospitable. Trust enables individuals to form meaningful connections with others from whom they can derive an array of assets, including access to jobs and knowledge of job opportunities, money, friendship, moral and social support, care, transportation, and physical and mental health.

ETHICAL DECISION-MAKING MODEL

Although several models have been proposed for ethical decision-making, they all contain key components or steps for inclusion in the decision-making model (Table 2-4). Possessing knowledge of issues related to the law and of issues related to ethics in dental hygiene is critical in assisting the dental hygienist

Table 2-4. *Key Components of an Ethical Decision-Making Model*

Step 1	Identify the ethical dilemma or problem. This is the most critical step in the decision-making model. There has to be recognition whether an ethical problem or dilemma exists. If it is determined that an ethical dilemma does not exist after considering that the problem is not in conflict with ethical principles, then it stops here in terms of working through the rest of the model. If, in fact, it is determined that an ethical dilemma exists and is in conflict with ethical principles, then it becomes necessary to work through the ethical decision-making model. Questions to consider: • Who are the concerned parties? • Is there a conflict with ethical principles? • Is there a conflict with standards of care? • Is there a conflict with the American Dental Hygienists' Association, Canadian Dental Hygienists' Association, or International Federation of Dental Hygienists Codes of Ethics?
Step 2	*Gather the facts.* To make good decisions, the decision maker needs to be well informed. Gathering credible resources and facts is critical in this process. Codes of ethics, standards of care, professional liabilities, and legal regulations are important tools and resources, and an understanding of them is crucial. Beyond the facts, values are another source of information that is necessary for informing the decision maker. Bringing these resources to bear upon the relevant issue will ensure a good faith effort to weigh what would be an appropriate and reasonable response to an ethical dilemma.
Step 3	*List the options/alternatives.* Although one straightforward answer would be the easiest route, in ethics that is seldom the case. Brainstorming through possible options and alternatives can help in seeing the situation through multiple lenses. Context is extremely important because each ethical dilemma or problem that presents is encased in its own specific context. These special circumstances must be factored in when determining options and alternatives to come up with the best option for that particular situation.
Step 4	*Apply the ethical principles to the options.* A good strategy for closing in on the best option is to apply the ethical principles and facts that have been gathered to each option. Develop a list of pros and cons for each of the options that illustrates how each option holds up when weighed against the ethical principles and facts. By examining the options carefully and thoughtfully, it often becomes obvious which is the best solution to the ethical dilemma or problem.
Step 5	*Choose the best option and implement the decision.* Step 4 should have been instructive as to which option is best given the facts known at the time. In this step the decision maker must make a final decision of which option to choose and then act on it.
Step 6	*Evaluate.* As with the dental hygiene process of care, which involves assess, diagnose, plan, implement, and evaluate, the final step in ethical decision-making is evaluation. A question to consider is: If I had a chance to do it all over again, would I make the same decision?

to think through step 1 in the ethical decision-making model. Step 1 is the most critical step in the model. Being able to identify whether a problem exists is key to what will be an appropriate response. Determining whether an ethical dilemma exists involves considering whether the problem is in conflict with ethical principles or the law. Questions to consider asking oneself when attempting to determine whether an ethical dilemma exists are provided in Table 2-4. If it is determined that an ethical dilemma or problem exists, work through steps 2 to 6 in the ethical decision-making model.

Step 2 can be thought of as evidence-based decision-making in that the dental hygienist needs to gather credible resources and facts about the ethical dilemma or problem in question to make an appropriate and reasonable decision about what the response will be. Without an understanding of ethical principles, codes of ethics, standards of care, professional liabilities, and legal regulations, the dental hygienists lacks the knowledge to make a well-informed decision. Step 3 is a deliberate effort to brainstorm what possible actions or options and alternatives could help in seeing the ethical dilemma or problem through multiple lenses. Step 4 then involves closing in on the best option by applying the ethical principles and facts or evidence to the various options determined in step 3. By working through this process, the best solution to the ethical dilemma or problem will often become obvious. Once the best solution has been determined, step 5 involves implementing the decision. Again, drawing on one's knowledge of evidence-based decision-making, the dental hygienist in step 6 will evaluate the outcome of the decision. A good question to consider is: If I had a chance to do it all over again, would I make the same decision?

It is impossible to be part of a people-centered profession such as dentistry and dental hygiene and not confront ethical dilemmas and problems. Having tools to assist and inform decision-making is important in helping dental health professionals critically think through these dilemmas and problems as they arise and arrive at an ethical decision. The process of decision-making is dynamic as each situation has its own unique features, making this a complex process. In addition, new information and knowledge is evolving constantly and requires consideration when it comes to ethical decision-making.

Case Study

Ann, a recent dental hygiene graduate, has been working temporarily in different offices as she attempts to find a permanent position. Dr. Thurlow's office manager called and asked Ann to work a couple of days while the current hygienist is out of town. Ann arrives on Monday morning and the dental assistant shows her the operatory where she will be working. The office is beautiful and full of the latest technology. The assistant tells Ann that she and Dr. Thurlow have worked together for 15 years. Ann also learns that the receptionist has been there for 10 years and that Susan, the office manager, is new. Ann's first reaction is, "Wow, not too much turnover; this would be a great place to work." As the day progresses, Ann seats a new patient and begins the appointment. When she goes to find Dr. Thurlow for the new patient examination, she looks in his operatory and office but cannot locate him. Just as Ann comes around the corner, she hears the receptionist talking to Dr. Thurlow in an overflow operatory. As she steps up to the door to let him know her patient is ready, she notices Dr. Thurlow reclined in the dental chair. The receptionist is seated next to the nitrous oxide tank and states that she is adjusting the flow of gas. The receptionist then gets up and leaves Dr. Thurlow and heads up to the front desk to talk with Susan, the new office manager. She did not see Ann back around the corner.

Case Study Exercises
1. What action, if any, should Ann take?
   A. Confront Dr. Thurlow.
   B. Discuss the situation with the office manager.
   C. Report Dr. Thurlow to the state dental board.
   D. Discuss the situation with Dr. Thurlow and give him an opportunity to report himself to the state dental board.

2. Ann's responsibility is to:
   A. Dr. Thurlow
   B. The patients of the office
   C. The law
   D. B and C

3. Which of the following core values might Ann find MOST helpful in determining how to respond to this situation?
   A. Societal Trust—Dental hygienists value patient trust and understand that public trust in their profession is based on their actions and behaviors.
   B. Confidentiality—Dental hygienists respect the confidentiality of patient information and relationships as a demonstration of the value they place on individual autonomy. Dental hygienists acknowledge their obligation to justify any violation of a confidence.
   C. Justice—Dental hygienists value justice and support the fair and equitable distribution of health-care resources. They believe all people should have access to high-quality, affordable oral health care.

4. Many dental and dental hygiene regulating bodies have established Well-Being Committees to address the issue of impaired providers. As a profession, dental hygienists honor their obligation to society through the establishment and work of such committees. This is referred to as:
   A. Justice
   B. Veracity
   C. Paternalism
   D. Self-regulation

Review Questions

1. The model for health care practiced today is referred to as paternalistic.
   A. True
   B. False

2. Which of the following terms captures the elements of disclosure, understanding, and permission giving?
   A. Beneficence
   B. Justice
   C. Nonmaleficence
   D. Informed consent

Review Questions—cont'd

3. It is in the best interests of the dental hygiene profession in those instances where they are regulated by state dental boards consisting predominantly of dentists to have the practice acts revised through rulemaking versus statutory law.
   A. True
   B. False

4. The *primary* message highlighted in the U.S. Surgeon General Report on Oral Health and the Canadian Oral Health Strategy was:
   A. Oral health is essential to the general health and well-being of individuals.
   B. The two leading dental diseases are caries and periodontal disease.

C. The fluoridation of water was one of the most significant public health measures in the 20th century.
   D. General risk factors such as tobacco use and poor dietary practices affect oral and craniofacial health.

5. Common findings in both the U.S. Surgeon General Report on Oral Health and the Canadian Oral Health Strategy include the issues of disparity and access.
   A. True
   B. False

Active Learning

1. Most state dental hygiene associations organize legislative lobby days for their members each year. Lobby Day provides an opportunity for dental hygiene students to travel to their respective state capitols to see for themselves firsthand how the legislative process actually works. Contact your state dental hygiene association to find out when the next Lobby Day event will take place and make plans to attend.

2. Interview two to three practicing dental hygienists about ethical dilemmas that they have encountered during their years in practice. Bring these dilemmas back for a class discussion.

3. Find the practice acts for the state/province that you plan to practice in upon graduation by searching the Internet and finding the regulatory body for dentistry and dental hygiene.

4. Using the ethical dilemmas identified by the practicing dental hygienists, review the state practice act, and use the ethical decision-making model to determine whether the practice act has any impact on determining the appropriate course of action. ■

REFERENCES

1. Menikoff J. *Law and Bioethics: An Introduction.* Washington, DC: Georgetown University Press; 2001:1.

2. Schackman B, Gebo K, Walensky R, et al. The lifetime cost of current immunodeficiency virus care in the United States. *Med Care.* 2006;44(11):990-997.

3. HIV transmission. Atlanta, GA: Centers for Disease Control and Prevention. http://www.cdc.gov/hiv/resources/qa/transmission.htm#10. Updated March 25, 2010. Accessed October 29, 2010.

4. Enforcing the ADA: looking back on a decade of progress. Washington, DC: U.S. Department of Justice. http://www.ada.gov/pubs/10thrpt.htm#anchor30598. Updated July 2000. Accessed October 29, 2010.

5. Recommendations for preventing transmission of human immunodeficiency virus and hepatitis B virus to patients during exposure-prone invasive procedures. Atlanta, GA: Centers for Disease Control. http://www.cdc.gov/mmwr/preview/mmwrhtml/00014845.htm. Updated July 1991. Accessed December 2, 2010.

6. Code of ethics. Chicago, IL: The American Dental Hygienists' Association. http://www.adha.org/downloads/ADHA-Bylaws-Code-of-Ethics.pdf. Adopted June 28, 2010. Accessed October 29, 2010.

7. Code of ethics. Ottawa, ON: The Canadian Dental Hygienists' Association; 2002. http://www.cdha.ca/pdfs/Profession/Resources/CDHA_Code_of_Ethics_public.pdf. Accessed October 29, 2010.

8. Code of ethics. Victoria, Australia: The International Federation of Dental Hygienists; 2003. www.ifdh.org/dt/ifdh_Code_of_Ethics.pdf. Accessed October 29, 2010.

9. *Standards for Clinical Dental Hygiene Practice.* Chicago, IL: American Dental Hygienists' Association; 2008. http://www.adha.org/downloads/adha_standards08.pdf. Accessed October 29, 2010.

10. *The Americans with Disabilities Act and the Rights of Persons with HIV/AIDS to Obtain Occupational Training and State Licensing.* Washington, DC: U.S. Department of Justice. http://www.ada.gov/qahivaids_license.pdf. Accessed October 29, 2010.

11. *Dent v State of West Virginia* 129 U.S. 114 (WV Supreme Ct 1898).

12. Gadbury-Amyot C, Brickle C. Legislative initiatives of the developing advanced dental hygiene practitioner. *J Dent Hyg.* 2010;84(3):110-113.

13. Regulatory authorities in Canada. Ottawa, ON: The Canadian Dental Hygienists' Association. http://www. cdha.ca/cdha/Career_folder/Regulatory_Authorities/ CDHA/Career_Regulatory_Authorities/Regulatory_ Authorities.aspx. Accessed October 29, 2010.

14. Oran D, Tosti M. *Oran's Dictionary of the Law.* 4th ed. Independence, KY: Cengage Learning–Delmar; 2007.

15. Leeuw W. *Maintaining Proper Dental Records.* Cincinnati, OH: Crest Oral-B; 2010. http://www.dentalcare.com/ en-US/dental-education/continuing-education/ce78/ ce78.aspx?ModuleName=introduction&PartID=-1 &SectionID=-1. Accessed June 20, 2012.

16. Zarkowski P. Ethical and legal decision-making. In: Darby ML, Walsh MM, eds. *Dental Hygiene Theory and Practice.* Philadelphia, PA: WB Saunders; 2003:1107-1134.

17. Edelstein L. The Hippocratic oath: text, translation and interpretation. In: Temkin O, Temkin CL, eds. *Ancient Medicine: Selected Papers of Ludwig Edelstein.* Baltimore, MD: John Hopkins University; 1967:6.

18. Position paper: guidelines for periodontal therapy. Chicago, IL: American Academic of Periodontology; 2001. *J Periodontol.* 2001;72:1624-1628. http://www. perio.org/resources-products/pdf/33-therapy.pdf. Accessed October 29, 2010.

19. Fones AC. The origin and history of the dental hygienists. *J Dent Hyg.* 2013;87(Suppl 1):58-62.

20. Oral health in America: a report of the Surgeon General. Rockville, MD: U.S. Department of Health and Human Services, National Institutes of Health, National Institute of Dental and Craniofacial Research; 2000. http://www. nidcr.nih.gov/DataStatistics/SurgeonGeneral/ Documents/hck1ocv.@www.surgeon.fullrpt.pdf. Accessed October 29, 2010.

21. National call to action to promote oral health. Rockville, MD: U.S. Department of Health and Human Services, National Institutes of Health, National Institute of Dental and Craniofacial Research; 2003. http:// www.nidcr.nih.gov/DataStatistics/SurgeonGeneral/ NationalCalltoAction/nationalcalltoaction.htm. Accessed October 29, 2010.

22. A Canadian oral health strategy. Montreal, QC: Federal, Provincial, and Territorial Dental Directors; 2005. http://www.fptdwg.ca/English/e-cohs.html. Accessed October 29, 2010.

23. Beauchamp TL, Childress JF. *Principles of Biomedical Ethics.* 5th ed. New York: Oxford University Press; 2001.

24. Lindhe J, Socransky S, Nyman S, Haffajee A, Westfelt E. Critical probing depths in periodontal therapy. *J Clin Periodontol.* 1982:9:323-336.

25. Alves RV, Machion L, Casati MZ, Nociti FH, Sallum AW, Sallum EA. Attachment loss after scaling and root planing with different instruments. A clinical study. *J Clin Periodontol.* 2004;31(1):12-15.

26. Health Information Portability and Accountability Act (HIPAA) Privacy Rule. Washington, DC: U.S. Department of Health & Human Services; 2003. http://www. hhs.gov/ocr/privacy/hipaa/administrative/privacyrule/ index.html. Accessed November 4, 2010.

27. HIPAA Privacy Rule and Public Health: Guidance from CDC and the U.S. Department of Health and Human Services. *MMWR Morb Mortal Wkly Rep.* 2003;52:1-12. http://www.cdc.gov/mmwr/preview/mmwrhtml/ m2e411a1.htm.

28. Welch MR, Rivera RE, Conway BP, Yonkoski J, Lupon PM, Glancola R. Determinants and consequences of social trust. *Social Inquiry.* 2005;75:453-473.

Chapter 3 | Communication Skills

Stacy McCauley, RDH, MS

KEY TERMS

ambivalence

closed-ended questions

motivational interviewing (MI)

nonverbal communication

open-ended dialogue

proxemics

reflective listening

two-way communication

verbal communication

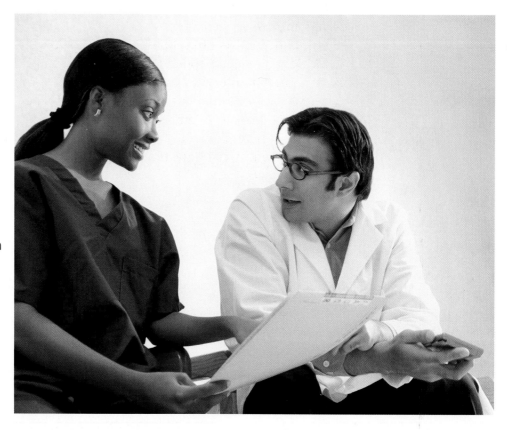

LEARNING OBJECTIVES

After reading this chapter, the student should be able to:

3.1 Discuss strategies for impactful communication throughout the dental hygiene process of care.

3.2 Outline ideal proxemics for optimal patient communication.

3.3 Describe various communication strategies for eliciting comprehensive information from a patient.

3.4 Detail the principles of motivational interviewing and how to apply them to clinical care.

3.5 Give examples of language strategies to create value for the dental hygiene process of care.

3.6 Discuss cultural differences and how they might apply to the dental hygiene process of care.

KEY CONCEPTS

• Communication skills are highly individualized from person to person.

• Some of the best communicators are first and foremost good listeners.

• Reflective listening is a critical skill that allows the dental hygienist to gather important information related to the individual patient.

- In addition to oral communication skills, current technology trends and generational preferences have spawned a new era of communication that uses platforms such as e-mail communication, text messaging, and social media websites.
- Communication proxemics is essential skills used during the dental hygiene appointment.
- Dental hygienists can set patients up for success while creating value for the dental hygiene appointment through compelling word choices.
- Motivational interviewing is a new strategy for enhancing the relationships between clinician and patient to better achieve adherence with treatment plans and long-term oral care protocols.
- With the increasingly diverse landscape of culture across the United States, cultural competency awareness is necessary for all dental hygiene professionals.

RELEVANCE TO CLINICAL PRACTICE

Communication is the cornerstone of almost every aspect of the dental hygienist's career. Productive, healthy communication occurs between the dental staff and the dentist, between individual staff members, between clinicians and patients, and between clinicians and patient caregivers (i.e., parents of minors, spouses, home health aides, among others). For behavior change to occur, patients must feel a connection with the dental professional. Connections are made through strategic, purposeful listening and dialogue tactics that allow for clinicians to establish common ground with patients, essentially humanizing themselves to break through the sterile relationship of health-care provider and patient.

WHAT IS COMMUNICATION?

Definition

Gary Schwartz defines communication as "the imparting or interchange of thoughts, opinions, or information by speech, writing, or signs."[1] Although communication can involve a one-way approach, this chapter emphasizes two-way communication. **Two-way communication** is the primary mode of communication for dental hygienists in the professional setting. From this point forward in this chapter, the term *communication* will carry the connotation of the two-way model.

Types of Communication

Communication is divided into two main categories: verbal and nonverbal. **Verbal communication** can be further divided into written and oral communication. Oral communication can be in person and face-to-face, or it can occur in an alternative setting such as communicating over the phone or communicating via voice over the Internet. Oral communication is heavily influenced by voice tone, inflection, volume, word selection, speed, and clarity. Early research into the science of communication revealed three major components that convey meaning in face-to-face verbal communication: body language, tone of voice, and word use. Dr. Albert Mehrabian concluded from his research that when we assess oral communication, the listener relies on the following cues to interpret what the speaker has said: 55% of the impact is determined by the speaker's body language (posture, gestures, and eye contact), 38% by the tone of voice, and 7% by the content or words spoken.[2] Proper proxemics, detailed later in this chapter, is a key component for impactful communication. If a dental hygienist strictly communicates while multitasking (i.e., while donned in mask, gloves, and safety glasses, washing hands, looking down at the chart, or scaling with the ultrasonic), the patient is not in the ideal situation to assess the clinician's body language (i.e., postures, gestures, and eye contact).

Verbal communication can also be in the written form. Examples of written communication are text messages, e-mails, and letters/postcards via traditional mail. The effectiveness of written communication depends on the type of written communication preferences of the receiver, the appropriateness of the vocabulary used, grammar, and conciseness. Examples of different models of communication are listed in Table 3-1. Which one would be more appropriate for everyday communication with patients?

Nonverbal communication is the body language of the speaker, including facial expressions, posture, use of hand gestures, body movements, and even the type of handshake given. Patients will likely make snap judgments about your intelligence, your professionalism, and your clinical skill, simply by assessing your nonverbal communication. This nonverbal communication assessment begins when you walk out into the reception area to greet your patient. Consider how you present yourself to your new patient. Are you smiling? Do you extend your hand to offer a friendly yet firm handshake? Is your gate brisk and confident, or are you slouching and walking without confidence? Cultural norms influence many aspects of nonverbal communication. They are discussed later in this chapter. Another type of nonverbal communication that is commonly used in the dental hygiene process of care is the use of pictorial representations (such as a picture of the progression of periodontal disease or a poster showing black lungs caused by smoking).

Proxemics is also discussed when researchers study nonverbal communication. As early as 1966, anthropologist Edward T. Hall described **proxemics** as the study of set measurable distances between people as they interact (Fig. 3-1).[3]

Hall's research revealed that body spacing and posture were natural human unconscious reactions to perceived fluctuations in the sound and pitch of a person's voice. During communication, Hall found that study subjects varied their proxemics (body spacing and posture) constantly because of varying degrees of changes in the conversation. Hall also described various degrees

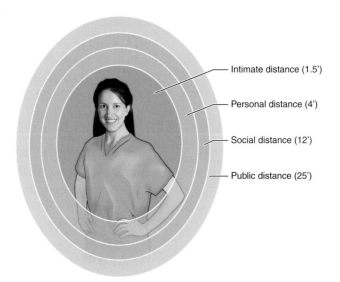

Intimate distance (1.5')
Personal distance (4')
Social distance (12')
Public distance (25')

Figure 3-1. Edward Hall's proxemics personal space.

of proxemic distance depending on the type of communication, the relationship of the communicators, and the content of the message. Below are the types and descriptions of the various types of distance that were defined by Hall. During dental hygiene instrumentation, the clinician is most frequently in the patient's intimate and personal distance:[3]

- *Intimate distance* for embracing, touching, or whispering
  - Close phase: less than 6 inches
  - Far phase: 6 to 18 inches
- *Personal distance* for interactions among good *friends* or *family members*
  - Close phase: 1.5 to 2.5 feet
  - Far phase: 2.5 to 4 feet
- *Social distance* for interactions among acquaintances
  - Close phase: 4 to 7 feet
  - Far phase: 7 to 12 feet

Table 3-1. *Examples of Interpreting Two-Way Communication*	
Two-Way Communication Sending Professional, Concise Message Chairside	**Two-Way Communication Sending Professional, Concise Message Chairside**
Example of oral message: "I am concerned about the moderate bone loss between the molars on the upper right. At your next periodontal maintenance appointment, I will be carefully evaluating the disease progression."	Example of oral message: "I found a tiny bit of bone loss today. We'll keep an eye on it. By the way, make sure you bring that recipe you told me about to your next checkup. I love Thai food!"
Two-Way Communication Sending a Mixed-Message Chairside	**Two-Way Communication Sending a Mixed Message as Follow-up**
Written message appointment confirmation: "Your oral health is important to us. We have reserved time just for you. Please consider this your confirmation of your preventive maintenance appointment with our hygienist, Kristen, on May 20th at 9:50 a.m.	Written message appointment reminder: "Don't forget! Your checkup and cleaning is just around the corner. We hope to see you and your teeth then ☺ LOL! Just remember you only have to floss the ones you want to keep... ROTFL!!!

- *Public distance* used for public speaking
  - Close phase - 12 to 25 feet
  - Far phase - 25 feet or more

The dental hygienist is entering into the intimate and personal distance zone during dental hygiene treatment. Based on what we know about those typically allowed in this intimate distance, one can imagine how intrusive and uncomfortable this invasion of personal space might feel to some patients. Therefore, clinicians should save intimate distance for instrumentation only. When a clinician wants to communicate an important message, the patient should be repositioned at a personal distance or social distance (Fig. 3-2).

Hall notes that different cultures maintain different standards of personal space. For example, in Latin cultures, distances are smaller, and people tend to be more comfortable standing close to each other.[3] In many Native American tribe cultures, direct eye contact is a sign of disrespect and moments of silence after being asked a question is a sign of respect. Later in this chapter, cultural communication strategies will be discussed in detail.

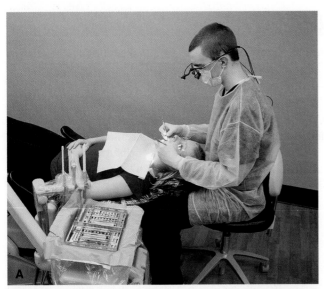

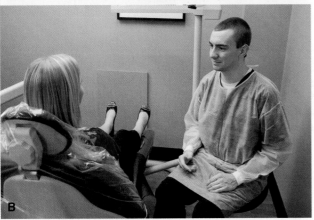

Figure 3-2. Examples of varying distances during dental hygiene treatment. (A) Intimate distance is appropriate for instrumentation. (B) A more appropriate distance is used during patient education.

WHY DO WE HAVE COMMUNICATION BREAKDOWNS?

Communication is deemed successful only when both parties in the two-way communication loop process correctly understand the message sent and received. Common barriers must be addressed before the "source/dental hygienist" sends a message to the "receiver/patient." The dental hygienist must plan the message before sending it. It is imperative to construct a concise, well-planned message. What are some common mistakes in this first step of communication? If your message (e.g., oral hygiene instructions) is too lengthy, too complex, contains grammatical errors, uses objectionable or culturally insensitive language, or is inaudible, the patient will not decode your message with the context you intended. Therefore, when the patient returns to the dental hygiene clinic 3 months later, it may seem as if the patient has not followed recommendations such as using a recommended power toothbrush. Effective communicators use the KISS (Keep It Simple and Straightforward) principle.

Good communication must be efficient and effective to be successfully processed. One common mistake in communication is not to know your audience (the patient). Your message of oral hygiene instructions will be constructed very differently based on your audience. For example, during a dental hygiene appointment, you would precode your message related to oral hygiene instructions with more scientific terminology if you are dealing with a 55-year-old pharmacist. Your message will be coded very differently for your next patient, who is a 17-year-old boy with Asperger disorder and who also suffers from a severe dental phobia. This message is coded in more teen-friendly, layperson, soft-spoken, slower-paced language. Failure to understand who you are communicating with will result in delivering messages that are misunderstood and will result in failed communication.

Customizing the message and sending it is only one part of the communication process. How do you know if the patient understood you correctly? A common mistake that can shut down the two-way communication process is to follow up your message with a question such as, "Do you have any questions?" or "Do you understand?" Questions worded in this fashion can be perceived as condescending or challenging. For effective two-way communication, dental hygienists could rephrase "Do you understand?" like this, "Kelly, I have had other patients tell me they are confused about the various options for orthodontic treatment I have just explained. Tell me what might have been unclear and I will be happy to go over anything I may not have explained well." Phrasing the question in this fashion lets the patient know it is acceptable to ask questions because other patients have had the same confusion. It also tells the patient that the hygienist takes responsibility for not being clear, taking away any of the embarrassment the patient may feel about asking a question. Table 3-2 shows patient communication scenarios regarding precoding the message.

Another key aspect of communication is the ability to deliver a form of communication that the individual patient prefers. As you consider the generational differences in your patient population, would an adolescent prefer scenario A or scenario B in Table 3-3?

In January 2010, the Kaiser Family Foundation revealed research showing the average child, aged 8 to 18 years, connects with media (music, TV, Internet, video games) an average of 75 hours per week.[4] That estimate did not include the hour and a half spent text messaging each day, and the half hour spent talking on a cell phone. The research also revealed that children spent only 38 minutes a day reading books (read primarily during required reading at school). Technology and brevity are imperative for the adolescent and teen patient. Conversely, an elderly patient will likely prefer an eye-to-eye, one-on-one verbal conversation with plenty of time for asking questions.

DIALOGUING WITH THE PATIENT

The process of dental hygiene care is comprehensive and holistic. At the dawn of dental hygiene, clinicians focused solely on what they saw in the patient's mouth during the dental hygiene appointment. Within recent years, the dental hygiene process of care is now increasingly comprehensive. Adding to this comprehensive approach is the changing landscape of the demographics of health in this country. Dental hygienists treat more complex, medically compromised patients than ever before. To ascertain the holistic nature of the patient, the dental hygienist must be able to gather in-depth personal details surrounding the patient's medical history, social history, oral care behaviors at home, and individual patient wants and needs regarding long-term oral health.

One strategy for getting a patient to open up and allow the dental hygienist to gather accurate, comprehensive information for better assessment and treatment planning is to try to incorporate **open-ended dialogue** during patient communication (Table 3-4).

Table 3-2. *Patient Communication Scenarios: Precoding the Message*		
Scenario	**Critical Thinking Questions**	**Feedback**
Scenario A: Celia is a 29-year-old single mother with four children. She works full-time as a bus driver for the city transit department and there are rumors that the city will be cutting jobs in her department by the end of the year. She has a history of severe depression and was hospitalized twice in the past for attempted suicide. Her two older children, ages 12 and 11, spent most of their early years in and out of foster care while Celia was being treated for severe depression. Two years ago, Celia regained full custody of her four children. Today, Celia has brought her youngest son, age 3, in for his first dental visit because she noticed his "upper teeth are rotting." Another issue to consider is Celia's own dental history: Celia is an extremely fearful dental patient with a history of abscessed teeth and dental extractions.	How would you precode Celia's message? What level of language would you use? What type of tone, volume, and nonverbal communication strategies would you use?	In this instance, less is more for this single mother who is overwhelmed, dental phobic, and medically complicated. Keep the oral hygiene instruction very basic, use helpful language, ask permission to show her how to implement new strategies for better brushing, and avoid asking her questions that might be interpreted as questioning her competence as a mother.
Scenario B: Pedro is a 33-year-old attorney specializing in medical malpractice. Pedro has maintained a perfect record of seeing the dental hygienist every 3 months for his periodontal maintenance appointments over the past 8 years. Pedro has recently undergone a "smile makeover" where the dentist placed 12 beautiful porcelain veneers on Pedro's maxillary teeth. He is a self-proclaimed "health nut" and is very well-read on both homeopathic medicine and emerging trends in biomedical science. On the weekends, Pedro also performs stand-up comedy during amateur hour at the local comedy club.	How would you precode Pedro's message? What level of language would you use? What type of tone, volume, and nonverbal communication strategies would you use?	Pedro exhibits a high level of science and health knowledge. His dental history leads us to believe he is very committed to keeping his mouth as healthy as possible. Pedro is highly educated and has a jovial personality. A more lighthearted, yet science-based tone would be appropriate for this patient.

Table 3-3. *Patient Communication Scenarios: Precoding the Message for Generational Differences*

Scenarios	Critical Thinking Questions	Feedback
Scenario A: The patient is an 11-year-old boy. The dental hygienist spends 10 minutes discussing the caries disease process using an in-depth, face-to-face explanation communication approach where the adolescent patient spends 95% of the time listening to the hygienist talk about "a bunch of technical stuff."	Based on your knowledge of precoding the message to the intended end user, which scenario is most appropriate for this patient?	Scenario B is definitely the more appropriate choice for this 11-year-old boy.
Scenario B: In this scenario with the 11-year-old boy, the dental hygienist puts a laptop computer in the child's lap and the child is introduced to a 45-second, interactive computer game that diagrams the caries disease process using computer-generated animation.		

Table 3-4. *Open-Ended Dialogue Versus Closed-Ended Questions*

Examples of Closed-Ended Questions	Examples of Open-Ended Dialogue
"Have you been flossing?"	"Tell me what you are doing on a daily basis to take care of your teeth and gums."
"Have you had any changes in your health history?"	"Please share with me what has been going on with your health, medications, hospitalizations, and so forth since your last visit."
"You're not still putting cola in her sippy cup, are you?"	"Mom, share with me a typical day for Ava regarding food preferences, drink choices, and snacking."
"Did you fill that prescription for fluoride?"	"Tell me how it's going with the fluoride rinse Dr. Greenberg prescribed at your last appointment."

Closed-ended questions are answered with "yes" or "no." An example of a closed-ended question would be, "Have you been flossing?" or "Have there been any changes to your medical history?" Closed-ended questions are fine when the clinician does not need an in-depth explanation. However, they do not allow the patient to elaborate. When the dental hygienist is attempting to construct a comprehensive overview of the individual patient, open-ended dialogue is the best strategy. Open-ended questions/dialogue cannot be answered with a simple yes or no.

Many patients feel apprehensive during a dental hygiene visit and might withhold information for the following reasons: (a) They do not feel that it is necessary to elaborate on the topic because they feel it is probably not pertinent to the dental hygiene appointment; (b) they are embarrassed about sharing their private information with you; or (c) they have not had to answer these types of questions in the past, so they do not understand why they need to share personal information now. Many patients hold this opinion: "I don't see why it's any of their business that I'm taking an antidepressant; it's just a cleaning appointment. It's not like I'm at the doctor's office." Patients do not always understand the complexities of the mouth–body connection, or the impact of certain

Application to Clinical Practice

Open-ended questions and the principles of motivational interviewing (MI) are appropriate for all aspects of human communication. Although deeply seated in the professions of counseling and psychiatry, MI is also being embraced by all facets of medicine and dentistry. Can you think of a time when you have been a patient and you have not felt comfortable with sharing everything with your doctor, nurse practitioner, or even dental hygienist?

MI and open-ended questioning are even being used in family and marriage counseling. For example, instead of a wife asking her husband, "Did you buy that pool table even though it was far over our budget?" MI strategies would have posed the question in a much less threatening and defensive-response fashion. Think about this response instead of the response to the previously asked question: "Tell me how things are going with your search for a pool table?" Whether talking about our own personal relationships or our relationships with our patients, MI is the key for open discussion and nonjudgment. ■

prescription and over-the-counter medications or certain social behaviors on their oral health, and the clinician's rationale for making assessment, treatment planning, and long-term oral care recommendations.

One of the pitfalls of wording a question in a closed format is the potential for the patient to simply say no and the conversation stops. The open-ended format puts the onus on the patient to provide more information. Another potential pitfall of asking a closed-ended question is the potential for the patient to interpret your question as accusatory in tone. "Did you fill that prescription for fluoride?" can make the patient defensive, especially if she did not fill the prescription. In that instance, the patient may feel that she has failed and let you down. The patient might also fear she will be reprimanded by you and the dentist. So, to avoid this potentially negative situation, the patient might: (a) lie and tell you she filled the prescription and is doing fine with it; or (b) tell you "No!" and say nothing else, all while exhibiting strong nonverbal communication that she does not want to be reprimanded about it.

The open-ended dialogue strategy puts the question in a positive tone of assumption that the patient has already been successful. The following sentence is not in the form of a question; the sentence is purposefully worded in a statement that assumes the patient was adherent: "Tell me how it's going with the fluoride rinse Dr. Greenberg prescribed at your last appointment." In this example, the hygienist carefully preplanned his dialogue in a supportive tone. Through strategic word choices, the hygienist is alluding to the fact that he is confident that the patient was adherent with the recommendation for the use of prescription fluoride. Even if the patient did not fill the prescription, the clinician has created a nonthreatening, supportive tone of conversation and the patient is more likely to be honest about not adhering to the dentist's recommendation. The conversation can continue without a wall of defensiveness. Hygienists may try to persuade patients to change and patients may resist these pleas with excuses and reasons they are unable to follow the recommendations.[5] If clinicians can adopt open-ended dialogue into their patient interactions, this no-win power struggle can be avoided.

MOTIVATIONAL INTERVIEWING: STRATEGIES TO ELICIT REAL CHANGE

Smoking is bad for you; so why don't people quit? Adherence to prescribed medication is critical to maintain safe blood pressure; so why are people noncompliant? Adhering to periodontal maintenance protocols is essential for controlling the periodontal disease process; so why do some patients stop coming to their appointments? Across all disciplines of health

Teamwork

You are helping another dental hygiene student document a patient's periodontal assessment data in clinic today. You notice that the student, Logan, is using with her patient today the skills she learned in this communication skills chapter. After she finished charting, she asked her patient about the xylitol rinse that was recommended and noted in the previous chart notes. Logan said to the patient, "Tell me how it's going with the xylitol rinse our clinic dentist recommended at your last appointment." In this example, Logan has carefully preplanned her dialogue in a supportive tone. Through strategic word choices, Logan is alluding to the fact that she is confident that the patient was adherent with the recommendation for the use of the xylitol rinse. Even if the patient did not comply with the dentist's recommendations for using the rinse, she has created a nonthreatening, supportive tone of conversation and the patient is more likely to admit to not adhering with the dentist's recommendation and the conversation can continue without a wall of defensiveness. While Logan steps away from her operatory to process her radiographs, the patient turns to you, and says, "I was afraid she was going to scold me for not buying that rinse the dentist recommended. I'm glad she didn't make me feel bad about it." Later, while you are helping her clean her operatory, you compliment Logan on her use of MI language strategies. ■

care, there are widespread challenges for adherence to professional recommendations. One strategy to assist the dental hygienist in avoiding some of the resistance to adherence challenges is the concept of **motivational interviewing (MI).** Steven Rollnick, in his book *Motivational Interviewing in Healthcare,* defines MI as "a collaborative, person-centered form of guiding to elicit and strengthen motivation for change."[6] Traditional oral health education consists of advice giving and persuasive approaches.[7] The current assessment of this traditional oral health education model reveals an enormous failure in the system. Education and information transferred to the patient does not equate to health-care recommendation adherence. The dental hygienist can present the information to the patient, explain the diagnosis, and discuss the treatment plan options, but that does not mean the patient will adhere to the recommendations. The patient must feel the need for change.

MI is a communication strategy that can be easily integrated into the dental hygiene process of care. MI is a patient-centered interaction, a brief counseling technique in which negation guides behavior change.[8] Through a series of open-ended questions, the clinician can help guide the conversation to help a patient

Spotlight on Public Health

Using an MI approach in patient education can be helpful. In a public health setting, where individuals might not have received routine dental care, the benefits of MI are numerous. The MI approach is nonthreatening and uses patient-driven cues to help guide the clinician in evoking patient-initiated change. The traditional education-based approach is ultimately unsuccessful, especially in a dental-phobic or dentally unaware (low dental IQ) patient population. For example, MI would be an appropriate technique for communicating the information regarding early childhood caries with a parent in a public health clinic. If a clinician strictly uses education and authority to drive her messaging, the parent will likely become defensive and will not be open to change. ■

express how he feels about a certain behavior (flossing, spit tobacco habit, drinking excessive amounts of soda, etc.). Clinicians most always know the answer to the patient's problem (e.g., patient needs to adhere to oral hygiene recommendations). It would be so easy to give the patient the solution (e.g., "You wouldn't have chronically sore, bleeding gums if you adhered to proper flossing!"). But remember, patients typically *know* the solution and they are not doing it. They have to hear themselves come up with the answer. Lasting change comes from within.

The Spirit of Motivational Interviewing: Three Pillars

Autonomy, collaboration, and evocation form the three pillars of MI (Fig. 3-3). In the traditional approach of hygienist-to-patient education, the hygienist feels compelled to force the patient into compliance with change. In the spirit of MI, the hygienist honors the patient's autonomy, realizing that people can and do make choices about the course of their lives and it is ultimately up to the patient to decide what to do regarding behavior change. The hygienist is encouraged to inform, advise, and even warn patients about risky behaviors and behavior change, but ultimately to respect the fact that change must be patient driven to be successful in the long term.[6]

Read the case study of Bob, a patient with a smoking addiction, later in this chapter. The dental hygienist

in scenario A of the case study fell into the trap of being perceived as confrontational. Even though her intentions were well-meaning, the patient immediately felt like he was being attacked. The spirit of MI focuses on collaboration as the second pillar. MI is successful only if the dynamic between the patient and the hygienist is one of cooperation and collaboration. If the dynamic shifts into a perceived confrontation, then the likelihood for a partnership to develop is ultimately compromised. Bob perceived the dental hygienist's line of questioning as accusatory and demeaning in tone from the first sentence in scenario A. In scenario B, Bob perceived the dental hygienist as one who is caring and understanding. She listened to Bob and let him know that she is willing to wait for him to signal when it is time to collaborate on smoking cessation.

The final pillar of the spirit of MI is the concept of evoking change from within the patient. A patient will not change a behavior simply because you tell him it is bad for him. The only long-term hope for behavior change comes from the health-care professional eliciting and evoking a response from the patient in self-identifying the personal need for change. When the patient and dental hygienist can discuss personal goals, values, dreams, and aspirations, the patient is set up for success because he can see how this particular behavior change fits in with what he wants for himself. In scenario A, the dental hygienist assuming the tactic of saying, "You want to live long enough to see your grandkids graduate high school, don't you?" was enough to get Bob motivated to change. In scenario B, Bob self-identifies the dissolution of his marriage as a major reason he failed at his last smoking cessation attempt. He did not mention his grandchildren as a reason to change. Therefore, the dental hygienist's threat of not seeing his grandkids graduate fails to compel Bob to attempt to quit again.

Listening, specifically reflective listening, is a key component of MI. **Reflective listening** is a two-way feedback loop of communication.[6] Box 3-1 illustrates patient–clinician reflective listening.[6]

The practice of dental hygiene can be frustrating when patients fail to heed our professional recommendations and experience disease progression . . . despite our best efforts, patients with progressive disease fail to change behaviors and end up losing teeth unnecessarily. It is critical to understand that all behavior change (whether related to weight loss, increased exercise, tobacco cessation, adherence to medications or improved oral hygiene) involves some level of **ambivalence.** In MI, the role of the dental hygienist is to engage the patient in meaningful interaction where the patient has the opportunity to explore their values and beliefs about oral/dental health, examine pros and cons related to changing oral health behavior and articulate and resolve ambivalence to change in

A	C	E
Autonomy vs. Authority	Collaboration vs. Confrontation	Evocation vs. Education

Figure 3-3. Three pillars of motivational interviewing.

Box 3-1. *Example of Reflective Listening*

Dental Hygienist: "You mentioned you were worried about seeing the oral surgeon to have that area under your tongue biopsied."

Patient: "I'm beyond worried—I'm scared he'll tell me I have cancer."

Dental Hygienist: "It sounds like the fear of a serious diagnosis has you really scared."

Patient: "Yes, if I go for the biopsy, I know it could be benign and my life will continue on just as it is now. However, if my diagnosis is bad, I'm scared to death I won't be around for my family."

Dental Hygienist: "Being around for your family is the most important thing to you."

Patient: "My family means everything to me. I am tempted to just wait it out to see if that sore under my tongue disappears. Who knows, maybe it will go away on its own."

Dental Hygienist: "It sounds like you don't know what to do. If you have the biopsy and you have a good outcome, that would be a good thing, right?"

Patient: "I suppose. I'm just not sure."

Dental Hygienist: "It sounds like you just don't know what to do. This is not an easy decision for anyone. I have had other patients express the same concern when we discovered an area needing biopsy. From what you're saying today, it sounds like the fear of how this will impact *your family* is actually far more concerning than what an actual cancer diagnosis would mean *to you*. Does that sound about right?"

Patient: "I would say that is right on the money! I know the decision is up to me. I know the best thing to do is to get this checked out. It really helped to talk through this with someone who has dealt with this kind of thing before." ■

---

a nonjudgmental environment. Ultimately, this strategy elicits the patient's own motivation toward behavior change and allows them to become invested in the change process. **It is only when patients are invested in their own behavior that optimal oral health can be achieved.**[5]

The preceding excerpt mentions the term **ambivalence.** What is ambivalence and how does it factor into your strategies for patient communication?

Ambivalence = "I want to, but I don't want to."
"I want to brush better, but I am always in a hurry."
"I know I should brush twice a day, but I am too tired before I go to bed."
"I know I should floss, but it gets shredded and stuck in my teeth so I don't do it."
"I should stop smoking, but I just can't seem to do it."

The "but" in the middle of the statements is a strong sign of ambivalence. It is as though the statements on either side of the "but" cancel each other out so nothing happens—the patient is stuck in a no-change situation. How does a clinician overcome a patient's ambivalence? The clinician can use open-ended or guiding questions to overcome ambivalence.

"I want to brush better, but I am always in a hurry."
Traditional response: "Brushing only takes 2 minutes! You're telling me you can't find 2 little minutes out of an entire day to brush?"
MI type of response: "Many of my patients have the same issue regarding busy schedules. May I introduce you to a way to better clean your teeth that will not take any longer in your busy schedule?"
"I know I should brush twice a day, but I am too tired before I go to bed."
Traditional response: "Why don't you try and brush right after dinner instead of right before bed?"

MI type of response: "I know exactly what you mean; bedtime is so busy, especially with four young kids. Can you tell me your routine after dinner and before bedtime? Maybe you can find a few spare minutes that are not too close to bedtime."
"I know I should floss, but it gets shredded and stuck in my teeth so I don't do it."
Traditional response: "Here is a sample of shred-free floss. I'm sure this will do the trick."
MI type of response: "That must be frustrating; tell me more about where the floss catches between your teeth."
"I should stop smoking, but I just can't seem to do it."
Traditional response: "I know it's probably hard to quit, but you really need to try again."
MI type of response: "How do you see your life being different when you do quit smoking?"

CREATING VALUE FOR THE DENTAL HYGIENE APPOINTMENT THROUGH COMMUNICATION

Competence in mastering the clinical skills of dental hygiene is essential for optimal patient care. However, clinical care is only one aspect of long-term oral health. Long-term oral health is also achieved when the clinician achieves adherence with patient behavior change at home. Motivating communication strategies are critical for compelling the patient to adopt new home care routines. In addition, communication strategies for creating value for the dental hygiene appointment are equally as important. According Linda Miles and associates, "The number one reason a patient fails to keep an appointment for a dental hygiene visit is the fact that they are unaware of their need for keeping it."[9] The hygienist must communicate value for the patient to be compelled to return for future treatment. Review the following two scenarios. Kevin, the hygienist, is communicating with Hank, a routine prophylaxis patient. As the appointment concludes, Kevin removes the patient's bib and says:

Scenario A: "Hank, it was great seeing you today. Make sure you bring your vacation pictures with you when I see you in 6 months! I've heard so many wonderful things about Alaskan cruises. When you check out at the front desk, Mary will make your next cleaning appointment. Bye!"

Scenario B: "Hank, I am so glad you came in for your appointment today so I could carefully evaluate everything. It looks like you have been really stepping things up at home with your brushing and flossing—keep up the good work. However, I am still quite concerned about the bleeding you have on the lower right. The lower right also has the area of slight gum recession. Hank, over the next 6 months, I want you to continue to be mindful of this area. I am going to make a note in your chart so I am sure to evaluate the area carefully, to assess the bleeding, at your next preventive maintenance visit. I would like to set aside time especially for you. Would you like to see me at 11:00 on the 9th of June or 10:30 on the 13th of June?"

Which scenario creates a compelling reason for Hank to value his next dental hygiene appointment with Kevin?

Scenario B creates value multiple times. First, Kevin creates value by telling Hank he was glad he came in for the appointment so he could carefully evaluate Hank's condition. Second, Kevin compliments Hank's attempts at improving his home care routine. However, Kevin follows up these positive comments with very specific feedback regarding Hank's current oral condition. By calling attention to site-specific concerns, Kevin is signaling to Hank the need for more adherence to oral hygiene at home to potentially improve the tissue health on the lower right. Kevin is using communication to create value for the next preventive maintenance visit by saying, "I'm going to make a note in your chart so I am sure to evaluate the area carefully, to assess the bleeding, at your next preventive maintenance visit." Kevin also creates value by using the word choices of "set aside time especially for you," and by personally making Hank's appointment's with a definite choice of two concrete dates and at set times. As a result of Kevin's communication strategy, Hank is more likely to make a committed choice for his next preventive maintenance visit because Kevin has limited him by giving Hank only two choices in scheduling. Compare this strategy with the one used in scenario A where Kevin said, "When you check out at the front desk, Mary will make your next cleaning appointment. Bye!" Finally, for this concept of creating value for the patient to be solidified, Kevin must follow through with what he told Hank. The June appointment should

begin with an evaluation of the tissue response to assess bleeding on the lower right, as well as an evaluation of the recession. This will clearly signal the value of maintaining the preventive maintenance visits for this patient.

PRACTICING DENTAL HYGIENE IN A MULTICULTURAL SOCIETY

The United States has been known as a melting pot of cultures for generations. This presents an exciting opportunity for dental professionals, but it can also be a source of frustration. Unless we are educated on the cultural nuances among various ethnic/cultural/religious groups, it may be a source of potential miscommunication. Intercultural communication principles guide the process of exchanging meaningful and unambiguous information across cultural boundaries in a way that preserves mutual respect and minimizes antagonism.[10]

The Dutch sociologist Gerard Hendrik Hofstede conducted much of the early research examining cultural differences. His work describes five key dimensions of culture (Table 3-5):[11]

1. **Power/Distance (PD):** This refers to the degree of inequality that exists—and is accepted—among people with and without power. A high PD score indicates that society accepts an unequal distribution of power and people understand their place in the system. Low PD means that power is shared and well dispersed. It also means that society members view themselves as equals.
   Clinical Application: According to Hofstede's model, a patient from a high PD country such Mexico may not respond well to direction from the dental assistant. They may be more likely to adhere to recommendations if they come directly from the dentist.

2. **Individualism (IDV):** This refers to the strength of the ties people have to others within the community. A high IDV score indicates a loose connection with people. In countries with a high IDV score, there is a lack of interpersonal connection and little sharing of responsibility beyond family and perhaps a few close friends. A society with a low IDV score would have strong group cohesion, and there would be a large amount of loyalty and respect for members of the group. The group itself is also larger and people take more responsibility for each other's well-being (see Table 3-5).
   Clinical Application: Hofstede's analysis suggests that in cultures from countries where the IDV scores are very low, a clinician who emphasizes how oral health of the parents can negatively impact the oral health of the child would be very impactful. In high IDV cultures, the impact on others is not considered as important. Therefore, patient communication must be primarily focused on how this solely impacts the patient.

Table 3-5. *Hofstede's Research Surrounding Cultural Values, Behaviors, Intuitions, and Organizations*

Five Key Dimensions of Culture	Characteristics	Clinical Implications
Power/Distance (PD)—refers to the degree of inequality that exists, and is accepted, among people with and without power		
High PD Cultures (e.g., Russian, Mexican)	• Strong hierarchies • Large gaps in compensation, authority, and respect	• Respect for hierarchy • Be aware that you may achieve greater patient adherence if the dentist is directly involved in making recommendations
Low PD Cultures (e.g., Israeli, Austrian)	• Everyone is on a level playing field—in the workplace, supervisors and employees are considered almost as equals	• Use teamwork • Involve as many people as possible in decision-making
Individualism (IDV)—refers to the strength of the ties people have to others within the community		
High IDV (e.g., American, British)	• High valuation on people's time and their need for freedom • An enjoyment of challenges, and an expectation of rewards for hard work • Respect for privacy	• Acknowledge the patient's accomplishments • Do not ask for too much personal information • Encourage dialogue and expression of patient's own ideas
Low IDV (e.g., Pakistani, Guatemalan)	• Emphasis on building skills and becoming masters of something • Work for intrinsic rewards • Harmony more important than honesty	• Show respect for age and wisdom • Suppress feelings and emotions to work in harmony • Respect traditions and introduce change slowly
Masculinity (MAS)—how much a society sticks with, and values, traditional male and female roles		
High MAS (e.g., Japanese, Hungarian)	• Men are masculine and women are feminine • There is a well-defined distinction between men's work and women's work	• Be aware that people may expect male and female roles to be distinct • Male patients are not likely to make decisions based on emotion
Low MAS (e.g., Swedish, Norwegian)	• A woman can do anything a man can do • Powerful and successful women are admired and respected	• Avoid an "old boys' club" mentality • Ensure job design and practices are not discriminatory to either sex • Treat men and women equally
Uncertainty/Avoidance Index (UAI)—degree of anxiety society members feel when in uncertain or unknown situations		
High UAI (e.g., Greek, Portuguese)	• Very formal business conduct with lots of rules and policies • Need and expect structure • Sense of nervousness spurs high levels of emotion and expression • Differences are avoided	• Be clear and concise about your expectations and parameters • Plan and prepare, communicate often and early, provide detailed plans and focus on the tactical aspects of a treatment plan • Express your emotions through hand gestures and enthusiastic voice inflection

Table 3-5. *Hofstede's Research Surrounding Cultural Values, Behaviors, Intuitions, and Organizations—cont'd*

Five Key Dimensions of Culture	Characteristics	Clinical Implications
Low UAI (e.g., Jamaican, Swedish)	• Informal business attitude • More concern with long-term strategy than what is happening on a daily basis • Accepting of change and risk	• Do not impose rules or structure unnecessarily • Minimize your emotional response by being calm and contemplating situations before speaking • Express curiosity when you discover differences
Long-Term Orientation (LTO)—refers to how much society values long-standing, as opposed to short-term, traditions and values		
High LTO (e.g., Chinese, Taiwanese)	• Family is the basis of society • Parents and men have more authority than young people and women • Strong work ethic • High value placed on education and training	• Show respect for traditions • Do not display extravagance or act frivolously • Reward perseverance, loyalty, and commitment • Avoid doing anything that would cause another to "lose face"
Low LTO (e.g., Canadian, American)	• Promotion of equality • High creativity, individualism • Treat others as you would like to be treated • Self-actualization is sought	• Expect to live by the same standards and rules you create • Be respectful of others • Do not hesitate to introduce necessary changes

3. **Masculinity (MAS):** This refers to how much a society adheres to, and values, traditional male and female roles. High MAS scores are found in countries where men are expected to be tough, the provider, assertive, and strong. If women work outside the home, they have separate professions from men. Low MAS scores do not reverse the gender roles. In a low MAS society, the roles are simply blurred. Women and men work together equally across many professions. Men are allowed to be sensitive and women can work hard for professional success. Clinical Application: Japan is highly masculine, whereas Sweden has the lowest measured value of masculinity. According to Hofstede's analysis, if you work as a dental hygienist in a practice with a large number of patients who are Japanese businessmen, you might have greater success in gaining adherence if a male coworker or if the male dentist reinforces your treatment plan recommendations. Conversely, an immigrant from a country like Sweden would not consider gender whatsoever in how he or she receives information regarding his or her treatment plan.

4. **Uncertainty/Avoidance Index (UAI):** This relates to the degree of anxiety society members feel when in uncertain or unknown situations. High UAI-scoring nations try to avoid ambiguous situations whenever possible. They are governed by rules and order, and they seek a collective "truth." Low

UAI scores indicate the society enjoys novel events and values differences. There are few rules and people are encouraged to discover their own truths. Clinical Application: Hofstede's Cultural Dimensions imply that when discussing a treatment plan with a patient from a country with a high UAI, such as Portugal, you should be concise when you present the treatment plan, but be sure to have very detailed information available in case the patient has questions.

5. **Long-Term Orientation (LTO):** This refers to how much society values long-standing, as opposed to short-term, traditions and values. This is the fifth dimension that Hofstede added in the 1990s after finding that Asian countries with a strong link to Confucian philosophy acted differently from Western cultures. In countries with a high LTO score, delivering on social obligations and avoiding "loss of face" are considered very important. Clinical Application: According to Hofstede's analysis, people in the United States and Canada have low LTO scores. This suggests that you can pretty much expect anything in this culture in terms of creative expression and novel ideas. American and Canadian patients might be more willing to adapt to new dental office protocols and nonessential dental procedures such as whitening and veneers compared with a high LTO patient.

Case Study

Scenario A

Dental hygienist says: "Bob, has anyone ever talked with you about smoking cessation before?"

Patient is thinking: *Duh, of course everyone tries to lecture me about how bad it is for me . . . doesn't she know I wish I could have stopped smoking years ago?*

Patient says: "Oh no! You aren't going to start nagging me like my wife, are you?"

Dental hygienist is thinking: *Here we go again . . . another patient resistant to smoking cessation!*

Dental hygienist says: "Gee, Bob, you really need to start thinking about quitting. You want to live long enough to see your grandkids graduate high school, don't you?"

Patient is thinking: *How could she be so insensitive! Of course I don't want to die early! Doesn't she know I've tried to quit and have failed a million times before? I am obviously just too weak and stupid to kick the habit!*

Patient says: "I'm not paying for a lecture today! Please just cut the guilt trip and clean my teeth!"

Scenario B: Using a Motivational Interviewing Approach

Dental hygienist says: "Bob, now that I've finished your dental examination, I would like to check in with you regarding your current smoking status, if I may. I know we've been through this conversation before, but it's important for me to stay current with how things are going for you. Could you share with me how smoking cessation is fitting into your life right now?"

Patient is thinking: *It sounds like she understands that smoking cessation isn't always convenient to fit into my life during certain stressful times.*

Patient says: "You might have heard through the grapevine that Alice and I are getting a divorce. I was really doing well with quitting until I got served with the divorce papers."

Dental hygienist is thinking: *Sounds like things are really stressful for him right now. I'm so proud to hear that Bob actually had a period of success with smoking cessation. I think I'll focus on his period of success while acknowledging that this period of stress must be almost unbearable.*

Dental hygienist says: "I'm so sorry to hear about the divorce. I must, however, applaud what you said earlier. I'm thrilled to hear you had a successful streak where you stopped smoking. With your permission, I'd like to talk with you more about that point in time to find out more about what you did to be so successful with your quitting."

Patient is thinking: *I'm relieved she didn't scold me for going back to smoking.*

Patient says: "I guess I was able to relieve my cravings over the summer because I was involved with my volunteer work and I was playing tennis about three to four nights a week. However, right now, I just can't deal with trying again. Maybe when my divorce is final I'll give it yet another try."

Dental hygienist is thinking: *Right now, I'll just focus on the next attempt and won't stress him out with a lecture on smoking cessation today.*

Dental hygienist says: "It sounds like you had some great success with quitting when you were really involved with your volunteer work and your tennis league. Bob, I am confident you'll be back on track very soon. With your permission, I'd like to check in with you again at your next appointment to see how you're doing with quitting. Would that be okay?"

Case Study Exercises

1. Which scenario seemed to elicit a confrontational and defensive tone by both parties beginning with the opening sentence?
   A. Scenario A
   B. Scenario B
2. Which scenario best demonstrated reflective listening, a key component of MI?
   A. Scenario A
   B. Scenario B
3. Which scenario best demonstrated being comfortable with the patient being the driver of the decision to change on his own terms and at his own time?
   A. Scenario A
   B. Scenario B
4. Scenario B demonstrated which of the following techniques key for MI?
   A. Open-ended questions
   B. Reflective listening
   C. Noting a "bad attitude" in the patient's chart
   D. Both B and C
   E. Both A and B
5. The dental hygienist's final comment in scenario A and scenario B vary dramatically. Identify the MI technique(s) used by the dental hygienist in scenario B.
   A. "It sounds like you had some great success with quitting when you were really involved with your volunteer work and your tennis league."
   B. "Bob, I am confident you'll be back on track very soon."
   C. "With your permission, I'd like to check in with you again at your next appointment to see how you're doing with quitting."
   D. "Would that be okay?"
   E. All of the above

Review Questions

1. According to the proxemics research by Hall, and considering proper patient-operator positioning, which of the following dental hygiene procedure(s) is/are appropriate for the patient's intimate space?
   1. Periodontal probing
   2. Updating medical history
   3. Explaining treatment plan
   4. Demonstrating use of power toothbrush on a dentiform during oral hygiene instruction
   A. 1 only
   B. 2, 3, 4 only
   C. 2 only
   D. All of the above

2. The spirit of MI encompasses three pillars. All of the following are correct EXCEPT which one?
   A. The spirit of MI uses autonomy versus authority.
   B. The spirit of MI uses education versus evocation.
   C. The spirit of MI uses evocation versus education.
   D. The spirit of MI uses collaboration versus confrontation.

3. A hygienist concludes the dental hygiene appointment by saying, "Pat, I'm so glad you came in for your appointment today so I could carefully evaluate everything. It looks like you have really been stepping things up at home with your brushing and flossing—keep up the good work. However, I am still quite concerned about the moderate inflammation you have on the lower right. The lower right also has the area of tooth sensitivity and gum recession. Pat, over the next 6 months, I want you to continue to be mindful of this area. I'm going to make a note in your chart so I am sure to evaluate the area carefully. I will be evaluating the inflammation and examining the sensitivity and recession in that area at your next preventive maintenance visit. I would like to set aside time especially for

you. I know you typically like morning appointments. I have a 10:00 on the 9th of December or a 9:00 on the 13th of December. Which would you prefer?" By ending the appointment with this dialogue, the hygienist has created _____ for the appointment and compels the patient to return for his next appointment.
   A. Validity
   B. Fear
   C. Value
   D. Scare tactics
   E. None of the above

4. Chad, a recent dental hygiene graduate, is applying for a job with a periodontist. Chad has included training in motivational interviewing (MI) on his résumé. The periodontist is not familiar with MI. Which of the following would best describe MI to the periodontist?
   A. MI is a self-taught interviewing technique devised to try and convince patients they need to listen to the expert's opinion.
   B. MI is a collaborative, patient-centered form of guiding to elicit and strengthen motivation for change.
   C. MI is a strategy dentists can use to get patients to say yes to expensive treatment plans.
   D. MI is a communication style that is only used in dentistry and has no application to any other aspects of life.
   E. All of the above

5. Carl is here today for his 3-month periodontal maintenance visit. Maya, the dental hygienist, asks Carl the following question: "Carl, have you had any changes in your health history?" What type of question is this?
   A. Open-ended question
   B. Closed-ended question

Active Learning

1. In groups of three, role-play a dental hygiene appointment. One student is the patient, one student the dental hygienist, and the other student the observer. The hygienist asks a closed-ended question related to any changes in the patient's health history (see Table 3-4). The observer should note how many words and how much useful information is gained using a closed-ended question.
2. The patient and hygienist now switch roles. The new hygienist uses open-ended questions to elicit information

about changes in the patient's health history. The observer should note how many words and how much useful information is gained using an open-ended technique.
3. Discuss the pros and cons of using closed- and open-ended communication strategies with the class. Was it difficult coming up with a question in an open-ended format? Is it ever appropriate to use closed-ended questions? ■

REFERENCES

1. Schwartz GE, Simon WL, Carmona R. *The Energy Healing Experiments.* New York: Simon & Schuster; 2008.
2. Mehrabian A, Ferris S. Inference of attitude from nonverbal communication in two channels. *J Consult Psychol.* 1967;31:248-252.
3. Hall ET. *The Hidden Dimension.* Garden City, NY: Doubleday; 1966.
4. Rideout V, Foehr U, Roberts D. Generation M2: media in the lives of 8- to 18-year-olds. Kaiser Family Foundation Report. http://www.kff.org. Accessed January 20, 2010.
5. Williams K. Motivational interviewing: application to oral health behaviors. *J Dent Hyg.* 2010;84(1):6-9.
6. Rollnick S, Miller W, Butler C. Motivational interviewing in health care: helping patients change behavior. New York: The Guilford Press; 2008.
7. Weinstein P, Harrison R, Benton T. Motivating parents to prevent caries in their young children, one-year findings. *J Am Dent Assoc.* 2004;135(6):731-793.
8. Miller W, Rollnick S. *Motivational Interviewing: Preparing People to Change Addictive Behavior.* New York, NY: Guilford; 1991.
9. Inspired Hygiene. Full today, no-show tomorrow: stop the roller coaster. http://www.inspiredhygiene.com/full-today-no-show-tomorrow-stop-the-roller-coaster/. Accessed March 10, 2010.
10. Singelis T, Brown M. Culture, self, and collectivist communication linking culture to individual behavior. *Hum Commun Res.* 2010;21(3):354-389. http://www3.interscience.wiley.com/journal/118533486/home?CRETRY=1&SRETRY=0. Accessed March 10, 2010.
11. Hofstede G. *Culture's Consequences: Comparing Values, Behaviors, Institutions and Organizations Across Nations.* Thousand Oaks, CA: Sage Publications; 2001.

Part II

The Dental Hygienist's Role in the Delivery of Health Care

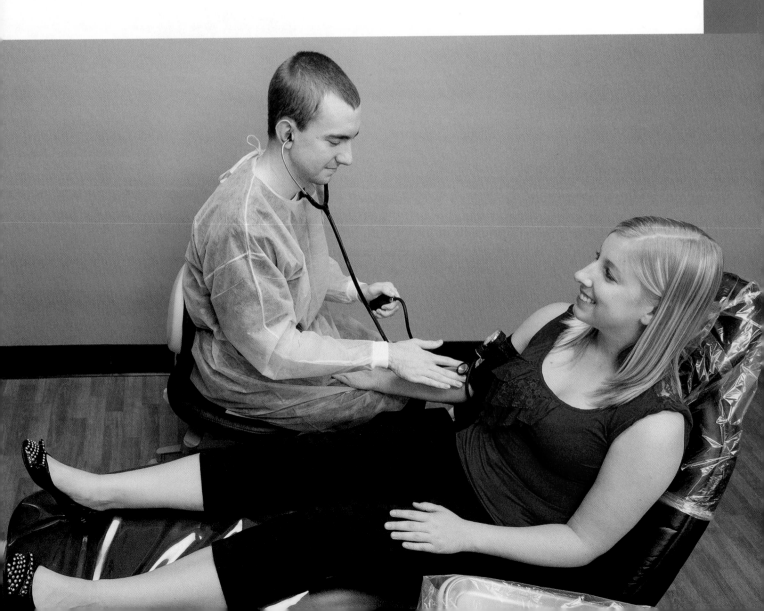

Chapter 4 | Health Education and Promotion

Shirley Beaver, RDH, PhD

KEY TERMS

external locus of control
health
health disparities
health education
health promotion
holistic
internal locus of control
locus of control
paternalism
self-efficacy
wellness

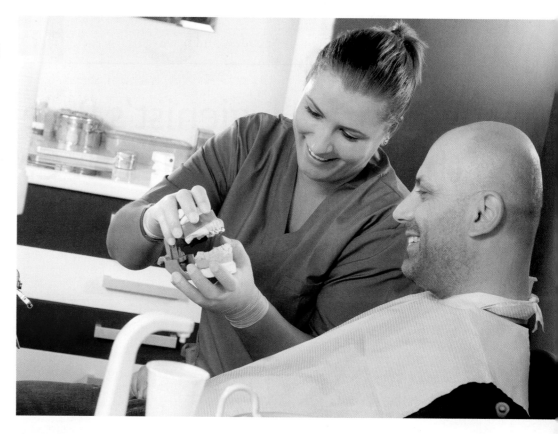

LEARNING OBJECTIVES

After reading this chapter, the student should be able to:

4.1 Discuss disparities in oral health care.

4.2 Distinguish between health and wellness.

4.3 Explain similarities and differences between education for prevention and education for promotion.

4.4 Compare and contrast health-promotion strategies.

4.5 Assess, plan, implement, and evaluate oral health behavior change using health-promotion strategies.

4.6 Differentiate health-promotion strategies for the child, adolescent, and adult.

4.7 Implement tobacco cessation strategies as appropriate.

KEY CONCEPTS

- Dental hygienists contribute to their patients' health and wellness by providing holistic care.
- Dental hygienists help patients achieve optimal health and wellness through health promotion and education.
- In the United States, the cost of health care and lack of health insurance coverage limits accessibility to health care for a large number of people. The

Affordable Care Act makes dental insurance coverage available to all children and does not require parents to enroll children to gain coverage. For adults, some health plans will include dental coverage and some will not.

- Health education and health-promotion models include Maslow's hierarchy of needs, the learning ladder, the health belief model, and the transtheoretical model. To be effective, dental hygienists must be comfortable with a variety of models and use the model most appropriate for individual patients and their needs.
- Health education and promotion can be applied to every step of the dental hygiene process of care.
- Prevention and health-promotion models can be adapted to any age group. When providing health education, it is important to evaluate the motivating factors that are relevant to that age and to use age-appropriate language.
- Behavior modification models are effective for encouraging patients to adopt positive health behaviors and to eliminate negative health behaviors such as smoking. Patients must make the decision and commit to change to be successful.

RELEVANCE TO CLINICAL PRACTICE

Many systemic and oral diseases in the United States could be prevented with lifestyle changes. Modifying lifestyle by daily exercise, improving dietary habits, and decreasing tobacco use would help prevent many of the diseases that cause premature death and would decrease the prevalence of oral diseases.[1] As preventive oral health professionals, dental hygienists identify their patients' health risks and provide health education, motivation, and health promotion. The dental hygiene appointment offers an opportunity to discuss the relationship among the patient's oral conditions, what was reported on the medical history, and other information provided. As respected professionals in the community, dental hygienists also provide health education and health-promotion services at schools, health fairs, or other community events.

HEALTH AND WELLNESS

Individuals may define *health* and *wellness* differently based on personal experience and expectations. However, the World Health Organization (WHO) defines **health** as "a state of complete physical, mental, and social well-being and not merely the absence of disease or infirmity."[2] The National Wellness Institute defines **wellness** as "an active process through which people become aware of and make choices toward a more successful existence."[3] Wellness is multidimensional and often includes social, occupational, spiritual, physical, intellectual, and emotional dimensions, as well as environmental, cultural, financial, medical, and mental dimensions.[3,4] Wellness is also related to the patient's functional ability. For example, the patient may be able to explain correct brushing and flossing techniques, but not be able to implement them in the oral cavity because of arthritis or other conditions.

Individuals must take responsibility for their own health and wellness. They must determine what actions they will take to create total health by achieving a balance between body and mind, theory and practice. Dental hygienists contribute to their patients' health and wellness by providing **holistic** care—that is, treating the whole patient, not just individual parts. If the patient needs to make a change such as quitting smoking, the dental hygienist assesses the patient's motivation to change, plans patient education regarding the need to change, collaborates with the patient to set goals for implementing changes when the patient expresses the desire to quit, and follows up with the patient to evaluate the patient's progress.

HEALTH PROMOTION

Optimal health is a balance of physical, emotional, social, spiritual, and intellectual health. Factors that influence health include an individual's ability to eliminate risk behaviors; improve healthy behaviors; change knowledge, attitudes, and skills; and assume personal responsibility for his or her own health. Other factors that influence health are social inequities, empowerment of individuals and communities, access to health care, and environmental issues.[5] Dental hygienists help patients achieve optimal health and wellness through health promotion and education. **Health promotion** is defined by the WHO as "the process of enabling people to increase control over their health and its determinants, and thereby improve their health."[5] **Health education** is defined as "any planned combination of learning experience designed to predispose, enable, and reinforce voluntary behavior conducive to health in individuals, groups, and communities."[5] Simply providing written information to patients to motivate them to change is not effective. Instead, health education must be a planned, evidence-based, patient-centered combination of information and activities that provide the patient with the opportunity to make an informed choice to change his or her behavior. **Paternalism** (the act of telling a person what to do like a father manages a child) is not appropriate. As discussed in Chapter 2, the ethical principle of autonomy states that each person has the right to make personal choices for himself or herself as long as those choices do not injure anyone else. Informed consent and informed refusal are critical in patient education as the patient makes decisions he determines is the best course of action for him based on the best available information.

U.S. HEALTH-CARE SYSTEM

The current ranking of the world's health-care systems was completed by the WHO in 2000. The WHO has indicated another ranking will not be done because of the complexity of the task. Although much disagreement exists over the validity of the report, the United States ranked 37th in the world in quality of health care.[5] As a country, the United States has developed some of the most sophisticated medical treatments in the world. However, the cost of health care and lack of health insurance coverage limits the accessibility to health care for a large number of people. With the implementation of the Affordable Care Act (ACA), dental coverage is available to all children. Parents do not have to enroll their child in dental coverage. For adults, some health plans include dental coverage and some do not. For those with health-care plans that do not include dental coverage, separate, optional dental plans are available.[6]

Health Disparities

The U.S. Department of Health and Human Services states: "The term **health disparities** refers to population specific differences in the presence of disease, health outcomes, quality of health care and access to health care services – that exist across racial and ethnic groups."[7] A review of the literature revealed a variety of circumstances that contribute to disparities in access to health care, as well as in quality of health and health care. Variables are related to disparities in health and health care for all ethnic groups. Health insurance, socioeconomic status, level of education, and peer pressure all influence health-promotion and disease prevention practices. Also, varying exposure to adverse conditions, varying vulnerability among groups and/or individuals, incidence of disabilities, and lack of access to health care because of living in medically underserved areas, whether urban or rural, have an impact on utilization and effectiveness of the health-care system. However, when all factors were considered, minority groups tended to experience a higher incidence of unmet medical/dental needs than any other group.[8,9] Also, a number of people who have insurance and easy access to dental-care providers do not receive regular oral health care. This may be because of fear or not placing importance on oral health care.

Socioeconomic conditions in the United States have contributed to a decrease in oral prevention and health-promotion activities. When economic conditions are not favorable and there is loss of jobs with resulting loss of dental insurance, oral health care becomes a lower priority. Between 1997 and 2009, the percentage of adults 18 to 64 years of age who did not receive dental care because of the cost increased from 11% to 17% of the population. For the group of individuals who had not had insurance for more than 12 months, the percentage of adults who did not receive health care increased to 43.7%.[8]

In addition to socioeconomic conditions, additional barriers exist to the implementation of prevention and health-promotion activities, as well as health care. These include lack of access to transportation, inability to take time off from work, not having a dental home (an ongoing relationship with a dental care provider that provides for all the patient's dental needs), inability to pay the required copayment, cultural factors, and language barriers. Lower-income families may have access to dental care through Medicaid. However, it is often difficult to find a dental provider who will accept the lower rates paid by Medicaid.

Healthy People 2020

In Healthy People 2020, the U.S. Department of Health and Human Services set national objectives for improving the health of all Americans. See Spotlight on Public Health 1 for a list of the objectives.

Spotlight on Public Health 1

Dental hygienists have the education and information to provide health education and health-promotion activities throughout the world to show the relationship between oral health and general health.

Suggestions for how dental hygienists can be instrumental in achieving the Healthy People 2020 objectives follow each objective in parentheses.

ORAL HEALTH OF CHILDREN AND ADOLESCENTS

OH-1 Reduce the proportion of children and adolescents who have dental caries experience in their primary or permanent teeth. (Dental hygienists can educate pregnant women and new mothers about the transmissibility of the bacteria that cause dental decay. They can also educate all age groups about methods for preventing dental decay, such as the use of fluoride, good nutrition, and good oral hygiene habits.)

OH-2 Reduce the proportion of children and adolescents with untreated dental decay. (Dental hygienists can organize a day on a regular basis [every 3, 6, 9 months] where dentists, dental hygienists, and dental therapists offer free preventive and restorative services to those in need of care.)

ORAL HEALTH OF ADULTS

OH-3 Reduce the proportion of adults with untreated dental decay. This includes those over the age of 75 who have root caries. (Dental hygienists can volunteer to train the aids in a local nursing or retirement facility to assist the residents with their oral care needs. This could include prevention, oral cancer screening, and referral to a dentist or dental therapist for restorative care.)

OH-4 Reduce the proportion of adults who have ever had a permanent tooth extracted because of dental caries or periodontal disease. (Dental hygienists can present information at a local senior center to educate the seniors about oral prevention and self-care techniques. Provide toothbrushes and toothpaste donated from corporate entities. Raffle off a donated power toothbrush.)

OH-5 Reduce the proportion of adults aged 45 to 74 years with moderate or severe periodontitis. (Dental hygienists can prepare a 60-second public service announcement [PSA] on prevention of periodontal disease.)

OH-6 Increase the proportion of oral and pharyngeal cancers detected at the earliest stage. (Dental hygienists can work with a community or church group to present a free oral cancer screening event.)

ACCESS TO PREVENTIVE SERVICES

OH-7 Increase the proportion of children, adolescents, and adults who used the oral health-care system in the past year. (Dental hygienists can work with the local public health department to set up school screenings.)

OH-8 (Dental hygienists can) Increase the proportion of low-income children and adolescents who received any preventive dental service during the past year.

OH-9 (Dental hygienists can) Increase the proportion of school-based health centers with an oral health component. This would include education, dental care, sealants, fluoride.

OH-10 (Dental hygienists can) Increase the proportion of local health departments and Federally Qualified Health Centers (FQHCs) that have an oral health program.

OH-11 (Dental hygienists can) Increase the proportion of patients who receive oral health services at Federally Qualified Health Centers (FQHCs) each year.

ORAL HEALTH INTERVENTIONS

OH-12 (Dental hygienists can) Increase the proportion of children and adolescents who have received dental sealants on their molar teeth.

OH-13 Increase the proportion of the U.S. population served by community water systems with optimally fluoridated water. (Dental hygienists can advocate for optimally fluoridated water in their communities.)

OH-14 (Dental hygienists can) (Developmental) Increase the proportion of adults who receive preventive interventions in dental offices. This includes tobacco cessation, cancer screening, those tested and referred for glycemic control.

MONITORING, SURVEILLANCE SYSTEMS

OH-15 (Dental hygienists can) (Developmental) Increase the number of States and the District of Columbia that have a system for recording and referring infants and children with cleft lips and cleft palates to craniofacial anomaly rehabilitative teams.

OH-16 (Dental hygienists can) Increase the number of States and the District of Columbia that have an oral and craniofacial health surveillance system.

PUBLIC HEALTH INFRASTRUCTURE

OH-17 (Dental hygienists can) Increase health agencies that have a dental public health program directed by a dental professional with public health training. This includes the Indian Health Service. ■

BEHAVIORAL CHANGE MODELS

How can dental hygienists motivate patients and the community to incorporate positive health practices into their daily lives? There are many different models for health education and promotion, including Maslow's hierarchy of needs, the learning ladder, the health belief model, and the transtheoretical model. To be effective, dental hygienists must be comfortable with a variety of models and use the model most appropriate for individual patients and their needs.

Maslow's Hierarchy of Needs

Maslow's hierarchy of needs, visualized as a pyramid, has been influential in increasing understanding of readiness to change behavior (Fig. 4-1). Beginning at the bottom of the pyramid, the needs in each category must be satisfied before an individual can fulfill needs on the next level. Basic physiological needs have to be met before an individual can focus on other needs. The person who is lacking shelter, food, sleep, or sex will not be able to concentrate on higher-level needs. Once those needs are met, physical and psychological safety must be achieved and so on until self-actualization is possible.

Oral health may not be a high priority for an individual who is homeless and does not know when food will next be available. Oral health could become important at the safety level where general health becomes a need or it may not be a priority until higher levels are achieved.

What the dental hygienist desires for the patient and what the patient wants or is able to accomplish may not be the same.

Learning Ladder

The learning ladder provides a model to evaluate the stage where an individual is on a continuum related to making a behavioral change (Fig. 4-2). The belief is that each rung of the ladder has to be accomplished before the patient can move to the next rung of the ladder.[10]

On the first rung the individual is unaware of any problem or any reason to make a behavioral change. An example is a person who has high blood pressure but is not aware of it. At the next level, the person becomes aware of a condition that may require a change in behavior. Awareness may result from education by a health-care worker, a public service program on television, or an article in a magazine. During the preventive appointment with the dental hygienist, a blood pressure assessment is completed and the patient is aware she has high blood pressure.

The third rung is self-interest. This is where the aware person contemplates how this new information applies to her. She considers how high the blood pressure is and whether she should do something about it. What will happen if she does not do anything about it? She may decide to do nothing or she may move to the next stage, involvement. The person realizes that high blood pressure is related to heart disease, stroke, and other systemic conditions and that some action needs to be taken. In the action stage the new information is incorporated into behavior change. The change may be seeking medical advice, researching the condition on the Internet, starting an exercise program, evaluating her diet, or a combination of actions. When the new actions are practiced consistently, they become a habit or a permanent change. The length of time it takes to form a habit depends on the behavior and the person. Generally it seems that a behavior change maintained for 3 weeks is considered a habit.

True learning results in belief change that leads to a behavioral change. If a person verbalizes a change in beliefs but does not change his or her behavior, the new belief has not really been learned.[10] For example, the dental hygienist who tells patients they should floss every day but does not floss every day himself has not learned that flossing is important.

Both Maslow's hierarchy of needs and the learning ladder move in a progressive manner from the bottom up. The following models are not progressive and the person may relapse at any time.

Locus of Control

Locus of control is an individual characteristic that may influence all of the models for behavior change. **Locus**

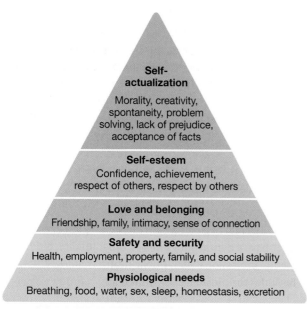

Figure 4-1. Maslow's hierarchy of needs.

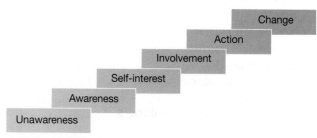

Figure 4-2. Learning ladder.

of control refers to an individual's beliefs about what factors determine his or her rewards or outcomes in life.[11] This trait can be mapped on a continuum from internal to external with many people exhibiting characteristics of both. **Internal locus of control** is the term used to describe the belief that control of future outcomes resides primarily in oneself. Individuals with an internal locus of control are more likely to be successful at making behavior changes because they believe they are in control of what happens to them. A person with an internal locus of control does not need rewards for accomplishing a goal because the achievement of the goal is enough of a reward. Self-accountability, success in life, higher socioeconomic status, and aging tend to increase internal locus of control. **External locus of control** refers to the belief that control of outcomes is outside of oneself, either in the hands of powerful others or due to fate or chance. The person with an external locus of control does not really believe she can make a change but will be more willing to try if a reward is offered. A person with an external locus of control has possibly grown up without a role model who has achieved success based on her own endeavors or seems to have bad experiences she feels she does not control.[12]

Theory of Reasoned Action/Planned Behavior

The theory of reasoned action/planned behavior focuses on the individual's intent. The person decides to change a behavior and with intention based on knowledge, he makes the change. Behavioral beliefs and evaluation of behavioral outcomes form the individual's attitude toward behavior. Normative beliefs and motivation to comply merge to provide a subjective norm. Beliefs regarding control and perceived power provide perceived behavioral control. Attitude toward behavior, subjective norms, and the perceived degree of behavioral control merge to provide the individual's intent to make a behavioral change.[13]

Social Learning and Social Cognitive Theories

Although most of the behavioral change models progress in a linear fashion, the social learning theory is multidirectional and based on environment, information, and behavior. Interaction among these three aspects is continually changing to influence behavior. Social learning theory and social cognitive theory are closely related. Social cognitive theory emphasizes personal accountability more than the environment. As the three elements of environment, information, and behavior interact with positive outcomes, the person will develop self-efficacy, the ability to take charge and make decisions.

According to Albert Bandura, **self-efficacy** is "the belief in one's capabilities to organize and execute the courses of action required to manage prospective situations."[14] Self-efficacy is at the core of the social cognitive theory. As the feeling of self-efficacy grows, the person will be more likely to have an internal locus of control. This person will be more successful at making behavioral changes once she has acquired information related to such a need.[14]

Social cognitive theory is based on the belief that behavior changes occur most readily due to social pressures combined with knowledge. The theory is especially applicable to adolescents. Expert opinions differ on exactly what separates social cognitive theory from the more general social learning theory. In general, however, the following principles can be used to define social cognitive theory: People learn through their own experiences and also by observing others. Although learning can have an effect on behavior modification, people do not always apply the information. Choices are often made on a personal decision of perceived outcome of the behavior. People tend to model behavior that is exhibited by someone they admire or respect. Self-efficacy then plays an important part if the decision is to set a goal. The goal will be set only if the individual believes he can achieve it. This theory is used in advertising to facilitate identification of the target group with the actors. For example, advertisements of specific products are targeted to the audience who will be watching a television show. This relates to peer pressure. Peer pressure plays a large role in decisions that individuals make regarding health and safety.[15]

HEALTH-PROMOTION MODELS

Health-promotion models, such as the health belief model and the transtheoretical model, help dental hygienists understand patients' motivation and readiness for change, and plan appropriate interventions.

Health Belief Model

The health belief model was constructed by the social psychologists Hochbaum, Rosenstock, and Kegels in the 1950s. They were trying to determine why people did not take advantage of programs to detect and prevent disease such as free radiograph screenings for tuberculosis.[16] The model was based on four constructs that influence an individual's decision to take action to prevent, screen for, or control a health condition (Fig. 4-3):

- Perceived susceptibility—the individual's beliefs about the probability of development of a condition, such as heart disease
- Perceived severity—the individual's beliefs about how serious a condition is if it does develop
- Perceived barriers—the individual's beliefs about how difficult it will be to make a behavior change
- Perceived benefits—the individual's beliefs about how effective making a change will be

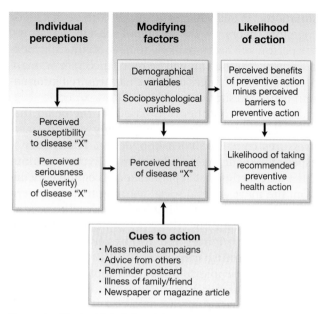

Figure 4-3. The health belief model. (From National Institutes of Health, Bethesda, MD.)

Researchers subsequently expanded the health belief model to include the following constructs:

• Cues to action—exposure to information that motivates the individual to act
• Self-efficacy—the individual's belief in his or her ability to take action

The combination of the individual's perceived susceptibility and perceived severity determines the perceived threat. The decision regarding whether the perceived threat is low or high influences the decision to take action. Modifying factors that affect final decisions include age, sex, ethnicity, social class, peer pressure, and knowledge about the disease. Cues to action may be advice from significant others or a physician, a friend or colleague who is diagnosed with a serious disease, a television special that highlights the disease, or a magazine article. The individual evaluates the pros and cons of preventive action and decides whether to follow the recommendations. Self-efficacy influences change because people who feel they will not be successful with preventive action will not implement it.[16]

Transtheoretical/Stages of Change Model

The transtheoretical model, which was published by Prochaska in 1979, was initially used for smoking cessation, as well as drug and alcohol addiction, but it is also appropriate for implementing positive behavior such as flossing.[17] This model incorporates six stages with regard to an individual's readiness to change for improved health. Once the individual's level of readiness is determined, appropriate interventions can be determined.

1. Precontemplation: The person is not thinking about change.
2. Contemplation: The person starts to think about a change.

3. Preparation: The person decides to make a change and makes action plans.
4. Action: The person implements an action plan.
5. Maintenance: The action plan is in effect, but the person struggles with the possibility of relapse. At this stage relapse is common. Encouragement from the dental hygienist is needed if there is relapse.
6. Termination: Success. The change is permanent. There will be no temptation to relapse.[17]

Other models have a similar philosophy with a different number of steps or different names for the stages, or both. The Cancer Prevention Research Center lists 10 processes of change.[18] The theory of self-efficacy is influential in many of the models. In all models there is a period when the individual is more likely to have a relapse. It is important to work with patients and assure them that relapse is not failure and they still can achieve success with behavior change. Many factors contribute to relapse. Peer pressure can have a negative or positive effect at any stage of the behavioral change process. Guilt techniques should never be applied if the person has a relapse.

Motivational Interviewing

In the past, oral health-care providers believed that if patients were told what to do to improve their oral health, their behavior would change. That style of education was not successful. Motivation is the key to behavior change. If patients are motivated, informed decision-making can occur regarding oral care. To change behavior, it is critical that patients internalize the desire to change their behaviors. Motivated patients will use their personal problem-solving abilities and critical thinking skills to incorporate a new habit and then develop the skills necessary to maintain that habit.[19]

Motivational interviewing (MI) is a health-promotion technique that has shown a positive relationship to behavior change. MI incorporates a modified version of the stages of change model used in the transtheoretical model.[20] Refer to Chapter 3 for detailed information on MI; more information about can also be found online at: http://motivationalinterviewing.org/.

DENTAL HYGIENE PROCESS OF CARE

Health education and promotion can be applied to every step of the dental hygiene process of care (assessment, dental hygiene diagnosis, planning, implementation, evaluation, and documentation).

Assessment

The assessment phase begins with observing the way the patient walks into the operatory, the way she is breathing, and the color of her skin, and continues with reviewing the medical history, and what the intraoral and extraoral examination reveal about the individual's health. Each component of the assessment provides information about what may need to be addressed through education and health promotion.

Dental Hygiene Diagnosis

The assessments are used to determine issues that need attention. For example, the patient may not brush daily, may have a family history of diabetes but not have been evaluated by his family physician, may have a family history of heart disease but be overweight, or may have areas on the skin that should be evaluated by a physician.

Planning

Collaboration with the patient is critical in the planning phase. Telling someone to stop smoking, go on a diet, or have a blood sugar evaluation will probably not produce positive results. It is best to discuss health issues that require behavior change with the patient and let him or her decide what to do.

Implementation

Educate the patient during treatment and involve the patient in formulating goals to accomplish with specific time limits. For example, while performing quadrant scaling, encourage the patient to floss every other day at the next appointment, and every day at the third appointment.

Evaluation

Using measurable criteria, evaluate the patient's progress toward achieving goals, and communicate the outcomes to the patient, dentist, and other health-care providers. Collaborate with the patient on determining next steps and revising goals as necessary.

Documentation

Document each step of dental hygiene process of care, including all assessment information, dental hygiene diagnoses, planning, implementation, and evaluation. Include information about all interactions with the patient, including office visits and telephone calls.

PREVENTION AND PROMOTION FOR SPECIFIC POPULATIONS

Prevention and health-promotion models can be adapted to any age group. When providing health education, it is important to look at the motivating factors that are relevant to that age and to use age-appropriate language.

Infants and Children (Birth to 12 Years)

The American Academy of Pediatric Dentistry (AAPD) recommends the concept of a dental home for infants, children, adolescents, and persons with special needs. This originated with the American Academy of Pediatrics concept of the medical home. The dental home provides a stable facility where the patient feels welcome and familiar with the health-care providers. Comprehensive family-centered care is provided with an emphasis on health education and promotion for health and wellness. For example, the hygienist at the dental home might provide guidance to caregivers about the use of pacifiers. Cultural differences are considered in the dental home. Children who participate in a dental home are more likely to receive regular preventive care. The infant can have the first dental appointment as early as 6 months and no later than 12 months. Clinicians recommend the frequency of subsequent visits based on their risk assessment of the child. By establishing a schedule for visits, the clinicians are able to provide preventive maintenance and counseling, and promote health and wellness. The AAPD reaffirmed the policy on the dental home in 2010.[21] For more information on the definition of a dental home see Chapter 46.

Adolescents (13–18 Years)

Adolescents are tasked with developing a sense of self and personal identity. Family interactions, age, and biological development influence how adolescents

Teamwork

Dental hygienists collaborate with other members of the dental team and other health-care professionals to provide health education and promotion. The patient may ask the dental hygienist if they really need a treatment the dentist has recommended. Or, they may ask the receptionist whether quadrant scaling and root planing really make a difference. The dental hygienist may not be qualified to provide in-depth education in some areas and may refer the patient to other health-care providers. For example, the hygienist can make recommendations for a person with uncontrolled diabetes, but a referral to a dietitian is required for in-depth nutritional counseling.

BRIGHT FUTURES

Bright Futures is a national health-promotion initiative developed by the American Academy of Pediatrics based on the principle that every child should be healthy. Through its Bright Futures health-promotion initiative, the American Academy of Pediatrics offers health-promotion materials for parents from pregnancy through adolescence. The health-promotion materials are available for all aspects of health and wellness.[31] A resource of particular interest to dental hygienists is *Bright Futures in Practice: Oral Health Pocket Guide*, developed by the National Maternal and Child Oral Health Resources, which provides a variety of educational and motivational programs. This initiative also encourages oral health screenings and application of fluoride varnish for all children.[31] ■

view themselves. Peer pressure is a major influence during this stage of development. Most adolescents do not believe anything bad will happen to them, so risk-taking is at a peak. Adolescents with highly developed self-efficacy (belief that they can influence what happens to them) will be able to take setbacks in stride and move forward.[22]

Brukiene and Aleksejuniene[23] conducted an evidence-based search of the last four decades of literature related to adolescent health care. The results of this study indicated that very little research in promotion of health care for adolescents has been conducted. The authors believed that the results of that research would have little meaning for the adolescent of today. Their research showed that habits related to smoking, oral care, and health are established in adolescence and become difficult to change in adulthood. It may be difficult to establish good health behaviors during this time because teenagers do not believe they are vulnerable to disease. Oral health is of less importance than general health.[23]

The dental hygienist should adapt prevention and promotion models to the adolescent's stage of development. It is suggested that health promotion would be more effective if the emphasis were placed on social consequences rather than health consequences. "Appearance, fresh breath and kissability" become important during the teen years.[23,24] The Bright Futures Initiative provides motivational information for use with adolescents.

Elderly

The current cohort of elderly is unlike any previous cohort. The baby boomers (those born between 1946 and 1964) have begun turning 65 years old and expect to live longer, healthier lives including maintenance of good oral health. The connection between systemic health and oral health takes on increasing significance as people age. More than 500 medications cause xerostomia and many elderly take these medications. Some elderly persons will have increased oral health problems and may not have access to oral care because of cost, mobility, and lack of motivation. The dental team must be prepared to provide care to both segments of the elderly population.[25,26] Prevention and health-promotion models will be effective with the elderly when the education is relevant and individualized. Everyone ages differently, and patient education must be based on each individual's mental, physical, psychological, and sociological functional status.

SMOKING CESSATION

Behavior modification models are effective for encouraging the adoption of positive health behaviors and eliminating negative health behaviors. As with any of the prevention and health-promotion concepts, the patient must make the decision and internalize the desire to quit using tobacco. MI works well with tobacco cessation as the hygienist listens and facilitates movement of the patient through a serious of steps until the patient makes the decision to quit. See Chapter 3 for more information on MI.

Dental hygienists should ask each patient the following two questions: "Do you use tobacco products?" and "Do you want to quit?" With patients who say they do not want to quit, ask if they have thought about quitting. Discuss the negative outcomes of tobacco use along with the pros and cons of tobacco cessation, but avoid telling patients they should stop. Let them know that you are available for assistance should they decide to quit. This approach instills the idea in patients' minds and leaves it open for discussion at the next recall/recare appointment.

5 A's of Tobacco Cessation

Many tobacco users who express the desire to quit may need extra motivation or assistance to actually quit. Five Major Steps to Intervention ("5 A's") is a clinical practice guideline established by the U.S. Public Health Service as a framework for health-care providers to use with patients who use tobacco products (Box 4-1). The 5 R's of Motivation—Relevance, Risks, Rewards, Roadblocks, and Repetition—are part of MI and are used effectively with the 5 A's of tobacco cessation.

Ask. Advise. Refer.

A variety of sources use the 5 A's or a modification of them. At http://www.smokefree.gov it is suggested that the patient write down all of the reasons he wants to stop smoking and then carry that list with him, perhaps in the place where he usually carries tobacco. Once the individual has decided to quit, the following START process is suggested:

S = Set a date he will quit.
T = Tell everyone he sees on a regular basis that he is quitting.
A = Anticipate and identify obstacles he may encounter.
R = Remove all tobacco products from his environment.
T = Talk to his health-care provider regarding help. This could be a physician, dental hygienist, dentist, or public health nurse.[27]

In 2008, a consortium of federal government and nonprofit organizations completed an update to *Treating Tobacco Use and Dependence*. The information was developed using a systematic review and meta-analysis of 11 topics and thousands of articles, and includes information on new, effective clinical treatments for tobacco dependence.[28] The full article and many educational materials including a PowerPoint presentation for implementing the recommendations are

Box 4-1. *The 5 A's of Tobacco Cessation*

ASK—Ask the patient about tobacco use at every appointment. Ask how long the patient has been using tobacco, what kind of tobacco, how much is used, and what situations trigger tobacco use. Ask if the patient has thought about quitting. Document this information in the chart.

ADVISE—Urge the patient to quit. Emphasize that quitting smoking is the best thing the patient could do for his or her health. Personalize the reasons why the patient should quit.

ASSESS—Assess readiness to quit. The patient must want to quit. Is he ready to try to quit within the next 14 to 30 days? If he is not, review the 5 R's of motivation. If the patient still is not ready to quit, document that in the chart and continue the process at the next appointment.

ASSIST—If the patient is ready to quit, collaborate with the patient to set a quit date. Work with the patient to determine the method of quitting and provide resources for the method she chooses. This could be referral to a support group, nicotine replacement therapy or other approved pharmacology, a hot line, or a combination of resources.

ARRANGE—Follow up with a phone call or personal visit within a week of the quit date. Congratulate the patient's successes. Anticipate challenges. Provide support should the patient relapse. Never use guilt techniques should the patient relapse. Provide support at every visit.[28,29] ■

available online at http://www.ahrq.gov/professionals/clinicians-providers/guidelines-recommendations/tobacco/index.html.

Smoking Cessation for Adolescents

Cigarette smoking declined among middle- and high-school youth between 2000 and 2011. However, use of electronic cigarettes doubled in those age groups from 2011 to 2012, and use of hookahs increased among high-school students. Youth are more likely to smoke if they:

- Are exposed to advertising and movies that portray smoking as the social norm
- Have peers or parents who use tobacco
- Are anxious, depressed, or experiencing stress
- Associate positive outcomes such as controlling weight with smoking
- Lack parental support
- Have low self-esteem
- Lack resources to resist pressure to smoke
- Exhibit aggressive behavior
- Have low academic achievement

Higher academic achievement and goals, strong racial identity, and participation in religious activities translate to lower smoking levels.[29]

Ask concrete questions at each dental hygiene appointment to determine whether a teenage patient is using tobacco. For example, ask if the patient has smoked a cigarette in the past 30 days. If the patient has used tobacco, take the time to educate her about the dangers of tobacco use and suggest methods for quitting. Provide information in a nonjudgmental manner and avoid preaching. Follow up with the patient at each subsequent visit (see Spotlight on Public Health 2).

Changing Habits

In *The Power of Habit: Why We Do What We Do in Life and Business,* Charles Duhigg confirms through biological science that individuals could not function without habits because the brain would not be able to make a new decision for every action. That is why we lock the door as we leave for work or school without really realizing that we did. We have cues to action, then we do the action, and then we have a reward. This governs our behavior even though we do not realize it. Fortunately, with discipline, we can change our habits and reprogram ourselves with new habits. To change behavior, we have to change the cues that trigger the behavior and the reward.

Collaborate with the patient to determine what cues happen before the action that you are hoping to encourage or discourage and what reward follows. It can be going to bed without brushing and flossing, and needing to change the cues to action so that the patient brushes and flosses. Or it may be not having a cup of coffee after a meal because the coffee is a cue to action to have a cigarette.[30]

Dental hygienists may also want to change professional habits to improve access to care, help patients become motivated for health and wellness, and address the objectives for Healthy People 2020.

Spotlight on Public Health 2

In 2014, the U.S. Food and Drug Administration launched an antismoking initiative called "The Real Cost" to prevent and reduce tobacco use by youth aged 12 to 17 years. The campaign uses TV and print advertising, as well videos on Internet sites such as YouTube, to educate teens about the dangers of smoking and encourage them to avoid tobacco use. It also uses social media sites to provide teens opportunities to engage in peer-to-peer conversations. For more information about the campaign and additional resources, see http://www.fda.gov/newsevents/newsroom/pressannouncements/ucm384049.htm. ■

Case Study

The dental hygienist's 10:00 a.m. patient is a 45-year-old woman who is CEO of a Fortune 500 company. She has always prided herself on her appearance and can still wear the same-size clothes she did in high school. She smokes a pack of cigarettes each day, sleeps only 4 hours each night, and usually eats only one meal a day, which is dinner at 9:30 in the evening. She does not have time to work out. The hygienist notices signs of wear from bruxism when conducting the intraoral examination. She does not have any new carious lesions at this appointment.

Case Study Exercises

1. In the assessment phase of the dental hygiene process of care, the dental hygienist asks if the patient has considered quitting smoking. She answers yes, but she cannot quit because she cannot gain any weight because of her high-level position. Where is she with regard to the 5 A's of smoking cessation?
   A. The assist stage; the dental hygienist will collaborate with her to set a quit date.
   B. The arrange stage; the dental hygienist will call within a week to see if she has quit.
   C. The advise stage; the dental hygienist will personalize reasons why she should quit.
   D. The assess stage; the dental hygienist will ask if she is ready to try to quit within the next 30 days.

2. Based on her assessment of the patient's readiness to quit smoking, which of the following actions should the dental hygienist take?
   A. Call her before the next recall appointment to see if she has quit.
   B. Provide information regarding stopping smoking without gaining weight.
   C. Decide on a quit date and tell her how important it is for her to adhere to that date.
   D. Explain to her that her colleagues would prefer her to stop so that she does not smell of tobacco.

3. The patient states that because of the stress from her job she does not believe she will be able to stop smoking. This patient has an internal locus of control because she believes she has control over her personal outcomes.
   A. Both the statement and the reason are correct and related.
   B. Both the statement and the reason are correct but not related.
   C. The statement is correct, but the reason is not.
   D. The statement is not correct, but the reason is correct.
   E. Neither the statement nor the reason is correct.

4. Based on her assessment of the patient, what other health education and health-promotion areas should the dental hygienist discuss with this patient?
   A. The dental hygienist should reprimand her for eating only one meal a day.
   B. The dental hygienist should provide her with negative outcomes related to eating only one meal a day.
   C. The dental hygienist should have a discussion with the patient and ask her to suggest ideas for eating during the day.
   D. The dental hygienist should have the patient complete a 5-day diet diary to see if she is eating foods that cause carious lesions.

5. The patient says that she could try to cut down on the number of cigarettes she smokes each day. She is coming back for an evaluation appointment in 2 weeks. What would be the dental hygienist's appropriate response?
   A. That is terrific. What goal would you like to set to meet by the next appointment?
   B. That is terrific. I think you should cut the number of cigarettes you smoke down to three fourths of a pack per day.
   C. I am glad that you have decided to cut down, but that usually does not work. It is better if you totally stop.
   D. That is a really great idea. I think you should try to cut the number of cigarettes you smoke in half by the time you come for the next appointment.

Review Questions

1. Which of the following is NOT a part of the health belief model when evaluating the possibility of behavior change?
   A. The individual evaluates whether he believes he is susceptible.
   B. The individual evaluates whether she believes that the condition is serious.
   C. The individual evaluates whether the perceived benefits outweigh the perceived threats.
   D. The individual evaluates whether he is ready to set a date within the next 14 to 30 days for behavior change.

2. Patients with an internal locus of control exhibit which one of the following characteristics?
   A. They do not believe that anything bad will happen to them.
   B. They are confident that any behavior change will be successful.
   C. They will need external rewards to make a behavior change.
   D. They believe that making a behavior change will not make any difference.
   E. This is a characteristic of adolescents or younger adults.

3. On which rung of the learning ladder does the person internalize the information and make the decision to change his or her behavior?
   A. Unawareness stage
   B. Awareness stage
   C. Involvement stage
   D. Action stage
   E. Habit stage

4. In the health belief model, a cue to action usually decreases the likelihood of behavior change. Cues to action usually emphasize positive reasons for a behavior change.
   A. Both statements are true.
   B. Both statements are false.
   C. The first statement is true, the second is false.
   D. The first statement is false, the second is true.

5. Self-efficacy improves the chance that an individual will make positive behavior change and can be increased vicariously when the individual observes others having success with decision-making.
   A. Both the statement and the reason are correct and related.
   B. Both the statement and the reason are correct but not related.
   C. The statement is correct, but the reason is not.
   D. The statement is not correct, but the reason is correct.
   E. Neither the statement nor the reason is correct.

Active Learning

1. Prepare a PowerPoint presentation to teach parents about good self-care habits for them and their children.
2. Write and record a Public Service Announcement (PSA) about the dangers of candy containing sugar and acid, and suggest healthy alternatives. ■

REFERENCES

1. Danaei G, Ding EL, Mozffarian D, Taylor B, Rehm J, Murray CJ, Ezzati M. The preventable causes of death in the United States: comparative risk assessment of dietary, lifestyle and metabolic risk factors. *PLoS Med.* 2009;6(4):e10000058.
2. Preamble to the Constitution of the World Health Organization as adopted by the International Health Conference, New York, 19-22 June 1946; signed on 22 July 1946 by the representatives of 61 States (Official Records of the World Health Organization, no. 2, p. 100) and entered into force on 7 April 1948. The Definition has not been amended since 1948.
3. National Wellness Institute. The six dimensions of wellness. Stevens Point, WI: National Wellness Institute. http://www.nationalwellness.org/?page=Six_Dimensions. Accessed February 27, 2014.
4. Definition of Wellness Website. definitionofwellness.com. Accessed February 27, 2014.
5. The world health report 2000—health systems: improving performance. Geneva: World Health Organization; 2000. http://www.who.int/whr/2000/en. Accessed February 27, 2014.
6. Affordable Care Act, dental benefits examined. Chicago: American Dental Association; 2013. https://www.ada.org/news/8935.aspx. Accessed March 5, 2014.
7. Disparities in health. Washington, DC: National Conference of State Legislatures; 2014. Available from: http://www.ncsl.org/research/health/2014-health-disparities-legislation.aspx. Accessed March 5, 2014.

8. CDC health disparities and inequalities report—United States, 2011. Atlanta, GA: Centers for Disease Control and Prevention; January 5, 2012. Available from: http://www.cdc.gov/mmwr/preview/ind2011_su.html. Accessed March 5, 2014.

9. Braveman PA. A health disparities perspective on obesity research. *Prev Chronic Dis.* 2009;6(3):A91. Available from: http://www.cdc.gov/pcd/issues/2009/jul/09_0012.htm. Accessed March 5, 2014.

10. Gehrig JS, Willman DE. *Foundations of Periodontics for the Dental Hygienist,* 3rd ed. Philadelphia: Lippincott Williams & Wilkins; 2011.

11. Hollister MC, Anema MG. Health behavior models and oral health: a review. *J Dent Hyg.* 2004;78(3):5. Available from: http://jdh.adha.org/content/78/3/6.full.pdf. Accessed March 5, 2014.

12. Changing Minds. Locus of control. Available from: http://changingminds.org/explanations/preferences/locus_control.htm. Accessed March 5, 2014.

13. The theory of planned behavior. Boston: Boston University School of Public Health; 2013. Available from: http://sphweb.bumc.bu.edu/otlt/MPH-Modules/SB/SB721-Models/SB721-Models3.html. Accessed March 5, 2014.

14. Bandura A. Self-efficacy mechanism in human agency. *Am Psychol.* 1982;37(2):122-147. Available from: http://jamiesmithportfolio.com/EDTE800/wp-content/Primary Sources/Bandura3.pdf. Accessed March 5, 2014.

15. The social cognitive theory. Boston: Boston University School of Public Health; 2013. Available from: http://sphweb.bumc.bu.edu/otlt/MPH-Modules/SB/SB721-Models/SB721-Models5.html. Accessed March 5, 2014.

16. Hochbaum GM. Public participation in medical screening programs: a socio-psychological study (Public Health Service Publication No. 572). Washington, DC: Government Printing Office, 1958.

17. Prochaska JO. Decision making in the transtheoretical model of behavior change. *Med Decis Making.* 2008; 28:845-849. Available from: http://mdm.sagepub.com/content/28/6/845. Accessed March 5, 2014.

18. Transtheoretical model processes of change. Kingston, RI: University of Rhode Island Cancer Prevention Research Center. Available from: http://web.uri.edu/cprc/summary-overview/. Accessed March 6, 2014.

19. Freudenthal J. How to encourage change. *Dimens Dent Hyg.* 2010;8(9):60-65. Available from: http://www.dimensionsofdentalhygiene.com/2010/09_September/Features/How_to_Encourage_Change.aspx. Accessed March 5, 2014.

20. Rollnick S, Butler C, Kinnersley P, Gregory J, Mash B. Motivational interviewing. *BMJ.* 2010;340:c1900.

21. Policy on the dental home. Chicago: American Academy of Pediatric Dentistry; 2012. Available from: http://www.aapd.org/media/policies_guidelines/p_dentalhome.pdf. Accessed March 6, 2014.

22. Pajares F, Urdan T, eds. *Self-efficacy Beliefs of Adolescents.* Greenwich, CT: Information Age Publishing; 2006.

23. Brukiene V, Aleksejuniene J. Theory-based oral health education in adolescents. *Stomatologija.* 2010;12:3-9.

24. DiClemente, RJ, Santelli JS, Crosby, RA. Adolescent health: understanding and preventing risk behaviors. Hoboken, NJ: Jossey-Bass; 2009.

25. MacEntee MI. The educational challenge of dental geriatrics. *J Dent Educ.* 2010;74:13-19.

26. Dounis G, Ditmyer MM, McClain MA, Cappelli DP, Mobley CC. Preparing the dental workforce for oral disease prevention in an aging population. *J Dent Educ.* 2010;74(10):1086-1094.

27. It Doesn't Matter Where You Start, Just Start. Washington, DC: U.S. Department of Health and Human Services. Available from: www.smokefree.gov. Accessed March 6, 2014.

28. Treating Tobacco Use and Dependence: 2008 Update. Rockville, MD: Agency for Healthcare Research and Quality; 2008. Available from: http://www.ahrq.gov/professionals/clinicians-providers/guidelines-recommendations/tobacco/index.html. Accessed March 6, 2014.

29. Youth and tobacco use. Atlanta (GA): Centers for Disease Control and Prevention; 2014. Available from: http://www.cdc.gov/tobacco/data_statistics/fact_sheets/youth_data/tobacco_use/. Accessed June 5, 2014.

30. Duhigg C. *The Power of Habit: Why We Do What We Do in Life and Business.* New York: Random House; 2012.

31. Casamassimo P, Holt K, eds. 2014. Bright Futures in Practice: Oral Health—Pocket Guide (2nd ed.). Washington, DC: National Maternal and Child Oral Health Resource Center.

Chapter 5 | Immunology and the Oral Systemic Link

Maria Perno Goldie, RDH, BA, MS • Jessica Salisbury, RDH, MSA

KEY TERMS

active immunity
adaptive or acquired immune response
antigen–antibody complex
bacteremia
complement cascade
complement system
C-reactive protein (CRP)
cytokine
differential gene expression
glucometer
innate immune response
innate susceptibility
interleukin
lipoxin
matrix metalloproteinase (MMP)
meta-analyses
nosocomial pneumonia
passive immunity
periodontal medicine
polymorphonuclear neutrophil (PNM)
resolvins
risk factor
vaccination

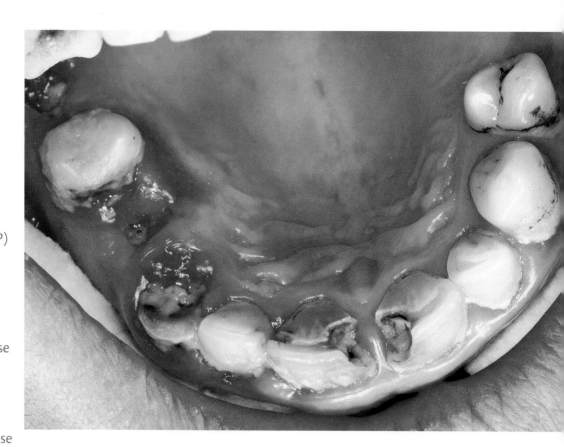

LEARNING OBJECTIVES

After reading this chapter, the student should be able to:

5.1 Describe the immune system and how it works.
5.2 Illustrate new concepts in the etiology and pathogenesis of periodontal diseases.
5.3 Distinguish the risk factors for periodontal disease.
5.4 Appraise the research regarding the connection between oral and systemic disease.
5.5 Examine the steps in co-management of periodontal and related systemic disease.
5.6 Enhance understanding of bacteremia associated with periodontal diseases.
5.7 Explain the link between oral and systemic disease to the patient.

KEY CONCEPTS

- Considerable epidemiological evidence supports the concept that poor oral health, especially the extent and severity of periodontal disease, may put patients at a significant risk for a variety of systemic conditions.
- There is increasing evidence that reducing the inflammatory component of periodontal tissue disease has potential systemic effects.

- Reducing the inflammatory burden in the periodontal tissues has been shown to improve the progression of periodontal diseases, improve hyperglycemic control in individuals with diabetes, and improve surrogate markers that may be of benefit in patients suffering from coronary heart disease.

RELEVANCE TO CLINICAL PRACTICE

Oral diseases and infections are a major public health problem worldwide, in spite of advances in understanding, prevention, and treatment of gingivitis and chronic periodontitis. They are still among the most prevalent microbial diseases of humankind.[1] As demographics change, and the number of people who retain their natural teeth increases, there is also an increased risk for periodontal disease (PD). The mouth is a significant contributor to the total burden of infection and inflammation and, consequently, to overall health and well-being. This chapter reviews the role the immune system plays in periodontal infection, the link between oral health and systemic health, and the theories that support this connection.

The term **periodontal medicine** refers to the role of systemic factors on PD and the association of PD with chronic diseases of aging such as diabetes and cardiovascular disease (CVD).[2] The relationship between oral health and general health has been increasingly recognized over recent years, and a number of epidemiological studies have now linked poor oral health with CVD, poor glycemic control in individuals with diabetes, respiratory diseases, rheumatoid arthritis, and osteoporosis. Systemic conditions may increase the susceptibility to PD and, conversely, periodontal infections may serve as risk factors for systemic illness. A **risk factor** is any attribute, characteristic, or exposure of an individual that increases the likelihood of developing a disease or injury. Some examples of the more important risk factors are underweight, unsafe sex, high blood pressure, tobacco and alcohol consumption, and unsafe water, sanitation, and hygiene.[3] The relationship between oral and general health is a significant issue, and it should lead to more aggressive prevention and management of PD and co-management of patients with other health-care professionals.

IMMUNE SYSTEM

The purpose of the immune system is to keep infectious microorganisms such as bacteria, viruses, fungi, and parasites out of the body and to destroy any that invade the body. Bone marrow, the soft tissue in the hollow center of bones, is the ultimate source of all blood cells, including lymphocytes. The immune system is made up of a complex and vital network of cells and organs that protect the body from infection (Fig. 5-1). The organs involved with the immune system are called the *lymphoid organs*, which affect growth, development, and the release of lymphocytes, a type of white blood cell. The blood vessels and lymphatic vessels are significant parts of the lymphoid organs because they carry the lymphocytes to and from different areas in the body. Each lymphoid organ plays a role in the production and activation of lymphocytes. Lymphoid organs include:

- Adenoids (two glands located at the back of the nasal passage)
- Appendix (a small tube that is connected to the large intestine)
- Blood vessels (the arteries, veins, and capillaries through which blood flows)
- Bone marrow (the soft, fatty tissue found in bone cavities)
- Lymph nodes (small organs shaped like beans, which are located throughout the body and connect via the lymphatic vessels)

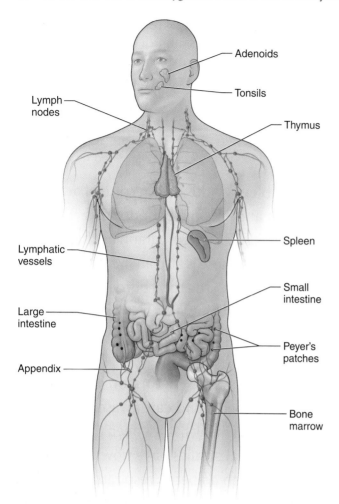

Adenoids

Lymph nodes

Tonsils

Thymus

Lymphatic vessels

Spleen

Large intestine

Small intestine

Appendix

Peyer's patches

Bone marrow

Figure 5-1. The immune system.

- Lymphatic vessels (a network of channels throughout the body that carries lymphocytes to the lymphoid organs and bloodstream)
- Peyer's patches (lymphoid tissue in the small intestine)
- Spleen (a fist-sized organ located in the abdominal cavity)
- Thymus (two lobes that join in front of the trachea behind the breastbone)
- Tonsils (two oval masses in the back of the throat)

The immune system has evolved to protect the host from pathogens while minimizing damage to "self" tissue. Central to the immune response is the ability to distinguish between "self" and "nonself." When immune defenders encounter foreign cells or organisms carrying markers that indicate "nonself," they quickly launch an attack. Anything that can trigger this immune response is called an *antigen*. An antigen can be a microbe such as a virus, or a part of a microbe such as a molecule. Tissues or cells from another person, except an identical twin, also carry nonself markers and act as foreign antigens, which is why tissue transplants may be rejected.

Innate and Acquired Immunity

Immune defenses are categorized as the **innate immune response,** or nonspecific immunity, and the

adaptive, or acquired, immune response. The innate immune response, the natural resistance with which a person is born, provides immediate protection against invading pathogens (Fig. 5-2). The adaptive, or acquired, immune response is not as instantaneous but confers specificity and long-lasting protection. Naturally acquired immunity occurs through *contact with a disease-causing agent,* when the contact was not deliberate, such as in measles, flu, cholera, plague, and hepatitis A. Artificially acquired immunity develops only through deliberate actions such as **vaccination.** Both naturally and artificially acquired immunity can be further subdivided depending on whether immunity is induced in the host or passively transferred from an immune host. **Passive immunity** is acquired through transfer of antibodies or activated T cells from an immune host; it is transient, usually lasting only a few months. **Active immunity** is induced in the host itself by an antigen and lasts much longer, sometimes for life.

Complement Cascade

Cells designed to become immune cells, like T cells and B cells, originate in the body's bone marrow from stem cells. **Cytokines** are varied and powerful chemical messengers secreted by the cells of the immune system. They are the chief communication signals of T cells and include **interleukins,** growth factors, and interferons. The **complement system** consists of a series of approximately 25 proteins that "assist" antibodies in destroying bacteria. The complement system also helps rid the body of **antigen–antibody complexes** or clear pathogens from an organism. Complement proteins cause blood vessels to become dilated and leaky, causing redness and swelling during an inflammatory response. Complement proteins circulate in the blood in an inactive form. The **complement cascade** is triggered when the first complement molecule, C1, encounters antibody bound to antigen in an antigen–antibody complex. Each of the complement proteins performs its specialized work, acting sequentially on the molecule next in line. The end product is a cylinder that

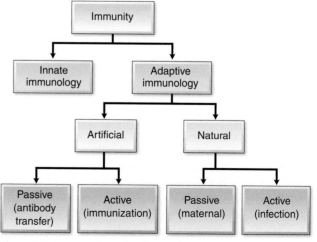

Figure 5-2. Innate and acquired immunity.

punctures the cell membrane and, by allowing fluids and molecules to flow in and out, kills the target cell.

Research

Although researchers have learned a great deal about the immune system, they continue to study how the body initiates attacks that destroy invading microbes, infected cells, and tumors while ignoring healthy tissues. New technologies for identifying individual immune cells are allowing scientists to determine rapidly which targets are triggering an immune response. Improvements in microscopy are permitting the observations of living B cells, T cells, and other cells as they interact within lymph nodes and other body tissues. Also, scientists are discovering the genetic blueprints that coordinate the human immune response, as well as those that dictate the biology of bacteria, viruses, and parasites. The combination of new technology and expanded genetic information will reveal more about how the body protects itself from disease.

PATHOGENESIS OF PERIODONTAL DISEASES, CHRONIC INFLAMMATION, AND RISK ASSESSMENT

Periodontal treatment planning is no longer based *only* on probing depths, mobility, occlusal abnormalities, mucogingival defects, and other clinical features. It is more often based on an understanding of the etiology and pathogenesis of, and patient susceptibility to, the disease. Susceptibility involves the interaction among host, bacterial, and environmental factors. It has become apparent that, although plaque biofilm is the cause of the disease, it is the **innate susceptibility** of the host that determines the ultimate outcome of the disease process.[4] It is important to understand the immunopathogenesis (the development of disease as affected by the immune system) of chronic periodontitis with respect to its possible clinical implications in terms of treatment planning and risk assessment. Identification of certain cytokine gene expressions in the peripheral blood and salivary RNA is now being studied as a possible marker of disease susceptibility. If this proves to be the case, a chairside salivary diagnostic could be developed in the near future.

Research has shown that in periodontitis, compared with gingivitis, immune response genes are differentially expressed, or expressed differently.[4] A total of 126 genes were upregulated (increased in response to a stimulus) in periodontitis compared with gingivitis and 55 genes were downregulated in periodontitis compared with gingivitis. These are considered pilot results, and it has yet to be determined whether susceptible patients can be identified on the basis of **differential gene expression.** However, differential gene expression offers exciting prospects for recognizing patients potentially at risk.[5]

The main features of PD are:

- The direct effects of the bacteria, such as proteases (collagenase) and cell toxins (leukotoxin)
- The host immunoinflammatory responses: lipopolysaccharide (LPS) triggers macrophages to produce **matrix metalloproteinases (MMPs),** which degrades collagen
- Disease modifiers: risk factors such as diabetes, which leads to a hyperinflammatory state and more inflammation
- Disease resolution: anti-inflammatory cytokines and oro-resolution molecules (resolvins) produced

Understanding risk factors for destructive PDs helps dental hygienists determine factors that are important in increased susceptibility or resistance to PDs, and provides the basis for interventions in prevention and management of PDs.

Even though plaque biofilm is the cause of PDs, it is the innate susceptibility of the host that determines the ultimate outcome of the disease process. Innate susceptibility is determined by the nature of the immune response to the specific periodontopathic (disease-causing) complexes comprising the plaque biofilm. All individuals have bacteria and biofilm in the mouth. As the biofilm matures, the concentration and virulence of the periodontal bacteria change.[6] It has been known for years that gingivitis develops over a period of several days in the presence of periodontal bacteria and that removal of the bacteria causes the gingival disease to resolve.[7] The body's response to the invading bacteria is the inflammatory process. This response includes the activation of immune system components, such as leukocytes, neutrophils, T lymphocytes, and plasma cells. This results in the release of antibodies, LPSs, and chemical inflammatory mediators that include cytokines, chemokines, and **C-reactive protein (CRP).** CRP is one of the acute-phase proteins that increase during systemic inflammation. CRP levels are increased in the presence of infection, in pregnancy, and during other events such as oral contraceptive use. The American Heart Association and U.S. Centers for Disease Control and Prevention have defined CRP risk groups as follows:

- Low risk: less than 1.0 mg/L
- Average risk: 1.0 to 3.0 mg/L
- High risk: greater than 3.0 mg/L

It has been suggested that testing CRP levels in the blood may be an additional way to assess CVD risk.[8]

LPSs are present in the gram-negative bacterial cell walls and act as powerful stimulants for the complex host response.[9] The early increased presence of neutrophils at the site is followed by the release of cytokines, which are released by both neutrophils and macrophages. Chemical mediators released include tumor necrosis factor alpha (TNFα), interleukin-1 (IL-1), and prostaglandins. The inflammatory process includes the stimulation of fibroblasts by IL-1 and the secretion of MMPs, of which collagenase is the most prominent, by **polymorphonuclear neutrophils (PNMs).** MMPs are responsible for increased collagen breakdown, and TNFα is primarily responsible for increased osteoclastic activity resulting in bone resorption. MMPs can also activate cytokines and chemokines, exacerbating the destructive process. Collagen production is inhibited by the reduced activity of fibroblasts in response to TNFα. The amount of periodontal destruction is dependent on the balance between destructive and protective inflammatory mediators. Although periodontal bacteria are required for infective PD, individual response determines disease progression. Individual reactions are affected by genetic signaling pathways that influence the expression of inflammatory mediators in response to bacterial LPSs.[10]

Most inflammation is principally protective. Acute inflammation usually resolves if the irritant is removed and if the resolution is not interrupted. The inflammatory response can become destructive, such as when an acute infection becomes chronic. The inflammatory response may not resolve and complete the repair phase.[11] The same outcome may result in some people if the inflammatory response is exaggerated when it is activated. Such exaggerated inflammatory responses may result from genetic differences among individuals or from other inflammatory diseases throughout the body.

Assessing a patient's risk for development of PD can have a significant impact on clinical decision making.[12] Modifiable risk factors include behavioral risk factors such as tobacco use and cigarette smoking. Cigarette smoking may account for half of the cases of advanced periodontitis in the United States.[13] Another significant behavioral risk factor is patient adherence, which includes many patient-centered behaviors such as attention to recommended oral hygiene practices and regular visits for dental care. Behavioral risk factors are modifiable, and the dental hygienist can use techniques such as motivational interviewing to encourage patients to change their behavior (see Application to Clinical Practice and Advancing Technologies).

Inflammation may also be destructive if the normal repair processes are disrupted, for example, as a result of smoking. It has been suggested that risk factors should be used to help identify patients who are more likely to have future destructive PD. The well-documented risk factors for future progression of periodontitis are smoking, diabetes, and certain genetic variations.[11]

Many clinical challenges exist in diagnosing and monitoring periodontal inflammation. Clinically, bleeding is often used as an indication of the level of inflammation in the periodontal tissue. However, bleeding on probing does not necessarily predict future disease activity; it has a low positive predictive value for the progression of periodontitis.[14] If decreasing the oral inflammatory load can support oral and systemic health, dental professionals must be able to accurately assess risk and disease, as well as detect changes in the inflammatory process. Currently, therapy consists of eliminating pathogenic bacteria that

Application to Clinical Practice

Translating didactic knowledge to practical experiences allows dental hygienists to look at the evidence and apply it to patients. Dental hygienists should explain to the patient that PDs are infections that trigger the immune response and the acute inflammatory response. This acute process helps to keep the body safe and attempts to wall off and destroy infectious agents (bacteria, viruses, fungi, and so on), and keep healthy and infectious organisms in the body in balance. When the acute inflammatory process becomes chronic, problems develop. The body's response to opportunistic pathogens also destroys healthy tissue, such as the periodontal ligament and the alveolar bone. Communicating to the patient that the infection must be treated and a healthy state be attained and maintained is critical to the long-term success of treatment. While communicating with patients, it is important to listen carefully and discern what is important to them. Motivational interviewing is a helpful tool to use. For detailed information on motivational interviewing, see Chapter 3: Communication Skills. ■

incite the inflammatory response through mechanical or chemical means to achieve a balance of bacteria that supports health.

Promising future approaches will rely more on modifying the inflammatory response itself, by limiting the activity of proinflammatory pathways and amplifying pathways that resolve inflammation.[15] Mechanisms being studied attempt to limit tissue destruction by directly blocking proinflammatory pathways without affecting bacterial accumulations, although continuing to reduce the bacterial burden to the point of a healthy balance is advised. Future therapy may function by modulating the inflammatory response earlier in the process of disease, interrupting the initial cascade of mediators that increase inflammation and bone resorption, or enhancing the resolution of inflammation.[16] The intricate proinflammatory pathways present many places where potentially therapeutic interventions could occur, either by inactivating effector cells or molecules or by limiting their activation or production.

Resolution of inflammation is also an active process mediated by specific resolution pathways.[17] Lipids made from fatty acids, such as **lipoxins** and **resolvins,** appear to be important in the resolution of inflammation. These anti-inflammatory lipids are made from omega-3 polyunsaturated fatty acids and omega-6 fatty acids such as arachidonic acid, which is also the precursor of some proinflammatory lipids.[15] Lipoxins can encourage the resolution of inflammation by limiting the migration of additional polymorphonuclear leukocytes (PMNs) into the site of inflammation, activating noninflammatory

Advancing Technologies

Tools for assessing a patient's risk for PD range from a low-technology guideline to sophisticated software:

- The "HealthPartners Dental Group and Clinics Periodontal Risk Assessment Guideline" can be used to identify patients at risk for development of PD, provide education and interventions, and standardize care according to the most recent research. It is available online from the U.S. Department of Health and Human Services (DHHS) Agency for Healthcare Research and Quality (AHRQ) at: http://www.guideline.gov/content.aspx?id=35131.

- PreViser analytic software (http://previser.com/) provides an easy-to-use, objective, and reproducible way to measure, understand, and communicate a patient's risk and disease level as simple numeric scores.

- MyPerioID PST is a test used to identify individual genetic susceptibility to PD and determine which patients are at increased risk for more severe periodontal infections because of an exaggerated immune response. The test is noninvasive and can be administered during the dental hygiene appointment. The patient swishes a saline solution in the mouth, expectorates into a collection tube, and the hygienist sends the sample to OralDNA Labs for analysis. This test can be used for patients with a family history of PD, patients with compromised immune systems, patients who have received therapy but continue with disease activity, patients who will receive implants and have lost teeth to PD, and adolescent patients (http://www.oraldna.com). OralDNA Labs also offers MyPerioPath test, a salivary test to determine the cause of periodontal infections, and OraRisk HPV test, a salivary test to determine who is at risk for human papillomavirus (HPV)–related oral cancers.

- Another tool for risk assessment for PD is the Florida Probe, a computerized probe that charts automatically (http://www.floridaprobe.com). Data are recorded by means of a foot switch. Other products include the GoProbe System, which enters data through a wireless keypad using any periodontal probe, and VoiceWorks, voice-activated software that uses a headset.

- Interleukin Genetics has the PerioPredict Genetic Test for PD susceptibility. It tests for a variation of the IL-1B gene, which was the most prevalent risk factor, affecting about one third of the population.[75] ■

development and progression of most of the chronic diseases of aging, diet and genetic variations interact to control differences in inflammation among individuals, inflammation is actively resolved by specific mechanisms that help to restore homeostasis, and there are ways to augment these processes.[18]

Acute inflammation is a protective attempt by the organism to remove the injurious stimuli and to initiate the healing process. Irritation, injury, or infection causes tissue redness (rubor), swelling (tumor), heat (calor), and pain (dolor). Prolonged inflammation, known as chronic inflammation, leads to a progressive shift in the type of cells present at the site of inflammation and is characterized by simultaneous destruction and healing of the tissue from the inflammatory process. Chronic inflammation can also lead to a host of diseases, such as hay fever, periodontitis, atherosclerosis, rheumatoid arthritis, and even cancer. Greater understanding of the complex pathways involved in inflammation may provide alternative therapeutic strategies to combat inflammation and chronic diseases potentially arising from it (see Teamwork).

Although an individual's genes do not change, the control of how certain genes are expressed in specific tissues can change substantially because of factors such as diet, stress, and bacterial accumulations. Visceral fat accumulation around the waist substantially increases the inflammatory burden on the body. Overexpression

Teamwork

Teamwork and interdisciplinary collaboration are essential to successful oral health care. The American Dental Education Association (ADEA) and several other national health profession associations and foundations are promoting interprofessional collaborative practice. Competencies and action strategies to be implemented in educational institutions in the United States, providing the foundation for improved patient care and services, are detailed in a report entitled *Core Competencies for Interprofessional Collaborative Practice* (available at: https://www.aamc.org/download/186750/data/core_competencies.pdf).[76] Building on this report, health-care leaders developed "Team-Based Competencies: Building a Shared Foundation for Education and Clinical Practice" (available at: http://www.aacn.nche.edu/leading-initiatives/IPECProceedings.pdf). These action strategies implement the Interprofessional Education Collaborative (IPEC) core competencies and provide a means of instilling collaboration among health professionals. (For more information, see *Collaborative Practice in Dentistry: Practice and Potential* [http://futurehealth.ucsf.edu/Content/29/2011-01_Collaborative_Practice_in_American_Dentistry_Practice_and_Potential.pdf].) ■

monocytes, and stimulating the removal of dead PMNs by macrophages.

An American Academy of Periodontology (AAP) workshop produced the following results: Inflammatory mechanisms appear to be critical factors in the of inflammation may be one of the key aspects of aging that influence and link different diseases in different individuals.

Numerous studies have demonstrated that the periodontitis lesion involves predominantly B cells and plasma cells, whereas the gingivitis lesion is primarily a T-cell–mediated response.[19] This led to the concept that the development of periodontitis involves a switch from a T-cell lesion to one involving large numbers of B cells and plasma cells.[20] It is also well recognized that control of this shift is mediated by a balance between the T helper type 1 (Th1) and Th2 subsets of T cells, with chronic periodontitis being mediated by Th2 cells. T regulatory (Treg) and Th17 cells have been confirmed in periodontal tissues, raising the possibility that these cells are also important in the immunoregulation of PD.

ORAL–SYSTEMIC CONNECTIONS

A large body of research has focused on the role periodontal health plays in systemic health and specifically how PD may be related to other conditions. Evidence for a link between PD and several systemic diseases is growing rapidly. The infectious and inflammatory burden of chronic periodontitis is thought to have an important systemic impact. Current evidence suggests that periodontitis is associated with an increased likelihood of coronary heart disease and may influence the severity of diabetes.[21]

A joint workshop organized by the European Federation of Periodontology (EFP) and the AAP aimed to establish a consensus knowledge base of the scientific evidence on the association between periodontitis and systemic diseases, specifically CVD, diabetes, and adverse pregnancy complications. Periodontal thought leaders from both Europe and the United States participated in the workshop, which was held in Segovia, Spain, on November 11 through 14, 2012 (http://www.perio.org/consumer/2012_EFP-AAP_Workshop). More than 70 experts in the specialty of periodontology were invited to participate in the workshop and were assigned to one of three workgroups: CVD and PD, diabetes and PD, and adverse pregnancy outcomes and PD. The workgroups were responsible for reviewing the scientific evidence in their respective areas and developing a consensus statement on each topic.

The introductory article scrutinizes the possible mechanisms that may play a role in the links between periodontitis and systemic conditions. Three basic mechanisms were hypothesized to play a role in these interactions: metastatic infections, inflammation and inflammatory injury, and adaptive immunity.[22] It was not a systematic or critical review, but rather an overview of the field to set the stage for the critical reviews in each of the working groups. It was stated that published evidence supports modest associations between periodontitis and some, although not all, of the diseases and conditions reviewed. Respiratory disease, chronic kidney disease, rheumatoid arthritis, cognitive impairment, obesity, metabolic syndrome, and cancer were reviewed. There is a need to reach a consensus on what constitutes periodontitis for future studies of putative associations with systemic diseases.[23]

Working group 4 reviewed the evidence for associations between periodontitis and various systemic diseases and conditions, including chronic obstructive pulmonary disease, pneumonia, chronic kidney disease, rheumatoid arthritis, cognitive impairment, obesity, metabolic syndrome, and cancer, and documented discussions of the state of each field.[24]

The group was unanimous that the reported associations do not imply causality, and establishment of causality will require new studies that fulfill the Bradford Hill or equivalent criteria. This includes statistical strength of association, consistency, specificity, temporal relationship (e.g., cause precedes consequence), biological gradient or dose–response relationship (e.g., more periodontitis leads to more atherosclerosis), biological plausibility, coherence, experimental reversibility, and analogy—other precedents.[25]

Working group 4 also stated that precise and community agreed-on case definitions of PD states must be implemented systematically to enable consistent and clearer interpretations of studies of the relationship to systemic diseases. Studies should focus on strong disease outcomes and avoid surrogate endpoints. It was concluded that because of the relative immaturity of the body of evidence for each of the purported relationships, gaps in knowledge are large.

Cardiovascular Diseases

Atherosclerotic cardiovascular diseases (ACVD) are a group of diseases that include fatal and nonfatal coronary heart disease (angina, myocardial infarction), ischemic cerebrovascular disease (stroke/transient ischemic attack), and peripheral arterial disease. Most recent research concludes that there is consistent and strong epidemiological evidence that periodontitis imparts increased risk for future CVD, and although in vitro, animal, and clinical studies do support the interaction and biological mechanism, intervention trials to date are not adequate to draw further conclusions. Well-designed intervention trials on the impact of periodontal treatment on prevention of ACVD with hard clinical outcomes are needed.[27]

In regard to the role of bacteria in the PD–CVD connection, there is support that periodontal pathogens can contribute to atherosclerosis.[28] It was reported that bacteria migrate from the oral cavity and settle on systemic vascular tissues; pathogens can be found in the targeted tissues, live within the new site, and create atherosclerosis in animal models of disease; noninvasive mutants of periodontal bacteria cause significantly reduced pathology in vitro and in vivo; and periodontal isolates from human atheromas can cause disease in animal models of infection.[28]

Regarding intervention, there is moderate evidence that periodontal treatment decreases systemic inflammation, as demonstrated by reduction in CRP. Also, there is some improvement of both clinical and surrogate measures of endothelial function. However, there seems to be no effect on lipid profiles, supporting specificity. Limited evidence shows improvements in coagulation, biomarkers of endothelial cell activation, arterial blood pressure, and subclinical atherosclerosis after periodontal therapy. The available evidence is consistent and speaks for a contributory role of periodontitis to ACVD. No periodontal intervention studies on primary ACVD prevention and only one feasibility study on secondary ACVD prevention have been reported.

Epidemiological data indicate that PD is an independent risk factor for myocardial infarction, coronary heart disease, diabetes, and other diseases and conditions.[29] Evidence supporting a causative role of chronic infection in coronary heart disease and other diseases is mostly circumstantial. The evidence supports the hypothesis that periodontitis leads to systemic exposure to oral bacteria. Cytokines and LPS produced in the infected periodontal tissues, which enter the bloodstream, are potential sources of systemic inflammatory mediators capable of initiating or worsening conditions associated with atherosclerosis and coronary heart disease. Cytokines produce their effects directly, whereas the LPS activates a systemic cascade of inflammatory cytokines capable of inducing effects associated with atherosclerosis and coronary heart disease. The continued systemic exposure to gram-negative bacteria and LPS results in a release of cytokines such as TNFα, IL-1β, and prostaglandin E_2, which may be a significant factor in the pathogenesis of coronary heart disease and stroke.

Studies to date discuss three possible justifications for the proposed epidemiological associations. One study theorizes that bacteria migrating to the bloodstream from the periodontal pocket (**bacteremia**) can attach to injured vascular endothelium and initiate or exacerbate the atherosclerotic disease process.[30] This hypothesis is supported by the demonstration of periodontal pathogens in atheromas taken from coronary and carotid arteries. Periodontal bacteria, and antibodies to the bacteria, have been found in the bloodstream and in atherosclerotic plaques.[31] *Streptococcus mutans* was the most frequently identified species in the cardiovascular specimens, followed by *Aggregatibacter actinomycetemcomitans*.[32] Regarding dental plaque biofilm specimens from patients who underwent cardiovascular operations, most of the tested periodontitis-related species, as well as oral streptococci, were detected at high frequencies. Also, the positive rate of *S. mutans* in cardiovascular samples from patients whose dental plaque specimens were also positive for *S. mutans* was 78%, which was significantly greater than any other tested species when the same analysis was performed. The study results propose that specific oral bacterial species, such as *S. mutans* and *A. actinomycetemcomitans*,

are related to bacteremia and may be etiologic factors for the development of CVDs.

Other studies connect inflammatory mediators from PDs to the increased risk for CVD.[33] Some researchers propose that risk factors common between the two diseases may be acting as a confounder in the analysis of association.[34]

We now have sufficient studies to conduct **meta-analyses,** which are analyses to determine whether the volume of evidence supports an association between the two diseases. The meta-analyses to date conclude that periodontitis is a significant and independent risk factor for ACVD.[35,36] At the same time, impressive evidence has emerged from the cardiovascular profession to suggest that the most reasonable explanation for this association with any chronic inflammatory disease, such as periodontitis, appears to involve the role of systemic inflammatory mediators that have been strongly implicated in ACVD events.

Research supporting oral-systemic links between periodontal infection and systemic disease includes studies on associations between periodontal status and CVD, diabetes, pulmonary disease, renal disease, and osteoporosis. Research suggests that the presence of periodontitis may increase the risk for cardiovascular events and severe periodontitis may increase the risk for cerebral ischemia or stroke.[37] Elevated CRP levels, inflammatory mediators associated with inflammation, are associated with PD, and long-term exposure to CRPs has been found to be associated with a threefold risk for CVD.[38] A meta-analysis found a significant association between PD and CVD after controlling for major co-contributors of CVD, such as smoking.[39]

Diabetes

According to the World Health Organization (WHO), the prevalence of diabetes worldwide is increasing at a rapid rate, from 171,000,000 cases in the year 2000 to an estimated 366,000,000 cases in 2030.[40] Figure 5-3 shows the prevalence of diabetes worldwide.

Diabetes and periodontitis are multifaceted chronic diseases with a recognized bidirectional relationship. There is long-established evidence that hyperglycemia in diabetes is associated with adverse periodontal outcomes. However, given the large presence of PDs and the developing global diabetes epidemic, it is appropriate to review the role of periodontitis in diabetes. Complications of diabetes contribute to significant morbidity and premature mortality. Over the last 20 years, reliable and strong evidence has shown that severe periodontitis adversely affects glycemic control in diabetes and glycemia in subjects without diabetes. In patients with diabetes, there is a direct and dose-dependent relationship between periodontitis severity and diabetes complications. Emerging evidence supports an increased risk for diabetes onset in patients with severe periodontitis.[41]

Systemic inflammation leads to type 2 diabetes and predisposes reduced pancreatic β-cell function, apoptosis

Prevalence of diabetes

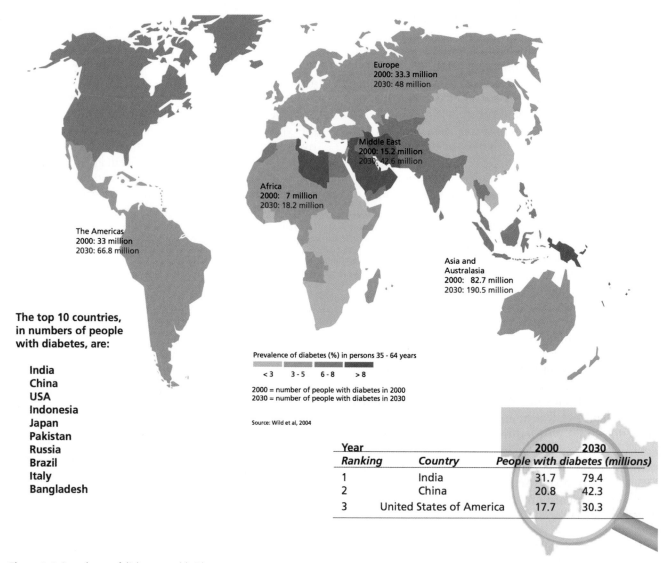

Figure 5-3. Prevalence of diabetes worldwide. (Reproduced, with the permission of the publisher, from *Traditional Medicine*. Geneva: World Health Organization; 2008.)

(programmed cell death), and insulin resistance. Research supports elevated systemic inflammation, as evidenced by acute-phase and oxidative stress biomarkers, resulting from the entry of periodontal organisms and their virulence factors into the circulation, providing biological plausibility for the effects of periodontitis on diabetes. Virulence factors are often responsible for causing disease in the host. Advanced glycation end products–receptor for advanced glycation end products interactions and oxidative-stress-mediated pathways provide believable mechanisms in the diabetes-to-periodontitis direction.

Randomized controlled trials (RCTs) dependably prove that mechanical periodontal therapy results in about a 0.4% reduction in hemoglobin (Hb) A_{1c} at 3 months, a clinical impact equivalent to adding a second drug to a pharmacological regime for diabetes. Hb A_{1c} is a laboratory test that shows the average level of blood sugar (glucose) over the previous 3 months. No current evidence supports adjunctive use of antimicrobials for periodontal management of patients with diabetes.

Studies have shown that TNFα induced from periodontal pathogens may increase insulin resistance, which may lead to a risk for CVD.[34] Periodontal infections were also shown to contribute to elevated systemic CRP levels.[42] Deep pockets were closely related to current glucose tolerance status and the development of glucose intolerance.[43] Severe periodontitis is associated with metabolic syndrome in middle-aged individuals.[44] PD is a complication of diabetes mellitus, and patients who suffer from both PD and diabetes have poorer glycemic control than those diabetics with little or no PD. Treatment of PD in diabetes mellitus enhances glycemic control. Periodontal treatment to remove bacteria appears to reduce circulating TNFα levels.[45] Nonsurgical periodontal treatment is associated with improved glycemic control in patients with type 2 diabetes mellitus.[46] Also, lower frequency of teeth brushing is related to greater prevalence of diabetes mellitus, hypertension, and high triglyceride and/or low high-density lipoprotein cholesterol in both men and women. Maintaining good oral hygiene by regular teeth brushing may prevent type 2 diabetes, hypertension, and dyslipidemia.[47]

Using guidelines established by the American Diabetes Association, one study determined that 93% of subjects who had PD (compared with 63% of those without the disease) were considered to be at high risk for diabetes and should be screened for the disease.[48] The guidelines recommend that diabetes screening should be conducted in people who are 45 years or older who have a body mass index of 25 or greater and at least one additional risk factor. In Strauss et al's study,[48] additional risk factors such as high blood pressure and a first-degree sibling with diabetes were reported in a significantly greater number of subjects with PD than in subjects without PD. Dental hygienists can screen patients for diabetes by evaluating them for risk factors. These include overweight, belonging to a high-risk ethnic group (African American, Latino, Native American, Asian American, or Pacific Islander), having high cholesterol, having high blood pressure, having a first-degree relative with diabetes, having had gestational diabetes mellitus, or having given birth to a baby weighing more than 9 pounds. Also, use of a **glucometer** (a glucose meter or medical device for determining the approximate concentration of glucose in the blood) in the dental office or clinic to evaluate blood samples is suggested. Diabetes mellitus accelerates atheromas, a mass or plaque of degenerated thickened arterial intima, occurring in atherosclerosis, increasing the risk for a stroke. Compared with the 5% atheroma rate reported among healthy individuals, rates were significantly greater in patients with diabetes mellitus. Clinicians treating patients with diabetes mellitus may see atheromatous lesions on panoramic radiographs and refer them for treatment[49] (see Evidence-Based Practice).

A small body of evidence supports significant adverse effects of PD on glycemic control, diabetes complications, and development of type 2 (and possibly gestational) diabetes. Although current research proposes that PD adversely affects diabetes outcomes, further longitudinal studies are needed.[50]

Evidence-Based Practice

A bidirectional relationship exists between periodontal infection and systemic conditions such as diabetes. Treating periodontal infection is not only important for oral health, but can affect overall health, such as blood sugar levels in people with diabetes. Also, uncontrolled blood sugar levels can exacerbate PDs. The evidence regarding treatment of periodontitis in affecting systemic conditions is stronger in some cases than in others. However, it is important to remember that treatment of periodontal infection can improve oral health and affect the immune system, so unless someone is immunocompromised and requires special treatment, treating oral infection is defensible. ■

Respiratory Infections

It has been hypothesized that poor oral health may predispose high-risk patients to oral colonization by respiratory pathogens. The method is that respiratory pathogens may colonize in the oral pharyngeal tissues, and these pathogens may be released and aspirated into the lower airway to cause pneumonia. It has also been shown that plaque control may reduce the risk for **nosocomial pneumonia** (also known as hospital-acquired pneumonia or health-care-associated pneumonia), which is acquired in a hospital or health-care setting such as a nursing home. Nosocomial pneumonia is often caused by bacteria that are not common members of the oropharyngeal flora such as *Pseudomonas aeruginosa, Staphylococcus aureus,* and enteric gram-negative bacteria. These organisms populate the oral cavity in certain settings, such as in institutionalized subjects and in people living in areas served by unsanitary water supplies.[51] It is likely that oral and respiratory bacteria in the dental plaque are shed into the saliva and are then aspirated into the lower respiratory tract and the lungs to cause infection.[52] Cytokines and enzymes from the periodontally inflamed tissues by the oral biofilm may also be transferred into the lungs where they may stimulate local inflammatory processes preceding colonization of pathogens and the actual lung infection. In a healthy patient, the respiratory tract has the ability to protect against aspirated bacteria. Patients with reduced salivary flow, decreased cough reflex, swallowing disorders, less aptitude to perform good oral hygiene, or other physical disabilities have a high risk for pulmonary infections. Oral bacterial load increases during intubation, and higher dental plaque scores increase the risk for pneumonia.[53]

Cariogenic bacteria and periodontal pathogens in saliva or dental plaque are found to be risk factors for aspiration pneumonia in nursing home patients. It is recognized that the teeth and gingival margin are places that favor bacterial colonization, and periodontal pockets may serve as reservoirs for potential pathogens for pneumonia.[54]

Improved oral hygiene has been shown to reduce the occurrence of nosocomial pneumonia, in both mechanically ventilated hospital patients and nonventilated nursing home residents. Hospitalized intensive care unit (ICU) patients were shown to benefit from daily oral cleaning. Studies have shown that the use of oral topical chlorhexidine reduces pneumonia in mechanically ventilated patients and may even decrease the need for systemic IV antibiotics or shorten the duration of mechanical ventilation in the ICU.[55] Mechanical oral care in combination with povidone-iodine has been shown to significantly decrease pneumonia in ventilated ICU patients.[56] Toothbrushing combined with a topical antimicrobial agent is a promising method for oral cleansing of mechanically ventilated patients.

Professional debridement by a dental hygienist once a week significantly reduced the prevalence of fever and fatal pneumonia in 141 elderly patients in nursing homes.[57] A weekly professional oral cleaning also significantly reduced influenza infections in an elderly population.[58]

Poor oral health, inability to perform daily oral hygiene, oral colonization of periodontal and respiratory pathogens, and the presence of periodontitis are linked to nosocomial pneumonia. A direct causal relationship between periodontitis and pneumonia has not been established; however, oral hygiene will assume an even more important role in the care of patients in the hospital ICU and elderly patients (see Spotlight on Public Health).

Pregnancy

Pregnancy sometimes has adverse outcomes including low birth weight (less than 2,500 g), preterm birth (less than 37 weeks), growth restriction, pre-eclampsia, miscarriage, and/or stillbirth. Maternal periodontitis directly or indirectly has the potential to influence the health of the fetal–maternal unit. Low birth weight, preterm birth, and pre-eclampsia have been associated with maternal periodontitis exposure. However, the strength of the observed associations is modest and seems to vary according to the population studied, the means of periodontal assessment, and the PD classification used.[59] Although periodontal therapy is safe during all trimesters of pregnancy and leads to improved periodontal conditions in pregnant women, case-related periodontal therapy, with or without systemic antibiotics, does not reduce overall rates of preterm birth and low-birth-weight newborns. Further investigation is still necessary to fully translate the findings of basic research into clinical studies and practice. In the meantime, the California Dental Association provides evidence-based guidelines for dental care during pregnancy (http://www.cdafoundation.org/Portals/0/pdfs/poh_guidelines.pdf).

Clinical studies on the effects of periodontal infection on preterm birth/low-birth-weight newborns began to appear in 1996 with Offenbacher et al's study.[60] No consensus has been reached about the influence of PD on preterm low birth weight. Part of the reason for the ambivalence is that no consensus exists on a uniform definition of PD in studies on PD and preterm low birth weight.[61]

Several studies found positive associations between PD and preterm low birth weight.[60,62–68] In one study, the hypothesis that PD is a risk factor for undesirable pregnancy outcomes was rejected. Unlike other studies on the topic, clinical measures relating to PD were not associated with low birth weight, preterm birth, and preterm birth and low birth weight.[69] Evidence of no association between PD and preterm low birth weight in this study was also reported by others.[70–73] According to the authors, heterogeneity in diagnostic criteria for PD in previous studies is an important source of discrepancies.[61] The strength of their study is that a wide range of measures of PD was used to avoid objections about measuring PD. In conclusion, PD is not a risk factor for low birth weight, preterm birth, and preterm birth and low birth weight.

Maternal periodontitis is modestly but independently associated with adverse pregnancy outcomes, but the findings are impacted by periodontitis case definitions. It has been suggested that future studies use both continuous and categorical assessments of periodontal status. Further use of the composite outcome preterm low birth weight is not encouraged. Further studies using women with established PD, effective periodontal therapies that resolve the disease, and proper adverse pregnancy outcomes, such as spontaneous abortion, are needed.[74]

IMPROVING OUTCOMES

Disorders or diseases can occur concurrently or develop consecutively where progression or exacerbation of one disease may affect another disease. The suggestion that PD is a significant risk factor for coronary, respiratory, and other systemic diseases such as diabetes demands a new outlook on oral health. In the future, PD may be added to the factors used to assess patients' risk profiles for coronary heart disease, stroke, diabetes, and other diseases. In addition, treatment of PD should become a standard part of therapy for patients with coronary, respiratory, and other systemic diseases.

Considerable epidemiological evidence supports the concept that poor oral health, especially the extent and severity of PD, may put patients at a significant risk for a variety of systemic conditions. There is increasing evidence that reducing the inflammatory component of the disease in the periodontal tissues has potential systemic effects. Reducing the inflammatory burden in the periodontal tissues has been shown to improve hyperglycemic control in individuals with diabetes, reduce the prevalence of adverse pregnancy outcomes, and improve surrogate markers that may be of benefit in patients suffering from coronary heart disease.

Spotlight on Public Health

Lessons abound from this chapter regarding public health benefits from dental hygiene interventions. Dental hygienists or dental hygiene students can organize projects to (within the confines of the law): work in long-term care facilities, perform periodontal and oral cancer screenings, assist with self-care instructions and oral care with patients in long-term care facilities, train-the-trainer regarding oral health of the home-bound and those in long-term care facilities, volunteer to label dentures, and other public health projects. Presenting courses to consumers and having a booth at a health fair are other public health activities that could benefit the community. ■

Case Study

Mrs. Brown arrives at the dental office for a "cleaning" because her gums are bleeding and she has strange swelling between #8 and #9. #8 and #9 are overlapped, the "swelling" is about 8 mm and reddish purple, and her oral hygiene is fair. She is a patient of record, has type 2 diabetes, and during the medical history, Mrs. Brown divulges that she is 3 months pregnant. Her gingival tissue is red and easy to bleed, and periodontal pockets are 3 to 4 mm. No bone loss is present on her radiographs. She says that she heard that bleeding gums could cause her to have problems with her pregnancy, and she also heard that any dental or dental hygiene treatment during pregnancy was not advised. She is unsure of how to proceed.

Case Study Exercises

1. The dental hygiene process of care should be implemented. The dental hygienist should inform Mrs. Brown that although there is no conclusive evidence to suggest that hormonal gingivitis could harm the fetus and that treating the infection may or may not be beneficial to the fetus, débridement will help the oral condition and *may* have a positive effect on the fetus.
   A. Both statements are true.
   B. Both statements are false.
   C. The first statement is true, the second is false.
   D. The first statement is false, the second is true.

2. What factors must be considered while making a dental hygiene diagnosis for Mrs. Brown?
   A. Her periodontal condition
   B. Her pregnancy
   C. Her control (or lack thereof) of her type 2 diabetes
   D. All of the above

3. Each of the following statements regarding dental hygiene treatment during pregnancy is appropriate EXCEPT:
   A. There is no conclusive evidence to suggest that hormonal gingivitis could harm the fetus.
   B. Treatment of periodontitis in pregnant women improves periodontal disease and is safe.
   C. Treatment of periodontitis in pregnant women improves rates of preterm birth, low birth weight, or fetal growth restriction.
   D. The swelling present could be a pregnancy granuloma.

Review Questions

1. Order the steps in the complement cascade.
   _____ A. The target is killed.
   _____ B. There is a cylinder that punctures the cell membrane.
   _____ C. The complement molecule, C1, encounters an antigen–antibody complex.
   _____ D. Each of the complement proteins performs its specialized work, acting sequentially on the molecule next in line.
   _____ E. Fluids and molecules flow in and out.

2. All of the following are correct about lipoxins, EXCEPT:
   A. They are proteins that encourage the resolution of inflammation.
   B. They work by limiting the migration of polymorphonuclear leukocytes (PMNs) into the site of inflammation.
   C. They activate noninflammatory monocytes.
   D. They stimulate the removal of dead PMNs by macrophages.
   E. They are made from omega-3 polyunsaturated fatty acids.

3. Oral diseases and infections are not major public health problems worldwide, like diabetes. However, they are still among the most prevalent microbial diseases of humankind.
   A. Both statements are true.
   B. Both statements are false.
   C. The first statement is true, the second is false.
   D. The first statement is false, the second is true.

4. The purpose of the immune system is to keep infectious microorganisms such as bacteria, viruses, fungi, and parasites out of the body, and to destroy any that invade the body. Bone marrow, the soft tissue in the hollow center of bones, is the ultimate source of all blood cells.
   A. Both statements are true.
   B. Both statements are false.
   C. The first statement is true, the second is false.
   D. The first statement is false, the second is true.

5. The organs involved with the immune system are called the *lymphoid organs*. They affect growth, development, and the release of erythrocytes, a kind of white blood cell.
   A. Both statements are true.
   B. Both statements are false.
   C. The first statement is true, the second is false.
   D. The first statement is false, the second is true.

Active Learning

1. Divide the classroom into three groups. Each group will develop a PowerPoint presentation on the oral–systemic link to be delivered to the one of the following audiences: nurses, the general public, or nursing home aids. Share the presentation with the class.
2. Develop a 60-second Public Service Announcement on the oral–systemic link to be delivered on the radio. Present it to the class.
3. Outline the main points of this chapter to create study notes. ■

REFERENCES

1. Seymour GJ, Ford PJ, Cullinan MP, Leishman S, West MJ, Yamazaki K. Infection or inflammation: the link between periodontal and cardiovascular diseases. *Future Cardiol.* 2009;5(1):5-9.
2. Genco RJ, Williams RC. *Periodontal Disease and Overall Health: A Clinician's Guide.* Yardley, PA: Professional Audience Communications, Inc.; 2010:48.
3. World Health Organization. Risk factors. Available from: http://www.who.int/topics/risk_factors/en. Accessed May 27, 2014.
4. Ohlrich EJ, Cullinan MP, Seymour GJ. The immunopathogenesis of periodontal disease. *Austral Dent J.* 2009;54(suppl 1):S2-S10.
5. Gilbert SF. *Developmental Biology.* 6th ed. Sunderland, MA: Sinauer Associates; 2000. Available from: http://www.ncbi.nlm.nih.gov/books/NBK10061. Accessed May 27, 2014.
6. Socransky SS, Haffajee AD, Cugini MA, et al. Microbial complexes in subgingival plaque. *J Clin Periodontol.* 1998;25:134-144.
7. Loe H, Theilade E, Jensen SB. Experimental gingivitis in man. *J Periodontol.* 1965;36:177-187.
8. American Heart Association. Inflammation, heart disease and stroke: the role of C-reactive protein. *Circulation.* 2003;108:e81-e85.
9. Serio FG, Duncan TB. The pathogenesis and treatment of periodontal disease. IneedCE.com. Chesterland, OH: PennWell. Available from: http://www.ineedce.com/coursereview.aspx?url=1686%2fPDF%2fPathogenesisandTreatment.pdf&scid=14046. Accessed August 6, 2013.
10. Barksby HE, Nile CJ, Jaedicke KM, et al. Differential expression of immunoregulatory genes in monocytes in response to Porphyromonas gingivalis and Escherichia coli lipopolysaccharide. *Clin Exp Immunol.* 2009;156(3):479-487.
11. Richards DW. An interview with Dr. Kenneth Kornman. *CDA J.* 2010;38:259-262.
12. Page RC, Martin J, Krall EA, Mancl L, Garcia R. Longitudinal validation of a risk calculator for periodontal disease. *J Clin Periodontol.* 2003;30(9):819-827.
13. Tomer JL, Asma S. Smoking-attributable periodontitis in the United States: findings from NHANES III. National Health and Nutrition Examination Survey. *J Periodontol.* 2000;71(5):743-751.
14. Lang NP, Joss A, Orsanic T, Gusberti FA, Siegrist BE. Bleeding on probing. A predictor for the progression of periodontal disease. *J Clin Periodontol.* 1986;13:590-596.
15. Schonfeld SE. Strategies for managing periodontal inflammation. *CDA J.* 2010;38:272-282.
16. Graves D. Cytokines that promote periodontal tissue destruction. *J Periodontol.* 2008;79(8 suppl):1585-1591.
17. Van Dyke T. The management of inflammation in periodontal disease. *J Periodontol.* 2008;79(8 suppl):1601-1608.
18. American Academy of Periodontology (AAP). Inflammation and periodontal diseases, Special Supplement. *J Periodontol.* 2008;79:1501-1614. Available from: http://www.joponline.org/toc/jop/79/8s.
19. Orozco A, Gemmell E, Bickel M, Seymour GJ. Interleukin-1beta, interleukin-12 and interleukin-18 levels in gingival fluid and serum of patients with gingivitis and periodontitis. *Oral Microbiol Immunol.* 2006;21:256-260.
20. Mosmann TR, Cherwinski H, Bond MW, Giedlin MA, Coffman RL. Two types of murine helper T cell clone. I. Definition according to profiles of lymphokine activities and secreted proteins. *J Immunol.* 1986;136:2348-2357.
21. Nakajima T, Ueki-Maruyama K, Oda T, et al. Regulatory T-cells infiltrate periodontal disease tissues. *J Dent Res.* 2005;84:639-643.
22. Van Dyke TE, van Winkelhoff AJ. Infection and inflammatory mechanisms. *J Periodontol.* 2013;84(4 suppl):S1-S7.
23. Linden GJ, Lyons A, Scannapieco FA. Periodontal systemic associations: review of the evidence. *J Periodontol.* 2013;84(4 suppl):S8-S19.
24. Linden GJ, Herzberg MC, on behalf of Working Group 4 of the Joint EFP/AAP Workshop. Periodontitis and systemic diseases: a record of discussions of working group 4 of the Joint EFP/AAP Workshop on Periodontitis and Systemic Diseases. *J Periodontol.* 2013;84(4 suppl):S20-S23.
25. Höfler M. The Bradford Hill considerations on causality: a counterfactual perspective. *Emerg Themes Epidemiol.* 2005;2:11.
26. Williams RC, Barnett AH, Claffey N, et al. The potential impact of periodontal disease on general health: a consensus view. *Curr Med Res Opin.* 2008;24(6):1635-1643.
27. Tonetti MS, Van Dyke TE, on behalf of Working Group 1 of the Joint EFP/AAP Workshop. Periodontitis and atherosclerotic cardiovascular disease: consensus report of the Joint EFP/AAP Workshop on Periodontitis and Systemic Diseases. *J Periodontol.* 2013;84(4 suppl):S24-S29.
28. Reyes L, Herrera D, Kozarov E, Roldan S, Progulske-Fox A. Periodontal bacterial invasion and infection: contribution to atherosclerotic pathology. *J Periodontol.* 2013;84(4 suppl):S30-S50.
29. Karnoutsos K, Papastergiou P, Stefanidis S, Vakaloudi A. Periodontitis as a risk factor for cardiovascular disease: the role of anti-phosphorylcholine and anti-cardiolipin antibodies. *Hippokratia.* 2008;12(3):144-149.
30. Pihlstrom B, Michalowicz B, Johnson N. Periodontal diseases. *The Lancet.* 2005;366:1809-1820.
31. Kozarov EV, Dorn BR, Shelburne CE, Dunn WA Jr, Progulske-Fox A. Human atherosclerotic plaque contains viable invasive Actinobacillus actinomycetemcomitans and Porphyromonas gingivalis. *Arterioscler Thromb Vasc Biol.* 2005;25(3):e17-e18.

32. Nakano K, Nemoto H, Nomura R, et al. Detection of oral bacteria in cardiovascular specimens. *Oral Microbiol Immunol.* 2009;24:64-68.

33. Nakajima T, Yamazaki K. Periodontal disease and risk of atherosclerotic coronary heart disease. *Odontology.* 2009;97:1618-1647.

34. Genco R, Offenbacher S, Beck J. Periodontal disease and cardiovascular disease: epidemiology and possible mechanisms. *J Am Dent Assoc.* 2002;133(suppl): 14S-22S.

35. Humphrey LL, Fu R, Buckley DI, Freeman M, Helfand MJ. Periodontal disease and coronary heart disease incidence: a systematic review and meta-analysis. *J Gen Intern Med.* 2008;23:2079-2086.

36. Bahekar AA, Singh S, Saha S, Molnar J, Arora R. The prevalence and incidence of coronary heart disease is significantly increased in periodontitis: a meta-analysis. *Am Heart J.* 2007;154:830-837.

37. Lee H, Garcia RI, Janket S, et al. The association between cumulative periodontal disease and stroke history in older adults. *J Periodontol.* 2006;77(10):1744-1754.

38. D'Aiuto F, Parkar M, Andreou G, et al. Periodontitis and systemic inflammation: control of the local infection is associated with a reduction in serum inflammatory markers. *J Dent Res.* 2004;83:156.

39. Bahekar AA, Singh S, Saha S, et al. The prevalence and incidence of coronary heart disease is significantly increased in periodontitis: a meta analysis. *Am Heart J.* 2007;154(5):830-837.

40. WHO Diabetes Programme. Country and regional data. Available from: http://www.who.int/diabetes/facts/world_figures/en. Accessed August 5, 2013.

41. Chapple ILC, Genco R, on behalf of Working Group 2 of the Joint EFP/AAP Workshop. Diabetes and periodontal diseases: consensus report of the Joint EFP/AAP Workshop on Periodontitis and Systemic Diseases. *J Periodontol.* 2013;84(4 suppl):S106-S112.

42. Noack B, Genco RJ, Trevisan M, Grossi S, Zambon JJ, De Nardin E. Periodontal infections contribute to elevated systemic C reactive protein level. *J Periodontol.* 2001;72:1221-1227.

43. Saito T, Shimazaki Y, Kiyohara Y, et al. The severity of periodontal disease is associated with the development of glucose intolerance in non-diabetics: the Hisayama study. *J Dent Res.* 2004;83:485-490.

44. D'Aiuto F, Sabbah W, Netuveli G, et al. Association of the metabolic syndrome with severe periodontitis in a large U.S. population-based survey. *J Clin Endocrinol Metab.* 2008;93:3989-3994.

45. Iwamoto Y, Nishimura F, Nakagawa M, et al. The effect of antimicrobial periodontal treatment on circulating tumor necrosis factor-alpha and glycated hemoglobin level in patients with type 2 diabetes. *J Periodontol.* 2001;72:774-778.

46. Singh S, Kumar V, Kumar S, Subbappa A. The effect of periodontal therapy on the improvement of glycemic control in patients with type 2 diabetes mellitus: a randomized controlled clinical trial. *Int J Diabetes Dev Ctries.* 2008;28(2):38-44.

47. Fujita M, Ueno K, Hata A. Lower frequency of daily teeth brushing is related to high prevalence of cardiovascular risk factors. *Exp Biol Med.* 2009;234:387-394.

48. Strauss SM, Russell S, Wheeler A, Norman R, Borrell LN, Rindskopf D. The dental office visit as a potential opportunity for diabetes screening: an analysis using NHANES 2003-2004 data. *J Public Health Dent.* 2010;70(2):156-162.

49. Dolatabadi MA, Motamedi MHK, Lassemi E, Talaeipour AR, Janbaz Y. Radiographs of dental patients with diabetes. *CDA J.* 2010;38:187-191.

50. Borgnakke WS, Ylostalo PV, Taylor GW, Genco RJ. Effect of periodontal disease on diabetes: systematic review of epidemiologic observational evidence. *J Periodontol.* 2013;84(4 suppl):S135-S152.

51. Scannapieco FA. Role of oral bacteria in respiratory infection. *J Periodontol.* 1999;70:793-802.

52. Scannapieco FA, Wang B, Shiau HJ. Oral bacteria and respiratory infection: effects on respiratory pathogen adhesion and epithelial cell proinflammatory cytokine production. *Ann Periodontol.* 2001;6:78-86.

53. Munro CL, Grap MJ, Elswick RK Jr, et al. Oral health status and development of ventilator-associated pneumonia: a descriptive study. *Am J Crit Care.* 2006;15:453-460.

54. Paju S, Scannapieco FA. Oral biofilms, periodontitis, and pulmonary infections. *Oral Dis.* 2007;13(6):508-512.

55. Koeman M, van der Ven AJ, Hak E, et al. Oral decontamination with chlorhexidine reduces the incidence of ventilator-associated pneumonia. *Am J Respir Crit Care Med.* 2006;173:1348-1355.

56. Mori H, Hirasawa H, Oda S, et al. Oral care reduces incidence of ventilator-associated pneumonia in ICU populations. *Intensive Care Med.* 2006;32:230-236.

57. Adachi M, Ishihara K, Abe S, Okuda K, Ishikawa T. Effect of professional oral health care on the elderly living in nursing homes. *Oral Surg Oral Med Oral Pathol Oral Radiol Endod.* 2002;94:191-195.

58. Abe S, Ishihara K, Adachi M, et al. Professional oral care reduces influenza infection in elderly. *Arch Gerontol Geriatr.* 2006;43:157-164.

59. Sanz M, Kornman K, on behalf of Working Group 3 of the Joint EFP/AAP Workshop. Periodontitis and adverse pregnancy outcomes: consensus report of the Joint EFP/AAP Workshop on Periodontitis and Systemic Diseases. *J Periodontol.* 2013;84(4 suppl):S164-S169.

60. Offenbacher S, Katz V, Fertik G, et al. Periodontal infection as a possible risk factor for preterm low birth weight. *J Periodontol.* 1996;67(10 suppl):1103-1113.

61. Vettore MV, Lamarca GA, Leão AT, Thomaz FB, Sheiham A, Leal MC. Periodontal infection and adverse pregnancy outcomes: a systematic review of epidemiological studies. *Cad Saude Publica.* 2006;22: 2041-2053.

62. Offenbacher S, Lieff S, Boggess KA, et al. Maternal periodontitis and prematurity. Part I: obstetric outcome of prematurity and growth restriction. *Ann Periodontol.* 2001;6:164-174.

63. López NJ, Smith PC, Gutierrez J. Higher risk of preterm birth and low birth weight in women with periodontal disease. *J Dent Res.* 2002;81:58-63.

64. Radnai M, Gorzó I, Nagy E, Urbán E, Novák T, Pál A. A possible association between preterm birth and early periodontitis. A pilot study. *J Clin Periodontol.* 2004; 31:736-741.

65. Dörtbudak O, Eberhardt R, Ulm M, Persson GR. Periodontitis, a marker of risk in pregnancy for preterm birth. *J Clin Periodontol.* 2005;32:45-52.

66. Jarjoura K, Devine PC, Perez-Delboy A, Herrera-Abreu M, D'Alton M, Papapanou PN. Markers of periodontal infection and preterm birth. *Am J Obstet Gynecol.* 2005 Feb;192(2):513-519

67. Marin C, Segura-Egea JJ, Martinez-Sahuquillo A, Bullon P. Correlation between infant birth weight and mother's periodontal status. *J Clin Periodontol.* 2005;32:299-304.

68. Moliterno LF, Monteiro B, Figueredo CM, Fischer RG. Association between periodontitis and low birth weight: a case-control study. *J Clin Periodontol.* 2005;32:886-890.

69. Vettore MV, Leal M, Leão AT, Monteiro da Silva AM, Lamarca GA, Sheiham A. The relationship between periodontitis and preterm low birthweight. *J Dent Res.* 2008;87:73-80.

70. Davenport ES, Williams CE, Sterne JA, Murad S, Sivapathasundram V, Curtis MA. Maternal periodontal disease and preterm low birthweight: case-control study. *J Dent Res.* 2002;81:313-318.

71. Lunardelli AN, Peres MA. Is there an association between periodontal disease, prematurity and low birth weight? A population-based study. *J Clin Periodontol.* 2005;32:938-946.

72. Rajapakse PS, Nagarathne M, Chandrasekra KB, Dasanayake AP. Periodontal disease and prematurity among non-smoking Sri Lankan women. *J Dent Res.* 2005;84:274-277.

73. Michalowicz BS, Hodges JS, DiAngelis AJ, et al. Treatment of periodontal disease and the risk of preterm birth. *N Engl J Med.* 2006;355:1885-1894.

74. Ide M, Papapanou PN. Epidemiology of association between maternal periodontal disease and adverse pregnancy outcomes—systematic review. *J Periodontol.* 2013;84(4 suppl):S181-S194.

75. Giannobile WV, Braun TM, Caplis AK, Doucette-Stamm L, Duff GW, Kornman KS. Patient stratification for preventive care in dentistry. *J Dent Res.* 2013;92(8):694-701.

76. Interprofessional Education Collaborative Expert Panel. *Core Competencies for Interprofessional Collaborative Practice: Report of an Expert Panel.* Washington, DC: Interprofessional Education Collaborative; 2011.

Chapter 6 | Evidence-Based Care

Susan Badanjak, RDH, ADH • Deborah Finnegan, RDH

KEY TERMS

best practice

bias

biomedical database

blinding

case–control study

case report

case series

empirical evidence

evidence-based care (EBC)

evidence-based decision-making (EBDM)

evidence-based dental hygiene practice

intervention

in vitro

levels of evidence

literature review

primary research

randomization

randomized controlled trial

reference citation

reliability

secondary research

statistical significance

systematic search

validity

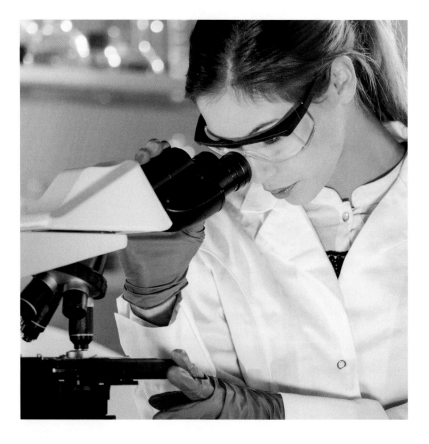

LEARNING OBJECTIVES

After reading this chapter, the student should be able to:

6.1 Define *evidence-based care.*

6.2 Discuss the principles of evidence-based care.

6.3 Describe the methods of the evidence-based process.

6.4 Explain the importance and hierarchy of the evidence-based process.

6.5 Apply evidence-based decision-making to patient care.

6.6 Perform a basic search for and evaluation of scientific literature.

6.7 Write a basic scientific paper.

KEY CONCEPTS

- Evidence-based care (EBC) is based on three tenets and is considered to be actively in use only when *all* three tenets have been incorporated into the process of care.
- The three tenets are: (a) the best available scientific evidence; (b) a clinician's skill, judgment, and experience; and (c) consideration for the patient's needs, preferences, values, and beliefs. Evidence alone does not replace sound clinical judgment. However, the hierarchical levels of quality and valid evidence aid in the clinical decision-making process. The dental hygiene process of care is based on a critical thinking model, and the focus is on provision of patient-centered, comprehensive care.

- As dental hygienists perform the roles of clinician, educator, researcher, manager, and advocate to prevent oral disease and promote overall health, it is imperative that they remain scientifically up to date to answer the needs of their patients.

RELEVANCE TO CLINICAL PRACTICE

Dental hygienists are required to make informed decisions about patient care. Careful examination of scientific research allows clinicians, together with their patients, to make **best practice** decisions about that care. **Evidence-based care (EBC)** is a patient-centered approach to care, merging the best available research with clinical expertise and patient preferences.[1–6] It serves as a blueprint for health professionals as they make patient care decisions to ensure the best health outcomes. **Evidence-based decision-making** requires critical thinking and research skills.[1–7] Dental hygienists must be proficient at locating, interpreting, and appropriately applying scientific evidence to support their patient care decision-making.

Patients look to oral health professionals not only for clinical care but for answers to questions and to verify information obtained via the Internet or other sources. Due to the vast number of research articles published annually, it can be difficult for oral health professionals to keep abreast of current research findings.[8] The amount of new research may cause variations in dental hygiene practice. Variations can occur from the lack of integration of new knowledge into practice, reliance on traditional passive methods of continuing education and the absence of active searches for **empirical evidence,** incorrect interpretation or evaluation of new information, and poor or lack of scientific evidence required to answer specific clinical questions.[9–11] The same technological advancements have changed the way oral health-care professionals seek and gather information. Knowing how to efficiently and effectively conduct searches for scientific evidence and critically appraising it will yield valid information for answering clinical and patient questions, and providing the best care to patients.

Evidence-based dental hygiene care requires the skills of efficient, systematic literature searches and application of the rules of evidence to critically evaluate the clinical literature. A **systematic search** is a strategized tactic for locating answers to clinical and other questions by mining scientific and biomedical databases.[7,9,12] A good clinical question starts the process.[3,12–16] It formally introduces the patient, who presents with a problem. Second, it promotes more questioning, which helps to formulate the principal question and pinpoints the issue. Finally, a good clinical question defines and refines the evidence search strategy. The purpose of a systematic literature search is to identify potentially relevant articles. Evaluating the evidence critically reveals the validity and pertinence of a study.[7,16,17] Clinically relevant research that has been conducted using reliable methodology provides the best evidence.[7,16,17]

WHAT IS EVIDENCE-BASED CARE IN DENTAL HYGIENE PRACTICE?

Evidence-based dental hygiene practice is the combined use of current, relevant, scientifically sound evidence and professional clinical judgment to evaluate information to determine and provide optimal patient-centric comprehensive oral care, with consideration for the patient's point of view (Fig. 6-1).[1–7]

THE EVIDENCE-BASED PROCESS

There are six steps in the evidence-based process[3,18] (Fig. 6-2):

1. Assess.
2. Ask.
3. Acquire.
4. Appraise.
5. Apply.
6. Auto-evaluate.

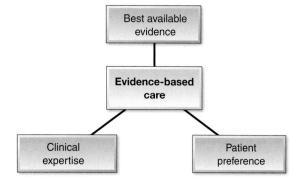

Figure 6-1. Three tenets of the evidence-based process.

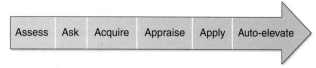

Figure 6-2. Evidence-based process.

Remember that the evidence-based process of care always begins and ends with the patient (Table 6-1).

GOOD CLINICAL QUESTION FRAMEWORK

A good clinical question provides the structure for the research strategy. The PICO mnemonic is used to formulate a question pertaining to the problem (Fig. 6-3).[9,13,15] The *P* stands for patient or problem. This may include a patient with a certain condition or a specific presentation of disease. The *I* stands for intervention. The intervention is what treatment or diagnostic testing the provider will offer. The *C* stands for comparison. The comparison is an alternative treatment or choice. The *O* stands for outcome. The outcome is how you will measure how the result or effect of the treatment. The following scenario describes how the PICO question is derived.

Scenario A

Mrs. Takahashi, a 50-year-old woman, presents for her re-care appointment. She is on 3-month re-care because of generalized, moderate-to-severe, chronic periodontal disease induced by hepatitis C virus (HCV) infection. She states that she keeps getting sores on the inside of her cheek. The dental hygienist performs an intraoral examination and discovers a lesion that resembles Wickham's striae of oral lichen planus (OLP). It may be helpful to work through the PICO question when deciding on further diagnosis and treatment for this patient. Figure 6-4 illustrates how the PICO question is formulated.

PICO Question

In a patient with recurrent sores on the buccal mucosa that resemble OLP lesions and who is HCV positive, is there any evidence-based association between HCV and OLP that would explain the recurrent OLP? Figure 6-5 illustrates this question.

Scenario B

Mr. Edwards, a 59-year-old man who is new to the dental office, presents for his dental hygiene appointment.

Table 6-1. *Six Steps of the Evidence-Based Process*	
ASSESS the patient.	A clinical problem or question arises from and/or during the process of patient care.
ASK the question(s).	Compose a pertinent, accurate, and specific question regarding the problem or question.
ACQUIRE the evidence.	Select the appropriate resource(s) and conduct a search for evidence-based literature.
APPRAISE the evidence.	Evaluate the validity and applicability of the evidence.
APPLY the evidence.	Discuss the findings with the patient; integrate and apply the evidence through clinical expertise and conscious awareness of patient considerations.
AUTO-EVALUATE.	Self-evaluate the evidence-based process of care, the patient's outcomes, and the clinical execution.

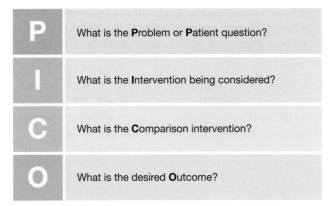

Figure 6-3. Formulating the PICO question.

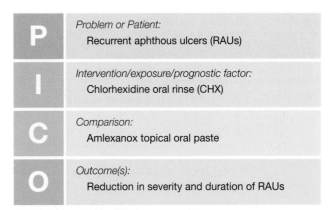

Figure 6-6. Formulating the PICO question: scenario B.

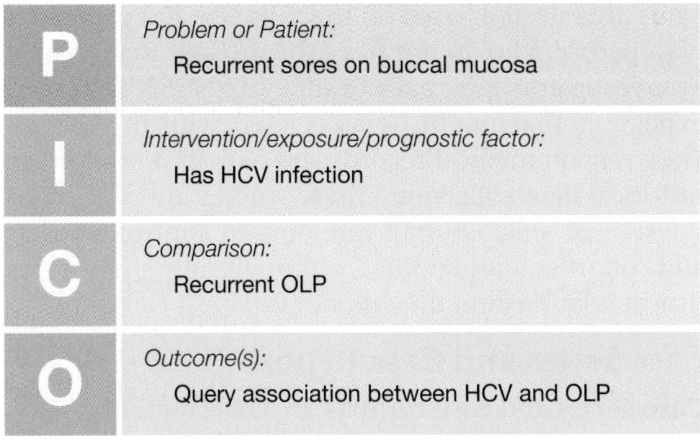

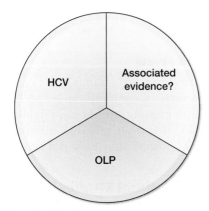

Figure 6-4. Formulating the PICO question: scenario A.

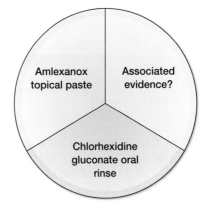

Figure 6-7. Scenario B pie chart.

LEVELS OF EVIDENCE

Information gathered to answer the clinical question should be valid and scientifically supported. Search results can be evaluated for quality by determining where the research study design is located in the design hierarchy.[16,19] Thinking of a pyramid shape, as shown in Figure 6-8, can be helpful when considering the hierarchy of **levels of evidence** and research study design. Understanding the differences between research study designs will bolster critical appraisal skills. The closer the study design is to the top of the pyramidal hierarchy, the stronger the level of evidence.[16,19]

Meta-analysis

A meta-analysis thoroughly examines a number of valid studies on a topic and combines the results using accepted statistical methodology to report the results as if they were one large study.[16] The Cochrane Collaboration is an excellent source for meta-analyses and systematic reviews.[20]

Systematic Review

Systematic reviews focus on a clinical topic to answer a specific question. An extensive literature search on the topic is conducted to identify studies with sound methodology. Studies without sound methodologies are rejected. The remaining studies are reviewed,

Figure 6-5. Scenario A pie chart.

His chief concern is the pain and discomfort associated with recurrent aphthous ulcers (RAU). He has been using chlorhexidine gluconate (CHX) oral rinse as recommended by his previous dentist, which provides slight relief. Mr. Edwards states his friend uses amlexanox topical paste for RAU. Mr. Edwards wonders if amlexanox would be a better choice for treating his RAU than rinsing orally with CHX. Figure 6-6 illustrates how the PICO question is formulated. *PICO Question:* Will the recurring RAU occur less frequently and lessen in severity if treated with amlexanox topical oral paste than with CHX? Figure 6-7 illustrates the question.

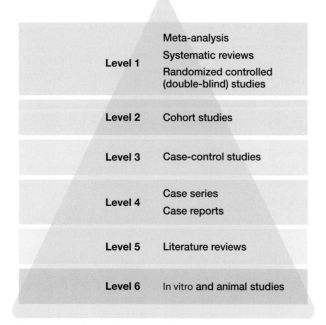

Level 1	Meta-analysis Systematic reviews Randomized controlled (double-blind) studies
Level 2	Cohort studies
Level 3	Case-control studies
Level 4	Case series Case reports
Level 5	Literature reviews
Level 6	In vitro and animal studies

Figure 6-8. Levels of evidence pyramid.

assessed, and the results summarized according to the predetermined criteria of the review question.[16] A concise and exhaustive summary of the literature, systematic reviews are usually performed by authors with highly developed database searching, critical assessment, and statistical interpretation skills.

Randomized Controlled Trial

A **randomized controlled trial** is a carefully planned study in which at least one group of participants receives some sort of **intervention,** or treatment, whereas the other group receives a placebo, or standard of care.[16] Researchers use randomization and blinding to reduce the potential for **bias** (error introduced by favoring one answer, outcome, or value over another) and to allow for comparison between the groups.[16,21] **Randomization** is a study control method by which researchers assign trial participants to an experimental or control group by chance.[16,21] Randomization is not a haphazard assignment; it is performed using a carefully planned strategy.[16,21] **Blinding** is another type of control method. In a single-blind study, the participant is unaware of what the intervention will be.[21] A double-blinded study signifies that neither participant nor researcher is informed about the intervention.[21] A nonblinded study, commonly known as open-label, means both the participant and the researcher are cognizant of the intervention.[21] A randomized controlled trial can provide sound evidence of cause and effect, because participants are assigned exposures and are then followed to an outcome (end result of the trial).

Cohort Study

A cohort study examines a large population of participants based on common factors such as exposure status or treatment and follows them through time.[16] The

outcomes are then compared with a similar population that has not been exposed to or affected by the treatment being studied.[16] There are two types of cohorts for observational studies:

1. A prospective cohort study starts with the exposure and follows patients forward to an outcome.[16]
2. A retrospective cohort study starts with the outcome and goes back in time to the moment of exposure.[16]

Because cohort studies observe two populations that may differ in ways other than the variable being studied, they are not as reliable as randomized controlled trials.[16]

Case–Control Study

Case–control studies are studies in which participants are selected based on their disease and compared with people who do not have the disease. Researchers or investigators look back in time to identify factors or exposures that might be associated with the illness. They rely on medical records and patient recall for the historical data collection. These studies are often considered less reliable than randomized controlled trials and cohort studies because, although they show a statistical relationship, they do not establish causality.[16]

Case Series and Case Report

Case series and **case reports** are collections of reports on the treatment of individual patients, or on one single patient. This information is generally considered anecdotal because they are reports of cases and do not use control groups with which to compare outcomes. Case series and case reports are said to have no statistical validity.[16]

Literature Review

Literature reviews are an important component in scientific research. A comprehensive, preliminary investigation into existing studies can establish what direction to take, if further research is required. It can also answer questions that may not require further research.[22]

In Vitro and Animal Studies

In vitro and animal studies are experimental studies without human participants. They are used primarily to evaluate safety, toxicity, and potential therapeutic effects.[23]

Two additional components should be considered to further refine the search for evidence: the type of question and the best type of study to answer the question[14] (Table 6-2).

LITERATURE SEARCH

Primary research is often referred to as clinical or basic research. The information arising from primary research may yield new information or it may validate results from prior studies. Basic research is

Table 6-2. Choosing the Study to Fit the Question

Type of Question	Best Type of Study
Dental hygiene diagnosis	Prospective, blind comparison with a gold standard
Dental hygiene therapy	RCT, cohort, case–control, case series
Dental hygiene prognosis	Cohort study, case–control, case series
Harm/etiology	RCT, cohort, case–control, case series
Dental hygiene prevention	RCT, cohort study, case–control, case series
Dental hygiene clinical examination	Prospective, blind comparison with a gold standard

RCT, randomized controlled trial.

conducted to gain knowledge and understanding of a subject. It involves information-gathering and the analysis of that information. Clinical research refers to studies related to human beings; it may be observational or involve trials to evaluate the efficacy of a particular intervention.[23,24] **Secondary research** includes literature reviews and meta-analyses.[24]

Peer-Reviewed Articles

Peer-reviewed articles have been thoroughly evaluated for quality of content. If an article has not been peer-reviewed, be wary and reconsider the source.[7,25]

RESOURCES

Dental hygienists must be able to determine the relevance and validity of Internet search results when conducting research. Becoming familiar with research databases and different types of literature will aid in distinguishing between strong and weak sources of materials. Many Internet search results are considered to be weak because they contain erroneous or unsupported information. Searching specific literature databases, such as a **biomedical database,** listed in Table 6-3, will yield valid results.[5,7,19,21,24]

EVIDENCE EVALUATION

Having gathered relevant and scientifically supported information, the next step is to read and evaluate the studies. When evaluating the evidence, four questions need to be answered for every type of study, including randomized controlled studies:

1. Are the results of the study valid and reliable?
2. What are the results, and are they statistically and clinically significant?
3. Will the results help in caring for my patient?
4. Does my patient meet the inclusion criteria of the study?

The first query prompts questioning and critical review of the important elements that help in judging the validity and reliability of the findings.[21] These elements are found in the methodology and results of the study. The second question addresses the clinical and statistical significance of the results by evaluating the size and the precision of the effect.[21] **Statistical significance,** expressed as p value, refers to the level of significance; it is the level of probability that an association between two or more variables occurred by chance alone.[21,26] Arbitrarily chosen, the commonly accepted p value is (0.05.[21,26] If $p \leq 0.05$, the probability that the observed results occurred entirely by chance is less than 0.05, or less than 5 in 100 or 1 in 20.[21,26] Question 3 raises the issue of outcomes and of reporting adverse effects to determine which patients may best benefit from the new intervention.[21] The final question evaluates the relevance and pertinence of the study in relation to the patient. The following hypothetical example clarifies the evaluation process.[21]

Table 6-3. Electronic Biomedical Database

American Dental Association (ADA)	ADA Center for Evidence-Based Dentistry	http://ebd.ada.org
PubMed	National Center for Biotechnology Information	https://pubmed.gov
MedlinePlus	U.S. National Library of Medicine	https://www.nlm.nih.gov/medlineplus
Scopus*	Peer-reviewed literature	http://www.info.sciverse.com/scopus
CINAHL*	Health-care literature	http://www.cinahl.com
Cochrane Library	Health-care literature	http://www.thecochranelibrary.com
ERIC	Educational Resources Information Center	http://eric.ed.gov
Google Scholar	Scholarly literature	http://scholar.google.com

* Require subscription.

Evidence Evaluation Example

A new product, an adjunct to nonsurgical periodontal therapy (NSPT) for adult patients with chronic periodontitis and with pocket depths ≥5 mm, becomes available. The results of the randomized, placebo-controlled, double-blinded study showed that the product, in combination with NSPT, statistically reduces pocket depth compared with NSPT alone. The average pocket depth reductions from baseline probing depths were 1.2 and 1.3 mm, respectively. That is, use of the product with NSPT reduced the pocket by 0.1 mm more than scaling alone. Statistical analysis showed that this reduction was significant, with $p = 0.04$.

Are the results of the study valid? **Validity** in a study refers to the extent to which a study measures what it actually intended to measure.[14,17,27] In this example, it is pocket reduction when the product is used adjunctively with NSPT, in adults with chronic periodontitis and pocket depths ≥5 mm. The results may be valid; however, to obtain such small probing measurements would require highly sophisticated measuring equipment. **Reliability,** in a study or clinical context, means the extent to which a method or a measurement repeatedly and consistently produces the same outcome or results performed under identical conditions.[14,17,27] How does one repeatedly and consistently measure a 0.1-mm pocket reduction in a clinical setting, using a standard probe? Although a 0.1-mm reduction in pocket depth was deemed to be statistically significant ($p = 0.04$), is the result clinically significant?[21,26,28] The answer is no. Will the results have an impact on the periodontal health of patients?[21,26,28] In all likelihood, no; had the reduction been 1.0 mm, that would probably have made a difference in periodontal treatment planning in a patient with baseline pockets of 5 mm that measured 4 mm after combination therapy.

EVIDENCE APPLICATION

Using evidence-based clinical recommendations or best practice guidelines is essential when considering treatment options and providing advice to patients on making good oral health choices. Because they are based on reviewed, published, and current scientific knowledge, the presence of recommendations may improve patient confidence in making informed treatment decisions. Recommendations do not constitute standard of care; they must be considered along with oral health-care expertise and the needs and preferences of the patient in EBC decision-making.

OUTCOME EVALUATION

The evidence-based process is recursive; as previously stated, it begins and ends with the patient. The final step in the evidence-based process is to evaluate the applied care, patient's outcome, and clinical performance. If the outcomes are not satisfactory, the six steps of the evidence-based process and the PICO process are repeated.

PARTS OF A SCIENTIFIC PAPER

Scientific papers are arranged in a particular format. Although there may be slight differences in the format, each paper typically contains a title, abstract, introduction, materials/methods, results, discussion/conclusion, conflicts of interest, acknowledgments, and references.[29,30]

Title

The title is usually the first part of a paper that readers see, whether searching a database or looking at the first page of a scientific paper. It should contain information pertinent to the topic. A good title is informative and succinct, and catches the reader's eye, enticing the reader into learning more about the topic.[29,30]

Abstract

The abstract portion of a scientific paper is a short summary of the paper. It includes the study purpose, hypothesis, procedure, population, results, and conclusions. An abstract can help readers determine whether they wish to delve further into the full article.[29,30]

Introduction

The introduction section contains the study background. It states the study's purpose, objectives, hypothesis, and relevance. The introduction section may also include references to previous studies on the same subject.[29,30]

Materials/Methods

The materials and methods section includes information on the study design and how researchers conducted the study. The authors should include enough methodology to enable others to replicate the study. Identifying the type of study design and locating it in the hierarchy of the levels of evidence pyramid provided in Figure 6-8 will help determine the strength of the study design.[29,30]

Results

The results section contains a summary of the research results or findings. It may also include tables or graphics, which provide a visual description of the research data.[29,30]

Discussion/Conclusion

The discussion/conclusion section provides an interpretation of the study results and any potential implications or applications. Results may be conclusive or inconclusive.[29,30]

Conflicts of Interest

Authors should disclose any conflicts of interest. Readers should be aware of the potential for bias in a study funded by organizations or companies that may have financial or other interests in the outcome. Be wary of conflicts of interest, and reconsider the source.

Acknowledgments

Authors who wish to thank those who may have provided expertise or guidance may do so in the acknowledgments section.

References

The reference section contains the list of references cited by the authors throughout the paper. A **reference citation** is a numbered or annotated section of text within a manuscript that refers to or cites the source of information and corresponds to the author's (or authors') published or unpublished work listed in the references.[25,29,30] The references are formatted according to the citation style preferred by the editors of the publication or by professors of an academic institution. The reference list allows readers to locate the sources cited by the authors for further information on the topic.[29,30]

INTRODUCTION TO WRITING A SCIENTIFIC PAPER

Writing well is an acquired skill. It is important to understand that it is a multistep process. Much of the process involves editing, rewriting, and revision of various drafts (Box 6-1). Writing a scientific paper differs from other forms of writing in that authors must follow specific guidelines and adhere to certain writing and citation styles. Scientific papers should be written in a clear, concise style using the active voice and organized into formats, as previously discussed. When writing for a publication, determine which format and citation style is preferred. Each journal or publication will have its own specific rules for article length, layout, and citation style. Authors may refer to guidelines available on the journal's website or by contacting the publishers. Three citation styles common to scientific papers are identified in Table 6-4.[30]

Formulate the Idea and Conduct Research

The writer may generate an idea for the paper or it may be an assigned topic. Once the subject matter has been decided on, the writer researches the topic. The research process is described earlier in this chapter.

Box 6-1. *Phases of the Writing Process*[30]

1. Formulate the idea and conduct research.
2. Write the first draft.
3. Edit: Choose precise words and use proper grammar.
4. Edit: Ensure continuity and flow; vary sentence length.
5. Revise and proofread. ■

Table 6-4. *Citation Styles Often Used in Scientific Literature*

Type	Published by	Webpage
Vancouver	International Committee of Medical Journal Editors (ICMJE)	www.icmje.org
AMA	American Medical Association	www.amamanualofstyle.com
APA	American Psychological Association	http://apastyle.org

Write the First Draft

After evaluating literature on the topic, determine the main point or objective of the scientific paper. Construction of a thesis statement is essential to convey the objective of the paper to the reader. The paper will be developed around the thesis, using the evidence-based literature collected to support the statement. Formulating a thesis statement starts with a proposal question.[30] For example, "Is halitosis strictly a cosmetic problem?" The question is then converted into a thesis statement such as, "Halitosis is/is not strictly a cosmetic problem." A thesis statement can and should be revised after investigation and review of the literature, and based on research findings, may read as follows: "Halitosis: An important cosmetic, dental, and medical problem."

Creating an outline helps to organize thoughts and ideas—a roadmap of sorts. Writing the first draft is an opportunity to organize the layout of the paper and your thoughts on your topic. The first draft is a starting point to work with and expand on. Slight editing may be done while writing the first draft; however, the majority of rewriting and revision is conducted in the next phase.

Editing: Choosing Precise Words and Using Proper Grammar

The editing phase of revision and rewriting takes place once the first draft has been completed. Review the draft and examine word choice and grammar. Scientific writing must clearly convey the intended message, using precise scientific terms, rather than colloquial terms, to ensure there is no chance for reader misunderstanding. Proper grammar is essential to a professional writing style. Complete sentence fragments, revise run-on sentences, and correct punctuation. Although word-processing programs are helpful in locating some editing errors, do not rely on spell-check and grammar-check tools exclusively.[30]

Continuity, Sentence Length, and Flow

The draft must be evaluated for message continuity and sentence flow. To avoid monotony, consider sentences of varying lengths. Similarly constructed sentences have the same cadence. Well-written paragraphs include sentences that create ebb and flow patterns, which are more pleasing to the reader than repetitive sounding sentences of similar lengths and styles.[30]

Plagiarism

Plagiarism is a very serious breach of academic and personal ethics. Plagiarism is defined as the use of another's work or ideas without giving credit to that person. Credit must be given by citing the source, to allow readers and researchers to locate and retrieve the information. Paraphrasing by substituting words and/or word order is unacceptable, even if cited, and is simply another form of plagiarism. Plagiarism is dishonest and fraudulent behavior; it may result in severe punishment. Disciplinary actions may include academic expulsion, and loss of personal and professional reputation.[30] Table 6-5 provides online resources for more information on plagiarism.

Table 6-5. *Online Resources for Avoiding Plagiarism*

Author	Topic	Website
OWL (Purdue University Online Writing Lab)	Avoiding plagiarism	http://owl.english.purdue.edu/owl/resource/589/1
OWL (Purdue University Online Writing Lab)	Quoting, paraphrasing, and summarizing	http://owl.english.purdue.edu/owl/resource/563/1
The Writing Center at the University of North Carolina	Plagiarism pdf is available for download	http://writingcenter.unc.edu/handouts/plagiarism
Plagiarism.org	Learning About and Checking for Plagiarism	http://plagiarism.org

Case Study

A patient brings in an article she found on the Internet about how rinsing the mouth with a new product can help reduce the recurrence of apthous ulcers. The dental hygienist reads the article with the patient. The patient seems very excited that there is a rinse that might help with the problem she has had for so many years. The patient asks the hygienist if he thinks it will help her recurrence of aphthous ulcers.

Case Study Exercises

1. To provide the patient with an evidence-based recommendation, the dental hygienist needs to:
   A. Read the full article that the patient brought and decide if he thinks it might help alleviate the recurrence of aphthous ulcers.
   B. Complete a systematic search in a biomedical database and determine whether the product has been shown to be effective.
   C. Rely on anecdotal evidence from friends and colleagues.
   D. Conduct his own scientific experiment to determine whether the rinse will reduce recurrence.
2. As the dental hygienist searches for information about the rinse, which type of study would be considered the highest level of evidence?
   A. Case–control study
   B. Literature review

C. Case report
D. Systematic review
3. Statistical significance of the results of a study is often expressed as a _____ value.
   A. *v*
   B. *s*
   C. *p*
   D. *t*
4. The hygienist finds a study that compared the rinse with a placebo and found a statistical significance of $p = 0.04$. This means that:
   A. The probability that the observed results occurred entirely by chance is less than 0.05 or less than 1 in 20.
   B. The measurement can be repeated correctly 40% of the time.
   C. The probability that the observed results occurred entirely by chance is less than 0.04 or 1 in 25.
   D. The results were not statistically significant.
5. The dental hygienist finds several short summaries of articles that include the study purpose, hypothesis, procedure, population, results, and conclusions. This summary is called the
   A. Abstract
   B. Introduction
   C. Methods
   D. Results

Review Questions

1. A patient wants a professional opinion on which power toothbrush to buy. Evidence is gathered to answer the patient's question regarding power toothbrushes. Using the levels of the evidence pyramid, where would the most robust evidence be found?
   A. Meta-analyses
   B. Literature reviews
   C. Systematic reviews
   D. Randomized controlled trials

2. What is the correct order of the six steps in the evidence-based process?
   A. Auto-evaluate, acquire, assess, ask, appraise, apply
   B. Apply, acquire, assess, appraise, ask, auto-evaluate
   C. Assess, ask, acquire, appraise, apply, auto-evaluate
   D. Ask, apply, assess, acquire, auto-evaluate, appraise

3. What does the mnemonic PICO stand for?
   A. Prevention, intervention, comparison, outcome
   B. Patient/problem, intervention, comparison, outcome
   C. Patient/problem, intervention, comparison, oral hygiene instruction
   D. Prevention, instruction, clinical intervention, outcome

4. The evidence-based process involves the following:
   A. Best research evidence and clinical judgment
   B. Clinical expertise, best research evidence, and patient values and preferences
   C. None of the above
   D. All of the above

5. A literature search for information on prevention of root caries and root sensitivity is conducted. The results are listed. Considering the hierarchy of levels of evidence, which study is likely to be lowest on the hierarchal pyramid?
   A. Drebenstedt S, Zapf A, Rödig T, Mausberg RF, Ziebolz D. Efficacy of two different CHX-containing desensitizers: a controlled double-blind study. *Oper Dent.* 2012;37(2):161-171.
   B. Tan HP, Lo ECM, Dyson JE, Luo Y, Corbet EF. A randomized trial on root caries prevention in elders. *J Dent Res.* 2010;89(10):1086-1090.
   C. Baca P, Clavero J, Baca AP, Gonzalez-Rodriguez MP, Bravo M, Valderrama MJ. Effect of chlorhexidine-thymol varnish on root caries in a geriatric population: a randomized double-blind clinical trial. *J Dent.* 2009;37(9):679-685. doi: 10.1016/j.jdent.2009.05.001
   D. Anand V, Govila V, Gulati Minkle, Anand B, Jhingaran R, Rastogi P. Chlorhexidine-thymol varnish as an adjunct to scaling and root planing: a clinical observation. *J Oral Biol Craniofac Res.* 2012;2(2):83-89.

Active Learning

HINT: Librarians are a valuable resource when researching; ask questions to optimize search strategies.

1. Reread scenario A in this chapter. Using a database from Table 6-3, locate and retrieve the following scientific articles. Considering the hierarchy of levels of evidence, which study or studies are likely to be highest on the hierarchal pyramid?
   A. Cruz-Pamplona M, Margaix-Munoz M, Sarrion-Perez MG. Dental considerations in patients with liver disease. *J Clin Exp Dent.* 2011;3(2):e127-e134. doi:10.4317/jced.3.e127
   B. Nagao Y, Sata M. A retrospective case-control study of hepatitis C virus infection and oral lichen planus in Japan: association study with mutations in the core and NS5A region of hepatitis C virus. *BMC Gastroenterol.* 2012;12:31-230X-12-31. doi: 10.1186/1471-230X-12-31

   C. Jayavelu P, Sambandan T. Prevalence of hepatitis C and hepatitis B virus infection(s) in patients with oral lichen planus. *J Pharm Bioallied Sci.* 2012;4 (Suppl 2):S397-S405. doi: 10.4103/0975-7406.100302
   D. Lodi G, Pellicano R, Carrozzo M. Hepatitis C virus infection and lichen planus: a systematic review with meta-analysis. *Oral Dis.* 2010;16(7):601-612. doi: 10.1111/j.1601-0825.2010.01670x

2. Reread scenario B in this chapter. Using a database from Table 6-3, locate and retrieve the following scientific articles. Considering the hierarchy of levels of evidence, which study or studies are likely to be highest on the hierarchal pyramid?
   A. Messadi DV, Younai F. Aphthous ulcers. *Dermatol Ther.* 2010;23(3):281-290.
   B. Meng W, Dong Y, Liu J, et al. A clinical evaluation of amlexanox oral adhesive pellicles in the treatment

Continued

Active Learning—cont'd

of recurrent aphthous stomatitis and comparison with amlexanox oral tablets: a randomized, placebo controlled, blinded, multicenter clinical trial. *Trials.* 2009;10(1):30.

C. Bailey J, McCarthy C, Smith RF. Clinical inquiry. What is the most effective way to treat recurrent canker sores? *J Fam Pract.* 2011;60(10):621-623.

D. Elad S, Epstein JB, von Bültzingslöwen I, Drucker S, Tzach R, Yarom N. Topical immunomodulators for management of oral mucosal conditions, a systematic review; Part II: miscellaneous agents. *Expert Opin Emerg Drugs.* 2011;16(1):183-202. ■

REFERENCES

1. About EBD. Chicago: ADA Center for Evidence-Based Dentistry; 2013. Available from: http://ebd.ada.org/about.aspx. Accessed May 6, 2013.
2. EBD Educational Tutorials. Series on evidence-based dentistry. Chicago: ADA Center for Evidence-Based Dentistry; 2013. Available from: http://ebd.ada.org/VideoTutorials.aspx. Accessed May 6, 2013.
3. Guyatt G, Meade MO. How to use the medical literature—and this book—to improve your patient care. In: Guyatt G, Rennie D, Meade MO, Cook DJ, eds. *User's Guide to Medical Literature: A Manual for Evidence-Based Clinical Practice.* 2nd ed. Toronto, ON: McGraw-Hill; 2008:1-4.
4. Centre for Evidence-Based Medicine. Oxford, U.K.: University of Oxford; 2011. Available from: http://www.cebm.net/index.aspx?o=1914. Accessed September 30, 2013.
5. Ross T. Evidence-based practice. In: *A Survival Guide for Health Research Methods.* New York: McGraw-Hill; 2012:5-19.
6. What is evidence-based practice (EBP)? Durham, NC: Introduction to Evidence-Based Practice; 2013. Available from: http://guides.mclibrary.duke.edu/content.php?pid=431451&sid=3529499. Accessed September 30, 2013.
7. Selecting the resources. Durham, NC: Introduction to Evidence-Based Practice; 2013. Available from: http://guides.mclibrary.duke.edu/content.php?pid=431451&sid=3530457. Accessed September 30, 2013.
8. Bastian H, Glasziou P, Chlamers I. Seventy-five trials and eleven systematic reviews a day: how will we ever keep up? *PLoS Med.* 2010;7(9):1-6.
9. Faggion CM Jr. The development of evidence-based guidelines in dentistry. *J Dent Educ.* 2013;77(2):124-136.
10. Marshal TA, Straub-Morarend CL, Qian F, Finkelstein MW. Perceptions and practices of dental school faculty regarding evidence-based dentistry. *J Dent Educ.* 2013;77(2):146-151.
11. Palcanis KG, Geiger BF, O'Neal MR, Ivankova N, Retta RE, Kennedy LB, Carera KW. Preparing students to practice evidence-based dentistry: a mixed methods conceptual framework for curriculum enhancement. *J Dent Educ.* 2012;76(12):1600-1614.
12. Acquiring the evidence. Durham, NC: Introduction to Evidence-Based Practice; 2013. Available from: http://guides.mclibrary.duke.edu/content.php?pid=431451&sid=3530449. Accessed September 30, 2013.
13. Asking the well built clinical question. Durham, NC: Introduction to Evidence-Based Practice; 2013.

Available from: http://guides.mclibrary.duke.edu/content.php?pid=431451&sid=3529524. Accessed September 30, 2013.
14. Type of question. Durham, NC: Introduction to Evidence-Based Practice; 2013. Available from: http://guides.mclibrary.duke.edu/content.php?pid=431451&sid=3530451. Accessed September 30, 2013.
15. Centre for Evidence-Based Medicine. Oxford, U.K.: University of Oxford; 2009. Available from: http://www.cebm.net/index.aspx?o=1036. Accessed September 30, 2013.
16. Type of study. Durham, NC: Introduction to Evidence-Based Practice; 2013. Available from: http://guides.mclibrary.duke.edu/content.php?pid=431451&sid=3530453. Accessed September 30, 2013.
17. Evaluating the validity of a therapy study. Durham, NC: Introduction to Evidence-Based Practice; 2013. Available from: http://guides.mclibrary.duke.edu/content.php?pid=431451&sid=3718368. Accessed September 30, 2013.
18. Welcome to the introduction to evidence-based practice tutorial. Durham, NC: Introduction to Evidence-Based Practice; 2013. Available from: http://guides.mclibrary.duke.edu/content.php?pid=431451&sid=3529491. Accessed September 30, 2013.
19. Guyatt G, Haynes B, Jaeschke R, Meade MO, Wilson M, Montori V, Richardson S. The philosophy of evidence-based medicine. In: Guyatt G, Rennie D, Meade MO, Cook D, eds. *User's Guide to Medical Literature: A Manual for Evidence-Based Clinical Practice.* 2nd ed. Toronto, ON: McGraw-Hill; 2008:5-16.
20. Langendam MW, Akl EA, Dahm P, Glasziou P, Guyatt G, Schünemann HJ. Assessing and presenting summaries of evidence in Cochrane reviews. *Syst Rev.* 2013;2(81).
21. Estellat C, Torgerson DJ, Ravaud P. How to perform a critical analysis of a randomised controlled trial. *Best Pract Res Clin Rheumatol.* 2009;23(2):291-303.
22. Levy L. Review of the literature. In: Blessing JD, Forister JG, eds. *Introduction to Research and Medical Literature for Health Professionals.* 3rd ed. Burlington, MA: Jones and Bartlett Learning; 2013:99-107.
23. Blessing JD, Forister JG. Introduction. In: Blessing JD, Forister JG, eds. *Introduction to Research and Medical Literature for Health Professionals.* 3rd ed. Burlington, MA: Jones and Bartlett Learning; 2013:3-9.
24. Neutens JJ. Critical review of the literature and information sources. In: Neutens JJ, Rubinson L, eds. *Research Techniques for the Health Sciences.* 5th ed. Montreal: Pearson; 2014:26-45.

25. Cawley JF. Writing and publishing in the health professions. In: Blessing JD, Forister JG, eds. *Introduction to Research and Medical Literature for Health Professionals.* 3rd ed. Burlington, MA: Jones and Bartlett Learning; 2013:231-251.

26. Brignardello-Peterson R, Carrasco-Labra A, Shah P, Azarpazhooh A. A practitioner's guide to developing critical appraisal skills: what is the difference between clinical and statistical significance? *J. Am. Dent. Assoc.* 2013;144(7):780-786.

27. Bork CE, Jarski RW, Forister JG. Methodology. In: Blessing JD, Forister JG, eds. *Introduction to Research and Medical Literature for Health Professionals.* 3rd ed. Burlington, MA: Jones and Bartlett Learning; 2013:111-127.

28. Matthews D. Local antimicrobials in addition to scaling and root planning provide statistically significant but not clinically important benefit. *Evid. Based Dent.* 2013;14(3):87-88.

29. Neutens JJ. Communicating your research. In: Neutens JJ, Rubinson L, eds. *Research Techniques for the Health Sciences.* 5th ed. Montreal: Pearson; 2014:286-306.

30. Terryberry K. *Writing for the Health Professions.* Clifton Park, NY: Delmar Cengage Learning; 2005.

Part III

Infection Control

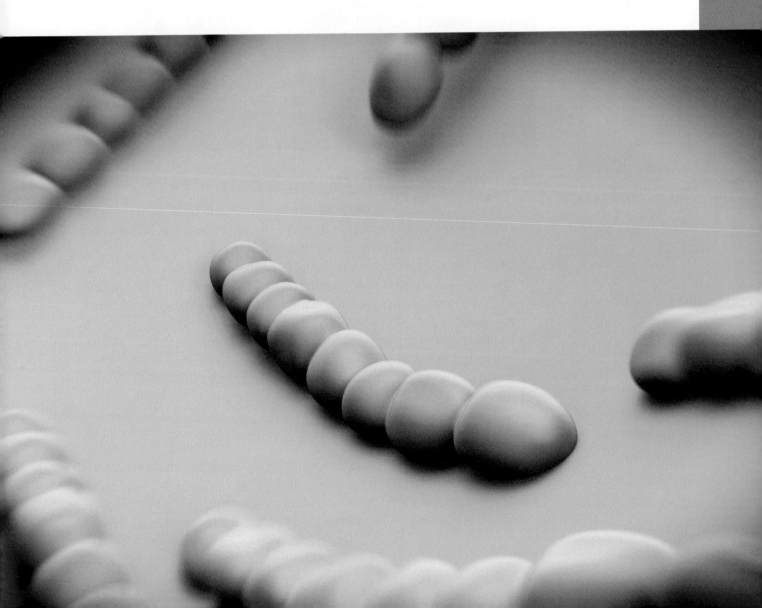

Chapter 7 | Exposure and Infection Control

Maureen Vendemia, RDH, MEd • Suzanne Smith, RDH, MEd

KEY TERMS

active immunization

aerosol

AIDS

autoinoculation

bioburden

biofilm

carrier

coinfection

convalescent stage

cross-contamination

disinfectant

engineering controls (EC)

germicide

hepatitis

human herpesvirus

latent period

opportunistic infection

passive immunization

pathogenic

personal protective equipment (PPE)

primary prevention

prodromal stage

recrudescence

residual

secondary prevention

seroconversion

spatter

standard precautions

sterilization

substantivity

superinfection

surfactants

tertiary prevention

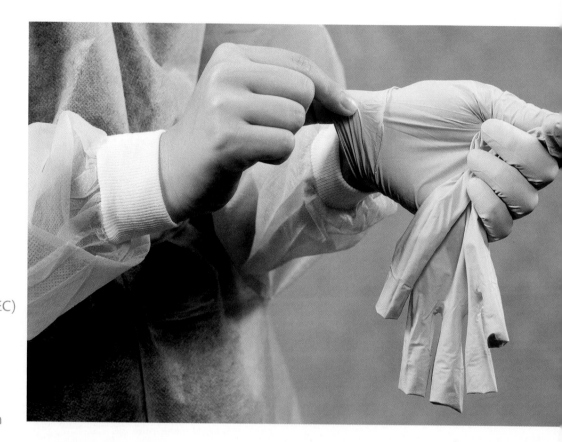

LEARNING OBJECTIVES

After reading this chapter, the student should be able to:

7.1 Discuss infectious diseases in terms of the infectious disease process and interventions to prevent disease transmission.

7.2 Outline initial intervention procedures of an occupational exposure, screening tests, and postexposure prophylaxis for HIV, hepatitis B, and hepatitis C.

7.3 Use critical thinking skills in the implementation of infection-control practices.

7.4 Explain the difference between nonregulated and regulated medical waste and infectious waste.

7.5 Integrate the environmentally responsible choices into infection-control practices.

KEY CONCEPTS

- Preventing disease transmission through the use of standard precautions is the responsibility of the dental hygienist.
- Work-related risk assessment, engineering controls, and work-practice controls are necessary in reducing occupational exposures.

titer

tuberculosis (TB)

universal precautions

work practice controls
(WPC)

- Ethics plays a role in infection-control practices when providing dental hygiene care.

RELEVANCE TO CLINICAL PRACTICE

Dental hygienists may come in contact with communicable diseases when providing dental hygiene care to their patients. It is important for hygienists to understand transmissible diseases and how to prevent their transmission in the dental environment. Previously, dental health-care personnel (DHCP) followed **universal precautions** that were based on the concept that all blood and body fluids were infectious. In 1996, **standard precautions** were introduced by the Centers for Disease Control and Prevention (CDC) and expanded to include pathogens that can spread by blood or any other body fluid, excretion, or secretion.[1] Standard precautions apply to: (a) contact with blood; (b) all body fluids, secretions, and excretions excluding sweat; (c) nonintact skin; and (d) mucous membranes.[1] Both universal precautions and standard precautions were instituted to protect both DHCP and patients.

TRANSMISSIBLE DISEASES

It is an ethical responsibility of dental hygienists to treat all patients without discrimination. This includes those patients who may have a transmissible disease. It is also the responsibility of dental hygienists to correctly implement procedures to prevent disease transmission. Failure to do either is a breach of the code of ethics.

Many **pathogenic** (disease-producing) microorganisms are of concern in the dental health-care setting. DHCP not only have to be concerned about transmission to themselves but also to their patients. Transmission can be direct contact with body fluids, indirect contact with contaminated surfaces or items, droplets such as **spatter** (biological contaminants that are greater than 50 μm in diameter and may be visible) or inhalation of **aerosols** (invisible biological contaminants less than 50 μm in diameter).[2]

There are five stages of disease: incubation, prodrome, clinical, decline, and recovery. The incubation stage is considered the **latent period.** This is the time from when the infectious agent enters the body until the time when the first symptoms emerge. The **prodromal stage** is when general symptoms such as fever, nausea, and headache occur. This stage is communicable. Next is the clinical stage. This is considered the peak and there are characteristic symptoms of the disease at this point. Next is the decline stage when the

symptoms begin to disappear and the patient begins to recover. Relapses are possible if the patient does not temporarily limit activities. Last is the **convalescent stage,** when the body begins to restore itself. However, in this stage it is possible that the patient remains a **carrier;** that is, the infectious agent can still be transmitted to others despite the absence of signs or symptoms of the disease.[3] Examples of diseases that have a carrier state are hepatitis B and hepatitis C.

The infectious process takes place through a series of six events involving the infectious agent, reservoir, port of exit, mode of transmission, port of entry, and susceptible host. The infectious agent is the invading organism and the reservoir is where the organism lives and multiplies. Examples of reservoirs are people, equipment, and instruments. The port of exit is the mode of escape from the reservoir, for example, saliva and blood. The mode of transmission is the means by which contact occurs and is described as either direct (physical contact or a droplet from an infected individual to a susceptible host) or indirect (infected individual to intermediary object to susceptible host). The port of entry or mode of entry is the access site for the infectious agent to pass through open skin or mucous membranes of the host. The susceptible host is someone who does not have immunity to the infectious agent (Fig. 7-1).[4] Interventions such as standard precautions can prevent the spread of disease.

Prevention is of significant importance, and there are three levels of prevention: primary, secondary, and

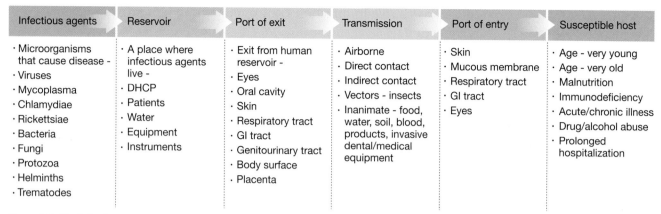

Infectious agents	Reservoir	Port of exit	Transmission	Port of entry	Susceptible host
· Microorganisms that cause disease - · Viruses · Mycoplasma · Chlamydiae · Rickettsiae · Bacteria · Fungi · Protozoa · Helminths · Trematodes	· A place where infectious agents live - · DHCP · Patients · Water · Equipment · Instruments	· Exit from human reservoir - · Eyes · Oral cavity · Skin · Respiratory tract · GI tract · Genitourinary tract · Body surface · Placenta	· Airborne · Direct contact · Indirect contact · Vectors - insects · Inanimate - food, water, soil, blood, products, invasive dental/medical equipment	· Skin · Mucous membrane · Respiratory tract · GI tract · Eyes	· Age - very young · Age - very old · Malnutrition · Immunodeficiency · Acute/chronic illness · Drug/alcohol abuse · Prolonged hospitalization

Figure 7-1. The infectious process.

tertiary. **Primary prevention** is when measures such as vaccinations are used to prevent a disease from occurring. Clinical screening and self-examinations facilitate early detection and treatment of diseases to prevent further progression. This is considered **secondary prevention.** Lastly, **tertiary prevention** occurs with chronic diseases or following advanced disease states in which rehabilitation is necessary to regain optimal health.[5]

Several diseases are of concern for DHCP. In most cases, transmission can be prevented when standard precautions are applied consistently. However, when DHCP are in a communicable stage of a disease or are a carrier, there may be suggested restrictions.

HIV/AIDS

HIV causes an infection that destroys the immune system. The late stage of the HIV infection is known as **AIDS.** The AIDS diagnosis is related to the development of one or more **opportunistic infections.**[6] These infections are caused by microorganisms that are only capable of producing disease due to the impairment of the immune system from the HIV. There are two types of HIV: type 1 (HIV-1) and type 2 (HIV-2). HIV-1 is the most common type in the United States and around the world.

HIV is found in varying concentrations or amounts in blood, semen, vaginal fluid, breast milk, saliva, and tears.[7] Exposure to saliva, tears, and sweat of an HIV-infected person has not resulted in transmission of the virus.[7]

No vaccine is available to prevent HIV transmission.[8] HIV is spread by sexual contact with an infected person or by sharing needles and/or syringes (primarily for drug injection) with someone who is infected. HIV-infected women may infect their babies before or during birth or through breastfeeding after birth.[7]

HIV is less commonly transmitted through transfusions of infected blood or blood-clotting factors. This achievement is the result of rigorous testing of the U.S. blood supply using HIV-1 and HIV-2 antibody detection laboratory tests.[9] In fact, HIV does not survive well outside the body. Dried blood or body fluids have a reduced risk for transmission. Furthermore, HIV cannot reproduce outside of the host. Therefore, it is unlikely that HIV will be transmitted through environmental surfaces.[7]

It is imperative that postexposure prophylaxis (PEP) be started as soon as the source is determined to be positive for HIV. Rapid HIV tests are available to expedite this process. The focus of drug regimens is to inhibit HIV enzymes and, therefore, suppress HIV replication (Table 7-1).[10,11]

These drugs have potential toxicities and are only recommended when the source is HIV-positive.[12] When the status of the source is unknown, there are three considerations that must be evaluated before a decision is made about PEP:

- Type of exposure
- Known risk characteristics of the source
- Prevalence in the setting concerned[13]

More information regarding treating patients with HIV/AIDS can be found in Chapter 43.

HEPATITIS

Hepatitis refers to inflammation of the liver. Five viruses that cause viral hepatitis are discussed in this chapter: hepatitis A, B, C, D, and E. Hepatitis F and G are unclassified and are not discussed. Hepatitis can also be caused by nonviral means such as excessive alcohol consumption.

Hepatitis A and E are transmitted through contaminated food and water. Hepatitis B, C, and D are bloodborne and are transmitted through direct or indirect contact with infectious body fluids.

Symptoms for all types of viral hepatitis are similar. Usually one or more of the following are experienced:

- Fever
- Fatigue
- Loss of appetite
- Nausea
- Vomiting
- Abdominal pain
- Dark urine
- Clay-colored bowel movements

Table 7-1. *Recommended HIV Postexposure Prophylaxis for Percutaneous Injuries*

		Infection Status of Source			
Exposure Type	**HIV-Positive, Class 1***	**HIV-Positive, Class 2***	**Source of Unknown HIV Status†**	**Unknown Source‡**	**HIV-Negative**
Less severe§	Recommend basic two-drug PEP	Recommend expanded ≥3-drug PEP	Generally, no PEP warranted; however, consider basic two-drug PEP¶ for source with HIV risk factors–	Generally, no PEP warranted; however, consider basic two-drug PEP¶ in settings in which exposure to HIV-infected persons is likely	No PEP warranted
More severe**	Recommend expanded three-drug PEP	Recommend expanded ≥3-drug PEP	Generally, no PEP warranted; however, consider basic two-drug PEP¶ for source with HIV risk factors–	Generally, no PEP warranted; however, consider basic two-drug PEP¶ in settings in which exposure to HIV-infected persons is likely	No PEP warranted

*HIV-positive, class 1—asymptomatic HIV infection or known low viral load (e.g., less than 1,500 ribonucleic acid copies/mL). HIV-positive, class 2—symptomatic HIV infection, AIDS, acute seroconversion, or known high viral load. If drug resistance is a concern, obtain expert consultation. Initiation of postexposure prophylaxis (PEP) should not be delayed pending expert consultation, and because expert consultation alone cannot substitute for face-to-face counseling, resources should be available to provide immediate evaluation and follow-up care for all exposures.

†For example, deceased source person with no samples available for HIV testing.

‡For example, a needle from a sharps disposal container.

§For example, solid needle or superficial injury.

¶The recommendation "consider PEP" indicates that PEP is optional; a decision to initiate PEP should be based on a discussion between the exposed person and the treating clinician regarding the risks versus benefits of PEP.

–If PEP is offered and administered and the source is later determined to be HIV-negative, PEP should be discontinued.

**For example, large-bore hollow needle, deep puncture, visible blood on device, or needle used in patient's artery or vein.

Source: Panlilio AL, Cardo DM, Grohskopf LA, Heneine W, Ross CS; U.S. Public Health Service. Updated U.S. Public Health service guidelines for the management of occupational exposures to HIV and recommendations for postexposure prophylaxis. *MMWR Recomm Rep.* 2005;54(RR09):1-17. Available from: http://www.cdc.gov/mmwr/preview/mmwrhtml/rr5409a1.htm.

- Joint pain
- Jaundice

Hepatitis A

The disease caused by the hepatitis A virus (HAV) was previously known as infectious hepatitis. Depending on conditions, HAV can live outside the body for months. The virus is found in feces and is spread from person to person through the fecal–oral route (ingestion of something fecally contaminated). Transmission can also be the result of eating contaminated shellfish.

According to the CDC, 70% of HAV-positive children who are younger than 6 years are asymptomatic. If illness does occur, jaundice is not typical in this age group. However, infection is symptomatic in older children and adults with jaundice, occurring in more than 70%.[14]

The incubation period is 15 to 50 days, with the average being 28 days, before the onset of symptoms. DHCP should refrain from patient contact until 7 days after the onset of jaundice.[1] There is no chronic carrier state. Primary prevention involves good sanitation, good personal hygiene, and vaccination.[14]

The hepatitis A vaccine, which is an **active immunization,** meaning the body produces its own antibodies, became available in 1995 and is now recommended in childhood after the age of 12 months. The available vaccines are HAVRIX and VAQTA, and they are administered in two doses. Twinrix, a combination vaccine for hepatitis A and hepatitis B intended for use in persons aged 18 years and older, is administered in three doses. Postvaccination testing is not recommended because of the high rate of response to the vaccine. Protection from the vaccine is expected to last 25 years for adults and 14 to 20 years in children.[14]

An injection of immune globulin will create **passive immunization** by delivering antibodies to the HAV into the body. This will last up to 3 months. For maximum protection, immune globulin needs to be administered within 2 weeks of being exposed to HAV. It can also be administered before exposure. In 2007, the U.S. guidelines were revised to also allow for a single dose of single-antigen hepatitis A vaccine to be used within 2 weeks of exposure in healthy individuals, aged 1 to 40 years. This is now preferred over immune globulin due to the ease of administration, long-term protection, and the equivalency of the vaccine to immune globulin. When there are intermediate or high rates of HAV, either immune globulin or the hepatitis A vaccine, or both, can be administered.[14]

Hepatitis B

Transmission of the hepatitis B virus (HBV) can be through percutaneous or mucosal exposure to HBV infectious blood or body fluids. HBV is highest in blood and is in lower quantities in other body fluids such as saliva and semen. Several other body fluids contain the hepatitis surface antigen (HBsAg); however, transmission through other body fluids is not as likely as blood.[1]

At room temperature, the HBV can be viable for 7 days or longer on environmental surfaces.[15] Because of this, it provides an opportunity for direct or indirect contact transmission through an opening in the skin or on mucosal surfaces.

Transmission of the HBV occurs when a source is HBsAg-positive. The risk for transmission also depends on the source's hepatitis B e antigen (HBeAg) status. The HBeAg is a protein from the HBV found in the blood serum during the acute and chronic stages of HBV infection. The presence of this protein is a marker that indicates that the virus is replicating and that the source is at an increased level of infectiousness.[1]

After 6 months, if the HBsAg is still detected, it indicates that the exposed individual is a carrier of HBV. This means that there will be lifelong shedding of HBV.

Hepatitis B has been considered an occupational risk. However, when a DHCP is vaccinated against HBV and **seroconversion,** the development of antibodies, has occurred, the risk can be nonexistent. This form of active immunization for hepatitis B has been available since the early 1980s. It is administered in three injectable doses: the initial dose, followed by injections 1 month and 6 months after the initial dose. Prevaccination serological testing (blood test to determine levels of HBeAg and HBsAg) is not generally recommended; however, postvaccination testing is suggested. Serological testing will determine whether there has been seroconversion, and it is recommended 1 to 2 months after the third dose of the hepatitis B vaccine. When there is seroconversion, the results will indicate an HBV antibody response (anti-HBs). If a DHCP has an inadequate response to the three-injection series (less than 10 mIU/mL), either a second series of three injections or serological testing to determine whether the DHCP is HBsAg-positive is recommended. If a second series is administered, the DHCP should be retested for antibodies. If at that time seroconversion has not occurred and the DHCP is HBsAg-negative, passive immunization with hepatitis B immune globulin would have to be considered in the event of an occupational exposure. There is no antiviral PEP for HBV.[15]

Although antibodies to HBV diminish over time, studies indicate that long-term protection is present. Consequently, when there has been an adequate initial response to the HBV vaccine and the individual is immunologically strong, revaccination or serological testing is not recommended. However, if serologic monitoring indicates a need, immunocompromised individuals should receive a booster dose.[16]

A DHCP who is active or chronic with HBV should refrain from performing exposure-prone procedures until consultation with a review panel is completed. The panel must be knowledgeable about state and local regulations, recommendations, or both. If the procedures under question can be performed, standard precautions must be followed. It would also be important to restrict work until the HBeAg results are negative.[1]

Hepatitis C

Hepatitis C infection is caused by the hepatitis C virus (HCV), which is widely considered to be the most serious of the hepatitis viruses. Shared needles during illegal, intravenous drug use commonly facilitate indirect contact transmission of blood contaminated with this virus. Most infected individuals are unaware of the infection for decades because of a lack of symptoms. Viability of the HCV in the environment is not exactly known, but it is at least 16 to 23 hours.[17,18] Hepatitis C can be an acute illness, but more commonly it is a chronic infection that leads to cirrhosis or cancer of the liver. HCV infection becomes chronic in approximately 75% to 85% of cases.[19] The risk for exposure through occupational means has been low. The prevalence of HCV infection among dentists, surgeons, and hospital-based health-care personnel (HCP) is similar to the general population, which is approximately 1% to 2%.[20] However, baseline and follow-up testing should be considered, especially if the donor is known to be positive for hepatitis C.[21] Blood screening for hepatitis C became available in 1992. Blood banks now screen for HCV, and the risk is considered to be less than 1 chance per 2 million units transfused.[22]

Hepatitis D

Hepatitis D (also called delta hepatitis) is caused by the hepatitis D virus (HDV) and can only replicate itself if HBV is present. It can be acute or chronic. Transmission is through percutaneous or mucosal contact with infectious blood. It can be acquired either as a **coinfection,** that is, HBV and HDV develop simultaneously, or as a **superinfection** where there is already an existing high **titer,** the concentration of a substance (antigen) in a solution (blood), of HBsAg when HDV is introduced. No vaccine exists to prevent hepatitis D; however, the hepatitis B vaccine will provide indirect protection against hepatitis D.

Hepatitis E

Hepatitis E is caused by the hepatitis E virus (HEV) and is similar to hepatitis A. Spread of the virus is through the fecal–oral route. It is usually associated with countries that have inadequate sanitation such as fecally contaminated drinking water. In developing countries, older adolescents and adults are more likely to encounter symptoms in 15 to 60 days after exposure to HEV.[23] Children usually have mild or no symptoms. Pregnant women are most likely to experience severe illness and also have a higher mortality rate. The disease is fatal in 10% to 30% of women in their third trimester of pregnancy.[23]

Antiviral therapy is not available for hepatitis E. It usually resolves on its own; however, it can become chronic. Chronic HEV is rare and has been limited to patients with organ transplantation. China has registered the first vaccine for hepatitis E, and it has been available in that country since 2011.[24] In the United States, there is no U.S. Food and Drug Administration (FDA)–approved vaccine for HEV, and immune globulin is not effective.[23] Fortunately, the disease is not common in the United States.

HUMAN HERPESVIRUSES 1 TO 8

There are eight **human herpesviruses** (HHVs; Fig. 7-2). There is no cure for herpes infections; however, the drug acyclovir (Zovirax) can reduce the severity and duration of the infections.

Human Herpesviruses 1 and 2

HHV type 1 (HHV 1), also known as herpes simplex virus type 1 (HSV-1), is generally referred to as herpes labialis when it appears on the lip. HSV-1 has also been known to cause infections around the mouth and nose, inside the mouth on the gingiva and palate, in the eye, and on the skin and genitals. Herpes simplex virus type 2 (HSV-2) is referred to as genital herpes. However,

HSV-2 can be transmitted to the oral area through oral-genital sex.

Herpetic gingivostomatitis, an uncommon form of herpes simplex, involves the mucosa throughout the oral and pharyngeal areas. Generally, the first outbreak of herpes is subclinical to mild in severity. As a result, more than 80% of individuals infected with HSV-1 or HSV-2 are unaware of their infection.[25] This primary gingivostomatitis is seen predominately in children younger than 6 years, although it may occur at any age. Other manifestations of primary gingivostomatitis may include anorexia, fever, lymphadenopathy, and malaise.

The incubation period for HSV-1 and HSV-2 ranges from 2 to 12 days.[26] Primary outbreaks can be either asymptomatic or symptomatic. For symptomatic episodes, itching and tingling usually occur first as part of the prodrome (initial or premonitory symptoms) followed by vesicles. The vesicles rupture, coalesce, and crust. Until complete healing of oral or perioral lesions, dental or dental hygiene procedures should not be performed. Patients should be informed that viral shedding can still occur after complete healing.

In addition to sunlight and fever, stress and trauma from dental procedures have been known to be triggers for HSV. A study published in 2004 showed that **recrudescence,** or becoming reactivated after a period of inactivity, was decreased by valacyclovir prophylaxis. The clinical implication is that antiviral therapy could be considered before procedures to reduce the risk for a recurrence and, in turn, lessen the possibility of transmission.[27]

Human Herpesvirus 3

HHV 3, also called *varicella zoster virus* (VZV), causes chickenpox and shingles. The primary infection is chickenpox and usually occurs in children. Shingles, which is considered the recurrent disease, usually occurs in medically compromised individuals and adults aged 50 years and older.[28]

The incubation period of VZV ranges from 10 to 21 days. Chickenpox may be accompanied by a fever before or when the rash begins to appear. The lesions first appear like an insect bite that soon blisters. The disease is spread by coughing, sneezing, direct contact with the lesions, and aerosols produced from the lesions. It is highly communicable, and the disease tends to be more serious in immunocompromised infants, adolescents, and adults. Serious complications such as infections, encephalitis, and pneumonia can occur as a result of chickenpox.

Shingles is a reactivation of VZV and is extremely painful. There is usually itching and tingling followed by a rash. The rash is unilateral, meaning it usually appears on the right or left side of the body, because it follows a nerve pathway. Common areas for the rash are the face and trunk of the body. The rash usually clears within 2 to 4 weeks.[28] Other accompanying symptoms tend to be flu-like such as fever, chills, headache, and upset stomach. Complications have been rare but can include pneumonia, hearing problems,

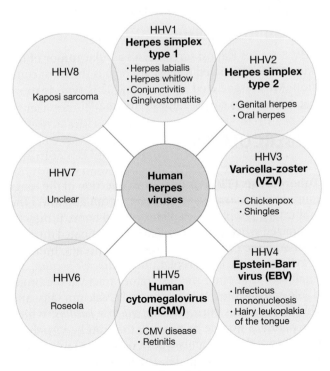

Figure 7-2. Herpes virus types 1 through 8.

blindness, encephalitis, or even death. Postherpetic neuralgia can also occur, which means that an individual can experience pain after the rash has disappeared. Furthermore, patients with shingles can give chickenpox to someone who does not have a history of chickenpox, and possibly give chickenpox to someone who has not been immunized with the chickenpox vaccine. Shingles cannot be transmitted from person to person.

There is a vaccination for both chickenpox and shingles. The chickenpox vaccine is administered in two doses. Although even vaccinated individuals may contract chickenpox, it is recommended for anyone who has not had the disease because the disease tends to be milder in those who have been vaccinated. The shingles vaccine is recommended for adults who are 60 years or older. It is administered in a single dose and can reduce a person's risk for shingles by 51%.[28]

Human Herpesvirus 4

HHV 4, or Epstein–Barr virus, causes infectious mononucleosis. Infection with Epstein–Barr usually occurs during adolescence and young adulthood. It has been known as the "kissing disease" because it is usually spread through saliva. The incubation period is from 4 to 6 weeks.[29] Fever, sore throat, malaise, and swollen lymph nodes are common symptoms of mononucleosis. Enlargement of the liver and spleen have occurred. In rare cases, there have been problems with the heart and the central nervous system. The EBV identified on the tongue of an HIV-infected person is known as hairy leukoplakia.[30]

Symptoms of the disease usually resolve within 1 to 2 months;[29] however, the virus can remain latent indefinitely. The virus can reactivate, but it usually does not cause symptoms. There is no vaccine and there are no antiviral drugs to treat the disease. Steroids have been used to decrease swelling of the throat and tonsils. When illness lasts more than 6 months, the infection has been called *chronic Epstein–Barr virus infection*.[29]

Human Herpesvirus 5

HHV 5 causes cytomegalovirus (CMV) disease. In the United States, CMV infects 50% to 80% of adults by the age of 40 years.[31] The virus is found in all body fluids (urine, saliva, breast milk, blood, tears, semen, and vaginal fluids). It can be transmitted congenitally, sexually, and possibly through the respiratory system.[32] The incubation period is 3 to 12 weeks. Most infections cause no symptoms. An acute infection of CMV may appear similar to infectious mononucleosis, hepatitis, or pneumonia. However, the infection in pregnant women is a major concern because it can cause disease and serious birth defects.[32] According to the CDC, approximately 1 in 750 children is born with or develops permanent disabilities caused by CMV.[33]

Some temporary symptoms caused by congenital CMV are liver, spleen, and lung problems, low birth weight, jaundice, purple skin splotches, and seizures. Permanent symptoms or disabilities can be hearing and vision loss, mental disability, microcephaly (small head

size), lack of coordination, and seizures.[34] Death can also be a result of the disease.

Currently, experimental vaccines are being tested that are aimed at protecting women of childbearing age. Immunocompromised individuals may benefit from antiviral therapy to prevent CMV infection; however, it is still being tested and is used only in severe cases. Conscientious hygiene is the best practice for prevention of CMV. Pregnant women should also avoid contact with the tears and saliva of infants and young children. Despite the fact that HCP have the greatest opportunity for exposure to CMV, standard precautions make the actual risk very low.[32]

Human Herpesviruses 6 and 7

HHV 6 causes roseola. The disease usually occurs in infants and young children between 6 months and 3 years of age. The incubation period is about 5 to 15 days.[35] Symptoms are a high fever (greater than 103°F [39.4°C]) followed by a rash that begins on the trunk and spreads to the face and extremities. This rash consists of small, pink sores that are slightly raised and it does not itch. There may be a white ring around some of the spots. Less common symptoms are runny nose, sore throat, and upset stomach. Sometimes lymph nodes are enlarged in the neck and back of the scalp.[36] The rash subsides within a few hours to a few days. The disease usually resolves on its own, although children may be treated for symptoms with bedrest, fluids, and fever-reducing drugs. In severe cases, especially children with compromised immune systems, antiviral drugs are used.[37]

HHV 7 currently has no other name. Some evidence suggests a link to roseola infantum.[35] No vaccine to prevent roseola exists. Careful and frequent hand washing as well as isolation of infected individuals prevent the spread of HHV 6 and HHV 7.[38]

Human Herpesvirus 8

HHV 8 causes Kaposi sarcoma, a vascular tumor of the skin. AIDS-associated Kaposi sarcoma is the most common AIDS-associated malignancy. This type is more aggressive than classic Kaposi sarcoma.[39]

TUBERCULOSIS

Tuberculosis (TB) is primarily an infection of the lungs caused by *Mycobacterium tuberculosis*. It can also infect the oral cavity, lymph nodes, kidneys, and bone. It may be contracted when a person inhales contaminated droplets from an infected person who coughs, sneezes, breathes heavily, or sings. The droplet nuclei, *tubercle bacillus*, are small rods that enter the respiratory tract via the bronchiole and alveolus. White blood cells, calcium salts, and fibrous materials surround the *tubercle bacillus*, which forms a hard nodule or tubercle that can be visualized on radiographs. TB can be latent or active (Table 7-2).

In the latent stage of TB, the patient has no symptoms and is not infectious. However, despite the lack of symptoms, the patient must be treated to prevent

Table 7-2. *Difference Between Latent Tuberculosis Infection and Tuberculosis Disease*

Person With Latent TB Infection	Person With TB Disease
• Has no symptoms	• Has symptoms that may include: • A bad cough that lasts ≥3 weeks • Pain in the chest • Coughing up blood or sputum • Weakness or fatigue • Weight loss • No appetite • Chills • Fever • Sweating at night
• Does not feel sick	• Usually feels sick
• Cannot spread TB bacteria to others	• May spread TB bacteria to others
• Usually has a skin test or blood test result indicating TB infection	• Usually has a skin test or blood test result indicating TB infection
• Has a normal chest radiograph and a negative sputum smear	• May have an abnormal chest radiograph, or positive sputum smear or culture
• Needs treatment for latent TB infection to prevent active TB disease	• Needs treatment to treat active TB disease

TB, tuberculosis.

Source: Centers for Disease Control and Prevention (CDC). Tuberculosis (TB) fact sheet: The difference between latent TB infection and active TB disease. Atlanta, GA: CDC; 2012. Available from: http://www.cdc.gov/tb/publications/factsheets/general/ltbiandactivetb.htm. Accessed May 27, 2013.

progression to the active form of the disease. The recommended drug regimen to treat latent TB is isoniazid, which is taken daily for 9 months.[40]

The incubation period for TB ranges from 2 to 12 weeks. Active TB may present as low-grade fever, loss of appetite and weight, cough, and productive sputum. This may progress to a persistent cough, temperature elevation, and night sweats. Several drugs are used for 6 to 9 months to treat TB disease: isoniazid (INH), rifampin (RIF), ethambutol (EMB), and pyrazinamide (PZA).[41]

Airborne droplets infected with *M. tuberculosis* bacterium can hang in the air for hours, and surgical masks do not prevent inhalation of the droplet nuclei. Nonetheless, prolonged exposure is necessary to contract TB from an individual with the active form of the disease. Immunocompromised individuals and those living in densely populated quarters are at increased risk for TB infection.[1] Following diagnosis, medications must be taken as prescribed to treat the disease and to avoid resistance to the drugs. Drug-resistant TB is more difficult and more expensive to treat.[42]

To further protect DHCP, both the CDC and the American Dental Association (ADA) recommend that elective dental treatment is not provided in the dental office for patients with suspected active TB until a physician consultation determines that the patient is noninfectious. For emergency dental procedures, the CDC recommends the use of a disposable particulate respirator mask (PRM) by the DHCP in a setting equipped for airborne infection isolation.[1,43]

For early detection, the Mantoux tuberculin skin test (TST) is used. Purified protein derivative is injected into the skin of the inner surface of the forearm. The test must be read within 48 to 72 hours. Skin interpretation depends on the size of the induration in millimeters, the person's risk for being infected, and risk for progression to disease if infected.[44] Two-step testing is recommended especially in HCP who will be periodically tested. Two-step testing involves administering a second test after the first test results in a negative response. CDC guidelines are established for HCP dependent on risk category.

The QuantiFERON-TB Gold test (QFT-G) is a whole blood test for use as an aid in diagnosing *M. tuberculosis* infection, including latent TB infection (LTBI) and TB disease. This test was approved by the FDA in 2005. Laboratory testing must be completed within 12 hours of collecting the blood sample. This test is not affected by the bacille Calmette-Guérin vaccination. This vaccine is not recommended in the United States.[45]

OTHER DISEASES AND CONDITIONS

Beyond those diseases identified previously, several other infectious diseases and conditions are summarized in terms of causative agent, modes of transmission, incubation period, and vaccine availability in Table 7-3. In addition, Table 7-4 outlines work restrictions for HCP infected with or exposed to several major infectious diseases.[46]

Table 7-3. *Summary of Infectious Diseases*

Disease or Infection	Causative Agent	Mode of Transmission	Incubation Period	Vaccine
Conjunctivitis		Droplets, fomites, and hand-to-eye inoculation		No
Viral	Adenovirus, Enteroviruses		5–12 days	
Bacterial	*Staphylococcus aureus, Streptococcus pneumoniae, Haemophilus* sp., *Chlamydia trachomatis, Neisseria gonorrhoeae*		12 hours to 14 days	
Cytomegalovirus infection	CMV human herpesvirus type 5	Blood, body fluids, or transplanted organs	9–60 days	No
Hepatitis A	Hepatitis A virus	Fecal-oral contamination, food, water, shellfish	15–50 days	Yes
Hepatitis B	Hepatitis B virus	Blood, semen, and other body fluids	45–160 days	Yes
Hepatitis C	Hepatitis C virus	Blood	14–180 days	No
Herpes simplex	HSV-1, HSV-2	Saliva, direct contact, sexual contact	2–12 days	No
Herpes labialis				
Genital herpes				
Herpetic whitlow	HSV- 1	Saliva, direct contact	2–20 days	No
Mumps	Paramyxovirus	Direct contact with saliva, airborne droplets, blood, urine, cerebrospinal fluid if CNS involvement	14–24 days	Yes
Bacterial meningitis	*Neisseria meningitidis*	Direct contact with respiratory secretions	3–7 days	Yes
Rubella (German measles)	Rubella virus	Respiratory droplets	14–21 days	Yes
Rubeola	Rubeola virus	Secretions from nose, throat, mouth, airborne droplet	7–14 days	Yes
Staphylococcus aureus	*Staphylococcus aureus*	Direct contact	4–10 days	No
Streptococcal Group A	*Streptococcus pyogenes*	Direct contact, respiratory droplets	1–3 days	No
Tuberculosis	*Mycobacterium tuberculosis*	Saliva, sputum, droplets	2–10 weeks	Yes
Chickenpox (varicella)	Varicella zoster virus	Direct contact, droplets	10–21 days	Yes
Shingles (herpes zoster)	Varicella zoster virus	Direct contact	None	Yes

Table 7-4. *Examples of Suggested Work Restrictions for Health-Care Personnel Infected With or Exposed to Major Infectious Diseases in Health-Care Settings, in the Absence of State and Local Regulations*

Disease/Problem	Work Restriction	Duration	Category
Conjunctivitis	Restrict from patient contact and contact with patient's environment	Until discharge ceases	II
Diarrheal diseases			
Acute stage (diarrhea with other symptoms)	Restrict from patient contact, contact with the patient's environment, or food handling	Until symptoms resolve	IB
Convalescent stage, *Salmonella* spp.	Restrict from care of high-risk patients	Until symptoms resolve; consult with local and state health authorities regarding need for negative stool cultures	IB
Herpes simplex			
Genital	No restriction		II
Hands (herpetic whitlow)	Restrict from patient contact and contact with patient's environment	Until lesions heal	IA
Orofacial	Evaluate for need to restrict from care of high-risk patients		II
Meningococcal infections	Exclude from duty	Until 24 hours after start of effective therapy	IA
Streptococcal infection, Group A	Restrict from patient care, contact with patient's environment, or food handling	Until 24 hours after adequate treatment started	IB

Source: Bolyard EA; Hospital Infection Control Practices Advisory Committee. Guidelines for infection control in health care personnel, 1998. *Am J Infect Control.* 1998;26:289-354. Available from: http://www.cdc.gov/hicpac/pdf/InfectControl98.pdf.

RESOURCES AND REFERENCES FOR INFECTION CONTROL

The CDC is part of the Department of Health and Human Services. Its mission statement is "to protect America from health, safety and security threats, both foreign and in the United States. Whether diseases start at home or abroad, are chronic or acute, curable or preventable, human error or deliberate attack, CDC fights disease and supports communities and citizens to do the same."[47] "Guidelines for Infection Control in Dental Health-Care Settings—2003"[1] is one of many valuable resources available through the CDC. Twenty-four-hour assistance is available. See Box 7-1 for contact information for the CDC and other agencies discussed in this section.

The National Institute for Occupational Safety and Health (NIOSH) is a federal agency that is part of the CDC. It is responsible for conducting research and making recommendations for the prevention of work-related injury and illness. It also provides information, education, and training. Twenty-four-hour assistance is available for further information.

The Occupational Safety and Health Administration (OSHA) is in the U.S. Department of Labor. It is responsible for developing and enforcing workplace safety and health regulations. There are no standards specifically written for dentistry; however, there are several standards regarding bloodborne pathogens, hazard communication, **personal protective equipment (PPE),** hand protection, sanitation, and medical services and first aid that can be applied to dentistry. Both NIOSH and OSHA were created as a result of the Occupational Safety and Health Act of 1970.

The American National Standards Institute (ANSI) is a private, not-for-profit agency. Its mission statement is "to enhance both the global competitiveness of U.S. business and the U.S. quality of life by promoting and facilitating voluntary consensus standards and conformity assessment systems, and safeguarding their integrity."[48] ANSI's accreditation program includes personal protective and safety equipment.

The Environmental Protection Agency (EPA) has a mission "to protect human health and the environment."[49] One of its many responsibilities is to issue regulations that require testing of chemicals to determine their effects on health and the environment.

Box 7-1. *Contact Information for Infection-Control Resources*

Centers for Disease Control and Prevention (CDC)
  1600 Clifton Rd., Atlanta, GA 30333
  http://www.cdc.gov
  1–800-CDC-INFO (1-800-232-4636)
  TTY 1-888-232-6348

National Institute for Occupational Safety and Health (NIOSH)
  1600 Clifton Rd., Atlanta GA 30333
  http://www.cdc.gov/niosh/about.html
  1-800-CDC-INFO (1-800-232-4636)
  TTY 1-888-232-6348

Occupational Safety and Health Administration (OSHA)
  200 Constitution Ave. NW, Washington, DC 20210
  http://www.osha.gov/SLTC/dentistry/index.html
  1-800-321-OSHA (1-800-321-6742)
  TTY 1-877-889-5627

American National Standards Institute (ANSI)
  1899 L Street, NW, 11th Floor, Washington, DC 20036
  http://www.ansi.org
  202-293-8020

Environmental Protection Agency (EPA)
  Headquarters: Ariel Rios Bldg., 1200 Pennsylvania Ave. NW, Washington, DC 20460
  http://www.epa.gov

202-272-0167
TTY 202-272-0165
Specific Regional/Laboratory Addresses and Phone numbers:
http://www2.epa.gov/aboutepa/mailing-addresses-and-phone-numbers

U.S. Food and Drug Administration (FDA)
  10903 New Hampshire Ave., Silver Spring, MD 20993
  http://www.fda.gov
  1-888-INFO-FDA (1-888-463-6332)
  Specific Phone Numbers and Email Addresses:
  http://www.fda.gov/AboutFDA/ContactFDA/default.htm

Organization for Safety and Asepsis Protocol (OSAP)
  839 Bestgate Road Suite 400 Annapolis, Maryland 21401
  http://www.osap.org
  1-800-298-6727

State Dental Licensing Boards
  http://www.dentalwatch.org/org/boards.html

American Dental Association (ADA)
  211 E. Chicago Ave., Chicago, IL 60611
  http://www.ada.org
  312-440-2500 ■

The FDA is in the U.S. Department of Health and Human Services. Its mission is "protecting consumers and enhancing public health by maximizing compliance of FDA-regulated products and minimizing risk associated with those products."[50] One responsibility is to clear sterilants and high-level **disinfectants** for the processing of reusable medical and dental devices.[51] Additional information about the responsibilities of the FDA and reporting emergencies and nonemergencies can be found on the website.

The Organization for Safety and Asepsis Protocol (OSAP) is a nonprofit organization whose mission is "to be the world's leading advocate for the safe and infection-free delivery of oral healthcare."[52] The organization provides publications, educational tools, and programs and answers to questions regarding infection control and safety. An example of an educational tool available in the OSAP online store (www.osap.org) is the "If Saliva Were Red Training DVD."

The practice of dentistry is regulated by a state board of dentistry, dental hygiene, or a specified central agency. Infection-control requirements are often addressed. Usually inspections can be conducted with or without notice. Boards or agencies have the responsibility of disciplining licensees for any violations of their state Dental Practice Act.

The ADA provides resources, such as research, evidence-based position papers, and educational information for dental professionals and the public. Some of the issues discussed are bloodborne pathogens including HIV, dental unit water lines, and postexposure evaluation and follow-up requirements.

The *Merck Manual of Diagnosis and Therapy* is a reference book for health-care professionals. It provides information on medical disorders and is divided by organ systems. Major diseases of each system are discussed in terms of diagnosis, prognosis, and treatment.

ENGINEERING AND WORK PRACTICE CONTROLS

Engineering controls (ECs) and **work practice controls (WPCs)** are meant to prevent or reduce the HCP's exposure to bloodborne pathogens. These controls should be evaluated on a regular basis. Replacements of ECs or revisions to practices should be made as necessary.

According to OSHA, ECs are controls to isolate or remove bloodborne pathogen hazards from the workplace. Examples of ECs are a sharps container, instrument cassette, and needle recapping device. WPCs are controls that reduce the risk for exposure by changing the way that a task is performed. For example, a WPC would be recapping a needle using the one-handed scoop technique rather than the two-handed technique (this procedure is illustrated in Chapter 33). The two-handed technique puts DHCP at risk for an exposure (see Application to Clinical Practice). Implementation of ECs and WPCs followed by strict compliance is necessary in the dental setting.

PERSONAL PROTECTIVE EQUIPMENT

PPE must be worn by DHCP to prevent disease transmission. Attire consists of protective clothing, protective eyewear, mask, and appropriate gloves for the procedure being performed. Face shields, bouffant surgical caps, and surgical shoe covers are optional.

Protective Clothing

A protective covering such as a gown or laboratory coat must be worn (Fig. 7-3). It must have sleeves that will protect the forearms. Ideally, protective clothing should

Application to Clinical Practice

Upon providing dental hygiene care, the patient is experiencing a significant amount of sensitivity and moderate bleeding. The patient requests that she be anesthetized. You had not anticipated the need for anesthesia, but you are qualified to administer it. What ECs and workplace practices regarding infection control should be incorporated to provide a safe environment for you and the patient? ■

have a closed front with no pockets and should be long enough to cover the clinician's knees. This style provides more protection especially in the chest area as well as the thigh area. Both areas are vulnerable to spatter and aerosols. Gowns should be changed daily or sooner if they are visibly soiled. Employees must remove protective clothing before leaving work. According to OSHA, DHCP are not permitted to take protective clothing home for laundering. Employers are responsible for either laundering the gowns in the office or having a third-party service. Disposable gowns are acceptable but are not part of an environmentally friendly program because they create more waste.

Protective Eyewear

Protective eyewear should be designed to prevent: (a) exposure to bloodborne pathogens and other potentially infectious body material, (b) trauma from loose debris such as calculus, and (c) contact with chemicals. If protective eyewear meets the standards of the ANSI, ANSI Z87.1 will be imprinted on the frame or lenses. There are numerous styles of ANSI Z87.1 protective eyewear. The most protective style is the goggle type because it fits up against the skin and encloses the eye area on the top, sides, and bottom (Fig. 7-4).

DHCP should select a style that has adequate side shields and is close fitting to the face so there is less potential for an exposure incident or an eye injury. They should also be comfortable because of the amount of time that the eyewear will be worn. Eyewear is required during any procedure that has the potential for eye exposures or injuries. If it is uncomfortable, it is less likely to be worn. Many DHCP choose to wear

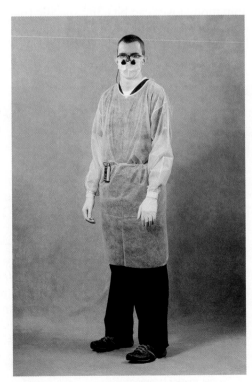

Figure 7-3. Personal protective equipment (PPE).

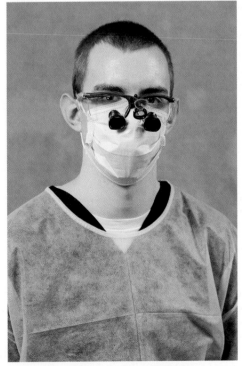

Figure 7-4. Protective eye wear on dental health-care personnel.

magnification loupes instead of basic protective eyewear. Magnification loupes may meet the ANSI standard, but this should be confirmed with the manufacturer.

Personal eyeglasses do not provide adequate protection. DHCP who require prescription lenses can either select a protective eyewear that will fit over the glasses or have prescription glasses made by an optometrist that meets the ANSI standard. Polycarbonate lenses are more impact resistant than glass, but both can meet the standard.

Patients should also be provided with safety eyewear for the same reasons as DHCP. An additional reason for the patient is protection from the possibility of an instrument being accidentally dropped in the eye area. Protective eyewear can be worn over a patient's prescription glasses or alone (Fig. 7-5).

Protective eyewear for either DHCP or patients should be placed before hand washing and donning of gloves by the DHCP. This eyewear should be washed with soap and water, rinsed, and dried. If heavily contaminated, a disinfectant, used according to manufacturer's instructions, may be considered.

Masks

Masks should have greater than 95% bacterial filtration efficiency, protect the nose and mouth of DHCP from exposures to aerosols and spatter, and be fluid resistant. The mask should be placed and adjusted before hand washing and donning of gloves by the DHCP. It is important for the DHCP to make sure that the bendable nose piece is adjusted to conform to the bridge of the nose, and the bottom of the mask needs to be fully under the chin to create a seal around the bridge of the nose and completely cover the mouth. The entire border of the mask should fit snugly to the face. Masks are secured by either ties or elastic and should be fully in place during clinical procedures. Masks should not be worn longer than 20 minutes in a wet, heavy aerosol, or spatter environment, no longer than 1 hour in a dry environment, and a new mask should be worn for each patient being treated.[53] Contaminated masks should never be worn under the chin or around the neck following procedures (Fig. 7-6). Removal of a mask should be accomplished using bare hands and by grasping the elastic strap or ear loops rather than touching the contaminated mask itself.

PRMs rather than surgical, medical, or dental masks can be used when greater filtration is needed. These masks provide a tight seal around the face and must be fit-tested and NIOSH-approved with a filtration of 95% (N95). A PRM is needed if a patient has an actively infectious disease such as TB. These masks should be worn once and properly disposed of immediately after use.

Face Shields

Face shields are not a substitute for protective eyewear or masks (Fig. 7-7). They can be used for additional protection in combination with a disposable mask. They should be cleaned or disposed of according to the manufacturer's instructions.

Gloves

Four types of gloves are used in the dental environment: nonsterile examination gloves, sterile surgeon's gloves, utility gloves (overgloves), and heavy-duty utility gloves. The FDA regulates examination and sterile surgeon's gloves.

Examination gloves can be hand specific (right- and left-handed) or ambidextrous. Ambidextrous gloves are available in bulk but may not fit well. Ambidextrous

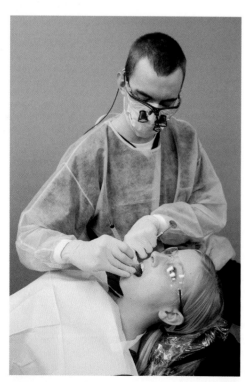

Figure 7-5. Protective eyewear on patient and dental health-care personnel.

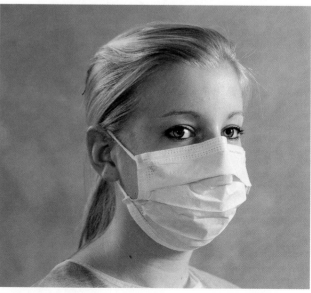

Figure 7-6. Proper mask placement.

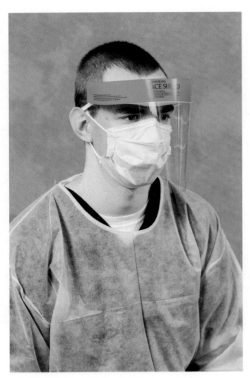

Figure 7-7. Face shield.

gloves may pull and put undue stress on the hand, especially on the thumb, causing musculoskeletal injury. An examination glove that fits properly will not pull over the palm or between the thumb and index finger. Examination gloves should be donned and removed in front of patients.

Examination gloves are made of latex, vinyl, nitrile, or chloroprene. DHCP should be aware that the integrity of certain gloves can be compromised, for example, by chemicals used in dentistry, hand lotions, and petroleum-based products, including lip balm. If hand sanitizers are used, hands should be dry before gloving, because the alcohol may affect glove integrity. Manufacturers of gloves can be consulted regarding the specifics of what compromises glove integrity.

Torn, cut, tacky, or punctured gloves need to be removed immediately on discovery of the defect. Hands should be thoroughly washed with soap and water. Maintaining short, well-manicured fingernails, removing jewelry, and handling sharps appropriately will protect glove integrity.

Sterile surgeon gloves are donned specifically for surgical procedures and are more expensive than examination gloves. They are sterile and usually packaged individually as right- and left-handed gloves. Double gloving may be considered for additional protection particularly for oral surgical procedures or procedures lasting longer than 45 minutes. The highest incidence rate of perforation (10%) of the outer glove occurs during oral surgery.[1]

Neoprene and polynitrile are used for heavy-duty utility gloves. They are bulky but usually puncture resistant. These gloves are used for general cleaning,

disinfecting, and handling instruments. They can be washed or disinfected and reused. Some can be autoclaved, but autoclaving may cause them to deteriorate faster. Regardless of the method chosen to prepare them for reuse, gloves should be checked for tears and cracks each time before gloving.

Overgloves are thin and made of vinyl or copolymer. They are known as food-handler gloves and are used by DHCP. During procedures when paperwork must be completed, overgloves are slipped on over the examination gloves. Paperwork and writing utensils can then be handled. In the case of electronic records, the computer keyboard should be covered by a plastic barrier for use during patient treatment. The mouse may be covered by a plastic barrier or handled with overgloves on gloved hands. Use of these gloves can prevent disease transmission from contaminated examination gloves. CDC recommendations for using overgloves can be found in the "Guidelines for Infection Control in Dental Health-Care Settings—2003" (available online at: www.cdc.gov).

When degloving examination gloves or surgeon's gloves, it is important to handle gloves by touching "clean-to-clean" and "contaminated-to-contaminated" surfaces. For example, the outside of the right examination glove is contaminated, so it can be touched only by the contaminated left glove. The right hand should pinch and cuff the left hand glove (Fig. 7-8A). The left hand should pinch below the edge of the right-hand glove near the wrist and remove the glove, turning the contaminated side inside and holding in the left palm (Fig. 7-8B and 7-8C). The right hand, which is glove free, should touch only the clean part of the left cuff (side that touched skin); pinch and pull off and over the right glove (Fig. 7-8D and 7-8E). Gloves should be disposed of properly. This method will help avoid contamination.

Overgloves can be removed by pulling off the right glove with the left glove. The right contaminated examination glove can go inside the left overglove and scoop the left glove off.

Latex gloves can cause contact dermatitis or latex hypersensitivity. Hand hygiene products, chemical exposure, and gloves can cause either irritant or allergic contact dermatitis. Dry, itchy, irritated skin is the result. Allergic contact dermatitis is also referred to as type 4 hypersensitivity and is characterized by a delayed reaction. Products used in the manufacture of gloves such as accelerators and other chemicals can cause a reaction that usually occurs hours after contact.

When gloves are powdered, more latex proteins contact the skin. DHCP with repeated exposure to latex protein can become sensitized to it. Gloving and degloving sends latex proteins in the air. Practices should be latex free to protect patient and dental office personnel from serious allergic reaction or be prepared for a medical emergency.

Latex allergy, also known as type 1 hypersensitivity to latex proteins, can cause a serious systemic allergic reaction. This type of reaction can occur within minutes

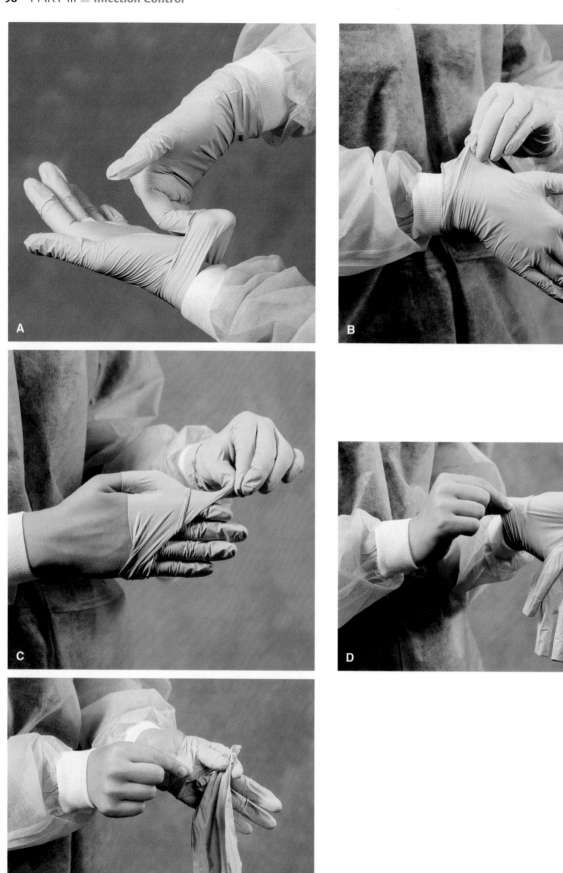

Figure 7-8. Degloving. (A) With the right hand, pinch and cuff the left-hand glove. (B) With the left hand, pinch under the edge of the right-hand glove near the wrist. (C) Remove the right-hand glove. (D) With the right hand, pinch the clean part of the left-hand glove. (E) Pull the left-hand glove off and over the right-hand glove.

of exposure or it can occur hours later. Runny nose, sneezing, itchy eyes, scratchy throat, hives, and itchy burning skin sensations are examples of some of the less severe reactions. A more severe reaction is the development of asthma with difficulty breathing, coughing, and wheezing. Cardiovascular and gastrointestinal ailments may occur. Anaphylaxis and even death can result, but it is rare.

INFECTION CONTROL IN THE PATIENT CARE AREA

Numerous steps must be taken to prevent disease transmission in the patient care area. Responsibilities must be completed at the beginning of the day, between patients, and at the end of the day (Table 7-5).

Table 7-5. *Infection Control in the Patient Area*

At the Beginning of the Day	Between Patients and After the Last Patient of the Day	At the End of the Day
Clean and disinfect equipment and surfaces unless plastic barriers are going to be used. • Treatment area: countertops and surfaces surrounding the area such as partitions, cupboards, and drawers • Patient chair, switches, and light assembly • Delivery systems (chair mounted or cart) including top, handpiece holders, and nonsterilizable handpieces/tubing • Low- and high-volume evacuator handpieces • View box • Sink • Radiograph unit • Operator and assistant stools Place clean barriers. Items to be considered are areas that are difficult to clean and disinfect: • Patient chair specifically, headrest and chair back that includes switches • Delivery systems (chair mounted or cart) especially top where instruments are placed, handpiece holders, and nonsterilizable handpieces/tubing • Light handles and on/off switch • Computer keyboard and mouse • Dispensers Attach sterilized air/water syringe and tip and high- or low-speed handpiece(s), or both. Fill water bottle and follow water treatment protocol for self-contained water system according to manufacturer's instructions. Prepare waste containers for regulated and nonregulated medical waste. Acquire patient treatment supplies such as the patient bib and holder, protective eyewear, sterilized instruments with disposables such as gauze, cotton rolls, and cotton swabs, and other supplies necessary during treatment such as prophy paste, floss, fluoride trays/varnish, and a cup for mouthrinse. Nonsterilized items must be kept separate from sterilized items. Products that will be dispensed must be dispensed without contaminating the container or product. Examples are toothpaste, fluoride, and mouthrinse. Overgloves may be considered in some situations. Patient education models and materials can also be acquired. Contamination must be avoided. Paper, pens, and charts, including contents, should not be contaminated. Clean hands should be used to handle them. In some cases, overgloves may need to be considered.	Remove and dispose of barriers, low-/high-volume evacuator tips, and other disposables in proper waste containers. Remove from the treatment area equipment that requires sterilization (air/water syringe and tip and high- and low-speed handpieces) and instruments. Clean and disinfect appropriate equipment and surfaces. Discharge water for 20–30 seconds from dental unit water lines after every patient. Place clean barriers and low-/high-volume evacuator tips. Attach sterilized air/water syringe and tip and high- or low-speed handpiece(s), or both. Check level of water in bottle of self-contained water system. Refill and follow water treatment protocol. Prepare a regulated medical waste container. Acquire necessary supplies and products that are mentioned in the beginning of the day.	Follow manufacturer's instructions for maintaining dental unit water lines and self-contained water systems. Run an evacuation cleaner through low- and high-volume evacuation lines according to manufacturer's instructions. Properly dispose of regulated and nonregulated medical waste. Follow manufacturer's instructions for proper chemical disposal.

Clinical Contact Surfaces and Housekeeping Surfaces

In preparing for patient care, environmental surfaces should be divided into clinical contact surfaces and housekeeping surfaces. Clinical contact surfaces have the potential to transmit diseases, whereas housekeeping surfaces are less likely to transmit disease (Table 7-6).

Clinical contact surfaces can be directly contaminated by direct spray or spatter generated during dental procedures or by contact with the DHCP's gloved hands. According to the CDC, strategies for cleaning and disinfecting surfaces in patient care areas should consider the following factors: (a) potential for direct patient contact; (b) degree and frequency of hand contact, and (c) potential contamination of the surface with body substances or environmental sources of microorganisms (e.g., soil, dust, or water).[1]

Cleaning and Disinfection

Cleaning is an essential part of the disinfection process and the first step in it. This procedure will remove debris such as organic matter, salts, and visible soils that interfere with microbial inactivation. A substantial number of microorganisms can be removed through scrubbing with detergents and **surfactants,** which are surface-active agents that reduce surface tension so that soil can be more easily rinsed away.

When a surface is cleaned, a **germicide,** an agent that destroys microorganisms, can be more effective. A germicide for environmental surface use is referred to as a *disinfectant.* This is the second step of the disinfection process.

This distinct two-step process of cleaning and disinfecting must take place between patients if barrier techniques are not used. For cleaning to be accomplished, the surface must be visibly clean. A scrubbing motion is used, and the presaturated wipe or gauze, with the cleaning agent applied to it, must be changed as it becomes soiled. Disinfecting may begin immediately after cleaning. Clinical surfaces should appear wet with the disinfectant and remain wet for the length of time specified on the product label.

A single product may be selected for both cleaning and disinfection as long as the label supports its efficacy for both steps. This is recommended by OSAP in addition to several other product qualities including EPA registration; labeled as a "hospital disinfectant"; compatibility with surfaces and staff; low allergenicity; ease of use; simple instructions; 10 minutes or less contact time; acceptable storage/disposal requirements; and acceptable shelf life. Housekeeping surfaces require less rigorous methods of decontamination in comparison with clinical contact surfaces.

Surface Barriers

Surface barriers are single-use disposable items that are impervious to moisture (Fig. 7-9). Many styles are available for use such as plastic wrap, bags, sheets, tubing (some specifically designed for dental equipment), plastic-backed paper, and other materials that are impervious to moisture. Barriers can be used without disinfecting equipment or in conjunction with disinfection before placement of the barrier. Barriers are especially useful for difficult-to-clean clinical contact surfaces and should be placed with clean hands. Contaminated barriers should be removed with gloved hands after each patient. Protected surfaces should be disinfected at the end of each day or if contamination is evident.[54]

Dental Radiograph Equipment and the Darkroom

Dental radiograph equipment and the darkroom are often neglected in terms of infection control. Panoramic bite sticks and film-holding devices are semicritical items, and **sterilization** after each use is recommended if instruments are heat tolerant. Furthermore, any part

Table 7-6. *Clinical Contact and Housekeeping Surfaces*

Clinical Contact Surfaces	Housekeeping Surfaces
Light handles	Floors
Switches	Walls
Dental radiograph equipment	Sinks
Dental chairside computers	
Reusable containers of dental materials	
Drawer handles	
Faucet handles	
Countertops	
Pens	
Telephones	
Doorknobs	

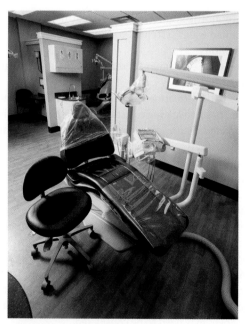

Figure 7-9. Surface barriers on patient chair and delivery system.

of radiograph equipment that will be touched during exposure of films is considered a clinical contact surface and should be either cleaned and disinfected or covered with a barrier (Fig. 7-10).[54] Examples of barriers for intraoral radiograph units include a clear plastic bag or plastic wrap to cover the position-indicating device and the tube head and plastic wrap covering the control panel. The use of digital radiography also necessitates a protective plastic barrier on the sensor and plastic wrap placed across the computer keyboard. Examples of barriers for extraoral radiograph units would be a plastic sandwich bag covering the chin rest and activation button, plastic sleeves covering the temple supports, and plastic wrap covering the control panel.

Films can be transported to the darkroom in a disposable cup or on a reusable tray that can be sterilized. If barrier film was used, examination gloves can be used to open the barrier and drop the film packet on a clean surface (Fig. 7-11). Once all barrier film packets are open, examination gloves can be removed. Bare hands can be used to open the uncontaminated film packets and place films in the automatic processor or on a film rack for manual processing. If barrier film was not used, examination gloves should be used to open the film packet and pull the black paper that surrounds the film from the packet. The film should be dropped to a clean surface to avoid contamination. The lead foil should be dropped into a recycling container, and the black paper and outer covering should be disposed of in a waste container. Gloves should be removed, and with bare hands, the film can be inserted in the automatic processor or placed on the film rack for manual processing.

The darkroom should be cleaned and disinfected throughout the workday. Waste should be disposed of

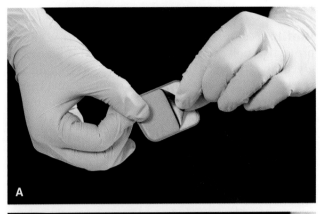

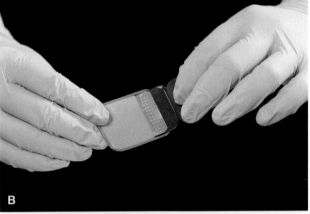

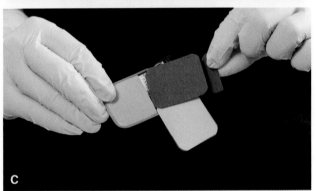

Figure 7-11. Wearing examination gloves, open the radiograph film packet and drop it onto a clean surface.

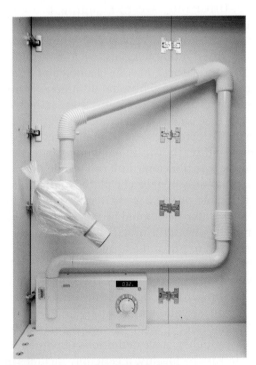

Figure 7-10. Barriers on radiograph tube head.

properly at the end of the day. It is important to comply with local, state, and federal infection-control and bloodborne pathogen standards.

If a daylight loader is used, DHCP should be conscientious not to contaminate the hand opening of the daylight loader. This can be done by lifting the lid above the daylight loader compartment and placing a clean cup, clean examination gloves, and the cup with the contaminated films in the compartment. Once the lid is closed, DHCP can put their clean hands in the opening, glove, and follow the procedure for either barrier film packets or nonbarrier film packets. Once films are placed in the processor with ungloved hands, the hands can be removed from the daylight loader. Hands should be washed and regloved. The lid to the daylight loader compartment can be opened and all contents removed and disposed of in appropriate containers.

Dental Unit Water Lines

Biofilm, colonization of microorganisms within a protective polysaccharide slime layer also known as glycocalyx, forms within dental tubing. Biofilm is a reservoir for free-floating microorganisms that can be delivered through dental unit water.[1] This is measured in colony-forming units (CFU), and the recommended value for safe drinking water is 500 CFU/mL or less.

Self-contained water systems combined with chemical treatment and inline microfilters have maintained the recommended value of 500 CFU/mL or less (Fig. 7-12).[1] Self-contained water systems using tap water alone have not been effective. In-office testing kits are available and there are nationwide laboratories that test water quality.[55] The manufacturer's instructions for maintaining self-contained water systems must be followed (see Evidence-Based Practice).

Antiretraction valves in dental units prevent the retraction of oral fluids. However, older dental units may

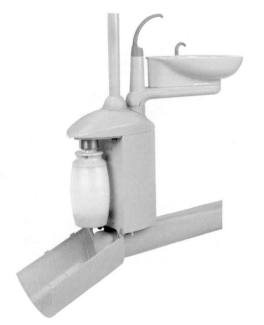

Figure 7-12. A-dec delivery system with self-contained water bottle. (Courtesy of A-dec)

Evidence-Based Practice

Safety of dental unit water lines has been a concern for years. Biofilm has been the culprit. Flushing of the water lines was recommended in 1993 by the CDC to reduce microbial load.[1] However, studies determined that this practice did not affect the biofilm nor did it significantly improve the water quality. Other strategies must be used to obtain values of 500 CFU/mL or less. Self-contained water systems do not solve the problem unless biofilm is controlled by treatment with germicides. ■

have valves that require maintenance. The manufacturer's instructions should be consulted to ensure that they are operating properly. Even with the valves, water and air should be discharged from water lines for 20 to 30 seconds between patients.[1] This includes air/water syringes, high-speed handpieces, and ultrasonic scalers.

DHCP should not permit patients to close their lips around the saliva ejector during suctioning. When a seal is created in this way, backflow of previously suctioned fluids have the potential to be retracted into the patient's mouth. This is more likely to occur if the suction tubing is held above the patient's mouth or if the low-volume suction is used simultaneously with the high-volume suction in another operatory. Although no adverse health effects are known to have occurred, this practice is not recommended. Possible suggestions are to use the high-volume suction when possible, to allow the patient to expectorate into a disposable paper cup or a funnel attachment for the high-volume suction, or to use the low-volume suction without the patient closing his or her lips around the tip.[56]

Evacuation Systems

An evacuation system cleanser should be run through the high- and low-volume evacuation lines at the end of each day following the manufacturer's instruction. The solids waste filter should also be cleaned or replaced. Both will reduce debris accumulation.[57]

Dental Laboratory

The dental laboratory also requires procedures to prevent disease transmission. All items used during patient treatment should be handled with care to avoid contamination. In addition, contamination of equipment and environmental surfaces must be avoided. DHCP must wear PPE during procedures in the laboratory.

Dental prostheses, appliances, impressions, and other prosthodontic materials, such as articulations, case pans, and lathes, must be cleaned and disinfected with an EPA-registered hospital disinfectant with a tuberculocidal claim. Sterilize items that can be sterilized and dispose of single-use packets.

If patients' prostheses and appliances need to be cleaned in-office, they must be handled with examination gloves. The ultrasonic unit can be filled with water; the prosthodontic item can be placed in a sterile beaker or a disposable plastic bag with an approved product. If a beaker is used, it should be placed into the beaker holder of the ultrasonic unit. If a bag is used, the opening is secured to prevent leakage and the bag is placed into the basket of the ultrasonic unit.[57] The unit must be covered. Manufacturer's instructions must be followed with regard to length of time for use and rinsing of the prosthesis following cleaning.

Most laboratory waste is not regulated medical waste. Although specific definitions of regulated medical waste vary by locality, it generally includes materials saturated with blood or other infectious fluids.

Sharp items such as scalpel blades and burs used in the laboratory must be placed in puncture-resistant containers.[1,57]

ENVIRONMENTAL PROTECTION

"Going green" is a concept that needs serious consideration in the dental setting. The purpose is to improve the environment through practices such as the use of new technology and environmentally safe products. Safety and health should be an essential component in a green training program.

Transitioning to electronic patient records and digital radiographs can positively impact the environment. Paper can be reduced in the patient chart, with one result being that there is less need to remove examination or overgloves to handle paper. This is also a plus for infection-control practices. Digital radiographs can eliminate chemicals used in processing films and lead foil from film packets. Manual or automatic processing chemicals and lead foil should be recycled if the office does not use digital radiography.

Instrument preparation can also be more eco-friendly. Steam sterilization does not involve chemicals and does not require special ventilation. It can also accomplish sterilization within a short period using less electricity. Office equipment such as ultrasonics, sterilizers, computers, and automatic processors can be unplugged to save electricity. Solutions used in ultrasonic cleaners before sterilizing are becoming more biodegradable. Reusable sterilization cassettes and reusable fabric sterilization pouches can be used instead of disposable bags or pouches. If cassettes are immediately used at the end of the sterilization cycle, they do not need to be wrapped.[1] If they do need to be wrapped, a biodegradable product should be used. Larger and smaller cassettes are available. The size should be determined based on the number of instruments that require sterilization. If smaller cassettes can be used, less wrapping material will be required.

Disinfection involves the use of chemicals and disposables such as gauze or the use of chemical wipes. Wipes minimize chemicals released in the air. However, they need to be evaluated for their ability to biodegrade. Disinfectant wipe packets manufactured as refills for reusable plastic containers may be available in the near future. Reusing these containers would result in a substantial reduction of plastics being put into the environment as waste. Surface barriers can be used to lessen the amount of chemicals used in disinfection. Barriers are also a concern because they are plastic and not biodegradable; however, they may be recyclable if they are not considered regulated medical waste. If paper tray covers are used, alternatives should be considered. If necessary, they can be made from chlorine-free pulp.

An in-office Energy Star (an energy performance rating system administered by the EPA) washer and drier can be purchased for laundering gowns and other reusable linens. Reusable linens, such as cloth bibs, small towels, and headrest covers, can also be purchased to limit the use of disposables. If disposable gowns and barriers are used, they should be selected based on their biodegradability.

There are challenges in "going green" in dentistry; however, DHCP should embrace new technology as it becomes available (see Advancing Technologies). Protecting the environment may not only save the environment for future generations but also may be cost saving.[58]

INSTRUMENT PROCESSING

Area

A specific area in the dental practice should be designated as the instrument processing area. The area should be divided into receiving, cleaning and decontamination, preparation and packaging, sterilization, and storage. Areas designated as clean should never be contaminated by unclean instruments or equipment.

Transportation

PPE must be used along with heavy-duty utility gloves for instrument transportation and processing. Instruments should be transported from the clinical treatment area to the instrument processing area by an EC such as a cassette. Instruments can remain in the cassette during the entire processing procedure, from removal from the treatment area, through processing and return to the treatment area. If cassettes are not used, then a puncture-resistant closed container should be used to transport instruments. This will prevent **cross-contamination,** or passing harmful substances indirectly between patients through unsterile equipment, procedures, or products. It will also prevent occupational exposure incidents. The container should be designated as biohazardous either by the color red or the biohazard symbol.

Advancing Technologies

As dental offices try to become eco-friendly, infection-control practices pose a challenge. Alternatives are still limited, but advances are anticipated. Manufacturers are aware of the need to "go green." It behooves them to develop products that are biodegradable, reusable, and recyclable, especially for DHCP who are conscientious and concerned about the environment. When purchasing products for the office, DHCP should determine which products are the best alternatives. It is anticipated that eco-friendly disinfectants, packaging, and other infection-control products will become available in the near future. ■

Cleaning and Decontamination

Once in the processing area, cleaning is the first step to removing **bioburden,** the number of viable organisms in or on an object or surface. Not removing it can interfere with microbial inactivation. If cleaning will be delayed, instruments should be placed in a puncture-resistant container or ultrasonic unit with a detergent or enzymatic cleaner to prevent body fluids and debris from drying on them. Otherwise, they should be immediately cleaned in an ultrasonic cleaner, instrument washer, or washer-disinfector (see Teamwork).

Ultrasonic cleaners are commonly used in private practices. They use electrical energy to generate sound waves that travel through the liquid (ultrasonic cleaner). Tiny bubbles are formed and continually burst or implode. This process disrupts the bonds that hold debris on the instruments.

Ultrasonic cleaners come in different sizes to accommodate individual instruments or instrument cassettes. Ultrasonic cleaners should be filled with cleaner before placing instruments and should never be turned on without liquid in them, because the unit could be damaged. Solution must cover the items being cleaned and should be changed at least daily. Visible debris indicates a need to change the solution sooner. When in operation, the lid needs to be on the unit to limit aerosols. The time needed to ultrasonically clean loose instruments is generally 3 to 6 minutes and is less than the time needed to clean instruments contained in cassettes, approximately 10 to 20 minutes. These times vary by manufacturer. Whether using a small unit or a large unit, instruments need to be rinsed, inspected, and dried.

Ultrasonic cleaners can be checked periodically for proper functioning. Manufacturers usually suggest holding aluminum foil in the ultrasonic cleaner vertically 1 inch above the bottom while activating the unit for 20 to 60 seconds. Upon examination, the foil should appear pitted. Areas that lack this effect may indicate a need for servicing.

Instrument washers may become a more acceptable method as dentistry moves toward being "eco-friendly." These units use water and can process more instruments. Washer-disinfectors have a high-temperature cycle to achieve high-level thermal disinfection and cleaning. Both types are regulated by the FDA.

Although hand-scrubbing instruments is not recommended because it creates more potential for injury and exposure, there are times when this method is unavoidable. DHCP should take steps to ensure safe instrument handling. In addition to PPE, heavy-duty gloves should be worn and a long-handled brush should be used to reduce spatter. The instruments should be scrubbed under clear water so they can be seen during the cleaning process.

Preparation, Packaging, and Sterilization Monitoring

After cleaning, instruments are prepared by visually inspecting them for cleanliness and drying them before being packaged. A variety of packaging materials such as bags, pouches, and wraps are available. They are usually plastic, paper, or a combination of both. Packaging must be suitable for the selected method of sterilization. Instrument packages should always be marked with the date and, in practices with more than one sterilizer, the sterilizer used.

Three types of monitoring should take place to ensure sterilization has occurred. The first is mechanical monitoring, which should take place with each load of instruments. This is the observation of the time, temperature, and pressure displays on the sterilizer.

The second type is internal and external chemical monitoring. An internal chemical indicator strip must be placed in each package or cassette (Fig. 7-13A). External chemical indicator tape should be placed on the outside packaging (Fig. 7-13b) if the internal strip cannot be viewed. Alternatively, packaging is available for purchase that has both internal and external chemical indicator markings incorporated into the package itself. Chemical indicators use sensitive chemicals to assess physical conditions during the sterilization process. The physical parameters that must be achieved for sterilization to occur may include temperature, time at the temperature, and pressure. The exact parameters vary depending on the method of sterilization used. Indicator strips used to monitor sterilization may test only one parameter or multiple parameters and should be selected according to the type of sterilizer used.[54,59] These strips should be inspected for color change following the sterilization cycle and then discarded. They **do not** verify sterility; rather, they indicate only that the packages have been through the process. These indicators provide immediate feedback and if they indicate a problem, the

Teamwork

The dental office employs two dental assistants. They primarily remove instrument cassettes, clean, disinfect, set up the dentist's operatories between patients, as well as assist the dentist. Today one of the assistants is out sick. The dentist's and hygienists' schedules are completely filled. In addition, two patients called the office with dental emergencies that need to be worked into the dentist's schedule. One of the hygienists notices that the assistant has not had time to sterilize cassettes or clean and disinfect one of the dentist's operatories. He tells the assistant that he has time to help with one of those chores. The assistant responds that the next patient has already been kept waiting and that preparing the operatory is currently the higher priority. The dental hygienist agrees to clean and set up the dentist's operatory so the assistant can take care of the instruments. ■

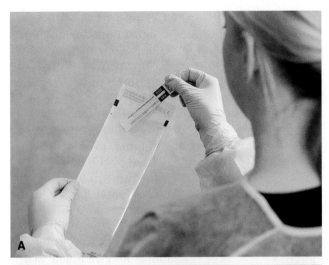

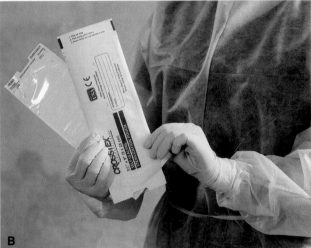

Figure 7-13. (A) Chemical indicator strip is placed in an autoclave bag. (B) External chemical indicator tape is placed on the exterior packaging.

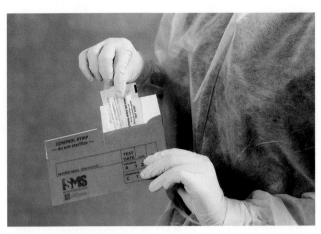

Figure 7-14. Spore check.

instruments in that load should be rewrapped and sterilized again.[59]

The third type of monitoring uses biological indicators or spore tests that are specific for each method of sterilization (Fig. 7-14). Moist heat: steam under pressure and chemical vapor sterilization use the microorganism *Geobacillus stearothermophilus;* it can come in vials, ampules, or strips for steam under pressure and in strips for chemical vapor. The biological indicator for dry heat is *Bacillus atrophaeus,* which comes in a strip.

Testing with biological indicators must be conducted weekly and documented. In addition, a control must be used. Equipment can be purchased to conduct in-office tests or an off-site monitoring service can be used. Off-site services will mail reports to the dental office for record-keeping purposes and notify the office immediately by phone if failure is indicated. In the event of a positive spore test, a review of all sterilization equipment and procedures should be conducted to identify and correct problems. Follow-up procedures are mechanical, chemical, and three consecutive biological monitoring tests in an empty sterilization chamber. Once the sterilizer has passed all testing it may return to routine use.[1,59]

Sterilization

After preparation and packaging, instruments are sterilized. Sterilization is the destruction or removal of all forms of life, specifically microorganisms, from materials or objects. Methods of sterilization used in dental offices are moist heat (steam under pressure), dry heat, and chemical vapor. The FDA regulates sterilization equipment.[54]

Moist Heat: Steam Under Pressure

Moist heat: steam under pressure, also known as autoclaving, destroys microorganisms by inactivation of essential cellular proteins or enzymes through coagulation. This method of sterilization is for items that are not sensitive to heat or moisture. Sterilization is achieved by the heat and steam; pressure serves only to attain high temperature. Distilled or deionized water is used to prevent mineral buildup in the sterilizer. Saturated steam must contact all items in the sterilizer at the required temperature and pressure for all microorganisms to be killed. Because of this, instruments must be carefully arranged and the autoclave should not be overloaded (Fig. 7-15). Manufacturer's operating

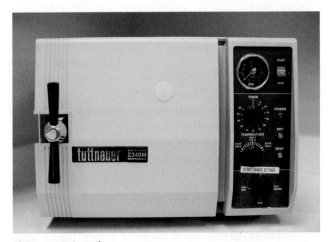

Figure 7-15. Autoclave.

temperatures and times should be followed. Common settings are 250°F (121°C) for 15 to 30 minutes or 270°F (132°C) for 3 to 10 minutes. Extra time must be allowed for warm-up and cool-down of the autoclave. Manufacturer's instructions should be consulted regarding heavy loads, different wrapping materials, and the nature of materials being sterilized. Daily maintenance includes checking the water level and washing trays and the interior of the chamber with a mild detergent. The filter or strainer should also be cleaned according to manufacturer's instructions. Weekly cleaning usually consists of flushing the chamber discharge system with a cleaning solution such as hot trisodium phosphate or a commercial cleaner. Instructions for its use should be carefully followed.

There are two types of steam sterilizers: gravity displacement and prevacuum steam sterilizers. Until recently, gravity displacement sterilizers were the most commonly used. However, the prevacuum steam sterilizer is becoming more popular in dental offices because of its smaller size.

In the gravity displacement sterilizer, steam is self-generated or is created by a steam generator. Because of the possibility of cool air pockets, some sterilizers have pressure-pulsing techniques to help remove air from the chamber before the cycle begins along with gravity-displacement techniques. Some models have a prevacuum cycle that removes air before the steam enters.

Prevacuum steam sterilizers have a pump that creates a vacuum in the chamber before steam enters. If an air-removal test is recommended for daily testing, it should be conducted before the first load is run to ensure it is working properly. This type of sterilizer is faster and allows more thorough steam penetration throughout the load. There is also a poststerilization vacuum cycle that facilitates faster drying.

Sterilized packages must be dry and cool before they are handled. Touching them before this can result in damage to the packaging and affect sterility. Covered or closed cabinets are recommended for storage to maintain the integrity of the packaging. Examine the wrapping before using the instruments. The instruments will remain sterile unless the packaging has become soiled or perforated, in which case the instruments should not be used until they have been cleaned, prepared, packaged, and resterilized. This is referred to as event-related shelf life. Another option is to use a date-related shelf life otherwise known as the "first in-first out" rule.[1]

Moist heat: steam under pressure has advantages. It is economical and efficient. Also, a variety of instruments can be sterilized by this method. Disadvantages are that the steam may cause corrosion or dulling of some instruments.

Dry-Heat Sterilization

Dry-heat sterilization uses dehydration to sterilize. Sterilization occurs when there is a transfer of heat energy to objects. This method is used for items that cannot be sterilized with moist heat: steam under pressure. The process requires higher temperatures and longer exposure to heat. Items must be thoroughly dried before they are placed in the sterilizer.

The two types of dry-heat sterilizers are static air and forced-air dry-heat sterilizers. The static-air sterilizer is oven-like and has heating coils on the bottom or in the sides. Heat rises through natural convection. This type of sterilizer requires 1 to 2 hours for sterilization at 320°F (160°C). The forced-air or rapid heat-transfer sterilizer circulates the heated air at a high velocity, allowing for a more rapid energy transfer from the air to the instruments. This shortens the time required for sterilization to 6 minutes at 375°F (190°C) for unpackaged items and to 12 to 20 minutes for packaged items. For either type, the times do not include warm-up or cooling. Similar to the autoclave, items should be carefully arranged with adequate space between packs. Manufacturer's instructions should be followed carefully. An advantage of this method is that dry heat is suitable for sharp instruments at the proper time and temperature. In addition, there is no corrosion as with moist heat: steam under pressure. Disadvantages are long exposure for static air and high heat for both types.

Chemical Vapor Sterilization

Unsaturated chemical vapor sterilizers use a mixture of chemicals and heat to sterilize instruments in a closed pressurized chamber. The chemicals used, including alcohols, water, and formaldehyde, are available through the manufacturer. Instruments must be dry before placing them in the sterilizer. The recommended time and temperature is usually 20 minutes at 270°F (132°C). Packages must be wrapped loosely so that the vapors can adequately penetrate. An advantage is that this method can sterilize in a relatively short period. There is a decreased possibility of corrosion and rusting because a small percentage of water is used in the mixture. Disadvantages are formaldehyde is considered a carcinogen, adequate ventilation is needed because of the chemicals, and there is a slight odor. Material safety data sheets (MSDSs) should be checked regarding the chemicals, and state and local regulations should be followed for proper disposal.

CHEMICAL DISINFECTANTS

Chemical disinfectants are regulated by the EPA and the FDA. Classification of these products is based on the level of germicidal activity and is described as high, intermediate, and low level. The level of disinfection necessary is determined by the manner in which an item is used and the degree of risk for cross-contamination. The Spaulding classification scheme helps put inanimate objects such as dental equipment into one of three categories: critical, semicritical, or noncritical (Table 7-7).

Table 7-7. *Classification of Dental Instruments and Equipment*

Category	Definition	Risk for Transmission	Sterilization or Disinfection	Examples
Critical	Instruments that penetrate soft tissue and bone	High	Heat sterilization	Curets Scalers Explorers Probes Scalpels
Semicritical	Instruments that contact but do not penetrate soft tissue and bone	Moderate	Heat sterilization (for heat-sensitive instruments high-level disinfection)	Radiograph film holding devices Dental mirrors Air/water syringe Ultrasonic scaler handpiece
Noncritical	Instruments or equipment that do not come in contact with mucous membranes but may contact skin	Low	Intermediate or low-level disinfection	Dental radiograph equipment (position indicating device) Lead apron Safety glasses Light handles Blood pressure cuff

Source: Adapted from Table 4 in Kohn WG, Collins AS, Cleveland JL, Harte JA, Eklund KJ, Malvitz DM; Centers for Disease Control and Prevention (CDC). Guidelines for infection control in dental health-care settings—2003. *MMWR Recomm Rep.* 2003;52(RR-17):1-61. Available from: http://www.cdc.gov/mmwr/preview/mmwrhtml/rr5217a1.htm#top

Critical items, as well as semicritical items that can withstand heat, are required to be heat-sterilized.[1]

High-level disinfectants inactivate spores, bacteria, fungi, and viruses. These products can be used as a sterilant or as a high-level disinfectant depending on the amount of time that the product is in contact with the instruments. The use of high-level disinfectants as cold sterilants is necessary for heat-sensitive, semicritical items (Table 7-8).[1] The FDA website provides a list of FDA-cleared products for processing reusable medical and dental instruments (http://www.fda.gov/MedicalDevices/DeviceRegulationandGuidance/ReprocessingofSingle-UseDevices/ucm133514.htm).

The manufacturer's instructions should be followed to determine the criteria needed for sterilization versus disinfection for a specific product. A disadvantage of chemical sterilization is that it is technique sensitive. The time recognized for sterilization on the label is for a specific temperature. Items must be completely submerged. Extended amounts of time are necessary to

Table 7-8. *Germicidal Activity for Disinfectants*

CDC Classification	FDA or EPA Registered Labeling	Recommendation	Examples
High	FDA sterilant or high-level disinfectant	Heat-sensitive items	Glutaraldehyde
Intermediate*	EPA hospital disinfectant with tuberculocidal claim	Surfaces that have been contaminated: dental unit surfaces and operatory countertops	Chlorine-containing compounds Iodophors Phenolics
Low*	EPA hospital disinfectant	General housekeeping purposes: floors and walls	Detergents

*The Environmental Protection Agency (EPA) does not use the terms *intermediate-* and *low-level disinfectants.*

CDC, Centers for Disease Control and Prevention; FDA, U.S. Food and Drug Administration.

Source: Adapted from Appendix C in Kohn WG, Collins AS, Cleveland JL, Harte JA, Eklund KJ, Malvitz DM; Centers for Disease Control and Prevention (CDC). Guidelines for infection control in dental health-care settings—2003. *MMWR Recomm Rep.* 2003;52(RR-17):1-61. Available from: http://www.cdc.gov/mmwr/preview/mmwrhtml/rr5217a4.htm

achieve sterilization with disinfection requiring less time. The product degrades with time and must be changed on a strict schedule, 5 to 30 days as indicated by the manufacturer's instructions, and biological monitoring is not possible. After removal from the chemical sterilant, items must be thoroughly rinsed, dried, and stored in clean packaging or a sterile container. For these reasons, heat-tolerant or disposable, semicritical items may be preferable.[60]

Intermediate disinfectants do not inactivate spores, but they will inactivate all other microorganisms such as mycobacteria, viruses, fungi, and vegetative bacteria. The EPA awards the term *hospital disinfectant* to any product in this category that has documented its ability to kill *Staphylococcus aureus*, *Salmonella enterica*, and *Pseudomonas aeruginosa*. Some products registered as hospital disinfectants by the EPA are also tuberculocidal and should be selected for use in dentistry.[1]

The low-level disinfectants destroy vegetative bacteria and lipid or medium-sized viruses. They do not destroy spores, mycobacteria, nonlipid or small viruses, or fungi. Low-level and intermediate-level disinfectants are used for noncritical items as well as environmental surface disinfection.[1]

The ideal disinfectant is broad and fast-acting across the antimicrobial spectrum, not affected by organic matter such as blood and saliva, nontoxic and nonallergenic, does not compromise equipment integrity, and has a residual antimicrobial effect on treated surfaces, meaning it remains effective for some time after contact.

The label on chemical disinfectants must state the shelf life, use life, and reuse life.

The shelf life is the date the product expires without opening the container. This means the product is no longer effective. The use life is the length of time the product will be effective after activation without being used for contaminated items. Lastly is the reuse life, which means the amount of time a product can be used and reused while it is challenged with contaminated instruments. The reuse life differs from the use life because it takes into account that instruments are wet and covered with bioburden.

DISPOSAL OF WASTE AND SHARPS

Dental practices generate regulated and nonregulated medical waste. It is important for DHCP to be knowledgeable about who regulates the waste at the national, state, and local levels.

The majority of waste generated in dental practices can be disposed of and managed as ordinary waste. Therefore, PPE (disposable gowns, masks, gloves), disposables or single-use items (lightly soiled gauze and cotton rolls, prophy angles, saliva ejectors, high-volume evacuator tips), and environmental barriers (plastic bags or wrap to cover equipment) can be disposed of in a regular office wastebasket.

Regulated medical waste is a small percentage of the total waste generated in a dental practice. A few examples of regulated waste are gauze saturated and dripping with blood or saliva, extracted teeth, surgically removed hard and soft tissues, scalpel blades, and needles. State and local regulations need to be consulted regarding disposal of extracted teeth that have amalgam restorations in them.

Sharps such as scalpel blades, needles, lancets, instruments, and broken glass must be disposed of in an approved sharps container that is puncture resistant, leak proof, and clearly labeled with the biohazard symbol (Fig. 7-16). These containers should be located close to the area where the items are used.

Nonsharp disposable items that are heavily soiled with body fluids should be disposed of in a biohazard bag, labeled, and prepared for disposal. This type of waste is usually removed, neutralized, and disposed of by a regulated medical waste hauler for an additional cost. It is important to check the credentials of the hauler to ensure proper handling of the waste.

Blood or other body fluids can usually be suctioned or poured down a utility sink, sewer, or toilet. Appropriate PPE should be worn by DHCP when either procedure is carried out. State and local regulations should be consulted to determine whether pretreatment is necessary for body fluids and if there is a limit on volume.[1]

An office waste management plan should be developed. The plan should clearly outline the following issues: (a) who will oversee the program, (b) who must be trained about handling and possible hazards, (c) what waste is nonregulated and regulated, (d) what PPE is needed for handling, (e) location for waste disposal, (f) proper packaging and labeling, (g) storage and disposal, and (h) record-keeping.[61]

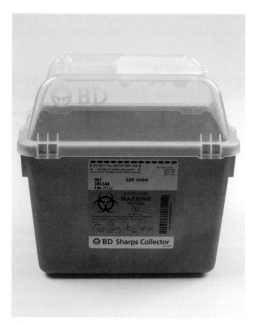

Figure 7-16. Biohazard symbol on a sharps container.

PREVENTIVE STEPS

Patient

Each patient's medical/dental history must be reviewed before providing any dental hygiene care. In some cases, a consult with a medical professional may be necessary. Some symptoms may be indicative of transmissible disease. If active disease is present, postponement of care may be necessary. Less aerosol-producing procedures may need to be considered for patients who are carriers of disease.

In addition to reviewing medical/dental histories, oral examinations should be performed. The presence of lesions may also be indicative of transmissible disease, for example, HSV. Because it is transmissible, a decision must be made to either treat or postpone treatment. Ideally, if it is not an emergency, treatment should be postponed. The rationale for deferral of treatment is to reduce the risk for **autoinoculation,** or spreading the disease to other areas on the patient's skin, eyes, and nostrils/nose.[62]

An antimicrobial mouthrinse is recommended before dental procedures especially when using ultrasonic scalers. The intention of a preprocedural rinse is to reduce the number of microorganisms in aerosols and spatter created during the appointment. This will also decrease contamination of clinical contact surfaces. It is unclear whether this practice decreases the number of microorganisms introduced into the bloodstream during invasive procedures.[1]

DENTAL HEALTH-CARE PERSONNEL

Health Maintenance

It is important for DHCP to maintain their health. By eating a nutritious diet, getting adequate sleep, exercising, and being up to date with vaccinations, DHCP are in a better position to resist disease and infection (Table 7-9).[63]

Hair

Hair is easily contaminated through procedures that produce aerosols and spatter. Hair must be kept away

---

Table 7-9. *Vaccination Recommendations for Health-Care Personnel*

Vaccines	Recommendations in Brief
Hepatitis B	If you do not have documented evidence of a complete hepatitis B vaccine series, or if you do not have an up-to-date blood test that shows you are immune to hepatitis B (i.e., no serological evidence of immunity or prior vaccination), then you should: • Get the three-dose series (dose 1 now, dose 2 in 1 month, dose 3 approximately 5 months after dose 2). • Get anti-HBs serological tested 1–2 months after dose 3.
Flu (influenza)	Get one dose of influenza vaccine annually.
MMR (measles, mumps, and rubella)	If you were born in 1957 or later and have not had the MMR vaccine, or if you do not have an up-to-date blood test that shows you are immune to measles or mumps (i.e., no serological evidence of immunity or prior vaccination), get two doses of MMR (one dose now and the second dose at least 28 days later). If you were born in 1957 or later and have not had the MMR vaccine, or if you do not have an up-to-date blood test that shows you are immune to rubella, only one dose of MMR is recommended. However, you may end up receiving two doses, because the rubella component is in the combination vaccine with measles and mumps. For health-care workers born before 1957, see the MMR Advisory Committee on Immunization Practices vaccine recommendations.
Varicella (chickenpox)	If you have not had chickenpox (varicella), if you have not had varicella vaccine, or if you do not have an up-to-date blood test that shows you are immune to varicella (i.e., no serological evidence of immunity or prior vaccination), get 2 doses of varicella vaccine, 4 weeks apart.
Tdap (tetanus, diphtheria, pertussis)	Get a one-time dose of Tdap as soon as possible if you have not received Tdap previously (regardless of when previous dose of Td was received). Get Td boosters every 10 years thereafter. Pregnant health-care workers need to get a dose of Tdap during each pregnancy.
Meningococcal	Those who are routinely exposed to isolates of *N. meningitidis* should get one dose.

Source: Recommended vaccines for healthcare workers. Atlanta, GA: CDC; 2014. Available from: http://www.cdc.gov/vaccines/adults/rec-vac/hcw.html. Accessed September 25, 2014.

from the face. If longer than collar length, hair should be pulled back and secured to prevent it from falling toward the patient and instruments in the care delivery area. Securing the hair eliminates the temptation to push back the hair while wearing examination gloves. Surgical bouffant caps can be worn to protect the hair. Facial hair such as beards and mustaches should be groomed to fit completely under a facial mask or shield. It is suggested that DHCP thoroughly wash their hair at the end of each workday because it is a source of cross-contamination.

Jewelry

Jewelry, especially watches and rings, should not be worn during clinical procedures. The only jewelry considered professionally acceptable is small earrings. There have been variable findings in studies on whether jewelry can transmit pathogenic microorganisms. However, wrist and finger jewelry can make it difficult to wash hands thoroughly and also don gloves efficiently and effectively. The jewelry can not only alter glove integrity while donning gloves, but also while performing procedures. Tears and small holes that are sometimes not visible can occur, providing an opportunity for body fluids to pass through the gloves. This can put DHCP at risk for disease transmission.

Hand Care: Fingernails and Skin

Hand care is especially important in the prevention of disease transmission. Proper hand-washing techniques must be used often during the workday. The majority of flora on the hands is found under and around the fingernails. Nails should be short enough to easily clean under them and well-manicured. Long nails have more surface area to keep clean and can have an effect on glove integrity. Hangnails can be a port of entry for pathogenic microorganisms.

Artificial nails and extensions are discouraged because they have been associated with fungal and bacterial infections. If worn, nail polish should be freshly applied to short nails. Chipped nail polish has been known to harbor microorganisms.

The skin is an effective barrier to prevent disease transmission. However, repeated hand washing and hand sanitizing can damage the skin, providing another port of entry for pathogenic microorganisms. Hands should be thoroughly rinsed and dried after washing with either a nonantimicrobial or an antimicrobial soap. Hands should be completely dry after hand sanitizing with an alcohol-based hand rub. These steps should be followed before donning gloves and after glove removal.

Hand Lotions

Lotions can reduce dermatitis and other skin irritations. However, the ingredients of any lotion should be evaluated carefully. To determine whether a product will cause interactions with other products used in dentistry, consult the manufacturer or obtain an MSDS. Some products may interfere with glove integrity. Petroleum-based products have been known to weaken latex and make them permeable to body fluids. Because lotions may affect gloves, it is best to apply them at the end of the day.

Selection, Storage, and Dispensing of Hand Hygiene Products

DHCP should select hand hygiene products that are effective, not offensive in smell, and less irritating to the skin. The selected products need to be protected from contamination. Containers for liquid products should be either disposable or washable containers. Washable containers impact the environment less in terms of waste. Hand hygiene products should not be added to, or "topped off," when partially full because of the possibility of microbial contamination. Instead, the container should be emptied, thoroughly washed, and dried before refilling. Manufacturer's instructions must be followed regarding appropriate use, storage, and dispensing of the product.

Nonantimicrobial or antimicrobial hand hygiene products should be selected according to need. Nonantimicrobial soap can be used to remove soil, transient microorganisms, and glove powder from the skin. The purpose of antimicrobial agents is to remove or destroy transient microorganisms and reduce resident flora of the skin. Products made with active ingredients that have **substantivity,** the ability to remain on the skin after rinsing and drying to inhibit the growth of bacteria, are beneficial and provide an additional barrier.

Active ingredients that have been used in hand hygiene agents are alcohol, chlorhexidine gluconate, chloroxylenol parachlorometaxylenol (PCMX), hexachlorophene, iodine and iodophors, quaternary ammonium, and triclosan. When selecting an agent, performance activity should be evaluated. Agents should be broad spectrum, persistent (i.e., extended activity that prevents or inhibits survival of microorganisms after the product is applied), and fast-acting.[1,64]

Alcohol-containing preparations containing between 60% and 95% ethanol or isopropanol are most effective. An alcohol-based hand rub should only be used when hands are not visibly soiled. They are germicidal but do not provide a **residual** or persistent effect. To achieve a persistent effect, they should include an antiseptic.

Chlorhexidine gluconate was introduced into the United States in the 1970s. It has substantial residual activity and for the most part has been used safely. There is no or minimal absorption through the skin. Skin irritation has been concentration dependent, and allergic reactions have been uncommon. Protective eyewear should be in place when using the product because it can cause conjunctivitis and severe corneal damage if a splash occurs.

Chloroxylenol PCMX has been widely used in the United States. It is available in 0.3% to 3.75% concentrations. It has been minimally affected by the presence of organic debris. PCMX is absorbed through the skin, but allergic reactions are uncommon.

Hexachlorophene 3% was used in the 1950s and 1960s as a hygienic hand wash and surgical scrub and for routine bathing of infants. It has a residual effect, but it has been known to cause neurotoxicity in infants. In 1972, the FDA said that it could no longer be used to bathe infants.

Iodine is one of the oldest antiseptics; however, it has drawbacks. It can be irritating and produce allergic reactions. Iodophor has replaced iodine as an active ingredient in hand hygiene preparations. The preparations contain between 7.5% and 10% povidone-iodine. Even with iodophor there are more cases of contact dermatitis than with other preparations.

Quaternary ammonium has been seldom used for hand antisepsis during the past 15 to 20 years in the United States. It tended to be well tolerated, but contamination was an issue. More research is needed on newer formulations that are being considered for HCP.

Triclosan was introduced in the 1960s and is used in concentrations ranging from 0.2% to 2%. It has been well tolerated, but contamination has been a concern. The FDA and the EPA are planning to collaborate on studies to further understand endocrine-related effects, toxicologic effects, human relevance, and the doses at which any effects occur. This research is needed to determine the continued use of the agent in hand hygiene products.[65]

Hand Hygiene Methods

There are four different methods for hand hygiene: routine hand wash, antiseptic hand wash (Box 7-2), antiseptic hand rub, and surgical antisepsis. Both the routine hand wash and the antiseptic hand wash (Fig. 7-17) are performed using water for 15 seconds; plain soap is used for the routine hand wash and antimicrobial soap is used for the antiseptic hand wash. The antiseptic hand rub is performed with an alcohol-based agent and the hands

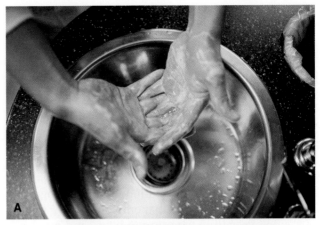

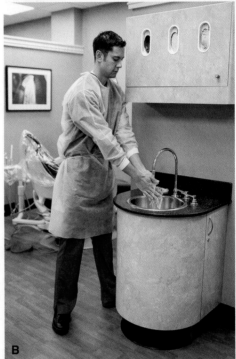

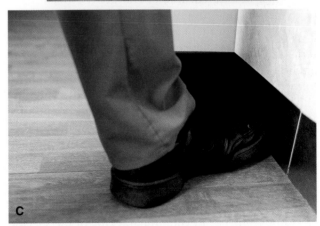

Figure 7-17. Antiseptic hand wash at foot-controlled sink.

are rubbed until the agent is dry. Surgical antisepsis is performed for 2 to 6 minutes with either water and antimicrobial soap, or water and nonantimicrobial soap followed by an alcohol-based surgical hand-scrub product with persistent activity.[1]

Box 7-2. *Antiseptic Hand Wash*

Remove jewelry from hands and wrists. Using cool, running water, premoisten nails, fingers, and hands. Following application of antimicrobial soap, achieve a lather and clean under all nails, then vigorously rub hands together interlacing fingers for 15 seconds. Thoroughly rinse antimicrobial soap from nails, fingers, and hands. Using disposable paper towels, dry each hand completely. Discard each paper towel directly into a waste container immediately after use. To maintain the antiseptic technique, the last paper towel used should be used to turn off the faucet if a hands-free mechanism is not available.[1] ■

DHCP should select the method that is most appropriate for the procedure being performed and the degree of contamination. Some procedures may indicate a need for persistent antimicrobial action on the skin; therefore, an antimicrobial agent that will provide a persistent effect should be selected. Manufacturer's instructions should be consulted.

EXPOSURE CONTROL PLANS

OSHA standard 1910.1030, Bloodborne Pathogens,[66] details the responsibilities that employers have to protect employees from exposure to blood and other potentially infectious materials. The key requirement of the standard is the preparation of an exposure control plan. Critical elements of the plan include:

1. Exposure determination
2. Office personnel or an appointed staff person must determine which employees have a high, medium, or low risk for occupational exposure. Risk is determined without considering any protection the employee may be provided.
3. A description of how the provision of the standards will be implemented, including a schedule of when each step will occur. Included are:
   a. Methods to prevent contact with blood or other potentially infectious materials, including general steps to prevent transmissions along with specific task-related methods of eliminating or minimizing employee exposure. The latter includes ECs and WPCs. PPE must be provided by the employer.
   b. Hepatitis B vaccination
   c. Office personnel who have occupational exposure must be offered, free of charge, the hepatitis B vaccination series
   d. Exposure incident reports
   e. When an employee has been exposed to blood or other potentially infectious material, she must clean the wound and report the incident immediately to her employer (Table 7-10). The employer must document the circumstances under which the exposure occurred. This incident report must include the manner by which the employee was exposed, the protective barriers worn at the time, and the specific actions of the employee at the time of exposure. The employee is directed to a health-care professional for evaluation and testing.[1,11,13,67–70] Beyond the tracking of the specific event, review of incident reports provides valuable insights for both additional training and potential revision of WPCs.

Training of employees is required and must be conducted by a qualified individual on an annual basis. Employees must be informed of possible hazards from body fluids and how they can protect themselves by wearing PPE. When training is conducted, participants must be provided an opportunity to discuss and ask questions. Training must be conducted for new employees before working.[71]

RECORD-KEEPING AND DOCUMENTATION

OSHA requires that employee training and medical records be kept for all employees subject to occupational exposure. Documentation of training must include the dates of training, content of the sessions, names and qualifications of those conducting the training, and names and job titles of all employees attending the session.

Each dental office must also maintain medical records of employees, including:

1. Name and social security number
2. Hepatitis B vaccination status, including the dates of all the hepatitis B vaccinations and any medical records relative to the employee's ability to receive vaccination
3. A copy of all results of examinations, medical testing, and follow-up procedures related to exposure incidents

These medical records must be kept confidential. They cannot be disclosed or reported without the employee's express written consent to any person within or outside the workplace except as may be required by law. The office must maintain these records for at least 30 years beyond the employee's last date of service.[66]

Other infection-control documents and records include the following:

- A TB infection-control plan is recommended by the CDC. The plan must ensure prompt detection, airborne precautions, and treatment of persons who have suspected or confirmed TB disease.[72]
- State and local regulations must be followed regarding sterilization. A sterilization log must be maintained for the office. Each sterilizer should be identified by serial number, and malfunctions and repairs need to be documented. A protocol is needed for the management of sterilization failures. In addition, mechanical and chemical monitoring must be performed daily. Biological monitoring should be performed and documented weekly to ensure effectiveness of sterilization. The person conducting the testing must be identified.[73]
- Records for the treatment and final disposal of regulated waste must be maintained. Offices should confirm that the waste transporter is EPA approved. Also, paperwork should include the identifying contractor

Table 7-10. *Exposure Incident*

Disease	Initial Intervention, Baseline and Follow-up Testing	Screening Test	PEP	Risk From Occupational Exposure
HIV	**Urgent medical concern** If stuck by a needle or other sharp, or get blood or other potentially infectious materials in eyes, nose, mouth, or on broken skin: • Immediately flood the exposed area with water and clean wound with soap and water or a skin disinfectant if available. • Report this immediately to employer. • Seek immediate medical attention.	Blood Rapid test is available HIV-antibody testing by enzyme immunoassay should be used to monitor HCP for seroconversion for more than 6 months after occupational HIV exposure	Basic 4-week regimen: • Two drugs for most HIV exposures • Three drugs for expanded regimen for HIV exposures that pose an increased risk for transmission HCP with occupational exposure to HIV should receive follow-up counseling, postexposure testing, and medical evaluation regardless of whether they receive PEP.	Low
Hepatitis B	National Clinicians' PEP telephone hotline: 888-448-4911 After baseline testing at the time of exposure, follow-up testing should be considered at: • 6 weeks • 12 weeks • 6 months	Blood	If not previously vaccinated or inadequate vaccine response, hepatitis B immune globulin and/or hepatitis B vaccine should be considered.	23%–62% if not vaccinated
Hepatitis C	Risk for infection if exposed depends on: • Inoculums size • Route of exposure • Susceptibility of DHCP	Blood	No recommended PEP Refer to specialist for medical management. If HCV is detected early, consideration may be given to antiviral therapy.	Low*—average incidence of seroconversion after percutaneous exposure from HCV-positive source is 1.8%

*Risk is low if there is not a large volume of blood.
DHCP, dental health-care personnel; HCP, health-care personnel; PEP, postexposure prophylaxis.

number. Receipts from the hauler for removal of waste should be kept on file. The waste-removal company should inform the office about the treatment and the final site of disposal.[74]

• Every office should have a written hazard communication program. OSHA's Hazard Communication Standard specifies that certain information must be included on an MSDS. A 16-section MSDS is becoming the international norm, and ANSI recommends a format in which the information of greatest concern to employees is at the top of the sheet.[75] OSHA 1910.1200(g)(6)(i) and 1910.1200(g)(7)(i) mandate that chemical manufacturers, importers, and distributors ensure that employers are provided an MSDS with the initial shipment and the first shipment following an update.[76] Often, companies also make them available on their websites. MSDSs should be obtained for all hazardous chemicals in the office and maintained in a binder located in a common area. Furthermore, a list of chemicals kept in the office should be compiled and the chemicals should be labeled. All employees should receive formal training.[77]

Case Study

Dr. William Jones recently obtained his dental license. He is about to purchase a practice and is interviewing you for a dental hygiene position. If hired, you would also be the compliance officer. You would need to develop the exposure control plan for the office and be knowledgeable about infection-control guidelines for dentistry.

Case Study Exercises

1. Which of the following statements is correct according to OSHA's Bloodborne Pathogens Standard?
   A. You can use the exposure control plan already present in the office from the previous dentist.
   B. You should develop an exposure control plan, then review and update it annually.
   C. As the compliance officer for the facility, you should keep the document in your possession and staff should ask you if they have questions.
   D. You should develop an exposure control plan, then review and update it when the CDC releases updated infection-control guidelines.

2. As a Registered Dental Hygienist, one of your qualifications to be the compliance officer is that:
   A. You look at the medical histories of all of the patients.
   B. You have a college degree in a health-related discipline.
   C. You provide direct patient care and are potentially exposed to injuries from contaminated sharps.
   D. You have time to review the plan regularly when patients cancel or break their appointments.

3. Implementation of a one-handed, scoop method of needle recapping is which type of control?
   A. Work-practice control
   B. Engineering control
   C. Universal control
   D. Standard control

4. In the Spaulding classification, a Gracey curette fits which category?
   A. An environmental item
   B. A noncritical item
   C. A semicritical item
   D. A critical item

5. An employee has punctured a gloved finger with a sharp scaler when caring for a patient and is experiencing heavy bleeding. What is the appropriate postexposure protocol?
   A. Remove the gloves, rinse the finger with water, place a bandage on it, and reglove.
   B. Call 911, remove the gloves, wash with soap and water, bandage the finger, and wait for paramedics to arrive.
   C. Remove the gloves, wash your hands with soap and water, and refrain from providing further care for the day.
   D. Remove the gloves, wash the finger thoroughly, bandage the finger, ask the patient if he or she is willing to be tested for HIV, hepatitis B, and hepatitis C, and depending on the patient's response, determine the next step.

Review Questions

1. Which of the following hepatitis viruses has no available vaccine (directly or indirectly) to prevent its transmission?
   A. Hepatitis A
   B. Hepatitis B
   C. Hepatitis C
   D. Hepatitis D

2. The Occupational Safety and Health Administration (OSHA) protects:
   A. The environment
   B. Employers
   C. Employees
   D. Water reservoirs

3. Which of the following agencies provides guidelines for exposure control plans?
   A. Occupational Safety and Health Administration (OSHA)
   B. Centers for Disease Control and Prevention (CDC)
   C. Organization for Safety and Asepsis Procedures (OSAP)
   D. Environmental Protection Agency (EPA)

4. Microbial load or organic material on a surface or object before disinfection or sterilization is called:
   A. Germicide
   B. Asepsis
   C. Resident flora
   D. Bioburden

5. Which statement is true for chemical indicators?
   A. Verify that sterilization has occurred.
   B. Assess time and temperature but do not verify sterilization.
   C. They are not necessary in every package of instruments.
   D. They are not necessary if a biological indicator is used once a week.

Active Learning

1. Place aluminum foil in the ultrasonic cleaner to comprehend the bubbles imploding debris.
2. Take a picture of a patient care area and mark each area that needs to be cleaned or disinfected and/or requires a barrier.
3. Design an instrument processing area and outline the steps to be accomplished in each area.
4. Watch "If Saliva Were Red Training DVD" (available online at: www.osap.org).
5. Develop an exposure control plan. ■

REFERENCES

1. Kohn WG, Collins AS, Cleveland JL, Harte JA, Eklund KJ, Malvitz DM; Centers for Disease Control and Prevention (CDC). Guidelines for infection control in dental health-care settings—2003. *MMWR Recomm Rep.* 2003;52(RR-17):1-61. http://www.cdc.gov/mmwr/preview/mmwrhtml/rr5217a1.htm#top.
2. Harrel S, Molinari J. Aerosols and splatter in dentistry: a brief review of the literature and infection control implications. *J Am Dent Assoc.* 2004;135:429-437. http://jada.org/cgi/content/full/135/4/429.
3. Hamann B. *Disease Identification, Prevention, and Control.* 3rd ed. Boston: McGraw Hill; 2007:42.
4. Hamann B. *Disease Identification, Prevention, and Control.* 3rd ed. Boston: McGraw Hill, 2007:40.
5. Cottrell R, Girvan J, McKenzie J. *Principles and Foundations of Health Promotion and Education.* 4th ed. San Francisco: Pearson Benjamin Cummings; 2009:20.
6. National Institute of Allergy and Infectious Diseases (NIAID). HIV/AIDS: what are HIV and AIDS? Bethesda, MD: NIAID. http://www.niaid.nih.gov/topics/HIVAIDS/Understanding/Pages/whatAreHIVAIDS.aspx. Updated April 3, 2012. Accessed May 19, 2013.
7. Centers for Disease Control and Prevention (CDC). HIV transmission. Atlanta, GA: CDC. http://www.cdc.gov/hiv/basics/transmission.html. Updated May 14, 2013. Accessed May 19, 2013.
8. National Institute of Allergy and Infectious Diseases (NIAID). HIV/AIDS: prevention. Bethesda, MD: NIAID. http://www.niaid.nih.gov/topics/hivaids/understanding/prevention/Pages/prevention.aspx. Updated April 28, 2009. Accessed May 19, 2013.
9. Centers for Disease Control and Prevention (CDC). Blood safety. Atlanta, GA: CDC. http://www.cdc.gov/bloodsafety/basics.html. Updated January 31, 2013. Accessed May 19, 2013.
10. Beers M, Porter R, Jones T, Kaplan J, Berkwits M, eds. *The Merck Manual.* 18th ed. Whitehouse Station, NJ: Merck Research Laboratories; 2006:1625.
11. Panlilio AL, Cardo DM, Grohskopf LA, Heneine W, Ross CS; U.S. Public Health Service. Updated U.S. Public Health Service guidelines for the management of occupational exposures to HIV and recommendations for postexposure prophylaxis. *MMWR Recomm Rep.* 2005;54(RR09):1-17. http://www.cdc.gov/mmwr/preview/mmwrhtml/rr5409a1.htm. Accessed May 19, 2013.
12. The Body, the Complete HIV/AIDS Resource. Side effects chart. http://www.thebody.com/content/art1210.html. Updated March/April 2012. Accessed May 19, 2013.
13. Chapman LE, Sullivent EE, Grohskopf LA, et al; Centers for Disease Control and Prevention (CDC). Recommendations for postexposure interventions to prevent infection with hepatitis B virus, hepatitis C virus, or human immunodeficiency virus, and tetanus in persons wounded during bombings and similar mass-casualty events—United States, 2008. *MMWR Recomm Rep.* 2008;57(RR06):1-19. http://www.cdc.gov/mmwr/preview/mmwrhtml/rr5706a1.htm. Accessed May 19, 2013.
14. Centers for Disease Control and Prevention (CDC). Hepatitis A FAQ's for health professionals. Atlanta, GA: CDC. http://www.cdc.gov/hepatitis/HAV/HAVfaq.htm#general. Updated August 4, 2011. Accessed May 19, 2013.
15. Centers for Disease Control and Prevention (CDC). Hepatitis B information for health professionals. Atlanta, GA: CDC. http://www.cdc.gov/hepatitis/HBV/HBVfaq.htm#overview. Updated January 31, 2012. Accessed May 19, 2013.
16. Leuridan E, Van Damme P. Hepatitis B and the need for a booster dose. *Clin Infect Dis.* 2011;53:68-75. http://cid.oxfordjournals.org/content/53/1/68.full.pdf+html. Accessed May 19, 2013.
17. Kamili S, Krawczynski K, McCaustland K, Li X, Alter MJ. Infectivity of hepatitis C virus in plasma after drying and storing at room temperature. *Infect Control Hosp Epidemiol.* 2007;28:519-524.
18. Patel PR, Larson AK, Castel AD, et al. Hepatitis C virus infections from a contaminated radiopharmaceutical used in myocardial perfusion studies. *JAMA.* 2006;296:2005-2011.
19. Centers for Disease Control and Prevention (CDC). Hepatitis C FAQ's for the public. Atlanta, GA: CDC. http://www.cdc.gov/hepatitis/hepatitis/c/cfaq.htm#cFAQ36. Updated October 22, 2012. Accessed May 29, 2013.
20. Molinari JA, Harte JA. *Practical infection control in dentistry.* 3rd ed. Philadelphia, PA: Lippincott Williams & Wilkins; 2010.
21. Centers for Disease Control and Prevention (CDC). Hepatitis C FAQ's for health professionals. Atlanta, GA: CDC. http://www.cdc.gov/hepatitis/HCV/HCVfaq.htm#f1. Updated May 7, 2013. Accessed. May 19, 2013.
22. Centers for Disease Control and Prevention (CDC). Hepatitis C FAQ's for health professionals. Atlanta, GA: CDC. http://www.cdc.gov/hepatitis/HCV/HCVfaq.htm#b1. Updated May 7, 2013. Accessed May 19, 2013.
23. Centers for Disease Control and Prevention (CDC). Hepatitis E FAQ's for health professionals. Atlanta, GA: CDC. http://www.cdc.gov/hepatitis/HEV/HEVfaq.htm#. Updated September 17, 2012. Accessed May 19, 2013.
24. World Health Organization. Hepatitis E. Geneva: WHO. http://www.who.int/mediacentre/factsheets/fs280/en. Updated 2012. Accessed May 19, 2013.
25. Centers for Disease Control and Prevention (CDC). Genital herpes–CDC factsheet. Atlanta, GA: CDC. http://www.cdc.gov/std/herpes/STDFact-herpes-detailed.htm. Updated February 13, 2013. Accessed May 19, 2013.
26. Hamann B. *Disease identification, prevention, and control.* 3rd ed. Boston: McGraw Hill, 2007.

27. Miller C, Cunningham L, Lindroth J, Avdiushiko S. The efficacy of valacyclovir in preventing recurrent herpes simplex virus infections associated with dental procedures. *J Am Dent Assoc.* 2004;35:1311-1318. http://jada.ada.org/cgi/reprint/135/9/1311?maxtoshow=&hits=10&RESULTFORMAT=1&author1=miller&author2=cunningham&andorexacttitle=and&andorexacttitleabs=and&andorexactfulltext=and&searchid=1&FIRSTINDEX=0&sortspec=relevance&resourcetype=HWCIT. Accessed March 29, 2010.

28. Harpaz R, Ortega-Sanchez IR, Seward JF; Advisory Committee on Immunization Practices (ACIP) Centers for Disease Control and Prevention (CDC). Prevention of herpes zoster recommendations of the Advisory Committee on Immunization Practices (ACIP). *MMWR Recomm Rep.* 2008;57(Early Release):1-30. http://www.cdc.gov/mmwr/preview/mmwrhtml/rr57e0515a1.htm. Accessed May 19, 2013.

29. Centers for Disease Control and Prevention (CDC). Epstein-Barr virus and infectious mononucleosis. Atlanta, GA: CDC. http://www.cdc.gov/ncidod/diseases/ebv.htm. Updated May 16, 2006. Accessed May 19, 2013.

30. Walling D. Oral hairy leukoplakia: an Epstein-Barr virus-associated disease of patients with HIV. http://www.thebody.com/content/art16898.html. Published December 2000. Accessed May 19, 2013.

31. Centers for Disease Control and Prevention (CDC). Cytomegalovirus (CMV) and congenital CMV infection. Atlanta, GA: CDC. http://www.cdc.gov/cmv/overview.html. Updated December 6, 2010. Accessed May 19, 2013.

32. Mayo Clinic. Cytomegalovirus (CMV) infection. Bethesda, MD: Mayo Clinic. http://www.mayoclinic.com/health/cmv/DS00938/DSECTION=prevention. Updated April 30, 2011. Accessed May 19, 2013.

33. Centers for Disease Control and Prevention (CDC). Cytomegalovirus: protect your baby. Atlanta, GA: CDC. http://www.cdc.gov/features/cytomegalovirus/. Updated June 18, 2012. Accessed May 19, 2013.

34. Centers for Disease Control and Prevention (CDC). Congenital CMV infection. Atlanta, GA: CDC. http://www.cdc.gov/cmv/congenital-infection.html. Updated December 6, 2010. Accessed May 19, 2013.

35. Beers M, Porter R, Jones T, Kaplan J, Berkwits M, eds. *The Merck Manual.* 18th ed. Whitehouse Station, NJ: Merck Research Laboratories; 2006:1612.

36. Mayo Clinic. Roseola: symptoms. Bethesda, MD: Mayo Clinic. http://www.mayoclinic.com/health/roseola/DS00452/DSECTION=symptoms. Updated June 29, 2012. Accessed May 19, 2013.

37. Mayo Clinic. Roseola: treatment and drugs. Bethesda, MD: Mayo Clinic. http://www.mayoclinic.com/health/roseola/DS00452/DSECTION=treatments-and-drugs. Updated June 29, 2012. Accessed May 19, 2013.

38. Mayo Clinic. Roseola: prevention. Bethesda, MD: Mayo Clinic. http://www.mayoclinic.com/health/roseola/DS00452/DSECTION=prevention. Updated June 29, 2012. Accessed May 19, 2013.

39. Beers M, Porter R, Jones T, Kaplan J, Berkwits M, eds. *The Merck Manual.* 18th ed. Whitehouse Station, NJ: Merck Research Laboratories; 2006:1024.

40. Centers for Disease Control and Prevention (CDC). Tuberculosis (TB) fact sheet: treatment options for latent tuberculosis infection. Atlanta, GA; CDC. http://www.cdc.gov/tb/publications/factsheets/treatment/LTBItreatmentoptions.htm. Updated January 20, 2012. Accessed May 27, 2013.

41. Centers for Disease Control and Prevention (CDC). Tuberculosis (TB) fact sheet: treatment of drug-susceptible tuberculosis disease in persons not infected with HIV. Atlanta, GA; CDC. http://www.cdc.gov/tb/publications/factsheets/treatment/treatmentHIVnegative.htm. Updated June 15, 2012. Accessed May 27, 2013.

42. Centers for Disease Control and Prevention (CDC). Tuberculosis (TB) fact sheet: the difference between latent TB infection and active TB disease. Atlanta, GA: CDC; 2012. http://www.cdc.gov/tb/publications/factsheets/general/ltbiandactivetb.htm. Reviewed September 1, 2012. Accessed May 27, 2013.

43. American Dental Association (ADA). Statement on the treatment of patients with infectious diseases of uncertain transmission. Chicago: ADA. http://www.ada.org/1858.aspx. Published 2012. Accessed May 27, 2013.

44. Centers for Disease Control and Prevention (CDC). Tuberculosis (TB) fact sheet: tuberculin skin testing. Atlanta, GA: CDC. http://www.cdc.gov/tb/publications/factsheets/testing/skintesting.htm. Reviewed 2012. Accessed May 27, 2013.

45. Centers for Disease Control and Prevention (CDC). Tuberculosis (TB): testing & diagnosis. Atlanta, GA: CDC. http://www.cdc.gov/tb/topic/testing/. Updated 2013. Accessed May 27, 2013.

46. Bolyard EA; Hospital Infection Control Practices Advisory Committee. Guidelines for infection control in health care personnel, 1998. *Am J Infect Control.* 1998;26:289-354. http://www.cdc.gov/hicpac/pdf/InfectControl98.pdf.

47. Centers for Disease Control and Prevention (CDC). About CDC: CDC organization. Atlanta, GA: CDC. http://www.cdc.gov/about/organization/cio.htm. Updated April 14, 2014. Accessed July 21, 2014.

48. American National Standards Institute (ANSI). About ANSI: overview. Washington, DC: ANSI. http://www.ansi.org/about_ansi/overview/overview.aspx?menuid=1. Accessed May 27, 2013.

49. Environmental Protection Agency (EPA). About EPA. Washington, DC: EPA. http://www2.epa.gov/aboutepa. Updated May 16, 2013. Accessed May 27, 2013.

50. U.S. Food and Drug Administration (FDA). Inspections, compliance, enforcement, and criminal investigations vision/mission/values. Silver Spring, MD: FDA. http://www.fda.gov/ICECI/Inspections/IOM/ucm124442.htm. Updated February 29, 2012. Accessed May 27, 2013.

51. U.S. Food and Drug Administration (FDA). Medical devices: FDA-cleared sterilants and high level disinfectants with general claims for processing reusable medical and dental devices—March 2009 . Silver Spring, MD: FDA. http://www.fda.gov/MedicalDevices/DeviceRegulationandGuidance/ReprocessingofSingle-UseDevices/ucm133514.htm. Updated April 26, 2009. Accessed May 27, 2013.

52. Organization for Safety and Asepsis Protocol. About OSAP. Annapolis, MD: OSAP. http://www.osap.org/?AboutOSAPAbout. Accessed May 27, 2013.

53. Molinari JA, Harte JA. *Practical Infection Control in Dentistry.* 3rd ed. Philadelphia, PA: Lippincott Williams & Wilkins; 2010:111.

54. Centers for Disease Control and Prevention (CDC). Guideline for disinfection and sterilization in healthcare

facilities, 2008. Atlanta, GA: CDC. http://www.cdc.gov/hicpac/pdf/guidelines/disinfection_nov_2008.pdf. Accessed May 27, 2013.

55. American Dental Association (ADA). Statement on dental unit waterlines. Chicago: ADA. http://www.ada.org/1856.aspx. Updated April 2012. Accessed May 27, 2013.

56. Centers for Disease Control and Prevention (CDC). Infection control in dental settings: saliva ejector. Atlanta, GA: CDC. http://www.cdc.gov/oralhealth/infectioncontrol/faq/saliva.htm. Reviewed September 22, 2009. Accessed May 27, 2013.

57. USAF Dental Evaluation and Consultation Service. USAF guidelines for infection prevention & control in dentistry. http://www.afms.af.mil/shared/media/document/AFD-130404-207.pdf. Published January 2012. Accessed May 27, 2013.

58. Molinari J. Infection control going green: oncoming reality? Part 2. RDH. http://www.dentaleconomics.com/articles/print/volume-99/issue-4/columns/emerging-infection-control-challenges/infection-control-going-green-oncoming-reality-part-2.html. Published April 29, 2009. Accessed May 27, 2013.

59. Centers for Disease Control and Prevention (CDC). Infection control in dental settings: sterilization—monitoring. Atlanta, GA: CDC. http://www.cdc.gov/oralhealth/infectioncontrol/faq/sterilization_monitoring.htm. Modified September 9, 2011. Accessed May 27, 2013.

60. Miller CH, Palenick CJ. *Infection Control and Management of Hazardous Materials for the Dental Team.* 4th ed. St. Louis, MO: Mosby Elsevier, 2010:163-166.

61. Molinari JA, Harte JA. *Practical Infection Control in Dentistry.* 3rd ed. Philadelphia: Lippincott Williams & Wilkins; 2010.

62. Siegel MA. Diagnosis and management of recurrent herpes simplex infections. *J Am Dent Assoc.* 2002;133:1245-1249. http://jada.ada.org/cgi/reprint/133/9/1245. Accessed March 29, 2013.

63. Recommended vaccines for healthcare workers. Atlanta, GA: CDC. http://www.cdc.gov/vaccines/adults/rec-vac/hcw.html. Updated April 15, 2014. Accessed September 25, 2014.

64. Boyce JM, Pittet D; Healthcare Infection Control Practices Advisory Committee; HICPAC/SHEA/APIC/IDSA Hand Hygiene Task Force. Guideline for Hand Hygiene in Health-Care Settings Recommendations of the Healthcare Infection Control Practices Advisory Committee and the HICPAC/SHEA/APIC/IDSA Hand Hygiene Task Force. *MMWR Recomm Rep.* 2002;51(RR16):1-44. http://www.cdc.gov/mmwr/preview/mmwrhtml/rr5116a1.htm. Accessed May 27, 2013.

65. Environmental Protection Agency (EPA). Pesticides reregistration: triclosan facts. Washington, DC: EPA. http://www.epa.gov/oppsrrd1/REDs/factsheets/triclosan_fs.htm. Updated May 9, 2012. Accessed May 27, 2013.

66. U.S. Department of Labor, Occupational Safety and Health Administration. Standard 29 CFR Part 1910.1030. Occupational Safety and Health Standards, Toxic and Hazardous Substances, Bloodborne pathogens. 56 FR 64004, Dec. 06, 1991, as amended at 57 FR 12717, Apr 13, 1992; 57 FR 29206, Jul 1, 1992; 61 FR 5507, Feb. 13, 1996; 66 FR 5325 Jan., 18, 2001; 71 FR 16672 and 16673, Apr 3, 2006; 73 FR 75586, Dec. 12, 2008; 76 FR 33608, June 8, 2011; 76 FR 80740, Dec. 27, 2011; 77 FR 19934, April 3, 2012. http://www.osha.gov/pls/oshaweb/owadisp.show_document?p_table=STANDARDS&p_id=10051. Accessed May 27, 2013.

67. U.S. Department of Labor, Occupational Safety and Health Administration. Bloodborne pathogens and needlestick prevention post-exposure evaluation. http://www.osha.gov/SLTC/bloodbornepathogens/evaluation.html. Accessed May 27, 2013.

68. Smith DK, Grohskopf LA, Black RJ, et al; U.S. Department of Health and Human Services. Antiretroviral postexposure prophylaxis after sexual, injection-drug use, or other nonoccupational exposure to HIV in the United States. *MMWR Recomm Rep.* 2005;54(RR02):1-20. http://www.cdc.gov/mmwr/preview/mmwrhtml/rr5402a1.htm. Accessed May 27, 2013.

69. Glick M. Rapid HIV testing in the dental setting. *J Am Dent Assoc.* 2005;136(9):1206-1208. http://jada.ada.org/cgi/reprint/136/9/1206?maxtoshow=&hits=10&RESULTFORMAT=1&author1=glick&andorexacttitle=and&andorexacttitleabs=and&andorexactfulltext=and&searchid=1&FIRSTINDEX=40&sortspec=relevance&resourcetype=HWCIT. Accessed March 29, 2010.

70. Centers for Disease Control and Prevention (CDC). Recommendations for prevention and control of hepatitis C virus (HCV) infection and HCV-related chronic disease. *MMWR Recomm Rep.* 1998;47(RR-19):1-39. http://www.cdc.gov/mmwr/preview/mmwrhtml/00055154.htm. Accessed May 27, 2013.

71. American Dental Association (ADA). Post-exposure evaluation and follow-up requirements under OSHA's standard for occupational exposure to bloodborne pathogens. http://www.ada.org/sections/professionalResources/pdfs/post-exposure_prophylaxis.pdf. Accessed May 27, 2013.

72. Centers for Disease Control and Prevention (CDC). Tuberculosis (TB): infection control in health-care settings. Atlanta, GA: CDC. http://www.cdc.gov/tb/topic/infectioncontrol/default.htm. Updated March 29, 2012. Accessed May 27, 2013.

73. Molinari JA, Harte JA. *Practical Infection Control in Dentistry.* 3rd ed. Philadelphia: Lippincott Williams & Wilkins; 2010:166.

74. Miller C, Palenik CJ. *Infection Control and Management of Hazardous Materials for the Dental Team.* 4th rev. ed. St. Louis, MO: Mosby Elsevier; 2010:222.

75. Occupational Safety & Health Administration (OSHA). Occupational Safety & Health Administration: recommended format for materials safety data sheets (MSDSs). Washington, DC: OSHA. http://www.osha.gov/dsg/hazcom/msdsformat.html. Accessed May 27, 2013.

76. U.S. Department of Labor, Occupational Safety and Health Administration. Standards-29 CFR Part 1910.1200. Occupational Safety and Health Standards, Toxic and Hazardous Substances, Hazard Communication. Washington, DC. http://www.osha.gov/pls/oshaweb/owadisp.show_document?p_table=standards&p_id=10099. Accessed May 27, 2013.

77. Miller C, Palenik CJ. *Infection Control and Management of Hazardous Materials for the Dental Team.* 4th rev. ed. St. Louis, MO: Mosby Elsevier; 2010:270.

Part IV

Assessment

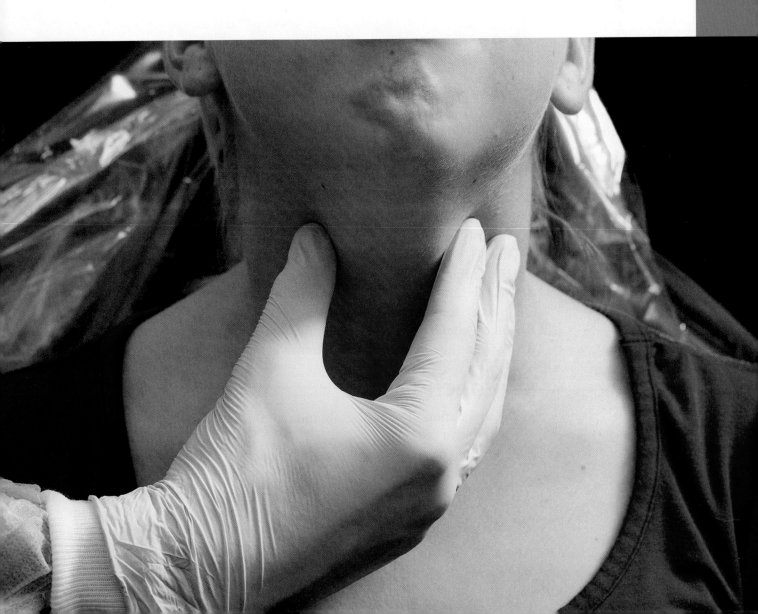

Chapter 8 | Comprehensive Medical and Oral Health History

JoAnn R. Gurenlian, RDH, PhD

KEY TERMS

blood pressure
body mass index (BMI)
chief complaint
diastolic blood pressure
dyspnea
functional capacity
hypertension
hyperventilation
hypotension
infective endocarditis
metabolic equivalents
orthopnea
orthostatic hypotension
pulse
respiration
sinus bradycardia
systolic blood pressure
tachyarrhythmia
tachycardia
tachypnea

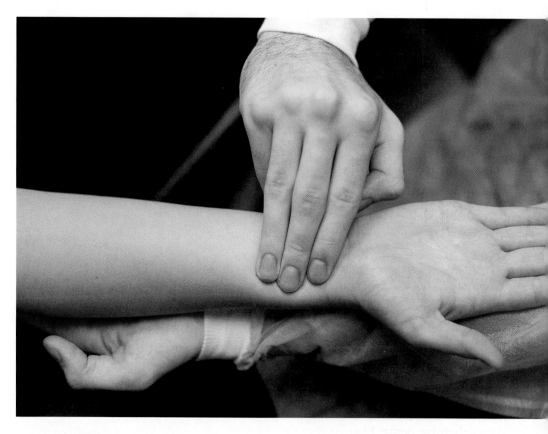

LEARNING OBJECTIVES

After reading this chapter, the student should be able to:

8.1 Identify key components of comprehensive medical and dental histories.
8.2 Use probing questions to elicit accurate information.
8.3 Search sample health histories and customize appropriately to a clinical practice setting.
8.4 Take a comprehensive history and vital signs for each patient.
8.5 Explain the need for a comprehensive and accurate history.

KEY CONCEPTS

- The foundation of patient evaluation and risk assessment is the patient health history.
- Performing a comprehensive health history is vital to determining general and oral health status, determining whether rendering care is appropriate, and avoiding potential medical emergencies.
- As part of the Standards for Clinical Dental Hygiene Practice developed by the American Dental Hygienists' Association, dental hygienists are

expected to conduct a thorough assessment of each patient with respect to oral and general health status and patient needs.

- Vital signs are taken at each appointment as a means to identify signs of an infection, as a baseline measure to anticipate and/or prevent a medical emergency, or to identify a diagnosed or undiagnosed systemic condition.

RELEVANCE TO CLINICAL PRACTICE

Every patient who appears for a dental hygiene appointment presents with a unique set of circumstances and physical, mental, social, and emotional health states. Conducting a health history is the first phase of the assessment component of the dental hygiene process of care. Taking the time to perform a comprehensive health history is vital to determining general and oral health status, determining whether rendering care is appropriate, and anticipating potential medical emergencies.

ROLE AND IMPORTANCE OF THE PATIENT HISTORY

The foundation of patient evaluation and risk assessment is the patient health history. This is typically supplemented by a comprehensive clinical examination, laboratory and other diagnostic tests, radiographic studies, and medical consultation. Thorough personal, medical, oral, and drug histories are used as part of comprehensive dental hygiene care to:

- Determine an accurate dental hygiene diagnosis.
- Plan treatment with greater dental hygienist and patient awareness.
- Obtain an informed consent.
- Determine whether proposed treatment is appropriate or if modifications are indicated.
- Decide whether a medical or other health professional consult is needed.
- Identify undiagnosed systemic conditions.
- Identify causative factors that contribute to general and oral health.
- Provide insight into cultural beliefs, ethnic influences, emotional and psychological factors, and attitudes that may affect risk for general and oral diseases.
- Determine whether the patient has the functional capacity to tolerate treatment.
- Anticipate medical emergencies during the course of care (see Spotlight on Public Health).

Patient Interview

In general, the dental hygiene care provider has three format options for interviewing each patient: open-ended,

Spotlight on Public Health

In every setting, we cannot make assumptions about the needs of the patient. Using the medical and dental histories is a starting point that helps to provide a profile of the patient and the support of his family in providing care. In long-term care facilities, oral neglect may readily occur. Dental hygienists need to show caregivers at the facility and the patient's family members how to provide better care by addressing all of the patient's needs. Having complete information about the health status of the patient, disease conditions, medications used, and oral complaints is an essential component of being able to create a comprehensive treatment plan and implement one that is of value to the patient and her community. It is important to remember that the patient is connected to a family who is connected to a community.

Further, with health care focused on treating the underserved and improving access to care, dental hygienists may be encountering greater oral health and general health challenges than from those patients who have presented to a school clinic or one in a practice setting that tends to have patients who present in good health. Before care is provided, the medical and dental histories can guide the dental hygienist in determining a priority for treatment and coordinating resources for providing both medical and oral health care to those who are underserved or have limited access to health care. ■

closed-ended, or a combination format. In the open-ended format, the dental hygienist asks the patient a series of predetermined questions, recording the patient's responses on a blank sheet of paper. The patient and the dental hygienist engage in continuous dialogue throughout this process, and additional questions are posed to clarify and obtain further significant information.

The closed-ended format uses a preprinted questionnaire that the patient uses to respond to medical and oral health items. Although convenient and efficient, this format tends to limit dialogue between the patient and the practitioner. Further, the patient may not understand some of the questions or choose not to provide answers for the items he deems unnecessary or too personal.

A combination format is frequently used in dental practice settings. Patients are offered a questionnaire to complete to the best of their ability. The dental hygiene provider then reviews the responses and asks follow-up questions to clarify and obtain additional details. As with the open-ended format, the dental hygienist is primarily responsible for the information and analysis of the significance of the data obtained. This combination format is relatively efficient and allows for greater communication to occur than the closed-ended format.

Types of Record Forms

A variety of health history forms are available that can be used in the dental hygiene practice setting. Some forms are commercially prepared, whereas others can be loaded onto a computer and customized for the practice (see Advancing Technologies). Practitioners

who use customizable forms are able to add items as new information about systemic and oral diseases is uncovered, provide information in other languages appropriate to the patient population served, change the font size for those with vision impairments, and provide additional space needed for those with lengthy and complicated general health or drug histories, or both. Some patients may be taking multiple medications that require more than an inch of space to note the name of medication, dosage, frequency, use, and so on. Having the flexibility to modify health history forms provides options that enhance clinical practice.

With greater emphasis on risk assessment for systemic and oral conditions, offices may want to design their own forms or use commercially prepared supplementary forms that identify risk factors for various conditions. Assessing risk for cardiovascular disease diabetes mellitus, tobacco use, caries, periodontal disease, xerostomia, and oral cancer can be conducted as part of a comprehensive health history. These supplementary forms can be used for patient education purposes, encouraging the patient to make lifestyle changes to improve health. They can be updated when the patient returns for continuing care appointments.

In addition, clinical practice settings are converting to Electronic Dental Records (EDR). This change will allow dental hygienists to readily review and update health information at each patient appointment.

History-Taking Preparation

Conducting a health history requires preparation and teamwork from the office staff. When a patient telephones the office to schedule his initial appointment, the receptionist has an opportunity to ask some screening questions to determine whether further information is needed before arranging the appointment. Inquiring about general health status, recent hospitalizations, and key health conditions (i.e., cardiovascular, diabetes, stroke, cancer, among others) will help to determine the length of the initial appointment, if an appointment will need to be postponed, or if antibiotics will need to be prescribed before treatment. Advance notice of these situations facilitates efficiency and comprehensive care for both the provider and the patient.

As a means of having more complete information readily available at the time of the appointment, many medical practices and some dental practices are mailing the health history home to the patients in advance of their appointments. In some cases, these forms can also be accessed online. The purpose of this process is to help patients obtain the necessary information in the comfort of their home where they can set the pace for answering the health questionnaire. Patients can collect their medication bottles and provide complete information, locate their family practitioner's name or phone number, and use their personal records to identify hospitalizations, surgical procedures, allergies, and adverse effects of medications. Another benefit to this procedure is that the patients are completing the health

Advancing Technologies

Students of this newer generation have a benefit over older dental hygienists in that they understand and use technology better, faster, and more widely than those who grew up in a different era. Technology will allow these future practitioners to use electronic forms and modify them as needed based on patient population groups. Forms can be printed in larger print for those individuals with vision challenges. Forms can be translated into various languages for those patients who prefer to use English as a second language. Translation of these documents will help the dental hygienist have a more accurate picture of the patient's medical and oral health conditions. In addition, using technology can enable the dental hygienist to contact the patient's family physician, nurse practitioner, or health-care specialist when more information is needed about care to be provided, precautions needed, and whether consent to treat is required. This technology can speed the process of treatment without having to reschedule the patient for another appointment. ■

history in their own words. When they bring the completed health questionnaire to their initial appointment, the dental hygiene care provider can enter the information into the EDR, review the information, and ask follow-up questions as needed to gain specific details to assist with further assessment, diagnosis, and treatment planning.

If the dental hygiene care provider wants to ensure that the health history obtained is as complete and accurate as possible, she must be skilled at establishing a rapport with each patient. Interviewing the patient may require assistance from a parent, family member, or translator. The interview should occur in a private area so that the patient does not feel that others in the reception area can overhear the discussion of his health information. If the dental hygienist is limited to using the dental operatory for reviewing the health history, she should make sure that the patient is seated in an upright position in the dental chair and that the patient is at eye level when discussing health-related questions. It is important to convey an attitude that is open, interested, accepting, and nonjudgmental. Thoughtful and direct questions need to be asked, and adequate time needs to be set aside to allow the patient to answer each question and complete his thoughts.

Focus of Health Histories

Health histories may be designed based on a particular focus. For example, some histories are based on a review of systems. Questions related to the gastrointestinal system, cardiovascular system, pulmonary system, and so on are created and then related to specific diseases, treatment, and outcomes. The systems-oriented approach is comprehensive and provides the patient and dental hygienist an opportunity to relate signs and symptoms to specific diseases whether known or undiagnosed. Follow-up questions can be related to the severity of symptoms, date noticed, duration, and treatment rendered. The dental hygienist can then determine what adaptations to treatment may be indicated based on these findings.

Many health histories use a disease-oriented focus that asks patients to identify whether they have or have had a history of diseases such as asthma, hepatitis, diabetes, and periodontal treatment. The diseases or conditions may be arranged based on body organs or systems, or appear alphabetically. The dental hygienist can ask follow-up questions as noted previously.

Some patients may not be aware that they have a particular disease or condition. Using a symptoms focus to the health history may help to uncover a systemic disease. For example, inquiring whether the patient has experienced flu-like symptoms, weight loss, persistent cough for 3 weeks, or coughing of blood may indicate the patient has tuberculosis. The patient can be referred for further evaluation and rescheduled after clearance has been obtained by the physician of record.

Another approach to the health history is to use a cultural focus. For some patients, their cultural and ethnic beliefs, values, and attitudes will influence the way they participate in completing the health history. In some cultures, a male family member will answer questions for the female patient. In other cultures, privacy is meant to be honored. Some cultures do not subscribe to western medicine and prefer to use herbal supplements and other approaches to health care. The dental hygienist is challenged to respect and adapt to cultures while eliciting accurate information to make sound clinical decisions about treatment and interactions.

Samples of Health Histories

In March 2008, the American Dental Hygienists' Association (ADHA) published the Standards for Clinical Dental Hygiene Practice.[1] These standards represent a framework for clinical practice so that patient-centered and evidence-based care can be provided. The standards are based on the dental hygiene process of care including assessment, diagnosis, planning, implementation, and evaluation. Another component reflected in these standards is the importance of complete and accurate documentation.

As part of the clinical standards, dental hygienists are expected to conduct a thorough assessment of each patient with respect to oral and general health status and patient needs. As detailed in the standards, a patient history is to be conducted that includes[1]:

- Recording personal profile information such as demographics, values and beliefs, cultural influences, knowledge, skills, and attitudes
- Recording current and past dental and dental hygiene oral health practices
- Collecting the patient's health history data, including:
  - Current and past health status
  - Diversity and cultural considerations (e.g., age, sex, religion, race, and ethnicity)
  - Pharmacological considerations (e.g., prescription, recreational, over the counter [OTC], herbal)
  - Additional considerations (e.g., mental health, learning disabilities, phobias, economic status)
  - Vital signs and comparison with previous readings
  - Consultations with appropriate health-care provider(s) as indicated

Many health histories are available for use in clinical practice. The American Dental Association (ADA) has a two-page health history form that can be accessed online (www.ada.org). This form addresses most conditions of concern related to oral health care. However, this form is limited in terms of providing vital sign information, following up in key areas related to health status, and contributing to decision-making about the influence of medication management with oral treatment. An alternative form, developed and used by the College of Registered Dental Hygienists of Alberta (CRDHA), incorporates more vital sign information, critical thinking, an analysis based on the drug history, and a risk classification system developed by the American Society of Anesthesiologists (Fig. 8-1). It also

The Dental Offices of
Dr. Davis W. Ford, DDS

Health History Questionnaire

☐Mr. ☐Mrs. ☐Miss ☐Ms. ☐Dr.

Last: First: Middle:

Date of Birth _____ / _____ / _____
Year   Month   Day

Address/Home: Phone: Occupation:

City: Postal Code: Business Phone:

Height: Weight: Blood Pressure: Pulse: Resp:

In case of emergency, we should notify: Name: Relationship: Phone:

Family Doctor: Phone: Medical Specialist: Phone:

Other Health Provider: Area of Specialty: Address/Phone:

Your safety and optimal oral health are our priorities. The following information enables us to provide you with the best oral health care services safely and effectively. **Please complete the entire form.** During your visit, you will be asked questions regarding your questionnaire responses. All information is confidential and treated in accordance with applicable provincial and federal privacy legislation.

A. DENTAL INFORMATION

1. Do your gums bleed when you brush?	Y	N	
2. Have you ever had orthodontic or orthotropic treatment (e.g., braces)?	Y	N	
3. Have you had any periodontal (gum) treatment?	Y	N	
4. Are your teeth sensitive to hot, cold, sweets, or pressure?	Y	N	
5. Have you ever had an injury to your head, face, or jaw?	Y	N	
6. Do you suffer from frequent headaches?	Y	N	
7. Do you have earaches or neck pains?	Y	N	
8. Do you have removable dental appliances? Implants?	Y	N	

9. Are you nervous during dental treatment?   Y   N

10. What is the reason for your dental visit?

11. Date of last dental examination:

12. Date of last dental x-rays:

Please explain any YES answers:

B. GENERAL INFORMATION

1. When was your last medical checkup? Date:	Y	N
2. Are you being treated for any medical condition or have you been treated within the past year?	Y	N
3. Has there been any change in your general health in the past year?	Y	N
4. Have you ever been hopitalized for any illness or operations?	Y	N
5. Do you have a prosthetic or artificial joint?	Y	N
6. Have you ever been advised to take antibiotics before dental treatment?	Y	N
7. Have you ever had a particular or adverse reaction, including allergies, to any medications or injections?	Y	N
8. Do you have any allergies to any foods or materials (e.g., latex or metals)?	Y	N
9. Do you have any other allergies?	Y	N
10. Cancer?	Y	N
11. Dry mouth?	Y	N

Do you have or have you ever had?

12. Ear or hearing problems?	Y	N
13. Eye problems (e.g., require corrective lenses, glaucoma)?	Y	N
14. Sleep disorders?	Y	N

WOMEN

15. Are you or could you be pregnant? If yes, expected delivery date:	Y	N
16. Are you breastfeeding?	Y	N
17. Are you taking hormone replacement therapy?	Y	N

Please explain any YES answers:

18. Are you taking medications of any kind? Include prescription drugs, over-the-counter medications (e.g., cold and flu remedy), natural health products (e.g., vitamins, herbal, and diet supplements). If yes, please list.

Drug Name	Amount, Dose, Frequency	Reason	Date Prescribed and Prescriber

Figure 8-1. Health history questionnaire. (Reprinted courtesy of the College of Registered Dental Hygienists of Alberta [CRDHA])

C. CARDIO/RESPIRATORY

Do you have or have you ever had:

	Y	N
1. Cardiovascular diseases? If yes, specify below:	Y	N

Angina	Heart attack
Arteriosclerosis	Heart murmur
Artificial heart valves	High or low blood pressure
Congenital heart defects	High or low cholesterol
Congestive heart failure	Mitral valve prolapse
Coronary artery disease	Pacemaker/defibrillator
Damaged heart valves	Rheumatic heart disease/fever

	Y	N
2. Chest pains upon exertion?	Y	N
3. Shortness of breath?	Y	N
4. Asthma?	Y	N
5. Chronic bronchitis or emphysema?	Y	N
6. Sinus trouble or nasal congestion?	Y	N
7. Tuberculosis?	Y	N
8. A persistent cough for more than 3 weeks?	Y	N
9. Cough that produces blood?	Y	N

Please explain any YES answers:

D. ENDOCRINE/DIGESTIVE

Do you have or have you ever had:

	Y	N
1. Malnutrition?	Y	N
2. Eating disorder?	Y	N
3. Dietary restrictions (self-imposed or doctor perscribed)?	Y	N
4. Night sweats?	Y	N
5. Slow healing or recurrent infections?	Y	N
6. Thyroid or parathyroid disease?	Y	N
7. Diabetes? If yes, indicate type:	Y	N

Please explain any YES answers:

E. GASTROINTESTINAL/GENITOURINARY

Do you have or have you ever had:

	Y	N
1. Hepatitis, jaundice, or liver disease?	Y	N
2. Difficulty swallowing?	Y	N
3. G.E. reflux/persistent heartburn?	Y	N
4. A stomach ulcer?	Y	N
5. Gallbladder problems?	Y	N
6. Kidney or bladder trouble?	Y	N
7. Excessive urination?	Y	N

Please explain any YES answers:

F. HEMATOLOGIC

Do you have or have you ever had:

	Y	N
1. Prolonged or abnormal bleeding with a simple cut or following surgery, extraction, or an accident?	Y	N
2. A blood transfusion? if yes, date:	Y	N
3. A tendency to bruise easily?	Y	N
4. Any blood disorder (e.g., anemia or hemophilia)?	Y	N

Please explain any YES answers:

G. IMMUNE SYST./INFECTIOUS DIS.

Do you have or have you ever had:

	Y	N
1. Systemic lupus erythematosus?	Y	N
2. Painful swollen joints or rheumatoid arthritis?	Y	N
3. HIV/AIDS?	Y	N
4. Other diseases or conditions that affect your immune system (e.g., sarcoidosis, Epstein-Barr, radiotherapy, chemotherapy, steroid therapy)?	Y	N
5. A blood transfusion? if yes, date:	Y	N

Please explain any YES answers:

H. NEURO/MUSCULOSKELETAL

Do you have or have you ever had:

	Y	N
1. A stroke?	Y	N
2. Convulsions or seizures (e.g., epilepsy)?	Y	N
3. Mental health disorders?	Y	N
4. Arthritis?	Y	N
5. Osteoporosis or osteopenia?	Y	N
6. Chronic pain?	Y	N

Please explain any YES answers:

I. OTHER

	Y	N
1. Do you smoke, chew, or snort tobacco products?	Y	N
If yes: Frequency (daily, weekly)?		
Number of years use?		
Have you ever tried to quit?	Y	N
Are you interested in quitting?	Y	N
2. Do you have a drug or alcohol dependency?	Y	N
3. Other diseases or medical problems that run in your family?	Y	N
4. Other conditions or medical problems not listed?	Y	N
5. Other special needs that will affect your dental care?	Y	N

Please explain any YES answers:

To the best of my knowlege, the above information is correct.

Parent/Guardian Signature: _____   Date: _____

Reviewed by: _____ (DDS, RDH)   Date: _____

Figure 8-1.—cont'd

Continued

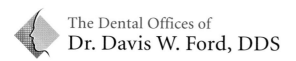

The Dental Offices of
Dr. Davis W. Ford, DDS

Fundamental Questions within the Dental Hygiene Process of Care
FOR COMPLETION BY DENTAL HYGIENIST

Date: _____ Client Name: _____

1. Why is the patient taking the medication(s) (See reasons listed for question #18 of Health History Questionnaire) _____

_____

2. What are the adverse effects of this drug? _____

_____

3. Are there potential drug interactions? _____

_____

4. Is there a problem with drug dosage? _____

_____

5. How is the patient managing his or her medication? _____

_____

6. Will any oral side effects of this medication require intervention? _____

_____

7. Are the patient 's symptoms caused by a known or unknown condition, or are the symptoms possible side effects of a drug that the client is taking? _____

_____

_____

8. Given the data obtained from the drug profile review and other assessment data, what are the risks of treating this patient? _____

_____

_____

Notes   ASA Classification: I   II   III   IV   V   E

Comments on patient interview concerning health history.

_____

_____

_____

Significant findings from questionnaire or verbal interview.

_____

_____

_____

Considerations for the care plan.

_____

_____

_____

Figure 8-1.—cont'd

The Dental Offices of
Dr. Davis W. Ford, DDS

Health History Updates

Please review your previous medical history (dated: _____/_____/_____) and advise us if there are anyy changes.
Year   Month   Day

Height:	Weight:	Blood Pressure:	Pulse:	Resp:

1. Has there been any change in your health, such as serious illnesses, surgeries, hospitalizations, or new allergies?

   ☐ YES   ☐ NO   ☐ NOT SURE

   If yes, please explain: _____

   _____

2. Are you taking any new medications (both prescription and non-prescription) or has there been any change in your medications?

   ☐ YES   ☐ NO   ☐ NOT SURE

   If yes, please explain: _____

   _____

3. Have you had a heart murmur diagnosed or had any change in an existing cardiac problem or murmur?

   ☐ YES   ☐ NO   ☐ NOT SURE

   If yes, please explain: _____

   _____

To the best of my knowlege, the above information is correct.

Patient /Parent/Guardian Signature: _____   Date: _____

Reviewed by: _____ (DDS, RDH)   Date: _____

Figure 8-1.—cont'd

includes a section for updating the health history at each appointment with key questions related to significant changes in health and medication use.

If the dental hygienist prefers to customize a health history form and favors the review-of-systems approach, examples of items that can be used for this type of health history are shown in Figure 8-2.

As can be seen by the review-of-systems style of health history presentation, the forms will be lengthy. Many practitioners prefer something that is less involved. However, this method does provide opportunities for learning more about the patient's general health status. If this type of health history form is mailed in advance, the patient can complete most of these items at his leisure and the dental hygiene practitioner can review it and conduct further probing questions as needed. In the medical profession, the review of systems is used routinely. Because patients have experience with this form, the transition can be made to oral health care with some advance preparation for the patient. In addition, the dental hygienist may want to combine elements of the health history form provided by the CRDHA to encompass the oral history, vital signs and background information, and drug history components to complement the review of systems, making the form more comprehensive (see Professionalism).

Professionalism

As part of professionalism, it is important to embrace the concept of lifelong learning. As health-care providers, we have the opportunity to learn from each other. One way to continue to improve on the medical and dental histories is to form study clubs with area practices. Case presentations can be provided that will allow each dental hygienist the chance to see how the histories were taken, what other probing questions could be asked, and whether prophylactic antibiotics or referrals were indicated. Individuals can research and present new models of medical, dental, and drug history forms that dental hygienists can review and then determine whether these models are appropriate for their practice settings. ■

ELEMENTS OF THE HEALTH HISTORY

Biographical Data

The initial part of the health history usually begins with biographical information. The patient's name, address,

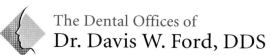

The Dental Offices of
Dr. Davis W. Ford, DDS

Health History Updates

Constitutional symptoms
- ☐ Good general health lately
- ☐ Recent weight change
- ☐ Fever/chills/sweats
- ☐ Fatigue
- ☐ Headaches
- ☐ Other, specify _____

Mouth/throat
- ☐ Mouth sores (ulcers, canker sore, fever blisters)
- ☐ Bleeding gums
- ☐ Bad breath or bad taste
- ☐ Sore throat or voice change
- ☐ Dry mouth
- ☐ Swollen glands
- ☐ Other, specify _____

Cardiovascular
- ☐ Shortness of breath
- ☐ Difficulty walking distances/stairs
- ☐ Fainting spells
- ☐ Chest pain or pressure
- ☐ Angina
- ☐ Swollen ankles
- ☐ Low blood pressure
- ☐ Orthostatic hypotension
- ☐ High blood pressure
- ☐ Rheumatic fever/heart disease
- ☐ Mitral valve prolapse
- ☐ Congenital heart disorder
- ☐ Heart murmur
- ☐ Abnormal heartbeat/rhythm
- ☐ Pacemaker or defibrillator
- ☐ Congestive heart failure
- ☐ History of endocarditis
- ☐ Myocardial infarction/heart attack
- ☐ Arteriosclerosis/atherosclerosis
- ☐ Heart valve problem or artificial valves
- ☐ Stroke or transient ischemic attack
- ☐ Taking blood thinners
- ☐ Coronary artery bypass/stent/angioplasty
- ☐ Other, specify _____
- ☐ Has your physician recommended premedication?
    If yes, type _____

Eyes
- ☐ Eye disease or injury
- ☐ Wears glasses/contact lenses
- ☐ Blurred or double vision
- ☐ Drooping eyelids
- ☐ Cataracts
- ☐ Glaucoma
- ☐ Blindness
- ☐ Other, specify _____

Integumentary (skin, breast)
- ☐ Rash or itching
- ☐ Hives
- ☐ Bruise easily
- ☐ Eczema, psoriasis, seborrhea
- ☐ Varicose veins
- ☐ Change in skin color
- ☐ Change in hair or nails
- ☐ Skin cancer, moles, or melanoma
- ☐ Allergic/adverse reactions to latex, medication, bees, foods, metals
- ☐ Breast pain
- ☐ Breast lump
- ☐ Breast discharge
- ☐ Other, specify _____

Respiratory
- ☐ Acute or chronic coughing
- ☐ Difficulty breathing
- ☐ Coughing of blood
- ☐ Wheezing or asthma
- ☐ Bronchitis or emphysema
- ☐ Tuberculosis
- ☐ Pneumonia
- ☐ Seasonal allergies
- ☐ Other, specify _____

Neurologic
- ☐ Frequent or recurring headaches
- ☐ Light-headed or dizziness
- ☐ Fainting spells
- ☐ Memory loss
- ☐ Balance/coordination problems
- ☐ Convulsions or seizures
- ☐ Epilepsy or seizure disorder
- ☐ Numbness or tingling sensations
- ☐ Speech problems
- ☐ Tremors
- ☐ Head injury
- ☐ Paralysis or stroke
- ☐ Alzheimer disease
- ☐ Muscular dystrophy
- ☐ Lyme disease
- ☐ Parkinson disease
- ☐ Transient ischemic attack (TIA)
- ☐ Stroke (CVA)
- ☐ Other, specify _____

Ears/nose
- ☐ Hearing loss or ringing of ears
- ☐ Vertigo
- ☐ Hearing aids
- ☐ Earaches or drainage
- ☐ Chronic sinus problems/rhinitis
- ☐ Nose bleeds
- ☐ Other, specify _____

Musculoskeletal
- ☐ Joint pain
- ☐ Joint stiffness/swelling
- ☐ Difficulty walking
- ☐ Arthritis or rheumatism
- ☐ Weakness of muscles or joints
- ☐ Muscle pain or cramps
- ☐ Fibromyalgia
- ☐ Lupus, scleroderma, Sjögren syndrome
- ☐ Back/neck pain
- ☐ Bone deformity
- ☐ Gout
- ☐ Osteoporosis
- ☐ Cold extremities
- ☐ Prosthetic joints
- ☐ Other, specify _____
- ☐ Has your physician recommended premedication?
    If yes, type _____

Genitourinary
- ☐ Frequent urination
- ☐ Burning or painful urination
- ☐ Blood in urine
- ☐ Difficulty controlling urine
- ☐ Kidney infections
- ☐ Bladder infections
- ☐ Kidney stones
- ☐ Renal or kidney dialysis
- ☐ Change in force of strain when urinating
- ☐ Incontinence or dribbling
- ☐ Enlarged prostate
- ☐ Sexual difficulty
- ☐ Sexually transmitted infection/disease
  Female
    - ☐ Pain with periods
    - ☐ Irregular periods
    - ☐ Vaginal discharge
    - ☐ Pelvic infection
    - ☐ Pregnant, which trimester ___
    - ☐ # of pregnancies ____
    - ☐ # of miscarriages ____
    - ☐ Perimenopausal
    - ☐ Post menopause

Figure 8-2. Sample sections to include in a review of systems.

Endocrine

- ☐ Glandular or hormone problem
- ☐ Excessive thirst or urination
- ☐ Heat or cold intolerance
- ☐ Skin becoming dryer
- ☐ Change in glove or hat size
- ☐ Diabetes mellitus, type _____
- ☐ Adrenal gland problems
- ☐ Enlarged thyroid
- ☐ Hypothyroid
- ☐ Hyperthyroid
- ☐ Steroid use
- ☐ Other, specify _____

Psychiatric

- ☐ Nervousness or anxiety
- ☐ Difficulty sleeping
- ☐ Depression
- ☐ Memory loss or confusion
- ☐ Bipolar disorder
- ☐ Emotional problems
- ☐ Considered suicide
- ☐ Other, specify _____

Hematologic/lymphatic

- ☐ Slow to heal after cuts
- ☐ Bleeding or bruising tendency
- ☐ Anemia
- ☐ Blood transfusion
- ☐ Enlarged glands/lymph nodes
- ☐ Hemophilia
- ☐ Leukemia
- ☐ AIDS/HIV positive
- ☐ Cancer
- ☐ Other, specify _____

Other conditions

Please use the space below to describe any other diseases, conditions, or problems not listed above.

_____

_____

_____

_____

_____

Figure 8-2.—cont'd

telephone numbers, e-mail address (if available), date of birth, sex, ethnicity or racial background, marital status, and occupation may be reported. These personal data are obtained to help manage appointment scheduling and financial aspects of the oral health care provided, to be able to answer questions or concerns when the patient contacts the office and the dental care provider is unavailable to attend to a call at that moment, to identify the need for approval of care for a minor patient or one with impairment or disability, and to determine culturally relevant communication approaches. Learning the patient's occupation may contribute to evaluating the patient for occupational oral hazards, as well as understanding opportunities for oral health care in work settings. Some individuals may be reluctant to provide personal information for fear of misuse or identity theft. Explanations of patient confidentiality will need to be reinforced to obtain appropriate information. All practices must conform to the Health Insurance Portability and Accountability Act (HIPAA) to provide protection of confidential information. Chapter 2 provides detailed information about HIPAA.

The biographic section should also include the patient's current physician's name, address, telephone number, fax number, and e-mail information. Most health histories do not provide sufficient room for recording these data, but it is essential for the dental hygienist to know key health provider information. When patients provide their family practitioner data, it is important to note how often they visit their doctor, reasons for visits, diagnoses and treatments rendered, and date of most recent appointment. Including specialist provider data will give the dental hygienist an opportunity to contact the specialist for consultations. Physician information is useful for seeking assistance when disease symptoms are identified on the health history form and follow-up is needed for definitive diagnosis; when medication, premedication, or both are indicated; and during an emergency situation. Knowing that a patient is receiving medical care for a specific condition will help the practitioner determine whether there could be a risk for medical problems during oral health care, if there might be medication interactions or adverse effects, oral side effects of medical treatment or the condition itself, and potential for cross-contamination. Those patients who schedule regular appointments with their family physician or specialist, or both, may place a higher value on their health and health care. Individuals who report that they do not have a family physician may be presenting with undiagnosed conditions and should be carefully assessed.

Chief Complaint

The **chief complaint,** or chief concern, is the reason why the patient has presented for oral health care. Not every patient will have a complaint; they may be attending a routine continuing care appointment. Other patients may have a toothache, an abscess, one or more ulcers, gingival bleeding, or an esthetic concern such as stains on their teeth. An easy way to garner information about the chief complaint is to ask the patient a question such as "What brings you to this appointment today?"

The chief complaint should be noted in the patient's own words in quotation marks in the dental record. For example, "I noticed that my front upper tooth appears to be moving" or "I woke up with pain on the side of my tongue and it looks like there is an ulcer there."

Discussion of the chief complaint occurs at the beginning of the appointment during the patient interview. This process communicates that the patient's concern will be taken seriously and that the treatment plan will incorporate this concern. If the chief complaint appears to be urgent, the dental hygienist will need to modify the treatment plan to address this concern first. Satisfying the patient's real or perceived immediate need will build trust and confidence in the oral health-care provider.

As with every aspect of the health history, follow-up questions will need to be conducted to learn more about this chief complaint. For the patient who presents with ulcers along the side of the tongue, the dental hygienist should include a complete description by asking the following questions:

- When did you first notice this ulcer?
- Is it painful or annoying?
- Can you tolerate foods and liquids?
- Do you have any other symptoms (e.g., sore throat, swollen glands, ulcers elsewhere on the body)?
- What makes this condition feel better? Feel worse?
- Have you had ulcers in your mouth before? How long did they last? What treatment was used? Was it effective?

For those patients who present for routine continuing care, follow-up questions may include:

- How often do you have routine dental hygiene appointments?
- What kind of treatment has been provided?
- Were you satisfied with your treatment?
- Did you experience any problems during treatment (e.g., stress, pain, bleeding, emergency, among others)?

In many cases, the patient's response to follow-up questions will help the dental hygienist diagnose the problem or determine other diagnostic studies that will need to be conducted. In addition, it may help the dental hygienist learn more about the patient's level of involvement in and attitude toward oral health care.

General Health

Questions related to general health include broad concerns relevant to the patient's past and current medical

health, a family history to identify problems for which the patient may be predisposed, and a review of systems to assess the patient's current state of health in relation to each major body system. Examples of general health questions appear in section B of the health history questionnaire designed by CRDHA. As can be seen from this health history, the patient will be asked about recent medical conditions, hospitalizations, antibiotic premedication, allergies, and adverse reactions. These general items help the dental hygiene care provider determine the significance of health information in relation to oral health care and whether modifications in treatment may be indicated.

Many health histories include a component related to the history of the family. This family history alludes to oral and general health conditions that may have a known genetic etiology. Examples of oral health problems that may be inherited include malocclusion, cleft lip and palate, unusual appearance of teeth, and in some cases, periodontal disease. Examples of general health conditions with a familial tendency may include cancer, cardiovascular diseases, diabetes, allergies, asthma, arthritis, and sickle cell anemia. If there is not a section on the medical history form related to the family history, the dental hygienist can pose questions such as:

- Do you have a family history of cancer, heart disease, diabetes, or blood disorders?
- Do you have a family history of allergies to medications, bees, foods, or other products and/or asthma?
- Are there any other general health problems in your family?
- Do you have a family history of oral health problems, for example, clefts, too many teeth, not enough teeth, crowded teeth, gum disease?

Examples of medical conditions that are associated with a review of systems and oral treatment considerations are listed in Table 8-1, which highlights key conditions but is not exhaustive. Students and practitioners interested in learning more about systemic health should consult oral medicine texts.

Oral History

The patient's oral history or dental history provides the dental hygiene care provider an opportunity to explore previous dental experiences, motivation, and attitudes and beliefs toward oral health. A review of this aspect of the health history includes the present chief complaint, previous dental and dental hygiene treatment, knowledge of oral health care, personal daily oral health practices, emergency treatment needed, and any relevant attitudes or cultural beliefs that influence oral and general health care.

A review of key elements of the oral history appears in Table 8-2. As shown in Table 8-2, the dental hygienist can discover significant information that may impact preventive programs, treatment, and patient education. *(Text continued on page 138)*

Table 8-1. *Review of Systems Health History Considerations for Oral Health Care*

Review of Systems Category	Medical Considerations	Oral Health Treatment Considerations
Constitutional	• Evaluate outward appearance of patient (gait, body habitus, posture, odors, difficulty breathing, etc.).	• Assess body odors for signs of diabetes, renal failure, respiratory infection, alcohol use. • Assess for potential to withstand treatment (i.e., cachexic, lethargic). • Assess for potential for infection or other systemic conditions.
Eyes	• Eyes may indicate systemic disease (hyperthyroidism, xanthomas, hepatitis, sicca syndrome, allergy, infection).	• If patients are sensitive to light, offer sunglasses. • Ensure operatory area is safe for patients with low vision, double vision, blindness. • Escort patient to and from operatory. • If visually impaired, ensure patient can perform oral hygiene measures. • Avoid use of anticholinergics in patients with glaucoma.
Ears/Nose	• Inspect for signs of skin cancer. • Identify whether patient has hearing loss. • Discuss nasal conditions—sinusitis, upper respiratory infection, seasonal allergies. • Identify medications used for nasal problems. • Note nosebleeds, frequency, potential causes.	• Speak clearly and close to patient if patient is hearing impaired; face patient while talking. • Refer patient if skin changes are noted. • Review systemic and oral effects of antihistamines, decongestants with patient. • Advise patients to rinse after use of inhalers to prevent candidiasis. • Assess for bleeding disorder, anemia, etc.
Mouth/Throat	• Inspect neck and thyroid for enlargement and asymmetry. • Evaluate for goiter, tumors, infections, cysts, lymphadenopathy, or vascular changes. • Note frequency and duration of oral complaints (i.e., ulcers, bad breath, dry mouth, bleeding gingival, pain, sensitivity).	• Refer patient for further evaluation for neck and throat concerns. • Evaluate for potential for infection transmission. • Defer treatment if viral infection is present (herpes labialis, herpetic gingivostomatitis). • Review over-the-counter and prescription medications to treat mouth complaints.
Integumentary	• Identify changes in nails and skin (skin cancer, petechiae/ecchymosis for blood dyscrasias, cyanosis and clubbing of fingers for cardiac or pulmonary disorders, yellow for liver disease, splinter hemorrhages from bacterial endocarditis). • Discuss treatment for specific conditions. • Identify itching, rash, hives, swelling, wheezing, etc. that may be attributable to allergic response. • Identify substances that may cause allergic reaction (i.e., latex, anesthetics, antibiotics, foods, iodine, bees).	• Refer to appropriate specialist for further evaluation. • Review adverse effects of medication used to treat condition. • Review oral effects of medications used. • Determine whether oral treatment should be deferred. • Avoid use of latex products if allergic. • Avoid prescribing drug allergens (antibiotics, analgesics). • Anticipate potential medical emergency anaphylaxis.

Continued

Table 8-1. *Review of Systems Health History Considerations for Oral Health Care—cont'd*

Review of Systems Category	Medical Considerations	Oral Health Treatment Considerations
Musculoskeletal		
Arthritis/Rheumatism	• Patient may be taking multiple medications (NSAIDs, aspirin, corticosteroids, immunosuppressives).	• Evaluate for bleeding tendencies or mucosal changes caused by medications used. • Provide pillows or alter chair position to support physical comfort. • Provide additional aides to assist with manual dexterity for oral hygiene home-care regimen. • Assess for temporomandibular joint involvement.
Artificial joints	• Assess for increased risk for infection because of bacteremia.	• Determine whether antibiotic premedication is warranted.
Osteoporosis	• Identify fractures, type, location. • Discuss medications and vitamins used.	• Assess operatory for risk for falls. • Escort patient to and from operatory for safety. • Evaluate patient for signs of bisphosphonate osteonecrosis of the jaws (BONJ). • Recommend computed tomography x-ray (CTX) study to determine risk for BONJ.
Cardiovascular		
Hypertension	• Identify medications used. • Identify symptoms—headaches, dizziness, visual changes.	• Take vital signs at each appointment. • Encourage adherence to medication regimen. • Use vasoconstrictors with caution. • Use stress-reduction protocol. • Assess for xerostomia caused by medication. • Assess for potential for postural hypotension based on medications used. • Defer treatment for patients with blood pressure ≥180/100 mm Hg.
Myocardial infarction	• Determine date of event, treatment rendered, medications used.	• Postpone elective treatment for 1 month after myocardial infarction. • Consult with cardiologist to discuss medications used and potential interactions with vasoconstrictors in local anesthetics, gingival hyperplasia, etc. • Take vital signs at each appointment. • Assess functional capacity; defer treatment if patient does not reach 4-MET level. • Use stress-reduction protocol and short appointments. • Do not take patient off anticoagulants unless advised by physician. • Identify INR (international normalized ratio) status if taking anticoagulants. • Assess for potential medical emergency. • Use cardiac dose of vasoconstrictor (2 cartridges 1:100,000). • Antibiotic premedication not indicated for those with stents, coronary artery bypass graft.
Angina pectoris	• Identify type of angina (stable vs. unstable), triggers, frequency of events, medications used.	• Use stress-reduction protocol and short appointments. • Take vital signs at each appointment. • Request patient bring nitroglycerin to appointment.

Table 8-1. *Review of Systems Health History Considerations for Oral Health Care—cont'd*

Review of Systems Category	Medical Considerations	Oral Health Treatment Considerations
		• Assess functional capacity; defer treatment if patient does not reach 4-MET level. • Use vasoconstrictions cautiously; use cardiac dose (2 cartridges 1:100,000). • Defer elective care for those with unstable or progressive angina. • Assess for potential medical emergency.
Heart failure	• Identify cause of condition—coronary artery disease, hypertension. • Identify medication used.	• Obtain consult with cardiologist to treat. • Adjust chair position to improve breathing. • Take vital signs at each appointment. • Assess functional capacity. • Use stress-reduction protocol. • Avoid vasoconstrictors if patient taking digoxin. • Assess for potential medical emergency—myocardial infarction, arrhythmias, acute heart failure, sudden death.
Arrhythmias	• Determine cause of condition—heart failure, ischemic heart disease, other medications. • Identify if patient has a pacemaker or defibrillator. • Identify medication used.	• Use stress-reduction protocol. • Take vital signs at each appointment. • Use local anesthetics with caution. • Assess for signs of oral effects of medication. • Postpone elective oral care in those with serious, symptomatic arrhythmias. • Antibiotic prophylaxis not required for those with pacemaker or defibrillator. • Considered to be at high risk for bacterial endocarditis; prophylactic antibiotics required.
Prosthetic heart valves	• Determine date of procedure, medications used.	• Antibiotic prophylaxis for invasive dental procedures is no longer recommended.
Other	• Other medical considerations are mitral valve prolapse, rheumatic fever, heart murmur caused by valvular disease.	
Respiratory		
Asthma	• Identify type, triggers, medication used. • Discuss need for emergency department treatment, date, length of hospitalization (if any), treatment rendered.	• Advise patient to bring inhalers to office. • Take vital signs and note respiratory sounds. • Use local anesthetic without vasoconstrictor if patient is allergic to sulfites. • Inform patient of need to rinse with water after inhaler use to avoid candidiasis. • Eliminate triggers in office. • Use stress-reduction protocol. • Avoid use of aspirin and NSAIDs, barbiturates, narcotics. • Obtain medical consult for severe persistent asthma cases.
Chronic obstructive pulmonary disease (COPD)	• Identify type of chronic disease, medications used, need for oxygen supplementation.	• Postpone treatment if upper respiratory infection is present. • Adjust chair position to upright. • Take vital signs and note respiratory sounds. • Avoid use of rubber dam in severe disease.

Continued

Table 8-1. *Review of Systems Health History Considerations for Oral Health Care—cont'd*

Review of Systems Category	Medical Considerations	Oral Health Treatment Considerations
		• Use pulse oximetry to monitor oxygen sedation. • Use low-flow supplemental oxygen when oxygen saturation drops to less than 95%. • Avoid use of barbiturates, narcotics, antihistamines, anticholinergics. • Avoid nitrous oxide/oxygen inhalation with severe COPD. • Ultrasonic and air-powder polisher contraindicated.
Tuberculosis	• Identify signs and symptoms of disease, active status, medications used. • Patient may be prescribed antibiotics for months.	• Defer treatment if active signs and symptoms. • Refer patient to specialist for treatment. • Postpone treatment until patient has had treatment for 3 weeks, is not coughing, has three consecutive negative sputum smears on 3 separate days. • Encourage adherence to medication regimen. • Safe to treat patients who have positive skin test but do not have active disease.
Gastrointestinal		
Gastroesophageal reflux disease	• Identify preventive measures and medications used to treat condition.	• Place patient in semisupine position as needed. • Avoid prescribing aspirin or NSAIDs for oral pain. • Examine teeth for signs of erosion; recommend daily fluoride therapy. • Schedule patient 3 hours after a meal. • Caution patient about timing of use of antibiotics.
Ulcers, Colitis	• Identify medications used to treat condition. • Determine diet restrictions and effect on health status.	• Avoid prescribing aspirin or NSAIDs for oral pain. • Evaluate need for antibiotics, which may worsen colitis. • Assess for xerostomia caused by medications used to treat condition.
Liver diseases	• Identify history of hepatitis, type, and carrier status (B, C, D). • Discuss treatment used for patients with cirrhosis or fatty liver disease.	• Assess potential for infection transmission. • Review laboratory studies with physician to determine carrier status, ability to metabolize analgesics and local anesthetics. • Evaluate for bleeding tendencies.
Genitourinary		
End-stage renal disease	• Patient may present with abnormal drug metabolism, hepatitis, infection, hypertension, heart failure, etc. • Patient may be on hemodialysis.	• Schedule appointments day after dialysis treatment. • Obtain medical consult with nephrologist. • Patients on dialysis do not require prophylactic antibiotics. • Take vital signs on opposite arm of shunt. • Review laboratory studies to identify potential for bleeding. • Evaluate for oral manifestations (uremic stomatitis, xerostomia, enlarged parotid glands, petechial hemorrhages, osteolytic lesions of jaws, periodontal disease). • Avoid aspirin and NSAIDs in cases of severe renal failure.

Table 8-1. *Review of Systems Health History Considerations for Oral Health Care—cont'd*

Review of Systems Category	Medical Considerations	Oral Health Treatment Considerations
		• Use of air polishing is contraindicated. • Maintain frequent continuing care appointments and encourage meticulous oral hygiene.
Sexually transmitted infections/diseases	• Identify type of infection (syphilis, gonorrhea, HIV, chlamydia, warts, human papillomavirus, etc.). • Note medications used for treatment.	• May have oral manifestations of disease. • Use universal precautions as disease can be transmitted to dental hygienist via direct contact with oral lesions or infectious blood. • Refer to physician and postpone treatment when oral lesions are present.
Pregnancy	• Identify trimester, any complications.	• Discuss preconceptional care and oral health care for infant and mother. • Time oral health treatment to support mother and any side effects from pregnancy (i.e., nausea, fatigue). • Adjust chair for comfort. • Take vital signs at each appointment to monitor for hypertension. • Use lidocaine in small doses (2 cartridges 1:100,000). • Do not prescribe tetracyclines. • Avoid prescribing NSAIDs, aspirin, codeine, barbiturates, benzodiazepines. • Schedule frequent appointments to maintain meticulous oral hygiene.
Endocrine		
Diabetes	• Identify type and medications used. • For those taking insulin, note peak activity of drug. • Discuss frequency of hypoglycemic episodes.	• Evaluate for oral signs of diabetes. • Evaluate for potential for medical emergency due to hypoglycemic episodes; have sugar source readily available. • Schedule morning appointments with breaks. • Advise patient to bring glucometer and healthy snack to appointment. • Schedule patients for frequent continuing care appointments to assist with achieving periodontal health. • Discuss need for meticulous home care. • Advise use of fluoride supplement to reduce caries incidence. • Refer patient to foot, eye, and pharmacist specialists for additional care.
Thyroid disease	• Assess for signs of hypothyroidism and hyperthyroidism. • Discuss treatment for condition (medication, surgery, radioactive iodine). • Identify if patient had any thyroid storm/crisis situations.	• Reinforce adherence to medication regimen for those with hypothyroidism. • Take vital signs at each appointment. • Use of vasoconstrictors are contraindicated for those with hyperthyroidism. • Avoid palpating thyroid gland in those with hyperthyroidism to avert thyroid storm. • Evaluate for potential for medical emergency. • Use stress-reduction strategies.

Continued

Table 8-1. *Review of Systems Health History Considerations for Oral Health Care—cont'd*

Review of Systems Category	Medical Considerations	Oral Health Treatment Considerations
Neurological		
Stroke/Transient ischemic attack (TIA)	• Identify risk factors (hypertension, diabetes). • Identify medication used. • Identify date of episode.	• Postpone elective oral health care for 6 months poststroke/TIA. • Schedule short, midafternoon appointments. • Take vital signs at each appointment. • Use vasoconstrictors with caution; no gingival retraction cord; use cardiac dose for local anesthesia. • Prolonged bleeding may occur with use of anticoagulant/antiplatelet medications. • Identify INR depending on medication used. • Use stress-reduction protocol. • Recommend oral health aides appropriate to residual impairment. • Assess panoramic films for plaques in the carotid arteries; refer to specialist as indicated.
Seizure disorders	• Identify history of seizures and degree of control. • Discuss potential triggers to avoid (bright lights, odors, sounds, etc.). • Verify patient is taking medication as prescribed.	• Obtain medical consult to determine disease control. • Assess for oral side effects of medications (gingival hyperplasia). • Reinforce need for adherence to prescribed medication. • Advise use of daily fluoride therapy if xerostomic. • Evaluate for potential for medical emergency.
Hematologic/Lymphatic		
Blood transfusion	• Determine reason for blood transfusions (bleeding disorder, surgical procedure, serious injury). • Identify date of transfusion(s).	• Assess risk for hepatitis B or C or HIV. • Consult with physician regarding status of liver function. • Use universal precautions/infection control.
Inherited bleeding disorders	• Identify type of bleeding disorder and treatment used.	• Assess risk for bleeding postperiodontal debridement; may need to apply direct pressure or local hemostatic agent after procedure. • Consult with physician or hematologist before treatment. • Review laboratory testing before treatment. • Assess potential for medical emergency.
Leukemia	• Determine type and treatment. • Discuss complications of treatment and bleeding tendencies. • Identify remission status.	• Assess for potential for bleeding complications, prolonged healing, or tendency toward infection. • Evaluate for signs of condition (petechiae, ecchymosis, spontaneous bleeding, skin pallor, gingival hyperplasia). • Consult with physician or hematologist before treatment.

Table 8-1. *Review of Systems Health History Considerations for Oral Health Care—cont'd*

Review of Systems Category	Medical Considerations	Oral Health Treatment Considerations
Psychiatric	• Identify type of psychiatric illness. • Note medications used for treatment. • Discuss behavioral management approaches that are helpful.	• Some psychiatric drugs act adversely with vasoconstrictors in local anesthetics—consult drug reference. • Medications may cause xerostomia; recommend daily fluoride therapy. • Other medication effects may complicate treatment—dystonia, tardive dyskinesia. • Patients who are anxious will require stress-reduction strategies.

Sources: Little JW, Falace DA, Miller CS, et al. *Dental Management of the Medically Compromised Patient.* 8th ed. St. Louis, MO: Mosby Elsevier; 2013:2-8; Goldberg C. A practical guide to clinical medicine. San Diego: University of California. https://meded.ucsd.edu/clinicalmed/introduction.htm. Accessed May 25, 2013; and Burgess J, Meyers AD. Dental management in the medically compromised patient. Medscape. http://emedicine.medscape.com/article/2066164-overview. Updated January 6, 2015. Accessed May 25, 2013.

Table 8-2. *Elements of the Oral History*

Items of Oral History	Prevention and Treatment Considerations
Chief Complaint • In own words • Type of complaint • Symptoms onset, duration, self-treatment performed	Need for emergency treatment or to reprioritize treatment Attitude toward oral health prevention and treatment
Prior dental/dental hygiene treatment • Date of last treatment • Service performed • Frequency of treatment • Bad experiences encountered • Emergencies occurred	Reveals patient's knowledge and value of regular oral health care Anticipate possible emergency
Family oral health history • Parental tooth loss • Regular oral health care	Attitude of family toward preventive care, saving teeth Cultural beliefs about oral health care Customary oral health practices
Radiation history • Dental and medical radiographs • Types, dates, reasons • Therapeutic treatment • Availability of previous radiographs	Amount of exposure Knowledge and value of using radiographs Need for radiographs given history and current clinical findings Attitude and knowledge of procedures
Anesthetic history • Local, general, nitrous oxide/oxygen • Adverse events/effects • Anxiety/nervousness during oral care	Choice of anesthetic Anticipate possible emergency
Past dental treatment • Restorative—frequency, procedures performed, referral to specialist • Periodontal—diagnosis, surgery, chemotherapeutics, current status • Orthodontic—age during treatment, type of treatment, habit correction, use of appliances • Endodontic—diagnosis, type of treatment, result • Prosthodontics—type of treatment, use of appliances	Knowledge and value of prevention Financial impact/considerations Negative outcomes Potential for emergency

Continued

Table 8-2. Elements of the Oral History—cont'd

Items of Oral History	Prevention and Treatment Considerations
• Oral and maxillofacial surgery—cause, type of treatment, dates, adverse events • Other—implants	
Oral diagnostics • Comprehensive oral examination • Adjunctive oral cancer screenings • Lasers for caries diagnosis • Periodontal examinations • Genetic testing • Salivary diagnostics	Understanding and value of oral diagnostics Need for follow-up care Need for referral Identification of genetic predispositions
Oral habits • Clenching, bruxism • Mouth breathing • Biting objects • Cheek or lip biting • Sucking on candies/chewing gum • Awareness of habits	Anxiety/tension of patient Interest in habit cessation if detrimental Potential for injury
History of injury to head or mouth • Date, cause, extent • Fractures/dislocations • Treatment rendered	Potential for further injury Attitude about risk behaviors Limitation of mouth opening Preventive care during treatment and healing
Temporomandibular joint • History of injury, discomfort, subluxation, dislocation, fracture, disease • Prior treatment—surgery, appliances, medications	Limitation of mouth opening Short appointments to prevent discomfort Referral to specialist—dental, physical therapist
Self-care practices • Daily biofilm removal—toothbrushing (type of brush, frequency of use, age of brush, brushing time, use of interdental aides) • Type of dentifrice (fluoride, antibacterial with fluoride, antibacterial and anti-inflammatory), reason selected • Dental aides (floss, water irrigation, interdental), frequency of use, reason selected • Chemotherapeutics (mouthrinses, host modulation therapy), frequency of use, reason selected • Fluoride—systemic or topical; community water; amount of fluoride in drinking water; frequency of use	Current practices Instruction provided Concerns about use of products New instruction needed Need for continued use Knowledge of benefits of preventive care and oral health Attitude and cultural beliefs

Personal Psychosocial History

A variety of nonmedical issues may impact the dental hygiene treatment plan. Personal information, social issues, and cultural beliefs are part of this aspect of the health history. These represent real-life issues that are important to the patient, and they help the care provider develop a relationship by demonstrating understanding and empathy.

Nutrition status is a concept to discuss with each patient. As noted previously, some patients may be overweight, obese, or morbidly obese. Other patients may be underweight or malnourished. Engaging in a conversation about typical diet patterns, healthy lifestyle practices, and weight management are important health topics to discuss. For some patients, dieting has been an unsuccessful way of life, and they may be less inclined to discuss another "diet plan" with the practitioner. Encouraging patients to complete a diet diary for 3 to 5 days and incorporating nutrition counseling is an invaluable health service. Chapter 16 includes more detailed information about nutrition assessment.

In addition, reviewing specific eating patterns such as snacking on foods with high sugar content and drinking acidic beverages is an important component of oral health education. Many individuals are not aware of the relationship between acidic carbonated beverages and dental erosion, whereas others have not made the connection between a refined carbohydrate diet and the dental caries process. Dietary modifications will need to be recommended based on each patient's diet history.

As part of a social history, the dental hygienist should discuss tobacco use, alcohol consumption, and use of recreational drugs. Determining use of these products and discussing oral and systemic implications is essential. The ADHA promotes a tobacco cessation program that can be accessed online (www.adha.org). Patients should be encouraged to quit smoking or using any form of tobacco to reduce the risk for oral and lung cancers. Those patients who have a history of alcohol abuse need to be educated about an increased risk for oral cancer, bleeding, and liver diseases. These individuals may have an inability to tolerate analgesics and anesthetics, may arrive at the practice inebriated, or may be nonadherent with oral health recommendations. In addition, those patients who indicate they are recovering alcoholics should be counseled to use nonalcoholic mouth rinses if indicated.

Oral effects are known to be apparent with the use of illicit substances. In addition, medical emergencies can occur in the dental office setting when patients have used recreational drugs. Patients should be counseled to avoid any drug use before an oral care appointment. Patients who smoke marijuana should be advised to refrain from using this product 1 week before an appointment in which local anesthesia containing a vasoconstrictor is planned. Likewise, when a patient admits to using cocaine, he or she should be cautioned to abstain for at least 18 hours before an appointment in which use of local anesthesia is planned. A person who uses methamphetamine should be cautioned to refrain from using for 24 hours before an appointment in which local anesthesia with a vasoconstrictor is planned.

Another aspect of the personal psychosocial history is information about the patient's occupation. Including this information serves several functions. First, the dental hygiene care provider can learn whether the patient has been exposed to any substances that may predispose him to systemic conditions or cancers. Discussing occupational considerations helps to establish rapport and determine the patient's commitment to and value of work. This attitude may translate to general and oral health. Further, this provides an opportunity to learn how busy someone is and whether she needs special consideration for scheduling appointments. Lastly, this information provides an opportunity to discuss financial matters and to determine how oral health care fits into the patient's budget and how her bills will be paid.

If cultural beliefs and attitudes have not been addressed during the family history, the personal history provides an opportunity to address any particular needs or concerns. In some cultures, looking a person in the eye is a sign of disrespect. The dental hygiene care provider needs to take the time to learn how the patient wishes to be treated, whether he is willing to accept proposed treatment, and whether he can trust the provider to maintain confidentiality when health history information is discussed.

Another aspect of this history relates to anxiety and stress. Stress has been shown to be associated with both periodontal disease and medical emergencies in practice settings. Patients may have other stressors besides concern or fear about dental hygiene treatment. He or she may be undergoing financial strain, experiencing a recent divorce or death in the family, moving to a new location, or taking a new job. Whatever the cause of stress, it is important for the dental hygienist to help the patient deal with stress to avoid medical emergencies such as syncope and hyperventilation.

Another area of concern for both the patient and the provider is the issue of access to care. Although some patients have an easy time getting to and from oral health appointments, others may have to rely on mass transportation or the kindness of a friend to transport them to the office. This may impact the time and day of availability for appointments. Likewise, some patients may have serious disabilities and need to schedule their visits around the caregiver's availability. The dental hygiene provider will need to demonstrate both understanding and flexibility to assist these individuals in acquiring oral health care.

Medication History

All of the medications or pills that a patient is taking, including herbal preparations and vitamins, should be identified on the health history. The dental hygienist is then responsible for identifying each medication for actions, adverse effects, potential drug interactions, and potential for an emergency in the operatory. Often, patients do not perceive over-the-counter drugs or herbal remedies as true medications and fail to mention them as part of the history. For some individuals, they will know the name of the medicine, but not the condition for which it is being used. Other patients will know the disease for which the medication is used, but not the name of the medication. They can describe the color and shape of the drug (e.g., purple pill), but cannot recall the name. Mailing the health history to the patient in advance allows the dental hygienist to obtain accurate information. This is especially important for those individuals who present with complex medical histories and are taking multiple medications (see Teamwork). It is important for the dental hygiene provider to have a reliable, current, comprehensive resource for drug information. Resources are available in print as well as online (Box 8-1).

Teamwork

Interacting with other health-care providers enriches dental hygiene practice. When considering opportunities available with respect to the medical and dental histories, dental hygiene providers can collaborate with local pharmacists. Pharmacists can assist dental hygiene specialists by reviewing a patient's drug history and assisting them with understanding adverse effects, side effects (including oral effects), and other medications that may be more effective and reduce side effects. This may be especially beneficial for those patients who present with multiple systemic conditions including cardiovascular disease and diabetes mellitus.

In addition, developing a collaborative team relationship with other specialists, including cardiologists, nephrologists, endocrinologists, and pulmonologists, may be useful when referring patients for further evaluation before treatment. Including these specialists as part of the practice, holding team sessions with them to learn the latest research in areas of systemic disease and medication management, may help provide better appreciation for and recognition of each person's respective knowledge, skills, and talents. ■

Box 8-1. Sources for Medication History Information

Texts

Wynn RL, Meiller T, Crossley HL. *Drug Information Handbook for Dentistry.* 15th ed. Hudson, OH: Lexi-Comp Inc.; 2010.

Pickett FA, Terezhalmy GT. *Dental Drug Reference with Clinical Implications.* Baltimore, MD: Lippincott Williams & Wilkins; 2009.

Skidmore-Roth L. *Mosby's Handbook of Herbs and Natural Supplements.* 4th ed. St. Louis, MO: Mosby; 2009.

La Gow B, ed. 2009. *PDR for Nonprescription Drugs, Dietary Supplements and Herbs.* Montvale, NJ: Thomson Healthcare.

Websites

HerbMed (subscription)
www.herbmed.org

RxList (Rx and herbal)
www.rxlist.com

WebMD (Rx and herbal)
www.webmd.com

PubMed
http://www.ncbi.nlm.nih.gov/pubmed

MedicineNet
www.medicinenet.com

Mayo Clinic
http://mayoclinic.com

Epocrates (Web-based research)
www.epocrates.com

Medscape (free subscription)
www.medscape.com

Natural Standard (subscription via academic library; evidence-based natural products database)
http://www.naturalstandard.com/ ■

The health history used by the CRDHA is unique in that it provides for a decision-making process about the patient's reported medications. The dental hygienist is posed questions about the rationale for the medication, adverse effects, drug interactions, dosage, how the patient is managing the medication, and oral side effects. The last step of this analysis is for the dental hygiene care provider to determine risks for treating this patient based on the medication profile. Further assessment and treatment should not proceed without this vital information.

Vital Signs

Vital signs that can be used in oral health assessment include height, weight, **body mass index (BMI)** (a measure of body fat calculated by a formula using an individual's height and weight), temperature, pulse, respiration, and blood pressure. In some circumstances, vital signs such as blood pressure and pulse may need to be repeated before treatment to ensure that normal values are obtained and it is safe to provide care.

Height, Weight, and Body Mass Index

Height, weight, and BMI are factors that, when taken together, may indicate patients who require counseling for being overweight, obese, or morbidly obese. These individuals may be at risk for diabetes mellitus, cardiovascular disease, metabolic syndrome, hypertension, stroke, gallbladder disease, osteoarthritis, sleep apnea, and cancers. It is estimated that approximately 154.7 million adults in the United States are overweight or obese.[2]

There is also concern about the growing number of children and adolescents who are overweight or obese. Reviewing these three values with patients and their families provides an opportunity to educate them about the importance of disease prevention and the need to take healthy lifestyle measures including weight management and exercise. Multiple resources for health professionals and the public regarding identification and treatment of overweight and obesity conditions are available online at: http://www.nhlbi.nih.gov/files/docs/guidelines/ob_gdlns.pdf.

Although most dental office settings do not have scales and devices for measuring height, approximations can be made and compared with a BMI table (Table 8-3). Established BMI categories[3] are:

- Underweight: <18.5
- Normal weight: 18.5–24.9
- Overweight: 25–29.9
- Obesity: ≥30

Table 8-3. Body Mass Index

Body Mass Index Table

Body Weight (pounds)

Height (Inches) BMI	Normal						Overweight					Obese										Extreme Obesity					
	19	20	21	22	23	24	25	26	27	28	29	30	31	32	33	34	35	36	37	38	39	40	41	42	43	44	45
58	91	96	100	105	110	115	119	124	129	134	138	143	148	153	158	162	167	172	177	181	186	191	196	201	205	210	215
59	94	99	104	109	114	119	124	128	133	138	143	148	153	158	163	168	173	178	183	188	193	198	203	208	212	217	222
60	97	102	107	112	118	123	128	133	138	143	148	153	158	163	168	174	179	184	189	194	199	204	209	215	220	225	230
61	100	106	111	116	122	127	132	137	143	148	153	158	164	169	174	180	185	190	195	201	206	211	217	222	227	232	238
62	104	109	115	120	126	131	136	142	147	153	158	164	169	175	180	186	191	196	202	207	213	218	224	229	235	240	245
63	107	113	118	124	130	135	141	146	152	158	163	169	175	180	186	191	197	203	208	214	220	225	231	237	242	248	254
64	110	116	122	128	134	140	145	151	157	163	169	174	180	186	192	197	204	209	215	221	227	232	238	244	250	256	262
65	114	120	126	132	138	144	150	156	162	168	174	180	186	192	198	204	210	216	222	228	234	240	246	252	258	264	270
66	118	124	130	136	142	148	155	161	167	173	179	186	192	198	204	210	216	223	229	235	241	247	253	260	266	272	278
67	121	127	134	140	146	153	159	166	172	178	185	191	198	204	211	217	223	230	236	242	249	255	261	268	274	280	287
68	125	131	138	144	151	158	164	171	177	184	190	197	203	210	216	223	230	236	243	249	256	262	269	276	282	289	295
69	128	135	142	149	155	162	169	176	182	189	196	203	209	216	223	230	236	243	250	257	263	270	277	284	291	297	304
70	132	139	146	153	160	167	174	181	188	195	202	209	216	222	229	236	243	250	257	264	271	278	285	292	299	306	313
71	136	143	150	157	165	172	179	186	193	200	208	215	222	229	236	243	250	257	265	272	279	286	293	301	308	315	322
72	140	147	154	162	169	177	184	191	199	206	213	221	228	235	242	250	258	265	272	279	287	294	302	309	316	324	331
73	144	151	159	166	174	182	189	197	204	212	219	227	235	242	250	257	265	272	280	288	295	302	310	318	325	333	340
74	148	155	163	171	179	186	194	202	210	218	225	233	241	249	256	264	272	280	287	295	303	311	319	326	334	342	350
75	152	160	168	176	184	192	200	208	216	224	232	240	248	256	264	272	279	287	295	303	311	319	327	335	343	351	359
76	156	164	172	180	189	197	205	213	221	230	238	246	254	263	271	279	287	295	304	312	320	328	336	344	353	361	369

Source: National Heart Lung and Blood Institute. Obesity Education Initiative: calculate your body mass index. https://www.nhlbi.nih.gov/about/org/oei. Accessed December 15, 2013.

Temperature

Body temperature is used as a screening tool for individuals who may present with a suspected infection or illness. For some patients, their concern about attending the oral health appointment supersedes their concern for a potential infection that could be transmitted throughout the dental office setting to other patients waiting in the reception area and to the practitioners. In addition, some individuals who present with oral infections may have increased body temperature. Those individuals with acute periodontal conditions including necrotizing gingivitis or periodontitis or periodontal abscesses may have elevated body temperature. During periods of flu epidemics, it is especially helpful to take body temperature as a means of identifying those who are contagious (Procedure 8-1). Normal body temperature for adults ranges from 96°F to 99.5°F (35.6°C–37.5°C). Children's temperatures may range from 98.0°F to 99.4°F (36.7°C–37.4). Because the human body has a circadian rhythm (biological activities that occur about the same time each day), body temperature may be lower in the morning and somewhat higher in the late afternoon and early evening.

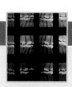

Procedure 8-1 Measuring Body Temperature

MATERIALS

| Thermometer (oral, electronic, ear, or forehead) | To determine body temperature |
| Protective sheath or sleeve | To reduce transmission of infection |

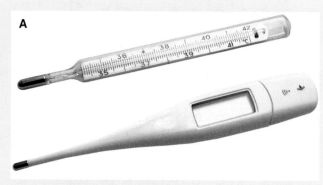

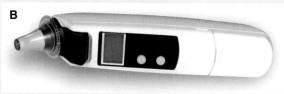

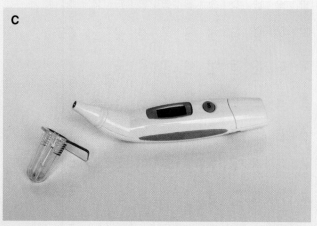

Thermometers: (A) oral, (B) electronic, and (c) ear. (Images from Thinkstock) ©Natalie Shmeliova ©Ruddi Hansen ©Amawasri

PREPROCEDURE

Patient Education

The patient or guardian, or both, must be educated on the importance of body temperature screening.

PROCEDURE

Oral

- Make sure the patient is able to breathe through the nose while keeping lips closed.
- Cover the thermometer with a protective sheath.
- Place the thermometer under the patient's tongue.
- Read the mercury column.
- Record the temperature on the patient's health history record.

Electronic

- Cover the thermometer with a protective sheath.
- Place the thermometer under the patient's tongue.
- Read the digital display.

Ear

- Cover the thermometer with a protective sheath.
- Insert the tympanic device gently into the ear canal.
- Digital display will record the temperature within several seconds.

Forehead

- Apply the chemical strip or wand across the patient's forehead.
- Color change on the strip shows the temperature or the digital display will reveal the temperature.

POSTPROCEDURE

After the temperature has been identified and recorded in the health history record, the patient or guardian, or both, should be informed of the results and advised of any changes needed based on the findings, such as postponing treatment until the body temperature is within normal limits.

Treat those patients who present with extremely elevated temperature readings (i.e., ≥105°F [40.6°C]) as a medical emergency, arrange for transport to a hospital for further medical care, and document the case in the patient record.

Pulse

The **pulse** reflects the count of the heartbeats. It is typically taken by palpating the radial artery for 1 minute and noting the force and regularity or quality of beats (Procedure 8-2). An even regular force and rate is referred to as normal. In adults, a normal pulse ranges from 60 to 80 beats per minute (bpm), although some texts may consider up to 100 bpm within normal limits.[4,5] Children's pulse rates may range from 80 to 120 bpm.

A slower heart rate may be a normal finding in athletes. However, a slower heart rate of less than 60 bpm may also represent a **sinus bradycardia.** This pulse rate may be associated with medications used to treat cardiovascular disease or systemic disorders such as hypothyroidism.

An unusually fast heart rate, more than 100 bpm in adults, is known as **tachycardia.** Atrial tachycardia is a fast, irregular pulse rate, also known as **tachyarrhythmia.** It represents a cardiovascular instability and may lead to cardiac arrest. A 60-second examination of the pulse is necessary to determine this abnormality.

Although some dental hygienists tend to monitor the pulse rate for 15 seconds and multiply by 4, in doing so they may be missing the changes in the pulse rate that would signal this abnormality. Other factors that may contribute to tachycardia include exercise, anxiety, anemia, medications, and hyperthyroidism. When a patient presents with a rapid pulse rate, a medical referral should be performed to determine the degree of cardiac health, and if any recommendations for oral treatment are warranted. If a patient presents with a pulse more than 120 bpm, elective oral health care should be delayed because a potential medical emergency may exist. Treatment can resume when the pulse rate returns to normal.

The radial artery is the most common site for taking a pulse. However, other sites can be used if necessary including the facial artery, temporal artery, and carotid artery. During a medical emergency, the carotid artery is typically used for determining the pulse in an adult, and the brachial artery is used for determining the pulse in an infant.[6]

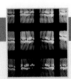

Procedure 8-2 Taking the Pulse

MATERIALS

A watch or clock with a second hand | To count pulse beats for 1 minute

PREPROCEDURE

- Inform the patient that the pulse will be taken.
- Make sure the patient is seated in a comfortable position with the palm down and the hand and arm supported.

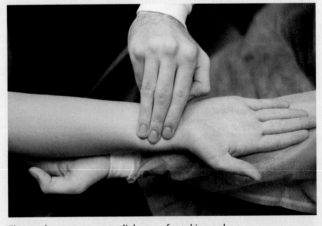

Finger placement over radial artery for taking pulse.

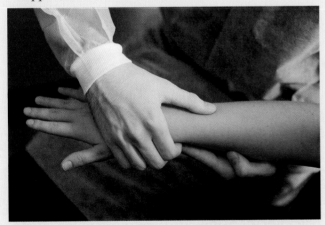

Patient's arm is extended palm down and supported when taking the pulse.

PROCEDURE

- Using the tips of three fingers (not the thumb, which has its own pulse), locate the radial pulse along the thumb side of the wrist.

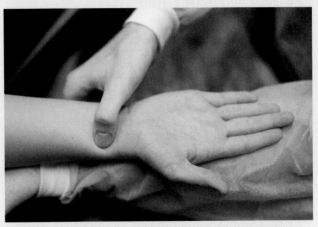

Incorrect taking of pulse using the thumb over the radial artery.

• Once the pulse is felt, count the beats for 1 minute using the second hand of a watch or clock. Note the rhythm (regularity of heartbeats) and the strength (strong, poor, weak, thready) of the heartbeats.

POSTPROCEDURE
• Record the date, pulse rate, rhythm, and strength on the patient's health history record.
• Inform the patient or guardian, or both, of the results.

Respiration is the inhalation and exhalation of air. Respiration functions to supply oxygen to the tissues and eliminate carbon dioxide. The respiration rate is measured as the number of times the chest rises in 1 minute (Procedure 8-3). A normal respiratory rate is 14 to 20 breaths per minute for adults, 20 to 24 breaths per minute for children, and up to 44 breaths per minute for infants. Variations in normal may be affected by age, gender, exercise, elevated body temperature, stress and anxiety, pain, hemorrhage, shock, odors, medications, and medical conditions. A respiration rate of 12 or less is subnormal in an adult and may be associated with medications or pulmonary insufficiency. Respiration rates greater than 28 breaths per minute in an adult represent an abnormal condition, and rates greater than 60 constitute a medical emergency.

Rapid breathing is referred to as **tachypnea.** Difficulty breathing is known as **dyspnea. Orthopnea** represents difficulty breathing while the patient is in a supine position. If this is noted to occur, place the patient in an upright position to provide dental and dental hygiene treatment. Deep, rapid, irregular breathing is known as **hyperventilation** and can be associated with a stress-related emergency or diabetic ketoacidosis. Observe the patient for signs of hyperventilation including facial perspiration, clutching the arms of the dental chair, or expressions of being frightened or feeling sick. In this instance, stress-reduction procedures are indicated to prevent a medical emergency.

Blood pressure refers to pressure that is exerted on the walls of the blood vessels. A measurement of blood pressure is affected by many factors including the muscular efficiency of the heart, blood volume and viscosity, age and health of the individual, and state of the vascular walls. The blood pressure provides a means of screening general health and is recommended for all who present for oral care, including children. It is not uncommon for practitioners to find that their patients do not have routine blood pressure measurements and are unaware that elevated blood pressure is associated with cardiovascular disease. The ADA advises that blood pressure be taken at continuing care appointments as a way to screen for undiagnosed or uncontrolled hypertension (Procedure 8-4).[7]

Systolic blood pressure (SBP) refers to arterial pressure when the heart muscle contracts and forces blood into the circulation. Normal SBP is less than 120 mm Hg. **Diastolic blood pressure** (DBP) represents the arterial pressure between heartbeats when the heart rests. Normal DBP is less than 80 mm Hg. The measurement is indicated as a fraction with the SBP over the DBP and millimeters of mercury (e.g., 120/80 mm Hg). Either arm can be used for blood pressure; however, measurements may vary as much as 10 mm

Procedure 8-3 Measuring Respiration

PREPROCEDURE
• Maintain the fingers over the radial pulse and count respirations. Do not advise the patient respiration is being measured because she may alter her breathing pattern.

PROCEDURE
• Count the number of times the chest rises during 1 minute.
• Note the depth of respiration (shallow, normal, deep).
• Note the rhythm as regular (evenly spaced) or irregular (unusual pauses between breaths).
• Note the quality of the respirations (strong, weak, labored, noisy). Sounds heard during respiration may indicate an airway obstruction. Determine what is causing the noise.

• Note the position of the patient on the health history form. In some cases, such as dyspnea associated with asthma, chronic obstructive pulmonary disease, or congestive heart failure, the patient will be using accessory muscles to aid in breathing. Note when the patient adjusts her position or asks to sit upright for improved breathing.

POSTPROCEDURE
• Record respiration findings in the patient's health history record.
• Inform the patient or guardian, or both, if irregular findings are identified. Determine whether it is sage to provide further care or if a referral for medical evaluation is needed.

Procedure 8-4 Taking Blood Pressure

MATERIALS

Stethoscope — Y-shaped instrument used to hear and amplify body sounds such as heartbeat, breaths, and air in the intestines

Sphygmomanometer — Instrument used for measuring arterial blood pressure

Cuff and gauge — Part of the sphygmo-manometer that inflates and shows blood pressure reading

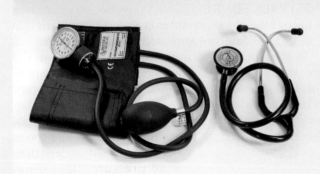

Sphygmomanometer with cuff and gauge.

PREPROCEDURE

• Inform the patient that the blood pressure will be taken and why.

• Ask the patient to loosen a tight sleeve, and adjust the shirt or blouse so that the upper arm is bare.

• Seat the patient in an upright position with the arm supported and at the level of the heart. Face the hand palm up. Legs should be uncrossed.

PROCEDURE

• Place the completely deflated cuff on the patient's arm supported at the level of the heart and not resting on the arm of the dental chair. Place the cuff over the brachial artery and fasten it so that it remains even and snug. The lower edge of the cuff should be about 1 inch above the antecubital fossa. Adjust the position of the gauge for ease of reading.

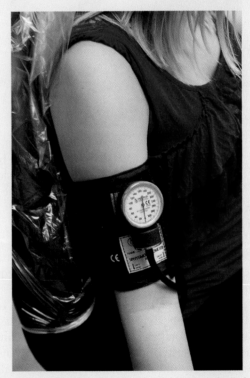

Blood pressure cuff in place over the brachial artery and 1 inch above the antecubital fossa.

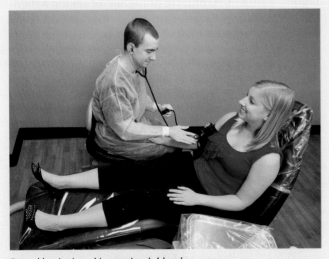

Dental hygienist taking patient's blood pressure.

- Locate the brachial pulse and place the stethoscope over this area. Position the stethoscope in the ears with the tips facing forward.

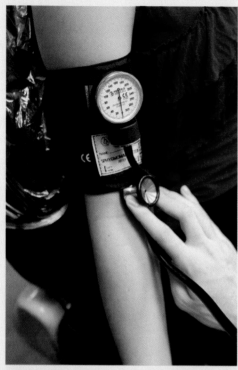

Stethoscope in place over the brachial artery.

- Close the needle valve attached to the control bulb, place the fingers over the brachial pulse, and slowly inflate the cuff until the pulse can no longer be felt.

Note the level on the dial at which the pulse cannot be felt. Pump an additional 20 to 30 mm Hg beyond this point, referred to as the maximum inflation level (MIL).

- Slowly release the air lock and deflate the cuff at a steady rate (approximately 2–3 mm/sec). Listen for the first sound and note the level on the dial. This is the systolic pressure.
- Continue to slowly release the pressure until the sound becomes muffled and then disappears. Note the number on the dial where the last sound occurred. This number is the diastolic pressure.
- Release the rest of the air rapidly. Let the patient rest for several minutes and repeat the process. The average of the two readings represents the final measurement.

POSTPROCEDURE

- Record the blood pressure on the patient's chart noting the date and arm used.

  If abnormal blood pressures are noted after the measurement has been repeated, advise the patient of this finding and refer for further evaluation as appropriate. A medical consult will need to be obtained before providing oral health care for those individuals presenting with stage 3 hypertension.

Hg from the right to left arm. For this reason, noting the arm used is important when taking subsequent measurements for comparison purposes.

Hypotension refers to an abnormally low blood pressure and may be associated with fasting, rest, syncope, shock, hemorrhage, medications such as antidepressants, and systemic diseases such as Addison's disease, hypothyroidism, anemia, and heart failure. **Orthostatic hypotension** is a form of low blood pressure that occurs when there is a sudden change from the horizontal position to the upright position or by prolonged standing resulting in syncope. A patient who stands up suddenly after being in the supine position in a dental chair may experience orthostatic hypotension. To prevent this situation from occurring, advise patients to remain seated for 1 minute before standing. The medical history may provide clues to anticipate this reaction. When patients are taking antihypertensive medications, tranquilizers, or narcotics, they may be prone to orthostatic hypertension.

Hypertension represents an abnormally elevated blood pressure. According to The Seventh Report of the Joint National Committee on Prevention, Detection, Evaluation, and Treatment of High Blood Pressure,[8]

hypertension is defined as a SBP of 140 mm Hg or higher, a DBP of 90 mm Hg or higher, or taking a medication to reduce blood pressure. A classification of blood pressure for adults with oral health treatment considerations appears in Table 8-4.[9] An elevated blood pressure may be associated with exercise, stress, and emotional disturbances, use of medications such as stimulants and birth control pills, and medical conditions including diabetes mellitus, metabolic syndrome, Cushing disease, coarctation of the aorta, and renal diseases.

Because children can present with hypertension, further evaluation can be determined as reported by Pickett and Kaelber[10] and based on the The Fourth Report on the Diagnosis, Evaluation, and Treatment of High Blood Pressure.[11] Pediatric hypertension is defined as having an SBP or DBP at or above the 95th percentile for sex, age, and height on three separate occasions. The Pickett and Kaelber model simplifies the Fourth Report model and uses age and sex as the basis of determining blood pressure status in children. Blood pressure is identified as normal (50th percentile), prehypertensive (90th percentile), stage 1 hypertension (95th percentile), or stage 2 hypertension (99th percentile) based on the age of the child. Adolescents with

Table 8-4. *Classification of Blood Pressure for Adults 18 Years or Older with Oral Health Treatment Considerations*

Category	Blood Pressure	Oral Treatment Considerations
Optimal	<120/<80	Provide routine treatment.
Normal	<130/<85	Provide routine treatment.
High-normal	130–139/85–89	Provide routine treatment. Remeasure BP at continuing care appointments to screen for hypertension.
Hypertension stage 1	140–159/90–99	Provide routine treatment. Remeasure BP after 5 minutes and patient has rested. Assess risk factors for hypertension. Refer for medical evaluation if patient has elevated BP on two separate appointments and has not been diagnosed with hypertension. Remeasure BP at continuing care appointment to screen for hypertension. Inform patient of elevated BP and recommend lifestyle changes.
Hypertension stage 2	160–179/100–109	Remeasure BP after 5 minutes and patient has rested. Assess for risk factors. If continued elevation, inform patient. Refer for medical evaluation; delay treatment if patient is unable to manage stress or if oral treatment planned will be lengthy. If using local anesthesia, limit to two cartridges of 1:100,000 vasoconstrictor. Routine treatment can be provided with stress-reduction protocol; keep appointment short.
Hypertension stage 3	≥180/ ≥110	Remeasure BP after 5 minutes and patient has rested. Assess for risk factors. Inform patient of results. Delay elective treatment until BP is controlled. Obtain a medical consult form approving oral health treatment. If emergency dental care is indicated, provide care in a setting in which emergency life support equipment is readily available.

BP, blood pressure.

Sources: Pickett FA, Gurenlian JR. *Preventing Medical Emergencies: Use of the Medical History.* 2nd ed. Baltimore, MD: Lippincott Williams & Wilkins; 2010; Chobian AV, Bakris GL, Black HR, et al. The seventh report of the Joint National Committee on Prevention, Detection, Evaluation, and Treatment of High Blood Pressure. National Heart, Lung and Blood Institute. The JNC 7 report. *JAMA.* 2003;289:2560-78; and National High Blood Pressure Education Program. Classification of blood pressure for adults age 18 or older. http://www.nhlbi.nih.gov. Accessed June 2, 2010.

values of 120/80 mm Hg or greater are considered prehypertensive and should be referred for medical evaluation. According to The Fourth Report, it is recommended that all children older than 3 years have their blood pressure measured using a cuff that accommodates the size of the upper arm.

Several types of devices are available for taking blood pressure. Aneroid manometers, electronic devices, and finger and wrist monitors have been developed. In dentistry, a mercury sphygmomanometer and stethoscope are the preferred tools for yielding accurate results. However, the practitioner must use the proper technique and an appropriate cuff size to obtain correct results. A standard cuff width is 12 to 14 cm. If a cuff is too small, falsely elevated levels will be obtained; if too large, falsely low values will occur. Narrower cuffs are available for use with children, and wider cuffs and thigh cuffs can be obtained for those patients who are large in size, overweight, or obese.

Decision-Making

Once the health history has been completed, the dental hygiene care provider is responsible for making decisions that impact the diagnosis and treatment plan. The dental hygienist may have to consult a physician to determine whether treatment is appropriate or needs to be postponed. If a patient presents with urgent cardiac symptoms, uncontrolled hypertension, or diabetes mellitus, immediate consultation is warranted. The patient may be referred for further medical care before considering offering oral health care. Once the patient is stabilized, a written consent form to begin treatment should be provided by the physician and placed in the patient's treatment record.

In some cases, treatment can proceed, but the practitioner feels the need to have a medical consultation. For example, if a patient presents with minor pulmonary complaints, such as intermittent difficulty breathing of unknown cause, but vital signs are within normal limits, the practitioner may begin performing assessment procedures. It is prudent to send a prepared medical consult form to the patient's pulmonologist or family practitioner to determine whether treatment should be modified. For those patients undergoing cancer therapy, a consult with the oncology team is warranted to establish baseline blood assay values, determine whether antibiotic premedication is indicated, and discuss coordination of oral health care with cancer care.

In addition, the health history may provide clues to an undiagnosed systemic condition, such as ongoing muscle and joint swelling and pain. The dental hygiene care provider is not expected to diagnose a systemic condition but should refer the patient for medical evaluation and diagnostic testing. A follow-up phone call to the patient reminding him to schedule this evaluation is helpful in reinforcing the need for additional medical care. Findings of this evaluation should be noted in the patient's record.

Premedication

Another decision that will challenge the dental hygiene practitioner is whether the patient requires prophylactic antibiotic therapy. Premedication has been used primarily to prevent **infective endocarditis** (IE), which is "an infection caused by bacteria that enter the bloodstream and settle in the heart lining, a heart valve, or a blood vessel."[12] Since 1955, the American Heart Association (AHA) has proposed recommendations for the prevention of IE. These recommendations are revised periodically. The most recent update to the guidelines was presented in 2007 with significant changes made based on evidence-based information (see Evidence-Based Practice). Research and literature reviews revealed that there is a very low incidence of IE. Bacteremias (the presence of bacteria in the blood) are more likely caused by daily activities than treatment performed during dental and dental hygiene appointments, and antibiotic premedication does not always prevent IE risk from occurring after invasive oral healthcare. Further, some patients are at risk for experiencing adverse effects from antibiotic therapy, whereas others may develop antibiotic resistance or a suprainfection.[12,13] Based on this information, the AHA revised their guidelines to limit antibiotic prophylaxis to particular cardiac conditions including artificial heart valves; a history of IE; serious congenital heart conditions such as unrepaired or incompletely repaired cyanotic congenital heart disease, including those with palliative shunts or conditions, a completely repaired congenital heart defect with prosthetic material or device during the first 6 months after the procedure, and any repaired congenital heart defect with residual defect; and a cardiac transplant that develops a heart valve problem. Prophylaxis is recommended by the AHA because endothelialization of prosthetic material occurs within 6 months after the procedure.[12] Antibiotic prophylaxis is recommended in patients with cardiac conditions for all dental procedures that involve manipulation of gingival tissues or the periapical region of teeth, or perforation of the oral mucosa. Antibiotic prophylaxis is not recommended for dental procedures or events such as routine anesthetic injections through noninfected tissues, taking dental radiographs, placement of removable prosthetic or orthodontic appliances, adjustment of orthodontic appliances, placement of orthodontic brackets, shedding of deciduous teeth, and bleeding from trauma to the lips or oral mucosa.[13] Prophylactic measures recommended by the AHA for oral procedures can be found online at: http://circ.ahajournals.org/content/116/15/1736/T5.expansion.html.

As the dental hygiene care provider is reviewing the findings of the patient history, it is also important to determine a general estimate of medical risk for the patient. The American Society of Anesthesiologists (ASA) developed a classification system for physical status that assesses risk even when anesthesia is not part of the planned treatment.[14] This status and oral implications are presented in Table 8-5.[14,15]

Although the ASA classification is helpful, it does not specify how treatment should be modified based on findings. Little and colleagues[4] have designed another system for assessing risk for treatment; their system is described in Table 8-6.

Evidence-Based Practice

With greater emphasis on providing care that is based on evidence, the dental hygiene practitioner can use this process when trying to make sound decisions about treatment needed. When a patient presents with a history of joint replacement, the dental hygienist can research current standards and guidelines for prophylactic antibiotics recommended by organizations based on evidence. In doing so, the dental hygienist may learn that there may be conflicts in the guidelines for prophylactic antibiotics. It will be up to the dental hygienist to review these guidelines and the evidence that supports them to determine the appropriate course of action for the patient. Further, the dental hygienist should then document the decision made and the rationale for making it in the patient record for future reference.

In addition, recommendations are made for when to provide care after a patient has had a cerebrovascular accident or a myocardial infarction. If the patient is challenging the provider's decision to delay treatment for a given period after recovery, the dental hygienist can show the patient the scientific evidence that supports this decision.

Evidence-based practice allows both the care provider and the patient an opportunity to learn more about each clinical situation and make sound decisions about best practice considerations. ■

Table 8-5. American Society of Anesthesiologists Physical Status Classification System With Oral Implications

Physical Status	Oral Implications
P1: a normal healthy patient	No treatment modification needed.
P2: a patient with mild systemic disease	Proceed with caution; these individuals are less able to tolerate stressful situations (e.g., smoking, obesity, substance abuse, anxiety or fear, well-controlled hypertension, or diabetes).
P3: a patient with severe systemic disease	Elective dental hygiene care is not contraindicated, but proceed with caution because the risk during treatment is increased (e.g., stable angina, postmyocardial infarction, morbid obesity).
P4: a patient with severe systemic disease that is a constant threat to life	Elective treatment should be postponed until the condition has improved and physical status classification has moved to P3 or better (e.g., recent history of myocardial infarction within the past 4 weeks or a stroke within the past 6 months, liver failure, end-stage renal disease).
P5: a moribund patient who is not expected to survive without the operation	No oral treatment should be rendered.
P6: a declared brain-dead patient whose organs are being removed for donor purposes	No oral treatment is indicated.

Sources: American Society of Anesthesiologists. ASA Physical Status Classification System. http://www.asahq.org/clinical/physicalstatus.htm. Accessed June 8, 2010; and Pickett FA, Gurenlian JR. *Preventing Medical Emergencies: Use of the Medical History.* 2nd ed. Baltimore, MD: Lippincott Williams & Wilkins; 2010:4-5.

Table 8-6. ABCs of Risk Assessment

Potential Concern	Follow-up Questions
Antibiotics	Will the patient need antibiotics, prophylactically or therapeutically? Is the patient currently taking antibiotics? For what purpose?
Analgesics	Is the patient taking aspirin or NSAIDS? For how long has the patient been using analgesic? What is the risk for bleeding during treatment? Will analgesics be needed after the procedure?
Anesthesia	Are any potential problems or concerns associated with the use of local anesthetics or with vasoconstrictors found in the local anesthetic?
Anxiety	Will the patient need a sedative or antianxiety medication?
Allergy	Is the patient allergic to anything that the dental hygienist may prescribe or with which he/she may come into contact in the clinical setting?
Bleeding	Is abnormal hemostasis a possibility?
Breathing	Doe the patient have any difficulty breathing, or is the breathing abnormally fast or slow?
Blood pressure	Is the blood pressure well controlled or is it likely to increase or decrease during treatment?
Chair position	Can the patient tolerate a supine chair position or is the patient likely to experience difficulty with rapid position changes?
Drugs	Have any potential drug interactions, adverse effects, or allergies been associated with any of the drugs being taken by the patient or with drugs that may be prescribed by the dental hygienist?
Devices	Does the patient have a prosthetic or therapeutic joint, coronary artery stent, pacemaker, or arteriovenous fistula that may require specific considerations during treatment?

Continued

Table 8-6. *ABCs of Risk Assessment—cont'd*

Potential Concern	Follow-up Questions
Equipment	Have any potential problems or concerns been associated with the use of dental equipment such as radiograph, ultrasonic devices, electrosurgery, or oxygen? Are devices such as a pulse oximeter, glucometer, or blood pressure monitor indicated?
Emergencies	Can any medical emergencies be encountered with this patient? If yes, how can they be prevented?
Follow-up	Is any follow-up care indicated? Should the patient be contacted at home to assess response to treatment?

Source: Adapted from Little JW, Falace DA, Miller CS, et al. *Dental Management of the Medically Compromised Patient.* 8th ed. St. Louis, MO: Mosby Elsevier; 2013:3.

Lastly, the level of **functional capacity** should be determined to assist the dental hygienist in deciding whether the patient can safely withstand oral care. The American College of Cardiology and the AHA created a method for determining cardiac risk based on the ability of the patient to perform basic daily activities.[16] Adequate functional capacity is defined as the individual being able to perform activities that meet a 4 metabolic level of endurance, also known as 4 **metabolic equivalents** (METs). A MET is a unit of measurement that represents the amount of oxygen consumption needed for physical activity and is another way to evaluate physical status. The following are examples of physical activities and their METs: sleeping, 0.9 MET; walking less than 2 mph on even ground, 2.0 METs; light or moderate calisthenics, 3.5 METs; and jogging, 7.0 METs.[16] The risk for a serious cardiac event occurring is increased when the patient is unable to meet a 4-MET demand during activities of daily living. Asking the patient whether he or she can walk on a treadmill, climb stairs with groceries, run a short distance freely, or golf will help indicate if the individual is at low risk for a cardiac emergency during oral hygiene treatment. The person who complains of shortness of breath, fatigue, chest tightness, or pain when doing these activities is at increased risk for cardiac emergency during dental hygiene treatment and should have a medical clearance provided in advance of treatment.

Updating the Health History

Although taking a comprehensive history is routine on new patients, it is equally important to update the health history at every follow-up appointment (see Application to Clinical Practice). A common mistake is to ask the patient if there have been any changes in his health since the last appointment. Most patients would be inclined to respond in the negative, not realizing or recalling that they had a recent illness or may be taking a new medication. Patients often do not perceive the importance of their medical history in relation to a dental hygiene or dental appointment, and may need to be prompted with key questions to elicit new information that is significant to clinical decision-making. Therefore, at each appointment, the dental hygiene care provider should be prepared to update the medical and dental histories noting

Application to Clinical Practice

In clinical practice, it is important to update the medical and dental histories at every appointment. It is easy to assume that little might have changed in a 1- or 3-month period. However, a patient could have had a stroke or myocardial infarction, been diagnosed with cancer, or developed caries, xerostomia, or an abscess. Neglecting to inquire about changes to a person's general and oral health places the practitioner in jeopardy of contributing to a medical emergency or a legal situation of malpractice. Providing best practice means providing best care at every patient appointment. Although some patients may just want the appointment to move along so they can get to the next part of their day, and would be pleased if all they were asked was "Has there been any change in your health since we saw you last?" it is important to educate them about how history-taking is a fundamental part of assessment. Holding high standards and gathering appropriate information is the hallmark of a licensed health-care professional. ■

any changes in health; recent illnesses, hospitalizations, or both; visits to physicians and outcomes; any laboratory or other diagnostic studies performed and the results; current medications and any adverse effects or oral side effects; and any changes in the oral cavity including pain, swelling, soreness, and bleeding.

In addition, vital signs should be taken at each appointment to note significant changes in weight (loss or gain), blood pressure, pulse, respiration, and body temperature. All findings should be documented on the health history form. If there are significant changes that warrant further medical attention, the patient should be referred for evaluation.

As with any history-taking event, the patient should sign the health history form certifying that she is providing correct information to the best of her ability. A parent or guardian should be asked to sign a child's health history form at initial and subsequent appointments.

Case Study

Mrs. Cynthia Berkowitz, a 66-year-old woman, presents to the practice for her routine comprehensive dental hygiene appointment. Her most recent visit occurred approximately 6 months ago, at which time she had indicated that she was in good health. At this appointment, Mrs. Berkowitz updated her health history and noted that she was recently diagnosed with hypertension. She states that she really did not have any symptoms and that her family doctor noticed her high blood pressure at a recent examination. She was prescribed lisinopril and she is feeling well. Upon further questioning about her health, the patient states that she was in the hospital for 3 days 2 weeks ago because she experienced a transient ischemic attack and a mild stroke. Her doctor prescribed clopidogrel (Plavix), but she is unsure why. She cannot recall the dosages of her medications but has "all that information at home." The patient states that she has no oral complaint and has not noticed any adverse effects of taking either medication. She wants her teeth cleaned so she will look nice at her granddaughter's wedding next week. The patient reports that she tends to drink a lot of tea throughout the day and does not want any stains on her teeth. In addition, she states that she is in a hurry today and wants to get her hair colored and permed before the wedding. Vital signs include: height, 5'5"; weight, 165 lb, BMI, 27.5; temperature, 98°F (36.7°C), pulse, 88 bpm; respiration, 18 breaths/min; and blood pressure, 150/95 mm Hg right arm.

Case Study Exercises

1. Using the medication history section that has the "Fundamental Questions Within the Dental Hygiene Process of Care" from the CRDHA health history form, answer items 1 through 6 based on the information provided in this case study.
2. Would you provide dental hygiene treatment for this patient? Why or why not?
3. Is antibiotic premedication indicated for dental hygiene treatment?
4. How would you explain your decision about providing care at this appointment to an elderly woman who appears to be very busy?

Review Questions

1. The first phase of the assessment process of dental hygiene care is:
   A. Performing a comprehensive oral examination
   B. Determining whether radiographic studies are indicated
   C. Conducting a health history
   D. Consulting with a physician

2. Thorough health histories are used to identify undiagnosed conditions, plan treatment, and anticipate medical emergencies. Health histories should be updated at each continuing care appointment.
   A. Both statements are true.
   B. Both statements are false.
   C. Statement one is true, statement two is false.
   D. Statement one is false, statement two is true.

3. The closed-ended format for health history questionnaires is a convenient and efficient way to obtain health information. Rapport and dialogue are easily established through this format.
   A. Both statements are true.
   B. Both statements are false.
   C. Statement one is true, statement two is false.
   D. Statement one is false, statement two is true.

4. Asking patients about changes in skin color, hair, or nails, bruising tendencies, rash, or itching is an example of which focus of a health history?
   A. Disease oriented
   B. Review of systems
   C. Cultural
   D. All of the above

5. Mr. Jones presents to the practice with a BMI of 27. He is:
   A. Underweight
   B. Normal weight
   C. Overweight
   D. Obese

Active Learning

1. While taking medical and dental histories, use visual cues with the patients to determine whether they are interested in the questions and providing accurate responses, if they have cultural issues that are important to them, if responses are supported by observed behaviors, and if the appearance of the person demonstrates any clues to general health.

2. During the history-taking process, take note of whether the patient can hear you so he can make appropriate responses, if he is articulate in his responses to follow-up questions, and if his tone of voice provides indications of how he feels about answering the questions.

3. Use the Internet and other medical textbooks to review samples of health histories. Identify any additional questions you would want to incorporate into the health history form used in your practice.

4. Practice taking vital signs (i.e., blood pressure, pulse, temperature, respiration) to develop skill and finesse with these procedures. ■

REFERENCES

1. *American Dental Hygienists' Association Standards for Clinical Dental Hygiene Practice.* Chicago: American Dental Hygienists' Association; 2008.

2. Go AS, Mozaffarian D, Roger VL, et al; on behalf of the American Heart Association Statistics Committee and Stroke Statistics Subcommittee. Heart disease and stroke statistics-2013update: a report from the American Heart Association. *Circulation.* 2013;127:e6-e245.

3. National Heart Lung and Blood Institute. Obesity Education Initiative: calculate your body mass index. https://www.nhlbi.nih.gov/about/org/oei. Accessed May 31, 2010.

4. Little JW, Falace DA, Miller CS, et al. *Dental Management of the Medically Compromised Patient.* 8th ed. St. Louis, MO: Mosby Elsevier; 2013.

5. Wilkins EM. *Clinical Practice of the Dental Hygienist.* 10th ed. Baltimore, MD: Lippincott Williams & Wilkins; 2009.

6. American Heart Association. *BLS for Healthcare Providers.* Dallas, TX: American Heart Association; 2006.

7. American Dental Association Council on Dental Health and Health Planning and Bureau of Health Education and Audiovisual Services. Breaking the silence on hypertension: a dental perspective. *J Am Dent Assoc.* 1985;10:781-789.

8. Chobian AV, Bakris GL, Black HR, et al. The seventh report of the Joint National Committee on Prevention, Detection, Evaluation, and Treatment of High Blood Pressure. National Heart, Lung and Blood Institute. The JNC 7 report. *JAMA.* 2003;289:2560-2578.

9. National High Blood Pressure Education Program. Classification of blood pressure for adults age 18 or older. http://www.nhlbi.nih.gov. Accessed June 2, 2010.

10. Pickett FA, Kaelber DC. Reducing kids' risk with blood pressure monitoring. *Dimens Dent Hyg.* 2010;8(2):20-25.

11. National High Blood Pressure Education Program Working Group on High Blood Pressure in Children and Adolescents. The fourth report on the diagnosis, evaluation, and treatment of high blood pressure in children and adolescents. *Pediatrics.* 2004;114(suppl):555-576.

12. American Heart Association. Endocarditis prophylaxis information. Dallas, TX: American Heart Association. http://www.americanheart.org/print_presenter. jhtml?identifier=11086. Published 2010. Accessed June 8, 2010.

13. American Heart Association. Antibiotic prophylaxis guidelines. http://www.qualitydentistry.com/dental/ information/abiotic.html. Published April 2007. Accessed June 8, 2010.

14. American Society of Anesthesiologists. ASA physical status classification system. http://www.asahq.org/ clinical/physicalstatus.htm. Accessed June 8, 2010.

15. Pickett FA, Gurenlian JR. *Preventing Medical Emergencies: Use of the Medical History.* 2nd ed. Baltimore, MD: Lippincott Williams & Wilkins; 2010.

16. Fleisher LA, et al. ACC/AHA 2007 guidelines on perioperative cardiovascular evaluation and care for noncardiac surgery: a report of the American College of Cardiology/American Heart Association Task Force on Practice Guidelines (Writing committee to revise the 2002 guidelines on perioperative cardiovascular evaluation for noncardiac surgery). http://circ. ahajournals.org. Accessed June 8, 2010.

Chapter 9 | Assessment Instruments

Rachel C. Kearney RDH, MS

KEY TERMS

assessment

assessment instruments

explorer

furcation probe

illumination

indirect vision

periodontal probe

retraction

transillumination

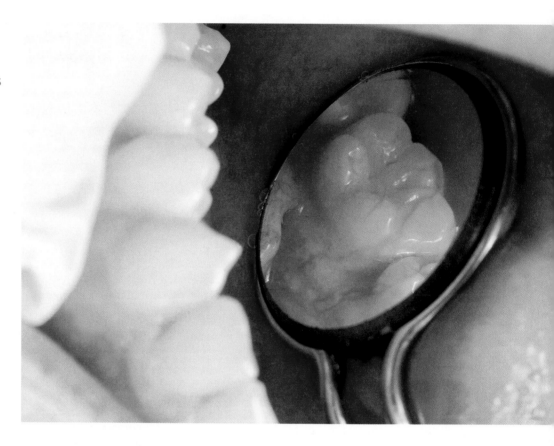

LEARNING OBJECTIVES

After reading this chapter, the student should be able to:

9.1 Describe the different types of assessment instruments.

9.2 Outline different types of mirrors, explorers, and probes and their uses.

9.3 Properly activate all assessment instruments.

9.4 Demonstrate correct technique in using assessment instruments.

KEY CONCEPTS

- Assessment instruments are essential tools used for dental hygiene care.
- There are numerous varieties and types of assessment instruments.
- Different types of instruments are better suited for certain purposes.

RELEVANCE TO CLINICAL PRACTICE

Assessment is a key step in providing optimal dental hygiene care to patients. **Assessment** can be defined as "the process of gathering information from the patient relative to general health and oral health status, medical history, medications, current needs and concerns."[1] The American Dental Hygienists' Association includes assessment in the Standards for Clinical Dental Hygiene Practice, a guide and expectation of the role dental hygienists play in the treatment of patients.[2] Being able to accurately and thoroughly complete assessments is an essential skill a dental hygienist must have. Assessments help to guide treatment options and help dental hygienists and patients make choices to obtain optimal oral health. In 2007 it was reported that dental hygienists spend 11.2 hours per week doing dental hygiene assessments, third to prophylaxis (21.4 hours) and patient education (11.8 hours).[3] This chapter discusses the basic instruments necessary to complete a clinical assessment. Other chapters within this textbook focus on periodontal, risk, nutritional, and caries assessments.

WHAT ARE ASSESSMENT INSTRUMENTS?

A variety of instruments are available to complete patient assessments. This chapter focuses on the mouth mirror, explorer, periodontal probe, and furcation probe and their roles in the assessment process.

Assessment instruments are instruments that help the dental hygienist collect data that are used to guide and determine treatment needs. Each instrument can serve a variety of different purposes when completing a clinical assessment, and the purposes of each instrument are discussed in this chapter. Each type of assessment instrument has many styles and brands available. It is impossible to highlight every option in this chapter, so it is important to try many brands and styles to find the right fit for you, your patients, and your practice needs.

MOUTH MIRROR

Purpose

Mouth mirrors have the most versatile uses of any assessment instrument. Mirrors are used for indirect vision, retraction, illumination, and transillumination.[4–6] Without the use of a mouth mirror there would be limited visualization of areas in the mouth and a hygienist's ergonomics would be severely compromised. Just try to look at the maxillary linguals of your patient's teeth without using a mirror.

Indirect vision is using a dental mirror to view an intraoral structure that cannot be seen directly.[4]

Indirect vision is most often used on the lingual surfaces, especially on the maxillary arch. Indirect vision is also often used in the posterior buccal surfaces. Mouth mirror indirect vision is not a skill that most people are proficient at naturally; it usually takes time and practice to become skilled in using indirect vision effectively (Fig. 9-1).

Mouth mirrors may also be used for **retraction.** The head of the mirror can be used to hold the patient's cheek, lip, or tongue out of the way of the hygienist's working area or field of vision. Using your finger for retraction is most comfortable for the patient, but using the mirror to retract tissue can be done comfortably. Most commonly the mirror is used for retraction of the tongue and the buccal mucosa on the hygienist's non-dominant hand side (Figs. 9-2 and 9-3).

Illumination is another helpful purpose of the mouth mirror. The mirror reflects light onto intraoral

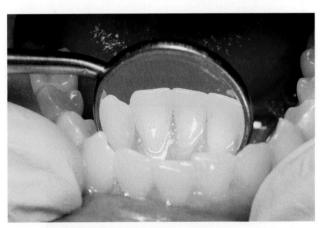

Figure 9-1. Dental hygienists use indirect vision to view intraoral structures such as lingual surfaces that cannot be seen directly.

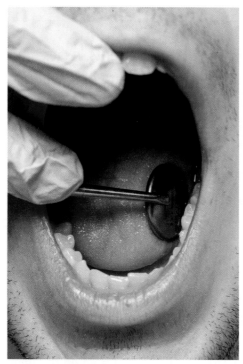

Figure 9-2. Using the mouth mirror to retract the patient's tongue allows the dental hygienist to view and access the working area.

surfaces that may otherwise be dark and more difficult to see (Fig. 9-4).

Transillumination uses illumination to direct light off of the mirror and through the anterior teeth. This creates light passing through the tooth. Transillumination can help to view calculus deposits, decay, and restorations on anterior teeth.[6]

Design

The parts of a mouth mirror are fairly simple and include the handle, shank, and mirror head or working end

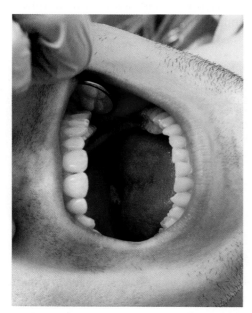

Figure 9-3. The mouth mirror used to retract the left-side buccal mucosa.

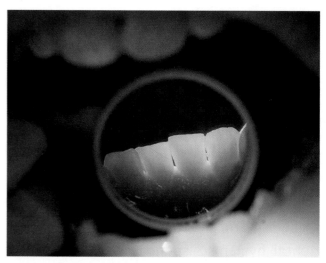

Figure 9-4. Illumination is helpful when viewing intraoral surfaces that would otherwise be dark.

(Fig. 9-5). With metal mouth mirrors, the mirror and shank portion may be threaded, allowing the mirror to screw into the handle. This design allows for replacement of the mirror as it scratches or wears. Other mirrors may be weld mounted or molded and are not removable.

Types

Endless varieties of mouth mirrors are available, and you will need to try different types to determine what works best for you and your patients. Some major differences in mirror types are outlined in the following subsections.

Disposable or Autoclavable

Most dental offices use autoclavable mirrors for dental hygiene procedures. To prevent scratching during ultrasonic cleaning and autoclaving, place the mirror in a cassette or cover the face of the mirror with gauze in a sterilization pouch.

Disposable mirrors are more appropriate for use in community events, such as screenings, or when using air abrasion techniques that can scratch the surface of a mirror. Disposable mirrors have a lower-quality

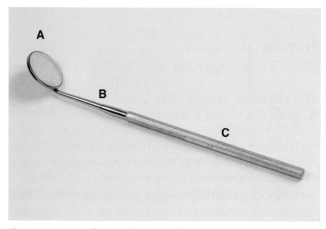

Figure 9-5. Parts of a mouth mirror: (A) working end, (B) shank, and (C) handle.

reflective surface and cost more than maintaining an autoclavable mirror.[5]

Mirror Surfaces

Mirror surfaces can be front surface, concave/curved, or plane/flat surface. The front surface mirror is most commonly used in dental mouth mirrors because it provides a clear, undistorted image. Concave/curved surfaces can create a magnified image, and plane/flat surface mirrors produce a double image.[4,6]

Size and Shape

A round mirror surface is most common, although rectangle and oval shapes are available from some manufacturers. Size four and five round mirrors are most common in dental mouth mirrors, and sometimes a size three mirror may be used if a smaller size is needed.[5]

Reflective Surface

Rhodium, a metal found in platinum ores, is historically and commonly what has been used to produce the reflective surface in mouth mirrors. As technology advances, other metal oxides have been used to create a sharper image on the reflective surface.

Single- or Double-Sided

Mirrors may be single- or double-sided. In providing dental hygiene treatment, a double-sided mirror can be convenient and more ergonomic than a single-sided mirror (Fig. 9-6).

Grasp

A mirror is held with a light, modified pen grasp in the nondominant hand with a fulcrum (Fig. 9-7). The mirror should be rotated in the finger grasp for better visualization.[4,5]

Retraction

The mirror can be used to retract the tongue or buccal mucosa to allow for better access or vision to specific areas in the mouth. When retracting with the mirror, ensure that light pressure is used so as not to cause discomfort at the commissures of the mouth or the tongue. Also take caution not to hit the mirror against the teeth, as this can cause discomfort for the patient.

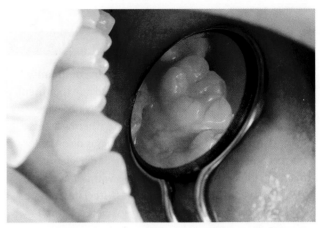

Figure 9-6. A double-sided mirror is convenient and more ergonomic than a single-sided mirror.

Clear Vision

Mirror fogging is a frustrating but common problem when using the mouth mirror. There are several ways to reduce fogging on your mouth mirror. The first and easiest is to run the face of the mirror over the buccal mucosa, warming and coating the mirror with saliva to prevent fogging. When the mirror is removed from the mouth and reinserted, this step should be repeated. This is a simple and easy technique but may not work in all circumstances, such as in a patient with extreme xerostomia.[5] Other solutions to fogging can involve running the mirror under warm tap water to bring it to a temperature closer to body temperature or coating the mirror with commercially available antifogging solutions that are safe for intraoral use.

EXPLORER

Purpose

An **explorer** is a flexible, thin assessment instrument that uses the clinician's tactile sense to evaluate tooth surfaces. The explorer allows the dental hygienist to

Advancing Technologies 1

Most dental mouth mirrors are made with rhodium, which gives the mirror the reflective property. Zirc makes a mirror out of three different metal oxides laid down in many different layers. The Crystal HD mirror has been reported to be more scratch resistant and create a clearer image for the clinician.[7] As technology improves, mirrors are sure to continue to have enhanced design features for the dental hygienist. Look at several brands and types of mirrors. Which one do you find is best for your needs? ▮

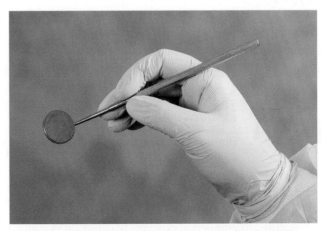

Figure 9-7. The mirror is held in the nondominant hand in a light, modified pen grasp. The mirror is rotated in the finger grasp for better visualization.

use tactile sensitivity, or the ability to perceive the sense of touch. Explorers are used to:

- Detect calculus
- Determine texture of tooth surface
- Examine tooth anatomy
- Detect decalcification and caries
- Evaluate margins of restorations

Explorers are essential in a dental hygienist's armamentarium of instruments. Explorers provide a way to evaluate the progress of calculus removal.

Design

Explorers are composed of a handle, shank, and working end. Explorers can be single- or double-ended (Fig. 9-8). The handle of an explorer can be different diameters and a wider diameter will aid in proper grasp, allowing for appropriate tactile sensitivity. Lightweight handles allow for better tactile sensitivity. The shank and working end of the explorer are thin and circular. The tip of the explorer is the last 1 to 2 mm of the working end; the sides of the tip are used to detect calculus and surface irregularities. The shank and working ends are thin and flexible to allow vibrations to be carried to the clinician's fingers.

Types

Many types of explorers are available, and each type of explorer is best suited for a specific task (Fig. 9-9). Table 9-1 lists the most common types of explorers used in dentistry and their applications.[4,9]

Evidence-Based Practice

Historically, explorers have been used to evaluate caries or suspected carious lesions. A new school of thought has emerged regarding being cautious about putting an explorer tip into a decalcified or suspected carious lesion.[8] Review some of the literature on using dental explorers to detect caries and decide what evidence-based technique you will use. ■

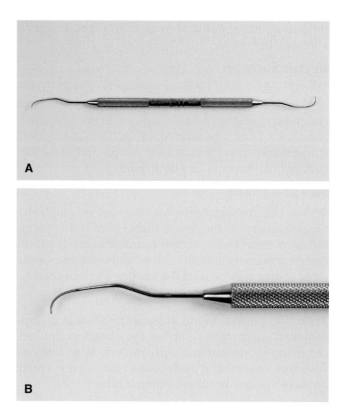

Figure 9-8. Explorers are single- (B) or double-ended (A).

Grasp

The grasp used with an explorer is a relaxed and light, modified pen grasp (Fig. 9-10). The middle finger should rest on the shank.

Activation and Technique

Although each explorer is designed differently, keep in mind some basic principles when using an explorer.

- Maintain a light grasp to aid in tactile sensitivity.
- Adapt the last 1 to 2 mm against the tooth surface.
- Apply only light pressure to the explorer.
- When using an explorer subgingivally, insert the explorer near a line angle working systematically over all surfaces of a tooth.
- Use light overlapping vertical, horizontal, and oblique strokes.

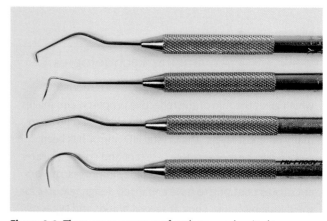

Figure 9-9. There are many types of explorers, each suited to a particular task.

Table 9-1. *Types and Uses of Explorers*

Types of Explorers	Uses
Shepherd hook explorer	Supragingival examination of caries and margins of restorations
Straight explorer	Supragingival examination of caries and margins of restorations
Curved explorer	Calculus detection in healthy pockets

Continued

Table 9-1. *Types and Uses of Explorers—cont'd*

Types of Explorers	Uses	
Pigtail explorer	Calculus detection in healthy pockets	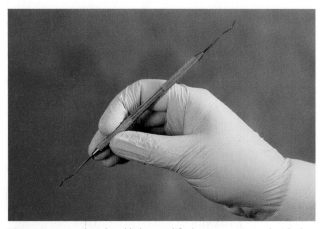
Right angle design explorer	Calculus detection on anterior root surfaces and facials and linguals of posterior teeth shallow or deep pockets	
Area-specific explorer	Supragingival and subgingival examination of posterior and anterior teeth in shallow or deep pockets	

Figure 9-10. A relaxed and light, modified pen grasp is used with the explorer. The middle finger rests on the shank.

- Always use a fulcrum.
- Wrist or digital activation is acceptable.

Exploring strokes should be used before, during, and after scaling to assess calculus deposits, assess progress, and evaluate complete calculus removal.

PERIODONTAL AND FURCATION PROBES

Purpose

A **periodontal probe** is an assessment instrument calibrated with millimeter markings that is used to evaluate the health of the periodontium. The periodontal probe may be used for:

- Measuring pocket depths
- Measuring clinical attachment loss
- Measuring width of attached gingiva
- Measuring the size of oral lesions
- Assessing the presence of bleeding or purulence[4]

A **furcation probe** is a type of periodontal probe used to evaluate the bone in areas of furcation on multirooted teeth. A complete discussion of periodontal assessments can be found in Chapter 11.

Types and Design

Both periodontal and furcation probes are designed with a handle and a blunted working end to allow for safe insertion into the pocket (Fig. 9-11). Periodontal probes have a 90-degree bend to allow for insertion into the sulcus. Furcation probes are curved to facilitate the examination of the furcation area between tooth roots.

Probes also are calibrated with millimeter markings to allow for recording measurements. Millimeter markings may be indicated by grooves, colored bands, or colored indentations.[4] Different probes have markings at different intervals (Fig. 9-12).

Grasp

Probes are grasped with a light, modified pen grasp.

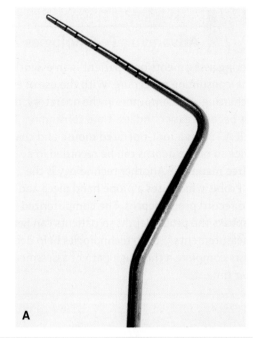

A

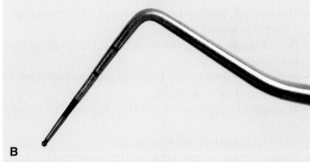

B

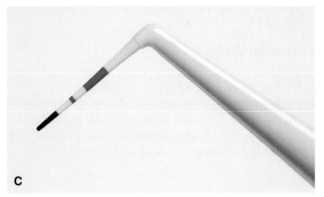

C

Figure 9-12. Probes are calibrated with millimeter markings to allow for recording measurements. A, Williams probe. B, PSR probe. C, Implant probe

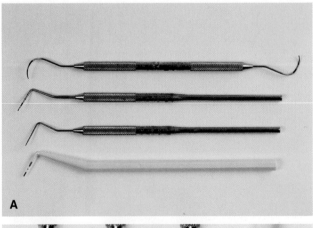

A

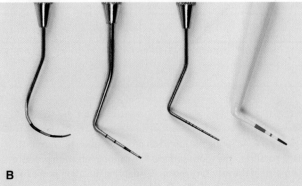

B

Figure 9-11. A, Furcation and periodontal probes have a handle and a blunted working end (B) to allow for safe insertion into the pocket.

Activation and Technique

Periodontal Probe

Periodontal probes are activated by walking the probe within the sulcus along the junctional epithelium. The walking stroke should cover the entire circumference of the tooth. The following is a description of proper technique used in activating the probe.

- Keep the probe tip against the tooth while probing.
- The probe should be kept parallel to the long axis of the tooth except when adapting to the proximal surface.

Advancing Technologies 2

Completing assessments on a patient is an essential but time-consuming procedure. With the use of electronic charting and computers in the operatory, this task has become easier and less time consuming. The Dental R.A.T. uses a foot-operated mouse and charting device so probe depths can be recorded in a hands-free manner.[10] Another technology is the Florida Probe, which uses a probe hand piece and foot pedal to record probe depths. The computerized probe speaks the probe depths so patients can hear their measurements.[11] Both technologies help dental hygienists complete a thorough patient assessment in a shorter time. ■

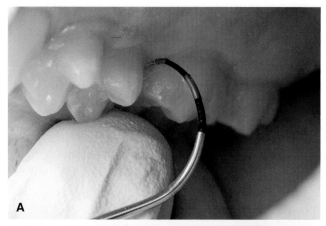

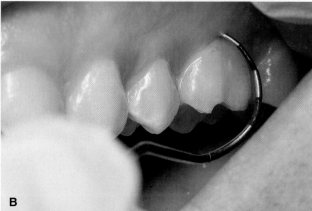

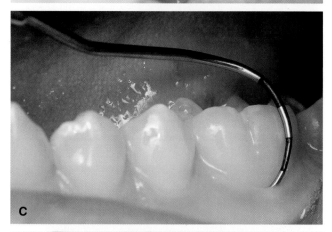

- The walking stroke should be 1 to 2 mm vertical and 1 mm horizontal.
- Do not remove the probe from the sulcus until moving to the next tooth.
- Pressure applied to the probe should be between 10 and 20 g of light pressure.
- The base of the pocket should feel soft and have some tension.
- Wrist or digital action is acceptable.
- As the probe is moved into the proximal surface, slant the probe so it reaches under the contact area (Fig. 9-13).

Furcation Probe

The clinician must select the proper working end of the furcation probe. The terminal shank should be positioned parallel to the tooth surface (Fig. 9-14).

To insert the furcation probe, slide the probe underneath the gingiva in the area of furcation (Table 9-2). Charting of furcations is discussed in Chapter 11.

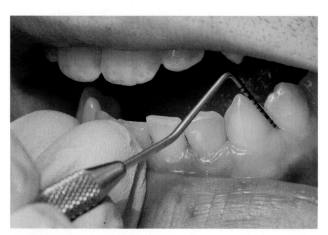

Figure 9-13. Adapting the probe to the proximal surface.

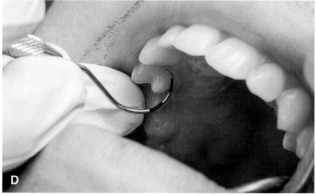

Figure 9-14. Adapting the furcation probe. Position the terminal shank parallel to the tooth surface. A, Adapting furcation probe to the mesial of the maxillary molar. B, Adapting furcation probe to the buccal of the maxillary molar. C, Adapting the furcation probe to the buccal of the mandibular molar. D, Adapting the furcation probe to the mesial of the maxillary first pre-molar.

Table 9-2. *Insertion Sites for Furcation Probe*	
Tooth	**Site**
Maxillary molars	Midbuccal, mesiolingual, distolingual
Mandibular molars	Midbuccal, midlingual
Maxillary first molars	Mesiolingual

Summary

Assessment instruments help the dental hygienist to gather data related to the health of the teeth and the periodontium. It is important that these data be recorded and properly documented within the patient chart. Documenting the assessment findings helps to create a proper dental hygiene diagnosis and treatment plan for the patient, and is an important step in maintaining professional liability.[12] Assessment instruments are essential tools for a dental hygienist, and proficiency and skill in using them is essential.

Case Study

A 53-year-old Hispanic man presents to the clinic because he "needs to have his teeth cleaned." His medical history indicates he has diabetes that is well controlled with Glucophage. You complete an intraoral and extraoral and periodontal assessment, and record your findings.

Case Study Exercises

1. Refer to the accompanying figure. The probe depth measurement you would record if this is the deepest measurement you identified on the buccal surface of tooth #30 is:
   A. 1 mm
   B. 2 mm
   C. 3 mm
   D. 4 mm

2. What instrument would best allow you to determine the amount of calculus present?
   A. Mirror
   B. Explorer
   C. Probe
   D. Furcation probe

3. If the probe is positioned in the incorrect position, the probe depth will likely be:
   A. Greater than the correct depth
   B. Less than the correct depth
   C. The same as the correct depth

4. The assessment data you have gathered will help you formulate:
   A. A dental hygiene diagnosis
   B. A dental hygiene treatment plan
   C. A complete patient record
   D. All of the above

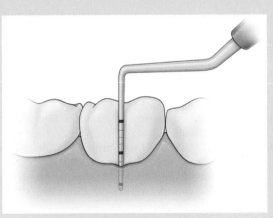

Review Questions

1. Mouth mirrors are used for all of the following EXCEPT:
   A. Retraction
   B. Subgingival calculus detection
   C. Indirect vision
   D. Transillumination

2. When using a mirror it should be held in the nondominant hand and should be used without a fulcrum.
   A. First part is true, and second part is true.
   B. First part is true, and second part is false.
   C. First part is false, and second part is false.
   D. First part is false, and second part is true.

3. The cross section of the working end of an explorer is in the shape of a
   A. Triangle
   B. Half circle
   C. Square
   D. Circle

4. The last 1 to 2 mm of an explorer's working end is called the
   A. Point
   B. Shank
   C. Tip
   D. Fulcrum

5. Assessment instruments use
   A. Wrist activation
   B. Digital activation
   C. Both wrist and digital activation
   D. None of the above

Active Learning

1. Use a probe on a scale and evaluate how much pressure 10 to 20 g really is.
2. Close your eyes and explore a typodont with calculus. Focus on what you are feeling.
3. Demonstrate how to use a furcation probe on extracted molars placed in plaster.

REFERENCES

1. Gibson-Howell J, Hicks M. Dental hygienists' role in patient assessments and clinical examinations in U.S. dental practices: a review of the literature. *J Allied Health.* 2010;39(1):e1-e5.
2. American Dental Hygienists' Association. Standards for clinical dental hygiene practice. March 10, 2008. Available from: http://www.adha.org/downloads/adha_standards08.pdf. Accessed February 12, 2010.
3. American Dental Hygienists' Association. Survey of dental hygienists in the United States, 2007: executive summary. 2009. Available from: http://www.adha.org/downloads/DH_practitioner_survey_Exec_Summary.pdf. Accessed on March 1, 2010.
4. Nield-Gehrig JS. *Fundamentals of Periodontal Instrumentation and Advanced Root Instrumentation,* 6th ed. Baltimore: Lippincott, Williams, & Wilkins; 2008.
5. Guignon AN. Comfort zone. Mouth mirror magic. *RDH.* 2007;27(5):90.
6. Kaiser K. Hygiene touch. Mirror image. *RDH.* 2006;36 (9):64.
7. Zirc Mouth Mirrors. Available from: http://www.zirc.com/Mouth_Mirors.asp. Accessed June 17, 2010.
8. Hamilton JC, Stookey G. Should a dental explorer be used to probe suspected carious lesions? *J Am Dent Assoc.* 2005;136:1526-1532.
9. Hodges K. Reconsidering the explorer. *Dimens Dent Hyg.* 2005;3(4):26-28.
10. Dental RAT. Available from: http://www.dentalrat.com/index.php. Accessed June 12, 2010.
11. Florida Probe Overview. Available from: http://www.floridaprobe.com/downloads/FP_Overview.pdf. Accessed May 2, 2010.
12. Armitage GC. The complete periodontal examination. *Periodontol 2000.* 2004; 34:22-33.

Chapter 10 | Extraoral and Intraoral Examination

Kathi R. Shepherd, RDH, MS • Kristina Okolisan-Mulligan, RDH, BS • Sara Gordon, DDS MSc

KEY TERMS

acquired condition

actinic cheilitis

ALARA

ankyloglossia

benign migratory glossitis

betel nut

biopsy

brush test

congenital condition

cytological smear

definitive diagnosis

denture-induced fibrous hyperplasia

differential diagnosis

dysplasia

epithelial dysplasia

epulis fissuratum

erythema migrans

erythroplakia

excisional biopsy

exfoliative cytology

exostosis

fibroma

fissured tongue

focal fibrous hyperplasia

Fordyce granules

geographic tongue

gingival epulis

gingival fibromatosis

grading

hairy tongue

human papillomavirus (HPV)

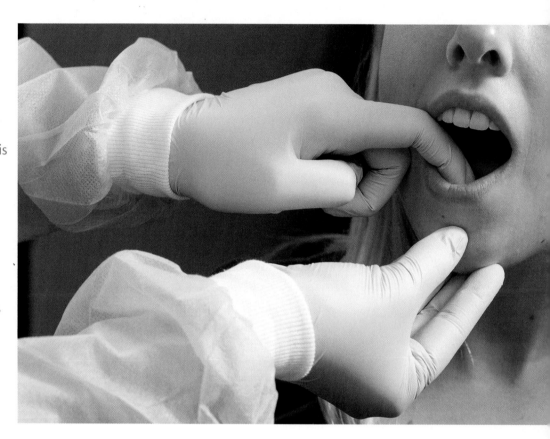

LEARNING OBJECTIVES

After reading this chapter, the student should be able to:

10.1 Perform a thorough, standardized extraoral and intraoral examination.

10.2 Identify clinical signs and symptoms of oral diseases and oral manifestations of systemic diseases.

10.3 Demonstrate a working knowledge of the language of oral pathology and an understanding of the etiology, pathogenesis, and structural and functional deviations resulting from the disease process.

10.4 Describe findings.

10.5 Select, obtain, and interpret information using a variety of diagnostic procedures consistent with medico-legal principles.

10.6 Develop a differential diagnosis derived from collected data consistent with medico-legal principles.

10.7 Recognize predisposing and causative risk factors that require intervention to prevent disease.

10.8 Discuss findings with dental and other health-care professionals, as well as with the patient, according to the standards of evidence-based dental hygiene care.

incisional biopsy

induration

inflammatory fibrous hyperplasia

inflammatory papillary hyperplasia

in situ

irritation fibroma

leukoedema

leukoplakia

linea alba

mandibular torus

metastasis

oral and maxillofacial pathology

palatal torus

paresthesia

peripheral giant cell granuloma

peripheral ossifying fibroma (POF)

pregnancy tumor

pyogenic granuloma

reactive conditions

speckled leukoplakia

squamous cell carcinoma

staging

tissue autofluorescence

tissue reflectance

toluidine blue dye

torus mandibularis

torus palatinus

traumatic fibroma

tumor board

vital tissue staining technology

wandering rash of the tongue

10.9   Explain how to use a variety of tools for early detection of oral cancer.

10.10 Make appropriate referrals for evidence-based care.

10.11 Use evidence-based decision-making to appraise and integrate emerging treatment modalities.

KEY CONCEPTS

- Knowledge of normal head and neck anatomy as well as skills necessary to perform a complete assessment of head and neck structures (extraoral and intraoral examination and oral cancer screening) are paramount to the early detection of head and neck abnormalities.
- Squamous cell carcinoma is the most common malignancy of the oral cavity. Knowledge of the cause, development, prevalence, risk factors, and characteristics of *all* oral lesions and pathology is critical in the development of a differential diagnosis.
- Developmental conditions may be congenital (present at birth) or may develop later in life, but once they have developed they are nonprogressive. They often require no intervention unless they interfere with normal function or esthetics.
- Reactive conditions occur in response to some type of environmental factor such as trauma. Underlying causes of these findings must be addressed to prevent recurrence.
- There are a number of commercial adjunctive techniques for detecting oral cancer, including vital tissue staining, visualization adjuncts, and exfoliative cytology (brush test); however, current dental literature has not provided evidence that they detect oral cancer earlier.
- The gold standard for a **definitive diagnosis** of any finding is a biopsy: an incisional biopsy for large lesions or lesions that are suspected to be cancerous, or both; and an excisional biopsy for small or harmless-appearing lesions, or both.

RELEVANCE TO CLINICAL PRACTICE

Published studies show that currently less than 15% of those who visit a dentist regularly report having had an oral cancer screening.[1] This is unfortunate when the greatest strides in combating most cancers have come from increased awareness and aggressive campaigns directed at early detection. Cancers of the head and neck, which include cancers of the oral cavity, larynx, pharynx, thyroid, salivary glands, and nose/nasal passages, account for approximately 6% of all malignancies in the United States.[2] An estimated 28,500 new cases (20,100 male and 8,400 female cases) of oral cavity and oropharyngeal cancer were diagnosed in 2009.[3,4] An estimated 6,100 people (4,200 male and 1,900 female individuals) will die of these cancers.[3]

Oftentimes the dental profession is the first line of defense in early detection of head and neck abnormalities including, but not limited to, head and neck cancer. One of the roles of a dental professional is to perform an examination of the head and neck region to recognize deviations from normal anatomy and structures so that proper referral to the appropriate health-care professional can be made if necessary.

The procedures and techniques involved with the extraoral and intraoral (head and neck) examination will be presented in this chapter. A discussion of oral lesions and pathology will serve as a foundation for recognizing variations from normal structures. Normal anatomy will be highlighted by way of photos and illustrations. A discussion on the manner in which this examination serves as an oral cancer screening as well as a tool for oral cancer prevention will also be provided.

OBJECTIVES OF THE EXTRAORAL AND INTRAORAL EXAMINATION

A thorough understanding of pathology and oral lesions, as well as normal palpation of head and neck structures, will enable the clinician to observe areas that deviate from normal. The cure rate of oral cancer is directly related to early detection. If found before the lesion size has exceeded 1.5 cm, the cure rate can be as high as 60%.[3] Many systemic conditions can also be detected by performing a head and neck examination. The intent of the examination is to provide early disease recognition. The examination may reveal abnormal conditions that require consultation. Findings of the examination also provide a means for documenting baseline data for subsequent comparison. Other purposes of the examination are to identify contraindications to treatment, assist in treatment planning, and provide documentation for legal records.

COMMON ORAL PATHOLOGY

Oral and maxillofacial pathology is the specialty of dentistry that deals with the etiology, pathogenesis, identification, and management of diseases that affect the oral and maxillofacial regions.[5] Pathology in the dental hygiene curriculum is the meeting ground for the basic and dental sciences, and it is also an important component of daily clinical dental hygiene. The knowledge gained from pathology is essential to understand clinical manifestations of the disease process and contributes enormously to the delivery of care, because treatment is ineffective unless it is based on the correct diagnosis.

The following findings are among the most common oral conditions that the dental hygienist will encounter in clinical practice. They are listed alphabetically and not in order of frequency.

Common Variations From Normal

Many common findings are considered variations from normal, rather than true disease states. This includes many developmental conditions, which are present for many years with little change. Some developmental conditions are **congenital,** or present from birth; others are **acquired,** or develop later in life. Developmental conditions include some conditions that are inherited from parents, but the cause of many of these conditions is incompletely understood.

- **Ankyloglossia:** This congenital condition, commonly referred to as "tongue-tied," occurs when the lingual frenulum attaching the tongue to the floor of the mouth or lingual gingiva is too short, thick, or tight, and often results in the inability to properly raise or extend the tongue. Ankyloglossia is a developmental variance that is present in about 4% to 10% of the population. In most cases, treatment is not required unless there are problems with function during infancy, especially maternal breast pain during breastfeeding, or later in life including speech, functional, or periodontal problems, in which a frenectomy (removal of the lingual frenum) may be performed.[6–8]

- **Exostosis** (*plural,* **exostoses**): Exostoses are bony outgrowths on the maxillary or mandibular alveolar ridges; they are usually asymptomatic. Most occur in adults and may slowly increase in size with age. No treatment is necessary unless traumatized or they interfere with fabrication of an appliance, in which case **excisional biopsy** could be considered. A **biopsy** is removal of a tissue for the purposes of obtaining a diagnosis. An excisional biopsy is the complete removal of the lesion for diagnosis.[9,10]

- **Fissured tongue:** Fissured tongue is a fairly common condition that affects the dorsum of the tongue in which multiple deep fissures or grooves are present (Fig. 10-1). The cause is unknown; however, a pattern of inheritance is commonly noted. No treatment is specified, but cleaning the tongue is highly recommended to keep food debris from collecting in the grooves and causing halitosis or irritation.[8]

- **Fordyce granules:** Fordyce granules are ectopic sebaceous glands that commonly occur on the labial and buccal mucosa, retromolar area, and anterior tonsillar pillar. Fordyce granules are present in about 80% of population and are most commonly found in adults. Clinically, they present as multiple yellowish white papules; they are usually asymptomatic. They are diagnosed simply by recognition of their characteristic clinical appearance, and no treatment is required.

- **Geographic tongue** (also called **benign migratory glossitis, erythema migrans, wandering rash of the tongue**): Geographic tongue is a benign inflammatory condition with an unknown cause, but nutritional deficiency, stress, and heredity may play roles (Fig. 10-2). Geographic tongue most commonly involves the dorsal and lateral portions of the tongue; it presents as single or multiple pink to red denuded areas of filiform papillae that are bordered by a white or yellowish rim (Fig. 10-2). The fungiform papillae remain intact. This condition changes its pattern from week to week (hence the names "geographic," "migratory," and "wandering") and is normally asymptomatic. Occasionally the patient may complain of mild burning irritation when eating hot, spicy, or acidic foods such as tomatoes. A palliative mouthwash may be soothing but not curative.[8]

- **Hairy tongue:** Hairy tongue occurs when the filiform papillae become abnormally elongated and give the dorsum of the tongue a hairlike appearance. Many contributing factors are related to this condition: smoking, medications, cancer therapy, poor oral hygiene allowing chromogenic bacteria to accumulate, and medications such as antibiotics all can play a role. The tongue may be densely white or become stained yellow, brown, and/or black. The filiform papillae occasionally grow to several millimeters in length. Hairy tongue is not a serious condition, but patients may find it cosmetically displeasing. They should clean the tongue by using a tongue scraper and discontinue causative factors if possible.[8]

- **Leukoedema:** Leukoedema is a variation of normal that affects nonwhite individuals, particularly African Americans more often than other populations. The cause is unknown, but the appearance is due to harmless accumulations of glycogen in the surface cells. It is asymptomatic. Leukoedema clinically appears bilaterally on the buccal mucosa as a grayish white opalescence that disappears when stretched. No treatment is required.[11]

- **Linea alba:** Linea alba is commonly found bilaterally on the buccal mucosa along the line of occlusion. Linea alba clinically appears as a thickened white line

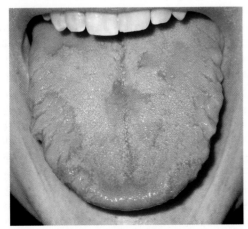

Figure 10-1. This tongue exhibits both fissured tongue and geographic tongue. These two common conditions are often seen in combination.

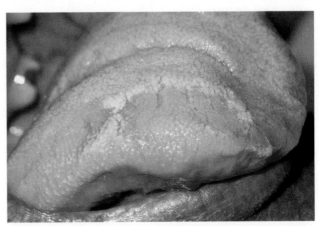

Figure 10-2. This tongue exhibits geographic tongue.

in response to friction. This condition requires no treatment and is diagnosed based on its appearance.

- **Torus mandibularis (mandibular torus)** (plural, **tori**): A torus is a common bony outgrowth, a form of exostosis, of unknown cause, although data suggest tori may be inherited. Mandibular tori are found bilaterally on the lingual aspect of the mandibular alveolar bone, most often in the premolar area. Tori are slow growing and usually develop after puberty. These lesions are usually asymptomatic unless they become very big or are traumatized. No treatment is necessary unless they are traumatized or they interfere with fabrication of an appliance, in which case excisional biopsy could be considered.[9,10,12]

- **Torus palatinus (palatal torus)** (plural, tori): A torus is a common bony outgrowth of unknown cause, although data suggest tori may be inherited. A palatal torus is a bony nodular growth present on the midline of the hard palate. Tori are slow growing and usually develop after puberty. These lesions are usually asymptomatic unless they become very big or are traumatized, but they can interfere with speech or prosthetic appliances. No treatment is necessary unless they are traumatized or they interfere with fabrication of an appliance, in which case excisional biopsy could be considered.[9,10,12]

Common Reactive Lesions

Reactive conditions are conditions that result from the reaction of tissues to mechanical trauma, heat, medications, or other environmental factors. A key factor in addressing reactive lesions is identifying and correcting the underlying environmental factor; otherwise, recurrence is more likely.

- **Epulis fissuratum** (also called **inflammatory fibrous hyperplasia, denture-induced fibrous hyperplasia**): Epulis fissuratum is caused by chronic trauma, most commonly from an ill-fitting denture. This lesion commonly occurs in the vestibular mucosa and clinically appears as folds of fibrous connective tissue. It ranges in size from less than a centimeter to massive lesions that involve most of the vestibule. Treatment consists of excisional biopsy and fabrication of a new denture.[13]

- **Fibroma** (also called **irritation fibroma** or **traumatic fibroma, focal fibrous hyperplasia**): The fibroma is the most common benign tumor-like growth in the oral cavity. Despite its name, it is not a true tumor, but a reactive hyperplasia of fibrous connective tissue in response to local irritation or trauma. The fibroma is usually less than 1 cm in diameter, but it may become larger. Fibromas are commonly located on the buccal mucosa, tongue, and lower lip (Figs. 10-3 and 10-4). Most fibromas are the same color as the adjacent tissue or a little lighter, especially if they are chronically traumatized. Trauma may also cause them to become ulcerated.

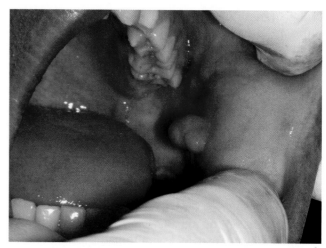

Figure 10-3. This fibroma in the buccal mucosa of a 36-year-old Dominican woman has been present for several years. She was relieved to have it removed because she thought it was cancer.

The treatment is excisional biopsy and removal of causative factors. Fibromas are not malignant.[14–16]

- **Gingival epulis** (plural, **epulides**): Epulis is a generic clinical descriptive term for a focal noninfectious enlargement or lump of the gingiva (Fig. 10-5). It is not a diagnosis but a category of lesions. The most common types of epulides are fibroma, pyogenic granuloma, **peripheral ossifying fibroma (POF),** and peripheral giant cell granuloma. Each of these lesions is discussed separately in this chapter. Biopsy is necessary to differentiate among these lesions.[14–17]

- **Gingival fibromatosis** (also called *gingival hyperplasia, gingival overgrowth*): This is an uncommon diffuse enlargement of the gingiva that is not caused by local inflammation or infection. It may become extensive enough to cover all or a major portion of the crowns of teeth in affected areas. It is frequently drug induced; associated medications include phenytoin, cyclosporin, and calcium channel blockers, which are drugs commonly associated with organ transplant, cardiovascular diseases, hypertension, and epilepsy (Fig. 10-6). It occasionally may be hereditary, either as an isolated problem or part of a number of syndromes. In some cases, the cause is unknown. Gingival fibromatosis is often aggravated by poor oral hygiene. Lesions are surgically excised (and a biopsy is taken to confirm the diagnosis) but may recur, especially if underlying causative factors cannot be controlled. An important differential diagnosis to consider is gingival enlargement secondary to leukemia, a blood cell malignancy. **Differential diagnosis** is the process of distinguishing a disease from other diseases with similar signs and symptoms.[15]

- **Inflammatory papillary hyperplasia** (also called *papillary hyperplasia of the palate, palatal papillomatosis*): Palatal papillomatosis is a common hyperplastic response to reactive tissue growth on the hard palate

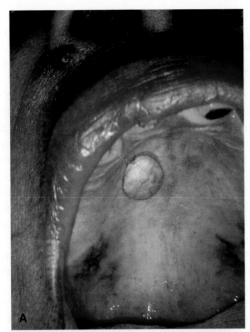

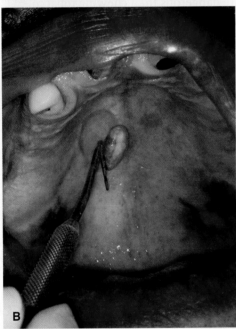

Figure 10-4. This large fibroma on the palate (A) is a type called a "leaf fibroma" because it hangs from a slender stalk like a leaf. (B) These fibromas are typically found on the hard palate under a denture.

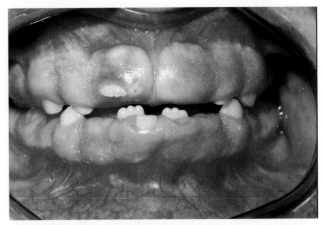

Figure 10-5. A biopsy was taken of this large epulis and it was diagnosed as a peripheral ossifying fibroma.

denture care to the patient and to stress the importance of removing the denture for a few hours each day.[13]

- **Peripheral giant cell granuloma:** This is an uncommon, but not rare, cause of focal gingival enlargement that is slightly more common in middle-aged patients. It occurs only on the gingiva. The cause is unknown, but it may represent a reaction to irritants trapped within the sulcus. Lesions are purple dome-shaped nodules on the gingiva, usually anterior to the molars, and are usually less than 1 cm. Treatment consists of excisional biopsy, and it is important to thoroughly scale the adjacent tissue to ensure all irritants are removed. The recurrence rate is 10% to 15%.[14,16,18,19]

- *POF:* This is an uncommon, but not rare, cause of focal gingival enlargement that occurs only on the gingiva. The cause is unknown, but it may represent a reaction to irritants trapped within the sulcus. The POF is most common in the anterior maxillary arch and colors range from red to pink or ulcerated from trauma. The POF is a pedunculated (attached by an

beneath the denture that may be caused by an ill-fitting denture, poor oral hygiene, and wearing a denture 24 hours a day. In many cases, a fungal infection is also present. Fungal infections, which are typically caused by *Candida albicans,* appear clinically as red mucosa with a nodular, pebbly, or papillary surface. The treatment usually begins with elimination of the *Candida* infection using oral or topical medications, improvement of denture fit, and meticulous self-care. Severe cases may require excisional biopsy of the hyperplastic tissue before fabrication of a new denture. It is important to provide instructions on proper

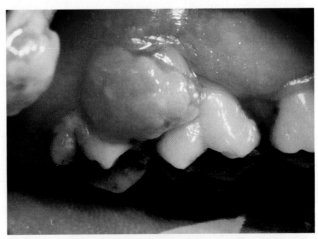

Figure 10-6. This 5-year-old child presented with generalized hyperplasia. The medical history revealed that the patient was taking phenytoin (Dilantin) for epilepsy. Biopsy confirmed medication-induced gingival fibromatosis.

elongated stalk of tissue) or sessile (attached directly, not by a peduncle) nodular mass. It can become quite large and interfere with eating or speaking. Treatment consists of excisional biopsy, and it is very important to thoroughly scale the adjacent tissue to ensure all irritants are removed because that can produce regrowth. About 20% of POFs recur.[15–17,19]

- **Pyogenic granuloma:** Pyogenic granuloma is an uncommon, but not rare, blood vessel proliferation in response to local irritation, trauma, or poor oral hygiene. Some cases appear to be influenced by high hormone levels such as at puberty or during pregnancy, hence the name **pregnancy tumor.** This lesion tends to be more common in female individuals. This lesion may appear as a smooth-surfaced or lobulated nodule, ranging in size from several millimeters to several centimeters, and its color is usually pink/ red/purple. Seventy-five percent of pyogenic granulomas develop on the gingiva, but they may also be found on the lips, tongue, buccal mucosa, and other parts of the body, including the fingers. The pyogenic granuloma is predominantly vascular and can bleed easily. Excisional biopsy is the treatment, although lesions occasionally recur.[14,16,17]

ORAL CANCER

The most common malignancy of the oral cavity is oral squamous cell carcinoma (OSCC), although the mouth can also experience malignancies of the salivary gland, blood cells, bone, melanocytes, or just about any other tissue (Fig. 10-7).[20]

How and Why Does Oral Cancer Arise?

Below are causes and risk factors of oral cancer.

- *Development:* OSCC, like carcinoma in other parts of the body, develops out of a precancerous lesion called **dysplasia.**[20,21]
- *Demographics:* OSCC is the sixth most common malignancy in males and the twelfth most common malignancy in females in North America, although in some parts of Asia it is the most common human cancer. Oral and pharyngeal **squamous cell carcinoma** (SCC) kill one patient every hour in the United States, and more than 35,000 patients develop OSCC annually in the United States.[3]

- *Age:* Dysplasia and OSCC are more common in older patients and in smokers, although patients of any age are potentially at risk. The average age of people diagnosed with oral cancer is 62 years. Approximately one third of oral cancers occur in patients younger than 55 years.[4,20–22]

- *Risk factors:* The cause of dysplastic transformation of oral epithelium is the development of specific genetic mutations; this is most strongly linked to tobacco use, especially smoked tobacco.

  - Approximately 90% of people with oral cavity and oropharyngeal cancer use tobacco, and the risk of developing these cancers increases with the amount smoked or chewed and the duration of the habit. No form of tobacco is safe, but smoking is even more dangerous than chewing tobacco.[2–4,20,22,23]

  - Chewing **betel nut** products (paan, quid), a common habit in parts of Asia, is also strongly linked to oral cancer. The betel nut is the fruit of the Areca catechu palm tree, which is native to Southeast Asia.[2–4,20,22–24]

  - On the vermilion border of the lip, the most important risk factor is sun exposure. More than 30% of patients with cancers of the lip have outdoor occupations associated with prolonged exposure to sunlight.[22]

- *Heavy alcohol use:* Seven of 10 patients with oral cancer are heavy drinkers (more than two alcoholic drinks per day). Oral cancers are approximately six times more common in drinkers than in nondrinkers. People who drink alcohol but do not smoke have a higher risk for cancer if they are particularly heavy drinkers. Heavy drinkers and smokers may have as much as a 100-fold increase in the risk of developing these cancers compared with people who do not smoke or drink. Recent research has questioned whether mouthwash with high alcohol content might be linked to a higher risk for oral and oropharyngeal cancers. This association has not been proved. Studying this possible link is complicated by the fact that smokers and frequent drinkers (who are already at increased risk for these cancers) are more likely to use mouthwash than people who neither smoke nor drink.[2–4,20,22–24]

- **Human papillomavirus (HPV):** HPV is a family of well more than 100 viruses. Many viruses cause harmless lesions such as warts and are spread readily through the environment. These types are not linked with cancer risk. However, a few sexually transmitted types of HPV (types 16, 18, and others) have been linked to pharyngeal, tonsillar, and some oral cancers, as well as cervical and rectal cancers. About 5% of tongue cancers are thought to be related to high-risk HPV, although a much greater

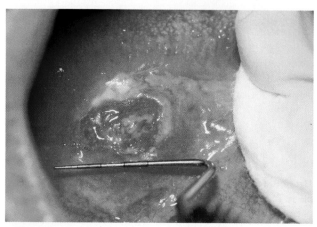

Figure 10-7. Oral squamous cell carcinoma.

percentage of tonsillar cancers are HPV related, and virtually all cervical cancers are believed to be caused by HPV. New vaccines exist that target these high-risk HPV types. The future impact of HPV vaccines on the incidence of oral cancer is currently unclear. HPV-positive disease could change the typical age groups afflicted by OSCC. Most oral cancer patients are still older smokers, but the use of tobacco products has declined in the United States every year for more than a decade. Nonsmoking patients younger than 50 years are the fastest growing segment of the oral cancer population.[1,22,25]

- *Less common causes:* Less common causes of precancerous transformation include genetics and other poorly defined risks that may include other infections, nutritional deficiencies, and immune deficiencies.[2–4,20,23–25]

What Is the Appearance of Oral Cancer?

Cancer and precancer can be detected clinically because of changes in color, contour, consistency, and function.

- *Color:* Dysplasia may begin as a very innocent-looking lesion but is most often apparent as a change in color to white, red, or a mixture (leukoplakia and erythroplakia are discussed in the following sublist). Dysplasia of the vermilion border of the lip is usually seen in combination with severe sun damage to the lip (**actinic cheilitis**), in which the lip becomes enlarged, blotchy, and the edge of the vermilion border becomes indistinct (Fig. 10-8).[20]
  - *White areas*—**leukoplakia:** Leukoplakia is a term that is used by some clinicians to describe a suspicious white oral area that may be at increased risk for oral cancer. The term *leukoplakia* is not synonymous with dysplasia or OSCC. It implies that dysplasia or OSCC may be detected if a biopsy of the area is taken, although biopsy of leukoplakia is more likely to show harmless changes. The World Health Organization defines leukoplakia as a "white patch on the oral mucosa that can neither

be scraped off nor classified as any other diagnosable disease." Thus, leukoplakia is not used to describe just any white spot in the mouth; it is a descriptive term when all potential diagnoses other than precancer or cancer have been considered and clinically deemed unlikely. About 10% to 15% of leukoplakias will develop into an oral precancer (**epithelial dysplasia**) or oral cancer (SCC) if left untreated. Red areas may clinically appear in a leukoplakia; this mixture of red and white is termed **speckled leukoplakia** and has a greater risk for malignancy. Management of leukoplakia consists of first determining the actual diagnosis by means of a biopsy (Figures 10-9, 10-10, and 10-11). Further treatment is then based on the biopsy-proven diagnosis.[20]

- *Red areas*—**erythroplakia:** Erythroplakia is a term that is used by some clinicians to describe a suspicious red oral area that may be at increased risk for oral cancer. Erythroplakia is not synonymous with dysplasia or OSCC. It implies that dysplasia or OSCC may be detected if a biopsy of the area is taken, although biopsy of erythroplakia may show harmless changes. The World Health Organization defines erythroplakia as a "chronic red mucosal macule that cannot be given another specific diagnostic name and cannot be attributed to traumatic, vascular, or inflammatory causes." Although erythroplakia is much less common than leukoplakia, it is much more dangerous, with biopsy revealing

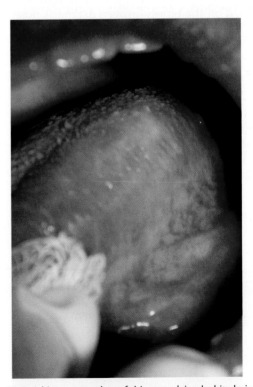

Figure 10-9. A biopsy was taken of this unexplained white lesion on the lateral tongue; it was diagnosed as hyperkeratosis. Hyperkeratosis is a benign thickening of the surface epithelium; in this case it was caused by chronic trauma, so no additional treatment was needed.

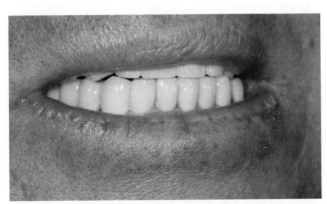

Figure 10-8. Actinic cheilitis is sun damage to the lips. This condition, which can lead to cancer, is seen in this patient as a blurring of the edge of the vermilion border of the lip and a red-and-white color to the lip itself.

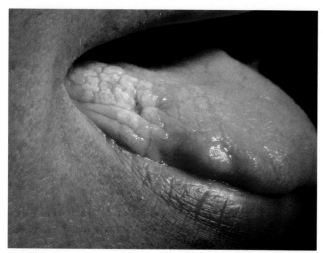

Figure 10-10. This unexplained rough white lesion is especially suspicious because it is in the high-risk area of the lateral tongue and because its rough surface suggests that the surface epithelium is growing faster than the underlying tissue. The patient was a heavy crack cocaine user and did not come back for his scheduled biopsy.

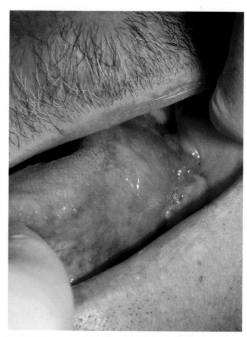

Figure 10-12. This unexplained red lesion on the lateral tongue is suspicious and must promptly undergo a biopsy because of the high risk for dysplasia or cancer. "See Red, Beware."

severe dysplasia or malignancy in 60% to 90% of cases. The saying "See Red, Beware" will remind you of this risk. It can occur in any mucosal site but is more likely in sites where oral cancer is more common, such as the lateral and ventral surfaces of the tongue or floor of the mouth (Fig. 10-12). Clinically, erythroplakia often occurs as a well-delineated red lesion with a velvety surface texture. A biopsy is of utmost importance due to its high risk for malignancy. Further treatment is then based on the biopsy-proven diagnosis. Recurrence is very common with erythroplakia, so long-term follow-up is extremely important.[26]

- *Contour:* The contour or shape of the lesion can become raised and rough. If tumor invades bone, there may be a poorly defined radiolucency. Some other warning signs of cancer are localized, poorly defined bone loss in one area of the jaw, when periodontal disease is minimal in all other areas; persistent nonhealing ulceration; or a nonhealing extraction socket.[20]
- *Consistency:* A cancerous area may change in consistency from soft to hard as the tumor invades, causing it to become fixed to adjoining tissues, a change that is referred to as **induration**.[20]
- *Function:* Changes in function may also develop as cancer invades nearby nerves and muscles (Fig. 10-13). Persistent hoarse voice or trouble swallowing are classic warning signs that can indicate cancer. **Paresthesia** is a sensation of numbness, tingling, or sharp, prickling pain that can signal compression of a nerve. If cancer spreads to adjacent lymph nodes, they may feel firm, fixed, and enlarged when palpated. Hemoptysis (coughing up blood) and unexplained weight loss are also signs of advanced disease.[5,23,27]
- *Location of OSCC:* OSCC can occur anywhere within the oral cavity, but some sites are more common than others. About half of OSCCs occur on the lateral or ventral surfaces of the tongue. OSCC originating on the dorsal surface of the tongue is rare. The second most common site is the floor of the mouth, where about a third of cases occur (Fig. 10-14).[20,21,26]

How Is Oral Cancer Diagnosed?

- A clinical examination is not sufficient to diagnose oral cancer; diagnosis requires a biopsy. Below are types of diagnoses and their descriptions.

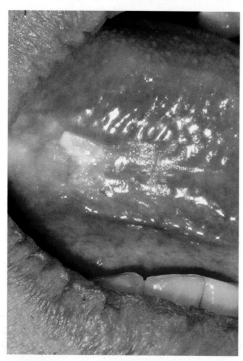

Figure 10-11. A biopsy was taken of this unexplained rough white lesion; it was subsequently diagnosed as carcinoma in situ. The entire lesion was excised and has not recurred.

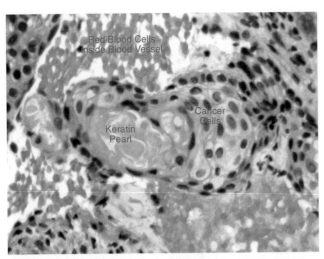

Figure 10-13. Microscopic view of well-differentiated oral squamous cell carcinoma that has invaded local blood vessels.

- *Diagnosis:* The diagnosis of OSCC or dysplasia is made on the basis of a biopsy. A dentist or surgeon takes a surgical sample of the suspicious lesion and submits it in a preservative solution to an oral pathologist for diagnosis.[1,17,20] This process is discussed in more detail later in this chapter.
  - *Dysplasia Versus OSCC:* In dysplasia, the precancerous transformed cells are strictly confined to the overlying epithelial surface; no invasion has occurred. As soon as the transformed cells begin to invade underlying tissue, OSCC has developed. This is an important difference because invasion potentially permits the cancer to spread to other parts of the body through blood vessels and the lymphatics, a process called **metastasis.**[20,21]
- **Grading** *of dysplasia:* Dysplasia is graded by the oral pathologist as mild, moderate, or severe, depending on how extensive the changes are in the affected cells and what proportion of the thickness of the epithelium has been altered.[20,21]

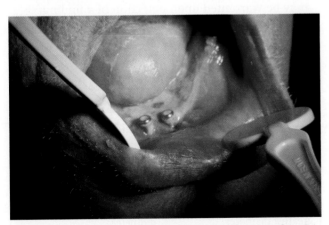

Figure 10-14. An elderly male oral cancer patient is shown after excision of cancer on the floor of the mouth, followed by radiation therapy. He has had extensive skin grafts. His mouth is very dry and will remain that way for the rest of his life because radiation therapy has destroyed the salivary glands. The patient is still suffering from radiation mucositis, so he has a large ulceration on the floor of his mouth.

- *Grading of OSCC:* OSCC is graded by the oral pathologist as well differentiated to poorly differentiated, depending on how well the cancer cells resemble normal squamous cells. An OSCC is called **in situ** if the process of invasion has not yet occurred, but it is apparent that the overlying epithelium looks cancerous.[20,21]

What Is the Treatment and Prognosis of Dysplasia and of Oral Cancer?

- *Dysplasia treatment and prognosis:* It is important to treat dysplasia so that it does not progress to cancer, although not all dysplasia is capable of progression. The treatment of dysplasia varies according to the size and grade of the lesion, the individual patient's health and wishes, and the clinician's preferences. However, moderate-to-severe dysplasia is usually surgically removed. Any patient habits such as tobacco use need to be discontinued, so the dental hygienist should assist with tobacco dependence education. Dysplasia may recur, especially if it is not totally excised, and the entire oral region is at risk for the development of additional new lesions; therefore, frequent recall and thorough examination at each visit is important.[20,21,24,28]
- **Staging** *of OSCC:* When OSCC has been diagnosed, the patient's next step is staging. Staging is a procedure that determines how large the cancer is and whether it has spread to other parts of the body. The cancer treatment team stages OSCC before the tumor treatment plan is finalized. The staging system currently used in North America is the TNM system, in which the tumor is assigned a number (0–4) based on its tumor size (T), whether lymph nodes are involved (N), and whether metastases have occurred (M). The tumor team may use advanced imaging procedures including radiographs, computed tomography scans, magnetic resonance imaging, and positron emission tomography scans to determine the patient's TNM stage (Box 10-1).[20,21,27]
- *Treatment of OSCC:* Treatment of OSCC is based on an individual treatment plan that takes into account the patient's wishes, medical status, tumor stage, and treatment availability. Usually treatment includes some or all of the following: surgical removal of the tumor, surgical removal of the lymph nodes of the neck (neck dissection), radiation therapy, and chemotherapy. Some newer therapies are also being developed. In many large hospitals, patient care is determined with the help of a multidisciplinary **tumor board,** which can include oral and general surgeons, radiologists, dentists, oral and general pathologists, speech pathologists, pharmacologists, social workers, and others.[20,21,27]
- *Prognosis of OSCC:* Early detection and treatment of dysplasia or OSCC is the patient's best chance at beating cancer. The lower the TNM stage, the lower the patient's estimated chance of dying from this disease within the next 5 years. The survival odds also depend on where the cancer is located; for example,

lower lip cancers have a good prognosis (about 90% 5-year survival), unlike cancers on the floor of the mouth. A patient with stage I SCC of the floor of the mouth has about a 70% chance of 5-year survival, but if the same patient is at stage IV, the 5-year survival rate declines to only 30%.[2,20,21,27,29,30]

- *Additional sites of involvement:* Fifteen percent of those individuals diagnosed with oral cancer will have another cancer in a nearby area or lung. Of those cured of the oral cancer, 10% to 40% will develop cancer later in one of these organs or will experience a second cancer of the oral cavity or oropharynx.[22]

EXTRAORAL AND INTRAORAL EXAMINATION

Principles of Examination

- The extraoral and intraoral examination are an essential part of providing dental care. The following are characteristics of a proper examination.
- *Examined structures:* The examination technique involves visual inspection and palpation of all structures in the region.
- *Systematic approach:* A thorough, systematic approach should be followed. Establishing a routine that you use every time with every patient will minimize the chance that you overlook any structure, as well as ensure that you provide a comprehensive assessment in a timely and efficient manner.
- *Good communication:* It is important to establish good rapport with the patient. Use tactful communication throughout the examination and speak with the patient at his or her level of understanding. Explain the purpose of the examination and inform the patient of any findings. Use questioning techniques that elicit applicable information that may lend itself to additional data contributing to a differential diagnosis of any finding. Educate the patient about the signs and symptoms of oral, head, and neck abnormalities, including cancer, and how to detect it at an early stage.[1] For more information on communication, see Chapter 3.

- *Thorough documentation:* All questionable findings must be documented. When documenting intraoral lesions, it is important to include: (a) the size in millimeters for both length and width (the probe is often used for measurement); (b) location, noting adjacent anatomical structures; (c) color; (d) morphological description differentiating whether the lesion is an ulcer (denoting loss of continuity in epithelium), macule (denoting that the lesion is flat), or the specific term for lesions appearing above the plane of mucosa (refer to Table 10-1 for a complete description of such lesions); and (e) history of lesion, including duration of lesion, familial history, and any symptoms the patient is exhibiting.

  When documenting nodes it is important to specify: (a) node chain or triangle; (b) single or multiple node involvement; (c) whether the node is fixed to underlying structures or moveable; (d) duration of node and whether it is tender or nontender; (e) symptoms patient is exhibiting or applicable health history finding such as acute infection; and (f) side of head or neck, or both, of detectable node.
- *Patient position:* The examination can be performed with the patient either supine (lying down) or seated upright. The intent is for the clinician to have the greatest amount of access to structures to thoroughly inspect and palpate each structure involved in the examination.
- *Barriers:* Gloves should be changed between the extraoral and intraoral examination.
- *Warning signals:* Throughout the extraoral/intraoral examination, the clinician should be aware of the following warning signals of head and neck cancer, as discussed previously: hoarseness, persistent coughing or feeling of a "lump in throat," a sore throat that does not heal or bleeds, dysphagia (difficulty in swallowing), paresthesia, any asymmetrical firm nodal enlargement or mass, bleeding, ulcer, thickening, and red or white patches lasting longer than 2 weeks. Pain is usually found in later stages of cancer. Detailed questioning regarding any of these conditions may be warranted upon detection of a finding.

Table 10-1. *Morphological Terminology for Lesions Above Mucosal Plane*

Tissue Lesions (nonblister form)	Fluid-Filled Lesions (blister form)
Papule: <5 mm in greatest diameter	Vesicle: <5 mm in greatest diameter
Nodule: >5 mm in greatest diameter	Bulla: >5 mm in greatest diameter
Plaque: broad, raised plateau-like "pasted-on" appearance, generally >5 mm	Pustule: contains pus having yellow appearance

• *Considerations when palpating nodes:* Nodes are not palpable unless they are enlarged. Nodes arising from acute inflammatory conditions (reactive nodes) tend to be tender, soft, enlarged, and freely moveable. Lymph node involvement due to malignant disease (neoplastic nodes) is often fixed to the surrounding structures (indurated), nontender, hard, and involves multiple nodes.

Examination Procedure

• *Equipment*
  • Gauze square
  • Mouth mirror
  • Tongue blade
  • Gloves (two pairs)
  • Probe
  • Good lighting source
  • Anesthetic spray for excessive gagging
• *Palpation:* Extraoral palpation consists of firm, gentle pressure, placing the fingers together and flat on the patient's skin. In a gentle manner, the examiner's fingertips are moved in a circular motion across the tissue. When palpating lymph nodes, lymph nodes are rolled against harder underlying structures. Intraoral palpation consists of application of fingers to the mucosa with firm, gentle pressure. There are four methods of palpation:
  • *Digital*—use of one finger when palpating the hard palate and lingual surface of the alveolar ridge
  • *Bidigital*—use of the thumb and one finger of one hand supporting a single structure (Fig. 10-15)
  • *Bimanual*—supporting tissue extraorally with the fingers of one hand while palpating the structure intraorally with the fingers of the other hand, using only the pads of the fingertips (Fig. 10-16)
  • *Bilateral*—simultaneous palpation/examination of a single area or structure on both sides of the head, neck, or both (Fig. 10-17)
• *Examination of the face, skin, voice, nose, eyes, and lips[23]:* The initial evaluation of the patient takes place when meeting the patient for the first time. The clinician should carefully note any signs of fatigue or weight loss in the face (Fig. 10-18). While taking the

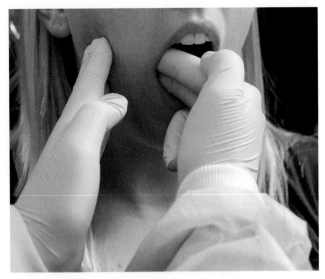

Figure 10-16. Bimanual palpation of buccal mucosa.

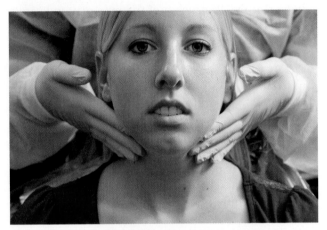

Figure 10-17. Bilateral palpation.

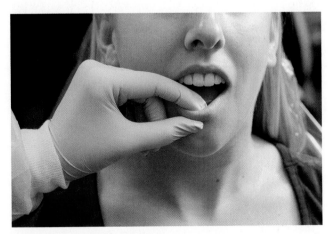

Figure 10-15. Bidigital palpation.

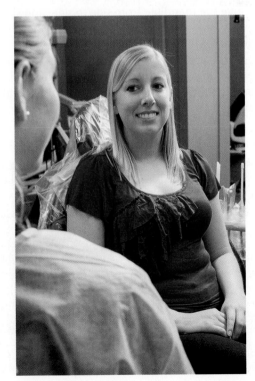

Figure 10-18. Examination of face.

patient's history, it is helpful to note any skin color deviation from normal; for example, a yellow appearance may indicate jaundice, whereas a bluish cast may indicate a respiratory deficiency. Facial asymmetry, masses, skin lesions, and facial paralysis should also be noted. A careful examination of the ears, particularly for male patients, is indicated due to this being a common area for skin cancer. Listening to the patient's voice while he or she is responding to questions may signal the presence of an oropharyngeal tumor. A raspy, hoarse voice could be the first sign of a laryngeal neoplasm.

The nose is a common site for skin cancer. Patients should also be assessed for the presence of unexplained nosebleeds, which can be a sign of cancer, hypertension, or allergies.

Any swelling of the eye or periorbital area should be noted and can be a late sign of a cancer that may have started in the palate, or the maxillary or ethmoid sinuses. Protrusion of the eyes may indicate a dysfunctional thyroid condition. Drainage from the lacrimal system may be a sign of an obstructing mass in the maxillary sinus, nose, or facial soft tissue. The eyes should also be inspected for color changes in the sclera; for example, as with skin color, a yellow appearance may indicate jaundice. Dilation of pupils may indicate a state of shock or drug use.

Inspection of the nose may reveal changes in the skin. Inspection of the lips can also be performed when greeting the patient in the reception area, during the interview, and when recording vital signs. Again, look for any asymmetry or gross lesions on the lips.

- *Bilateral palpation of temporomandibular joint (TMJ):* While using bilateral palpation on condyles, request that the patient: (a) open and close (Fig. 10-19), and (b) move the mandible from side to side, and slide the lower jaw forward. Note opening and any deviation to the left or right upon opening or closing in millimeters. Question patient about pain, headaches, or soreness when waking. Note any popping or clicking of jaw.
- *Bilateral palpation of auricular regions:* In bilateral, circular fashion, compress fingertips in front of and

behind ears in the area of the anterior and retroauricular nodes (Figure 10-20).

- *Bilateral palpation of the parotid region:* Extend bilateral, circular palpation from the tragus of the ear to the angle of the mandible in the area of the parotid gland and superficial parotid lymph nodes (Fig. 10-21).
- *Bilateral palpation of submandibular triangle:* Beginning at the symphysis of the mandible, compress the fingertips on the inferior border of the mandible while

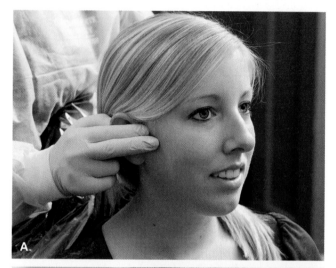

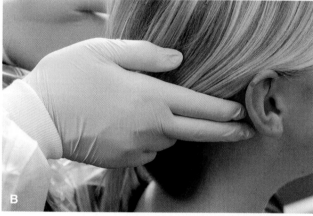

Figure 10-20. (A) Preauricular palpation. (B) Retroauricular palpation.

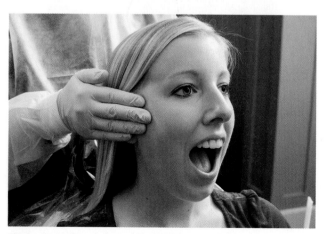

Figure 10-19. Temporomandibular joint palpation.

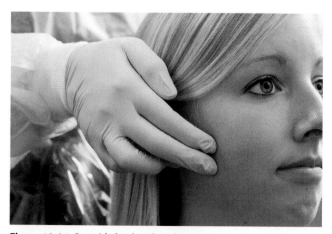

Figure 10-21. Parotid gland node palpation.

rolling laterally over the mandible. Proceed to the angle of the mandible (Fig. 10-22).

- *Palpation of submental triangle:* After requesting that the patient tilt his head downward, compress tissue with bimanual circular motion behind and beneath the symphysis of the mandible (Fig. 10-23).
- *Palpation of anterior midline:* Bidigitally palpate from the symphysis of the mandible to the hyoid bone. Proceed to the suprasternal notch. While palpating in the area of the thyroid cartilage, ask the patient to swallow (Fig. 10-24). The thyroid gland should move up and down without deviation. If the thyroid gland becomes enlarged, it will appear as a wide band of tissue across the trachea.
- *Palpation of sternocleidomastoid muscle (SCM):* Position the patient's head down and to the side. Expose the neck area. Use bidigital palpation of the right and left SCM grasping muscle starting at the mastoid process (Fig. 10-25). Proceed down the muscle to the clavicle.
- *Palpation of deep and superficial cervical lymph nodes:* Upon completion of SCM palpation, grasp the muscle between the thumb and index finger starting at the mastoid process and continuing down the muscle until the clavicle is reached, emphasizing palpation of the deeper, less accessible tissues (Fig. 10-26).
- *Palpation of supraclavicular nodes:* Compress fingers in a bidigital, circular motion above and along each

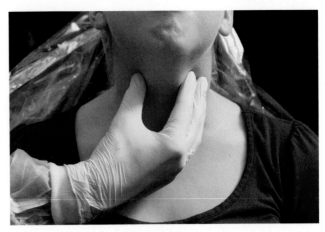

Figure 10-24. Anterior midline palpation.

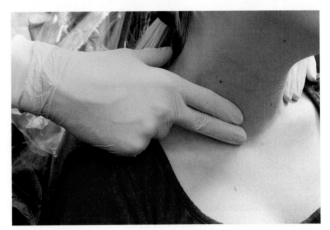

Figure 10-25. Sternocleidomastoid muscle palpation.

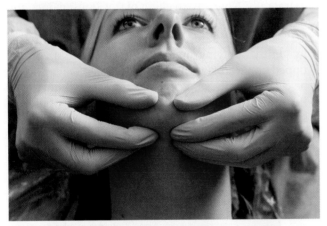

Figure 10-22. Submandibular triangle palpation.

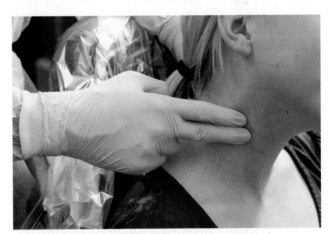

Figure 10-26. Deep cervical node palpation.

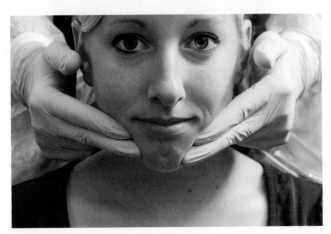

Figure 10-23. Submental triangle palpation.

clavicle (Fig. 10-27). Ask the patient to shrug the shoulders and roll them forward slightly to allow easier access to this area.

- *Palpation of posterior triangles:* Position the patient's head forward. Compress fingers in a bilateral, circular motion in the posterior triangles starting at base of the skull along the trapezius, clavicle, and SCM (Fig. 10-28). Zigzag across the triangle to ensure coverage of all areas.

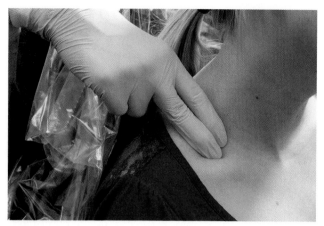

Figure 10-27. Supraclavicular node palpation.

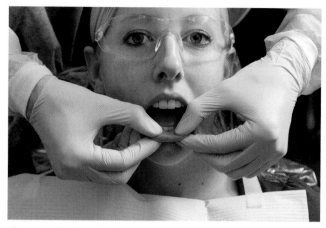

Figure 10-30. Lip palpation.

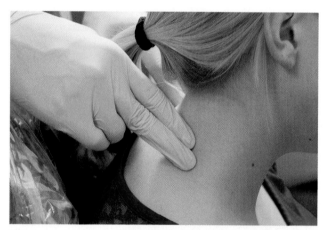

Figure 10-28. Posterior triangle palpation.

- *Visual inspection of oral cavity:* Using a good lighting source and mouth mirror for illumination, observe the oral cavity for changes in color, contour, consistency, and function as described in the earlier Oral Cancer section (Fig. 10-29). Look for unusual pigmentation, texture, scars, and lesions.
- *Palpation of lips, labial mucosa:* Palpate the lips in a bidigital, bilateral fashion starting at the midline and working toward the commissure noting any abnormalities in symmetry, color, and texture (Fig. 10-30). Note any palpable masses. Inspect the vermilion border of the lower lip, a common site for oral cancer.

Retract the lips to inspect the labial mucosa for any abnormalities in the mucosa.

- *Inspection of buccal mucosa:* Retract the buccal mucosa away from the teeth. Inspect the buccal mucosa from the commissure to the anterior tonsillar pillar for any irregularity in color or texture (Fig. 10-31).
- *Palpation of buccal mucosa:* Using bimanual palpation as noted in Figure 10-16, place two to three fingertips of one hand intraorally to palpate the buccal mucosa from the commissure to the anterior tonsillar pillar while the fingerpads of other hand support the tissue extraorally. Note any swelling of the Stensen duct, the duct of the parotid gland. Dry the parotid papilla with a 2 × 2 gauze square. Attempt to stimulate saliva flow by gently applying upward pressure with a cotton-tipped applicator or the mirror handle. Saliva should be clear. Refrain from covering the Stensen duct with the cotton-tipped applicator because it will absorb saliva and prevent proper assessment of salivary flow.

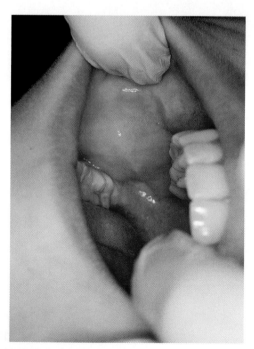

Figure 10-31. Buccal mucosa inspection.

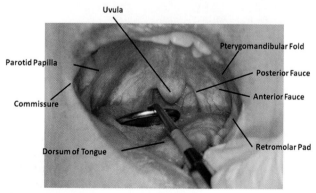

Uvula

Parotid Papilla

Commissure

Dorsum of Tongue

Pterygomandibular Fold

Posterior Fauce

Anterior Fauce

Retromolar Pad

Figure 10-29. Visual inspection of the oral cavity.

- *Inspection of gingiva:* Inspect all gingival tissues with a good light source and mouth mirror, noting any swelling or deviation from normal color (Fig. 10-32). Keep in mind that attached gingiva may exhibit melanin pigmentation, which is a deviation of normal for some patients.
- *Inspection of tongue:* Visually inspect the dorsum, ventral, and lateral borders of the tongue, keeping in mind that the tongue is the most frequent site of oral cancer. Note changes in color, loss of papilla, swelling, or palpable masses. Inspect the posterior tongue with a mirror (Fig. 10-33). Have the patient place the tongue against the palate to thoroughly inspect the ventral tongue.

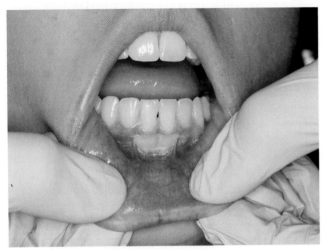

Figure 10-32. Inspection of the gingiva.

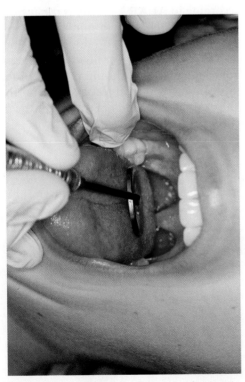

Figure 10-33. Inspection of dorsum of tongue with mirror/pharyngeal inspection.

- *Palpation of tongue:* Ask the patient to extend the tongue, wrap the tip with a 2 × 2 gauze square (Fig. 10-34), and palpate the dorsal surface with the other hand using digital palpation. Gently pull the tongue to one side to visually examine the lateral border before using bidigital palpation of that area (Fig. 10-35). Then pull the tongue in the opposite direction to palpate the other lateral border. After palpating both lateral borders, remove the gauze square and bidigitally palpate the tip. Palpate the entire body of the tongue. Not all clinicians palpate the base of the tongue, distal to the circumvallate papillae, but if possible this palpation is recommended.[13] To palpate the base of the tongue, ask the patient to stick her tongue out as far as possible. Gently but quickly insert the index finger past the circumvallate papillae and use a side-to-side pendulum sweep. Most clinicians cannot palpate further than about 1 cm distal to the circumvallate papillae. Patient gagging can be minimized by using a quick and gentle technique, asking the patient to breathe through the nose, distracting the patient by asking her to raise one foot in the air, and using topical anesthetic if all else fails.
- *Inspection of ventral surface of tongue and palpation of the floor of the mouth:* Ask the patient to lift the

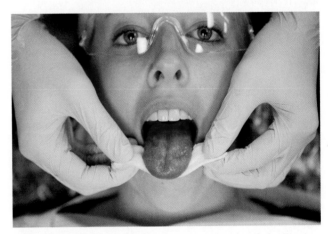

Figure 10-34. Tongue on gauze.

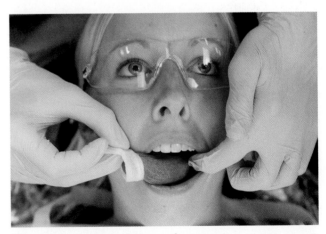

Figure 10-35. Palpation of dorsum of tongue.

tongue toward the roof of the mouth to allow in-spection of the ventral surface of the tongue. It may also be advisable to dry the salivary glands on the caruncles. Milk the ducts with a cotton-tipped applicator or the mirror handle, and dry with a 2 × 2 gauze pad. Oftentimes the salivary glands will spray as soon as they are dried. Then inspect the floor of the mouth with a mouth mirror. Ask the patient to relax the tongue to allow bimanual pal-pation of the floor of the mouth. Place one to two fingers of one hand intraorally while several fingers of the other hand support the tissue (Fig. 10-36). Use circular compressions, noting any enlarged masses or an enlarged submandibular gland.

- *Inspection of tonsillar/pharyngeal region:* Depress the posterior portion of the tongue with a mouth mirror or tongue blade and have the patient say "aah." The soft palate will rise. Inspect the tonsils and tonsillar pillars as well.
- *Inspection and palpation of palate:* Using digital palpation, palpate all regions of the hard palate, noting any swelling. Inspect the soft palate while depressing the tongue and asking the patient to say "aah" (Fig. 10-37).
- *Palpation of soft palate, tonsils, and posterior pharyngeal wall:* Not all clinicians palpate these areas, but if

possible this palpation is recommended.[13] To palpate the tonsils, gently but quickly insert the index finger past the lateral tongue to palpate laterally against the tonsil. Palpate each tonsil separately, letting the pa-tient recover briefly. Quickly palpate the posterior pharyngeal wall in a separate maneuver, and pal-pate the soft palate in the final maneuver, which is also the one most likely to cause the patient to gag. Patient gagging can be minimized by using a quick and gentle technique, asking the patient to breathe through the nose, distracting the patient by asking him to raise one foot in the air, and using a topical anesthetic if all else fails.

- *Inspection and palpation of alveolar ridges:* Palpate the alveolar ridges in bidigital fashion (Fig. 10-38).

The examination steps are summarized in Table 10-2.

DIAGNOSTIC AIDS

The thorough and thoughtful head and neck/oral ex-amination is the most powerful tool at the dental hy-gienist's disposal in the detection of abnormalities, including oral cancer.[8,13,20,23,26] A number of diagnostic aids are available in many offices, and it is important that the dental hygienist be a wise and critical con-sumer who keeps up to date on the independent re-search regarding the effectiveness of these techniques, not merely on persuasive advertising. These methods are summarized in Technology.

Use of Imaging for Screening

It is recommended that the use of radiographs be se-lected according to **ALARA** *(as low as reasonably achiev-able)* principles, which seek to minimize exposure to radiation. This means that all radiographs, including those to examine a patient for potential bone involve-ment from malignancies, should only be ordered on the basis of the patient's clinical history and the find-ings of the examination, and not simply for the purpose of screening for hidden disease.[13,17]

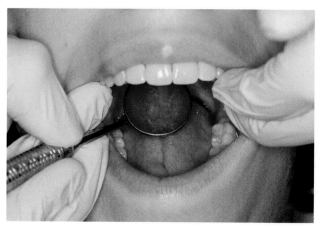

Figure 10-36. Palpation of the floor of the mouth.

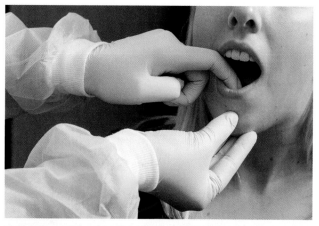

Figure 10-37. Hard and soft palate inspection.

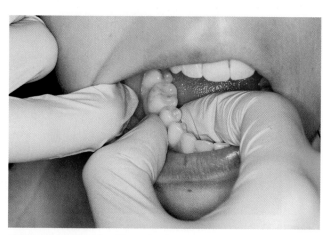

Figure 10-38. Alveolar ridge palpation.

Technology

Oral Cancer Screening Techniques

Technique and Common Trade Names	Approximate Cost to Dental Practice, Per Use	Results	Comments
Oral cancer examination	Chair time and disposables	Changes in color, contour, consistency, and/or function	• The classic and time honored way to detect abnormalities

Visualization adjuncts

Vital dye (toluidine blue, T-blue) Common trade names: ViziLite Plus *(T-blue + Vizilite)*	$20–$30 per kit	Proliferating tissues retain more dye—look bluer	• Tissues should be examined carefully in conjunction with use of these technologies
Tissue reflectance Common trade names: Microlux DL Orascoptic DK ViziLite Plus *(T-Blue + Vizilite)* ViziLite	$20–$30 per kit	Potentially abnormal tissue reflects more light—looks whiter	• Not proven to help or hinder the detection of oral cancer
Autofluorescence Common trade names: Velscope	$5000 to purchase unit + $5 per use	Potentially abnormal tissue loses normal fluorescence—looks darker	

Tissue sampling techniques

Exfoliative cytology Common trade names: Oral CDx brush test	$30–$40 per kit	Positive, negative, or atypical (categories)	• Patient costs include procedure and pathologist fees. • Not proved to be helpful in detecting cancer. • Recommended only for use on surface lesions that are *not at risk for oral cancer.*
Biopsy	Chair time and disposables	The only technique that results in definitive diagnosis.	• Gold standard • Patient costs include surgical and pathologist fees.

Table 10-2. Examination Steps: Examination at a Glance

Area	Palpation	Tips
Face	Inspection	Observe skin, eyes, nose, and lips.
Temporomandibular joint	Bilateral	Have patient open and close, then move mandible from side to side. Note opening and any deviation to right or left in millimeters.
Auricular/Parotid	Bilateral	Palpate in front and region behind ears then along.
Neck		
Submandibular	Bilateral	Palpate from posterior angle of mandible along border. Proceed to midline.
Submental	Bidigital	Palpate behind and beneath symphysis of mandible.
Anterior midline	Bidigital	Palpate anteriorly from chin to suprasternal notch, palpating thyroid cartilage area and having patient swallow to detect possible thyroid gland enlargement.

Continued

Table 10-2. *Examination Steps: Examination at a Glance—cont'd*

Area	Palpation	Tips
Sternocleidomastoid region	Bidigital	Palpate laterally from mastoid process to clavicle.
Deep/Cervical		Palpate deep anterior and posterior to muscle.
Supraclavicular nodes	Bilateral, bidigital	Have patient bend head forward and probe deeply with two fingers above the clavicle.
Posterior	Bilateral, bidigital	Palpate from occipital region anterior to and as far down the trapezius as possible.
Lips	Bidigital inspection	Palpate; observe for deviations from normal.
Labial mucosa	Inspection	Retract mucosa away from teeth. Inspect frenum areas.
Buccal mucosa	Bimanual	Palpate bidigitally intraorally with one hand while supporting tissue extraorally with several fingers of the other hand.
Gingiva	Inspection	Inspect all gingival tissues.
Tongue		Grasp extended tongue with gauze square.
Anterior: dorsal, ventral, and lateral surfaces	Index finger	Observe and palpate dorsal and lateral borders. For ventral surface: have patient place tongue against palate.
Posterior	Inspection	Use dental mirror to inspect.
Floor of mouth	Bimanual	While having patient place tongue on palate, observe all areas. Palpate with index finger of one hand intraorally while several fingers of the other hand support tissue extraorally.
Tonsillar/Pharyngeal region	Inspection	Depress mirror or tongue blade and have patient say "aah." Soft palate will rise.
Hard and soft palate	Index finger	Inspect while tongue still is depressed and then palpate.
Alveolar process	Bidigital	Palpate mandibular and maxillary ridges.
Occlusion	Inspection	Use mirror to retract buccal mucosa to view molar and canine relationships.

Vital Tissue Staining and Other Visualization Adjuncts

Some clinicians prefer to use adjunctive techniques as part of their screening examination. Despite their popularity, there is little current evidence that these techniques either help or hinder the detection of oral cancer and precancer. However, there is ongoing product development that could result in major future breakthroughs in these techniques. Common technologies include vital tissue staining and some special light sources that potentially highlight abnormal areas.

- **Vital tissue staining technology: Toluidine blue dye** is a dye that has an affinity for nucleic acids, which are more plentiful in actively dividing cells, including dysplastic and cancerous cells (Fig. 10-39). This dye can make it easier to see proliferating areas, but it does not distinguish between cells that are proliferating because of normal healing responses and those that are precancerous or cancerous.[16,20,24]

- *Other visualization adjuncts:* These technologies (of which there are several) operate on the principle that abnormal tissues absorb and reflect various forms of light differently (Fig. 10-40). Most of the commercial technologies make abnormal areas reflect extra light so that they appear more intensely white (**tissue reflectance**). At least one commercial technology makes abnormal areas appear black in contrast with the green-tinged fluorescence of normal tissues under that particular wavelength of light (**tissue autofluorescence**). However, false-positive results occur when these techniques fail to distinguish between cells that are proliferating because of normal healing responses and those that are precancerous or cancerous.[16,24]

- **Cytological smear:** The cytological smear is a simple technique in which tissues are wiped with a spatula, and the harvested cells are smeared on a glass slide. The slide is sprayed with a fixative, then stained and examined under the microscope. Although this technique has saved thousands of lives when used on the

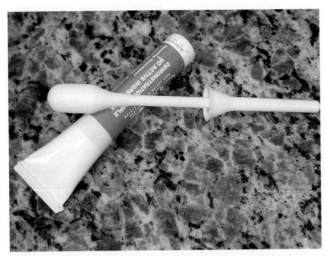

Figure 10-39. Toluidine blue is a dye that can be painted on the oral mucosa. The stain can make it easier to notice rapidly dividing areas, but a positive stain may happen because of normal healing, not just dysplasia.

uterine cervix as the Pap smear, it is not used in screening for oral cancer because it has been shown to be ineffective in the oral cavity for this purpose. It is used in the oral cavity primarily to detect oral Candidiasis. There is ongoing research on new ways to potentially harness this simple technique for oral pathology.[16,24,30]

- **Exfoliative cytology (brush test):** Exfoliative cytology is similar to a cytological smear in that it is used to examine individual cells under the microscope. However, there are some important differences between the techniques. In exfoliative cytology, the cells are harvested with a small brush that can penetrate to the basal cells of the epithelium, where dysplasia first develops. The slide is screened by a special computer system that is calibrated to pick up abnormal cells; then a pathologist

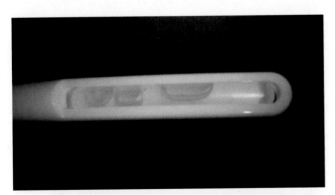

Figure 10-40. Tissue reflectance systems use a fluorescing disposable light source. These technologies operate on the principle that abnormal areas will reflect more light, and thus appear whiter than the surrounding areas. Such a light source is shown here. Many common benign conditions such as linea alba can give false-positive readings. Tissue autofluorescence systems operate on a different principle: They stimulate fluorescent light emissions from normal cells, but abnormal cells do not autofluoresce so they appear darker than the surrounding areas.

examines the slide. However, this technique does not result in a diagnosis in the same sense as a conventional biopsy does; it categorizes the findings as positive (definite abnormalities indicating neoplasia), atypical (abnormalities not necessarily denoting neoplasia), or negative (no abnormalities). However, false-positive results can create alarm for the patient. This technique does not replace the conventional biopsy, and it is best reserved for white surface abnormalities of the epithelium that are not considered at risk for oral cancer or dysplasia. It is not recommended for use in clinically suspicious lesions.[16,24]

BIOPSY TECHNIQUES

Types of Biopsies

Biopsies are performed by a licensed dentist or physician because they are surgical procedures. There are many different types of biopsy, but the most common categories of biopsy are incisional and excisional biopsies, which are explained in the following list. Biopsies can be performed with a number of different surgical techniques, but most dentists use a scalpel or a tissue punch to obtain the tissue. Diagnosis can also be determined by a number of different techniques, ranging from molecular analysis to gross examination, but most diagnoses are made by microscopic examination of the tissue.[16,24]

- **Incisional biopsy:** Incisional biopsy is defined as the removal of a representative portion of the lesion for diagnosis. It is the appropriate technique for suspected malignancies, as well as widespread and large lesions. It is indicated when removing a large section of tissue (as in excisional biopsy) may prove esthetically unappealing. More tissue will be removed if the biopsy is positive for precancer or cancerous lesions. This is a conservative technique designed to retain as much healthy tissue as possible. An elliptical, wedge-shaped incision is performed with a scalpel on the representative sample of the lesion. The sample is typically taken from the edge of the lesion with the surrounding normal tissue. Incisional biopsy is usually used for SCC, lichenoid lesions, large leukoplakic or erythroplakic areas, suspected dysplasias, ulcerations, erosions, and widespread inflamed conditions.
- *Excisional biopsy:* Excisional biopsy is defined as the complete removal of the lesion for diagnosis. This type of biopsy is indicated for small lesions, less than 1 cm in diameter, that are not suspected of malignancy, as well as for larger benign lesions that need to be removed for functional or esthetic reasons. Common lesions that are typically removed by excisional biopsy include epulis fissuratum, fibroma, lipoma, mucocele, pyogenic granuloma, small cysts,

and small, innocent-looking white lesions (Figure 10-41). A margin of approximately 3 to 5 mm and adequate depth of normal tissue surrounding the lesion is included with the specimen.

- *Punch biopsy:* A tissue punch can be used instead of a scalpel in both excisional and incisional biopsies. Tissue punches are sharp circular devices ranging in diameter from 2 to 10 mm. They cut a core of tissue, and the base of the tissue is separated using curved scissors or a scalpel. Punch biopsy is often used for widespread ulcerative conditions such as lichenoid mucositis, pemphigoid, or pemphigus.

Submitting a Biopsy

Oral biopsies should be immediately submitted to an oral pathology biopsy service. Oral and maxillofacial pathologists are dentists who undergo years of specialized training in pathology of the orofacial region, so they are uniquely trained and qualified to diagnose oral biopsies. Local oral pathology biopsy services can be identified through organizations such as the American Academy of Oral and Maxillofacial Pathology (http://www.aaomp.org).

The sequence of steps to submit a biopsy can be summarized as preserve, identify, submit.

- *Preserve:* To preserve the biopsied tissue so that it arrives at the biopsy service intact, the dentist must immediately place it into preservative, usually 10% buffered formalin (Fig. 10-42). It is very important to make sure that the preservative is in the office before the biopsy is performed, because as soon as the tissue is removed from the patient, it starts to decompose. A bottle of this preservative is part of a biopsy kit that is provided by the oral pathology biopsy service that will be performing the diagnosis. In an emergency situation in which the tissue is removed and no formalin is available, ethanol such as vodka or grain alcohol can serve as a lower-quality substitute, but rubbing alcohol is not an acceptable substitute for formalin. Occasionally, the patient needs a special biopsy, which requires a special type of fixative such as Michel Solution.
- *Identify:* The biopsy bottle must be clearly labeled with the patient's name and the name of the dentist who has performed the biopsy. A biopsy submission form, which is part of the biopsy kit supplied by the biopsy service, must also accompany the specimen, and it needs to be completely filled out.

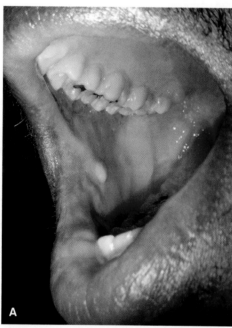

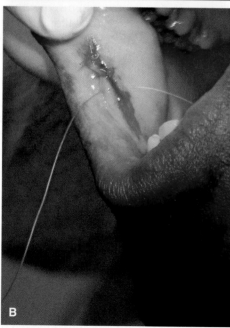

Figure 10-41. (A) A fibroma has been identified in the buccal mucosa. (B) An excisional biopsy has been completed, and sutures are being placed.

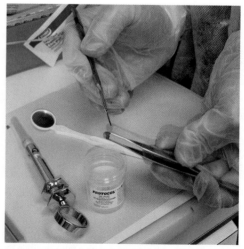

Figure 10-42. Excised tissue must be placed immediately into the bottle of formalin that is part of the biopsy kit. In this case, the fibroma in Figure 10-41 is being held in tissue forceps on its way to the fixative. The bottle must be immediately labeled with the patient's and surgeon's names.

- *Submit:* The biopsy in its labeled specimen bottle, with the accompanying paperwork, should be sent as quickly as possible to the oral pathology biopsy service, by courier or by mail. In very cold weather, care needs to be taken so that the specimen does not freeze in an outdoor pickup location. Freezing causes ice crystals to form, and these can ruin the specimen.

Generating a Pathology Report

An oral and maxillofacial pathologist will diagnose the biopsy and send a report to the submitting dentist. A number of steps need to take place in the pathology laboratory, and this typically takes about a week to complete. The report is often ready when the patient returns 1 week later to get sutures removed.

- *Grossing the specimen:* When the specimen arrives at the laboratory, a technologist or pathologist examines the specimen, makes a formal description, and

places the specimen in a small, labeled cassette for processing.
- *Processing the specimen:* The specimen is embedded in wax, sectioned into very thin slices that are mounted on labeled glass slides, and then stained.
- *Diagnosing the specimen:* The oral pathologist examines the specimen under the microscope and writes a formal report with diagnosis. Sometimes the oral pathologist needs to perform other special stains on the specimen or request consultations with other pathologists.
- *Reporting the diagnosis:* The formal report is generated and transmitted to the surgeon who performed the biopsy.

The patient should also be informed that the pathology service will bill the patient for the oral pathologist's professional fee and laboratory technical fees. These fees are in addition to the dentist's fee for performing the biopsy surgery. Pathology fees vary according to the complexity of the case.

Case Study

A patient presents for an initial visit to your office. He is a smoker, has two to three alcoholic drinks daily, and his chief complaints are a sore on the floor of his mouth (under his tongue) and discomfort in his TMJ.

Case Study Exercises

1. What steps should you follow with this patient?
   A. Immediately refer the patient to an oral surgeon.
   B. Perform an examination of the head and neck region.
   C. Use toluidine blue.
   D. Perform an intraoral examination and an examination of the head and neck region.
2. Is this patient at low, medium, or high risk for oral cancer? Why?
3. During the intraoral examination, you note a raised red lesion (erythroplakia) on the floor of the mouth. Should you tell the patient that he has oral squamous cell carcinoma (OSCC)?

4. When performing an intraoral and extraoral examination, all of the following are true EXCEPT:
   A. Patient position is upright.
   B. Gloves should be changed between the extraoral and the intraoral examination.
   C. Nodes are not palpable unless they are enlarged.
   D. Equipment includes gauze square, mouth mirror, tongue blade, gloves (two pairs), probe, good lighting source, and anesthetic spray for excessive gagging.
5. One of the patient's chief complaints is discomfort in the TMJ area. Is it necessary to perform an examination of the area, or is this the role of the dentist? If yes, what procedures should be followed?

Review Questions

1. What is the BEST way to distinguish between leukoedema and other similar conditions of the oral cavity?
   A. Stretching: Leukoedema disappears when stretched and the others do not.
   B. Brush biopsy: Leukoedema is negative and the others are positive.
   C. Diascopy: Leukoedema is negative and the others are positive.
   D. Scalpel biopsy: Leukoedema shows dysplasia and others do not.

2. This 28-year-old white male patient has a common condition of his tongue. What is it?

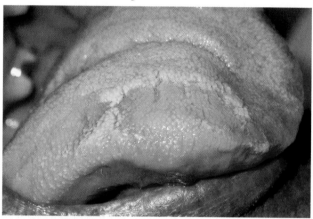

   A. Geographic tongue
   B. Fissured tongue
   C. Bifid tongue
   D. Ankyloglossia

3. Your 57-year-old white female patient has had a bony enlargement on the midpalate that has been unchanged for all of her adult life. It interferes with the planned removable partial denture for the maxilla, so it will be removed. What is its most likely diagnosis?
   A. Osteoma
   B. Osteoblastoma
   C. Osteosarcoma
   D. Palatal torus

4. Which of the following is the MOST APPROPRIATE technique to diagnose an oral epithelial lesion that is suspicious for malignancy?
   A. Exfoliative cytology brush test
   B. Tissue autofluorescence
   C. Incisional biopsy
   D. Cytological smear

5. Which of the following is the most likely origin for a soft lesion with a dome-shaped surface that is located in the buccal mucosa?
   A. Bone
   B. Fibrous tissue
   C. Surface mucosa
   D. Odontogenic epithelium

Active Learning

1. Pair off in groups of three. One person will act as a patient, the next will be the clinician, and the third will observe. Perform a thorough, standardized extraoral and intraoral examination. Take turns playing each role.

2. Prepare a public service announcement of 1 minute for a radio audience to help consumers identify clinical signs and symptoms of oral diseases and oral manifestations of systemic diseases. Be succinct and get across important messages.

3. Prepare a brief presentation to educate patients about procedures after a lesion is detected. This should include visualization adjuncts, biopsy procedures, and any other information patients will need to make an informed decision about their care.

4. Create a referral slip to a surgeon, including any information that should be included with a biopsy specimen. The referral slip should be a check-off list that is easy to complete in a short amount of time.

REFERENCES

1. Oral Cancer Foundation. The role of dental and medical professionals. http://www.oralcancerfoundation.org/dental/role_of_dentists.htm. Modified March 2014. Accessed June 9, 2010.
2. National Cancer Institute. Oral cancer screening PDQ. http://www.cancer.gov/cancertopics/pdq/screening/oral/HealthProfessional/page3. Accessed June 9, 2010.
3. National Cancer Institute. A snapshot of head and neck cancers. http://www.cancer.gov/aboutnci/servingpeople/snapshots/head-neck.pdf. Accessed June 9, 2010.
4. American Cancer Society. Detailed guide: oral cavity and oropharyngeal cancer. http://www.cancer.org/docroot/CRI/content/CRI_2_4_1X_What_is_oral_cavity_and_oropharyngeal_cancer_60.asp?rnav=cri. Accessed June 1, 2010.
5. American Academy of Oral and Maxillofacial Pathology. http://www.aaomp.org/about/index.php. Accessed June 1, 2010.
6. Patton LL, Epstein JB, Kerr AR. Adjunctive techniques for oral cancer examination and lesion diagnosis: a systematic review of the literature. *J Am Dent Assoc.* 2008; 139(7):896-905; quiz 993-4. http://jada.highwire.org/cgi/reprint/139/7/896. Accessed June 1, 2010.
7. Segal LM, Stephenson R, Dawes M, Feldman P. Prevalence, diagnosis, and treatment of ankyloglossia:

methodologic review. *Can Fam Physician.* 2007;53(6): 1027-1033. http://www.cfp.ca/cgi/content/full/53/6/ 1027. Accessed June 1, 2010.

8. Tewfik T. Congenital malformations, mouth and pharynx. eMedicine, Otolaryngology and Plastic Surgery Section. http://emedicine.medscape.com/article/ 837347-overview. Published March 4, 2010. Accessed June 1, 2010.

9. Jainkittivong A, Langlais RP. Buccal and palatal exostoses: prevalence and concurrence with tori. *Oral Surg Oral Med Oral Pathol Oral Radiol Endod.* 2000;90(1): 48-53.

10. Sawair FA, Shayyab MH, Al-Rababah MA, Saku T. Prevalence and clinical characteristics of tori and jaw exostoses in a teaching hospital in Jordan. *Saudi Med J.* 2009;30(12):1557-1562.

11. Reamy BV, Derby R, Bunt CW. Common tongue conditions in primary care. *Am Fam Physician.* 2010;81(5): 627-634. https://secure.aafp.org/login/. Accessed June 6, 2010.

12. Martin JL. Leukoedema: an epidemiological study in white and African Americans. *J Tenn Dent Assoc.* 1997; 77(1):18-21.

13. García-García AS, Martínez-González JM, Gómez-Font R, et al. Current status of the torus palatinus and torus mandibularis. *Med Oral Patol Oral Cir Bucal.* 2010;15(2): e353-360. http://www.medicinaoral.com/pubmed/ medoralv15_i2_p353.pdf. Accessed June 1, 2010.

14. Canger EM, Celenk P, Kayipmaz S. Denture-related hyperplasia: a clinical study of a Turkish population group. *Braz Dent J.* 2009;20(3):243-248. http://www. scielo.br/scielo.php?pid=S0103-64402009000300013 &script=sci_arttext. Accessed June 1, 2010.

15. Buchner A, Shnaiderman-Shapiro A, Vered M. Relative frequency of localized reactive hyperplastic lesions of the gingiva: a retrospective study of 1675 cases from Israel. *J Oral Pathol Med.* 2010;39(8):631-638.

16. Lederman DA, Fornatora ML. Oral fibromas and fibromatoses. eMedicine, Dermatology Section. http:// emedicine.medscape.com/article/1080948-overview. Published February 11, 2009. Accessed June 1, 2010.

17. Zhang W, Chen Y, An Z, et al. Reactive gingival lesions: a retrospective study of 2,439 cases. *Quintessence Int.* 2007;38(2):103-110.

18. Fatima G, Sandesh N, Ravindra S, Kulkarni S. Moving beyond clinical appearance: the need for accurate histological diagnosis. *Gen Dent.* 2009;57(5):472-477; quiz 478-9, 535-6. http://www.agd.org/support/articles/ ?ArtID=6204. Accessed June 6, 2010.

19. Allen C. Peripheral giant cell granuloma. eMedicine, Dermatology Section. http://emedicine.medscape.

com/article/1079711-overview. Published February 11, 2009. Accessed June 1, 2010.

20. de Marcos JA, de Marcos MJ, Rodríguez SA, et al. Peripheral ossifying fibroma: a clinical and immunohistochemical study of four cases. *J Oral Sci.* 2010;52(1): 95-99. http://jos.dent.nihon-u.ac.jp/journal/52/95.pdf. Accessed June 1, 2010.

21. Scully C. Cancers of the oral mucosa. eMedicine, Dermatology Section. http://emedicine.medscape.com/ article/1075729-overview. Published April 27, 2010. Accessed June 1, 2010.

22. Jerjes W, Upile T, Petrie A, et al. Clinicopathological parameters, recurrence, locoregional and distant metastasis in 115 T1-T2 oral squamous cell carcinoma patients. *Head Neck Oncol.* 2010;2(1):9. http://www.headand-neckoncology.org/content/pdf/1758-3284-2-9.pdf. Accessed June 6, 2010.

23. Tachezy R, Klozar J, Rubenstein L, et al. Demographic and risk factors in patients with head and neck tumors. *J Med Virol.* 2009;81(5):878-887.

24. Dyer TA, Robinson PG. General health promotion in general dental practice—the involvement of the dental team. Part 1: a review of the evidence of effectiveness of brief public health interventions. *Br Dent J.* 2006; 200(12):679-685; discussion 71. http://www.nature. com/bdj/journal/v200/n12/full/4813731a.html. Accessed June 6, 2010.

25. Stucken E, Weissman J, Spiegel JH. Oral cavity risk factors: experts' opinions and literature support. *J Otolaryngol Head Neck Surg.* 2010;39(1):76-89.

26. Marur S, D'Souza G, Westra WH, Forastiere AA. HPV-associated head and neck cancer: a virus-related cancer epidemic. *Lancet Oncol.* 2010;11(8):781-789.

27. Rethman M, Carpenter W, Cohen EWE, et al. Evidence-based clinical recommendations regarding screening for oral squamous cell carcinomas. *J Am Dent Assoc.* 2010; 141(5):509-520. http://jada.ada.org/cgi/ content/abstract/141/5/509. Accessed June 6, 2010.

28. Bagan J, Sarrion G, Jimenez Y. Oral cancer: clinical features. *Oral Oncol.* 2010;46(6):414-417.

29. Sklenicka S, Gardiner S, Dierks EJ, et al. Survival analysis and risk factors for recurrence in oral squamous cell carcinoma: does surgical salvage affect outcome? *J Oral Maxillofac Surg.* 2010;68(6):1270-1275.

30. Kujan O, Glenny A-M, Oliver R, et al. Screening programmes for the early detection and prevention of oral cancer. *Cochrane Database Syst Rev.* 2006;3:CD004150. http://www2.cochrane.org/reviews/en/ab004150.html. Accessed June 1, 2010.

Chapter 11 | The Periodontal Examination

Susan Long, RDH, EdD

KEY TERMS

acute inflammation

alveolar bone proper

alveoli

attached gingiva

bleeding on probing (BOP)

cementoenamel junction (CEJ)

chronic inflammation

clinical attachment level (CAL)

col

collagen

exudate

free gingiva

fremitus

furcation

gingival crevicular fluid

gingival recession

gingival sulcus

gingivitis

inflammation

mucogingival junction

papilla

periodontal disease

periodontal risk assessment

periodontal screening and recording (PSR)

periodontitis

periodontium

probe depth

refractory

suppuration

tooth mobility

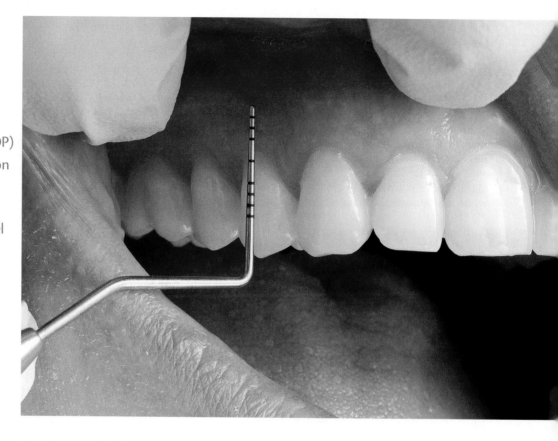

LEARNING OBJECTIVES

After reading this chapter, the student should be able to:

11.1 Describe the tissues of the periodontium.

11.2 State the difference between the periodontal screening and recording (PSR) and a comprehensive periodontal examination.

11.3 List and describe how to assess each component of a comprehensive periodontal examination.

11.4 Satisfactorily perform each of the components of a comprehensive periodontal examination.

11.5 Identify the clinical signs and symptoms of periodontal disease.

11.6 Recognize radiographic findings of periodontal disease.

11.7 Review current systems of classifications of periodontal diseases.

11.8 Accurately record the data collected during the periodontal examination.

KEY CONCEPTS

• A thorough assessment of the periodontium must be conducted to arrive at an accurate dental hygiene diagnosis, plan appropriate treatment, implement appropriate treatment, and adequately evaluate treatment outcomes.

- Periodontal diseases are a group of diseases typically characterized by bacterial infection of the periodontium. Although the initial bacterial challenge to a susceptible host begins with a local inflammatory reaction, most of the damage to the periodontium is due to the host's immune response to the predominantly gram-negative microorganisms.
- Radiographic assessment of the periodontium must accompany a periodontal examination because a periodontal diagnosis should be derived from a combination of sources.
- Adjunctive techniques such as microbial testing, gingival crevicular fluid assays, subgingival temperature, and/or genetic testing may be useful in risk assessment and screening.
- The American Academy of Periodontology (AAP) classification of periodontal diseases provides a general framework for studying the cause, pathogenesis, and treatment of periodontal diseases.

RELEVANCE TO CLINICAL PRACTICE

A thorough periodontal assessment includes evaluation of all aspects of the **periodontium** for signs of inflammation and resultant damage. Together with the medical and dental histories, extraoral and intraoral examination, and dental assessment, the periodontal assessment contributes to the comprehensive data required for diagnosis and treatment planning, as well as a basis for determining treatment plans and outcomes, subsequent treatment needs, and long-term monitoring of oral health.[1-3] The purpose of this chapter is to provide an overview of periodontal anatomy, itemize and describe the components of the comprehensive periodontal examination, and review the American Academy of Periodontology (AAP) classifications of **periodontal diseases** and conditions.[4]

INTRODUCTION TO PERIODONTAL ANATOMY

The periodontium (Greek *peri*, meaning "around," and *odontos*, meaning "tooth") is composed of the gingiva, cementum, periodontal ligament (PDL), and alveolar bone (Fig. 11-1). Together, they form the functional system of hard and soft tissues that surround and attach teeth to the bone and provide support, protection, and nourishment to the teeth.[5]

Gingiva

Gingival tissue is composed of stratified squamous epithelium, which consists of two layers: (a) an outer layer of closely packed flat cells arranged in multiple layers or sheets, with (b) a thin underlying mat of extracellular matrix called the *basal lamina*. Keratins are fibrous, structural proteins that make surface epithelial cells stronger and more resistant to insult. Examples of heavily keratinized epithelium are the palms of the hands and soles of the feet. Keratinized

epithelial cells have no nuclei, whereas nonkeratinized epithelial cells have nuclei and are softer and more flexible. The outer surface of epithelium may be nonkeratinized or keratinized. The oral epithelium of the labial and buccal mucosa, alveolar mucosa, floor

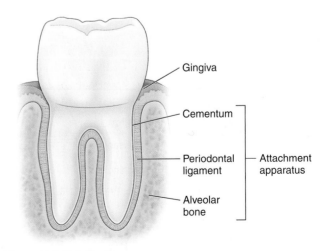

Figure 11-1. Periodontium.

of the mouth, ventral of the tongue, soft palate, sulcular epithelium, and the junctional epithelium are nonkeratinized, whereas the epithelium of the attached gingiva, hard palate, and labial aspect of the free gingiva are keratinized.[5,6]

The thin layers of epithelium rest on a foundation of connective tissue called the *lamina propria.* Because epithelium does not contain blood vessels, it receives nourishment from blood vessels in the underlying connective tissue. The majority of the lamina propria consists of collagen fibers along with fibroblasts, ground substance (a polysaccharide-protein complex), and nerve tissue.[6–8] **Collagen** is the most abundant protein in the body. It is a tough, flexible, white material that provides strength and resilience and is a major component of all connective tissue. Collagen fibers are bundled and grouped by location and direction with the primary function of maintaining the form for the free gingiva, attaching the junctional epithelium to the tooth and attaching gingiva to cementum and bone. The principal fiber groups include dentogingival, alveologingival, circular, dentoperiosteal, and trans-septal fibers (Fig. 11-2). The secondary or minor fiber groups are the periostogingival, interpapillary, transgingival, intercircular, intergingival, and semicircular fibers.[5–7] A review of the gingival fiber groups and their functions is provided in Table 11-1.

The gingival tissue forms a seal around the cervical portion of the tooth and covers the alveolar process of the maxilla and mandible (Fig. 11-3). It can be divided into four anatomical areas: free gingiva, gingival sulcus, attached gingiva, and interdental gingiva.

The **free gingiva,** or unattached gingiva, is the most coronal portion of gingival tissue, found in health close to the **cementoenamel junction (CEJ).** It is not attached to the tooth by gingival fibers and forms the soft tissue wall of the gingival sulcus. The margin of the free gingiva tapers to meet the tooth in a thin edge that can be described as knife-edged. The free gingiva is keratinized.[6]

The **gingival sulcus** is the space between the free gingiva and the tooth surface into which an instrument

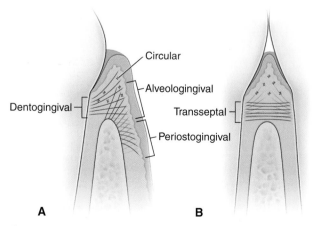

Figure 11-2. Principal gingival fiber groups.

Table 11-1. Principal Gingival Fiber Groups

The gingival fiber groups are a network of ropelike collagen fiber bundles located coronal to the crest of the alveolar bone. They provide rigidity to tissue and strengthen the junctional epithelium. Together, the junctional epithelium and gingival fibers are referred to as the *dentogingival unit.*

Classification and Function of Gingiva Fiber Groups

1. Alveologingival	Extend from the periosteum of the alveolar crest into the gingival connective tissue. Attach the gingiva to the bone.
2. Circular fibers	Encircle the tooth, coronal to alveolar crest. These fibers are *not* attached to cementum of tooth. Connect adjacent teeth to one another.
3. Dentogingival fibers	Embedded in cementum near the CEJ and fan out into the gingival connective tissue. Attach the gingiva to teeth.
4. Periostogingival	Embedded laterally from the periosteum of the alveolar bone. Attach the gingiva to the bone.
5. Trans-septal	Pass from the cementum of one tooth, over the rest of the alveolar bone, to the cementum of the adjacent tooth. Connect adjacent teeth to one another and secure alignment of teeth in the arch.
6. Intergingival	Extended in a mesiodistal direction along the entire dental arch and around the last molars in the arch. Link adjacent teeth into a dental arch unit.
7. Intercircular	Encircle several teeth. Link adjacent teeth into a dental arch unit.
8. Interpapillary	Located in the papillae coronal to the trans-septal fiber bundles. Connect the oral and vestibular interdental papillae of posterior teeth.
9. Transgingival	Extend from the cementum near the CEJ and run horizontally between adjacent teeth. Link adjacent teeth into a dental arch unit.

CEJ, cementoenamel junction.

such as a periodontal probe or curette can be inserted. Healthy sulcus depths range from 0.5 to 3.0 mm, with an average depth of 1.8 mm.[9] In health, the walls of the sulcus are created by the sulcular epithelium of the free gingiva and the tooth enamel. The base of the

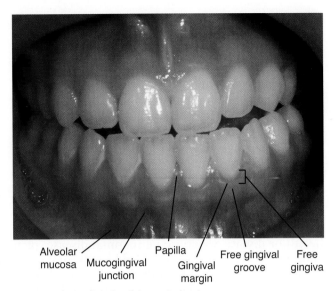

Figure 11-3. Landmarks of the periodontium.

Alveolar mucosa   Mucogingival junction   Papilla   Gingival margin   Free gingival groove   Free gingiva

sulcus is the junctional epithelium, a specialized type of nonkeratinized epithelium that attaches the gingiva to the tooth surface and varies in thickness from 15 to 30 cells in the coronal zone and 4 to 5 cells in the apical zone.[5–7] Being thin and nonkeratinized, the junctional epithelium is an easy point of entry for bacteria to invade into the underlying connective tissue.

The **attached gingiva** is the portion of the gingiva extending apically from the free gingival groove to the **mucogingival junction** where the attached gingiva meets the alveolar mucosa. Attached gingiva is keratinized and tightly knit to the underlying periosteum of the alveolar bone by collagen fibers, which results in its stippled texture. Attached gingiva is widest in the incisor and molar regions and is narrowest in the premolar regions; however, no absolute minimum width is required for periodontal health.[5–7]

The interdental gingiva, or **papilla,** is the portion of the gingival tissue that fills the interproximal space between the adjacent teeth. The interdental papilla is concave facial-lingually, creating a saucer-like depression called the **col.** The col area lies directly apical to the contact area of two adjacent teeth and is nonkeratinized. Location, anatomy, and lack of keratinization make the col area highly susceptible to periodontal breakdown.[5–7]

Cementum

Cementum is mineralized connective tissue that covers the root of the tooth and overlies dentin, sealing open dentinal tubules and protecting the underlying dentin. The cementum of the tooth root and the enamel of the tooth crown meet to create the CEJ. This junction can have one of three relationships: 60% of the time cementum overlaps enamel; 30% of the time the cementum and enamel meet; and 10% of the time the cementum fails to meet the enamel, creating a small gap. Covered by alveolar bone and gingiva, cementum is not normally exposed to the oral cavity except in the

case of **gingival recession.** A primary function of cementum is to anchor the tooth to the alveolus (tooth socket) and maintain occlusal relationships by means of the principle fibers of the PDL.[5,6,10] Cementum has no blood supply and receives nutrients from the PDL fibers that insert into it.

Periodontal Ligament

The PDL is a thin piece of fibrous connective tissue that surrounds the entire tooth root, fills the space between the root and the tooth socket, and connects to the tooth and bony wall of the alveolus. The PDL functions to suspend the tooth in the bony socket, transmit tactile pressure and pain sensations, and provide nutrients to cementum and bone. The PDL contains cementoblasts that produce cementum throughout the life of the tooth and osteoclasts that can resorb bone and cementum. Functioning as a unit, the alveolar bone, PDL, and cementum are referred to as the attachment apparatus.[5,6] The collagen fibers of the PDL are bundled into groups that are embedded into the cementum and bone and are classified by the location and direction of attachment (alveolar crest, horizontal, oblique, and apical; Fig. 11-4). A review of the principal PDL fiber groups and their functions is provided in Table 11-2.

Alveolar Bone

The alveolar process is the portion of the maxilla and the mandible that forms and supports the **alveoli** (bony sockets) of the teeth. It is divided into two parts based on function and adaptation: the alveolar bone proper and the supporting alveolar bone to include the cortical bone, cancellous bone, and periosteum. The **alveolar bone proper** is a thin layer of bone that supports the root and gives attachment to the PDL. This layer is also known as the lamina dura or cribriform plate, and it frequently contains Sharpey's fibers, collagen fibers from the PDL. Cortical bone is a layer of hard, compact bone

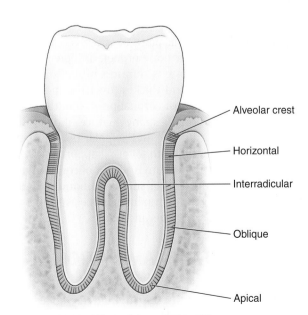

Alveolar crest

Horizontal

Interradicular

Oblique

Apical

Figure 11-4. Principal fibers of the periodontal ligament.

Table 11-2. *Periodontal Ligament Fiber Groups*

The five principal fiber groups of the periodontal ligament (PDL) surround the tooth root and connect it to the alveolar bone. They are classified by location and orientation.

Principal Fiber Groups of the PDL and Sharpey's Fibers	
1. Alveolar crest fibers	Extend from the cervical cementum, running downward in a diagonal direction to alveolar crest. Resists horizontal movements of the tooth.
2. Horizontal fibers	Located apical to the alveolar crest fibers. Extend from the cementum to the bone at right angles to the long axis of the root. Resist horizontal pressure against the crown of the tooth.
3. Oblique fibers	Located apical to horizontal group. Extend from cementum to the bone, running in a diagonal direction. Resists vertical pressures that threaten to drive root into its socket.
4. Apical fibers	Extend from apex of tooth to bone. Secures tooth in socket and resists forces that might lift the tooth out of socket.
5. Inter-radicular fiber group	Extend from cementum in the furcation area of multirooted tooth to the interradicular septum of alveolar bone. Help stabilize tooth in socket.
Sharpey's fibers	Ends of the PDL fibers that are embedded in the cementum and alveolar bone.

that forms the external plate of the alveolar process, surrounds the alveolar bone proper, and gives support to alveoli. Cortical bone is thinnest in incisor, canine, and premolar areas, and thickest over the molars. The alveolar crest is the most coronal portion of the cortical bone. Cancellous bone is spongy, lattice-like bone that lies between cortical bone and alveolar bone proper. It is oriented around the tooth to form support for alveolar bone proper. The periosteum is a layer of connective soft tissue that covers the outer surface of bone. It consists of collagen tissue with an inner layer of elastic fibers and a rich layer of blood vessels and nerves.[6,9]

PERIODONTAL EXAMINATION

The periodontal examination involves the collection of data designed to provide a comprehensive picture of the patient's periodontal health. Once collected and properly documented, the data should provide the clinician with a realistic picture of the patient's periodontal status. Along with radiographs, the data collected and properly documented demonstrate the patient's periodontal condition, but it is important to note that the data collected are not necessarily identifying an active disease process but the damage resulting from disease. The damage to the periodontium is the result of a bacterial infection of the periodontium (hard and soft tissues) with the majority of the damage predominantly from the host's immune response to the bacterial challenge.[1,7] Information gathered during the assessment provides data to be used to properly assess health or disease, diagnose periodontal disease, plan appropriate treatment, implement agreed-on treatment, and evaluate treatment outcomes. It also provides a baseline from which future disease activity can be compared.

Periodontal Risk Assessment

Risk is defined as "the probability that an event will occur in the future or the probability that an individual develops a given disease or experiences a change in health status during a specified interval of time."[11] According to Albandar, **periodontal risk assessment** assists in the identification of factors that may increase the onset, severity, and/or progression of periodontal disease. These contributing factors may be local or isolated to the oral cavity or systemic or intrinsic influences. Local contributing factors, such as dental calculus, faulty dental restorations, developmental defects, caries, patient habits, and occlusal trauma, are oral conditions that may increase an individual's susceptibility to periodontal infection in specific sites or contribute to disease already initiated by plaque biofilm. Eliminating or minimizing these factors may decrease the probability or severity of disease initiation, progression, or both. Systemic risk factors for periodontal disease include conditions, habits, or diseases that increase an individual's susceptibility to periodontal infection or contribute to the progression or severity of periodontal disease. Age, smoking, and diabetes mellitus have been correlated to an increased incidence of tooth loss caused by periodontal disease. Other contributing factors include patient sex, hormonal influences, genetics, nutritional state, psychosocial stress, blood dyscrasias, and certain diseases, such as osteoporosis and HIV infection.[11–13]

Formal risk assessment tools are available to assess and quantify an individual's risk for development of periodontal disease. PreViser's Oral Health Information Suite (OHIS) (previously called the RiskCalculator) uses the traditional oral assessment data collected during a comprehensive periodontal examination, together with other factors such as age, race, sex, habits, and medical history, to quantify the risk of developing periodontal disease through a risk score and the severity and extent of existing disease through a disease score. Quantifying these measures may assist in monitoring a patient's periodontal status, planning treatment, assessing treatment outcomes, and facilitating communication between provider and patient, collaborating health-care providers, and insurance companies.[14-16]

Periodontal Screening Examination

Introduced in 1992 and endorsed by the American Dental Association and the AAP as a mechanism for early detection of periodontal disease, the **periodontal screening and recording (PSR)** is a quick and easy screening tool used to identify the need for a comprehensive assessment. The PSR was adapted from the Community Periodontal Index of Treatment Needs (CPITN) of the World Health Organization; it is not intended to replace a comprehensive periodontal examination. Instead of using a traditional periodontal probe, a ball-tipped PSR probe (marked with a single color-coded zone from 3.5 to 5.5 mm) is used to measure the sulcus or pocket depth; however, no millimeter readings are noted. The clinician notes whether the gingival margin reaches or goes beyond the "colored zone." The clinician also notes the presence of calculus, as well as periodontal abnormalities such as furcation involvement, mobility, gingival recession, or other contributing factors. The mouth is divided into sextants, and a single code is recorded for each sextant based on the highest code number achieved for that specific sextant.[6] The PSR coding criteria is provided in Table 11-3. A code of 3 in a single sextant indicates the need for a complete periodontal probing of that sextant, whereas a code of 3 in two or more sextants or a code of 4 in any sextant requires a comprehensive periodontal examination.

Comprehensive Periodontal Assessment

A thorough clinical assessment includes evaluation of all aspects of the periodontium for signs of inflammation and resultant damage.[3] A comprehensive periodontal examination is not just periodontal probing. Probe depth measurements are just one piece of the puzzle and do not provide enough data from which to diagnose periodontal disease, plan appropriate treatment, or evaluate treatment outcomes. To get a clear picture of the patient's periodontal status, the clinician must gather all the pieces of the puzzle. Along with a thorough medical history, dental history, extraoral and intraoral examination, dental examination, and radiographic survey, the periodontal examination is the last component of the comprehensive evaluation of the patient's oral health[2,6,17] (see Application to Clinical Practice).

A thorough evaluation of the periodontium should include the following clinical assessments[2,6,17]:
• Gingival description
• Pocket probing depths
• **Bleeding on probing (BOP)**
• Level of the free gingiva (recession)
• **Clinical attachment level (CAL)**
• Furcation involvement
• Exudate

Application to Clinical Practice

You have just been hired by a recent dental school graduate as her new office's dental hygienist. She is counting on you to develop the practice's procedures for evaluating and monitoring the periodontal health of new and returning patients and treatment outcomes. What policy would you develop regarding periodontal examination of new patients? Continuing care patients? Nonsurgical periodontal therapy patients? Periodontal maintenance patients? What procedures would you include in your comprehensive periodontal evaluation of each of these categories of patients? ■

Table 11-3. Periodontal Screening and Recording Codes

Periodontal screening and recording (PSR) codes are based on the following system:

PSR Code	Description
Code 0	Colored area of probe remains completely visible in the deepest crevice in the sextant. No calculus or defective margins are detected. Gingival tissues are healthy with no bleeding after gentle probing.
Code 1	Colored area of probe remains completely visible in the deepest probing depth in the sextant. No calculus or margins are detected. There is bleeding after gentle probing.
Code 2	Colored area of probe remains completely visible in the deepest probing depth in the sextant. Supragingival or subgingival calculus and/or defective margins are detected.
Code 3	Colored area of probe remains partly visible in the deepest probing depth in the sextant.
Code 4	Colored area of probe completely disappears, indicating probing depth of greater than 5.5 mm.
Code *	Denotes clinical abnormalities including but not limited to furcation invasion, mobility, mucogingival problems, or recession extending to the colored area of the probe (≥3.5 mm).
Code X	Denotes edentulous sextant.

For example:

3*	2	2
2	1	X

- Mobility
- Fremitus
- Mucogingival defects
- Peri-implant assessment
- Oral hygiene assessment
- Presence of biofilm and calculus
- Contributing local factors
- Radiographic evaluation
- Microbial and/or genetic testing, as indicated

Required Instruments and Materials
- Two single-ended instruments or two cotton-tipped applicators, for mobility testing
- Implant probe—typically plastic (if the patient has an implant)

- Mouth mirror
- Periodontal explorer (ODU 11/12)
- Periodontal probe
- Nabers probe (furcation probe)
- Tri-syringe (for compressed air)
- Patient dental record—paper or electronic
- Colored pens or black pens—typically blue, red, and green (if using a paper chart)

Procedure

A thorough evaluation of the periodontium should include a variety of assessments. Table 11-4 provides a concise review of the assessments to be included in a comprehensive periodontal evaluation.

Table 11-4. *Overview of the Components of a Comprehensive Periodontal Examination*

Each of the following assessments should be performed and documented as appropriate when conducting a periodontal examination.

Assessments	Description	Measurement
Gingival description	The cardinal signs of inflammation include redness (erythema) and swelling (edema). The periodontal tissues are assessed for color, shape, consistency, and texture to assess clinical signs of inflammation.	In health, gingiva is coral to pale pink and is flat with a knife-edge, scalloped marginal contour. The gingival papillae are pointed and fill the embrasures between the teeth. Deviations from normal are to be noted.
Probing depths	Depth of the sulcus or pocket in millimeters. Sulcus implies a probe depth reading of 3 mm or less and is typically consistent with gingival health. Pocket implies a probing depth of more than 3 mm. The only method to detect and measure periodontal pockets is through the use of a periodontal probe.	Measured from the free gingival margin to the junctional epithelium. Depths are recorded in the nearest full millimeter. For example, 3.5 mm would be rounded to 4 mm. Six sites per tooth are recorded.
Bleeding on probing (BOP)	With gentle probing, the ulcerated soft tissue wall of an inflamed pocket/sulcus may bleed. Bleeding does not occur in health.	While probing, areas of bleeding are noted. It may be evident quickly upon probing or there may be a several-second delay. After probing, go back and look at the recently probed site to assess bleeding that occurred later.
Level of the free gingival margin	The gingival margin should be located at or slightly coronal to the CEJ. With inflammation, the gingival margin may be located farther coronal than normal. With gingival recession, the gingival margin is located apical to the CEJ.	Measured from CEJ to the free gingival margin. In the presence of gingival enlargement, the gingival margin may be coronal to the measurement if the gingival margin is coronal to the CEJ. In the presence of gingival recession, the gingival margin will be apical to the CEJ.
Clinical attachment level (CAL)	Measurement of the distance of the junctional epithelium from a fixed reference point, the CEJ. Best single measurement of tooth support.	Distance in millimeters from the CEJ to the junctional epithelium. Composed of a combination of two measurements: probe depth plus level of the free gingival margin. When no gingival recession or enlargement is present, the CAL and the probe depth are synonymous.
Furcation involvement	Bone loss between the roots of multirooted teeth.	A Nabers probe is typically used to assess the degree of involvement. The Glickman index grades the severity of furcation involvement from I to IV.

Table 11-4. *Overview of the Components of a Comprehensive Periodontal Examination—cont'd*

Assessments	Description	Measurement
Exudate or suppuration	A collection of dead white blood cells (neutrophils) that is indicative of infection. It may be a pearly white to a pale yellow.	May become apparent when probing or when applying pressure against the tissue with a digit. It may also be unprovoked.
Tooth mobility	Movement of a tooth that is greater than normal physiological movement. Teeth are held into the socket by fibers and have some normal movement. Horizontal mobility is facial-lingual movement. Vertical mobility is when the tooth can be depressed into the socket. To have vertical mobility, the tooth would typically have to have significant horizontal mobility.	Using the end of two single-ended instruments, pressure is applied in a back-and-forth motion (facial-lingual). The end of the instrument handle is placed on the occlusal/incisal surface with pressure applied to assess whether the tooth is depressible into the socket. Classified from 1 to 3.
Fremitus	Palpable or visible movement of a tooth when in function. Typically, the tooth in fremitus is occluding too hard against the opposing tooth in the opposite arch. Mobility is not due to bacterial infection as in periodontal disease but is due to hyperocclusion or traumatic occlusion.	Place a digit over the facial aspect of the tooth suspected and have the patient tap his or her teeth together in occlusion. A tooth "in fremitus" will wiggle as the opposing tooth makes contact.
Mucogingival defects	In cases of severe recession, the gingival margin may migrate very close or into the unattached mucosa. The width of attached gingiva, in this case, may be compromised, which may put the tooth at risk for bacterial insult.	Place the periodontal probe on the attached gingiva with the tip at the mucogingival junction. A measurement is taken from this point to the free gingival margin. Because this measurement includes both attached and free gingiva, the free gingiva, or sulcus/pocket depth, is subtracted from the measurement to determine the width of just the attached gingiva.
Peri-implantitis	Peri-implantitis is periodontal disease around a dental implant. It is caused by the same bacterial species and has the same progression as chronic periodontitis. Failure of a dental implant is most often caused by either occlusal trauma (biomechanical overload) or bacterial infection.	Evaluation of dental implants should include assessment of mobility (with/without prosthesis), testing for fluid percolation around the prosthesis, as well as sensitivity to percussion, occlusal analysis, periodontal probing, and the patient's biofilm removal.
Oral hygiene assessment	Periodontal disease is a bacterial infection of the soft and hard tissues of the periodontium. The amount and distribution of plaque biofilm can be measured on a patient's teeth for educational purposes. Calculus is mineralized plaque biofilm that contributes to the development of periodontal disease.	A plaque biofilm index, such as the plaque control record (O'Leary, Drake, and Naylor) or Plaque Index (Silness and Löe) can be used to quantify the amount and record the distribution of plaque biofilm. These data can be used as a patient education tool and an assessment of the patient's proficiency in biofilm removal.
Radiographic assessment	Radiographs have limited value in assessment of the soft tissue of the periodontium but may be helpful in evaluating the amount of bone present, condition of the alveolar crests, advanced bone loss in the furcation areas, width of the PDL space, local factors that can cause or intensify periodontal disease, root length and morphology, crown/root ratio, caries, apical lesions, and root resorption.	Although the diagnosis and determination of severity of periodontal diseases is based on clinical attachment level, a diagnostic full-mouth series of radiographs, including vertical bitewings, can be an important adjunct to the comprehensive periodontal examination.

Continued

Table 11-4. *Overview of the Components of a Comprehensive Periodontal Examination—cont'd*

Assessments	Description	Measurement
Local contributing factors	Local contributing factors promote periodontal infection by allowing bacterial plaque to accumulate easier.	Factors that may contribute to the accumulation of bacterial plaque include crowding, orthodontic appliances, overhang restorations, open contacts, poor prosthetic crown margins, etc.
Systemic contributing factors	Systemic contributing factors promote periodontal infection by altering the host response to the bacterial challenge.	Examples of systemic risk factors that may contribute to oral disease development include tobacco use, uncontrolled diabetes mellitus, pregnancy, psychosocial stress, genetic influences (interleukin-1 genotype, Down syndrome), HIV/AIDS, hematological disorders, chronic leukemia, and certain medications that may promote gingival enlargement, xerostomia, or both.

CEJ, cementoenamel junction.

Gingival Description

The gingival description differentiates soft tissue health from disease. In health, signs of gingival **inflammation** (redness, heat, edema, and pain caused by the body's response to injury) will be absent.[3] Plaque biofilm can initiate an inflammatory response that results in an increase in blood flow. The increased blood flow helps to deliver immune defenders to the site of injury. The immune defenders are responsible for the resulting redness and heat, whereas the leukocytes and plasma cells leaking from the capillaries into the tissues at the injury site can Contour result in edema and pain. These cells also have a direct role in initiating the host immune response. With an appropriate immune response, the tissue heals and inflammation is resolved. **Acute inflammation** (Fig. 11-5A) begins suddenly and is of short duration (≤2 weeks). **Chronic inflammation** (Fig. 11-5B) is a longer-lived response that continues for more than a few weeks because the body is unable to resolve the infection. With chronic periodontitis, there is a proliferation of collagen tissue, resulting in hard, fibrotic, overly stippled gingiva.[18]

The gingival description includes an assessment of the color, contour, consistency, and texture. A review of the terms used to describe the gingiva is provided in Table 11-5. The color of the gingiva is determined by the thickness of the epithelium, the amount of epithelial keratinization, the extent of vascularity in the underlying connective tissue, the amount of melanin pigment present, and subgingival deposits.[18] In health, the papillary, marginal, and attached gingiva is typically described as pink, pale pink, or coral pink, or it may be pigmented. Acutely inflamed gingiva typically appears as red, whereas chronically inflamed gingiva may appear with a bluish cast.

The contour of the gingiva is the form or shape of the gingival margin or border. The contour of the gingival margin may be influenced by the shape of the teeth, tooth position or alignment, location and size of the tooth contact areas, size of the embrasure spaces, and presence of inflammation. In health, the contour of the gingival margin may be described as scalloped and knife-edged. Knife-edged implies that the gingiva thins at the margin into a flat, thin edge. In health, this

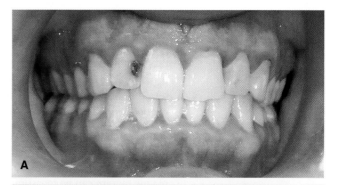
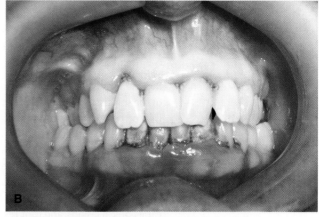

Figure 11-5. (A) Acute gingival inflammation. (B) Chronic periodontitis.

Table 11-5. *The Gingival Description*

The following terms can be used to describe the appearance of the gingiva:

Gingival Tissue	Health	Acute Inflammation	Chronic Inflammation
Color	Pale pink	Red	Bluish red
	Coral pink	Bright red	Bluish pink
	Pale coral		
	Pigmented		
Shape			
Gingival margin	Knife-edged	Rounded	Rounded
	Slightly rounded	Rolled	Rolled
Papillary	Pointed	Bulbous	Blunted
	Pyramidal	Smooth	Cratered
Texture	Stippled	Shiny	Missing
	Mattlike	Soft	Overstippled
Consistency	Firm	Spongy	Hard
	Resilient		Fibrotic

edge may also appear as slightly rolled.[19] The interdental papillae are flat and fill the embrasure spaces. When inflamed, the contour of the gingival margin may appear as rounded or rolled, promoting an exaggerated scalloping of the margin. The interdental papillae may appear as enlarged or bulbous. With long-standing inflammation, the interdental papillae may appear blunted or reduced, and the gingival margin may appear rolled with a diminished scalloped effect.

The consistency of the gingival tissue is determined by the cellular and fluid content and by the extent of collagen in the lamina propria beneath the epithelium. In health, the consistency of the gingiva is firm and resilient. When depressed by the side of a periodontal probe, the depression made in the tissue springs back quickly. When inflamed, the gingival tissue may appear soft or spongy. When depressed, the depression lingers in the tissue for a longer period. With chronic inflammation, gingival tissue may appear overly firm or even hard. This is due to the increased maturation of granulation tissue and excessive proliferation of collagen as a result of long-standing inflammation.

The surface texture of the gingiva is determined by the health of the epithelium–connective tissue interface. With the application of compressed air, healthy gingival tissue will appear slightly stippled, similar to the surface of an orange peel. The pattern and amount of stippling varies from person to person, as well as from one area in the mouth to another. Inflamed gingival tissue may appear smooth and shiny because of increased cellular fluid in the tissue; however, chronically inflamed gingiva may appear overly stippled because of the maturation of granulation tissue and proliferation of collagen.

Probing Depths

Periodontal probing provides an assessment of the severity of disease occurrence and is essential data to guide periodontal diagnosis and treatment planning. Together with clinical attachment and bone loss, periodontal probing is a cumulative measure of the damage of past disease activity.[19,20] **Probe depth,** or depth of the gingival sulcus, is determined by the distance from the edge of the free gingival margin to the junctional epithelium using a calibrated periodontal probe. The circumference of the sulcus around the tooth is probed at 1-mm intervals. Not every measurement is recorded. For recording purposes, the tooth is divided into six zones: distobuccal proximal to distobuccal line angle, distobuccal line angle to mesiobuccal line angle, mesiobuccal line angle to mesiobuccal proximal, mesiolingual proximal to mesiolingual line angle, mesiolingual line angle to distolingual line angle, and distolingual line angle to distolingual proximal. The deepest measurement in each zone is recorded with half measurements rounded up to next whole number.[3,6]

The term *sulcus* implies a probe depth measurement of 3 mm or less and is typically consistent with gingival health (Fig. 11-6). The term *pocket* implies that the probing depth is greater than 3 mm. The only method to detect and measure periodontal pockets is through the use of a periodontal probe.[9,20] With a true periodontal pocket, the increased probing depth is due to apical migration of the junctional epithelium. If this migration is above the crest of the alveolar bone, the pocket is a suprabony periodontal pocket. If the migration of the junction epithelium is below the alveolar bone crest, it is an infrabony periodontal pocket. If this

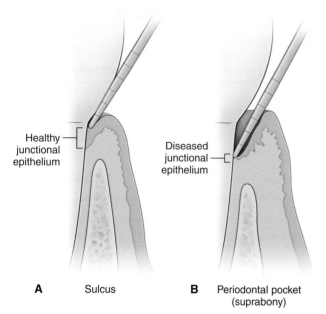

Figure 11-6. Periodontal probing.

increase in probing depth is not due to apical migration of the junction epithelium but rather enlargement of the gingival tissue due to inflammation, it is termed a *pseudopocket* or *gingival pocket.*

The validity and reliability of manual probing can be influenced by several factors such as diameter of the probe, angulation of the probe to the tooth surface, resiliency of the tissue, depth of the pocket, shape of the tooth crown, clinician experience, presence of subgingival calculus, and force used while probing.[18,20–23] Probing in the presence of inflammation can result in the tip of the probe penetrating into the underlying connective tissue, resulting in invalid pocket/sulcus depth measurements (see Evidence-Based Practice).[23] Clinicians should use 10 to 20 g pressure when probing so as not to penetrate the junctional epithelium.[24] With clinical practice and professional experience, one can

develop a consistent gentle probing technique. Computerized probes using a constant pressure, such as the Florida Probe, have been found to increase the reliability of probe depth measurements and standardize measurements between users.[1,23]

Bleeding on Probing

BOP may be the result of an ulcerated or inflamed epithelial wall of the sulcus or periodontal pocket (Fig. 11-7). Because epithelium does not contain blood vessels, the origin of the bleeding is the underlying connective tissue. Although not a strong indicator of periodontal breakdown, BOP can be correlated to gingival inflammation.[19,25,26] Although BOP has not been found to be a good predictor of future disease progression, the absence of BOP is typically viewed as a good indicator of gingival health and stability. However, it is notable that the absence of BOP is not necessarily indicative of health or absence of disease especially in patients who smoke.[27]

Level of the Free Gingiva

The level of the free gingiva is measured from the gingival margin to the CEJ. In health, the gingival margin is located at or slightly coronal to the CEJ; therefore, the measurement is zero. In the presence of inflammation, edema may result in a gingival margin that is coronal to the CEJ. If gingival recession is present, the gingival margin will be apical to the CEJ (Fig. 11-8). If the gingival margin is coronal to the CEJ, the distance from the CEJ to the gingival margin should be subtracted from the probe depth measurement when calculating the CAL. If the gingival margin is apical to the CEJ, the measurement from the gingival margin to the CEJ should be added to the probe depth when calculating the CAL.[6]

Clinical Attachment Level

The CAL is the distance from the junction epithelium to the CEJ (Fig. 11-9). Because the CEJ is a fixed reference point, this measure is considered the *best single estimate* of the periodontal support around the tooth.[1,3,18–20,28,29] Typically, two separate clinical

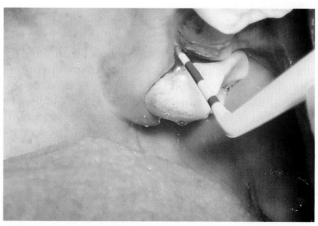

Figure 11-7. Bleeding on probing.

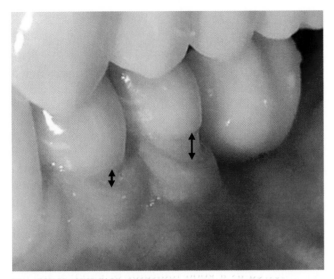

Figure 11-8. Gingival recession.

Furcation Involvement

Furcation involvement results from bone loss between the roots of multirooted teeth. The complex root morphology of the **furcation** puts the tooth at risk for greater attachment loss and a poorer prognosis after periodontal therapy than teeth without furcation involvement.[19] The average height of molar root trunks is 3.5 to 3.6 mm on the mesial aspect, 3.5 to 4.2 mm for the buccal aspect, and 4.1 to 4.8 mm for the distal aspect.[30] Therefore, furcation involvement should be suspected when the CAL on a multirooted tooth is 5 mm or greater. The instrument of choice to detect furcation involvement is a Nabers furcation probe (Fig. 11-10). Furcation involvement is classified using the Glickman furcation classification system.[6,29] A review of the Glickman furcation classification system is provided in Table 11-6.

measurements are added or subtracted to determine the CAL: probe depth plus/minus the level of the free gingiva. In the presence of gingival recession, the level of the free gingiva is added to the probe depth to achieve the CAL. In the presence of inflammation where the gingival margin is coronal to the CEJ, the level of the free gingiva is subtracted from the probe depth to achieve the CAL. When no gingival recession or enlargement is present, the CAL and the probing depth are synonymous.

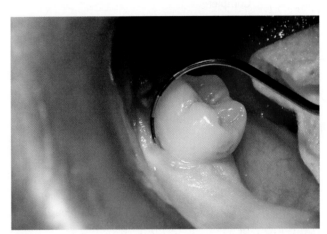

Figure 11-10. Nabers probe used to assess furcation involvement of a mandibular molar.

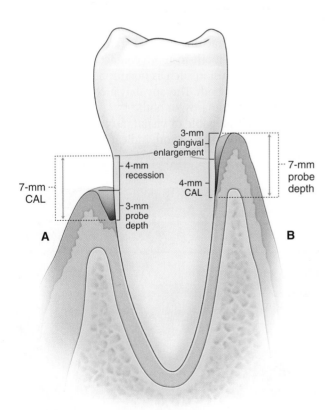

Figure 11-9. Clinical attachment level.

Table 11-6. *Glickman Furcation Classification System*		
Grade	**Description**	**Representation**
I	Incipient bone loss in the furcation area	Incipient bone loss in the furcation area.

Continued

Table 11-6. Glickman Furcation Classification System—cont'd

Grade	Description	Representation
II	Partial bone loss producing a cul-de-sac	Partial bone loss producing a cul-de-sac.
III	Complete bone loss resulting in a through-and-through opening in the furcation	Complete bone loss resulting in a through-and-through opening in the furcation
IV	Synonymous with grade III with recession of the gingival tissue that allows the furcation opening to be visualized	Synonymous with grade III with recession of the gingival tissue that allows the furcation opening to be visualized.

Suppuration

Suppuration, or purulent **exudate,** is an accumulation of dead or dying neutrophils that may appear spontaneously, upon probing, or by applying pressure with a digit to the area. Suppuration does not occur in healthy tissue and is indicative of an infection.

Mobility

All teeth have a limited amount of normal physiological movement because of the elasticity of the PDL. **Tooth mobility** is assessed by using two blunt-ended instruments or one blunt-ended instrument and a digit (Fig. 11-11). Horizontal movement is observed in a facial-to-lingual direction with the adjacent tooth observed as a point of reference. Vertical movement is observed in an up/down direction (pushing the tooth into the socket). Class 1 is slight tooth mobility up to 1 mm in a facial-lingual direction. Class 2 is moderate tooth mobility of more than 1 mm but less than 2 mm in a facial-lingual direction. Class 3 is severe tooth mobility of more than 2 mm in a facial-lingual direction or vertical displacement such as being pushed into the alveolus.[6,9,19] An electronic device (Periotest) is available to quantify tooth mobility and may reduce the inherent subjectivity of classifying tooth mobility. It may also be useful to document the progression of mobility over time.[9,19]

Trauma from occlusion can cause resorption of alveolar bone more rapidly if periodontal disease is present. Signs and symptoms of occlusal trauma include tooth mobility, sensitivity to pressure, migration of teeth, widening of the PDL space, and alveolar bone resorption. Primary occlusal trauma occurs when there are excessive occlusal forces on a healthy periodontium (e.g., high restorations, excessive force on abutment teeth from partial dentures). Signs and symptoms may include a widened PDL space, tooth mobility, and pain. These changes are typically reversible if the cause is removed. Secondary occlusal trauma is the result of abnormal occlusal forces on an unhealthy periodontium weakened by periodontitis, which may result in rapid bone loss and advancing clinical attachment loss. Parafunctional occlusal forces result from tooth-to-tooth contact made when not in functional occlusion such as nocturnal during clenching or grinding, or both. Therapy may include occlusal adjustment or night guards, or both.[6,9]

Fremitus is palpable or visual movement of a tooth when in functional occlusion, indicating that the tooth

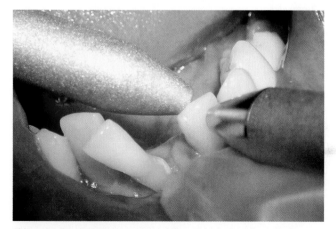

Figure 11-11. Assessing tooth mobility with the handle end of two single-ended instruments.

is in traumatic occlusion or hyperocclusion. To examine for fremitus, place a digit on the buccal aspect of the tooth while the patient taps his or her teeth in occlusion (Fig. 11-12). If the tooth is in fremitus, palpable movement will be detected.[6]

Mucogingival Involvement

Attached gingiva is tightly knit to the underlying cementum of the tooth and/or the periosteum of the alveolar bone. It is keratinized, giving it a pale pink color with a stippled surface texture. Attached gingiva extends apically from the free gingival groove to the mucogingival line. In contrast, the alveolar mucosa lining the vestibule is thin and nonkeratinized, causing it to appear a deeper pink than the attached gingiva. This junction of attached gingiva and alveolar mucosa, delineated by a distinct color change, is the mucogingival junction.[6]

In cases of moderate-to-severe gingival recession where it is apparent that attached gingiva is lacking, measuring the width of the remaining attached gingiva is desirable to monitor for further progression of the recession and for treatment planning. The periodontal probe is laid on the attached gingiva with the tip at the mucogingival line to measure the amount of attached gingiva present (width of attached gingiva). A measurement is taken from this point to the free gingival margin (Fig. 11-13). Because this measurement includes both attached and free gingiva, the free gingiva, or sulcus/pocket depth, is subtracted to determine the width of just the attached gingiva.[6]

Peri-implant Assessment

The supporting structures of a dental implant differ greatly from those of the periodontium of natural teeth. Endosseous implants lack a PDL and are osseointegrated, resulting in ankylosis of the implant in the alveolar bone. Without a PDL, dental implants have no physiological movement and little proprioceptive feedback; therefore, overloading dental implants can result in bone loss and implant failure. Made of titanium, the implant fixture also lacks a cemental surface to which gingival fibers can attach. Only vertical

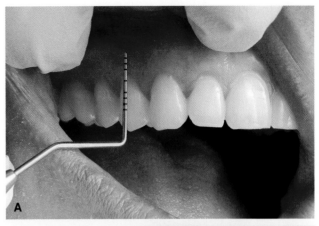

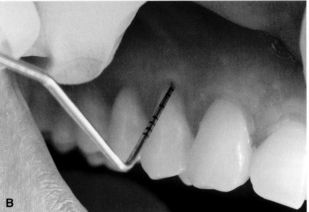

Figure 11-13. (A) First measurement for determining the width of attached gingival: mucogingival line to cementoenamel junction. (B) Second measurement for determining the width of attached gingival: junctional epithelium to gingival margin. Subtract measurement 2 from measurement 1 to determine the width of the attached gingival.

or circular gingival fibers form around the supracrestal portion of the implant. An epithelial attachment, called a *biological seal*, attaches to the titanium collar of the implant; however, there is no connective tissue attachment to the implant.

Failure of a dental implant (Fig. 11-14) is most often caused by either occlusal trauma (biomechanical overload) or bacterial infection (peri-implantitis). Peri-implantitis is caused by the same bacterial species as chronic periodontitis and has a similar progression. Notably, sulcus/pocket depth around dental implants is determined by type of implant and the height of abutment used. Probing depths around dental implants cannot be compared with those around natural teeth but should be used as a basis for comparison of that specific implant's health over time. While the 3 mm or less guideline for sulcus depths around natural teeth cannot apply to dental implants, it is desired that probe depths not exceed 4 to 5 mm. Periodontal evaluation of dental implants should include assessment of mobility (with/without prosthesis), testing for fluid percolation around the prosthesis, sensitivity to percussion, occlusal analysis, periodontal probing, and the patient's biofilm removal. Signs of implant failure may include erythema,

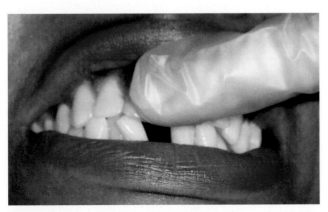

Figure 11-12. Assessing for fremitus by palpating the tooth while the patient occludes.

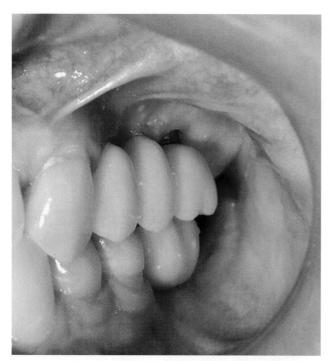

Figure 11-14. Implant failure. The gingiva surrounding tooth #14 is demonstrating signs of implant failure: erythema, edema, gingival recession, tissue retractibility, or pulling away from the implant surface. The implant also demonstrated class 2 mobility, and bone loss was evident in the radiographic survey.

edema, sensitivity to pressure, presence of exudate, gingival recession, tissue retractibility, and radiographic bone loss. Mobility of the implant fixture typically indicates implant failure, which requires removal of the implant.[9,31,32]

Oral Hygiene Assessment

The oral hygiene assessment includes determination of the presence and distribution of plaque biofilm or calculus, or both, in the dentition; this index can serve as a measure of the patient's oral hygiene proficiency and efforts. A plaque biofilm index, such as the plaque control record (O'Leary, Drake, and Naylor) and the Plaque Index (Silness and Löe), among others, can be used to quantify the amount and record the distribution of plaque biofilm.[6] Although the quantity of plaque biofilm cannot necessarily be directly correlated to the severity of disease present or predictive of future disease, it can be used as a patient education tool and an assessment of the patient's proficiency in biofilm removal. An abundance of plaque biofilm may be the result of a lack of ability to perform a particular skill to proficiency. Having patients demonstrate the skill in their own mouths may provide insight into their ability to sufficiently remove the biofilm. However, it may not be a matter of proficiency, but a lack of consistency in performing routine plaque biofilm removal. When coupled with the results of the gingival description, a plaque biofilm index can provide insight into the patient's short-term and longer-term plaque biofilm removal. For example, plaque biofilm accumulation in

the absence of signs of gingival inflammation may be indicative of a more recent or short-term insufficiency in plaque biofilm removal, whereas the presence of clinical signs of inflammation may indicate a longer-term absence of adequate plaque biofilm removal.

As mineralized plaque biofilm, dental calculus is a measure of long-term insufficiency, inconsistency, or both in plaque biofilm removal. The presence and location of dental calculus can also be used to guide patient education. Calculus indices record the distribution and quantity of dental calculus present and can be useful in monitoring a patient's oral hygiene efforts over time.[33]

Contributing Local Factors

Conditions within the oral cavity may contribute to the development of periodontal disease. Although these conditions alone are not the primary causative agent or cause of the disease process, they may contribute to a process already initiated by bacterial biofilm and the host response. These factors may increase the risk of developing disease or developing more severe disease and, therefore, should be eliminated or minimized.[3] Examples of local contributing factors include dental calculus, faulty dental restorations and appliances, developmental defects, dental caries, food impaction, occlusal trauma, and patient habits such as tongue thrusting, mouth breathing, and improper use of toothpicks and other interdental aids.

Contributing Systemic Factors

The medical history is a key element in the assessment of the periodontium. Many diseases, conditions, and medications may influence one's oral health and alter the course of treatment of periodontal disease. Examples of systemic risk factors that may contribute to oral disease development include tobacco use, uncontrolled diabetes mellitus, pregnancy, psychosocial stress, genetic influences (interleukin-1 [IL-1] genotype, Down syndrome), HIV/AIDS, hematological disorders, chronic leukemia, and certain medications that may promote gingival enlargement, xerostomia, or both.[19,34–38] See Chapter 5 for more information.

RADIOGRAPHIC EVALUATION OF THE PERIODONTIUM

Neither the clinical nor radiographic assessment alone provides the clinician with adequate data for diagnosis and treatment planning or evaluation of treatment outcomes, determination of subsequent treatment needs, and long-term monitoring of periodontal health. Although the diagnosis and determination of the severity of periodontal diseases are based on CAL, a diagnostic full-mouth series of radiographs, including vertical bitewings, can be an important adjunct to the comprehensive periodontal examination.[1,28] For example, a full-mouth radiographic series may be helpful in evaluating the amount of bone present, condition of the alveolar crests, advanced bone loss in furcation areas, width of the PDL space, local factors that can promote periodontal disease, root length and morphology, crown-to-root ratio, caries, apical lesions, and root resorption.[28]

Conventional dental radiographs can have a significant, but limited, contribution to a comprehensive clinical examination. Conventional radiographs provide a two-dimensional image of complex, three-dimensional anatomy, and superimposition often causes loss of the details of the bony architecture. They are limited in detecting early bone loss, the true topography of vertical osseous defects, the exact morphology of bone destruction, tooth mobility, and early furcation involvement.[1] Radiographs also have limited value in assessment of the soft tissue of the periodontium such as determining the level of the junctional epithelium; however, the use of diagnostic medical sonography may prove valuable in the future in the assessment of the soft tissues of the periodontium (see Advancing Technologies).

ADJUNCTIVE TECHNIQUES

Microbiological Testing

For patients with persistent periodontal disease that is unresponsive to treatment, microbiological testing may be helpful in detecting the presence of periodontal pathogens and guiding antimicrobial chemotherapy. Subgingival biofilm is collected and analyzed using phase-contrast or dark-field microscopy, bacterial enzyme analysis, immunoassay, DNA probes, polymerase chain reaction, or traditional microbiological culturing and sensitivity testing.[6,19] Chairside tests (Oratec, Oravital, MyPerioPath) are available to detect enzymes produced by bacterial pathogens (*Tannerella forsythia*, *Porphyromonas gingivalis*, and *Treponema denticola*) that are capable of hydrolyzing the synthetic peptide benzoyl-DL-arginine-naphthylamide (BANA). DNA probes of nucleic acid sequences and polymerase chain reaction technology are very sensitive tests that are also used to identify specific bacterial species. Although these tests provide useful information, only laboratory culturing and sensitivity testing can determine to which specific antibiotics bacteria are sensitive. Not indicated for general use, microbial analyses should be reserved for patients who have unusual forms of periodontal disease such as early-onset, refractory, or rapidly progressive disease.[17,18]

Biochemical Assays of Gingival Crevicular Fluid

Biochemical assays can be performed on the serum exudates in gingival crevicular fluid to detect and measure the biochemicals associated with inflammation. **Gingival crevicular fluid** is an inflammatory exudate that results from the increased vascular permeability of inflamed gingival tissue.[1,18] Prostaglandin E_2, cytokines, antibacterial antibodies, total protein, and acute-phase proteins are host inflammatory products and mediators of inflammation that have been examined as potential diagnostic markers of periodontal disease. In particular, prostaglandin E_2, the ILs (IL-1b, IL-6, and IL-8), and tumor necrosis factor-α have been identified as potential markers of disease progression.[6,39] Pyridinoline cross-links of carboxyterminal telopeptides to type I collagen (ICTP) has been demonstrated as a marker for bone collagen degradation.[40]

Aspartate aminotransferase, neutral protease, collagenase, β-glucuronidase, lactate dehydrogenase, neutrophil elastase, arylsulfatase, myeloperoxidase, and alkaline phosphatase are host-derived enzymes that may be associated with periodontal disease and serve as markers of periodontal inflammation. Because these enzymes are also found to be elevated in both **gingivitis** and nonprogressive **periodontitis,** the utility of gingival crevicular fluid testing to determine between sites that are breaking down and those that are not remains to be established.[1,6,41] Enzyme tests for aspartate aminotransferase (PocketWatch) and neutral proteases (Periocheck) are available as chairside gingival crevicular fluid tests and may serve as a means for rapidly screening for periodontal disease.[39,41]

Subgingival Temperature

An infrared thermometer (PerioTemp) can be used to measure subgingival temperature. Because temperature increases with the presence of inflammation, subgingival heat may serve as a diagnostic aid to identify an increased risk for clinical attachment loss.[1,19,42,43,44,45] However, because subgingival temperature varies

Advancing Technologies

Diagnostic medical sonography uses sound waves that reflect as echoes to produce images of structures within the body. A transducer converts electronic impulses into ultrasound waves that enter into tissues and are either absorbed, reflected, or scattered. The reflected waves return to the transducer where they are converted into an electronic impulse to produce an image.[58] Sonography of the periodontium has been used to evaluate gingival thickness before and after gingival grafting, connective tissue grafting, and placement of barrier membranes.[58] Sonography may provide a noninvasive diagnostic method for assessing the periodontium and accurate measurement of the dimensional relationship between hard and soft structures. Future research will focus on improving the quality of the soft tissue images produced and experimenting with changes in the equipment and its use to create a better image resolution.[59] ▪

throughout the oral cavity, overall differences in mean subgingival temperature in the mouth may be more predictive of future disease activity than temperatures from individual sites.

Genetic Tests

Genetic tests are available that analyze two IL-1 genes for variations that identify a host susceptibility or predisposition for overexpression of inflammation and risk for periodontal disease.[46–48] These tests examine the patient's DNA and look for the presence of specific genetic variations associated with IL-1 production.[49] IL-1 genetic susceptibility may not initiate or cause the disease, but rather may lead to earlier or more severe disease. In particular, the combination of these two IL-1 genes has been associated with severe disease in nonsmoking Caucasians. Studies have found an increased frequency of a different IL-1 genotype in people with advanced adult periodontitis compared with those with early or moderate disease.[19,50] Genetic tests are primarily a risk assessment tool for determining genetic susceptibility to the periodontal diseases and should not be considered a diagnostic test.[1,46–48,51]

CLASSIFICATION OF PERIODONTAL DISEASES

Periodontal disease is a group of diseases characterized by bacterial infection of the periodontium, including the gingiva, PDL, bone, and cementum. Although the initial bacterial challenge to a susceptible host begins with a local inflammatory reaction, most of the damage to the periodontium is due to a susceptible host's immune response to the predominantly gram-negative anaerobic microorganisms.[52] Chronic periodontitis is typically slow to progress, characterized by episodic bursts of activity, and is site specific. However, the intensity of the immune response to these periodontal pathogens varies considerably from one individual to another, as well as from one site to another within a patient's mouth.[1,52–55]

Based on the severity of attachment loss, periodontal diseases associated with plaque biofilm can be classified as either gingivitis or periodontitis. **Gingivitis** is inflammation localized to the gingival tissue with no apical migration of the junction epithelium. **Periodontitis** is inflammation of the structures of the periodontium marked by apical migration of the junctional epithelium. While all periodontitis begins as gingivitis, not all gingivitis progresses to periodontitis; therefore, the progression of the disease should not be assumed to be linear.[1,11,18,20] In 1999, the Workshop on Classification of Periodontal Diseases and Conditions revised the classification system for periodontal diseases. The system provides a general framework for studying the cause, pathogenesis, and treatment of periodontal diseases.[4] It groups similar diseases and conditions into general categories and is useful in evaluating an optimal treatment for a given group of patients. The revision of the classification system is not age dependent or based on the rate of progression. An outline of the 1999 AAP Classification of Periodontal Diseases and Conditions is provided in Table 11-7. The American Academy of Periodontology (AAP) Board of Trustees

Table 11-7. *Classification System for Periodontal Diseases and Conditions*

I. Gingival Diseases

A. Plaque biofilm–induced gingivitis
1. Gingivitis associated with plaque biofilm only
   a. Without local contributing factors
   b. With local contributing factors (see VIII.A)
2. Gingival diseases modified by systemic factors
   a. Associated with the endocrine system
      i. Puberty-associated gingivitis
      ii. Menstrual cycle–associated gingivitis
      iii. Pregnancy associated
         (1) Gingivitis
         (2) Pyogenic granuloma
         (3) Diabetes mellitus–associated gingivitis
   b. Associated with blood dyscrasias
      i. Leukemia-associated gingivitis
      ii. Other
3. Gingival diseases modified by medications
   a. Drug-influenced gingival diseases
      i. Drug-influenced gingival enlargements
      ii. Drug-influenced gingivitis
         (1) Oral contraceptive–associated gingivitis
         (2) Other

4. Gingival diseases modified by malnutrition
   a. Ascorbic acid–deficiency gingivitis
   b. Other

B. Non-plaque biofilm–induced gingival lesions
1. Gingival lesions of specific bacterial origin
   a. *Neisseria gonorrhoeae*–associated lesions
   b. *Treponema pallidum*–associated lesions
   c. *Streptococcal* species–associated lesions
   d. Other
2. Gingival diseases of viral origin
   a. Herpes virus infections
      i. Primary herpetic gingivostomatitis
      ii. Recurrent oral herpes
      iii. Varicella zoster infections
   b. Other
3. Gingival diseases of fungal origin
   a. *Candida* species infections
      i. Generalized gingival candidiasis
      ii. Linear gingival erythema
      iii. Histoplasmosis
      iv. Other

Table 11-7. Classification System for Periodontal Diseases and Conditions—cont'd

4. Gingival lesions of genetic origin
   a. Hereditary gingival fibromatosis
   b. Other
5. Gingival manifestations of systemic conditions
   a. Mucocutaneous disorders
      i. Lichen planus
      ii. Pemphigoid
      iii. Pemphigus vulgaris
      iv. Erythema multiforme
      v. Lupus erythematous
      vi. Drug-induced disorders
      vii. Other
   b. Allergic reactions
      i. Dental restorative materials
         (1) Mercury
         (2) Nickel
         (3) Acrylic
         (4) Other materials
      ii. Reactions attributable to the following:
         (1) Toothpastes and mouthwashes
         (2) Chewing gum additives
         (3) Foods and additives
      iii. Other allergic reactions
6. Traumatic lesions (factitious, iatrogenic, accidental)
   a. Chemical injury
   b. Physical injury
   c. Thermal injury
7. Foreign body reactions
8. Not otherwise specified

II. Chronic Periodontitis
A. Localized (≤30% of involved sites)
B. Generalized (>30% of involved sites)

III. Aggressive Periodontitis
A. Localized
B. Generalized

IV. Periodontitis Manifested by Systemic Disease
A. Associated with hematological disorders
   1. Acquired neutropenia
   2. Leukemias
   3. Other

B. Associated with genetic disorders
   1. Familial and cyclic neutropenia
   2. Down syndrome
   3. Leukocyte adhesion deficiency syndromes
   4. Papillon-Lefèvre syndrome
   5. Chédiak-Higashi syndrome
   6. Histiocytosis syndromes
   7. Glycogen storage disease
   8. Infantile genetic agranulocytosis
   9. Cohen syndrome
   10. Ehlers-Danlos syndrome
   11. Hypophosphatasia
   12. Other
C. Not otherwise specified

V. Necrotizing Periodontal Disease
A. Necrotizing ulcerative gingivitis
B. Necrotizing ulcerative periodontitis

VI. Abscess of Periodontium
A. Gingival abscess
B. Periodontal abscess
C. Pericoronal abscess

VII. Periodontitis Associated with Endodontic Lesions
A. Combined periodontal-endodontic lesions

VIII. Developmental or Acquired Deformities and Conditions
A. Localized tooth-related factors that modify or predispose to plaque biofilm–induced gingival or periodontal diseases
   1. Tooth anatomical factors
   2. Dental restorations and appliances
   3. Root fractures
   4. Cervical root resorption and cemental tears
B. Mucogingival deformities and conditions around teeth
   1. Gingival recession
   2. Lack of keratinized gingiva
C. Occlusal trauma
   1. Primary occlusal trauma
   2. Secondary occlusal trauma

Source: Adapted from Armitage GC. Development of a classification system for periodontal diseases and conditions. *Ann Periodontol.* 1999;4:1-6.

created a Task Force in 2014 to develop a clinical interpretation of the 1999 Classification of Periodontal Diseases and Conditions. This was done to address concerns expressed by the education community, the American Board of Periodontology, and the practicing community that the current Classification presents challenges for the education of dental students and implementation in clinical practice. An update to the 1999 Classification will begin in 2017. The July 2015 update focused on three explicit areas of the current classification: attachment level, chronic versus aggressive periodontitis, and localized versus generalized periodontitis.

The modifying term **refractory** can be added to any form of the disease to acknowledge disease that is relatively nonresponsive to repeated conventional treatment, such as "refractory aggressive periodontitis" or "refractory chronic periodontitis."[1,4] The extent or distribution of the disease is classified as either local (less than 30% of sites involved) or generalized (more than 30% of sites involved). Severity of disease involvement is classified by clinical attachment loss: slight (1–2 mm CAL), moderate (3–4 mm CAL), and severe (≥5 mm CAL).[28]

To assist with administrative and third-party reimbursement, the AAP along with the American Dental

Association have adopted a periodontal case typing system that classifies periodontal diseases into five broad case types based on severity of disease.[56] Case type 0 is health, and case type I is plaque biofilm–associated gingivitis. Chronic periodontitis is divided into three case types: mild periodontitis (class II), moderate periodontitis (class III), and severe periodontitis (class IV).[6] Mild periodontitis (class II) is characterized by the initiation of periodontal pocketing or attachment loss with the potential for slight bone loss. Moderate periodontitis (class III) typically presents with advancement of pocket depths or attachment loss with the potential of slight tooth mobility, bone loss, and grade I and/or grade II furcation involvement around multirooted teeth. Severe periodontitis (class IV) is characterized by further progression of attachment and major bone loss with mobility and furcation involvement a common finding. The term *refractory* can be applied to any case type to include patients who are not responsive to repeated conventional periodontal therapy and may benefit from microbial analysis.[6,19,56]

CHARTING EXAMINATION FINDINGS

During the periodontal examination, it is important that the data being gathered are documented appropriately. The periodontal chart provides a comprehensive graphical description of the health of a patient's mouth, and accurate documentation of the examination findings is critical to diagnosis, treatment planning, outcomes assessment, and monitoring the patient's long-term periodontal health.[3] Table 11-8 provides a review of the common symbols used to chart periodontal findings. Computerized charting software helps to standardize charting by recording the elements of the periodontal examination. This standardization results in charting that is more easily reproduced and more legible.[57] Charting of periodontal findings, either on paper or digitally, can be a time-consuming task. The help of an assistant can expedite charting; however, with practice, most dental hygienists become very efficient in this area (see Teamwork). A variety of systems is also available, some of which offer voice-activated charting commands, automated foot controls for charting, and/or automated probing. An example of a digital periodontal chart (Patterson Eaglesoft version 16) is provided in Figure 11-15

The periodontal examination is a fact-finding process designed to provide a comprehensive picture of the patient's periodontal health. It determines the lack of or presence (and degree or severity) of clinical and radiographic signs of inflammation caused by bacterial infection of the periodontium (hard and soft tissues) and the resultant damage. The data gathered form the basis for individualized treatment plans, provide data for outcomes assessment after nonsurgical periodontal therapy, and serve as a baseline from which future disease activity can be compared. Performing regular comprehensive periodontal examinations is standard of care, and it is expected that the prudent, ethical dental hygienist will provide this level of care to all patients for which it is indicated.

Table 11-8. *Charting of Periodontal Findings*

Charting of the data provided by a comprehensive periodontal examination is as follows:

Condition	Symbol	Explanation
Gingival description	Descriptive terms— see Table 11-5	Assessment of the color, shape, consistency, and texture of the gingiva
Probe depths	323 323 222 / 324 323 323 / Probe depths.	Six readings per tooth; recorded in millimeters, rounded up to the nearest whole number

Table 11-8. *Charting of Periodontal Findings—cont'd*

Condition	Symbol	Explanation
Bleeding on probing	 Bleeding on probing.	Red dot above the probe depth reading, circle the reading in red, or write the reading in red
Suppuration/Exudate	 Suppuration/Exudate.	Green dot above the probe depth reading, circle the reading in green, or write the reading in green
Furcation involvement	 Furcation involvement.	Draw in the following symbols in the furcation area or at the apices of the tooth roots:

Continued

Table 11-8. *Charting of Periodontal Findings—cont'd*

Condition	Symbol	Explanation
Height of the gingival margin	323 323 222 / 324 323 323 Height of the gingival margin.	Draw in a representation of the gingival margin to indicate the level of the margin and papillae
Mucogingival junction	323 323 222 / 324 323 323 Mucogingival junction.	Draw in a dashed line at the mucogingival junction
Mobility	Mobility.	N, 1, 2, 3 written on the crown forms

Table 11-8. *Charting of Periodontal Findings—cont'd*

Condition	Symbol	Explanation
Fremitus	222 212 212 212 F F 212 222 212 211 Fremitus.	"F" on the crown form
Frenum pull	222 212 212 212 √ 212 222 212 211 Frenum pull.	Place a checkmark (√) by the area

Teamwork

Sally's last patient of the day just canceled. The prospect of being able to leave work early and get a jump on the traffic is very appealing to her, but Sally quickly remembers that she is part of a team and remembers how much she appreciates the assistance that she receives from the other team members. Because the office does not have a voice-activated periodontal charting system, she knows that the other dental hygienist would be grateful for her assistance with periodontal charting. When a dental team member has time available to assist another member, assistance with periodontal charting, either on paper or digital, is always welcomed. ■

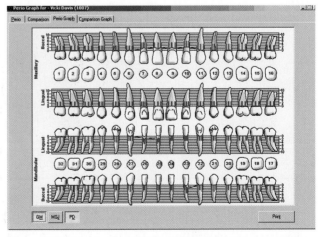

Figure 11-15. Sample of a digital periodontal chart. (Courtesy of Patterson Dental)

Case Study

Ms. Williams is a 37-year-old woman who has not had access to regular dental care. She takes 150 mg ibandronate sodium (Boniva) monthly for the prevention of osteoporosis. Her chief complaint is, "My front tooth is getting looser." The CAL ranges from 2 to 7 mm.

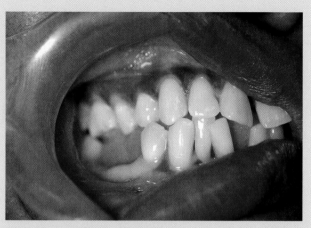

Intraoral image of right side occlusion.

Case Study Exercises

1. What is the cause of the patient's chief complaint?
2. What signs and symptoms would back up this differential diagnosis?
3. What clinical assessments would the hygienist perform to evaluate the patient's chief complaint?
4. What finding(s) on the radiograph support the patient's chief complaint?
5. What is the most likely form of periodontal disease exhibited by this patient?

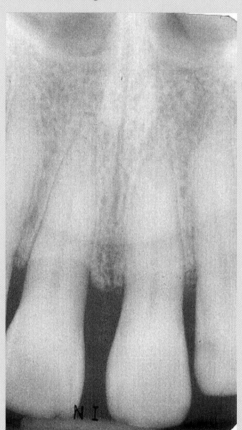

Periapical radiograph of maxillary anterior teeth.

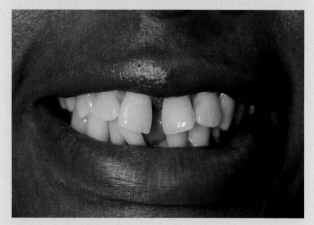

Intraoral image of central incisors.

Review Questions

1. The overhang margin on a dental restoration on the mesial of tooth #3 is the primary causative agent in the periodontal disease that is affecting that tooth, whereas the bacterial biofilm that collects on the restoration's margin is a contributing factor to the disease's progression.
   A. True
   B. False

2. You can palpate excessive mobility of your patient's maxillary central incisors when she taps her teeth together. This mobility is termed:
   A. Crepitus
   B. Fenestration
   C. Dehiscence
   D. Fremitus

3. After performing the PSR, you have the following codes. What is your next step?

4	2	2
2	1	2

   A. Nothing, the examination in complete.
   B. Probe the sextant with the code of 4.
   C. Probe the entire dentition.

4. Which of the following is the best single estimate of the periodontal support around a tooth?
   A. Probing depth
   B. Clinical attachment level
   C. Bleeding on probing
   D. Radiographic assessment

5. Periodontal case typing is primarily based on the severity of which of the following indicators?
   A. Probing depth
   B. Clinical attachment level
   C. Furcation involvement
   D. Radiographic bone loss

Active Learning

1. Draw the anatomy of the periodontium, the gingival fibers, and the PDL fibers.
2. Use index cards to create *Jeopardy!*-style questions using the chapter's key terms. Play a fun and educational game of *Jeopardy!* with a classmate.
3. List the order in which you will conduct a periodontal assessment.
4. Practice performing the various assessment procedures on a typodont.
5. Use a sensor probe (PDT Sensor Probe by Zila) to help maintain a consistent force of no more than 20 g pressure while probing. ■

REFERENCES

1. American Academy of Periodontology. Position paper: diagnosis of periodontal diseases. *J Periodontal.* 2003;74(8):1237-1247.
2. American Academy of Periodontology. Position paper: guidelines for periodontal therapy. *J Periodontal.* 2001;72(11):1624-1628.
3. Armitage GC. The complete periodontal examination. *Periodontol 2000.* 2004;34:22-33.
4. Armitage GC. Development of a classification system for periodontal diseases and conditions. *Ann Periodontal.* 1999;4:1-6.
5. Hassell TM. Tissues and cells of the periodontium. *Periodontol 2000.* 1993;3:9-38.
6. Serio FG, Hawley CE. *Manual of Clinical Periodontics: A Reference Manual for Diagnosis & Treatment.* 3rd ed. Hudson, OH: Lexi-Comp, Inc.; 2009.
7. Zappa U. Histology of the periodontal lesion implication or diagnosis. *Periodontol 2000.* 1995;7:22-38.
8. Mariotti A. The extracellular matrix of the periodontium: dynamic and interactive tissues. *Periodontolgy 2000.* 1993;3:39-63.
9. Newman MG, Takei H, Klokkevold PR, Carranza FA. *Carranza's Clinical Periodontology.* 11th ed. St. Louis, MO: Saunders; 2012.
10. Bosshardt DD, Selvig KA. Dental cementum: the dynamic tissue covering of the root. *Periodontol 2000.* 1997;13:41-75.
11. Albandar JM. Global risk factors and risk indicators for periodontal diseases. *Periodontol 2000.* 2002;29:117-206.
12. American Academy of Periodontology. Academy report: guidelines for the management of patients with periodontal diseases. *J Periodontal.* 2006;77:1607-1611.
13. Al-Shammari KF, Al-Khabbaz AK, Al-Ansari JM, Neiva R, Wang HL. Risk indicators for tooth loss due to periodontal disease. *J Periodontal.* 2005;76(11):1910-1918.
14. Douglass CW. Risk assessment and management of periodontal disease. *J Am Dent Assoc.* 2006;137(3):27S-32S.
15. Page RC, Martin J, Krall EA, Manel L, Garcia R. Longitudinal validation of a risk calculator for periodontal disease. *J Clin Periodontol.* 2003;30:819-827.

16. Page RC, Martin JA. Quantification of periodontal risk and disease severity and extent using Oral Health Information Suite (OHIS). *Perio*. 2007;4(3):163-180.

17. American Academy of Periodontology. Parameters of care supplement. Parameter on comprehensive periodontal examination. *J Periodontal*. 2000;72(11): 847-848.

18. Armitage GC. Clinical evaluation of periodontal diseases. *Periodontol 2000*. 1995;7:39-53.

19. Pihlstrom B. Periodontal risk assessment, diagnosis and treatment planning. *Periodontol 2000*. 2001;25:37-58.

20. Hefti AF. Periodontal probing. *Crit Rev Oral Biol Med*. 1997;8(3):336-356.

21. Buduneli E, Aksoy O, Kose T, Atilla G. Accuracy and reproducibility of two manual periodontal probes: an in vitro study. *J Clin Periodontol*. 2004;31(10):815-819.

22. Karpinia K, Magnusson I, Gibbs C, Yang MC. Accuracy of probing attachment levels using a CEJ probe versus traditional probes. *J Clin Periodontol*. 2004;31(3):173-176.

23. Khan S, Cabanilla LL. Periodontal probing depth measurement: a review. *Compend Contin Educ Dent*. 2009;30(1):12-14, 16, 18-21.

24. Alves RdeV, Machion L, Andia DC, Casati MZ, Sallum AW, Sallum EA. Reproducibility of clinical attachment level and probing depths of a manual probe and a computerized electronic probe. *J Int Acad Periodontol*. 2005;7(1):27-30.

25. Chaves ES, Wood RC, Jones AA, et al. Relationship of bleeding on probing and gingival index bleeding as clinical parameters of gingival inflammation. *J Clin Periodontal*. 1993;20(2):139-143.

26. Jahn C. Bleeding on probing: its significance in the prognosis and treatment of the periodontal diseases. *J Prac Hygiene*. 2001:42-45.

27. American Dental Assistants' Association, Council on Education. Gingival health—periodontal assessment. 2008. www.dentalcare.com. Accessed August 5, 2011.

28. Corbet EF, Ho DKL, Lai SML. Radiographs in periodontal disease diagnosis and management. *Australian Den J*. 2009;54(1 suppl):S27-S43.

29. Sweeting LA, Davis K, Cobb CM. Periodontal treatment protocol (PTP) for the general dental practice. *J Dent Hyg*. 2008;82(suppl 3):16-26.

30. Muller HP, Eger T. Furcation diagnosis. *J Clin Periodontol*. 1999;26:485-498.

31. American Academy of Periodontology. Parameters of placement and care of the dental implant. *J Periodontal*. 2000;7:870-872.

32. American Academy of Periodontology. Position paper: dental implants in periodontal therapy. *J Periodontal*. 2000;71:1934-1942.

33. Cobb CM. Microbes, inflammation, scaling and root planning, and the periodontal condition. *J Dent Hyg*. 2008;82(suppl 3):4-9.

34. American Academy of Periodontology. Parameter on periodontitis associated with systemic conditions. *J Periodontal*. 2007;71(5 suppl):876-879.

35. Carrillo-de-Albornoz FE, Herrera D, Bascones-Martinez A. Gingival changes during pregnancy: I. influence of hormonal variations on clinical and immunological parameters. *J Clin Periodontol*. 2010;37:220-229.

36. Carrillo-de-Albornoz FE, Herrera D, Bascones-Martinez A. Gingival changes during pregnancy: II. influence of hormonal variations on the subgingival biofilm. *J Clin Periodontol*. 2010;37:230-240.

37. Laxman VK, Sridhar A. Tobacco use and its effects on the periodontium and periodontal therapy. *J Contemp Dent Pract*. 2008;7(9):97-107.

38. Mealey BL, Oates TW. AAP commissioned review. Diabetes mellitus and periodontal diseases. *J Periodontol*. 2006;77(6):1289-1303.

39. Lamster IB, Ahlo JK. Analysis of gingival crevicular fluid as applied to the diagnosis of oral and systemic diseases. *Ann NY Acad Sci*. 2007;1098:216-229.

40. Risteli J, Elomaa I, Niemi S, Novamo A, Risteli L. Radioimmunoassay for the pyridinoline cross-linked carboxy-terminal telopeptide of type I collagen: a new serum marker of bone collagen degradation. *Clin Chem*. 1993;39:635-640.

41. Kaufman E, Lamster IB. Analysis of saliva for periodontal diagnosis. *J Clin Periodontol*. 2000;27:453-465.

42. Fedi PF, Killoy WJ. Temperature differences at periodontal sites in health and disease. *J Periodontol*. 1992;63:24-27.

43. Haffajee AD, Socransky SS, Goodson JM. Subgingival temperature. I. Relation to baseline clinical parameters. *J Clin Periodontol*. 1992;19:401-408.

44. Haffajee AD, Socransky SS, Goodson JM. Subgingival temperature. II. Relation to future periodontal attachment loss. *J Clin Periodontol*.1992;19:409-416.

45. Kung RTV, Ochs B, Goodson JM. Temperature as a diagnostic. *J. Clin Periodontol*. 1990;17:557-563.

46. American Academy of Periodontology. Academy report: informational paper. Implications of genetic technology for the management of periodontal diseases. *J Periodontol*. 2005;76(5):850-857.

47. Greenstein G, Hart TC. Clinical utility of a genetic susceptibility test for severe chronic periodontitis: a critical evaluation. *JADA*. 2002;133:452-459.

48. Greenstein GG. A critical assessment of inteleukin-1 (IL-1) genotyping when used in a genetic susceptibility test for severe chronic periodontitis. *J Periodontol*. 2002;73(2):231-247.

49. Lang NP, Tonetti MS, Suter J, et al. Effect of interleukin-1 gene polymorphisms on gingival inflammation assessed by bleeding on probing in a periodontal maintenance population. *J Periodont Res*. 2000;35:102-107.

50. Culliman MP, Westerman B, Hamlet SM, et al. A longitudinal study of interleukin-1 gene polymorphisms and periodontal disease in a general adult population. *J Clin Periodontal*. 2001;28:1137-1144.

51. Huynh-Ba G, Lang NP, Tonetti MS, Salvi GE. The association of the composite IL-1 genotype with periodontitis progression and/or treatment outcomes: a systematic review. *J Clin Periodontal*. 2007;34:305-317.

52. Armitage GC, Robertson PB. The biology, prevention, diagnosis and treatment of periodontal diseases: scientific advances in the United States. *JADA*. 2009; 140:36S-43S.

53. Dennison DK, Van Dyke TE. The acute inflammatory response and the role of phagocytic cells in periodontal health and disease. *Periodontol 2000*. 1997;14:54-78.

54. Ishikawa I, Nakashima K, Koseki T. Introduction of the immune response to periodontopathic bacteria and its

role in the pathogenesis of periodontitis. *Peridontol 2000.* 1997;14:79-111.

55. Offenbacher S. Periodontal disease: pathogenesis. *Ann Periodontol.* 1996;1L:821-878.

56. American Dental Association. Risk Management Series. *Diagnosing and Managing the Periodontal Patient.* Chicago, Ill. : American Dental Association 1986.

57. Balanoff WL, Duval C. *The Role of Technology in Periodontal Evaluation and Treatment Acceptance.* The Academy of Dental Therapeutics and Stomatology, PennWell, Tulsa, OK; 2007.

58. Bains VK, Mohan R, Gundappa M, Bains R. Properties, effects and clinical applications of ultrasound in periodontics: an overview. *Periodontal Practice Today.* 2008;5(4):291-302.

59. Brodala N. Beyond the probe: new technology and developments in periodontal assessment and diagnosis. *Dimens Dent Hyg.* 200;3(1):10-12, 14.

Chapter 12 | Hard Tissue Examination

Diane P. Kandray, RDH, MEd

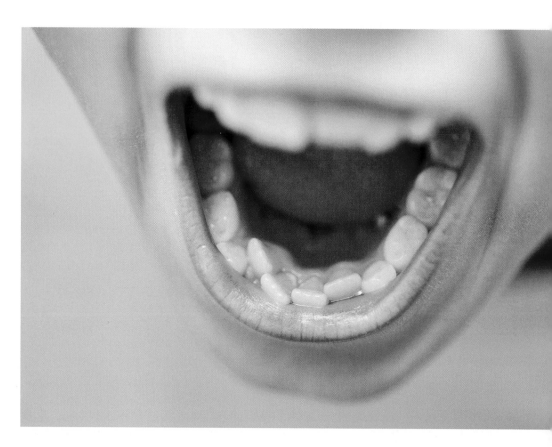

LEARNING OBJECTIVES

After reading this chapter, the student should be able to:

12.1 Assign the correct tooth designation using the appropriate numbering system.

12.2 Identify and chart normal and abnormal conditions of the dentition.

12.3 Properly classify the occlusion according to the Angle classification of occlusion.

12.4 Recognize new technology in the identification of carious lesions.

KEY CONCEPTS

• Accurate dental charting is an essential role of the dental hygienist.
• Teeth can be identified using a variety of numbering systems.
• Caries can be classified using a standard classification system.
• Dentitions can be classified using the Angle classification of occlusion.
• New technology exists to aid in the early detection of carious lesions.

RELEVANCE TO CLINICAL PRACTICE

Documenting an accurate record of the dentition is an integral part of the patient assessment process. The dental hygienist is often responsible for completing a dental chart at the initial patient visit and updating it on subsequent visits. A current and accurate dental chart is important for the quality planning of dental care, communication with other professions, legal documentation of dental treatment procedures, and forensics.

DENTAL CHARTS

Dental charting consists of recording normal and abnormal conditions, existing dental restorative treatments, and pathology. Dental charting must be done systematically to create a useful, accurate graphic representation of the dentition.

Many different types of charts exist. Each dental practice adopts a charting system for their needs and preferences. Dental charting can be done on paper forms, computer files, or both. Paperless dental charting has been increasing but is still not used exclusively.

TOOTH NUMBERING SYSTEMS

The dentition can be identified using several different numbering systems.[1]

Universal

The most common tooth designation system is the **universal numbering system** (Fig. 12-1). This system uses the numbers 1 to 16 for the maxillary arch beginning with the maxillary right third molar and ending with the maxillary left third molar. It continues with the mandibular left third molar, #17, and ends with the mandibular right third molar, #32. The primary dentition is identified using letters of the alphabet. A letter A is assigned to the maxillary right second molar and lettering continues sequentially around the upper arch to J, the second molar of the maxillary left quadrant. The letter K is the second molar of the mandibular left quadrant and lettering continues sequentially around the lower arch to T, the second molar of the mandibular right quadrant.

Palmer Notation

Some orthodontists use **Palmer notation,** a system in which a right-angle symbol (└) designates each quadrant. The right-angle symbol oriented right or left and up or down. The permanent teeth are then numbered sequentially starting at the midline with #1 and moving posterior to #8. The tooth number is placed in the right-angle symbol. Letters beginning with A are used in the symbol to identify primary teeth.

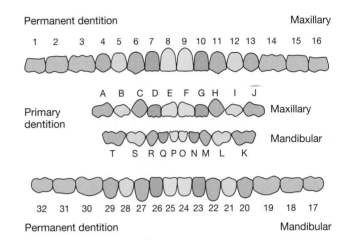

Figure 12-1. Universal numbering system for primary and permanent dentition. (From Prajer R, Grosso G. *DH Notes.* Philadelphia: F.A. Davis; 2011.)

International Standards Organization

The **International Standards Organization (ISO) designation system** may also be used for tooth numbering. This system uses a two-digit code to label teeth. The first number in the two-digit code indicates the quadrant, and the second number indicates the specific tooth in the quadrant. In this system, the digits 1 through 4 are used to depict the four permanent quadrants starting with the maxillary right, then maxillary left, mandibular left, and mandibular right, respectively. A second digit is used to identify the tooth number, beginning at the midline and sequentially numbering the teeth with number 1 for the central incisor to number 8 for the third molar. The numbers 5, 6, 7, and 8 are used to depict the four primary quadrants. This system was originally started by the Federation Dentaire Internationale. Figures 12-2 and 12-3 show comparisons of the numbering systems for permanent and primary teeth.

A dental chart can be presented as anatomically correct, showing several views of each tooth, or it can use symbols showing 2 rows of 16 circles each. Each circle represents a tooth and is divided to show five surfaces, a smaller round center and four outside surfaces. The round center represents the occlusal of posterior teeth, or the incisal of anterior teeth. The four surfaces surrounding the center represent the buccal (facial), mesial, lingual, and distal surfaces of the tooth (Fig. 12-4).

	Maxillary arch															
	Molars			Premolars		Canine	Incisors				Canine	Premolars		Molars		
Universal	1	2	3	4	5	6	7	8	9	10	11	12	13	14	15	16
Palmers notation	8	7	6	5	4	3	2	1	1	2	3	4	5	6	7	8
ISO	18	17	16	15	14	13	12	11	22	23	24	25	26	27	28	29

Right								Left								
Universal	32	31	30	29	28	27	26	25	24	23	22	21	20	19	18	17
Palmers notation	8	7	6	5	4	3	2	1	1	2	3	4	5	6	7	8
ISO	48	47	46	45	44	43	42	41	31	32	33	34	35	36	37	38
	Molars			Premolars		Canine	Incisors				Canine	Premolars		Molars		
	Mandibular arch															

Figure 12-2. Permanent tooth numbering systems.

	Maxillary arch									
	Molars		Canine	Incisors				Canine	Molars	
International	A	B	C	D	E	F	G	H	I	J
Palmers notation	E	D	C	B	A	A	B	C	D	E
ISO	55	54	53	52	51	61	62	63	64	65

Right						Left				
International	T	S	R	Q	P	O	N	M	L	K
Palmers notation	E	D	C	B	A	A	B	C	D	E
ISO	84	83	82	82	81	71	72	73	74	75
	Molars		Canine	Incisors				Canine	Molars	
	Mandibular arch									

Figure 12-3. Primary tooth numbering systems.

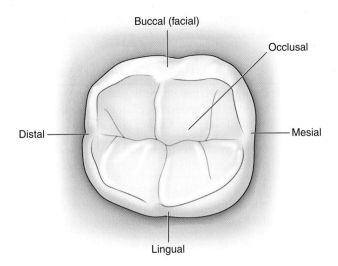

Figure 12-4. Surfaces of the teeth.

Small boxes are usually placed above and below the rows to allow coded notations for each tooth.

CHARTING DENTAL CONDITIONS

The hard tissue examination of the dentition includes a thorough recognition and documentation of normal and abnormal dental conditions. Careful examination and recording of dental conditions is important for the quality of planning further treatment.

Charting can be recorded on a paper chart or with the use of a computer software program (see Teamwork). A number of dental conditions such as missing teeth, rotated teeth, and unerupted teeth should be charted when charting on a paper chart. Common symbols are used to chart these existing conditions (Table 12-1). Existing and planned restorative procedures are also included on the chart.

Missing teeth are normally charted first, marked with an X or a single vertical line. Unerupted teeth may be completely circled, with the circle altered if necessary

Teamwork

Charting by hand and computer is most efficient with two people: one person performs the examination and the other records the findings on the chart. When a clinician working independently writes and draws findings on a dental chart, there are concerns about cross-contamination. If a computer is available in the treatment area, the clinician can cover the keyboard and mouse with plastic wrap to prevent cross-contamination. ■

Table 12-1. *Dental Charting Symbols*

Procedure/Condition	Pencil Color	Write in Tooth Box Above Tooth	Graphic/Drawing on Dental Chart
Amalgam	Blue		Outline restoration as accurately as possible and color in solid blue.
Anterior crowding	Lead pencil		Draw an arc from canine to canine on the lingual view and mark "ant cr" on the arc line.
Caries/decay	Red		Outline lesion and color in solid red.
Crown—porcelain/metal	Blue	PGVC PM	Outline ceramic crown in blue. Color metal portion solid blue. Write the type of crown in the tooth box above the tooth.
Defective restoration or poor margin integrity	Red		Outline the restoration in red.
Diastema	Lead pencil		Draw parallel lines at the location of the diastema on all views of the dental chart.
Edentulous arch	Lead pencil		Draw an X from the uppermost aspect of one third molar (#1) to the lowermost aspect of the third molar on the opposite side (#16). Indicate a denture by placing a checkmark in the appliance box.
Fixed partial denture (bridge—pontic, abutment)	Lead pencil	PGVC, PM, GC, etc.	Draw a horizontal line immediately above or below the crowns of the bridge on the lingual view. Place a checkmark in the appliance box.

Continued

Table 12-1. *Dental Charting Symbols—cont'd*

Procedure/Condition	Pencil Color	Write in Tooth Box Above Tooth	Graphic/Drawing on Dental Chart
Fixed retainer	Blue	NM	Draw the retainer on the lingual view as seen in the mouth. If applicable, chart any nonmetallic material and print NM in the tooth box.
Food impaction	Red		Draw an arrow on the lingual view of the chart to show interproximal areas of food impaction.
Fractured tooth	Red	RT	Draw a zigzag line on the tooth where the fracture occurred. Place an X over the entire crown if it is entirely fractured and root tip is retained.
Gold crown, gold foil, gold inlay, onlay	Blue	GC, GF, GI	Outline crown or restoration and draw diagonal lines.
Implant	Red	I	"X" out root in lead pencil; notate bridgework/crown as usual.
Incipient caries	Red		Outline areas in red.
Malposed tooth			
1. Drifting	Lead pencil		Place arrow in box indicating the direction the tooth has drifted.
2. Torsoversion	Lead pencil		Draw a curved arrow in the tooth box to indicate the proper direction the tooth is rotated.
3. Linguoversion, buccoversion, or labioversion	Lead pencil		Draw straight arrows in the tooth box to indicate the direction the tooth has moved.
4. Supraerupted or infraversion	Lead pencil		Place arrows on the lingual view of the tooth showing the direction of supraversion or infraversion.
Maryland bridge, cantilever and fixed bridge	Blue	PGVC, PM, PC	Draw a horizontal line immediately above or below the crown of the bridge on the lingual view.
Missing tooth	Lead pencil		If the tooth has been replaced by a fixed prosthesis, "X" out the root only. Draw an X through the root and crown if the root has been replaced by a removable prosthesis.
Mixed dentition	Lead pencil	PE UE	Draw an X through all missing deciduous teeth on the deciduous tooth chart. Write PE or UE in the tooth box of the permanent dentition.
Nonmetallic restoration	Blue	NM PC	Outline the restoration as accurately as possible. Write NM or PC in the tooth box.
Recession	Blue		Measure the amount of recession from the CEJ and draw a blue line indicating recession on the tooth root.
Removable partial denture	Lead pencil		Place a checkmark in the appliance box.
Retained deciduous tooth	Lead pencil	Print the letter of the deciduous tooth	"X" out the missing permanent tooth.
Root canal therapy	Blue	RC	Draw a line through the root canal on both the facial and the lingual views.
Sealants	Blue	S	Outline sealed areas in blue.

Table 12-1. Dental Charting Symbols—cont'd

Procedure/Condition	Pencil Color	Write in Tooth Box Above Tooth	Graphic/Drawing on Dental Chart
Supernumerary tooth	Blue		Draw on chart as close to their anatomic location and size as possible.
Temporary crown	Blue	TC	If temporary is metal.
Temporary restoration	Blue	T	Outline in blue pencil.
Unerupted or partially erupted tooth	Lead pencil	UE, PE	
Veneer	Blue	V	Outline restoration in blue if nonmetallic and color in solid.

CEJ, ementoenamel junction; GC, gold crown; GF, gold foil; GI, gold inlay; I, implant; NM, nonmetallic; PC, porcelain crown; PE, partially erupted; PGVC, porcelain gold veneer crown; PM, porcelain to metal crown; RC, root canal; RT, root tip if root tip is retained; S, sealants; T, temporary restoration; TC, temporary crown; UE, unerupted; V, veneer.

to show partial eruption. A fractured tooth is marked in red with a jagged line. Both carious lesions and restorations are marked by coloring the affected portion of the tooth, usually in different colors. For more precise charting, shadings, colors, or coded letters may be used to differentiate between types of restorations. Amalgam (i.e., silver) restorations might be colored blue, for instance, whereas composite (i.e., white) restorations might be outlined in blue. Gold crowns might be marked with a G (or designated with a blue outline and oblique lines), and porcelain crowns with a P. In addition, full-coverage crowns are usually marked by circling just the crown of the tooth on the chart in blue. Areas of decay or defective restorations are usually marked in red.

For the purposes of communication, tooth surfaces are referred to by their first initial. For instance, a restoration on the mandibular left first molar that covers the mesial and occlusal surfaces would be called an MO on #19. A carious lesion that extends from mesial to facial to incisal surface of the maxillary right lateral incisor would be an MFI on #7.

Endodontic (i.e., root canal) restorations can be marked with a black line extending up the length of the tooth root. The directions of malpositioned, drifted, and supererupted teeth can be indicated with arrows. Implants can be indicated in the appropriate box with the letter I. Fixed bridgework may be noted by using connecting lines joining the teeth in the bridge. Partial and complete dentures can be marked with brackets.

CLASSIFICATION OF DENTAL CARIES

A carious lesion is described as a demineralization of the tooth enamel that can occur in the pits, fissures, or smooth surfaces of a tooth. **G.V. Black classification of caries** is the most commonly used system to chart dental caries (Table 12-2). The classes refer to the tooth types and location or surface with caries. Restorations and lesions can also be classified according to location.

Table 12-2. G.V. Black Classification

Class	Description
Class I	Pits and fissures on the occlusal, buccal, and lingual surfaces of posterior teeth, and lingual surfaces of anterior teeth

Continued

Table 12-2. G.V. Black Classification—cont'd

Class	Description
Class II 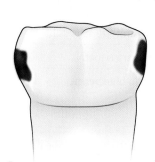	Proximal surfaces of posterior teeth and may include occlusal
Class III 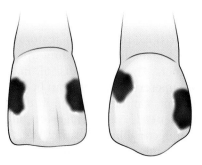	Proximal surfaces of anterior teeth, not including incisal edge
Class IV 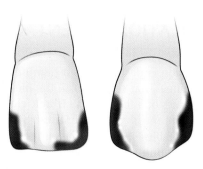	Proximal surfaces of anterior teeth that involve an incisal edge
Class V 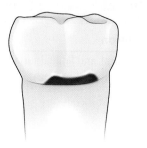 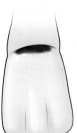	Gingival third (i.e., closest to the gum line) of the facial, buccal, or lingual surfaces of anterior and posterior teeth

Table 12-2. G.V. Black Classification—cont'd	
Class	**Description**
Class VI 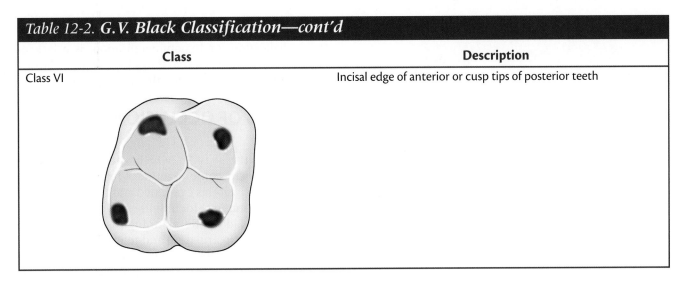	Incisal edge of anterior or cusp tips of posterior teeth

IDENTIFYING NONCARIOUS LESIONS

Noncarious lesions should also be identified and documented in the patient record. The following noncarious lesions can affect a single tooth or multiple teeth.

Abfraction

Abfraction is the flaking of facial enamel at the cervical third of the tooth (Fig. 12-5). It is thought to be the result of flexible forces at the cervix (neck) of the tooth. Excessive buccal or lingual occlusal forces may cause loss of tooth structure at the cement–enamel junction.

Abrasion

Abrasion is the mechanical wearing away of the tooth structure (Fig. 12-6). It may be caused by overaggressive tooth brushing. Abrasion typically looks like a V-shaped groove at the buccal or labial cervical part of the tooth.

Attrition

Attrition is the mechanical wearing down of the tooth structure resulting from bruxism or mastication (Fig. 12-7). Enamel is initially affected by the grinding

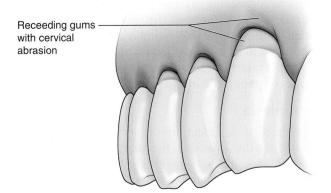

Receeding gums with cervical abrasion

Figure 12-6. Abrasion.

of the teeth but may proceed into the underlying dentin. The effects of attrition can be seen on the occlusal or incisal edges of teeth as wear facets or flattened surfaces.

Decalcification

Decalcification is the dissolution of enamel caused by acids produced by plaque biofilm or consuming acidic foods (Fig. 12-8). Decalcification initially appears as white spots on the teeth. These white spots can progress and lead to dental caries or be reversed and remineralized with proper oral hygiene.

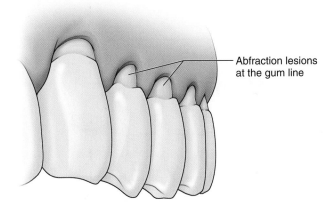

Abfraction lesions at the gum line

Figure 12-5. Abfraction.

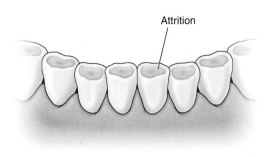

Attrition

Figure 12-7. Attrition.

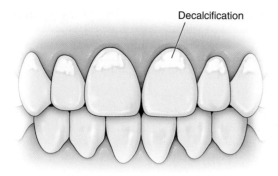

Figure 12-8. Decalcification.

Erosion

Erosion is the irreversible chemical wearing away of the enamel (Fig. 12-9). It is caused by some form of chemical dissolving of the tooth (acidic foods or chronic vomiting, bulimia, or gastroreflux). Erosion initially affects the enamel but may also progress to the underlying dentin. Clinical signs of erosion include a dull appearance of the usually shiny enamel. Erosion may lead to thinning of the enamel and sensitivity.

Hypoplasia

Hypoplasia is a defect in the enamel that occurs because of a disturbance in the quantity of enamel matrix during tooth development (Fig. 12-10). Hypoplasia results in white spots or a pitted appearance on the enamel surface.

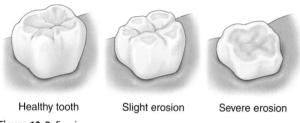

Healthy tooth   Slight erosion   Severe erosion

Figure 12-9. Erosion.

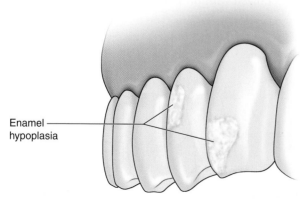

Enamel hypoplasia

Figure 12-10. Hypoplasia.

Hypocalcification (Hypomineralization)

Hypocalcification, or hypomineralization, is a lack of quality of the enamel matrix. It results in white or brown lesions of unknown origin on the tooth (Fig. 12-11).

ANALYSIS OF OCCLUSION

Occlusion is the way in which the maxillary and mandibular teeth come together when the mouth is closed. The occlusion is examined and recorded during the oral examination. Identifying and recording malocclusion can aid in the planning of dental hygiene care, home-care instruction, and referral to other dental professionals for comprehensive care. In addition to occlusion, several tooth relationships are important to record during the examination.

Recording occlusion begins with the recognition of the relationship between the maxillary arch and the mandibular arch. **Angle classification of malocclusion** was developed by Edward H. Angle in the early 1900s and is commonly used to record occlusion. The relationship of the maxillary first molar to the mandibular first molar is the key to occlusion, according to Angle. The relationship between the maxillary and the mandibular canines is also an important consideration in classifying occlusion, particularly when the first permanent molars are missing. A malocclusion occurs when the relationship is less than ideal. The classes and their associated facial profiles are described in the following subsections and are shown in Figure 12-12.

Class I

Class I malocclusion is described as neutroclusion. In this case, the mesiobuccal cusp of the maxillary first permanent molar is positioned in the mesiobuccal groove of the mandibular first molar. The maxillary canine occludes with the distal half of the mandibular canine and mesial half of the mandibular first premolar. The facial profile is mesognathic.

Class II

Class II or distoclusion occurs when the mesiobuccal cusp of the maxillary first molar lies mesial to the buccal groove of the mandibular first molar. The distal portion

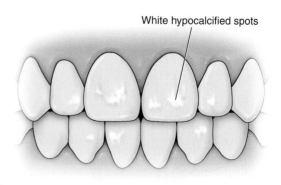

White hypocalcified spots

Figure 12-11. Hypocalcification.

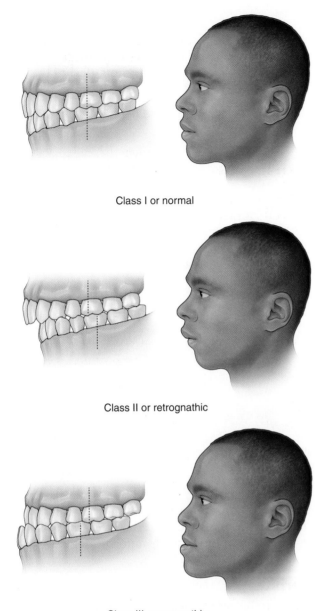

Class I or normal

Class II or retrognathic

Class III or prognathic

Figure 12-12. Classes of occlusion and associated facial profiles (mesognathic, retrognathic, and prognathic).

of the maxillary canine is mesial to the mesial portion of the mandibular canine by at least the width of a premolar. The facial profile is retrognathic. Class II has two divisions:

- **Division I** occurs when one or more maxillary anterior teeth protrude facially.
- **Division II** occurs when one or more maxillary anterior teeth are inclined lingually and a lateral incisor is positioned labially.

Class III

Class III or mesioclusion is when the mesiobuccal cusp of the maxillary first molar lies distal to the buccal groove of the mandibular first molar. The mesial portion of the maxillary canine is distal to the distal surface of the mandibular canine by at least the width of a premolar. The facial profile is prognathic.

A **tendency** occurs when the mesial cusp of the maxillary first molar is either mesial or distal to the central groove of the mandibular molar by less than the width of a premolar. Therefore, the classification is referred to as a "class I with a tendency toward a class II, or class III" as appropriate.[2]

The normal or desired occlusion of the primary dentition is known as the terminal plane. This can be observed as either a flush terminal plane, when the primary maxillary and mandibular second molars are in an end-to-end relationship, or a mesial step, when the primary mandibular second molar is in a position mesial to the maxillary molar. A less desirable relationship, known as a distal step, may occur in which the primary mandibular second molar is positioned distal to the maxillary second molar.

MALRELATIONS OF TEETH

An individual may have a normal relationship between the maxillary and the mandibular molars, but individual relationships between other teeth may classify him or her as having a malocclusion.

Anterior Crossbite

Anterior crossbite occurs when one or more maxillary incisors are lingual to the mandibular incisors (Fig. 12-13). Orthodontic treatment is usually required for correction of a crossbite.

Posterior Crossbite

Maxillary or mandibular posterior teeth are positioned either facial or lingual to their normal position (Fig. 12-14). This condition presents as bilaterally or unilaterally.

Edge-to-Edge Bite

With an edge-to-edge bite the incisal surfaces of maxillary teeth occlude with the incisal edges of mandibular teeth instead of overlapping (Fig. 12-15).

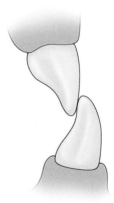

Figure 12-13. Anterior crossbite. (From Prajer R, Grosso G. *DH Notes.* Philadelphia: F.A. Davis; 2011.)

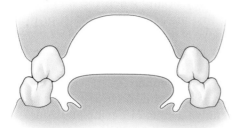

Figure 12-14. Posterior crossbite. (From Prajer R, Grosso G. *DH Notes*. Philadelphia: F.A. Davis; 2011.)

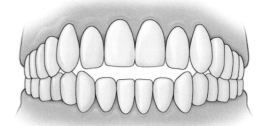

Figure 12-17. Open bite. (From Prajer R, Grosso G. DH Notes. Philadelphia: F.A. Davis; 2011.)

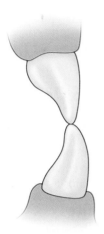

Figure 12-15. Edge-to-edge bite. (From Prajer R, Grosso G. *DH Notes*. Philadelphia: F.A. Davis; 2011.)

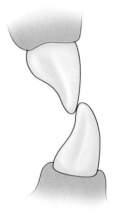

Figure 12-18. Underjet. (From Prajer R, Grosso G. *DH Notes*. Philadelphia: F.A. Davis; 2011.)

End-to-End Bite

An end-to-end bite means that molars and premolars occlude cusp to cusp (Fig. 12-16).

Open Bite

An open bite is the lack of occlusal or incisal contact between the maxillary and mandibular teeth. The teeth do not occlude (Fig. 12-17).

Underjet

Maxillary teeth are lingual to mandibular teeth (Fig. 12-18). An underjet occurs when the maxillary

anteriors are positioned lingually to the mandibular anteriors with excessive space between the labial of the maxillary anterior teeth and the lingual of the mandibular anterior teeth.

Overbite

Overbite is the vertical overlap of the maxillary anterior teeth with the mandibular anterior teeth, or the vertical distance by which the maxillary incisors overlap the mandibular incisors (Fig. 12-19). The list below describes the different types of overbite.

- Normal—incisal edges are within the incisal third of mandibular
- Moderate—within the middle third

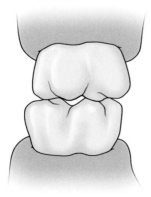

Figure 12-16. End-to-end bite. (From Prajer R, Grosso G. *DH Notes*. Philadelphia: F.A. Davis; 2011.)

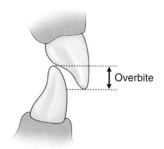

Figure 12-19. Overbite. (From Prajer R, Grosso G. *DH Notes*. Philadelphia: F.A. Davis; 2011.)

• Deep (severe)—incisal edges of maxillary are within the cervical third of the mandibular teeth

Overjet

Overjet is the horizontal distance between the labioincisal surfaces of the mandibular incisors and the linguoincisal surfaces of the maxillary incisors (Fig. 12-20).

MEASURING OVERBITE AND OVERJET

Overbite is the vertical overlap of the maxillary central incisors over the mandibular central incisors. To measure the amount of overbite (Fig. 12-21):

• With the patient's jaw closed, hold the probe vertically against the mandibular central incisors.
• As the patient slowly opens his or her mouth, measure the distance from the incisal edge of the mandibular central incisor to the facial surface of the mandibular incisor where the maxillary incisor overlaps.

To measure overjet (see Fig. 12-21):

• Hold the probe horizontally against the mandibular central incisor.
• Measure the horizontal distance the maxillary incisors overlap the mandibular.

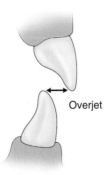

Figure 12-20. Overjet. (From Prajer R, Grosso G. *DH Notes*. Philadelphia: F.A. Davis; 2011.)

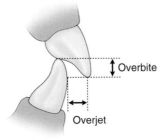

Figure 12-21. Measuring overbite and overjet.

MALPOSITION OF INDIVIDUAL TEETH

Malposition of individual teeth include:

• Buccoversion—buccal to normal
• Labioversion—labial to normal
• Linguoversion—position lingual to normal
• Supraversion—erupted beyond the occlusal plane
• Infraversion—depressed below the line of occlusion
• Torsoversion—turned or rotated

OCCLUSAL CONSIDERATIONS

Dental hygienists should be familiar with additional concepts related to occlusion. **Centric occlusion** is the voluntary position of the dentition that allows the maximum contact when the teeth occlude. Patients are instructed to bite on their molars to place the arches in centric occlusion.

Leeway space is the spacing that dentists preserve during the mixed dentition period to allow for adequate space for the permanent dentition to erupt. Primary teeth that are lost prematurely may decrease the leeway space and result in crowding of the permanent dentition.

The primary dentition ideally should have spacing between the maxillary lateral and canine and the mandibular canine and first molar. This **primate spacing** is essential to allow the larger permanent teeth to erupt without difficulty.

Teeth **curve of Spee** is an anatomic curvature of the occlusal alignment of the teeth, beginning at the cusp tip of the mandibular canine, following the buccal cusps of the premolars and molars, and continuing to the anterior border of the ramus.

PULP TESTING

Pulp testing is a clinical diagnostic aid to determine the vitality of a tooth. Pulp testing can be thermal or electrical. Both methods measure nerve activity in the tooth. An electrical impulse or ice or cold refrigerant is used on the tooth to be tested along with the adjacent teeth. Teeth that do not respond to the stimulation usually suggest pulpal necrosis or an abscess.

NEW TECHNOLOGY FOR IDENTIFICATION OF DENTAL CARIES

There are several ways to recognize caries in a clinical setting. The conventional methods to detect dental caries include visual inspection to observe changes in the color of the tooth, use of an explorer to locate demineralized areas of the tooth, and interpretation of traditional dental radiographs. These techniques, although easy to use, are relatively ineffective in discovering demineralization in the early stages. The use of an explorer is currently not a recommended method of caries detection. Explorers often present incomplete or inaccurate data and may actually disturb fragile, remineralizing enamel.

New technology is slowly replacing traditional methods in the detection of early dental carious lesions. Visual assessment may be improved by the use of magnification loupes and intraoral cameras. Computer and laser technology assist the dental professional to identify early caries that cannot be detected with conventional methods (see Technology).

As new advances in the early detection of dental caries continue to evolve, clinicians should not rely on one method to detect caries. Many factors must be considered in the assessment of an early carious lesion.

TECHNOLOGY

DIGITAL RADIOGRAPHY

Digital radiography creates a digital image that can be enhanced by altering the image brightness, contrast, and size. Digital radiography stores an image on the computer and can be used in future visits to compare the progression and severity of an incipient carious lesion. Dental hygienists may use digital radiography in place of traditional dental radiograph film techniques.

DIAGNODENT

The DIAGNOdent 2095 uses a laser light over the tooth surface to identify early carious areas of decay. No radiation is emitted, which makes this process safer than radiography. The results of the laser scan are measured and quantified by a number between 0 and 99. Readings greater than 20 to 25 indicate the possibility of demineralization on smooth surface and occlusal caries. The DIAGNOdent measures the amount of fluorescence on the tooth. The use of the laser is painless and when used in conjunction with other examination findings aids the dentist in developing the appropriate treatment plan for the individual. The DIAGNOdent is available in the classic model with a cord, as well as a wireless pen model. An advantage of the DIAGNOdent is the portability between operatories. The DIAGNOdent relies on a clean tooth surface to provide accurate results. Plaque, stain, dental anomalies such as hyperplasia, some dental materials, and arrested decay could result in a false-positive reading. Proper calibration before each use is required for accurate results.[3] This technology may be used by the dental hygienist to identify early carious lesions.

MIDWEST CARIES I.D. DETECTION HANDPIECE

The Midwest Caries I.D. detection handpiece uses LED fluorescence to detect decalcified enamel that may indicate caries. The unit is cordless and requires no calibration. The use of sound combined with light alerts the user to possible carious lesions. The unit shines a green light on the tooth and turns red when a carious lesion is detected. The audible sound speeds up and slows down as the decalcification of the tooth is decreased or increased. This battery-operated device is approved for use in detecting smooth surface, pit, fissure, and interproximal caries.[4] ■

Case Study

A 10-year-old patient in the dental hygiene clinic presents with interproximal caries on the mesial surface of the permanent mandibular right first molar (#30) and stained pits on the occlusal surface. The dental hygienist also records a type II, division I malocclusion.

Case Study Exercises

1. What is the G. V. Black classification for the restoration needed for tooth #30?
   A. Class I
   B. Class II
   C. Class III
   D. Class IV
   E. Class V

2. What preventive measures should be discussed with the parents to avoid further carious lesions?
   A. Use of a mouthguard
   B. Application of dental sealants
   C. Home fluoride rinse
   D. Both B and C

3. The 10-year-old child should be referred for an orthodontic consultation. The child's occlusion is not ideal and should be corrected.
   A. Both statements are true.
   B. Both statements are false.
   C. The first statement is true, the second is false.
   D. The first statement is false, the second is true.

Review Questions

1. Which of the following numbering systems was used to assign a permanent maxillary first molar a designation of #3?
   A. Palmer notation
   B. Universal
   C. International Standards Organization designation system
   D. Common dental terminology
   E. Standard

2. Which numbering system is used most commonly by orthodontists?
   A. Palmer notation
   B. Universal
   C. International Standards Organization designation system
   D. Common dental terminology
   E. Standard

3. What is the association between tooth #3 and tooth A?
   A. Tooth #3 replaces tooth A.
   B. Both are permanent teeth.
   C. Both are primary teeth.
   D. Tooth #3 erupts distal to tooth A.
   E. Tooth #3 erupts mesial to tooth A.

4. How many surfaces does every tooth have?
   A. Three
   B. Four
   C. Five
   D. Six
   E. Eight

5. Who devised the first practical classification of occlusion?
   A. Black
   B. Bolton
   C. Angle
   D. Wilhelm

Active Learning

1. Sketch a tooth and label its occlusal, buccal, mesial, lingual, and distal surfaces.
2. Prepare a slide show presentation explaining the different tooth numbering systems in use.
3. Take turns role-playing patient and dental hygienist, and measure overbite and overjet. ■

REFERENCES

1. Peck S, Peck L. A time for change of tooth numbering systems. *J Dent Educ.* 1993;57(8):643–647.
2. Gravely JF, Johnson DB. Angle's classification of malocclusion: an assessment of reliability. *Brit J Orthodontics.* 1974,1(3):79-86.
3. DIAGNOdent Pen. http://www.kavo.com/en/dental-instruments/diagnodent-pen. Accessed July 25, 2015.
4. Patel SA, Shepard WD, Barros JA, Streckfus CF, Quock RL. In vitro evaluation of Midwest Caries ID: a novel light-emitting diode for caries detection. *Oper Dent.* 2014 Nov-Dec;39(6):644-51. doi: 10.2341/13-114-L. Epub 2014 Aug 18.

Chapter 13 | Biofilm, Calculus, and Stain

Silvia A. Stefan, RDH, MHHS

KEY TERMS

acquired pellicle

biofilm

calculus

calculus ledges

calculus rings

calculus spicules

extrinsic staining

food debris

glycocalyx

halitosis

intrinsic endogenous stain

intrinsic exogenous stain

intrinsic staining

materia alba

pellicle formation

subgingival biofilm

subgingival (serumal) calculus

supragingival biofilm

supragingival (salivary) calculus

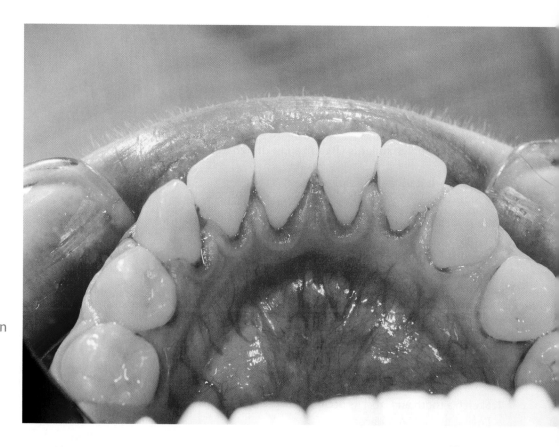

LEARNING OBJECTIVES

After reading this chapter, the student should be able to:

13.1 Define *biofilm* and *calculus*.

13.2 Identify the types of intrinsic and extrinsic stains.

13.3 Recognize the key microbes contained in bacterial biofilm.

13.4 List the different types of extrinsic stains and their cause.

13.5 Discuss the effects bacterial biofilm has on the oral cavity.

13.6 Give examples of different ways to detect calculus.

KEY CONCEPTS

- Reduction in biofilm growth will decrease the risk for periodontal disease and caries development.
- Accurate calculus detection and removal are important measures for an individual's overall health.
- The inflammatory process links periodontal disease to other chronic illnesses.

RELEVANCE TO CLINICAL PRACTICE

There are two types of deposits in the oral cavity: soft deposits (biofilm, pellicle, materia alba, and food debris) and hard deposits (**calculus**). All deposits can attach to teeth, soft tissue, prosthetics, and restorative materials. The dental hygienist should identify soft and hard deposits, upon careful initial assessment of the patient's intraoral cavity.

Poor or neglected oral hygiene and diet are the two most common risk factors for caries formation. The regular removal of dental plaque biofilm, which contains the bacteria responsible for caries formation, gingivitis, and periodontitis, is the basis for maintaining dental health.[1] Mechanical disruption of the community structure of biofilm is necessary before damaging effects develop on the soft and hard tissue. Methods to control caries formation and periodontitis should include the prevention of biofilm growth.

SOFT DEPOSITS

The four types of soft deposits are *nonmineralized;* that is, they have not yet hardened into dental calculus. The four types, the acquired pellicle, biofilm, materia alba, and food debris, are discussed below.

Acquired Pellicle

Acquired pellicle is a thin film that coats the tooth immediately on exposure to saliva. **Pellicle formation** is the preconditioning stage that defines reversible–irreversible attachment of the colonizing bacteria on the tooth surface.[2] Immediately after tooth cleaning, bacteria left on the tooth surface and bacteria attaching to the tooth surface from other parts of the oral cavity, such as the tongue, gingiva, and cheek mucosa, begin to regrow.[3] The acquired pellicle protects the tooth from acids that can cause demineralization of the enamel surface. However, bacteria can attach to the acquired pellicle, then feed off of the components of the pellicle, creating an environment for the development of biofilm plaque. The bacteria associated with acquired pellicle and biofilm formation are:

1. *Streptococcus mutans*
2. *Streptococcus sanguinis,* formerly known as *Streptococcus sanguis*
3. *Actinomyces viscosus*

Tooth brushing does not remove the acquired pellicle. The pellicle remains and creates a rough surface on the teeth, which attracts and encourages plaque formation.

Biofilm

Although dental biofilm cannot be eradicated, it can be controlled with oral hygiene measures that include a daily regimen of brushing, interdental cleaning such as flossing, and rinsing with antimicrobial mouth rinses.[2] Dental biofilm contains the bacteria responsible for caries formation, gingivitis, and periodontitis. Its regular removal forms the basis of dental health.[1] See Chapter 19 for detailed information on flossing and other interdental cleaning aids.

Dental **biofilm** is a soft, sticky deposit that adheres to the teeth as a natural occurrence in the oral cavity (Fig. 13-1). Formation of biofilm occurs in a series of steps. First is the growth of acquired pellicle. Next is the growth and accumulation of bacteria, and the final step is developed, mature biofilm.

Biofilm is an accumulation of microbial cells within an organic matrix, optimizing the use of the available nutritional resources.[1] Contained within the matrix are polysaccharides, proteins, and DNA. Polysaccharides are sticky and promote adhesion of biofilm to the teeth. As the biofilm develops, it may be thought of as an

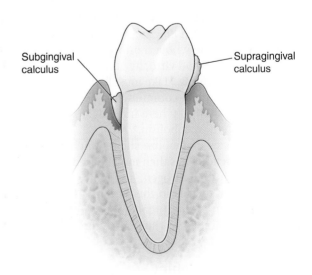

Figure 13-1. Supragingival and subgingival calculus.

ecosystem, containing many habitats and organisms.[1] Biofilm has organized structures that consist of numerous microorganisms and the sticky extracellular matrix they produce, the **glycocalyx,** which helps maintain the overall integrity of the biofilm.[4] The glycocalyx contains a network of channels and canals that exist within the biofilm, which allows for the exchange of nutrients between microbes and for the removal of their waste products.[4] Bacterial cells are continually transported to the pellicle-coated tooth surface through saliva, in association with dietary materials, or through other contact with the external environment. *S. sanguinis* has a stronger affinity for tooth enamel. Of all of the microbes present, the fewest numbers are of *S. mutans;* therefore, they have to compete for a tooth surface.[4] However, the only microorganisms that can colonize on the pellicle are those that can adhere to the pellicle-coated tooth surface or are in some other way retained.[4] Otherwise, saliva flow, chewing forces, and oral hygiene procedures would eliminate or clear them from the oral cavity.[4]

Supragingival biofilm accumulates on the clinical crown and **subgingival biofilm** is located within the periodontal pocket, or sulcus. Small amounts of supragingival biofilm can be difficult to detect clinically unless dyed using a disclosing solution or debriding the tooth surfaces with an instrument.[4]

In the gingival sulcus, an adherent, protected, and well-fed bacterial community accumulates and, eventually, biofilm forms on the tooth surface.[5] Gingivitis is the most common form of periodontal disease, and the most common form of gingivitis found in the general population is gingivitis associated with dental biofilm, also called *biofilm-associated gingivitis,* or gingivitis. This disease is directly related to the presence of bacterial biofilm.[1]

Cellular Communication of Biofilm

Although there are more than 400 species of bacteria in the oral cavity, only a few are associated with periodontal disease. Recent studies have shown that the bacteria in biofilm can communicate through chemical signals or, in some cases, with electric signals along so-called nanowires so that the whole community can coordinate its response to stress and virtually guarantee its predominance in all ecosystems.[5] Like most biofilm in the environment, the microbial communities in the oral cavity are polyspecies biofilm, where individual species differ in their respective metabolism.[5] Most *Streptococcus* and *Actinomyces* species metabolize sugars, such as glucose, to lactic acid. Lactic acid is then metabolized and broken down further into hydrogen, methane, and carbon dioxide by other species in the biofilm. The microbial community often forms broad food webs, in which nutrients are degraded to their basic components and turned into energy.[5]

Microbiology of Biofilm

Gingivitis is directly associated to the amount of biofilm and how long it has been present. So-called healthy biofilm contains gram-positive bacteria aerobes, which are usually not motile. However, when left undisturbed, the biofilm continues to mature and increase in size. The gram-positive bacteria begin to die, the plaque gets thicker, and the type of bacteria becomes gram-negative, anaerobic, and motile. When gram-negative bacteria die, the cells give off an endotoxin, increasing the inflammation process.

The biofilm in a healthy gingival crevice is typically dominated by relatively few bacteria of aerobe *Streptococcus* species, which require a fairly high oxygen level. Other species prefer a lower oxygen concentration, such as facultative anaerobe *Actinomyces,* anaerobic *Fusobacteria,* or *Capnocytophaga.* They are present in small numbers within the gingival sulcus.[5] The healthy microbial community in the gingival sulcus is in a permanent dynamic balance with the immune response of the host and his or her state of oral hygiene.[6,7] The increased amount of bacteria is accompanied by the growth of excreted bacterial metabolic by-products, which initiate the damage to the surrounding tissue and trigger inflammation.[8]

Materia Alba

Dental biofilm is distinguished from materia alba by the strength and adherence of the deposit.[1] **Materia alba** can be described as a loosely attached accumulation of bacteria that can be easily removed by mechanical actions such as vigorous rinsing or a strong spray of water. The color is generally white to yellow, and it has a thick, cottage-cheese-like texture.

Food Debris

Food debris is food that remains in the mouth after eating. Natural movement of the tongue and saliva flow will dislodge food to wash away. Rinsing with water or mouth rinse will also aid in removing debris.

ORAL MALODOR

Halitosis is an oral condition characterized by noticeable malodorous smell that is emitted during breathing or speaking. Halitosis can impact an individual's life socially and professionally. It can be caused by many factors, including oral conditions, as well as systemic factors. Also, particular foods (garlic and onions) and medications can be associated with bad breath. About 80% to 90% of cases are directly related to the hard and soft tissues of the oral cavity. Poor oral hygiene, including accumulated biofilm, materia alba, and food debris, coated tongue, extensive decay, periodontal disease, food impaction areas, and poorly contoured restorations can be associated with malodor in the oral cavity. Also, tonsilloliths (tonsil stones), air passages (sinuses, nostrils), gastrointestinal esophageal reflux disease, kidney disease, liver disease, and ketoacidosis associated with diabetes mellitus can all be associated with oral malodor.

HARD DEPOSITS

Hard deposits are calculus, which is biofilm that is mineralized, or calcified.

Calculus Formation

Calcium and phosphate salts are deposited into the biofilm that remains on the tooth surface. These salts occur naturally in saliva and gingival crevicular fluids. Although calculus contributes to gingivitis and periodontal disease, the cause of periodontal disease is biofilm. Calculus has been shown to have nonmineralized areas, which appear microscopically as channels that contain bacteria and other debris.[9] In turn, calculus provides a shelter for biofilm, which contains bacteria, holding it close to the tissues within the periodontal pocket. Calculus mineralization takes 24 to 72 hours; complete maturation, on average, is 12 days.

Calculus Location

Calculus is either supragingival or subgingival. It is often covered with plaque biofilm. **Supragingival (salivary) calculus** is defined as calculus located above the gingival margin. It appears creamy white to yellow and changes color as it is exposed to foods and tobacco products. Where large amounts of supragingival calculus are present, removal of these deposits will also be necessary for effective personal oral hygiene to be achieved. **Subgingival (serumal) calculus** is defined as calculus that forms apical to the gingival margin. It is usually dark to black, due to the blood pigment, hemosiderin. It is not visible through an oral examination but is often seen with a radiographic examination. The inorganic makeup is primarily calcium; the organic makeup contains no salivary protein, only serum protein. If not removed, gingival enlargement can occur as a response to irritation caused by calculus, or plaque, repeated friction or trauma, fluctuations in hormone levels, or the use of some medications. Calculus, a local risk factor, may increase the risk for periodontal diseases. One study showed that deposits of subgingival calculus covered with biofilm were directly related to more than 60% of pocket wall inflammation as measured by increased redness of the pocket epithelium. This was in comparison with biofilm alone.[10]

Forms of Calculus

There are three forms of calculus: (a) **Calculus rings** are a layer of calculus that encircles the buccal or lingual surface of the tooth, either subgingival or supragingival; (b) **calculus spicules** are small, needle-like or pointed pieces of calculus at the line angle that appear on the mesial and distal surfaces of the tooth; and (c) **calculus ledges** are subgingival, shelf-like pieces of calculus that accumulated parallel to the cementoenamel junction of the tooth.

Calculus Detection

Calculus detection is very important for the prevention of periodontal disease. Calculus can be detected through clinical examination, radiography, and by exploration. During an assessment of the patient, it is essential to determine the type, amount, and location of calculus for it to be effectively removed (Table 13-1).

Supragingival calculus can be identified visually or by gently blowing a stream of compressed air on the deposit. However, subgingival calculus is not visible, so the clinician must rely on the use of an explorer for detection. It is important for the dental hygienist to have strong knowledge of tooth anatomy to be able to recognize irregularities on the tooth surface and not cause damage to the tooth (see Professionalism).

The explorer is used before, during, and after periodontal debridement. An explorer is an assessment instrument with a flexible, wirelike working end, which quivers or clicks as it is moved over tooth surface irregularities such as dental calculus. Several types of explorers may be used for subgingival calculus detection. The most common are the curved explorer, pigtail or cowhorn explorer, and the 11/12 explorer. The curved explorer is used for calculus detection in normal sulci or a shallow pocket. The pigtail or cowhorn explorer is used for normal sulci or a shallow pocket extending no deeper than the cervical third of the root. The 11/12 explorer is used in normal sulci or shallow pockets, as well as in deep periodontal pockets.[11] See Procedure 13-1: Calculus Detection.

Professionalism

Participation with the American Dental Hygienists' Association (ADHA) is an important aspect of professionalism. Knowing and following the organization's code of ethics is the dental hygienist's professional responsibility. According to the ADHA, the practicing dental hygienist is responsible for three levels of care: (a) prevention, (b) therapeutic scaling and root planing, and (c) supportive periodontal maintenance. Patient education is an essential area of the profession of dental hygiene. Having the knowledge to improve the patient's quality of life and decrease health disparities is vital. ■

Table 13-1. Calculus Detection

Type of Calculus	Amount of Calculus	Location of Calculus
Rings	Mild	Subgingival
Spicules	Moderate	Supragingival
Ledges	Heavy	Generalized
		Localized

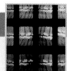

Procedure 13-1 Calculus Detection

MATERIALS AND PREPARATION

Gather and organize the necessary materials before the patient's arrival.

Materials

Mirror	Air/water syringe tip
For direct or indirect vision of supragingival calculus deposits	Personal protective equipment
Subgingival explorer	For rinsing and drying tooth surface during exploration
To detect calculus deposits	

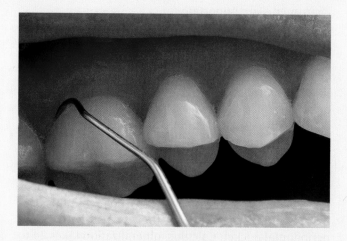

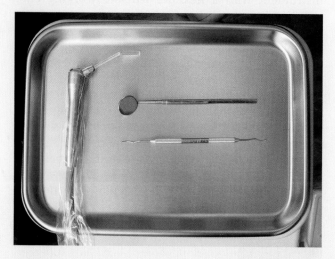

Preprocedure

Consider having the patient rinse with a product containing an antimicrobial product such as chlorhexidine gluconate, essential oils, or povidone iodine, which reduce the level of oral microorganisms generated in aerosols or spatter during routine dental procedures with rotary instruments. They can decrease the number of microorganisms introduced into the patient's bloodstream during invasive dental procedures. The American Heart Association recommends that patients at risk for bacterial endocarditis use an antimicrobial mouth rinse before dental treatment. However, more studies are needed to determine whether a preprocedural mouth rinse can reduce the risk for bacteremia caused by oral procedures and the relationship of bacteremia to disease.

PATIENT EDUCATION

Explain the procedure for calculus detection and answer any questions the patient or caregiver poses.

Procedure

1. Put on personal protective equipment.
2. Place the working end of the explorer above the gingival margin, flush with the tooth.

3. Keeping the explorer modified to the tooth surface, lightly slide the tip under the gingival margin.
4. Gently move the explorer to the base of the pocket. At all times be attentive for "quivers" or a "clicking" sound of the explorer, indicating calculus deposits.
   - Assess the base of the pocket first.
   - Move the explorer to the middle third of the tooth within the pocket.
   - Then move the explorer closest to the gingival margin.
5. Move the explorer in small up-and-down or "walking" strokes, 2 to 3 mm at a time, keeping the tip constantly adapted to the tooth.
6. Move the explorer across the entire root surface, covering every area. Do not continually remove the explorer from the pocket and reinsert it, because this can cause trauma or otherwise injure the tissue.
7. Use the side of the tip of the explorer for assessment of the mesial and distal surfaces of the tooth.
   - Insert the explorer on the mesial or distal surface from the buccal surface to the base of the pocket, continuing halfway through to the lingual surface.
   - When exploring mesial or distal surface from the lingual, continue halfway through to the buccal surface. This ensures that all areas of the interproximal sulcus will be explored.
8. Record subgingival calculus deposits on the assessment form.

Postprocedure

- Discuss the findings with the patient or caregiver, or both.
- Document the procedure in the patient's record.

Calculus Removal

Ultrasonic devices, electrical instruments, and hand instruments are important for calculus removal. Along with supragingival scaling, root planing and subgingival scaling are necessary. Removing calculus reduces the rough surface and, in turn, reduces the amount of biofilm that can attach to the tooth. However, it is not the intention to deliberately remove tooth substance. Although the goal is to mechanically remove microbial plaque and calculus without any intentional removal of the root surface, it is accepted that because root surface instrumentation is conducted blind in most cases, some removal of the root surface cementum may inadvertently occur. See Spotlight on Public Health.

THE BODY'S RESPONSE TO BIOFILM AND CALCULUS

Inflammation is the end result of biofilm that remains in the oral cavity. Gingivitis, periodontal disease, and tooth decay are all diseases associated with plaque biofilm. The body responds to plaque biofilm with an inflammatory response. If not removed, plaque biofilm can cause chronic inflammation, which leads to destruction of alveolar bone, as well as gingival and connective tissue. Also, chronic inflammation has been associated with a host of chronic health conditions.

Recently, a great deal of emphasis has been placed on the association between the oral cavity and the overall health of the individual. Clinical research shows a direct link between chronic inflammatory conditions such as periodontal disease, heart and lung disease, premature birth, low birth weight, and diabetes. The primary bacteria responsible for periodontal disease are present in saliva and can be passed from one individual to another. It is the responsibility of the dental hygienist to recognize if a patient has periodontal disease, to provide the appropriate treatment, and to prevent future systemic complications. More information on this topic can be found in Chapter 5.

STAINING AND TOOTH DISCOLORATION

Teeth can be discolored by intrinsic or extrinsic stains. Some stains can be removed to improve appearance, whereas others cannot be treated.

Intrinsic Stains

Intrinsic staining is a discoloration of the teeth from within. The tooth shade cannot be altered through scaling, root planing, or polishing procedures. The dental hygienist recognizes the patient's concerns and educates him or her on possible options for shade alterations.

Intrinsic endogenous stain occurs during tooth development and is incorporated into the structure of the tooth. Dental fluorosis, tetracycline (and related antibiotics), nonvital pulp, tooth trauma, defective tooth development, and endodontic therapy are all common reasons for intrinsic endogenous stain. The use of the antibiotic tetracycline in pregnant women and children younger than 12 years is strongly advised against.

Intrinsic exogenous stain is staining that occurs within the tooth because of changes from outside sources. Extrinsic stains such as those caused by smoking and use of smokeless tobacco products, such as chewing tobacco, dissolvable tobacco, and snuff, can alter the intrinsic shade of teeth. Also included are patients with a tendency to accumulate green stain. Green stain has a clinical appearance of yellowish green to dark green and is primarily found on children's maxillary anterior teeth at the cervical line. Its exact cause is unknown, but after it is removed, usually self-care can prevent its reoccurrence. Dental caries can also discolor the tooth chalky white to brown-black. Tooth-colored restorations can be stained by extrinsic factors and alter the intrinsic color of the tooth. Metals such as amalgam, an alloy of mercury with various metals used for dental fillings, can alter the color to gray. As individuals age, their teeth tend to darken or become more yellow in appearance because enamel becomes thinner with age and the dentin, which is darker, begins to show through.

Spotlight on Public Health

A direct association exists between socioeconomic status and oral health. Individuals of a low socioeconomic status have a greater risk for untreated caries and periodontal disease. According to the World Health Organization World Oral Health Report 2003, "Because of high prevalence and incidence in all regions of the world, oral disease is a major health problem."[12] Advancements have been made to increase access to care throughout the world. Currently, within the United States, many states are introducing the mid-level oral health practitioner that will enable the dental hygienist to practice unsupervised in a public health-care setting, bridging the gap of health disparities. The American Dental Hygienists' Association (ADHA) has defined a mid-level oral health practitioner as follows: "A licensed dental hygienist who has graduated from an accredited dental hygiene program and who provides primary oral health care directly to patients to promote and restore oral health through assessment, diagnosis, treatment, evaluation, and referral services. The mid-level oral health practitioner has met the educational requirements to provide services within an expanded scope of care and practices under regulations set forth by the appropriate licensing agency."[13] ■

Extrinsic Stains

Extrinsic staining on teeth occurs generally because of external factors. The most common attributing factor for extrinsic stain is poor oral hygiene. The inability to prevent stain-producing materials from attaching to teeth contributes to the accumulation of stain. Smoking/tobacco use, certain foods, coffee, tea, colas, red wine, stannous fluoride, chlorhexidine 0.12% rinses, betel nut, and minerals from some water systems contribute to extrinsic stains (Table 13-2). See Chapter 30 for detailed information on stains and their treatment.

Table 13-2. Extrinsic Stains

Stain	Cause of Stain
Brown stain	Occurs readily after prophylaxis, chemical alteration of pellicle, smooth.
Black line stain	Usually follows the gingival margin, pits and fissures. Black stain is recognized as microorganisms in an intermicrobial substance. It can occur in all age groups and is more common in children.
Orange/red stain	Usually seen on the cervical third of the tooth. Although recognized, it is not common. Most frequently seen on facial and lingual surfaces of the anterior teeth.
Yellow stain	Caused by cigarettes, cigars, pipes, and tobacco chewing. The stain can occur on any tooth surface. It is seen as thick, tenacious, and light to dark brown, even black.
Betel leaf stain	Caused primarily by microorganisms that are mineralized on the tooth surface. This stain is dark brown, almost black; it can be thick, hard, smooth, and rough; it occurs in all ages; and it is found more often in Eastern countries.

Case Study

Mr. Smith has a history of cigarette smoking, drinking coffee, and poor oral hygiene. Documented on his chart from his last visit were moderate subgingival and supragingival calculus, moderate yellow-brown extrinsic stain, and posterior bleeding on probing. Chlorhexidine 0.12% rinse was prescribed to reduce the bleeding, and Mr. Smith was scheduled for a re-evaluation in 6 weeks. Mr. Smith canceled the appointment and advised the front office manager that he would call to reschedule. That was 18 months ago. When asked why he did not return to the dental office as recommended, Mr. Smith replies that he lost his dental insurance because of cutbacks at work. Money is tight and he made an appointment only because he has noticed recent generalized sensitivity. Upon her intraoral examination of Mr. Smith, the dental hygienist notices his oral cavity is worse than she suspected. He now has heavy subgingival and supragingival calculus. The stain appears to be heavier than before, black in the anterior region and dark brown elsewhere. She notices generalized recession, especially in the anterior region, and localized mobility in the maxillary and mandibular anterior areas. She feels frustrated.

Case Study Exercises

1. What is most likely the reason for the increase in sensitivity?
   A. Mr. Smith has heavy calculus and needs his teeth cleaned
   B. The localized mobility in the anterior region
   C. The generalized recession
   D. Both A and B
2. Why is there an increase in the amount of stain on Mr. Smith's teeth?
   A. It has been 18 months since his last prophylaxis
   B. He has a history of poor oral hygiene
   C. The past use of chlorhexidine
   D. All of the above
3. Why is there more bleeding on probing in the posterior than the anterior region?
   A. Because there is more calculus in the posterior region.
   B. Mr. Smith has a history of smoking and the tissue in the anterior area is keratinized.
   C. Mr. Smith only flosses the anterior teeth.
   D. None of the above.

Case Study—cont'd

4. What is the most effective way to detect the subgingival calculus?
   A. Through a visual examination
   B. Through radiographs
   C. Exploring subgingival with an Exp. 11/12 explorer
   D. Both B and C

5. What would be the dental hygienist's most effective use of time at this visit?
   A. Use the ultrasonic scaler to remove stain and large pieces of calculus so Mr. Smith can see how nice his teeth can look.
   B. Scold Mr. Smith for canceling his last appointment.
   C. Take and develop a complete series of radiographs; complete a new periodontal charting including periodontal probing, recession, and mobility; and explain to Mr. Smith the severity of his periodontal disease.
   D. Reprobe Mr. Smith's mouth.

Review Questions

1. Hard and soft deposits can attach to:
   A. Teeth
   B. Soft tissue
   C. Prosthetics
   D. Restorative material
   E. All of the above

2. The preconditioning stage of biofilm attachment is considered:
   A. Materia alba
   B. Acquired pellicle
   C. Glycocalyx
   D. None of the above

3. The primary purpose of acquired pellicle is to:
   A. Encourage bacterial biofilm to attach to the teeth
   B. Stimulate absorption of fluoride ions into the teeth
   C. Protect the teeth from potential acid attacks
   D. All of the above

4. Which of the following is NOT a primary bacterium associated with biofilm formation?
   A. *Streptococcus mutans*
   B. *Streptococcus sanguinis*
   C. *Actinomyces viscosus*
   D. *Streptococcus viscosus*

5. Plaque biofilm is a hard deposit that adheres to teeth as a natural occurrence. Formation of plaque biofilm occurs in one distinct step.
   A. First statement is true, but second statement is false.
   B. Both statements are true.
   C. Second statement is true, but first statement is false.
   D. Both statements are false.

Active Learning

1. Working with a partner, take turns practicing the calculus detection procedure detailed in this chapter. Evaluate each other for preparation, thoroughness in completing all steps, and patient education and communication.

2. Prepare a brief PowerPoint presentation explaining the differences among biofilm, materia alba, and food debris and their effects on dental health. ■

REFERENCES

1. Gorur A, Lyle D, Schaudinn C. Biofilm removal with a dental waterjet. *Compend Contin Educ Dent.* 2009;30 (Spec No 1):1-6.
2. Thomas J, Nakaishi L. Managing the complexity of a dynamic biofilm. *J Am Dent Assoc.* 2006;137:10S-15S.
3. Stoody P, Wefel J, Gieseke A, deBeer D, von Ohle C. Biofilm plaque and hydrodynamic effects on mass transfer, fluoride delivery and caries. *J Am Dent Assoc.* 2008;139:1182-1190.
4. Perry D, Beemsterboer P. *Periodontology for the Dental Hygienist.* 4th ed. St. Louis, MO: Saunders; 2013:63-123.
5. Costerton J, Schaudinn C. The secret life of biofilm. *Dimens Dent Hyg.* 2011(suppl):2-22.

6. Slots J. Microflora in the healthy gingival sulcus in man. *Scand J Dent Res.* 1977;85:247-254.

7. Listgarten MA. The structure of dental plaque. *Periodontol 2000.* 1994;5:52-65.

8. Rateitschak KH, Rateitschak Elanten EM, Wolf E. *Farbatlanten der Zahnmedizin.* Stuttgart/New York: Thieme Verlag; 1984. *Parodontologie*; vol 9.

9. Grenwell H, Armitage GC, Mealey BL. Local contributing factors. In: Rose LF, Meaaley BL, eds. *Periodontics: Medicine, Surgery, and Implants.* St. Louis, MO: Mosby; 2004:117-130.

10. Wilson TG, Harrel SK, Nunn ME, Francis B, Webb K. The relationship between the presence of tooth-borne subgingival deposits and inflammation found with a dental endoscope. *J Periodontol.* 2008;79(11):2029-2035.

11. Nield-Gehrig J. *Fundamentals of Periodontal Instrumentation & Advanced Root Instrumentation.* 7th ed. Philadelphia: Lippincott Williams & Wilkins; 2012:162-274.

12. Petersen PE. The World Oral Health Report 2003: continuous improvement of oral health in the 21st century – the approach of the WHO Global Oral Health Programme. Community Dentistry and Oral Epidemiology, Volume 31, Issue Supplement s1, pages 3–24, December 2003.

13. American Dental Hygienists' Association. Oral Preventive Assistant (OPA) Background. February 19, 2015. https://www.adha.org/resources-docs/OPA_Memo_2-18-2015.pdf. Accessed July 25, 2015.

Chapter 14 | Indices

Christine Charles, RDH, BS

KEY TERMS

calibration

data

dichotomous scale

index

irreversible index

mean score

ordinal scale

reliability

reversible index

Russell periodontal index

validity

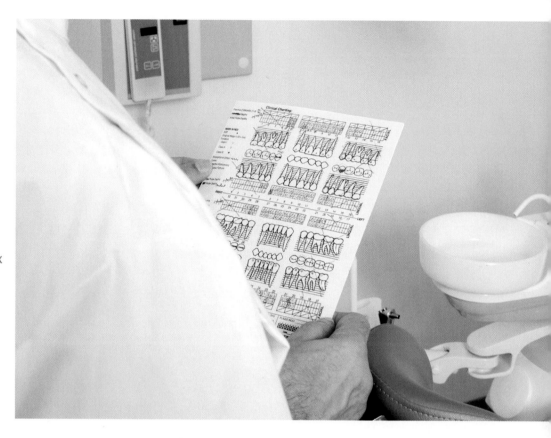

LEARNING OBJECTIVES

After reading this chapter, the student should be able to:

14.1 Describe the characteristics of a suitable or ideal index.

14.2 Explain the advantages and disadvantages of a useful index and indicate if it is appropriate for monitoring dental hygiene patients.

14.3 Choose a periodontal assessment tool for a new patient to determine: (a) periodontal problem, (b) treatment plan, (c) risk factors for future disease, (d) patient education plan, and (e) sequence of appointments.

14.4 Explain how indices are useful as an epidemiological tool.

14.5 Discuss the relationship of indices to evidence-based practice.

KEY CONCEPTS

- Oral indices translate a clinical picture into a numerical tool for comparisons of interest to characterize oral health status and provide evidence-based dental and dental hygiene care.
- Oral indices are helpful tools in risk assessment and needs assessment.
- Selection of an index depends on the question of interest or the purpose of evaluation.
- Indices provide feedback that determines success of care or opportunities for modifying patient care.

RELEVANCE TO CLINICAL PRACTICE

Assessment of the oral condition of the dental patient is essential to determine his or her current status of health and cleanliness, and it serves as the basis for problem identification or diagnoses and therapeutic interventions (see Application to Clinical Practice 1). One of the tools for oral health assessment is a clinical **index,** which is simply a scoring system or measuring device. For example, the periodontal probe can be used like a ruler to measure the height of calculus on the six mandibular lingual incisor teeth (Volpe-Manhold Index [VMI]) or to measure the depth of the gingival sulcus (clinical probing depth). An index used for oral health assessment can be a tool for evaluating, educating, and motivating the patient; it can be used to create a treatment plan and to monitor changes over time to measure the success of personal disease-control efforts. Indices can be used to help a patient recognize an oral problem, reveal the proficiency of current oral hygiene procedures, motivate a patient to eliminate or control oral disease, and evaluate the success of patient and professional treatment over a period. Indices are also an important tool for documentation and recordkeeping. Indices may also provide some measure of the dental hygienist's capability, not only as an educator or motivator but also as a clinician. Indices can be a reflection of the success of types of services provided.

Application to Clinical Practice 1

Dental indices (data created by clinical observations that are translated into numbers) provide an oral health assessment record so the entire dental and health-care team can make informed decisions based on evidence to provide the best outcome for the patient. ■

WHAT ARE INDICES?

An index is a method of converting the observed severity of a parameter of interest into a numerical form that is amenable to statistical analysis. For an index to be considered useful, there must be an established relationship between severities (of the index of interest) and actual clinical changes accompanying the progression or regression of disease.

The famous British mathematician and physicist Lord Kelvin (1824–1907) remarked, "Until you can count it, weigh it, or express it in a quantitative fashion, you have scarcely begun to think about the problem in a scientific fashion." This really is the essence of indices. Indices are the pillar of epidemiological studies and dental product and procedure evaluations.

A suitable or ideal index should be simple to use, and the criteria describing the scores should be clear and easily understood. The index scores should be equally sensitive throughout the range of the index, indicate the clinical stages of disease, and be amenable to statistical analysis. An index should also be acceptable to the study subject, valid, reliable, quick and practical, and clinically significant to the researcher or clinician.

Indices are used in private practice and in clinical research, public health surveys, and industry, and no single index has universal application or acceptance.[1] An index is appropriate only if it can achieve the goals of accurate assessment and documentation of the individual patient or the objective(s) of the clinical trial in which it is used.[2] First, an examiner needs to be trained on the index and then establish **calibration,** or agreement with an experienced user of the index; for example, the trainer scores a gingival unit as 3 and the learner also scores 3—this is agreement. Another consideration when using indices, especially for research purposes, is establishing examiner **reliability,** or repeatability. Analysis of the individual index scores between examiners, or within repeated measurements by one examiner, will determine the degree of agreement. When an examiner or clinician is calibrated, agreement with the trainer is reached and then reliability should be determined. Observations and measurements need to be objective, precise, and reproducible, as summed up by this quote from Fleiss in 1986: "The most elegant design of a clinical study will not overcome the damage caused by unreliable or imprecise measurement."[3]

When more than one examiner is used in a longitudinal clinical trial or a large epidemiological survey, interexaminer reliability (between-examiner agreement) is key to the success of the study so that all examiners are using the index scale in the same way. Individual repeatability or intraexaminer reliability (within-examiner agreement) should be established. Just like buying paint, if someone needs to purchase a second can in the same color, he or she wants to know that the color of the second can will match perfectly with that of the first. An examiner or clinician should be repeatable in his or her interpretation and use of the index over the course of the research study or over the course of time. For example, if a patient is seen every 6 months, and an index of oral hygiene is determined on that patient at each visit, to have confidence in that index score as representing the clinical condition, the hygienist should be able to replicate the way the index was used and the conditions under which the **data** were collected each time the patient is seen. Otherwise, any change in the numerical index could either be reflective of the patient's oral health status or could be a change in how the clinician applied the index. Furthermore, the hygienist should document which index is used each time, because a score of 2 in one index may reflect a very different condition than a score of 2 using another index. If treatment decisions are based on that data, it is important to know variability of the examiner or clinician collecting the data, as well as the description of the scores used. It is important to remember that indices are just one of many procedures for patient assessment, such as medical history, vital signs, intraoral and extraoral examination, radiographs, microbiological or salivary diagnostic tests, and when indicated, brush biopsy. Selection of an index is based on your question of interest and what you wish to measure. Indices used in practice may be very different from what a researcher or epidemiologist may choose (see Professionalism).

TYPES OF CLINICAL INDICES

Clinical indices are similar to thermostats or gas gauges in that they are tools to help make decisions, to help determine whether a patient's oral condition is on the healthy side or more on the diseased side. The hygienist's observations may be refined by translating a patient's clinical picture into numbers, which then may be helpful in making treatment, product, and oral and lifestyle recommendations, as well as for patient records and documentation purposes (see Teamwork).

Clinical indices have many uses, including:

- Assessing individual patients
- Evaluating agents or procedures for prevention, reduction, or control of oral diseases or conditions as part of clinical trials
- Quantifying the amount or severity, or both, of a disease or condition in communities or populations
- Contributing to overall oral disease risk assessment

Clinical indices can be as simple as those based on a **dichotomous scale,** which is a measurement based on two variables only. This is when the variable of interest (e.g., bleeding or plaque) is either

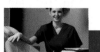

Professionalism

Dental professionals from the private practice clinician to the researcher use indices to benefit patients. The hygienist may use a plaque index to impress upon a patient the need for better oral hygiene, whereas the researcher may use the same index to assess the home-care practices of a population. Indices will continue to be important and necessary tools for dental professionals. As a professional, it is important to keep abreast of the literature that can provide an evidence base for your recommendations and for your practice of dental hygiene. In addition, when reviewing literature, advertisements, or professional sales materials, it is helpful to be able to recognize some commonly used indices. The hygienist needs to be knowledgeable in assessing this information so that he or she can answer questions that patients raise and feel comfortable making evidence-based recommendations for patients' home care. ■

Teamwork

Your colleague is busy handling an emergency in the office, so you seat her patient, review the patient's chart, review the indices recorded at the last visit, update the medical history, and conduct an indices assessment. When your colleague is ready to see her patient, you can quickly paint a verbal picture of the oral condition changes by comparing the indices over the last three visits. Your colleague can now start thinking about the visit treatment and patient education needs based on the summary of indices. She is very grateful and acknowledges your contribution to the office team in caring for her patient. ■

present or absent, with no concern for quantifying any further. Clinical indices can also be more complex and use an **ordinal scale,** where the variable of interest is quantified by severity or extent (e.g., periodontal indices), and there are distinct definitions for each score in the graduated scale with upper and lower limits. Clinical indices can also be reversible or irreversible. **Reversible indices** are those that measure reversibility, or what damage or factors can be reversed, including, for example, some plaque biofilm and debris indices, gingival indices, and some bleeding indices. These indices are frequently used in the dental office to illustrate patient progress at recall appointments but can also be used in epidemiological surveys and in clinical research studies.

The DMFT (decayed, missing, filled teeth) or DMFS (decayed, missing, or filled teeth/surfaces) index is a very commonly used index for evaluating caries status and risk, and it is used in the private office, research, and population surveys. It is considered an **irreversible index.** This index has been used in large populations and caries trials to demonstrate the benefits of water fluoridation or fluoride-containing dentifrices and mouth rinses.

Dental Caries Indices

The most widely used index to assess the dental caries experience in a person or population is the DMFT or the more detailed DMFS index.[4] Both of these indices provide a past and present caries status on all permanent teeth excluding third molars or unerupted teeth (for primary dentition, scoring is referred to as *deft* or *defs*[5] and used for 7- to 12-year-olds). In a mixed dentition situation, the index is determined separately for the permanent and the primary teeth or surfaces. A mirror, explorer, and adequate light are needed and preferably an assistant to record the scores for the examiner.

Evidence-Based Practice

It is important to understand the hierarchy of evidence-based medicine or dentistry, with meta-analysis and systematic reviews at the top of the pyramid, followed by randomized controlled clinical trials, and with decreasing quality of evidence to the base of the pyramid with laboratory studies and opinions. Therefore, a basic understanding of clinical indices that will be found in reading the dental literature helps the dental hygienist to transfer evidence into clinical recommendations or practice and to monitor the benefit that his or her services and recommendations may be having on a patient's oral health at each visit. ■

The scores[6] are assigned as follows:

0—Sound crown or root, showing no evidence of treated or untreated decay (caries)

1—A definite decay (temporary fillings and teeth that are sealed but also decayed are also scored 1)

2—Filled teeth, with additional decay

3—Filled tooth with no decay or crowned tooth due to prior decay (if crowned for other reason it does not count as filled)

4—Missing tooth as a result of decay

5—Missing tooth for any other reason than decay (e.g., extractions for orthodontic or periodontal disease reasons, congenitally missing teeth)

6—Teeth with sealants placed

7—Tooth that is part of a fixed bridge, teeth with veneers or laminates covering the facial surface

8—Space with an unerupted permanent tooth where no primary tooth is present (these are excluded from the calculation of caries)

9—Erupted teeth that cannot be examined, for example, because of orthodontic banding

T—Indicates trauma, for example, when crown is fractured and some of surface is missing but with no evidence of decay

The DMFT calculation is performed as follows: D = all teeth scored 1 or 2, M = all teeth scored 4 in subjects younger than 30 years and scored 4 or 5 in subjects older than 30 years. F = all teeth scored 3. All scores of 6, 7, 8, 9, or T are not included in DMFT calculation. To determine DMFT, determine the number of teeth with D, E (extracted), and F; for example, a patient with 2 areas of decay, 6 missing teeth, and 11 filled or crowned teeth has a DMFT of 19. Teeth that include both decay and fillings or crowns are given only a D.

The DMFS calculation is performed as follows: The DMFT calculation applies except that anterior teeth have 4 surfaces scored and posterior teeth have 5 surfaces scored such that a full dentition of 32 teeth has 128 surfaces. For a patient with 7 decayed surfaces, 20 missing surfaces, and 42 filled or crowned surfaces, the DMFS score is 69. When determining the index for a group, total the individual DMFT or DMFS and divide by the number of individuals; for example, if for 40 individuals the total DMFT is 360, then the group mean DMFT is 9.0.

The World Health Organization (WHO) developed the significant caries (SiC) index[6] in 2000. It is used when studying DMFT scores on a global basis. The SiC index isolates and highlights those individuals with the highest caries values in a particular population. Individuals are sorted according to DMFT values. The third of the population with the highest caries scores is isolated and a mean DMFT for this subgroup is calculated.

In epidemiological surveys, such as the National Health and Nutrition Examination Survey (NHANES), indices are used to assess the prevalence (total number of people manifesting a particular condition) and incidence (extent to which new cases exist within a population) of dental disease(s) in a given population, as well as risk factors for diseases. In addition, NHANES data are used as the basis for national standards of measurements such as height, weight, and blood pressure. Findings from the survey fuel additional health science research, including oral health research, and can be used to determine health policies. NHANES can be used to estimate future oral health needs, as well as treatment and preventive procedures. The data contribute to evidence-based dentistry and dental hygiene practice (see Spotlight on Public Health).[7]

Indices That Measure Oral Hygiene Status (Plaque Biofilm, Debris, and Calculus)

Indices used in dental hygiene practice provide a means of assessing oral hygiene status by measuring criteria such as the degree to which calculus has accumulated, plaque has built up on the teeth, and the degree or extent of extrinsic tooth stain that may be present. These indices provide a means not only to evaluate the oral cleanliness of a patient, but they serve as a means to educate and motivate the patient as well. Lifestyle factors that may affect a patient's oral health and pose risk for oral health problems can also be measured with indices. Clinical trials and other research studies also use indices as observational tools to evaluate oral health and efficacy of different products or treatment modalities. These indices can differ from indices used in practice in both intent and approach. Some commonly used indices that measure oral hygiene status are listed in Table 14-1.

Plaque Indices

Many indices are available to assess the location and quantity of plaque. Some indices are better suited for

Table 14-1. *Indices That Measure Oral Hygiene Status (Biofilm, Debris, and Calculus)*

Index	Purpose
Simplified oral hygiene index (OHI-S)[8]	To measure debris and calculus—one of the first indices developed
Plaque control record[9]	To record the presence of plaque biofilm on four surfaces of each tooth (mesial, distal, facial, lingual)—good for clinical practice
Rustogi modification of the Navy Plaque Index[10]	To determine plaque removal efficiency—good for research purposes
Silness Löe Plaque Index[11]	To assess thickness of plaque—good for clinical practice
Quigley-Hein Plaque Index[12–14]	To determine plaque area, especially the Turesky modification—good for research and clinical practice
Volpe-Manhold Index (VMI)[15–17]	To measure calculus—used in research
Lobene stain index[18]	To measure extrinsic tooth stain area and intensity—used in research, especially the MacPherson modification of the Lobene index

research, epidemiology studies, or clinical hygiene practice documentation or patient motivation. One of the original oral cleanliness indices is the oral hygiene index (OHI), which measures both debris and calculus[8] and has been used for surveys and patient evaluation. The OHI combines several variables into one index, as shown in Table 14-2. Even with changes in terminology (recently the term *plaque biofilm*, rather than *debris*, is preferred) and ways of evaluating patients (plaque biofilm and calculus are now evaluated separately, each with its own index), this is still a viable tool in clinical practice for characterizing the oral cleanliness of patients and comparing the index from visit to visit. The index is calculated as follows: Assess tooth surface area covered by plaque/debris on six teeth (#3, #8, #14, #19, #24, #30) by using tip of probe or explorer and record score for each tooth; total; and divide by the number of teeth scored. The same is done for presence of calculus. The dental hygienist can use each individually or add together.

Plaque Control Record

The Plaque Control Record[9] allows the therapist or the patient to determine where the plaque biofilm is present on the teeth and measure patient progress in

Table 14-2. *Oral Hygiene Index*

Debris Score	Calculus Score
0—No debris or stain present	0—No calculus present
1—Soft debris covering not more than one third of the tooth surface being examined, or the presence of extrinsic stains without debris regardless of surface area covered	1—Supragingival calculus covering not more than one third of the exposed tooth surface being examined
2—Soft debris covering more than one third but not more than two thirds of the exposed tooth surface	2—Supragingival calculus covering more than one third but not more than two thirds of the exposed tooth surface, or the presence of individual flecks of subgingival calculus around the cervical portion of the tooth
3—Soft debris covering more than two thirds of the exposed tooth surface	3—Supragingival calculus covering more than two thirds of the exposed tooth surface, or a continuous band of subgingival calculus around the cervical portion of the tooth

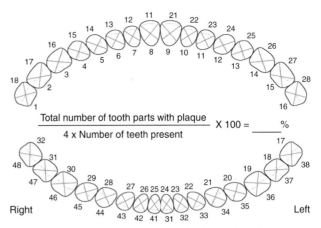

$$\frac{\text{Total number of tooth parts with plaque}}{4 \times \text{Number of teeth present}} \times 100 = \underline{\qquad} \%$$

Figure 14-1. Plaque control record. Divide the number of plaque-containing surfaces by the total number of tooth surfaces scored. In this example, 40 plaque-containing surfaces (4 surfaces of each of 10 teeth: 10×4) ÷ 40 tooth surfaces scored = 100%.

learning how to efficiently practice oral hygiene; it also can be used as a motivational tool. This examination system was developed to record the presence of plaque biofilm (a dichotomous scale) on four surfaces of each tooth—mesial, distal, facial, and lingual (Fig. 14-1). After disclosure of the plaque with a dye (usually a red food coloring; several disclosing solutions and tablets are available on the market), either the tip of an explorer or a probe is used to measure the presence of plaque biofilm, which is then recorded as present along the gingival margin on each of the four surfaces of the teeth. The index is derived by dividing the number of plaque-containing surfaces by the total number of tooth surfaces scored. The index can also be portrayed as percent of plaque-free surfaces or plaque-containing surfaces. The goal may be to achieve 10% or fewer of the tooth surfaces having plaque biofilm before periodontal surgical procedures may be initiated or the therapist considers the patient to have adequate plaque control.

Rustogi Modification of the Navy Plaque Index

Another example of a dichotomous plaque index is the Rustogi modification of the Navy Plaque Index (RMNPI),[10] which is commonly used in clinical research studies to measure the plaque removal effectiveness of different toothbrush designs. In this index, plaque is disclosed and each tooth is divided into 9

areas on both the facial and the lingual aspect of the tooth, totaling 18 surfaces scored per tooth (Fig. 14-2). Although the scale itself is simple, the complexity due to the number of surfaces evaluated can provide an interesting picture of plaque removal efficiency under controlled conditions of tooth brushing methods, brushing duration, or effectiveness of different toothbrush designs, either manual or powered. This scale also provides greater opportunity for the differentiation of the plaque-removing efficacy of toothbrushes. The clinician calls out the tooth areas with plaque to a recorder. The subject **mean score** is derived by the number of surfaces with plaque divided by the total surfaces scored. A mean score of 0.6 is usually required as a minimum plaque score to qualify for entry into a clinical research study to evaluate a toothbrush's plaque-removal ability, for example. Different regions of the mouth, different teeth, or different surfaces may be grouped for specific analyses when analyzing the data, such as those considered difficult to reach.

Silness Löe Plaque Index

An example of a plaque index that can be used without a disclosing solution is the classic Silness Löe

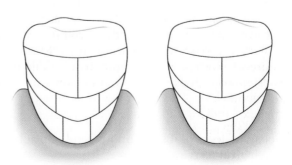

Figure 14-2. Division of tooth surface used by the Rustogi modification of the Navy Plaque Index.

Plaque Index,[11] which assesses the thickness of plaque around the tooth and is an example of an ordinal scale index. This can easily be done in the office as the dental hygienist conducts the oral examination and charting. The scores are described as follows:

0—No plaque in gingival area
1—Film of plaque adhering to free gingival margin and adjacent area of tooth; plaque may only be noticed by running a probe across tooth surface
2—Moderate accumulation of soft deposits within gingival pocket, on gingival margin, and/or on adjacent tooth surface, which can be seen by naked eye
3—Abundance of soft matter within gingival pocket and/or on gingival margin and adjacent tooth surface

The dichotomous or ordinal scale indices, which quantify amount or extent of plaque, can be used on selected teeth, rather than the whole mouth, as a measure of oral hygiene status. Often only partial mouth scoring is conducted for large population studies to generate more data in less time or so that more people can be evaluated. Generally recognized and used are the "Ramfjord teeth," which are #3, #9, #12, #19, #25, and #28. Dr. Sigmund Ramfjord selected these teeth when he developed oral health assessment tools for determining prevalence and severity of gingival and periodontal disease.

Turesky Modification of the Quigley-Hein Plaque Index

Another example of a plaque index with an ordinal scale is the Quigley-Hein Plaque Index (QHPI), later modified by Turesky (TMQHPI) to better define the lower end of the scale.[12,13] The TMQHPI is commonly used in clinical research studies and is widely recognized by professional and regulatory organizations responsible for reviewing clinical research to establish efficacy for product claims or advertising.

This index is used after disclosure of plaque, and it provides a single score on each of the facial and lingual aspects of the teeth. The modifications that have occurred with the QHPI provide an example of creating the right tool or right index to study a question and show the progression and adaptation of clinical indices to the question(s) of interest. The development of the Soparkar modification of the TMQHPI allows for further delineation of the facial and lingual aspects into a mesial, marginal, and distal score on each aspect, totaling six scores per tooth.[14] This index is commonly used in clinical research, particularly when proximal surfaces are of interest, for example, when evaluating brushes, mouth rinses, and floss. A description of the scores follows:

0—No plaque
1—Separate flecks or discontinuous band of plaque at the gingival (cervical) margin
2—Thin (up to 1 mm), continuous band of plaque at the gingival margin

3—Band of plaque wider than 1 mm but less than one third of surface
4—Plaque covering one third or more, but less than two thirds of surface
5—Plaque covering two thirds or more of surface

The index is derived by totaling the scores and dividing by the number of surfaces scored. A further modification of the TMQHPI is the plaque severity index, which measures the proportion of tooth sites rated with high TMQHPI scores (score ≥3).[19] The final result provides an assessment of how effective the test agent is on higher levels of plaque or more severe plaque accumulations.

Researchers develop dental indices to suit their particular needs, sometimes resulting in some duplication. Indices have become flexible, able to be adapted, modernized (especially in the case of periodontal indices), or simplified to fit different needs. Indices will continue to develop as those needs change again and as technology becomes available (see Application to Clinical Practice 2).

Calculus Indices

Calculus is usually measured in the mandibular anterior lingual surfaces using the VMI. The VMI has been correlated with photographic analysis of the calculus area.[15–17] The VMI uses a probe and measures the greatest height of calculus in three planes—mesial, distal, and lingual of each of the six anterior incisors—and the scores are totaled and divided by the number of teeth or surfaces. This index is generally used for research purposes to evaluate tartar-control products, such as toothpastes and mouthwashes. Other calculus indices include the simplified calculus index, which quantifies calculus by location and surface area; it is shown in Table 14-3.[8] The following teeth are scored: 3, 8, 14, 19, 24, and 30, with a single score on the buccal and a single score on the lingual surfaces. The calculus scores are totaled and divided by the number of surfaces scored. National Institute for Dental Research (NIDR) used a similar index for NHANES where the presence or absence of calculus both supragingival and

Application to Clinical Practice 2

Patients seek oral product recommendations or brushing technique recommendations from the dental hygienist, their preventive oral health expert. Therefore, it is essential for the hygienist to not only know how to read and critically evaluate the clinical research literature, but also to assess the materials that manufacturers' sales representatives provide, as well as critically evaluate the product advertisements that appear in professional journals. ■

Table 14-3. *Simplified Calculus Index*

Scores	Criteria
0	No calculus present
1	Supragingival covering not more than a third of the exposed tooth surface
2	Supragingival calculus covering more than one third but no more than two thirds of the exposed tooth surface or the presence of individual flecks of subgingival calculus around the cervical portion of the tooth, or both
3	Supragingival calculus covering more than two thirds of the exposed tooth surface or a continuous heavy band of subgingival calculus around the cervical portion of the tooth, or both

subgingival was assessed as part of the periodontal assessment and is further described as part of the periodontal index later in this chapter.

For clinical practice, the greater concern is to remove calculus, not to measure it; however, if a patient has a problem with calculus buildup, it might be worthwhile to measure the calculus with your chosen index and then recommend different home-care regimens or products to see what works best for that individual. A dental hygienist can conduct his or her own research in this way to provide better outcomes for each patient. This can be a way to teach patients what their score means and what a desirable goal would be and then re-evaluate at subsequent visits.

Indices That Measure Gingival and Periodontal Health Status

More than a half-dozen indices measure bleeding alone, whether using a dichotomous or an ordinal scale. An excellent review of bleeding indices by Barnett[2] discusses the objective and subjective aspects of evaluating bleeding. Selection of an appropriate index depends on the purpose.

In longitudinal studies, for example, perhaps only a visual assessment of gingival inflammation, rather than bleeding, as the measurement may be desired because of difficulty in calibrating examiners or in assessing the reliability of examiners. Replicate measurement increases the tendency for bleeding because of repeated probing, thus making it difficult to determine repeatability. Some studies include taking microbiological samples of plaque or sulcular fluids, which should be collected before bleeding or plaque measurements. This disruption can also affect the clinical indices, and these sites may be excluded from the data because of disrupting plaque at the margin and producing trauma to the gingiva.

Depending on the research question, if one is evaluating the effect of a treatment on inflammation or bleeding, then perhaps an ordinal scale is appropriate to measure changes in the amount or spontaneity of bleeding, as opposed to a dichotomous scale in which the number of sites bleeding, or not, is recorded. Again, depending on the question or the population being studied, one may consider sweeping a probe around the sulcus, as would be done in a patient with gingivitis, versus probing to the base of the pocket, as is done in a patient with periodontitis. Therefore, selection of the index to be used should be appropriate for the clinical condition and the research question.

For clinical practice, it may suffice to know if there is bleeding or not at a particular location or site in the mouth, and knowing the number of bleeding sites is a way to measure change over time. This is also useful for patient home-care motivation. Bleeding is something patients can see or taste during oral hygiene procedures, and so they know whether they experience bleeding. This way, they can see their own progress in achieving better oral health.

One may think a bleeding index is objective, but the subjectivity comes in with how the bleeding is elicited, which probe (manual or pressure-sensitive), where and how the bleeding is elicited, and quantifying the bleeding versus a simple yes or no value.

A probe, whether manual or pressure-sensitive, is used for most bleeding indices; however, the Eastman Interdental Bleeding Index, which uses a wooden Stim-U-Dent, has been shown to correlate with histological examination.[20] Bleeding sites contained a significantly greater degree of inflamed connective tissue than nonbleeding sites.[21] The gingival bleeding index uses floss to elicit bleeding and scores the presence or absence of bleeding in each interdental unit.[22] There are also ordinal bleeding indices such as the sulcus bleeding index with scales up to five values.[23]

Several indices are used to evaluate gingival inflammation. The modified gingival index (MGI) is strictly visual and noninvasive, whereas the gingival index (GI) uses a visual and a bleeding component.[24,25] Both of these gingival indices evaluate the marginal gingiva, are widely used in clinical research, and are recognized by professional bodies such as the American Dental Association (ADA) and the International Academy of Periodontology (IAP) and regulatory bodies such as the U.S. Food and Drug Administration (FDA). The MGI and GI are used to evaluate research for granting of a seal of acceptance (ADA), for approval of product claims of efficacy (ADA, FDA), and for marketing purposes (major networks such as ABC, NBC, CBS), science review boards, and the Federal Trade Commission. Using an experimental gingivitis model, researchers showed that the GI and two other bleeding indices significantly correlate with the purely visual MGI index, demonstrating that similar results can be found using different indices.[26]

The MGI provides greater differentiation than the GI at the lower end of the scale (in the mild inflammation category) to differentiate the extent of the inflammation. It is also a noninvasive index, thereby not disrupting plaque, which is useful when conducting clinical research when both indices are being used in the patient evaluation. MGI is highly correlated with the GI. Table 14-4 compares the MGI and GI.

Russell Periodontal Index

The first periodontal index, created by Russell, includes a composite of different variables. The **Russell periodontal index** measures the condition of the gingiva and the bone individually for each tooth and arrives at the average status of periodontal disease in a given patient.[27] This index has two scores for gingivitis, but it does not consider different degrees of inflammation; however, it does consider the extension of the marginal inflammation around a tooth. Fundamentally, this index records three stages in periodontal destruction: gingivitis (score 1, 2), pocket formation (score 5), and almost total breakdown

(score 8). It provides overall periodontal disease prevalence in a large population but is not recommended for measuring the effect of individual preventive and therapeutic procedures. For a strictly epidemiological study of variation in distribution of periodontal disease in a population, the Russell index is satisfactory. It has been used to characterize a population at the initiation of a clinical trial; however, it is no longer considered valid. It does not measure clinical attachment level and grades all pockets 3 mm or larger equally. It is included in this section to provide an understanding of the transformation and the creation of indices to suit the research question or the need of the clinician, or to be a quick, easy tool for large health surveys.

Periodontal Disease Index

The quality of the gingiva should be scored and the quantity of periodontal destruction measured in millimeters by probing pocket depth and attachment levels, to achieve a full understanding of the periodontal condition. The periodontal disease index (PDI) by Ramfjord was developed for the WHO and is a more sensitive version of the Russell periodontal index.[28] The PDI uses six teeth for examination—#3, #9, #12, #19, #25, and #28. These six teeth were selected by means of available data and clinical experience from practice and teaching to provide a valid indicator of the periodontal condition within the dentition. The PDI includes several scoring components, including the gingiva, attachment loss, calculus, tooth mobility, tooth contacts, and plaque.

Periodontal Screening Examination

The periodontal screening examination by O'Leary[29] divides the mouth into sextants—four posterior regions (premolars and molars) and two anterior regions (canines and incisors)—and records the highest score in each sextant. Bleeding, deposits, and pocket depth are considered.

Community Periodontal Index of Treatment Needs

The community periodontal index of treatment needs (CPITN), which was developed by the WHO in 1982, is a measure of treatment needs, not a measure of periodontitis.[30,31] Data are presented in categorical terms (0–4) rather than mean values, and individuals are placed into treatment groups based on the most severe oral finding. It is used for epidemiological surveys, and it uses O'Leary's sextants and 0 to 4 scale per sextant. It was modified into the CPI by WHO in 1994 to eliminate treatment need codes. It is considered a global standard for data on health planning. Three indicators of periodontal status are used in this assessment: gingival bleeding, calculus, and periodontal pockets. A special probe with a 0.5-mm ball tip is used and scored as follows: 0—healthy, 1—bleeding, 2—calculus detected,

Table 14-4. Comparison of the Modified Gingival Index With the Gingival Index

Modified Gingival Index (MGI)	Gingival Index (GI)
0—Absence of inflammation	0—Normal gingiva
1—Mild inflammation; slight change in color, little change in texture of any portion of but not the entire marginal or papillary gingival unit	
2—Mild inflammation; criteria as above but involving the entire marginal or papillary gingival unit	1—Mild inflammation—slight change in color, slight edema, *no bleeding on probing*
3—Moderate inflammation; glazing, redness, edema, and or hypertrophy of the marginal or papillary gingival unit	2—Moderate inflammation—redness, edema, and glazing; *bleeding on probing*
4—Severe inflammation; marked redness, edema, and/or hypertrophy of the marginal or papillary gingival unit; spontaneous bleeding, congestion, or ulceration	3—Severe inflammation—marked redness and edema, ulceration; *tendency to spontaneous bleeding*

3—pockets 4 to 5 mm, and 4—pockets 6 mm or larger. Its advantages include simplicity, international uniformity, and speed.

Periodontal Scoring and Recording Index

The CPITN was modified into the periodontal scoring and recording (PSR) index in the United States and was introduced by the ADA and the American Academy of Periodontology because none of the many periodontal indices is universally accepted or routinely used by most general practitioners for early detection of periodontal disease.[32] The PSR index is very similar to the CPITN. It is intended for use in individuals and is an early detection system for periodontal disease. It divides the mouth into six segments, recording the highest score in each sextant, and includes bleeding and probing depth measurements and serves as a screening tool, not intended to replace full periodontal charting. Landry concluded that the PSR is a simple, reliable, and reproducible periodontal index for screening purposes.[32] General dental practitioners and periodontists consider the PSR to be an effective tool for educating patients and facilitating communication between the dental professional and the patient, which is one of its most noted benefits.[33] It is simple, fast, and preferred by patients. Furthermore, Khocht et al.[34,35] have shown that PSR scores reflect periodontal status comparable with conventional periodontal examinations: The relationship of PSR scores and bone levels on radiographs showed significant associations with probing depths and attachment levels. Based on these findings, the PSR would appear to be a very useful tool for screening populations, as well as a quick measure of an individual patient's periodontal status, facilitating conversation with patients about their periodontal health. See Chapter 11 for more information on the PSR.

Periodontal Index

The periodontal index has been used for epidemiological surveys conducted in 1999 to 2000, 2001 to 2004, and NHANES III in the United States by the NIDR.[36,37] It assesses clinical evidence of gingival bleeding, presence of supragingival and subgingival calculus, and presence, extent, and severity of periodontal attachment loss. Two quadrants, one maxillary and one mandibular, are selected at random. The buccal and mesial sites only are examined on each tooth, and a periodontal probe #2-12 graduated in 2-mm intervals is used. Bleeding is scored as absent (0) or present (1) and calculus is scored as none (0), supra only (1), or subgingival or both subgingival and supragingival (2). Attachment level is also measured on the same teeth.[28] In the 2009 to 2010 cycle of the NHANES, a full-mouth assessment was conducted on six sites per tooth for all teeth present except third molars. Analysis of these data indicated that the prevalence of periodontitis was far higher than in previous epidemiological surveys in the United States, and it was concluded that bias resulted from the use of these partial-mouth recording systems with prevalence rate estimates of 19.5% to 27.1% compared with 47.2% based on full-mouth data.[38] This is another example of how tools change with more knowledge and experience, and the importance of indices. The impact of these prior data with an underestimation of the true prevalence of periodontitis affects the **validity** and inferences of all other periodontitis-related research based on the NHANES protocols and data.[39]

Indices Contribute to Oral Disease Risk Assessment

Indices provide a clinical snapshot at a moment in time, which numerically represent the results of the history of periodontal destruction or caries experience, for example. What these indices do not provide is an assessment of risk for future disease. Many factors including lifestyle are involved in risk assessment, in addition to the clinical indices. The assessment of risk for periodontal disease is an essential factor during treatment and maintenance phases of therapy. Many factors need to be considered and analyzed, which can lead to great variation in assessment of risk among general dentists and periodontists. There are computer-generated risk assessment models such as the Oral Health Information Suite (OHIS), the periodontal risk calculator, and PreViser, which is software that helps identify oral disease risk and severity.[40–42] There are risk assessments ranging from simple questionnaire-based tools to more complex tools that include clinical indices.[43] In addition to clinical indices to assess risk, there are microbiological tools that can also help assess disease risk.[44] If there is a preponderance of periodontopathic organisms, perhaps concomitant antibiotic therapy may be appropriate together with debridement techniques and oral hygiene instructions to achieve a healthier and more maintainable condition. Although these tools are diagnostic tests, they also use indices as part of the risk assessment.

Dental caries risk assessment should be a routine component of new and periodic examinations by oral health and medical providers, and it should be based on the child's age, biological factors, protective factors, and clinical findings. The Caries-Risk Assessment Tool (CAT) is a practical tool for assessing caries risk in infants, children, and adolescents based on a set of physical, environmental, and general health factors.[45] Dental and nondental health-care providers can use the CAT. With this assessment, the types and frequency of diagnostic, preventive, and restorative care can be determined for patient management of dental caries. The ADA has two questionnaires for caries risk assessment: one for children 0 to 6 years old and one for ages 6 to adult. The ADA criteria for caries risk assessment include contributing conditions (such as fluoride exposure, diet, and dental decay experience in family or caregiver), general health conditions (such as developmental, physical, mental, or medical special needs), and clinical condition of the child (deft or defs).[46] The parent interview provides the information, and overall caries risk (low, moderate, or high risk) is determined by adding up all the yes responses to the questionnaire. Both questionnaires are scored the same way to determine risk.[47]

Caries Management by Risk Assessment (CAMBRA) is another caries risk assessment tool, which is described fully in Chapter 21.[48] CAMBRA uses assessment forms for children 0 to 5 years old and also for ages 6 years to adult to assess risk as low, moderate, high, or extreme risk. CAMBRA clinical guidelines include use of over-the-counter and prescription products such as fluoridated toothpastes, xylitol, calcium phosphate, antimicrobials, and sealants.[49-51]

Use of the risk assessment tools over time may result in more uniform and accurate periodontal clinical decision-making, improve overall health, reduce the need for complex therapy, reduce health-care costs, and hasten the transition from a repair model to a wellness model of oral care (see Advancing Technologies).

Advancing Technologies

More refined and calibrated instrument probes are available for pocket depth and attachment level measurement. The different indices and their modifications over time contribute to the ability of the dental hygienist to refine oral assessments, thus providing better treatment, risk assessment, and home-care recommendations. Additional tools to enhance clinical oral assessment are now available as well, such as saliva-based diagnostics tests. The MyPerio-Path test[44] is a saliva test that identifies the type and concentration of specific periopathogenic bacteria that are known to cause periodontal disease. The results of DNA and polymerase chain reaction laboratory analysis of the salivary sample helps determine patient risk for periodontal disease and facilitates creation of personalized treatment options for more predictable patient outcomes.

MyPerioID PST determines genetic susceptibility for severe periodontal infections. The patient swishes a sterile solution, which is then expectorated into a container and sent to a laboratory for analysis. An exaggerated immune reaction elicited in the analysis indicates whether the patient is at increased risk for more severe periodontal infections, and thus permits the clinician to develop an individualized approach to therapy.[44] ■

Case Study

The dental hygienist works in a private practice that is interested in developing a plaque biofilm control program for patients with gingivitis. She has been asked to research the effects of mouthwashes on the reduction and prevention of plaque biofilm and gingivitis, and prepare a draft of a patient-education handout. She starts the project by visiting the websites of several mouthwash manufacturers where she finds the results of clinical trials conducted to evaluate the antiplaque and antigingivitis effects of the manufacturers' mouthwash products.

Case Study Exercises

1. What are some factors to consider when analyzing the results of clinical trials?
2. What criteria would the dental hygienist expect to find in the clinical trial results that would indicate that the studies and results are valid?
3. Describe the types of indices that the dental hygienist would expect to be used and explain why.

Review Questions

1. Which of the following does NOT apply to a suitable or ideal index?
   A. Simple to use and amenable to statistical analysis
   B. Scores are equally sensitive throughout the range of the index indicating the clinical stages of the disease
   C. Criteria describing the scores are clear and easily understood
   D. Index may not be acceptable to the patient
   E. Index should be sensitive and valid

2. The Silness Löe Gingival Index has universal application and acceptance. The Silness Löe Gingival Index is a noninvasive index.
   A. Both statements are true.
   B. Both statements are false.
   C. The first statement is false and the second is true.

3. DMFS (decayed, missing, or filled teeth/surfaces) is an irreversible index. DMFS is used to measure distal and mesial facial tooth surfaces covered with plaque.
   A. Both statements are true.
   B. Both statements are false.
   C. The first statement is true and the second is false.

4. Which of the following is NOT a reversible clinical index?
   A. Caries
   B. Periodontal disease
   C. Gingivitis
   D. Plaque
   E. VMI

5. An ordinal scale would be recommended for assessing presence or absence of plaque when conducting a survey of elementary student oral hygiene status. Selecting any two quadrants would be representative of the patient.
   A. Both statements are true.
   B. Both statements are false.
   C. The first statement is true and the second statement is false.

Active Learning

1. In groups of three (one as patient, one as examiner, and one as recorder), select a gingivitis, a plaque, and a calculus index, conduct the examinations, each taking a turn in each role, and calculate the indices. Discuss why you selected the indices you did.
2. View clinical photos and history and then calculate the DMFT and DMFS scores for the patient.
3. Design a dental screening event for a specific population. Decide what indices you will collect and justify your choices. ■

REFERENCES

1. Lobene RR. Discussion: clinical status of indices for measuring gingivitis. *J Clin Periodontal.* 1986;13:381.
2. Barnett ML. Suitability of gingival indices for use in therapeutic trials: is bleeding a sine qua non? *J Clin Periodontol.* 1996;23:582-586.
3. Fleiss JL. *The Design and Analysis of Clinical Experiments.* New York: John Wiley & Sons; 1986.
4. Klein H, Palmer CE, Knutson JW. Studies on dental caries 1. Dental status and dental needs of elementary school children. *Public Health Rep.* 1938;53:751.
5. Gruebbel AO. A measurement of dental caries prevalence and treatment service for deciduous teeth. *J Dent Res.* 1944;23:163.
6. Indices used for periodontal disease assessment. www.codental.uobaghdad.edu.iq/uploads/. . ./3%20PDD%20Indices.pdf. Accessed July 25, 2015.
7. U.S. Department of Health and Human Services Centers for Disease Control and Prevention National Center for Health Statistics. National Health and Nutrition Examination Survey, 2007-2008 overview. Published May 2, 2010. www.cdc.gov/nchs/njanes.htm. Accessed April 27, 2010.
8. Greene JC, Vermillion JR. The simplified oral hygiene index. *J Am Dent Assoc.* 1964;68:27-31.
9. O'Leary TJ, Drake RB, Naylor JE. The plaque control record. *J Periodontol.* 1972;43:38.
10. Rustogi KN, Curtis JP, Volpe AR, McCool JJ, Korn LR. Refinement of the Modified Navy Plaque Index to increase plaque scoring efficiency in gumline and interproximal tooth areas. *J Clin Dent.* 1992(suppl C):C9-C12.
11. Loe H. The gingival index, the plaque index and the retention index systems. *J Periodontol.* 1967;38:610-616.
12. Quigley GA, Hein JW. Comparative cleansing efficacy of manual and power brushing. *J Am Dent Assoc.* 1962;65:26-29.
13. Turesky S, Gilmore ND, Glickman I. Reduced plaque formation by the chloromethyl analogue of Victamine C. *J Periodontol.* 1970;41:41-43.
14. Lobene R, Soparkar M, Newman B. Use of dental floss—effect on plaque and gingivitis. *Clin Prev Dent.* 1982;4:5-8.
15. Volpe AR, Manhold JH, Hazen SP. In vivo calculus assessment. Part 1. A method and its examiner reproducibility. *J Periodontol.* 1965;36:292.
16. Volpe A, Charles CH, Cronin MJ, et al. Anticalculus efficacy of an antiseptic mouthrinse containing zinc chloride. *J Am Dent Assoc.* 2001;132:94-98.
17. Barnett ML, Charles CH, Gilman RM, et al. Correlation between Volpe-Manhold Calculus Index and calculus area measurements [abstract 920]. *J Dent Res.* 1989;68:296.
18. Lobene RR. Effects of dentifrices on tooth stains with controlled brushing. *J Am Dent Assoc.* 1968;77(4):849-855.
19. Palomo F, Wantland L, Sanchez A, DeVizio W, Carter W, Baines E. The effect of a dentifrice containing triclosan and a copolymer on plaque formation and gingivitis: a 14 week clinical study. *Am J Dent.* 1989;2:231-237.
20. Caton JG, Polson AM. The interdental bleeding index: a simplified procedure for monitoring gingival health. *Compend Contin Educ Dent.* 1985;6:88-92.
21. Abrams K, Caton JG, Polson AM. Histologic comparisons of interproximal gingival tissues related to the presence or absence of bleeding. *J Periodontol.* 1984;55:629-632.
22. Carter HG, Barnes GP. The gingival bleeding index. *J Periodontal.* 1974;45:801.
23. Muhlemann HR, Son S. Gingival sulcus bleeding—a leading sympton in initial gingivitis. *Helv Odontol Acta.* 1971;15:107.

24. Lobene RR, Weatherford T, Ross NM, Lamm RA, Menaker L. A modified gingival index for use in clinical trials. *Clin Prev Dent.* 1986;8(1):3-6.

25. Löe H, Silness J. Periodontal disease in pregnancy. I. Prevalence and severity. *Acta Odontol Scand.* 1963; 21:533.

26. Lobene RR, Mankodi SM, Ciancio SG, Lamm RA, Charles CH, Ross NM. Correlations among gingival indices: a methodology study. *J Periodontol.* 1989;60:159-162.

27. Russell AL. A system of classification and scoring for prevalence surveys of periodontal disease. *J Dent Res.* 1956;35(3):350.

28. Ramfjord SP. Indices for prevalence and incidence of periodontal disease. *J Periodontol.* 1959;30:51-59.

29. O'Leary T. The periodontal screening examination. *J Periodontol.* 1967;38(6 suppl):617-624.

30. Strohmenger L, Cerati M, Brambilla E, Malerba A, Vogel G. Periodontal epidemiology in Italy by CPITN. *Int Dent J.* 1991;41:313-315.

31. Miyazaki H, Pilot T, Lederq M. Periodontal profiles: an overview of CPITN data in the WHO global oral data bank for the age groups 15-19 years, 35-44 years. Geneva: World Health Organization; 1992.

32. Landry RG, Jean M. Periodontal Screening and Recording (PSR) index: precursors, utility and limitations in a clinical setting. *Int Dent J.* 2002;52:36-40.

33. Lo Frisco C, Cutler C, Bramson J. Periodontal screening and recording: perceptions and effects on practice. *J Am Dent Assoc.* 1993;124:226-229, 231-232.

34. Khocht A, Zohn J, Deasy M, Huang-Min C. Assessment of periodontal status with PSR and traditional clinical periodontal examination. *J Am Dent Assoc.* 1995;126: 1658-1665.

35. Khocht A, Zohn J, Deasy M, Huang-Min C. Screening for periodontal disease; radiographs vs. PSR. *J Am Dent Assoc.* 1996;127:749-756.

36. Dye BA, Tan S, Smith V, Lewis BG, Barker LK, Thornton-Evans G, et al. Trends in oral health status: United States, 1988-1994 and 1999-2004 [DHHS Publication No. (PSH) 2007-1698]. *Vital and Health Statistics,* Series 11, No. 248. Hyattsville, MD: U.S. Department of Health and Human Services, National Center for Health Statistics; 2007:1-92.

37. Dye BA, Barker LK, Selwitz RH, Lewis BG, Wu T, Fryar CD, et al. Overview and quality assurance for the National Health and Nutrition Examination Survey (NHANES) oral health component, 1999-2002. *Community Dent Oral Epidemiol.* 2007;35:140-151.

38. Papanou PN. The prevalence of periodontitis in the US: Forget what you were told. *J Dent Res.* 2012;91(10): 907-908.

39. Eke PI, Thornton-Evans GO, Wei L, Borgnakke WS, Dye BA, Accuracy of NHANES periodontal examination protocols. *J Dent Res.* 2010;89(11):1208-1213.

40. Page RC, Martin JA, Loeb CF. The oral health information suite (OHIS): its use in the management of periodontal disease. *J Dent Educ.* 2005;69(5):509-520.

41. Page RC, Martin J, Krall EA, Manci L, Garcia R. Longitudinal validation of a risk calculator for periodontal disease. *J Clin Periodontal.* 2003;30(9):819-827.

42. Emmott L. Previsor. Published April 6, 2005. http://emmottontechnology.com/general/previsor

43. American Academy of Periodontology. Comprehensive Periodontal Evaluation (CPE). https://www.perio.org/consumer/perio-evaluation.htm. Accessed July 25, 2015.

44. Oral DNA®Labs. Innovations in salivary diagnostics. Published April 27, 2010. http://www.oraldnalabs.com/OurTests/OralDNATests.aspx. Accessed April 27, 2010.

45. American Academy of Pediatric Dentistry. Guideline on caries risk assessment and management for infants, children and adolescents. Oral health policies adopted 2002. Revised 2006, 2010, 2011. Council on Clinical Affairs, Reference Manual 34:6;118-125. www.aapd.org

46. American Dental Association. ADA Council on Dental Practice. Published December 15, 2011. www.ada.org/sections/professionalResources/pdfs/topics_caries_educational_under6.pdf. Accessed April 30, 2013.

47. American Dental Association. ADA Council on Dental Practice. http://www.ada.org/sections/professional Resources/pdfs/topic_caries_over6.pdf. Accessed April 30, 2013.

48. Young DA, Featherstone JDB, Roth JR, et al. Caries management by risk assessment: consensus statement 2002. *J Calif Dent Assoc.* 2003;31(3):257-269.

49. Ramos-Gomez FJ, Crall J, Gansky S, Slayton R, Featherstone JD. Caries risk assessment appropriate for the age 1 visit (infants and toddlers). *J Calif Dent Assoc.* 2007;35(10):687-702.

50. Featherstone JD, Domejean-Orliaguet S, Jenson L, Wolff M, Young DA. Caries risk assessment in practice for age 6 through adult. *J Calif Dent Assoc.* 2007;35(10): 703-713.

51. Crystal YO, Creasey JS, Robinson L, Ramos-Gomez F. Successful business models for implementation of caries management by risk assessment in private practice settings, *J Calif Dent Assoc.* 2011;39(11): 795-805.

Chapter 15 | Radiology

Shawneen M. Gonzalez, DDS, MS

KEY TERMS

ALARA

analog

bitewing radiograph

collimation

complete mouth
  radiographic
  series (CMS)

computed
  radiography (CR)

contrast

density

deterministic effects

digital radiography (DR)

flat-panel detector

ionizing radiation

justification

latent image

lateral cephalometric
  skull radiograph

lead apron

nonionizing radiation

occlusal radiograph

optimization

pantomograph

periapical radiograph

photostimulable
  phosphor (PSP) plate

radiograph

radiolucent

radiopaque

sensor

sievert

stochastic effects

thyroid collar

x-ray

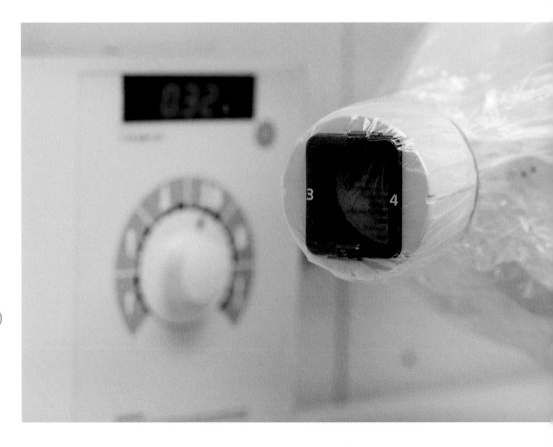

LEARNING OBJECTIVES

After reading this chapter, the student should be able to:

15.1 Describe properties of x-rays.

15.2 Describe and correctly use basic radiology terms when working with other dental professionals and patients.

15.3 Identify normal radiographic appearances of teeth and surrounding structures on radiographs.

15.4 Describe analog film versus digital imaging systems.

15.5 Describe ionizing radiation protection guidelines.

KEY CONCEPTS

- Basic radiographic terms are important when working with other dental professionals.
- Knowledge of the different types of imaging systems in dentistry is beneficial when working in a dental office.
- Responsible use of ionizing radiation is necessary to ensure patients are exposed to the least amount of radiation possible.

RELEVANCE TO CLINICAL PRACTICE

Radiographs show information including, but not limited to, location and quantity of calculus, bone defects, furcation involvement, and restorative margin defects. This information allows the dental hygienist to formulate optimum treatment plans for patients to aid in their efforts to improve or maintain their at-home oral health care.

ALARA

Radiation protection guidelines are important to minimize radiation exposure to both the patient and the operator. Estimations of risk associated with dental radiation dose levels are universally considered to be very small. Caution is appropriate because the biological effects associated with dental radiation cannot be distinguished from the same effects resulting from other environmental agents or associated with cases that arise spontaneously.

Radiation use is based on three related principles: ALARA, justification, and optimization.[1] The **ALARA** principle, radiation use **A**s **L**ow **A**s **R**easonably **A**chievable, seeks to minimize radiation exposure consistent with risk-benefit judgments (see Spotlight on Public Health). ALARA indicates you make the fewest number of radiographs to obtain the information necessary for treatment. For example, if an emergency patient comes in with a single tooth issue, a periapical radiograph of that tooth is typically recommended, and making bitewing radiographs at that appointment is excessive radiation exposure because that is not the reason the patient presented for care. The principle of **justification** states that radiographs are prescribed based on clinical findings and rejects radiographs prescribed on the basis of routine or a predetermined time interval. Justification indicates that you should evaluate each patient individually, taking into account their caries status and risk, oral hygiene status, and age, and not apply blanket policies that every patient is to receive a new set of bitewing radiographs every 6 months. The principle of **optimization** seeks to maximize diagnostic yield and to minimize patient exposure. An example of optimization is deciding whether a pantomograph or a periapical radiograph would be ideal to show an impacted mandibular third molar and its relationship to the mandibular canal on a patient who has a severe gag reflex. A periapical radiograph shows the apex and canal in detail; however, the likelihood of capturing this radiograph in one take is unlikely due to the patient's severe gag reflex and position of the image receptor for a posterior tooth. This results in unnecessary radiation to the patient when a pantomograph can be made with one take while not inducing the patient's gag reflex and limiting the patient's radiation exposure. This philosophy requires that the decision to use ionizing radiation for diagnostic purposes shall be made only after careful consideration of the patient's dental and general health needs as determined by medical and dental histories and a clinical examination.[2]

Spotlight on Public Health

The University of Nebraska Medical Center College of Dentistry in Lincoln, Nebraska, holds a sharing clinic that provides treatment to those unable to afford care at the surrounding community health centers. The clinic is staffed by volunteer faculty, dentists, students, and staff. This clinic is offered four to five times a year at the College of Dentistry clinics. All patients screened are asked whether they have had radiographs taken recently at another office. If so, every possible action is taken to acquire these images, thereby reducing unnecessary radiation exposure to the patient. This clinic has been providing care to those in the community since 2008, with more than 20 clinics held to date. ■

WHAT ARE X-RAYS?

Definition

There are two types of radiation: particulate and electromagnetic. Particulate radiation includes fast-moving particles that have both energy and mass and that travel in straight lines. Examples of particulate radiation are alpha particles, neutrons, protons, and electrons.[3] Electromagnetic radiation is electric and magnetic fields of energy that travel in pulsating waves. Each type of electromagnetic radiation is characterized by the overall energy and characteristics of the wave (wavelength and frequency). Wavelength is the distance between two crests of a wave. Frequency is the number of oscillations per second. A longer wavelength or lower frequency results in radiation with a lower energy, whereas a shorter wavelength or higher frequency results in radiation with a higher energy. Examples of electromagnetic radiation include radio waves, microwaves, visible light, ultraviolet light, and x-rays. **X-rays** produce ions as they travel through matter and are referred to as **ionizing radiation.** Not all energies on the electromagnetic spectrum are ionizing radiation.

History

The history of radiology started with Professor Wilhelm Röntgen, a German physicist who discovered x-rays by accident.[4] He was performing research using a cathode ray tube when he noticed a piece of barium platinocyanide glowing not far from the tube. He was unsure what new rays were causing this and proceeded to research them further. He called the new rays *x-rays* using the *x*, which represents unknown objects in algebraic equations. This was on November 8, 1895. He published his results on December 28, 1895, in an article entitled "On a New Kind of X Rays," which included the first radiograph, which was of his wife's hand. The exact exposure time for this radiograph has widely varied from 15 minutes up to 30 minutes.

The first radiograph in Europe was made only 10 days after the publication of the article on January 7, 1896; it was of a hand and was made in England by an electrical engineer. The first radiograph in the United States was made about 1 month later on February 3, 1896. A radiograph was made of a forearm on a patient in a hospital. The first dental radiograph was made by Otto Walkhoff, a German dentist, on January 12, 1896. He used himself as a patient, holding a photographic plate in his mouth and sitting still for a 25-minute exposure. The resulting image does not show much other than the outline of teeth, but it is the beginning of radiology in dentistry.

RADIOGRAPHIC TERMS

Definition

A **radiograph** is the resultant image after a patient or object is exposed to x-rays. Two groupings of radiographs are made in dentistry: intraoral, which refers to an image made with the image receptor in the patient's mouth; and extraoral, which refers to an image made with the image receptor placed outside the patient's mouth. The image receptor may be either analog film or a digital imaging system.

There are three types of intraoral radiographs: periapicals, bitewings, and occlusal radiographs. **Periapical radiographs** show an entire tooth on a single image (Fig. 15-1). They show the crown and root, including the surrounding bone of one jaw. These are most commonly made to evaluate the bone around the apex of a tooth to determine whether there is periapical pathosis. Periapical radiographs are identified by the location of the oral cavity shown. Three main identifications should be included when describing or prescribing a periapical radiograph: the jaw (maxilla or mandible), the side (left or right), and the specific teeth captured (molar, premolar, canine, etc.). See Teamwork.

Bitewing radiographs show the crowns of teeth of both the maxilla and the mandible on a single image

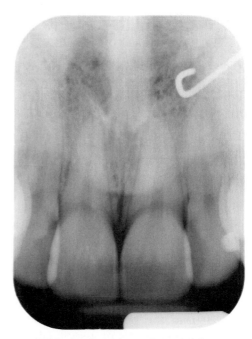

Figure 15-1. Periapical radiograph. Maxillary central incisors periapical.

Teamwork

Kathy is working in the radiology clinic during a busy Sharing Clinic. She is primarily setting up and cleaning the radiology cubicles. This aids the student operators by allowing more time for treatment. All the radiology cubicles are filled with patients and student operators. She notices Karen is struggling to take a maxillary molar periapical on an adult male with a severe gag reflex. She offers to help by pressing the x-ray exposure button once Karen has left the radiology cubicle so that the PSP plate is in the patient's mouth for as little time as necessary. With Kathy's help, Karen is able to capture the radiograph in one take. Some patients require a faster radiographic experience (placing image receptor in mouth, positioning x-ray unit, and pressing x-ray exposure button) to prevent possible reactions such as severe coughing or vomiting, or both. Working together facilitates the delivery of optimum patient care while obtaining the necessary radiographs. ■

(Fig. 15-2). These are most commonly made of the posterior teeth but can be made of the anterior teeth as well. Bitewing radiographs are used to evaluate for interproximal caries and adjacent bone levels. They are ideal for evaluating bone levels in relation to the teeth due to the near-perpendicular direction of the x-rays to the jaws. Horizontal bitewing radiographs are when

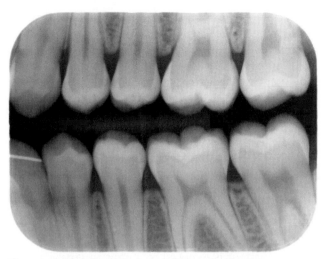

Figure 15-2. Bitewing radiograph. Left premolar bitewing.

Professionalism

You are in the radiology clinic to expose four bitewing radiographs on a 65-year-old woman. The patient has been dismissive and rude when going over her medical history insisting you do not need to know that information to clean or fix her teeth. She is visibly annoyed at having to have radiographs taken but agrees to them. You are about to position and expose the first bitewing when one of your classmates tries to strike up a conversation about an upcoming examination. You politely tell your classmate that you are busy with a patient and will discuss it at a later time. Your classmate leaves and you continue to expose the four bitewings focusing on proper technique. No retakes are necessary, and you take the patient back to the clinic chair to begin your prophylaxis. You notice your patient is very cooperative and no longer dismissive when you ask her questions about her oral hygiene. At the end of the appointment your patient thanks you for being so attentive when working with her. She states that during her last few appointments at the school she has felt ignored by the students treating her because they seemed more interested in talking with classmates then providing her care. She insists on seeing you the next time she comes back and thanks you once more. Professionalism when working with patients is important so that you are able to provide the best care possible. ■

loss. A common bitewing radiographic series consists of four radiographs: one molar bitewing radiograph and one premolar bitewing radiograph for each side. If the patient has fewer teeth, less than four radiographs may be necessary. Interproximal caries present as a radiolucent triangle in the enamel at the level just apical to the level of a contact with the point toward the dentin-enamel junction. Restorative materials have a range of appearances on radiographs from completely radiopaque (metal) to radiolucent (some composites). Bitewing radiographs are identified by the side and location. There is no jaw identification because both the maxilla and the mandible are captured on a single radiograph. See Professionalism.

A combination of periapical and bitewing radiographs, typically 18 to 20 radiographs, showing all the teeth in the oral cavity is referred to as a **complete mouth radiographic series (CMS)** or full-mouth series (sometimes abbreviated FMX). These radiographic series typically consist of four posterior bitewing radiographs, eight posterior periapical radiographs, and six to eight periapical radiographs (based on the preferences of the dental office). A CMS is frequently taken with a new patient examination, especially with multiple existing restorations or evidence of current carious lesions. This series shows detailed information of each tooth, allowing the dental practitioner to provide a thorough treatment plan for a patient.

Occlusal radiographs show an entire tooth, similar to periapicals; however, they are made with different angles, giving distorted images of those teeth (Fig. 15-3). Occlusal radiographs are identified by the jaw and the type.

Many different types of extraoral radiographs are available. The ones commonly seen in dentistry are pantomographs and lateral cephalometric skull radiographs. **Pantomographs** (also referred to as orthopantomographs and panoramic radiographs) are radiographs that show the entire maxilla and mandible

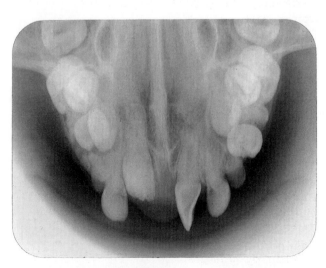

Figure 15-3. Occlusal radiograph. Maxillary standard occlusal.

the image sensor is placed such that the long axis is lateral. These are common with patients with minimal to no evident bone loss. Vertical bitewing radiographs are when the image sensor is placed such that the long axis is vertical. These are made when there is evident bone and surrounding structures superiorly to the orbits and inferiorly to the hyoid (Fig. 15-4). Pantomographs are made with the source of radiation and image receptor moving around the patient's head creating a focal trough around the jaws. **Lateral cephalometric skull radiographs** show a patient's anterior portion of the head from a lateral view (Fig. 15-5). These are made frequently in orthodontics to evaluate the position of the jaws in relation to each other and the skull base.

Four primary terms are used when describing radiographs: contrast, density, radiolucent, and radiopaque. Contrast and density refer to the amount of black, white, and gray on the final radiograph.[4] Radiolucent and radiopaque are descriptive terms used to identify the specific objects or anatomy, or both, seen on the final radiograph. The term **contrast** refers to the difference between two neighboring areas on the radiograph. This is how well the difference between two different gray areas on the radiograph can be distinguished. A radiograph with low contrast will be an overall gray image with little change in the grays throughout the image. A radiograph with high contrast will show obvious changes in the grays and have more black and white areas in the image (Fig. 15-6). **Density** is a property of the image receptor to block visible light. A radiograph with increased density appears blacker or darker.[5] A radiograph with decreased density appears whiter or lighter (Fig. 15-7). **Radiolucent** refers to areas that appear dark or black on the radiograph and is an adjective used to describe any part of the patient that allows the transmission of x-rays to the image receptor.[6] **Radiopaque** refers to areas that appear light or white on the radiograph and is an adjective used to describe any part of the patient that blocks the transmission of x-rays.

Relative Radiopacities/Radiolucencies

When a patient is exposed to x-rays to create a radiograph, certain anatomical and human-made entities will appear radiopaque, and certain anatomical and human-made entities will appear radiolucent. The most radiopaque entity on a radiograph is metal because it blocks the transmission of x-rays to the image receptor. Air, which allows for the transmission of nearly all the x-rays that pass through it, is the most radiolucent entity on a radiograph. Note that composites are listed twice in Table 15-1. Based on the manufacturer and when a composite was made, it may appear either radiopaque or radiolucent.

Normal Radiographic Appearances

Starting with the outermost visible portion of the tooth, enamel is a calcified structure and will appear radiopaque on radiographs. Dentin will also appear radiopaque but less so than enamel. The innermost

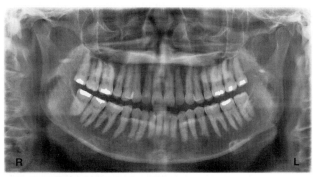

Figure 15-4. Pantomograph.

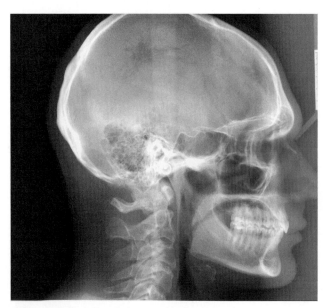

Figure 15-5. Lateral cephalometric skull radiograph.

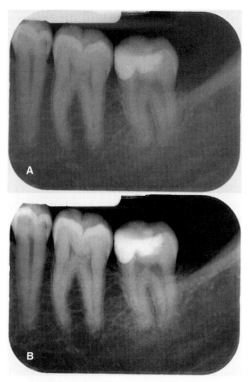

Figure 15-6. Radiographs with low contrast (A) and high contrast (B).

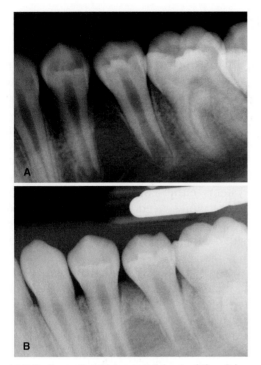

Figure 15-7. Radiographs with increased density (A) and decreased density (B).

portion of a tooth, the pulp chamber and root canal, is filled with soft tissue and will appear radiolucent on radiographs (Fig. 15-8). The periodontal ligament space surrounding the teeth is soft tissue and will appear radiolucent. The average size for this is 0.5 mm thick. The periodontal ligament space will not always be visible around every tooth. Around the periodontal ligament space is the bony socket referred to as *lamina dura*. This is hard tissue, specifically cortical bone, and will appear radiopaque on radiographs. The bone surrounding the teeth is hard tissue and will appear radiopaque on radiographs (Fig. 15-9).

A developing tooth will have a few key appearances on radiographs. The initial dental follicle is evident as a round/ovoid radiolucent area. The initial enamel formation in the shape of cusps will be the first radiopaque

component visible on radiographs (Fig. 15-10). As the tooth continues to form, the crown will complete formation first followed by the root. The entire root formation is not completed until 2 to 3 years after eruption of the tooth into the oral cavity. This root formation will appear as a widened root canal space near the apex of the tooth and should not be confused with periapical pathosis (Fig. 15-11).

DENTAL IMAGING SYSTEMS

Types

There are two primary forms of dental imaging systems: analog x-ray film and digital. **Analog** x-ray film is a type of photographic film used to visualize objects exposed to x-rays. Analog x-ray film comes in two different types: nonscreen film used for intraoral radiographs and screen film used for extraoral radiographs. Nonscreen analog x-ray film is contained in plastic or paper packets (film packets), protecting the film from visible light exposure and moisture from the oral cavity. Analog x-ray film is still in use due to the small silver grain making small changes, such as an incipient carious lesion, on the radiograph evident. Disadvantages of analog x-ray film include the storage and use of chemicals, which require special disposal.

Two digital imaging systems are used in dentistry: **computed radiography (CR)** and **digital radiography (DR).** CR is a digital imaging system that uses **photostimulable phosphor (PSP) plates** to capture an image, which is viewed on a computer after the PSP plate is scanned. PSP plates are made of "europium-doped" barium fluorohalide, which absorbs and stores energy when exposed by x-rays, creating a latent image. A **latent image** is an image that is created on either analog x-ray film or digital imaging (PSP plates and sensors) that is not visible to the naked eye until it is processed either via chemical (analog x-ray film) or by a computer (PSP plates and sensors). DR is a digital imaging system that uses

Table 15-1. *Relative Radiopacities/Radiolucencies*		
Radiopaque	**Radiolucent**	**Explanation**
Dentin Cementum		Under normal conditions, neither dentin nor cementum can be differentiated on a radiograph.
Cortical bone Cancellous bone Calculus		The cortical bone, cancellous bone, and calculus will appear similar under normal conditions. If a radiograph is made such that an edge of bone can be seen, the cortical bone appears more radiopaque compared with the cancellous bone.
	Soft tissues Body fluids Fat Radiolucent composites Air	On standard radiographic images, soft tissue and body fluids cannot be differentiated. They can be differentiated with more complex imaging modalities such as computed tomography (CT) and magnetic resonance imaging (MRI).

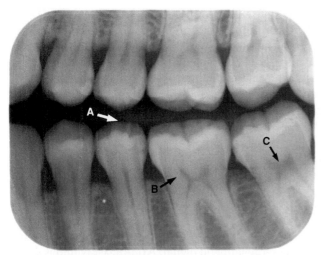

Figure 15-8. Normal radiographic appearances of a tooth: enamel (*A*), dentin (*B*), and pulp chamber/root canal space (*C*).

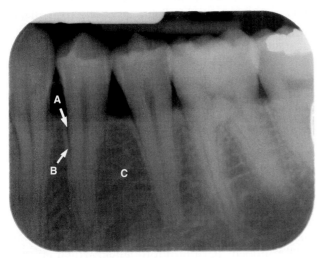

Figure 15-9. Normal radiographic appearances of anatomy surrounding a tooth: periodontal ligament space (*A*), lamina dura (*B*), and bone (*C*).

sensors and flat-panel detectors to capture images that are directly connected to a computer, providing a near-instantaneous image. **Sensors** are made of silicon crystals. These crystal bonds are broken when exposed to x-rays, creating a latent image on the sensor.

Flat-panel detectors are digital imaging sensors used for extraoral radiographs. CR and DR systems are covered with plastic barriers before being placed in the oral cavity to protect them from moisture. The plastic barrier also protects PSP plates from exposure to visible light. Advantages of digital imaging systems include ease of manipulation of the image (i.e., lightening/darkening, colorization) and ease of transfer of the data to other dental offices and insurance companies. A disadvantage of converting from an analog x-ray film office to a digital x-ray office is the expense of the systems, either PSP plates and scanners or sensors, both of which need computers in every operatory connected to a network joining them together along with computer software to capture and store the image.

Advantages of CR PSP plates compared with DR sensors are smaller size, increased flexibility, and absence of a wire. The main disadvantage of CR PSP plates is an increased processing time compared with DR.[3] This disadvantage is the primary advantage of DR sensors, which produce a nearly instant image. Some disadvantages of DR sensors compared with CR PSP plates include large size and a wire that makes positioning in the mouth difficult.[3] Both digital imaging systems use a shorter exposure time (compared with D and E speed analog film), resulting in reduction of radiation exposure to the patient. The specific amount of radiation exposure reduction varies based on the speed of the film and the digital imaging system type (Table 15-2).

Different sizes of image receptors are available that are labeled by their physical size (width and length). The sizes available are 0, 1, 2, 3, and 4. All five sizes (0, 1, 2, 3, and 4) are available in analog film and CR imaging systems. Three sizes (0, 1, and 2) are available in DR imaging systems. Analog film physical sizes are regulated by the American National Standards Institute (ANSI). Digital imaging systems size image receptors are not regulated by ANSI; they are determined by the manufacturer. CR PSP plates are similar physical size to analog film physical sizes. DR sensors vary in size and shape from analog film.[6] The different sizes have many uses in dentistry for children and adults (Table 15-3).

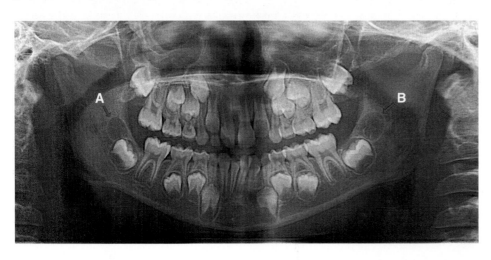

Figure 15-10. Developing tooth appearances: follicle (*A*) and follicle with enamel formation (*B*).

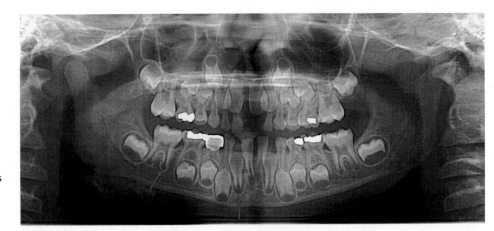

Figure 15-11. Developing root appearance. *Arrows* point to various stages of root development with the characteristic "open apex" appearance.

Table 15-2. Approximate Reduction of Radiation Exposure Times on Analog Film Versus Digital Imaging

Image Receptor	Computed Radiography (PSP plates)	Digital Radiography (sensors)
Film speed		
D	50%	75%
E	20%	60%
F	0% (no change in exposure time)	35%
Computed radiography (PSP plates)	—	50%
Digital radiography (sensors)	+50%	—
PSP, photostimulable phosphor.		

Analog Film

The two main components of nonscreen film are base and emulsion.[6] The base supports the emulsion and is flexible, aiding in ease of handling, and allows the film to withstand harsh processing chemicals. The emulsion is the film component that is sensitive to x-rays. There are two parts of the emulsion: silver bromide/silver halide grains (which are sensitive to x-rays and visible light) and a vehicle matrix. The vehicle matrix, a gelatinous material, suspends the silver bromide/silver halide grains. The vehicle matrix is flexible and covered with a thin overcoat to help prevent scratching or tearing of the emulsion. Screen film is used for extraoral radiographs and has a lower resolution compared with nonscreen film. Screen film is coated with dyes to increase sensitivity to visible light and must be placed in a cassette before it can be used.

Nonscreen film is contained in a packet that protects it from visible light and moisture. This "film packet" also contains a piece of black paper, lead foil, and one or two nonscreen films.[4] The black paper holds the film(s), aiding in extraction of the films from the packet. The lead foil is at the back side of the film packet and is used to prevent backscatter radiation from decreasing image quality. Duplicate film packets contain two films, creating an instant duplicate radiograph at the time of exposure. These duplicates are used for insurance purposes or to send to other dental offices for referrals. The film has a blue hue to ease eye strain when viewed by practitioners[7] and for improved diagnostic viewing (Fig. 15-12).[6]

Different sizes of silver bromide/silver halide grains are available. They are labeled as speeds of the film in accordance with ANSI standards. The film speeds are D, E, and F. The D speed film has the smallest silver bromide/silver halide grains and provides the highest resolution; however, it needs a longer exposure time because of the smaller grain size.[4] The F speed film has the largest silver bromide/silver halide grains and provides a lower resolution compared with D and E speed film. Due to the larger grain size, a shorter exposure time is required, thereby reducing radiation exposure to the patient.

Analog film processing occurs as the film is passed through a series of chemicals: a developer, a fixer, and a wash. The developer is the first step in analog film processing, reducing the exposed silver bromide/silver halide grains into black metallic silver. The areas of black metallic silver correlate to the radiolucent areas on the final radiograph. The fixer removes unexposed and undeveloped silver bromide/silver halide grains. The areas of grain removal correlate to the radiopaque areas on the final radiograph. The wash serves to remove the chemicals and prevent the film from continuing to

Table 15-3. Common Film Size Uses

Size	Physical Size (width × length)	Common Uses
0	13/16 × 1 3/8 inches 22 × 35 mm	Children (typically younger than 6 years) • Anterior/Posterior periapicals • Bitewings
1	15/16 × 1 9/16 inches 24 × 40 mm	Children • Anterior/Posterior periapicals • Bitewings Adults • Anterior periapicals
2	1 1/4 × 1 5/8 inches 31 × 41 mm	Children • Anterior/Posterior periapicals • Bitewings • Occlusal radiographs Adults • Anterior/Posterior periapicals • Bitewings
3	1 1/16 × 2 1/8 inches 27 × 54 mm	Adults • Bitewings
4	2 1/4 × 3 inches 57 × 76 mm	Adults • Occlusal radiographs

develop or fix. The wash is a moving water source. The final step is a drying step, which is achieved either with a fan or by hanging the film to dry.[4]

Computed Radiography

CR uses PSP plates for intraoral (Fig. 15-13) and extraoral imaging. The PSP plates are composed of "europium-doped" barium fluorohalide. When exposed to x-rays, valence electrons are created and trapped in the plate.[8] The plate has a latent image and must be processed in a scanner before the latent image is viewable. During processing, the scanner emits a red light (600 nm) toward the plate. This causes the plate to give off the energy where the electrons were trapped in the form of green light (300–500 nm). The specific energy of the green light emitted from the plate correlates to a gray level of the final image.[6] Before the plate can be used again it must be "washed" or erased of the previous image. This is done by exposing the plate to a bright light. Some scanners have a built-in erase function on the unit so that when the PSP plate comes out of the scanner the previous image has already been erased. For units that do not have a built-in wash, the light in a dental operatory can be used for several minutes or the PSP plates can be placed on a bright light box for a few minutes to erase the image.

Digital Radiography

DR uses sensors for intraoral radiographs (Fig. 15-14) and flat-panel detectors for extraoral radiographs. The

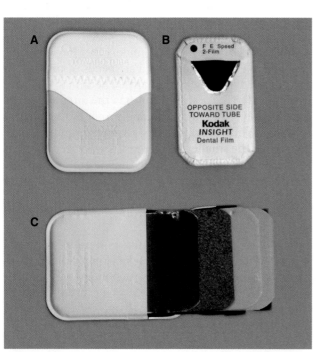

Figure 15-12. Analog film packets. (A) Size 2 plastic film packet. (B) Size 1 paper film packet. (C) Film packet contents (left to right): lead foil, black paper, and two analog films (blue).

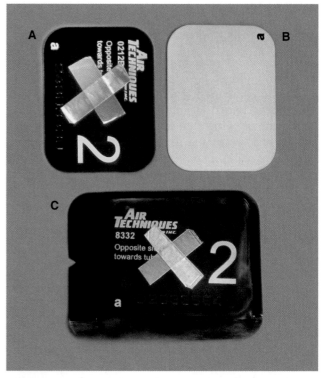

Figure 15-13. Photostimulable phosphor (PSP) plates. (A) Back side of PSP plate. (B) Sensitive side of PSP plate. (C) PSP plate in plastic protective barrier.

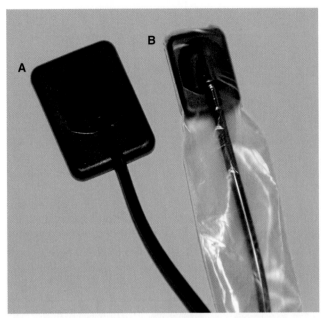

Figure 15-14. Digital radiography sensors. (A) Sensor. (B) Sensor in plastic protective barrier.

two types of sensors on the market are charge-coupled device (CCD) and complementary metal oxide semiconductors (CMOS). No research shows that one digital imaging system produces higher-quality images and both are of comparable diagnostic quality.[9,10] Flat-panel detectors are found on digital extraoral units such as pantomograph and lateral cephalometric skull x-ray units. The sensors are composed of silicon crystals. When an incoming x-ray interacts with the crystals, the bonds are broken. Where the bonds are broken, "charge packets" are created. Each charge packet is given a number based on the amount of broken bonds. These numbers correlate to a gray level on the computer resulting in a final image.[6] See Advancing Technologies.

Advancing Technologies

Cone beam computed tomography (CT) is a specialized CT unit for the maxillofacial region used in dentistry. Cone beam CT differs from traditional hospital-based CT units by showing only calcified tissues (such as bone, teeth, etc.), whereas a hospital-based CT unit is also able to differentiate soft tissues. This newer viewing modality shows three-dimensional views of the jaws and surrounding anatomy. Scans are made for many purposes including implant placement, impacted teeth, and lesions within the bone. Although cone beam CT use is increasing, it should still be used as a supplement to two-dimensional radiography such as intraoral and extraoral radiographs.[16–18] ■

IONIZING RADIATION PROTECTION GUIDELINES

Terminology

Several terms are used when describing aspects of ionizing radiation. Ionizing radiation is any type of radiation that can cause ionization of cells. Imaging systems that use x-rays or isotopes as the radiation source can cause ionization of cells. This includes dental radiography, computed tomography (CT), and positron emission tomography (PET). **Nonionizing radiation** is radiation that does not cause ionization of cells. The imaging systems capable of this are magnetic resonance imaging (MRI) and ultrasound. The SI unit of **sievert** refers to dose equivalent. An older term that is still occasionally used for dose equivalent is gray (1 gray = 1 sievert).

Effects on Biological Matter

Ionizing radiation has two different effects on biological matter: stochastic and deterministic.[5] **Stochastic effects** are all-or-nothing effects. This means that radiation-induced damage, such as cancer, either will or will not occur because of ionizing radiation exposure. This is a random effect, meaning not every ionizing radiation exposure will cause cancer; however, the greater the ionizing radiation exposure the higher the likelihood of a cancer developing.

Deterministic effects are dose-dependent effects. This means that a specific radiation dose must be received before the response will occur. With deterministic effects the radiation dose and response severity are proportional, meaning as the radiation dose increases, the severity of the response increases.[1] This is seen in acute radiation syndrome. Due to the randomness of stochastic effects on biological matter, each ionizing radiation exposure should be given using the lowest amount of radiation necessary to achieve the desired results.

Background Radiation Dose

The average radiation dose (background radiation) a person is exposed to in 1 year ranges from 360 to 620 mSv.[11] This exposure comes from external and internal sources of radiation. Examples of external radiation sources include cosmic, terrestrial (from the earth), radon, and human-made sources of radiation. Examples of internal radiation sources include digestion of foods and drinks. Radiation exposures for medical imaging such as plain film radiography, CT, and dental imaging are sources of external radiation. Radiation exposures in dentistry are so small that it accounts for less than 1% of the total average radiation dose.[11]

Lead Apron and Thyroid Collar

A lead apron has long been associated with radiation exposures in dentistry. A **lead apron** is a flexible shield placed over the thorax and pelvis of a patient with lead or lead equivalent thickness to block x-rays from exposing this area of the patient. Because every state law differs in the use of the lead apron, it is important to verify what your specific state laws are. Some states require the lead apron at all times and others follow the National Council on Radiation Protection and Measurements 145 (NCRP 145). According to the NCRP 145,[1] the lead (or lead equivalency) apron is not required as long as the dental office is in compliance with the following two recommendations:

- The office is using F speed film or a digital imaging system (CR or DR).
- All intraoral x-ray units use rectangular collimation.

A **thyroid collar** is a flexible shield with lead or lead equivalency that covers the neck, specifically the thyroid, blocking x-rays from exposing this area. The thyroid is more sensitive to radiation, especially in children compared with adults.[12] As with the lead apron, each state differs in the use of a thyroid collar and it is important to verify your specific state laws. According to NCRP 145, the thyroid collar shall be used on children and should be provided for adults regardless of the imaging system a dental office is using (analog x-ray film or digital). The only times a thyroid collar should not be used on an adult, according to NCRP 145, is when it will interfere with the path of x-rays and distort the final image.

Collimation

Collimation refers to shaping the x-ray beam to the area that is to be imaged. In dentistry, there are rectangular and round position-indicating devices (PIDs) or cones (Fig. 15-15). The PID/cone is the part of the x-ray unit where x-rays exit. Rectangular collimation creates a smaller x-ray beam that narrowly covers a size 2 analog film. Round collimation covers a much larger area of the patient than just the area to be imaged. Using a rectangular collimation with the same settings (mA, kVp, exposure time) as a round collimation results in a radiation exposure reduction to the patient by 60%.[6]

Radiation Exposure to the Operator

Operators can take several precautions to ensure that they are exposed to minimal, if any, amounts of ionizing radiation while exposing patients.

- The operator should be a minimum of 6 feet away from the source of radiation or behind a leaded (or lead equivalency thickness) barrier, typically a wall. Most dental operatories are designed such that the exposure button is in a location meeting this requirement.
- If the operator is not behind a barrier, but at a distance of 6 feet, he or she should be positioned 90 to 135 degrees to the x-ray beam to decrease any possible radiation exposure.[6]
- The operator should not hold the image receptor in the patient's mouth during exposure. Holding the image receptor in the patient's mouth results in direct exposure of the x-ray beam. This leads to an increased risk for radiation-induced damage.

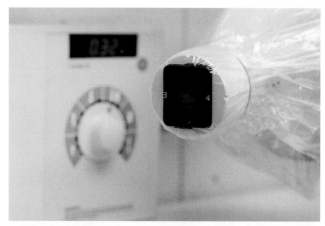

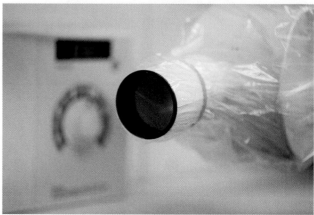

Figure 15-15. Rectangular collimation (A) and round collimation (B).

Prescription of Radiographs

Radiographs should be ordered and made only after reviewing the patient's medical history and a limited oral examination. A limited oral examination is the gathering of information from interview, medical and dental histories, observation, and clinical examination focusing on a specified issue. Radiographs should not be ordered on a routine basis. For new patients, efforts should be made to acquire radiographs from existing offices to aid in reduction of radiation exposure to that patient. The Food and Drug Administration (FDA) and American Dental Association (ADA) combined to create Guidelines for Prescribing Dental Radiographs[13] in 2004 to aid dental professionals in minimizing radiation exposure to patients (Table 15-4). It is necessary to review your state laws that determine who can order

Evidence-Based Practice

Research shows that the 2004 FDA/ADA Guidelines for Prescribing Dental Radiographs[13] are effective at providing minimal radiation exposure to patients with optimal diagnostic radiographs. By adhering to these guidelines, radiation exposure is limited, thereby decreasing the total lifetime radiation exposure for the patient.[19] ■

Table 15-4. Guidelines for Prescribing Dental Radiographs

Type of Encounter	Patient Age and Dental Developmental Stage				
	Child With Primary Dentition (before eruption of first permanent tooth)	Child With Transitional Dentition (after eruption of first permanent tooth)	Adolescent With Permanent Dentition (before eruption of third molars)	Adult, Dentate or Partially Edentulous	Adult, Edentulous
New patient being evaluated for dental diseases and dental development	Individualized radiographic examination consisting of selected periapical/occlusal views and/or posterior bitewings if proximal surfaces cannot be visualized or probed; patients without evidence of disease and with open proximal contacts may not require a radiographic examination at this time	Individualized radiographic examination consisting of posterior bitewings with panoramic examination or posterior bitewings and selected periapical images	Individualized radiographic examination consisting of posterior bitewings with panoramic examination or posterior bitewings and selected periapical images	Individualized radiographic examination consisting of posterior bitewings with panoramic examination or posterior bitewings; a full-mouth intraoral radiographic examination is preferred when the patient has clinical evidence of generalized dental disease or a history of extensive dental treatment	Individualized radiographic examination, based on clinical signs and symptoms
Recall patient with clinical caries and not at increased risk for caries	Posterior bitewing examination at 6- to 12-month intervals if proximal surfaces cannot be examined visually or with a probe	Posterior bitewing examination at 6- to 12-month intervals if proximal surfaces cannot be examined visually or with a probe		Posterior bitewing examination at 6- to 18-month intervals	Not applicable
Recall patient with no clinical caries and not at increased risk for caries	Posterior bitewing examination at 12- to 24-month intervals if proximal surfaces cannot be examined visually or with a probe	Posterior bitewing examination at 12- to 24-month intervals if proximal surfaces cannot be examined visually or with a probe	Posterior bitewing examination at 18- to 36-month intervals	Posterior bitewing examination at 24- to 36-month intervals	Not applicable

Source: From American Dental Association, U.S. Food and Drug Administration. The selection of patients for dental radiograph examinations. Revised 2012. http://www.fda.gov/Radiation-EmittingProducts/RadiationEmitting-ProductsandProcedures/MedicalImaging/MedicalX-Rays/ucm116504.htm. Accessed July 26, 2015.

radiographs. In most states, only a licensed dentist is legally able to prescribe radiographs. See Evidence-Based Practice.

RADIATION SAFETY

Radiation to children and pregnant women is frequently in the news as a developing fetus and child have increased susceptibility to ionizing radiation.[14] There are a few historical examples (Japan and Chernobyl) of large doses of ionizing radiation to pregnant women and children resulting in leukemia and various solid tumors both benign and malignant.[15] This overwhelming negative information about ionizing radiation can make it difficult to assure patients that radiographs are necessary to provide optimum care in a dental office.

Dental offices can help alleviate any concerns by establishing radiation protection guidelines and making these readily available to staff and patients. These procedures should include administration of the guidelines, criteria for exposure, and operating procedures. The administration of the guidelines determines who in the office is responsible for the x-ray–producing units. This is typically a dentist in the office. This person should create a quality-assurance program that monitors the images made and x-ray units to ensure that diagnostic-quality radiographs are being produced. The criteria for exposure should state whether the office follows the FDA/ADA Guidelines for Prescribing Dental Radiographs or a different set of guidelines as determined by the dentist(s) in the office. The operating procedures should include settings for x-ray units and other radiation safety precautions taken in the office including, but not limited to, the thyroid collar, lead apron, infection disease control, pregnancy, and past radiation exposure most commonly because of radiation therapy. Radiography is beneficial to patients, providing information to the practitioner not visible to the naked eye, but proper radiation protection guidelines must be followed with each exposure. See Application to Clinical Practice.

Application to Clinical Practice

You are volunteering for Dental Day, a day-long clinic serving children from underserved areas around the state. You have been assigned two patients aged 10 and 12 years. The 10-year-old patient has brought horizontal bitewing radiographs. The 12-year-old patient has not had radiographs in 3 years. A limited oral examination shows pink, stippled gingiva with no existing restorations or evident carious lesions. What radiographs will you recommend when discussing this case with the supervising dentist and why? ■

Case Study

Paul, a 7-year-old boy, presents with his mother as a new patient in the dental office. His last dental visit was 2 years prior. No recent radiographs are available. A limited intraoral examination reveals that Paul's oral hygiene is poor with red and swollen gingiva. The patient's mother notes that there is bleeding when he brushes and flosses. Generalized severe biofilm is present. There are restorations on the mandibular permanent first molars (#19 and #30), which are erupted onto the plane of occlusion. Large occlusal carious lesions are evident on the maxillary and mandibular primary second molars (A, J, K, and T). After discussing this case with the dentist, bitewing and periapical radiographs of the posterior teeth are recommended. The patient's mother is hesitant about the radiographs due to a recent news segment she saw involving over-radiation of children in a nearby state.

Case Study Exercises

1. What classification applies to this patient in the FDA/ADA Guidelines for Prescribing Dental Radiographs?
   A. Child with primary dentition, new patient
   B. Child with transitional dentition, new patient
   C. Child with primary dentition, recall patient
   D. Child with transitional dentition, recall patient
2. The radiographs prescribed by the dentist are in accordance with the FDA/ADA guidelines. The patient has overall poor oral hygiene.
   A. Both statements are true.
   B. Both statements are false.
   C. The first statement is true, but the second statement is false.
   D. The first statement is false, but the second statement is true.

Case Study—cont'd

3. What other permanent teeth are likely visible in the oral cavity?
   A. 24, 25
   B. 8, 9
   C. 23, 24, 25, 26
   D. 8, 9, 23, 24, 25, 26
4. Paul's mother's concern about radiation exposure is unfounded. The dental hygienist should discuss the necessity of radiographs with Paul's mother to obtain consent before exposures.
   A. The first statement is true, but the second statement is false.
   B. The first statement is false, but the second statement is true.
   C. Both statements are true.
   D. Both statements are false.
5. At what age should the primary mandibular molars (K and T) exfoliate?
   A. 6–8 years
   B. 7–9 years
   C. 10–12 years
   D. 13–15 years

Review Questions

1. Which of the following is NOT a type of digital radiography (DR)?
   A. CMOS
   B. CCD
   C. Flat-panel detector
   D. PSP plate

2. Which of the following is a type of intraoral radiograph?
   A. Cone beam CT
   B. Occlusal radiograph
   C. Lateral cephalometric skull
   D. Pantomograph

3. Collimation is the shaping of the x-ray beam. Rectangular collimation reduces radiation exposure by 60% compared with round collimation.
   A. Both statements are true.
   B. Both statements are false.
   C. The first statement is true, but the second statement is false.
   D. The first statement is false, but the second statement is true.

4. Density refers to the blacks, grays, and whites of a radiograph. An adjective used to describe any object/substance (part of the patient) that blocks the transmission of x-rays is radiolucent.
   A. Both statements are true.
   B. Both statements are false.
   C. The first statement is true, but the second statement is false.
   D. The first statement is false, but the second statement is true.

5. Medical imaging is a type of natural background radiation. Dental imaging accounts for less than 1% of the average annual radiation dose.
   A. Both statements are true.
   B. Both statements are false.
   C. The first statement is true, but the second statement is false.
   D. The first statement is false, but the second statement is true.

Active Learning

1. Find a dental operatory with an x-ray unit. Position it over the chair and measure out 6 feet to determine how far away this is from the unit. Make note of surrounding landmarks to use in the future.
2. Aim an x-ray unit at the wall opposite the direction you are facing. Determine where 90 to 135 degrees from the x-ray beam is.
3. View other radiographs in this textbook and online to visualize more examples of normal radiographic appearances including enamel, dentin, lamina dura, among others.
4. Discuss radiation safety with the members of the general public (not dental professionals) determining what they know or have heard about ionizing radiation or x-rays. Use this information to aid you when discussing radiation safety with patients and other dental professionals. ■

REFERENCES

1. Radiation protection in dentistry [National Council on Radiation Protection and Measurements (NCRP) Report No. 145]. Bethesda, MD: NCRP; 2003.

2. Rout J, Brown J. Ionizing radiation regulations and the dental practitioner: 1. The nature of ionizing radiation and its use in dentistry. *Dent Update.* 2012;39(3): 191-192, 195-198, 201-203.

3. Darby, Michelle L. *Mosby's Comprehensive Review of Dental Hygiene.* 7th ed. St. Louis, MO: Mosby; 2011.

4. Iannuci JM, Howerton LJ. *Dental Radiography: Principles and Techniques.* 4th ed. St. Louis, Mo: Elsevier; 2011.

5. Dietze G, Menzel HG. Dose quantities in radiation protection and their limitations. *Radiat Prot Dosimetry.* 2004;112(4):457-463.

6. White SC, Pharoah MJ. *Oral Radiology: Principles and Interpretation.* 6th ed. St. Louis, Mo: Mosby Elsevier; 2009.

7. Curry TS, Dowdey JE, Murray RC. *Christensen's Physics of Diagnostic Radiology.* 4th ed. Baltimore, MD: Lippincott Williams & Wilkins, 1990.

8. Kashima I. Computed radiography with Photostimulable phosphor in oral and maxillofacial radiology. *Oral Surg Oral Med Oral Pathol Oral Radiol Endod.* 1995; 80:577-598.

9. Luangjamekorn N, Williams N, Angelopoulos N. Digital panoramic radiography image quality: a comparison with film-based panoramic radiography. *Oral Surg Oral Med Oral Pathol Oral Radiol Endod.* 2005; 99(3):E25.

10. Paurazas SB, Geist JR, Pink FE, Hoen MM, Steiman HR. Comparison of diagnostic accuracy of digital imaging by using CCD and CMOS-APS sensors with E-speed film in the detection of periapical bony lesions. *Oral Surg Oral Med Oral Pathol Oral Radiol Endod.* 2000;89:356-362.

11. Ionizing radiation exposure of the population of the United States [National Council on Radiation Protection and Measurements (NCRP) Report No. 160]. Bethesda, MD: NCRP; 2009.

12. White SC, Mallya SM. Update on the biological effects of ionizing radiation, relative dose factors and radiation hygiene. *Aust Dent J.* 2012;57(suppl 1):2-8.

13. American Dental Association. Guidelines for Prescribing Dental Radiographs. Chicago, IL: American Dental Association. Updated November 2004. http://www.ada.org/sections/professionalResources/pdfs/topics_radiography_chart.pdf. Accessed October 2012.

14. Boice JD. Radiation epidemiology: a perspective on Fukushima. *J Radiol Prot.* 2012;32:N33-N40.

15. Krille L, Zeeb H, Jahnen A, Mildenberger P, Seldenbusch M, Schneider K, et al. Computed tomographies and cancer risk in children: a literature overview of CT practices, risk estimations and an epidemiologic cohort study proposal. *Radiat Environ Biophys.* 2012;51(2):103-111.

16. Fanning B. CBCT—the justification process, audit and review of the recent literature. *J Ir Dent Assoc.* 2011; 57(5):256-261.

17. American Academy of Oral and Maxillofacial Radiology executive opinion statement on performing and interpreting diagnostic cone beam computed tomography. *Oral Surg Oral Med Oral Pathol Oral Radiol Endod.* 2008; 106:561-562.

18. American Dental Association Council on Scientific Affairs. The use of cone-beam computed tomography in dentistry: an advisory statement from the American Dental Association Council on Scientific Affairs. *J Am Dent Assoc.* 2012;143(8):899-902.

19. Kim I, Mupparapu M. Dental radiographic guidelines: a review. *Quintessence Int.* 2009;40(5):389-398.

Chapter 16 | Dietary Assessment and Nutritional Counseling

Anne L. Hague, PhD, MS, RD, LD, RDH, CLT

KEY TERMS

cariogenic

cariostatic

dental erosion

dietary adequacy

dietary assessment

Dietary Guidelines for Americans, 2010

nutrient imbalance

nutritional counseling

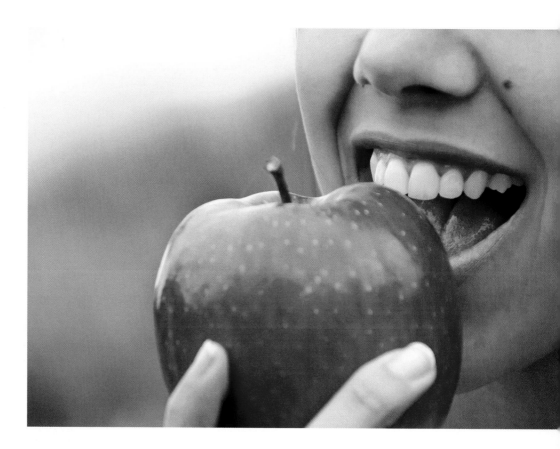

LEARNING OBJECTIVES

After reading this chapter, the student should be able to:

16.1 Recognize dietary factors that may increase a patient's risk for oral/dental conditions.

16.2 Recognize oral manifestations associated with nutrient imbalance.

16.3 Identify oral conditions that increase a patient's risk for nutrient imbalance.

16.4 Recognize the tools used to assess a patient's diet.

16.5 Demonstrate appropriate nutritional counseling procedures and communication skills.

16.6 Educate the patient about how diet impacts oral health and how oral health impacts diet.

16.7 Assist the patient in assessing the adequacy of his or her diet and the dietary risk factors to oral/dental health.

16.8 Recognize conditions that require a referral to a registered dietitian, physician, or both.

KEY CONCEPTS

- Oral/dental health affects diet and nutritional status.
- Diet and nutritional status affects oral/dental health.
- Diet screening, nutrition education, and guidance are essential components of clinical dental care.
- Good communication skills are critical to effective nutritional counseling.

RELEVANCE TO CLINICAL PRACTICE

Nutritional status, diet, and oral health are closely interrelated. A healthy dentition promotes good chewing function, and normal mastication is needed to support a healthy diet. Likewise, a healthy diet is needed to support and maintain optimal health of oral tissues. These relationships, along with the frequency of preventative dental care appointments, place the dental hygienist in an ideal position to screen patients for nutritional and oral health risk.

Dietary assessment or screening is considered an integral part of health promotion and disease prevention in comprehensive patient care.[1,2] Although all patients can benefit from dietary assessment, nutrition intervention is especially important when the patient's oral/dental conditions compromise dietary intake or the patient's diet represents an increased risk for oral/dental disease(s), or both.

IMPACT OF DIETARY RISK FACTORS ON ORAL HEALTH

Numerous dietary factors can increase or decrease oral health risks.

Oral Manifestations Associated With Nutrient Imbalance

Malnutrition represents an imbalance in the amount of energy and nutrients an individual obtains from his or her diet. This imbalance can be from an inadequate or excessive amount of energy and nutrient intake; impaired mastication, digestion, or absorption; and utilization of foods. Dental problems that interfere with normal chewing and swallowing can cause malnutrition. For example, a patient who suffers from chronic temporomandibular joint disorder is likely to select only soft foods and liquids, and avoid foods that require considerable chewing such as meats, fresh fruits, and vegetables. Such a diet may provide the calories needed to maintain body weight, but it may not provide an adequate amount of essential nutrients.

Malnutrition is not uncommon in the United States, particularly in the younger and older adult populations. Malnutrition has been reported to be as high as 10% for children younger than 5 years living in rural areas[3] and 5% to 10% of older adults living in areas without assisted care.[4] The oral health professional is likely to be the first health-care professional to detect a **nutrient imbalance** because clinical signs of malnutrition are often first observed in the oral cavity.[5] This is attributed to the more rapid turnover rate of oral soft tissues (3–7 days) and the increased immediate need for nutrients, compared with other tissues in the body.[6,7] Because clinical signs are evident only in advanced malnutrition, and specific testing is needed for diagnosis, the patient should be referred to a registered dietitian and physician for further assessment. Even though clinical signs are not present in less advanced stages, normal body functions are impaired. For instance, a malnourished patient undergoing oral surgery is at an increased risk for postoperative infection and diminished healing.[8,9]

When malnutrition is present, nutrient imbalance rarely occurs in isolation. Instead, malnutrition is usually associated with an imbalance in multiple nutrients. For instance, manifestations found in the oral soft tissues (i.e., tongue, mucosa, and gingiva) are usually associated with deficiencies in the B vitamins, vitamins A and C, zinc, and iron.[10–12] Hard tissue manifestations (i.e., teeth and bone) are usually associated with deficiencies in calcium, phosphorus, magnesium, fluoride, and vitamins A and D.[10–12] Nutrient imbalances associated with manifestations of the tongue, mucosa, periodontium, and teeth are provided in Table 16-1.

Table 16-1. Oral Signs Associated With Malnutrition

Condition	Nutrient Imbalance*
Manifestations of the Tongue	
Hypogeusia	Zinc, vitamins A, B_1, B_2, B_{12} (deficiencies)
Glossodynia	Iron, vitamins B_1, B_2, B_3, B_6, B_{12} (deficiencies)
Papillary atrophy	Iron, vitamins B_2, B_3 (deficiencies)
Pale tongue	Iron, vitamins folate, B_{12} (deficiencies)
Beefy red tongue	Vitamin B_3 (deficiency)
Glossitis	Iron, vitamins B_2, B_3, B_6, B_{12}, folate (deficiencies)
Manifestations of the Mucosa	
Angular cheilitis	Iron, vitamins B_2, B_3, B_6, B_{12}, folate, C (deficiencies)
Candidiasis	Iron, zinc, vitamins A, B_{12}, folate, C (deficiencies)
Delayed wound healing	Zinc, vitamins A, B_2, C (deficiencies)
Mucositis/ stomatitis	Vitamins B_1, B_3, B_{12}, folate (deficiencies)
Atrophic oral mucosa	Vitamin A, B_3, zinc (deficiencies)
Desquamation of oral mucosa	Vitamin A (deficiency)
Manifestations of the Periodontium	
Inflamed, bleeding gingiva	Vitamins B_2, B_3, B_{12}, folate, C, K (deficiencies)
Decreased alveolar bone integrity	Calcium, magnesium, vitamin D (deficiencies)
Manifestations of the Teeth	
Disturbed enamel development	Calcium, phosphorus, vitamins A, D (deficiencies)
Mottled enamel with pitting	Fluoride (excess)

*Vitamin B_1 (thiamin), vitamin B_2 (riboflavin), vitamin B_3 (niacin), vitamin B_6 (pyridoxine).

Sources: Deen D. Nutritional assessment of the oral cavity. *Nutr Clin Care.* 2001;4:28-33; Moynihan PJ, Lingstrom P. Oral consequences of compromised nutritional well-being. In: Touger-Decker R, Sirois D, Mobley C, eds. *Nutrition and Oral Medicine.* Totowa, NJ: Humana Press; 2005:107-127; Palmer CA, Papas AS. The minerals and mineralization. In: Cohen M, ed. *Diet and Nutrition in Oral Health.* Upper Saddle River, NJ: Pearson Prentice Hall; 2007:147-188; and Palmer CA, Papas AS. The minerals and mineralization. In: Cohen M, ed. *Diet and Nutrition in Oral Health.* Upper Saddle River, NJ: Pearson Prentice Hall; 2007. p.:147-188.

Malnutrition and Periodontitis

Periodontitis is an inflammatory response to dental biofilm infection. When nutrient deficiencies are present, the immune response is impaired. A compromised immune response can decrease the ability to effectively fight infection or can predispose an individual to infection.[13,14] The nutritional needs of a malnourished patient with periodontitis are further challenged because of the increased need for nutrients (e.g., antioxidant vitamins and minerals) when inflammation is present. It is important to note that an excess of select nutrients can alter the immune function as well. For instance, diets high in refined carbohydrates (glucose) can be a major cause of chronic inflammation. Subsequently, patients with periodontal disease should be counseled to consume a diet low in refined carbohydrates with emphasis on fruits, vegetables, and fish oil because these foods have been shown to provide anti-inflammatory effects.[15]

Malnutrition and Oral Tissue Development

Malnutrition also affects the development of oral tissues, causing abnormal tooth development (e.g., enamel hypoplasia), delayed eruption, altered salivary composition and volume, and diminished quantity and quality (i.e., density) of alveolar bone.[16] A single episode of mild-to-moderate malnutrition in the first year of life has been associated with an increased risk for dental caries in both the primary and permanent dentition.[17] This association is thought to be influenced by increased enamel solubility, hypoplastic grooves and/or pits in the enamel (causing a mechanical nidus, or point, for bacteria and food), and salivary gland hypofunction (causing reduced salivary flow rate and decreased antimicrobial proteins in the saliva).[18]

Fluid Imbalance and Xerostomia

Saliva is composed primarily of water. It is recommended that adults consume approximately 1 mL of water per kilocalorie of food consumed. Most water is obtained from foods and liquids. It is recommended for adults to consume approximately 8 cups of water daily.[19] Inadequate water intake can cause xerostomia (dry mouth), which is associated with an increased risk for dental caries and periodontal diseases. Optimal salivary flow reduces the risk for dental diseases via its antimicrobial activity, increased food clearance, buffering of acids (from bacteria), and promotion of remineralization of early carious lesions in enamel and cementum. Because stimulated saliva from chewing action has an even greater protective role (higher pH and buffer capacity) than nonstimulated saliva, fibrous foods and sugar-free chewing gum (e.g., sweetened with xylitol) are especially beneficial in reducing the risk for dental caries.[20]

Fermentable Carbohydrates and Dental Caries

Dental caries is a chronic site-specific disease that involves the presence of fermentable carbohydrates, select strains of bacteria in the dental biofilm (e.g., *Streptococcus mutans* and lactobacilli), and a susceptible tooth/host. Carbohydrates that are metabolized by the bacteria and reduce the plaque pH to less than 5.5, the critical level at which demineralization begins, are considered fermentable. Fermentable carbohydrates include sugars such as monosaccharides (glucose, galactose, and fructose), disaccharides (sucrose, maltose, and lactose), and cooked starches or polysaccharides. Sucrose is an important factor in the cause of caries because glucan (metabolic by-product of sucrose) facilitates the adherence of *Streptococcus mutans* to enamel and reduces plaque pH.[21] Although acid is produced at a slower rate for high-starch foods compared with other carbohydrates, the addition of sucrose to high-starch foods (e.g., sugar-sweetened cereals, cakes, cookies, pies, or pastries) makes them more **cariogenic** (likely to promote dental caries) because of greater food retention on tooth surfaces.[21,22] Examples of fermentable foods include cooked vegetables, most fresh fruits, ice cream, sweetened beverages, cookies, cakes, bread, rice, and slowly dissolving candies.[23]

Protective Foods and Beverages and Dental Caries

Select foods have anticariogenic, or **cariostatic,** properties. Foods high in protein and fat are considered cariostatic because they are not capable of causing a decline in pH to less than 5.5. For example, cheese and nonskim cow's milk contain protein (casein) and fat, as well as calcium and phosphorus. These nutrients help to buffer plaque acids, causing reduced demineralization and enhanced remineralization. Protective benefits are also obtained from raw fruits and vegetables and sugar-free chewing gum, via salivary stimulation.[23,24] Nutritive and non-nutritive sweeteners are also considered noncariogenic because the bacteria are unable to metabolize them (non-nutritive sweeteners) or metabolize them too slowly (sugar alcohols).[25] Xylitol is especially beneficial because it inhibits the growth of microorganisms, neutralizes plaque acids, and reduces bacterial adherence.[26,27]

Dietary Pattern and Dental Caries

Increased frequency in the consumption of fermentable carbohydrates is considered the primary dietary factor associated with increased caries activity.[28] Subsequently, it is recommended to reduce or avoid frequent consumption of fermentable carbohydrates, especially between meals.

Sequence of food consumption is also a strong determinant of caries risk (more than diet composition). For example, caries risk can be significantly reduced when a noncariogenic or cariostatic food (e.g., chewing gum sweetened with xylitol) is consumed at the end of a meal.[20,27] Caries risk can also be reduced by combining higher-risk foods with lower-risk foods such as cheese and crackers, peanuts and apple slices, and cottage cheese and bananas.

Consistency of Foods and Dental Caries

Fermentable carbohydrates that are retentive (e.g., cookies, crackers, and potato chips) or dissolve slowly in the mouth (e.g., hard candy) increase the risk for caries because of longer acid exposure or reduced oral clearance. Some foods have a high initial retention or stickiness (e.g., caramels, jelly beans, and raisins), but then are cleared quickly from the oral cavity because of increased salivary flow. Those foods that are retentive and have a slow oral clearance are considered especially cariogenic.[24,28] Fibrous foods that stimulate salivary flow increase oral clearance and may also help maintain supporting tissues of the teeth (i.e., bone and periodontal ligament). Although fibrous foods increase oral clearance, it is important to note that fibrous foods are not effective in removing dental biofilm. Therefore, eating an apple should not be considered "nature's toothbrush."

Dental Erosion

Dental erosion is a loss of tooth structure due to acid exposure from foods and beverages (exogenous sources) and/or gastric contents (endogenous sources). Unlike dental caries, dental erosion is due to a chemical process (rather than a bacterial process). Dental erosion is associated with the consumption of a number of different acidic (less than 5.5 pH) foods and drinks.[29] The recent increase in erosion, especially among children, has been attributed to a significant increase in soft drink (regular and diet) consumption.[30] Chronic exposure to acids (e.g., daily sipping of soft drinks) can weaken tooth integrity and increase the risk for caries.[14] Identifying the acid source (exogenous or endogenous) and other risk factors, such as reduced salivary flow, are critical in preventing further loss of tooth structure, pulp exposure, or both. Examples of high-acid foods include all fruits except figs, most tomatoes, pickled foods, jams, jellies, and fruit butters.[31]

IMPACT OF DENTAL/ORAL HEALTH ON DIET

Many oral conditions can affect a patient's diet and increase his or her risk for malnutrition (Fig. 16-1). Some of these conditions, such as oral pain and difficulty chewing and/or swallowing, not only alter the patient's diet but can increase the patient's need for nutrients (e.g., wound healing and infections). For example, common conditions in the older adult patient include active infections such as periodontitis and/or root caries, xerostomia, altered appetite, and edentulism. Xerostomia makes eating and swallowing more difficult, and missing teeth or dentures is associated with reduced chewing

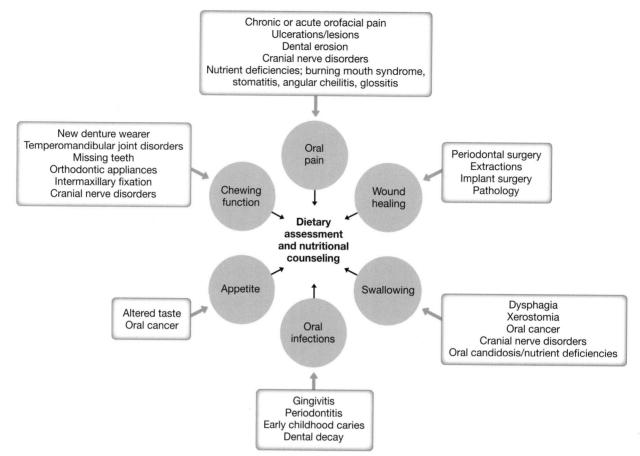

Figure 16-1. Oral conditions that affect diet.

function.[32] The chewing function of patients who wear dentures is approximately 20% of the chewing ability of a dentate individual with 20 or more teeth.[33] Compromised chewing function may result in the avoidance of difficult-to-chew nutrient-dense foods such as raw vegetables, fruits, whole grain breads, and meats.

Patients at increased risk for malnutrition because of compromised dental and oral conditions benefit greatly from dietary assessment and nutritional counseling. In fact, studies have shown that prosthetic rehabilitation without nutritional counseling failed to improve dietary intake.[34,35] For example, a patient with a new denture may be inclined to continue a soft diet and/or a diet with poor variety without nutritional counseling. Dietary improvements have been observed in older adults who received nutritional counseling with the provision of dentures.[36] Recognizing a patient who may be at risk for malnutrition because of existing dental and oral conditions is the first step in providing dietary assessment and nutritional counseling.

DIETARY ASSESSMENT PROCEDURES

Dietary assessment or screening should be provided to patients whose diet is negatively affecting their oral and dental health (e.g., nutrient imbalance, frequent consumption of fermentable carbohydrates, dental

erosion), as well as patients with oral condition(s) that are negatively affecting their diet (e.g., oral pain, oral/dental infections, altered chewing function). The role of the dental hygienist in **nutritional counseling** (ADA code D1310) is to:

1. Understand the patient's motivation and readiness to change.
2. Provide nutrition and oral health education.
3. Assist the patient in self-assessment of dietary and oral health risks.
4. Collaborate with the patient to determine appropriate dietary and lifestyle modifications.
5. Facilitate positive change via behavior modification.

The *Dietary Guidelines for Americans, 2010* should be used as the basis for patient education and guidance. These guidelines are recommendations for both healthy Americans and those at increased risk for chronic disease (age ≥ 2 years). The guidelines emphasize daily energy balance, physical activity, a healthy body weight, nutrient-dense foods, food safety, and healthy eating patterns that meet the nutritional needs for general and specific population groups (Box 16-1).[37] The *Dietary Guidelines for Americans, 2010* Executive Summary and Policy Document can be viewed at the U.S. Department of Agriculture (USDA) Center for Nutrition Policy and Promotion website (www.cnpp.usda.gov/DGAs2010-PolicyDocument.htm).

Table 16-2. *Sample 24-Hour Recall*

Mealtime	Food/Beverage Quantity	Location
Breakfast (7:10 a.m.)	0.5 large banana / 0.5 cup 2% cow's milk / 1 cup toasted whole grain oats cereal / 6 oz. fresh orange juice	Home
Snack (10:15 a.m.)	12 oz. bottled water	Classroom
Lunch (12:30 p.m.)	3 tbs. regular peanut butter / 2 tbs. strawberry jam / 2 slices wheat bread / 1 cup vanilla Greek yogurt / 2 homemade chocolate-chip cookies / 12 oz. regular cola	Cafeteria
Snack (4:30 p.m.)	1 oz. regular potato chips / 12 oz. regular cola	Work
Dinner (6:30 p.m.)	1 cup cooked spaghetti / 0.5 cup plain tomato sauce / 1 cup salad greens / 3 tbs. Italian dressing / 1 medium whole wheat roll / 2 tsp. butter / 1 cup 2% cow's milk / 1 cup regular chocolate ice cream	Home
Snack (9:15 p.m.)	2 cups tap water	Home

Dietary Assessment Tools

The primary purpose of dietary assessment for dental patients is to determine general **dietary adequacy** (number of servings in each food group) and usual eating habits and/or patterns of eating cariogenic foods and beverages. Dietary assessment tools that are commonly used include the 24-hour recall and the food record.

24-Hour Recall

The 24-hour recall is simple, quick (less than 20 minutes), and can show usual eating patterns and habits. For this reason, it is a useful tool for the evaluation of caries risk.[38] To complete a 24-hour recall, the patient is asked to recall all foods and drinks consumed from the previous 24-hour period. The patient is also probed for common omissions such as added items (e.g., sugar, dressings, butter) and nonfood items (e.g., lozenges, gum, supplements). These interviewing techniques require training and practice. The dental hygienist records the patient's responses, noting the patient's eating times and location, portion sizes, preparation method, and types and brand names of all foods and beverages consumed (Table 16-2). The format used for recording the 24-hour recall can be used for the food record, using multiple copies as needed.

Food Record

The multiple-day food record is more representative of usual intake than the 24-hour recall because it reflects day-to-day intake variability. For this reason it is a more appropriate determinant of dietary adequacy than the 24-hour recall. The same information obtained in the 24-hour recall is obtained in the food record except the food record is recorded by the patient at the time of consumption to minimize memory errors. Records are usually kept for a period of 3 to 7 days, including at least 1 weekend day. Three- to 5-day food records can help moderate the burden of recording foods and drinks for a full week and can help reduce potential bias (i.e., when usual intake is altered to streamline the recording process).

Effective Communication Skills

Nutritional counseling should be provided in a quiet, relaxed space that is separate from the clinical treatment area. A nonthreatening environment with teaching aids such as food models, brochures, and posters available is especially conducive to learning. The use of good communication skills is essential in this process (Fig. 16-2). To assist the patient in deciding what dietary and lifestyle changes to make, it is very important

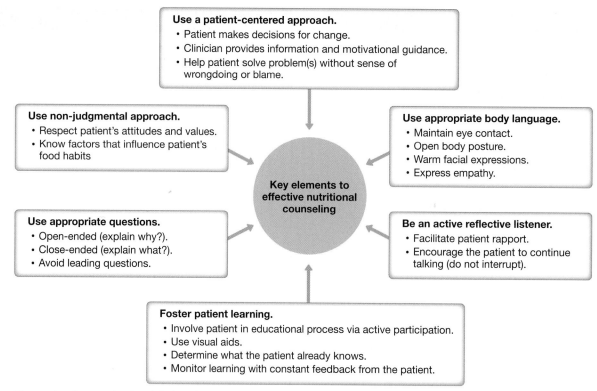

Figure 16-2. Communication skills for effective nutritional counseling.

the dental hygienist understands what factors influence the patient's food habits and food selection. Dietary influences often include timing, location, availability, dental and/or medical conditions, cultural values, as well as educational, economic, and psychological factors. Inquiry about the patient's typical daily activities and data from the Oral Health Evaluation form (Table 16-3) can help the dental hygienist gain insight into the patient's values, lifestyle, and dietary influences. A good understanding of these influences allows the dental hygienist to facilitate dietary and behavioral changes that are consistent with the patient's lifestyle and values. These considerations help contribute to the patient's success in long-term behavior modification.

Table 16-3. *Oral Health Evaluation Form*

Nutrition/Oral Health Evaluation

Patient Name: _____
Date: _____

Instructions: Please respond to the following questions by marking your answer in the appropriate column.

	Yes or How Many?	No or NA
Nutrition History*		
Are you on a special diet?		
Do you have any food allergies or restrictions?		
Have you recently lost or gained more than 10 pounds?		
Do you frequently vomit or experience indigestion?		
Do you chew regular gum or eat candy (including breath mints or hard candy)?		
Do you drink more than 3 alcoholic beverages daily?		
Do you usually eat snacks?		
Do you have difficulty shopping for or preparing food?		
Do you drink 6–8 cups of water each day?		

Table 16-3. *Oral Health Evaluation Form—cont'd*

	Yes or How Many?	No or NA
Do you chew sugarless gum?		
Are your feelings about food positive?		
Do you have a good appetite?		
How many times per day do you eat?		
How many times a day do you consume sugar-sweetened fruit drink/juice or soda (regular or diet)?		
How many times a day do you consume sugar-sweetened coffee or tea (hot or cold)?		
Dental History		
Do you have any dental problems that affect your chewing?		
Do you wear a denture or a partial denture?		
Do you wear your denture or partial denture regularly?		
Does your mouth feel "dry" most of the time or when eating a meal?		
Do you have difficulty swallowing foods?		
Do you use a fluoridated rinse or toothpaste?		
Do you have all of your natural teeth (with or without wisdom teeth)?		
How many times a day do you brush your teeth?		
How many times a day do you floss your teeth?		
Health History		
Do you have a medical condition?		
Are you pregnant?		
Do you have high blood pressure?		
Do you take prescription or over-the-counter medications on a regular basis?		
Do you experience any side effects from any medications you take?		
Do you use tobacco products?		
Do you take vitamin, mineral, herbal, or nutritional supplements?		
Exercise History		
Do you exercise regularly?		

*A positive response to boldface text requires follow-up with the patient.

NA, not applicable.

Twelve Steps to Dietary Assessment

The diet record is analyzed for adequacy, eating habits, and cariogenic potential using the following 12-step procedure. Emphasis is placed on the patient's self-assessment (for diet adequacy and dental caries), general nutrition education, and guidance by the dental hygienist (Box 16-2). A diet assessment can also be done using computer programs, such as the USDA Center for Nutrition Policy and Promotion MyPlate Super Tracker (available online at: www.choosemyplate.gov/super-tracker-tools/supertracker.html). The computer-assisted assessment can save time and provides good accuracy. However, it is important to note that neither approach (computerized or noncomputerized) should be used to determine whether dietary supplements are needed. Supplement recommendations should be determined via a more in-depth assessment.

Step 1: Provide Instructions to Complete the Food Record

Review the written instructions on how to record a dietary record with the patient and provide a copy for

Box 16-2. *Objectives of Nutritional Counseling*

- Use information from the patient histories (nutrition, dental, health, and exercise) to help the patient determine appropriate, individualized dietary and lifestyle modifications.
- Educate the patient about the *Dietary Guidelines for Americans, 2010* and the role of nutrition in general/oral health.
- Use the *Choose MyPlate Food Guidance System* to help the patient assess the adequacy of his or her diet.
- Educate the patient about dietary inadequacy or excess and its implications in general/oral health.
- Assist the patient in identifying unhealthy dietary and lifestyle habits and facilitate positive change via behavior modification.
- Determine whether the types of foods and beverages consumed and/or the pattern of food consumption, such as frequent snacking, increase the patient's risk for dental diseases. ■

his reference at home (Box 16-3). Use portion size estimates (Box 16-4) or multiple visuals, such as food models, household measures, and pictures of foods and utensils, to help the patient better estimate and understand portion sizes. The estimates need to be a reliable

indication of the amounts consumed because these are the determinants used for dietary adequacy and modifications. Comments about select foods that may bias the patient's recording also need to be avoided (e.g., "Be sure to record the amount correctly for healthy foods like whole grains as well as unhealthy foods like candy."). Such comments may cause the patient to alter her true recording to depict a more healthy diet. A follow-up appointment (steps 2–12) is scheduled for the diet assessment and nutritional counseling session after the patient completes the dietary record.

Step 2: Review Food Record

Review the food record with the patient to ensure completeness. Inquire about common omissions such as mayonnaise, salad dressings, butter or margarine, sauces, and milk, cream, or sugar in coffee or tea. Revisit the food models and household measures if the patient is uncertain about the amount(s) of food and drinks recorded.

Step 3: Review Patient Histories

Obtain nutrition, exercise, dental, and health history information (see Table 16-3). It is important to gather this information to help identify appropriate dietary and healthy lifestyle changes. For example, knowing the patient is following "a special diet" or has "food allergies or restrictions" (items 1 and 2 on the Oral Health Evaluation form in Table 16-3) will help the

Box 16-3. *Instructions to Complete a Food Record*

- Select days that are most representative of your usual intake (including a weekend day).
- Record *everything* consumed including water, supplements, lozenges, gum, and/or medications.
- Record food and drinks immediately after consumption to ensure *all* items are recorded.
- Include specific details (e.g., type of food and how it was prepared).
- List the food ingredients for combination foods individually (e.g., ham and cheese sandwich with lettuce, tomato, mayonnaise, and mustard).
- Provide accurate measurements. List the amounts in common household measures that you are familiar with (e.g., teaspoons, cups, pat, ounce, inch).
- Milk: Indicate whether milk is whole, low fat (1% or 2%), or skim. Include flavoring if used.
- Vegetables and fruits: Fresh whole fruits and vegetables should be listed as small, medium, or large. Be sure to indicate if the food was raw or cooked. Specify if sugar or syrup was added to fruit or if any margarine, butter, cheese, or cream sauce was added to vegetables. When recording salad, list items comprising salad and be sure to include if any dressing was used.

- Eggs: Indicate method of preparation (scrambled, fried, poached, etc.) and number eaten.
- Meat, poultry, fish: Indicate approximate size (e.g., 2" × 2" or 1") or weight in ounces of the serving. Be sure to include any gravy, sauce, or breading added.
- Cheese: Indicate kind, number of ounces, cubic inches, or slices, and whether it is made from whole milk, part skim, or is low calorie.
- Cereal: Specify kind, whether cooked or dry. Measure or estimate the amount in cups or ounces.
- Breads and rolls: Specify kind (whole wheat, enriched white, rye, etc.), number, size, and thickness of slices. Remember to include in your description any butter, margarine, or other condiment used on the bread and rolls.
- Beverages: Include every item you drink including water. Be sure to record cream and sugar used in coffee and/or tea. Indicate whether juices were sweetened or unsweetened and whether soft drinks were diet or regular.
- Fats: Remember to record all the butter, margarine, oil, and other fats used in cooking or added to foods. ■

Box 16-4. *Helpful Portion Sizes*

- 1 cup fruit ≈ size of a baseball
- ¼ cup dried fruit (e.g., raisins) ≈ size of a ping-pong ball
- 1 cup lettuce ≈ size of 4 leaves
- 1 cup cooked vegetables ≈ size of your fist
- 1 small fruit ≈ size of a tennis ball
- A medium potato ≈ size of a computer mouse
- 3 oz. meat ≈ size of a cassette tape
- 3 oz. grilled fish ≈ size of a checkbook
- 1 oz. cheese ≈ size of 4 stacked dice
- 1 oz. snack foods (pretzels, chips) ≈ size of a large handful
- 1 tsp. peanut butter/jam ≈ size of 1 dice
- A medium/average bagel ≈ size of 1 hockey puck
- ½ cup ice cream ≈ size of ½ tennis ball

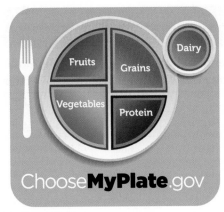

Figure 16-3. ChooseMyPlate.

dental hygienist assist the patient in identifying appropriate dietary and lifestyle modifications.

Step 4: Provide Nutrition Education

Explain MyPlate (Fig. 16-3) and how MyPlate represents the foundation of a healthy diet (i.e., meeting the recommended servings from each of the major food groups provides most of the nutrients needed daily). Review the key recommendations from the *Dietary Guidelines for Americans, 2010* (see Box 16-1) and explain that these recommendations promote health and lower the risk for chronic disease. Explain how MyPlate

and the Dietary Guidelines are used to plan nutritionally adequate diets and why an adequate diet is important in oral health.

Step 5: Examine Calorie Needs

Have the patient determine the amount of calories needed per day using the USDA Center for Nutrition Policy and Promotion *Estimated Calorie Needs per Day by Age, Gender, and Physical Activity Level* (Table 16-4). Refer to the definitions provided at the bottom of the table to determine the appropriate activity level.

Step 6: Examine Recommended Food Group Amounts

Have the patient use the daily recommended number of calories (step 5) to derive the recommended amount for each food group in Table 16-5.

Table 16-4. *Estimated Calorie Needs per Day by Age, Gender, and Physical Activity Level (Detailed)*

Estimated amounts of calories[a] needed to maintain calorie balance for various gender and age groups at three different levels of physical activity. The estimates are rounded to the nearest 200 calories. An individual's calorie needs may be higher or lower than these average estimates.

Gender/ Activity level[b]	Male/ Sedentary	Male/Moderately Active	Male/ Active	Female[c]/ Sedentary	Female[c]/Moderately Active	Female[c]/ Active
Age (years)						
2	1,000	1,000	1,000	1,000	1,000	1,000
3	1,200	1,400	1,400	1,000	1,200	1,400
4	1,200	1,400	1,600	1,200	1,400	1,400
5	1,200	1,400	1,600	1,200	1,400	1,600
6	1,400	1,600	1,800	1,200	1,400	1,600
7	1,400	1,600	1,800	1,200	1,600	1,800
8	1,400	1,600	2,000	1,400	1,600	1,800

Continued

Table 16-4. Estimated Calorie Needs per Day by Age, Gender, and Physical Activity Level (Detailed)—cont'd

Gender/ Activity level[b]	Male/ Sedentary	Male/Moderately Active	Male/ Active	Female[c]/ Sedentary	Female[c]/Moderately Active	Female[c]/ Active
9	1,600	1,800	2,000	1,400	1,600	1,800
10	1,600	1,800	2,200	1,400	1,800	2,000
11	1,800	2,000	2,200	1,600	1,800	2,000
12	1,800	2,200	2,400	1,600	2,000	2,200
13	2,000	2,200	2,600	1,600	2,000	2,200
14	2,000	2,400	2,800	1,800	2,000	2,400
15	2,200	2,600	3,000	1,800	2,000	2,400
16	2,400	2,800	3,200	1,800	2,000	2,400
17	2,400	2,800	3,200	1,800	2,000	2,400
18	2,400	2,800	3,200	1,800	2,000	2,400
19-20	2,600	2,800	3,000	2,000	2,200	2,400
21-25	2,400	2,800	3,000	2,000	2,200	2,400
26-30	2,400	2,600	3,000	1,800	2,000	2,400
31-35	2,400	2,600	3,000	1,800	2,000	2,200
36-40	2,400	2,600	2,800	1,800	2,000	2,200
41-45	2,200	2,600	2,800	1,800	2,000	2,200
46-50	2,200	2,400	2,800	1,800	2,000	2,200
51-55	2,200	2,400	2,800	1,600	1,800	2,200
56-60	2,200	2,400	2,600	1,600	1,800	2,200
61-65	2,000	2,400	2,600	1,600	1,800	2,000
66-70	2,000	2,200	2,600	1,600	1,800	2,000
71-75	2,000	2,200	2,600	1,600	1,800	2,000
76+	2,000	2,200	2,400	1,600	1,800	2,000

a. Based on Estimated Energy Requirements (EER) equations, using reference heights (average) and reference weights (healthy) for each age-gender group. For children and adolescents, reference height and weight vary. For adults, the reference man is 5 feet 10 inches tall and weighs 154 pounds. The reference woman is 5 feet 4 inches tall and weighs 126 pounds. EER equations are from the Institute of Medicine. *Dietary Reference Intakes for Energy, Carbohydrate, Fiber, Fat, Fatty Acids, Cholesterol, Protein, and Amino Acids.* Washington (DC): The National Academies Press; 2002.

b. Sedentary means a lifestyle that includes only the light physical activity associated with typical day-to-day life. Moderately active means a lifestyle that includes physical activity equivalent to walking about 1.5 to 3 miles per day at 3 to 4 miles per hour, in addition to the light physical activity associated with typical day-to-day life. Active means a lifestyle that includes physical activity equivalent to walking more than 3 miles per day at 3 to 4 miles per hour, in addition to the light physical activity associated with typical day-to-day life.

c. Estimates for females do not include women who are pregnant or breastfeeding.

Source: Britten P, Marcoe K, Yamini S, Davis C. Development of food intake patterns for the MyPyramid Food Guidance System. *J Nutr Educ Behav.* 2006;38 (6 Suppl):S78-S92.

Source: U.S. Department of Agriculture and U.S. Department of Health and Human Services. *Dietary Guidelines for Americans, 2010.* 7th ed. Washington, DC: U.S. Government Printing Office, December 2010.

Table 16-5. U.S. Department of Agriculture Food Patterns

For each food group or subgroup,[a] recommended average daily intake amounts[b] at all calorie levels. Recommended intakes from vegetable and protein foods subgroups are per week.
For more information and tools for application, go to ChooseMyPlate.gov.

Calorie level of pattern[c]	1,000	1,200	1,400	1,600	1,800	2,000	2,200	2,400	2,600	2,800	3,000	3,200
Fruits	1 c	1 c	1½ c	1½ c	1½ c	2 c	2 c	2 c	2 c	2½ c	2½ c	2½ c
Vegetables[d]	1 c	1½ c	1½ c	2 c	2½ c	2½ c	3 c	3 c	3½ c	3½ c	4 c	4 c
Dark-green vegetables	½ c/wk	1 c/wk	1 c/wk	1½ c/wk	1½ c/wk	1½ c/wk	2 c/wk	2 c/wk	2½ c/wk	2½ c/wk	2½ c/wk	2½ c/wk
Red and orange vegetables	2½ c/wk	3 c/wk	3 c/wk	4 c/wk	5½ c/wk	5½ c/wk	6 c/wk	6 c/wk	7 c/wk	7 c/wk	7½ c/wk	7½ c/wk
Beans and peas (legumes)	½ c/wk	½ c/wk	½ c/wk	1 c/wk	1½ c/wk	1½ c/wk	2 c/wk	2 c/wk	2½ c/wk	2½ c/wk	3 c/wk	3 c/wk
Starchy vegetables	2 c/wk	3½ c/wk	3½ c/wk	4 c/wk	5 c/wk	5 c/wk	6 c/wk	6 c/wk	7 c/wk	7 c/wk	8 c/wk	8 c/wk
Other vegetables	1½ c/wk	2½ c/wk	2½ c/wk	3½ c/wk	4 c/wk	4 c/wk	5 c/wk	5 c/wk	5½ c/wk	5½ c/wk	7 c/wk	7 c/wk
Grains[e]	3 oz-eq	4 oz-eq	5 oz-eq	5 oz-eq	6 oz-eq	6 oz-eq	7 oz-eq	8 oz-eq	9 oz-eq	10 oz-eq	10 oz-eq	10 oz-eq
Whole grains	1½ oz-eq	2 oz-eq	2½ oz-eq	3 oz-eq	3 oz-eq	3 oz-eq	3½ oz-eq	4 oz-eq	4½ oz-eq	5 oz-eq	5 oz-eq	5 oz-eq
Enriched grains	1½ oz-eq	2 oz-eq	2½ oz-eq	2 oz-eq	3 oz-eq	3 oz-eq	3½ oz-eq	4 oz-eq	4½ oz-eq	5 oz-eq	5 oz-eq	5 oz-eq
Protein foods[d]	2 oz-eq	3 oz-eq	4 oz-eq	5 oz-eq	5 oz-eq	5½ oz-eq	6 oz-eq	6½ oz-eq	6½ oz-eq	7 oz-eq	7 oz-eq	7 oz-eq
Seafood	3 oz/wk	5 oz/wk	6 oz/wk	8 oz/wk	8 oz/wk	8 oz/wk	9 oz/wk	10 oz/wk	10 oz/wk	11 oz/wk	11 oz/wk	11 oz/wk
Meat, poultry, eggs	10 oz/wk	14 oz/wk	19 oz/wk	24 oz/wk	24 oz/wk	26 oz/wk	29 oz/wk	31 oz/wk	31 oz/wk	34 oz/wk	34 oz/wk	34 oz/wk
Nuts, seeds, soy, products	1 oz/wk	2 oz/wk	3 oz/wk	4 oz/wk	4 oz/wk	4 oz/wk	4 oz/wk	5 oz/wk	5 oz/wk	5 oz/wk	5 oz/wk	5 oz/wk
Dairy[f]	2 c	2½ c	2½ c	3 c	3 c	3 c	3 c	3 c	3 c	3 c	3 c	3 c
Oils[g]	15 g	17 g	17 g	22 g	24 g	27 g	29 g	31 g	34 g	36 g	44 g	51 g
Maximum SoFAG[h] **limit, calories (% of calories)**	137 (14%)	121 (10%)	121 (9%)	121 (8%)	161 (9%)	258 (13%)	266 (12%)	330 (14%)	362 (14%)	395 (14%)	459 (15%)	596 (19%)

Continued

Table 16-5. U.S. Department of Agriculture Food Patterns—cont'd

[a]All foods are assumed to be in nutrient-dense forms, lean or low-fat prepared without added fats, sugars, or salt. Solid fats and added sugars may be included up to the daily maximum limit identified in the table. Food items in each group and subgroup are:

Fruits	All fresh, frozen, canned, and dried fruits and fruit juices: for example, oranges and orange juice, apples and apple juice, bananas, grapes, melons, berries, raisins.
Vegetables	
• Dark-green vegetables	All fresh, frozen, and canned dark-green leafy vegetables and broccoli, cooked or raw: for example, broccoli; spinach; romaine; collard, turnip, and mustard greens.
• Red and orange vegetables	All fresh, frozen, and canned red and orange vegetables, cooked or raw: for example, tomatoes, red peppers, carrots, sweet potatoes, winter squash, and pumpkin.
• Beans and peas (legumes)	All cooked beans and peas: for example, kidney beans, lentils, chickpeas, and pinto beans. Does not include green beans or green peas. (See additional comment under protein foods group.)
• Starchy vegetables	All fresh, frozen, and canned starchy vegetables: for example, white potatoes, corn, green peas.
• Other vegetables	All fresh, frozen, and canned other vegetables, cooked or raw: for example, iceberg lettuce, green beans, and onions.
Grains	
• Whole grains	All whole-grain products and whole grains used as ingredients: for example, whole-wheat bread, whole-grain cereals and crackers, oatmeal, and brown rice.
• Enriched grains	All enriched refined-grain products and enriched refined grains used as ingredients: for example, white breads, enriched grain cereals and crackers, enriched pasta, white rice.
Protein foods	All meat, poultry, seafood, eggs, nuts, seeds, and processed soy products. Meat and poultry should be lean or low-fat and nuts should be unsalted. Beans and peas are considered part of this group as well as the vegetable group, but should be counted in one group only.
Dairy	All milks, including lactose-free and lactose-reduced products and fortified soy beverages, yogurts, frozen yogurts, dairy desserts, and cheeses. Most choices should be fat-free or low-fat. Cream, sour cream, and cream cheese are not included due to their low calcium content.

[b]. Food group amounts are shown in cup (c) or ounce-equivalents (oz-eq). Oils are shown in grams (g). Quantity equivalents for each food group are:

• Grains, 1 ounce-equivalent is: 1 one-ounce slice bread; 1 cup ready-to-eat cereal flakes; ½ cup cooked rice, pasta, or cereal; 1 tortilla (6″diameter); 1 pancake (5″ diameter); 1 ounce ready-to-eat cereal (about 1 cup cereal flakes).

• Vegetables and fruits, 1 cup equivalent is: 1 cup raw or cooked vegetable or fruit; ½ cup dried vegetable or fruit; 1 cup vegetable or fruit juice; 2 cups leafy salad greens.

• Protein foods, 1 ounce-equivalent is: 1 ounce lean meat, poultry, seafood; 1 egg; 1 Tbsp peanut butter; ½ ounce nuts or seeds. Also, ¼ cup cooked beans or peas may also be counted as 1 ounce-equivalent.

• Dairy, 1 cup equivalent is: 1 cup milk, fortified soy beverage, or yogurt; 1½ ounces natural cheese (e.g., cheddar); 2 ounces of processed cheese (e.g., American).

[c]. See Appendix 6 for estimated calorie needs per day by age, gender, and physical activity level. Food intake patterns at 1,000, 1,200, and 1,400 calories meet the nutritional needs of children ages 2 to 8 years. Patterns from 1,600 to 3,200 calories meet the nutritional needs of children ages 9 years and older and adults. If a child ages 4 to 8 years needs more calories and, therefore, is following a pattern at 1,600 calories or more, the recommended amount from the dairy group can be 2½ cups per day. Children ages 9 years and older and adults should not use the 1,000, 1,200, or 1,400 calorie patterns.

[d]. Vegetable and protein foods subgroup amounts are shown in this table as weekly amounts, because it would be difficult for consumers to select foods from all subgroups daily.

[e]. Whole-grain subgroup amounts shown in this table are minimums. More whole grains up to all of the grains recommended may be selected, with offsetting decreases in the amounts of enriched refined grains.

[f]. The amount of dairy foods in the 1,200 and 1,400 calorie patterns have increased to reflect new RDAs for calcium that are higher than previous recommendations for children ages 4 to 8 years.

[g]. Oils and soft margarines include vegetable, nut, and fish oils and soft vegetable oil table spreads that have no *trans* fats.

[h]. SoFAS are calories from solid fats and added sugars. The limit for SoFAS is the remaining amount of calories in each food pattern after selecting the specified amounts in each food group in nutrient-dense forms (forms that are fat-free or low-fat and with no added sugars). The number of SoFAS is lower in the 1,200, 1,400, and 1,600 calorie patterns than in the 1,000 calorie pattern. The nutrient goals for the 1,200 to 1,600 calorie patterns are higher and require that more calories be used for nutrient-dense foods from the food groups.

Source: U.S. Department of Agriculture and U.S. Department of Health and Human Services. *Dietary Guidelines for Americans, 2010.* 7th Edition, Washington, DC: U.S. Government Printing Office, December 2010.

Step 7: Examine Amount Consumed for Each Food Group

Have the patient insert the recommended number of daily calories (step 5) and the respective amount for each food group (step 6) into the "Recommended Calories & Food Group Amounts" column in the Diet Analysis Form (Table 16-6). Assist the patient in determining the daily amount consumed for each food group from his dietary record and record the amount in the appropriate cells.

Step 8: Examine Adequacy of Diet

Have the patient assess her diet by comparing the daily average for each food group with the recommended food group amounts and indicate whether the recommended amounts were met. Reinforce good dietary habits and stress the importance of maintaining these habits. If the patient's daily average is excessive or deficient, explain the nutrition and oral health risks associated with an inadequate diet and the benefits of a healthy diet. Assist the patient in determining how and what changes can be made to improve dietary adequacy.

Step 9: Examine Dietary Risk(s) for Dental Caries

Review the general cause of caries and explain the role of diet in the caries process. Discuss the risks associated with the consistency (i.e., retentive versus nonretentive) and frequent consumption (i.e., between meal eating) of fermentable carbohydrates. Have the patient identify and circle high-risk foods and drinks in his dietary record. Review the Dietary Guidelines to Reduce Dental Caries Risk (Box 16-5) to help the patient devise recommendations and dietary modifications to reduce his caries risk.

Step 10: Guide Dietary and Lifestyle Modification(s)

Have the patient summarize the results obtained from the dietary and caries risk assessment and review the strategies to improve the patient's dietary and lifestyle changes.

Step 11: Document in Patient Record

Document in the patient's record the outcomes from the session including dietary discrepancies, caries risk factor(s), patient goal(s), and expected compliance.

Step 12: Evaluate Patient's Progress

Follow-up and evaluate the patient's progress at her next appointment as well as subsequent appointments if needed. Support and reinforce positive changes. If needed, clarify misconceptions and/or modify patient goals.

INTERDISCIPLINARY CARE

When patient needs are beyond the scope of dental hygiene practice, such as when dietary issues are related to underlying medical conditions, the patient should be referred to his or her physician and registered dietitian for a more in-depth assessment. The dental hygienist then plays an important role as part of an interdisciplinary team.

Some systemic conditions and related concerns (Table 16-7) often require an interdisciplinary health-care approach to facilitate optimal and efficient delivery of care to the patient.[39] The interdisciplinary model requires coordinated care and open communication among all team members, which include the patient, oral health professional(s), and other professionals pertinent to the patient's needs (see Teamwork).

Teamwork

Your assessment of a 23-year-old new female patient reveals multiple carious lesions, generalized moderate gingivitis, and moderate erosion, particularly on the maxillary anterior lingual surfaces. When you ask her about her usual dietary intake and habits, she indicates she snacks frequently throughout the day. Further probing reveals that most of her snacks are refined carbohydrates. Because the pattern of erosion is indicative of a possible eating disorder, you ask the patient if she has a history of an eating disorder. The patient is reluctant to answer but eventually shares with you that she does have a problem with food. She tells you she has never received treatment and is not sure she is ready to start. You convey trust and respect for her when you share your concern for her oral and general health. After speaking with you and the dentist, she agrees to a referral to an eating disorder specialist. You reassure her that you will follow up with her after her initial visit to the specialist, and that you and her dentist will be a part of her interdisciplinary team. ■

Table 16-6. Dietary Analysis Form

Food Groups	Serving Sizes	Day 1	Day 2	Day 3	Day 4	Day 5	Day 6	Day 7	Daily Average	Recommended Calories = _____ List Recommended Food Group Amounts Below	Needs Met?
Grains	1 oz.-eq = 1 slice bread, 1 cup ready-to-eat cereal or 1/2 cup cooked rice, pasta, or cooked cereal										
Vegetables	1 cup raw or cooked vegetables or veg-etable juice (2 cups raw leafy vegetables = 1 cup)										
Fruits	1 cup fruit or 100% fruit juice (1/2 cup dried fruit = 1 cup)										
Milk	1 cup milk or yogurt (1.5 oz natural cheese or 2 oz processed cheese = 1 cup)										
Meat and beans	1 oz.-eq = 1 oz. lean meat, poultry, or fish, 1 egg, 1 tbsp. peanut butter, ¼ cup cooked dry beans, or ½ cup nuts or seeds										
Water											
Oils											
Discretionary calories											

Box 16-5. Dietary Guidelines to Reduce Dental Caries Risk

- Added simple sugars: consume less than 55 g/day (1 tsp. = 4 g). Check your food labels for amounts.
- Natural sugars: limit consumption, especially fruit juice versus whole fruit.
- Frequency of meals and snacks: allow a minimum of 2 hours between eating occasions and limit the consumption of fermentable carbohydrates to mealtime.
- Avoid sticky foods: they increase retention and deter clearance of fermentable carbohydrates.
- Whole grain cereals and breads: increase salivary flow.
- Vegetables and crunchy fruits: increase salivary flow.

- Milk, yogurt, and cheese: increase salivary flow and contain calcium, phosphorus, and casein protein.
- Meat, poultry, fish, eggs, dry beans, and nuts: help to neutralize acids that cause dental decay.
- Water: helps to clear foods from the oral cavity. Recommend approximately 8 cups (64 oz.) per day.
- Sugar-free chewing gum: chew 1 stick after eating fermentable carbohydrates for 5–10 minutes.
- Combine select foods: consume higher-risk foods with lower-risk foods such as cheese and crackers, skim milk and cookies, peanuts and apple slices, bananas and cottage cheese, yogurt and granola, and peanut butter on celery. ■

Sources: Nappo-Dattoma (2009),[1] Zero, Fontana, and Martinez-Mier (2009),[21] Moynihan (2005),[24] Mobley (2007),[23] and Zero (2008).[25]

Table 16-7. Conditions Associated With Compromised Nutritional and Oral Health: Needing an Interdisciplinary Approach to Patient Care

Eating disorders	Salivary dysfunction
Dysphagia	Protein-energy malnutrition/wasting
Cardiovascular disease	Development disorders
Craniofacial anomalies	Musculoskeletal disorders
Diabetes	Osteoporosis
Disorders of taste and smell	Gastrointestinal disorders
End-stage renal disease	Infectious diseases
Systemic immunosuppressive therapy (e.g., organ transplant)	Neurodegenerative disorders that affect physical ability
Pathological immunosuppression (e.g., cancer, HIV infection, AIDS)	Oral or pharyngeal cancer and/or radiation therapy
Autoimmune disorders (e.g., Sjögren syndrome, lupus, rheumatoid arthritis)	Substance abuse (alcohol and/or drugs) or tobacco addiction

Sources: Touger-Decker R, Mobley CC. Position of the American Dietetic Association: oral health and nutrition. *J Am Diet Assoc.* 2007;107:1418-1428; and Kamer AR, Sirois DA, Huhmann M. Bidirectional impact of oral health and general health. In: Touger-Decker R, Sirois D, Mobley C, eds. *Nutrition and Oral Medicine.* Totowa, NJ: Humana Press; 2005:63-85.

SUMMARY

Nutrition and oral health have a synergistic, interdependent relationship. Dietary assessment can improve the patient's nutritional status, help prevent oral disease(s), and facilitate optimal treatment response. The dental hygienist has the responsibility to identify patients who are at risk and provide dietary assessment and nutritional counseling as a part of comprehensive patient care.

Case Study

Melanie Young is a 36-year-old single mother and new patient at the dental office. She works full-time third shift in the shipping department at a local business. Her dental history shows it has been approximately 5 years since her last dental examination and preventive prophylaxis. Her chief complaint is severe "hot and cold" sensitivity with occasional sensitivity to sweets, dry mouth, and bleeding gums. The patient reports a history of anxiety associated with dental care. Her medical history is not significant except for mild hypertension and the use of antihistamines due to environmental allergies. She was diagnosed with moderate generalized periodontitis, moderate-to-severe erosion (especially facial surfaces of maxillary anterior teeth), and six new carious lesions (interproximal and occlusal surfaces). The patient reports consuming a lot of diet soda and crackers and chips when she is at work. She never learned to cook, so most of the meals she prepares for her family are packaged, convenience foods. Her treatment plan includes dietary assessment and nutritional counseling, four quadrants of scaling and root planing, and restorative procedures. Her first appointment is scheduled to begin dietary assessment and scaling and root planing.

Case Study Exercises

1. It is most appropriate to use a 24-hour food record to assess Melanie's diet *because* she was diagnosed with multiple carious lesions and she is not at risk for malnutrition.
   A. Both statements are true.
   B. Both statements are false.
   C. The first statement is true and the second statement is false.
   D. The first statement is false and the second statement is true.

2. At the first appointment, the dental hygienist reviews the instructions on how to complete the diet record form. Which of the following should she do?
   A. Use visual aids to assist the patient in correct portion size.
   B. Provide nutrition education before reviewing the instructions.
   C. Tell Melanie to choose any days of the week she wants to record.
   D. Tell Melanie she will learn what foods/beverages are causing her oral health problems when she returns for nutritional counseling.

3. When Melanie returns for dietary assessment and counseling, the dental hygienist notices that not all food and beverage estimates or times were written down on the record. What should the dental hygienist do?
   A. Tell the patient that the record needs to be redone and reschedule the appointment.
   B. Tell the patient she can still provide dietary assessment/counseling without all the information recorded.
   C. Tell the patient she can fill in the omissions while the hygienist goes to the other room to get some educational materials for her.
   D. Review the omissions with the patient using visual aids to ensure proper estimates.

4. The dietary assessment reveals the patient is low in fruit, vegetable, milk, and water consumption and high in grains, meats, and beans. Which of the following would you recommend?
   A. Have the patient determine what dietary changes she could make to improve her diet.
   B. Provide wholesome recipes that she can prepare at home to help her improve her nutrient intake.
   C. Tell the patient to replace diet soda with coffee when she needs an "energy kick" at work.
   D. Increase water and fruit intake by eating more citrus fruit and apples between meals.

5. The dental hygienist should determine what Melanie already knows about diet and nutrition before providing nutrition education. The counseling should be provided in the dental operatory before beginning scaling and root planing.
   A. Both statements are true.
   B. Both statements are false.
   C. The first statement is true, but the second statement is false.
   D. The first statement is false, but the second statement is true.

6. Which of the following recommendations would you NOT include?
   A. Increase water consumption.
   B. Eat cariogenic foods with noncariogenic foods.
   C. Increase the consumption of fibrous foods to help remove biofilm.
   D. All of the above

Review Questions

1. A patient presents with six new interproximal lesions. Which of the following would the dental hygienist NOT recommend during nutritional counseling?
   A. Consume a noncariogenic food item such as cheese or peanuts after a cariogenic food item.
   B. Consume fibrous foods because they stimulate saliva, which buffers acids and aids in remineralization.
   C. Consume noncariogenic beverages such as diet soda.
   D. Limit simple sugar consumption to less than 55 g/day.

2. A synergistic effect occurs between sugar and starch. This is because starch contributes to the retentiveness of the food to increase its cariogenic potential.
   A. Both statements are true.
   B. Both statements are false.
   C. The first statement is true, but the second statement is false.
   D. The first statement is false, but the second statement is true.

3. Which of the following conditions may indicate the need for dietary assessment?
   A. Dental erosion
   B. Periodontitis
   C. Xerostomia
   D. All of the above

4. Which of the following is/are NOT true regarding oral signs and nutritional deficiencies?
   A. A vitamin B_2 (riboflavin) deficiency can cause angular cheilosis.
   B. A vitamin D deficiency will result in edematous, hemorrhagic gingivitis.
   C. A deficiency in a number of different B vitamins can contribute to a change in the size and/or color of the tongue.
   D. Nutrient imbalance rarely occurs in isolation.

5. A patient presents with xerostomia. Which of the following should the dental hygienist recommend?
   A. Increase the frequency of meals and snacks.
   B. Increase water consumption.
   C. Use hard candies such as mints to promote salivary flow.
   D. Answers A and B only
   E. Answers B and C only

Active Learning

1. Complete your own 3-day food record. Follow the instructions on how to complete the record and practice with food models and/or household items such as measuring cups and tablespoons. How does your 3-day average for each food group compare with the recommended number of servings? How do your diet and lifestyle compare with the *Dietary Guidelines for Americans, 2010*? What modifications can you make to improve your diet, lifestyle, or both?

2. Use the ChooseMyPlate Super Tracker to analyze your 3-day food record (www.choosemyplate.gov). How do the results from the computer analysis compare with your first (noncomputerized) analysis?

3. Use the dietary caries risk assessment form to determine your caries risk. What is your caries risk factor and what kind of dietary modifications can you make to improve this?

4. Write down the different conditions that can increase your patient's risk for malnutrition. Which of these conditions indicate your need to provide dietary assessment and nutritional counseling? Which conditions should be referred to a physician or registered dietitian, or both?

5. The skills required for effective nutritional counseling take practice. Role-play nutritional counseling with one of your classmates. Try to include at least six different skills when you practice (e.g., use active listening, maintain good eye contact, ask open-ended questions, monitor learning with constant feedback, help patient problem-solve, express empathy). ■

REFERENCES

1. Nappo-Dattoma L. Diet and dietary analysis. In: Koger B, ed. *Clinical Practice of the Dental Hygienist.* 10th ed. Philadelphia: Lippincott Williams & Wilkins; 2009: 521-543.

2. Touger-Decker R, Sirois DA. Approaches to oral nutrition health risk assessment. In: Touger-Decker R, Sirois D, Mobley C, eds. *Nutrition and Oral Medicine.* Totowa, NJ: Humana Press; 2005:287-297.

3. Shashidhar HR, Grigsby DG. Malnutrition. Published April 9, 2009. http://emedicine.medscape.com/article/985140-print. Accessed September 9, 2010.

4. Furman EF. Undernutrition in older adults across the continuum of care. *J Gerontol Nurs.* 2006;32:22-27.

5. Moynihan PJ. The relationships between nutrition and systemic and oral well-being in older people. *J Am Dent Assoc.* 2007;138:493-497.

6. Deen D. Nutritional assessment of the oral cavity. *Nutr Clin Care.* 2001;4:28-33.

7. Palmer CA, DePaola D. Nutrition as the foundation for general and oral health. In: Cohen M, ed. *Diet and Nutrition in Oral Health.* Upper Saddle River, NJ: Pearson Prentice Hall; 2007:1-13.

8. Badwall RS, Bennett J. Nutritional considerations in the surgical patient. *Dent Clin North Am.* 2003;47(2): 373-394.

9. Winkler M, Makowski S. Wound healing. In: Touger-Decker R, Sirois D, Mobley C, eds. *Nutrition and Oral Medicine.* Totowa, NJ: Humana Press; 2005:273-286.

10. Moynihan PJ, Lingstrom P. Oral consequences of compromised nutritional well-being. In: Touger-Decker R, Sirois D, Mobley C, eds. *Nutrition and Oral Medicine.* Totowa, NJ: Humana Press; 2005:107-127.

11. Palmer CA, Papas AS. The minerals and mineralization. In: Cohen M, ed. *Diet and Nutrition in Oral Health.* Upper Saddle River, NJ: Pearson Prentice Hall; 2007: 147-188.

12. Palmer CA. Vitamins today. In: Cohen M, ed. *Diet and Nutrition in Oral Health.* Upper Saddle River, NJ: Pearson Prentice Hall; 2007:189-229.

13. Enwonwu CO, Ritchie CS. Nutrition and inflammatory markers. *J Am Dent Assoc.* 2007;138(1):70-73.

14. Touger-Decker R, Mobley CC. Position of the American Dietetic Association: oral health and nutrition. *J Am Diet Assoc.* 2007;107:1418-1428.

15. Chapple ILC. Potential mechanisms underpinning the nutritional modulation of periodontal inflammation. *J Am Dent Assoc.* 2009;140(2):178-184.

16. Hayes C, Thornton K. Nutrition in the growth and development of oral structures. In: Cohen M, ed. *Diet and Nutrition in Oral Health.* Upper Saddle River, NJ: Pearson Prentice Hall; 2007:272-286.

17. Alvarez JO. Nutrition, tooth development, and dental caries. *Am J Clin Nutr.* 1995;61:410S-416S.

18. Psoter WJ, Reid BC, Katz RV. Malnutrition and dental caries: a review of the literature. *Caries Res.* 2005;39(6): 441-447.

19. Palmer CA. How the body uses fluids. In: Cohen M, ed. *Diet and Nutrition in Oral Health.* Upper Saddle River, NJ: Pearson Prentice Hall; 2007:138-146.

20. Stookey GK. The effect of saliva on dental caries. *J Am Dent Assoc.* 2008;139(5 suppl):11S-17S.

21. Zero D, Fontana M, Martinez-Mier EA. The biology, prevention, diagnosis and treatment of dental caries scientific advances in the United States. *J Am Dent Assoc.* 2009;140(9 suppl):25S-34S.

22. Klein MI, Duarte S, Xiao J. Structural and molecular basis of the role of starch and sucrose in Streptococcus mutans biofilm development. *Appl Environ Microbiol.* 2009;75:837-841.

23. Mobley C. Diet, nutrition, and teeth. In: Cohen M, ed. *Diet and Nutrition in Oral Health.* Upper Saddle River, NJ: Pearson Prentice Hall; 2007:287-306.

24. Moynihan PJ. The role of diet and nutrition in the etiology and prevention of oral diseases. *Bull World Health Organ.* 2005;83:694-699.

25. Zero DT. Are sugar substitutes also anticariogenic? *J Am Dent Assoc.* 2008;139:9S-10S.

26. American Academy of Pediatrics. Council on Clinical Affairs. Policy on the use of xylitol in caries prevention. Adopted 2006, Revised 2010. www.aapd.org/media/Policies_Guidelines/P_Xylitol.pdf. Accessed July 26, 2015.

27. Milgrom P, Ly KA. Mutans streptococci dose response to xylitol chewing gum. *J Dent Res.* 2006;85(2):177-181.

28. Mobley C. Nutrition and dental caries. *Dent Clin N Am.* 2003;47:319-336.

29. Gandara BK, Truelove EL. Diagnosis and management of dental erosion. *J Contemp Dent Pract.* 1999;1(1):16-23.

30. Lussi A, Jaeggi T. Erosion—diagnosis and risk factors. *Clin Oral Invest.* 2008;12(suppl 1):S5-S13.

31. Food List of Terms: P. Silver Spring, MD: US Food and Drug Administration. Updated February 28, 2014. Available from: http://www.fda.gov/food/foodscience research/toolsmaterials/ucm215845.htm. Accessed September 2, 2014.

32. Moynihan P. The interrelationship between diet and oral health. *Proc Nutr Soc.* 2005;64:571-580.

33. Michael CG, Javid NS, Collaizzi FA, Gibbs CH. Biting strength and chewing forces in complete denture wearers. *J Prosthet Dent.* 1990;63:549-553.

34. Moynihan P, Butler TJ, Thomason JM, Jepson NJ. Nutrient intake in partially dentate patients: the effect of prosthetic rehabilitation. *J Dent.* 2000;28(8):557-563.

35. Sahyoun N, Lin CL, Krall E. Nutritional status of the older adult is associated with dentition status. *J Am Diet Assoc.* 2003;103(1):61-66.

36. Bradbury J, Thomason JM, Jepson NJ, Walls AW, Allen PF, Moynihan PJ. Nutrition counseling increases fruit and vegetable consumption in the edentulous. *J Dent Res.* 2006;85(5):463-468.

37. U.S. Department of Agriculture and U.S. Department of Health and Human Services. *Dietary Guidelines for Americans, 2010.* 7th ed. Washington, DC: U.S. Government Printing Office; December 2010. http://www.cnpp.usda.gov/dietary-guidelines-2010. Accessed July 26, 2015.

38. Marshall T. Chairside diet assessment of caries risk. *J Am Dent Assoc.* 2009;140(6):670-674.

39. Kamer AR, Sirois DA, Huhmann M. Bidirectional impact of oral health and general health. In: Touger-Decker R, Sirois D, Mobley C, eds. *Nutrition and Oral Medicine.* Totowa, NJ: Humana Press; 2005:63-85.

Chapter 17 | Risk Assessment

Deborah Lyle, RDH, BS, MS

KEY TERMS

incidence
modifiable risk factor
nonmodifiable risk factor
odds ratio
prevalence
relative risk
risk
risk assessment
risk factor
risk indicator
risk marker

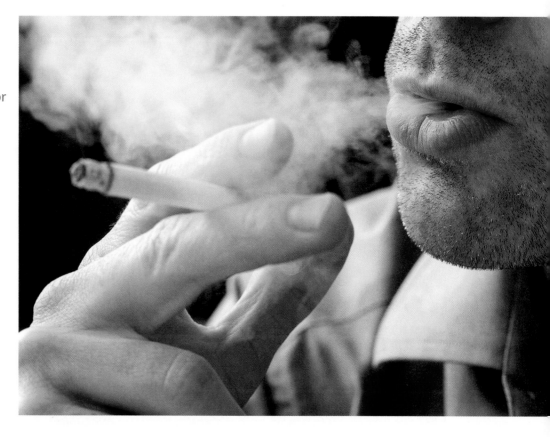

LEARNING OBJECTIVES

After reading this chapter, the student should be able to:

17.1 Discuss the relevance of risk assessment as part of dental hygiene practice.

17.2 Explain the difference among a risk factor, risk indicator, and risk marker.

17.3 Identify risk factors that affect the onset, severity, and progression of periodontal disease.

17.4 Differentiate between modifiable risk factors and nonmodifiable risk factors.

17.5 Explain the implications of a risk factor with a patient and implications for self-care regimen.

17.6 Discuss treatment recommendations for a patient who is genotype-positive.

17.7 Understand the difference between high-risk factors and low-risk factors.

17.8 Explain why diabetes, smoking, and genetics are significant risk factors.

17.9 Identify risk factors for oral cancer and dental caries.

17.10 Discuss the differences in risk for age, race, and genetics.

17.11 Develop a risk assessment form.

KEY CONCEPTS

- Risk assessment is the cornerstone to developing a patient-centered care plan.
- Risk factors modulate the onset, severity, and prognosis of periodontal diseases, dental caries, and oral cancer.
- The most significant periodontal risk factors are smoking, diabetes, and genetics.
- The most significant oral cancer risk factors are tobacco use, alcohol, and human papillomavirus.
- Reduction of risk factors improves therapy outcomes and prognosis.
- Patient compliance to self-care regimens and reduction of risk are important factors for the prevention or treatment of oral infectious diseases.

RELEVANCE TO CLINICAL PRACTICE

Preventing, eliminating, or managing oral inflammatory diseases depends on many factors: thorough documentation of clinical, historical, and biological data; patient behaviors and values; development of an individualized evidence-based care plan; and risk assessment. Risk assessment involves identifying patients who are at risk for developing oral disease such as periodontal disease, caries, and oral cancer. Assessing the patient's risk can have a significant impact on clinical decisions, interventions, and prognosis.[1–6]

Risk assessment, diagnosis, and presentation of a comprehensive care plan are the responsibility of the dentist and dental hygienist (see Professionalism). The patient's role is providing accurate and detailed information regarding medical and dental histories including personal habits and lifestyle behaviors, risk reduction by way of behavior change, incorporation of recommended self-care routine, and adherence to accepted care plan and continued care. This chapter discusses the impact of risk factors and the dental hygienist's role in patient assessment, education, and treatment planning.

Professionalism

The practice of dental hygiene is dynamic. Commitment to lifelong learning to maintain competence is essential. New information is disseminated through different channels including continuing education courses, peer-reviewed journals, electronic media, company representatives, and the American Dental Hygienists' Association. Dental hygienists are responsible and accountable for keeping up to date with information that impacts practice and decision-making. Staying abreast of the research on risk assessment is critical for optimum patient care. ■

ORAL RISK ASSESSMENT

Definitions

Risk is defined as the probability that loss, harm, or injury will occur if nothing is changed. For example, if a 50-year-old man who is overweight, smokes, and leads a sedentary lifestyle does not change these behaviors, he is at significant risk for heart disease. **Risk assessment** is the evaluation of the qualitative and quantitative information gained during the assessment and screening process. Levels of risk depend on the identification of risk factors, risk indicators, or risk predictors. A **risk factor** is a behavior or attribute that has a direct causal effect on the onset or progression, or both, of the disease.[3,5,6] Risk factors fall into two categories: **modifiable risk factors,**

those behaviors that *can* be changed, and **nonmodifiable risk factors,** personal attributes or genetics that *cannot* be changed (Box 17-1).[5,6]

A **risk indicator** is much like a risk factor except it does not meet the criteria of evidence. It is biologically plausible, but research has shown only an association with the disease. There are many risk indicators for periodontal disease because of the similar inflammatory response present in systemic diseases. Age, sex, and race are examples of risk indicators. A **risk marker** is a factor that has not demonstrated a causal or biological relationship with oral disease through research but has been associated with the disease when evaluating populations or data over a long period.[5,6]

Terms that refer to the proportion of disease noted in a specific population are prevalence and incidence. **Prevalence** is the number of cases of a disease or condition per population at risk at a particular point in time. **Incidence** is the number of new cases of a disease or condition over a specified period. Cross-sectional studies provide information about prevalence, and longitudinal studies assess incidence of a particular disease.[6]

Risk for oral disease is often reported in clinical studies as a relative risk or odds ratio. **Relative risk** is the probability of developing a disease if the person is exposed to the risk factor compared with a person who is not exposed to that same risk factor. An **odds ratio** is the odds of a person having the disease if he or she is exposed to the risk factor compared with having the disease if not exposed to that same risk factor.[6]

Modifiable Risk Factors

Smoking and Tobacco Use

Smoking is a well-established factor for oral disease, attributing to an increase in prevalence and severity of periodontal disease and the incidence of oral cancer.[7–9] Studies have shown that smokers can be at up to 20 times greater risk for periodontal disease than never smokers and nonsmokers.[10] A disproportionally high number of people diagnosed with periodontal disease are smokers. A large national study reported approximately 75% of patients with periodontal disease were smokers.[11] Smokers have more severe clinical findings (Box 17-2), and onset usually begins at an earlier age. The level of biofilm and inflammation present does not always correspond to the clinical measurements, with some smokers presenting with little biofilm but increased pocket depth and attachment loss.

The effects of smoking are cellular (host inflammatory response) and local (damage from heat and chemicals). Nicotine interferes with wound healing, undermining the inflammatory process by interfering with the normal release of inflammatory cytokines and neutrophil function. Nicotine can inhibit collagen production, which results in breakdown of connective tissue faster than it can be repaired and causes constriction of blood vessels, which limits blood flow to the gingival tissue.[12,13] The gingival tissue appears thickened, fibrotic, and pale with rolled margins (Figs. 17-1 and 17-2). Anterior regions, including maxillary lingual, may exhibit more destruction because of concentrated exposure to heat and chemicals.

Smokers do not respond as favorably to periodontal therapy as nonsmokers or never smokers, and this appears to be dose related, with heavy smokers exhibiting more attachment loss and worse prognosis than light smokers.[14–16] Attachment loss also increases with the

---

Box 17-1. *Risk Factors for Oral Disease*

Modifiable Risk Factors
- Smoking and tobacco use
- Oral health status and bleeding
- Biofilm and bacteria
- Local contributing factors
- Diabetes mellitus
- Osteoporosis
- Obesity
- Medications
- Xerostomia
- Immunosuppression

Nonmodifiable Risk Factors or Indicators
- Age
- Race
- Sex
- Genetics
- History of disease

Box 17-2. *Clinical Findings in Smokers*

- Greater alveolar bone loss
- Deeper periodontal pockets
- Greater recession
- Increased furcation involvement
- Increased tooth loss

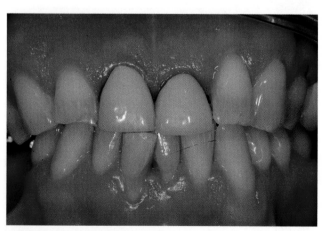

Figure 17-1. Rolled gingival margin seen in smokers. (Courtesy of Cecil White, Jr., DMD, MSD, Jacksonville, FL.)

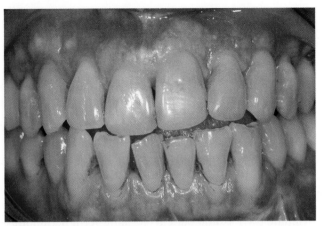

Figure 17-2. Fibrotic tissue seen in smokers. (Courtesy of Cecil White, Jr., DMD, MSD, Jacksonville, FL.)

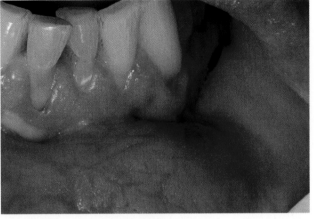

Figure 17-3. Gingival recession caused by smokeless tobacco use. (Courtesy of Cecil White, Jr., DMD, MSD, Jacksonville, FL.)

number of years a patient has smoked.[8] Subgingival pathogens are more difficult to eliminate, and the compromised immune system makes smokers less responsive to treatment.[9,10,17] Patients who quit smoking can have a similar response to periodontal therapy depending on the presence of other risk factors (see Evidence-Based Practice). Strategies for helping patients stop using tobacco are discussed in Chapter 4.

All patients should be screened for tobacco use. Children and adolescents who begin smoking or are exposed to secondhand smoke are also at risk for periodontal disease and other systemic disorders. Teens who smoke have more visible plaque, periodontal pockets of 4 mm or larger, and root surface calculus. Young adults have a higher prevalence and severity of periodontal disease.[17,18]

Smokeless tobacco, cigar, and pipe smoking are also significant risk factors for the initiation and progression of periodontal disease and tooth loss.[19] Smokeless tobacco users have a greater incidence of gingival recession, bone loss, and caries (Fig. 17-3).[19,20] It also causes leukoplakia in the area where it is held in the mouth (Fig. 17-4). Smoking, smokeless tobacco, and alcohol significantly increase the risk for oral cancer in the oral cavity and oropharynx. Pipe and cigar use increase the risk for lip cancer.[21] Chapter 45 provides information on different oral cancers, effects of radiation and chemotherapy on the oral cavity, and the dental hygienist's role and responsibility.

Oral Health Status and Bleeding

Periodontal disease affects all age groups and has a strong association with poor or inadequate oral hygiene. It is one of the easiest risk factors to eliminate and is a cornerstone in dental hygiene care. Patients will respond differently to the presence of biofilm because of genetics, systemic disease, oral findings or conditions, and other risk factors. Daily oral hygiene regimens help prevent oral infections and prolong the effects of professional dental hygiene care. Patients who practice good oral hygiene but still have clinical signs of inflammation or periodontitis need to be evaluated for other risk factors, such as undiagnosed diabetes, new prescription or over-the-counter drugs, xerostomia, accessibility to subgingival and interdental areas with current self-care routines, or modification to current care plan and continued care intervals.

Evidence-Based Practice

Research shows that smoking is one of the most significant risk factors for periodontal disease. Yet, no smoking cessation protocol is in practice. It is time to evaluate the office philosophy and patient focus. Discuss different ways this can be accomplished. One way is to provide referral services to local or state programs. Another way may be to expand the staff knowledge on smoking cessation by attending a continuing education program or reviewing the available resources on dental professional websites. A good place to start is the Ask, Advise, Refer website, an initiative of the American Dental Hygienists' Association in partnership with the Smoking Cessation Leadership Center.[57] ■

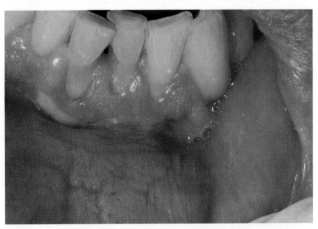

Figure 17-4. Leukoplakia in area where smokeless tobacco is used. (Courtesy of Cecil White, Jr., DMD, MSD, Jacksonville, FL.)

The effectiveness of periodontal treatment and self-care is often based on the presence or absence of bleeding. Bleeding alone is not a predictor of periodontal breakdown or future attachment loss. Bleeding in conjunction with other clinical signs of breakdown such as increased attachment loss or pocket depth does show a potential for continued periodontal destruction.[2,3] The absence of bleeding generally correlates with good periodontal health. A self-care intervention that the patient will comply with and that produces measurable outcomes (e.g., reduction of bleeding) provides a more favorable prognosis.

Biofilm and Bacteria

Specific bacteria have been identified in the initiation and progression of periodontal infections and caries. In the case of caries, the organisms are mutans streptococci and lactobacilli (acidogenic bacteria), and for periodontal infections, they include anaerobic gram-negative bacteria such as *Porphyromonas gingivalis, Aggregatibacter actinomycetemcomitans,* and *Tannerella forsythensis* (Box 17-3).[22,23] The presence of specific organisms increases the risk for infection, but the organisms require a susceptible host and the presence of other mitigating factors or risk factors for disease to occur. Periodontal pathogens fall into three categories: high risk, moderate risk, and low risk. Microbial assessments such as microarrays and genomic (DNA) probes are available and may provide information for clinical treatment decisions, especially if the patient does not respond to anti-infective therapy such as scaling and root planing, chemotherapeutic agents, local delivery drugs, and appropriate self-care methods. Caries risk assessment and management is covered in Chapter 21.

Local Contributing Factors

Biofilm will grow and mature in any area of the oral cavity. Areas that are inaccessible to daily cleaning are ideal places for biofilm to grow and mature, increasing the risk for infection. Local factors that contribute to the risk for periodontal disease include old or poorly placed restorations (open margins, overhangs, and crown or restoration margins placed subgingivally), orthodontic appliances and temporary anchor device, and removable partial dentures (Figs. 17-5, 17-6, and 17-7). Restorative problems can be corrected or replaced, eliminating the risk. Orthodontic appliances can be maintained by improved oral hygiene. Introduction of different cleaning methods, devices, and fluoride help minimize the risk. Permanent lingual retainers that cannot be effectively maintained by the patient may require a consultation with the orthodontist to evaluate the risk and benefits for long-term periodontal health (Fig. 17-8). Areas of risk for infection are documented and corrected to allow for adequate cleaning of the area and resolution of the periodontal infections.

Diabetes Mellitus

Diabetes is a well-documented risk factor for periodontal disease that affects both adults and children with type 1 or type 2 diabetes. The prevalence and severity

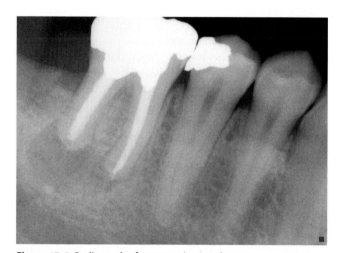

Figure 17-5. Radiograph of a restoration overhang. (Courtesy of Cecil White, Jr., DMD, MSD, Jacksonville, FL.)

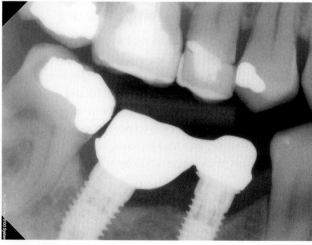

Figure 17-6. Open margin between two restorations. (Courtesy of Cecil White, Jr., DMD, MSD, Jacksonville, FL.)

> ### Box 17-3. *Bacteria Associated With Periodontal Disease*
>
> **Periodontal Pathogens (strong evidence)**
> - *Porphyromonas gingivalis*
> - *Tannerella forsythia*
> - *Aggregatibacter actinomycetemcomitans*
>
> **Putative Pathogens (moderate evidence)**
> - *Prevotella intermedia*
> - *Prevotella melaninogenica*
> - *Fusobacterium nucleatum*
> - *Peptostreptococcus micros*
> - *Eubacterium* spp.
> - *Eikenella corrodens*
> - *Prevotella nigrescens*
> - *Treponema denticola*
> - *Campylobacter rectus*

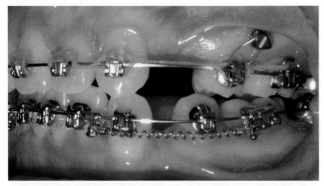

Figure 17-7. Temporary anchor device used in orthodontic treatment. (Courtesy of Daniel Bills, DMD, MS, New Jersey.)

of gingivitis and periodontitis is greater in individuals with diabetes, and individuals with poor or no glycemic control are at greater risk for periodontal infection. Increased levels of biofilm may not correlate with the severity of gingivitis or periodontitis in adults or children because of an exaggerated inflammatory response.[24] Children with diabetes had twice the amount of inflammation compared with children without diabetes with a similar level of biofilm. Children as young as 6 to 11 years had teeth with attachment loss and the incidence increased into adolescence (12–18 years of age).[25] In adults with similar biofilm and bacterial

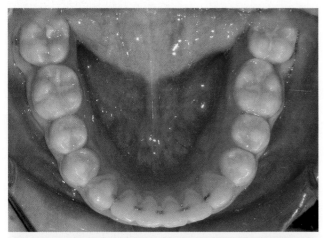

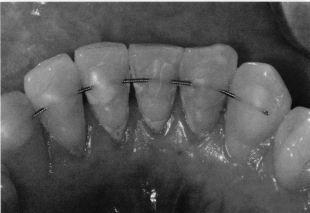

Figure 17-8. Permanent lingual orthodontic retainer. (Courtesy of Daniel Bills, DMD, MS, New Jersey.)

composition, gingival inflammation can develop more rapidly and be more severe. The bacterial microflora in either children or adults with periodontitis was similar between individuals with diabetes and those without diabetes.[24]

The increased susceptibility and severity of periodontal infection is linked to an altered immune response. Neutrophil, monocyte, and macrophage function is altered with an increase in the production of proinflammatory cytokines and mediators. The increased levels of attachment and bone loss are associated with alterations in connective tissue metabolism and impaired osseous healing and bone turnover.[26–28]

Periodontal disease can have a detrimental impact on the metabolic state in diabetes. Patients with diabetes with severe periodontal disease are six times more likely to have poor glycemic control over time.[29] The presence of severe periodontal disease has also been associated with an early onset of other complications, such as cardiovascular and renal disease, and increased mortality from these complications.[30,31]

Individuals with diabetes with good glycemic control respond similarly to periodontal therapy as individuals without diabetes. Patients with poor glycemic control are at risk for a rapid recurrence of deep pockets and a less favorable long-term prognosis.[24] Xerostomia has been reported in individuals with diabetes but may be a consequence of medication, age, or salivary dysfunction because no definitive association has been found. Regardless of cause, individuals with diabetes with xerostomia are at an increased risk for caries. Other oral lesions that have been reported in studies with patients with diabetes include lichen planus, recurrent aphthous stomatitis, and oral candidiasis. Chapter 42 provides information about the prevalence of diabetes and the dental hygienist's role and responsibilities.

Osteoporosis

Osteoporosis has been considered a potential risk factor for periodontal disease based on the premise that they are both bone resorptive diseases. Several cross-sectional studies have shown a correlation between reduced bone mineral density and increased severity of periodontal disease as measured by clinical attachment loss and alveolar bone loss. Some studies did not show a correlation, and the use of cross-sectional studies or the loss of teeth as a variable is not conclusive evidence. The presence of osteoporosis may impact the severity of alveolar bone loss in patients with periodontitis, especially in patients with pre-existing periodontal disease.[32]

Reports of osteonecrosis of the jaw associated with the use of bisphosphonate for the treatment or management of oncological conditions, metastatic malignancies, or osteoporosis was first reported in 2003. Subsequent reports provide a clearer picture of the association. Information about osteopenia, osteoporosis, and osteonecrosis is provided in Chapter 47.

Obesity

The relationship between obesity and periodontal disease has been the topic of several studies. The studies are cross-sectional but do provide early information. Increasing body mass index and waist/hip ratio was associated with risk for periodontal disease.[33] Two researchers used the National Health and Nutrition Examination Survey III (NHANES III) data to evaluate the relationship. One evaluation used waist circumference as the measure of obesity and found an association between periodontal disease in young adults but not middle-aged or older adults.[34] In contrast, another study used body mass index, waist/hip ratio, and multiple periodontal measures including attachment loss, pocket depth, bleeding, and calculus and found a significant relationship.[35] Obesity increases the inflammatory burden, and the relationship with periodontal disease needs to be evaluated in longitudinal studies (see Spotlight on Public Health).

Medications

Patients may not realize the impact medications can have on the oral cavity and may not report or document the information on the medical history form. Identifying medications, either prescribed or over the counter, is important in the assessment process. Some medications, such as antibiotics and nonsteroidal anti-inflammatory drugs, can have a positive effect on the microbial flora reducing inflammation and organisms. In some cases, these drugs may be prescribed to treat or manage aggressive or advanced periodontal infections.

Many drugs have oral side effects that can range from being a minor nuisance to debilitating for patients. There are more than 500 medications that cause xerostomia, the most commonly reported oral side effect. More than 80% of adults take at least one prescription medication.[36] Patients with drug-induced xerostomia suffer from reduced salivary flow and a change in both the nature and the quality of the saliva, resulting in less natural cleansing, biofilm adherence, and a more acidic pH.[37,38] This results in a greater risk for caries. It may also contribute to difficulty chewing, swallowing, mucositis, ulcerations, and burning mouth or tongue.[38] Some medications increase the risk for gingival hyperplasia and opportunistic infections, which can be severe in some cases. Complete disclosure of medications is needed to address the risk for oral complications or disease. Chapters 45, 47, and 48 provide more detail on the causes and effects of xerostomia and methods to prevent the risk for caries and periodontal disease.

Immunosuppression

Medical situations or autoimmune diseases, such as lupus, leukemia, chemotherapy, organ transplant, and HIV and AIDS, cause immunosuppression in patients and increase the risk for infection in the oral cavity or negatively impact the prognosis for therapy. Several oral manifestations have been documented in patients with HIV and AIDS, including candidiasis, necrotizing ulcerative gingivitis, linear gingival erythema, and Kaposi sarcoma (Fig. 17-9). With the introduction of highly active antiretroviral therapy, the incidence and severity of oral manifestations have been reduced. Collaboration with the medical team and compliance to treatment and self-care recommendations can result in effective management of oral complications and control or prevention of periodontal infections. Immunosuppressive disorders and dental hygiene management are covered in Chapters 43 and 45.

Spotlight on Public Health

Information about the relationship between systemic disease and oral health is communicated to the public regularly, especially after a 2004 article in *TIME* magazine addressed the common link: chronic inflammation. Over the past decade the association between periodontal disease and systemic diseases including cardiovascular disease, diabetes, Alzheimer disease, adverse pregnancy outcomes such as premature birth and low birth weight, stress, obesity, and arthritis has been reported in the news. The American Academy of Periodontology has a risk assessment tool for periodontal disease (www.perio.org/consumer/riskassessment). The American Dental Association provides a caries risk assessment form for dental care providers to use in determining the risk for caries in adults and children.[58,59] Other professional organizations have links to information about oral diseases to help individuals understand the risks of their behavior but do not quantify it with a measurement tool. Medical professionals are also including oral risk assessments in practice. The American Academy of Pediatrics provides online oral health risk assessment training for pediatricians and other child health professions. ■

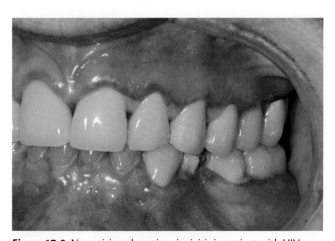

Figure 17-9. Necrotizing ulcerative gingivitis in patient with HIV.
(Courtesy of Cecil White, Jr., DMD, MSD, Jacksonville, FL.)

Nonmodifiable Risk Factors

Age, Race, and Sex

Periodontal disease is more prevalent in older populations. This is believed to be a result of cumulative tissue destruction and not an age-related risk factor. Over time, known risk factors such as smoking, pathogenic bacteria, xerostomia, and poor oral hygiene contribute to the increased incidence in older individuals. Individuals from a lower socioeconomic background are at greater risk for periodontal disease and other dental complications.[1,39] Smoking and alcohol use may be higher in these groups, increasing the risks for severe periodontal disease and oral cancer. Disparities in education and access to care contribute to the differences along with limited access to fresh fruits and vegetables for a healthy diet.

African Americans, Mexican Americans, and Native Americans have shown a higher incidence of periodontal disease, but this may be because of risk factors other than race, such as a greater incidence of diabetes, socioeconomic status, or limited access to care. A systematic review of the literature showed that men had a higher prevalence for destructive periodontal disease compared with women, but it did not show a greater risk for more rapid periodontal destruction.[40] Also, men are twice as likely as women to have oral cancer.[21] The long-term use of tobacco and alcohol are the contributing factors, but an increase in smoking by women may change this in the future.

Older individuals are at greater risk for oral cancer with estimates of half of all oral cancers diagnosed in people older than 68 years. The risk for oral cancer increases with the amount smoked or chewed and the duration of the habit. Ninety percent of patients with oral cancer use tobacco, and 75% to 80% drink alcohol frequently. Oral cancer is six times more frequent in alcoholic drinkers than nondrinkers.[21,41,42] Another risk factor for oral cancer is human papillomavirus (HPV). HPVs are a group of more than 100 viruses, are categorized as low risk and high risk, and are given a number, which is called an HPV type. HPV is a risk factor in about 20% to 30% of oral cancer cases. HPV can live only in squamous epithelial cells, which are found in the oral cavity and throat.[43] A case–control study found HPV-16 resulted in a 14 times greater risk for oral cancer and that the exposure to HPV preceded the appearance of the cancer by 10 years or more (Box 17-4).[44]

Women are at a greater risk for periodontal disease during pregnancy. Pregnancy complications are associated with increased inflammation, and the relationship between preterm low birth weight and periodontal disease has been studied. Links between the two inflammatory diseases have been identified, but intervention studies have not shown a decrease in the incidence of these adverse events.[45,46] The importance of good oral hygiene is still a key factor during pregnancy to prevent maternal periodontal complications and reduce the inflammatory burden.

Children and adolescents with a high consumption of soft drinks, juice, and other sweetened beverages are at risk for enamel erosion and caries. Children who

---

Box 17-4. Risks and Prevalence for Oral Cancer

Risks
- Smoking and tobacco use
- Alcohol use
- HPV

Prevalence
- Older individuals have a greater risk for oral cancer
- Men have twice the rate of oral cancer than women
- Oral cancer increases with the amount and duration of smoking
- Oral cancer is six times more frequent in persons with alcohol dependence
- Oral cancer is more common in people who drink alcohol and smoke
- HPV is associated with 20% to 30% of oral cancer cases

---

have higher milk consumption had a lower tendency for decay compared with children who consumed high amounts of juice. Primary teeth are at risk when young children consume high amounts of soft drinks, with a high intake at age 3 years being predictive of caries.[47–49] In a federal survey, nearly 28% of 2- to 5-year-olds had at least one cavity.[50] This represents a 4% increase from the previous report. For more information on caries risk assessment, see Chapter 21.

Genetics

Genetic and inherited disorders associated with impaired neutrophil function, connective tissue breakdown, collagen formation, and mineralization of bone are risk factors for periodontal disease, especially aggressive and early-onset types. Disorders include cyclic neutropenia, Chediak-Higashi syndrome, Ehlers-Danlos syndrome, trisomy 21 (Down syndrome), and Papillon-Lefèvre syndrome.[2,3]

Identifying individuals who are predisposed to periodontal disease is possible and marks a significant advancement in risk assessment and management. A genetic susceptibility test is commercially available and can be used to assess a patient's risk for developing severe chronic periodontal disease. The test is based on the identification of a gene group with a slight change in the genetic code (polymorphism) that is responsible for the production of proinflammatory mediators: interleukin-1 alpha (IL-1_) and interleukin-1 beta (IL-1β). A saliva sample is obtained and sent to a laboratory for analysis. A positive result (genotype-positive) means the patient has an increased risk for periodontal disease. A negative result (genotype-negative) means the patient has a normal risk for disease depending on assessment of other risk factors. It is estimated that approximately 30% of Caucasians will test positive for the disease.[51,52] In contrast, a Chinese population was only 2.3% genotype-positive and African Americans were

15% genotype-positive.[53,54] Some estimate the increased risk for severe periodontal disease in genotype-positive patients to be approximately 6.8 times greater than for genotype-negative patients. One study found that 67% of patients with severe periodontal disease were genotype-positive and 80% of those patients had two risk factors: being genotype-positive and smoking.[51,52]

This analysis is not a diagnosis for periodontal disease but provides information for better clinical decisions to reduce the risk in those individuals who are predisposed (see Advancing Technologies). Patients can be informed and put on a high-risk prevention program or they may be treated more aggressively to effectively arrest or manage the disease.

History of Disease

Patients who have a history of periodontal disease are at an increased risk for future attachment loss. The reasons for the past episode(s) are clues to identifying the need for changes in behavior, habits, and/or compliance. A history of smoking and poor oral hygiene may account for past disease. Present habits may include improved self-care, smoking cessation, and improved nutrition, which are considered in assessing the future risk for periodontal disease, oral cancer, and dental caries.

SYSTEMATIC APPROACH TO RISK ASSESSMENT

There are several steps to assessing a patient's risk for oral disease. The Standards for Clinical Dental Hygiene Practice published by the American Dental Hygienists' Association provides a framework for developing a systematic and comprehensive approach to gathering and assessing the data (Table 17-1).[55]

An oral risk assessment and evidence-based planning follow the dental hygiene process of care: assessment, diagnosis, planning, implementation, evaluation, and documentation. A risk assessment form or worksheet helps the dental hygienist identify risk factors. Modifiable risk factors can be addressed and outcome goals identified. These forms do not predict risk but identify areas that can be changed or modified to reduce risk based on current evidence of the odds for developing the oral disease. Effectiveness of treatment and need for continued care or different treatment options are assessed at each appointment.

Risk assessment transfers the focus from a medical model to a wellness model. Improving oral health can occur with attention to risk assessment. Dental hygienists are integral to this model, focusing on prevention and sustainable oral health (see Application to Clinical Practice and Teamwork).

Application to Clinical Practice

You plan to start a dental hygiene study club in your local area. Your goal is to recruit 6 to 10 hygienists from different offices to discuss how they are using risk assessment in practice. Some areas that you would like to cover include the benefits of risk assessment, personal philosophy, obstacles and challenges, and recent studies and available products. You want to make sure that the study club stays focused on the topic and that each person comes prepared to share information. What are some things you can do to meet this goal? ■

Advancing Technologies

New risk assessment devices will continue to be introduced to the profession. In many cases, these tools can be used by dental hygienists before and during treatment and continuing care in the practice. Current devices are available for oral cancer screening, periodontal risk assessment, and caries risk assessment. New studies are published regularly on the relative risk for disease and ways to assess risk, that is, salivary measures. Dental hygienists need to be cautious and understand the validity and accuracy of the devices or assessment tools. Oral infection is complicated and multifactorial. The dental hygiene profession should embrace evidence-based new diagnostics and technology even if it changes the current philosophy or paradigm. Transition to newer models of risk assessment may be slow due to cost and patient acceptance. Important questions to consider include: Will this assessment provide information that will impact diagnosis or treatment? Is it valid and accurate with appropriate research to support implementation? Can it realistically be implemented into practice? ■

Teamwork

Making a paradigm shift to using comprehensive risk assessment in practice requires cooperation and communication among the entire team. Each person has a role in making this change a success without creating a stressful environment. One way to improve success is regular staff meetings. These meetings should not just include announcements about practice protocols or changes but also include discussion and input from every member of the team. When the team is engaged and committed, the change will progress and every member will feel valuable and committed to patient care and the success of the practice. ■

Table 17-1. Systematic Process for Risk Assessment

Assessment	Gather and review patient data. This includes the written information provided by the patient, oral cancer screening, and comprehensive hard tissue and periodontal evaluation. Diagnostic tests may be performed at this time or later in the assessment process.
Analysis	Analyze the data for oral risk concerns or unfavorable outcome from treatment.
Dental hygiene diagnosis	The dental hygiene diagnosis is a component of the overall dental diagnosis and identifies the existing or potential oral health problems that a dental hygienist is licensed to treat[56]; for example, a 34-year-old white hispanic woman who is a patient of record in the office presents with generalized bleeding on probing and pockets 3–5 mm in posterior quadrants. This is unusual for the patient and started in the past 6 months. Medical and dental histories are negative for systemic disease, medications, and the patient does not smoke. The patient is overweight and she has not had a physical in 3 years. Her record reveals a history of excellent oral hygiene, and she insists she has not changed anything recently. Dental hygiene diagnosis is generalized gingivitis.
Plan	Identify outcome goals, patient-centered interventions, and changes in modifiable risk factors. Based on the diagnosis of generalized gingivitis, the primary goal is to eliminate bleeding on probing by identifying the cause and addressing how to manage. Interventions include supragingival and subgingival debridement and radiographs to compare bone level with baseline measures in file. Recommend a physical with blood work because the patient is obese and has not had one for 3 years. Modify her home-care routine to address better daily debridement of posterior pockets and schedule for an evaluation in 2–3 weeks. Other interventions may include microbial testing, referral to a periodontist, and local delivery of sustained-release antimicrobial agents.
Implementation	Deliver dental hygiene service and consultations.
Evaluation	Evaluate the outcomes and adjust or change plan as needed.
Documentation	Document all steps including changes in risk behavior and need for additional assessment tests, that is, microbial, genotype. Example documentation for the patient's chart: "Explained to patient the reasons for increased bleeding on probing including bacteria, change in medications, systemic disease, and poor oral hygiene. Discussed how diabetes may be an underlying factor in her case and the need for blood work to eliminate or confirm this possibility."

Source: Adapted from American Dental Hygienists' Association Standards for Clinical Dental Hygiene Practice.[56]

Case Study

Cathy is a 56-year-old woman who started her own consulting business 5 years ago when she lost her job in human resources as a trainer. She is divorced and has three adult children. Two of her children are self-supporting, but she is helping her youngest daughter finish her MBA. Cathy has been working many hours, skipping meals or eating whatever is available in the vending machines of her customers. Her last dental visit was 6 years ago when she still had dental insurance. She noticed her gums were bleeding when she brushed and became concerned. Upon examination, the hygienist finds generalized 4- to 5-mm pockets and severe bleeding. Only Cathy's third molars are missing and she has limited restorations, but several areas appear chalky white and have generalized moderate stain. Radiographically, there is early horizontal bone loss.

Case Study Exercises

1. Which risk factors or indicators might apply to Cathy?
   A. Diet
   B. Age
   C. Poor oral hygiene
   D. All of the above
2. What is the likely cause of the white spot areas?
   A. Smoking
   B. Poor oral hygiene
   C. Skipping meals
   D. Severe bleeding
3. Presence of gingival bleeding is indicative of clinical attachment loss. The absence of bleeding generally correlates with good periodontal health.
   A. The first statement is true, but the second statement is false.

Continued

Case Study—cont'd

B. The first statement is false, but the second statement is true.

C. Both statements are true.

D. Both statements are false.

4. What bacterial organisms would the dental hygienist expect to find in Cathy's mouth?

A. *Streptococcus mutans* and lactobacilli

B. *Porphyromonas gingivalis*

C. Acidogenic bacteria and periodontal pathogens

D. Motile rods and spirochetes

5. What risk factor or indicator may be affecting Cathy's oral health?

A. Smoking

B. Female sex

C. Poor nutrition

D. Diabetes mellitus

Review Questions

1. Which population has the highest risk for periodontal disease based on genotype-positive results?

A. Caucasians

B. African Americans

C. South Americans

D. Chinese

2. Why is diabetes mellitus considered a risk factor for periodontal disease?

A. Most people with diabetes have poor glycemic control.

B. Only type 1 is considered a risk factor for periodontal disease.

C. Presence of diabetes has been associated with the early onset of periodontal complications.

D. Individuals with diabetes with poor glycemic control respond favorably to periodontal therapy.

3. Risk assessment is the sole responsibility of the dental hygienists. Patients are only responsible for keeping their appointments.

A. The first statement is true, but the second statement is false.

B. The first statement is false, but the second statement is true.

C. Both statements are true.

D. Both statements are false.

4. The patient has adhered to all recommendations and modifiable risks have been eliminated. Why might the patient still have gingival bleeding?

A. Undiagnosed heart condition

B. Genotype-negative

C. Undiagnosed diabetes

D. Undisclosed smoking

5. The prevalence of oral cancer increases with which of the following risks?

A. Smoking, drinking alcohol, HPV-positive, male sex

B. Smoking, HPV-positive, smokeless tobacco, teenage boys

C. Drinking alcohol, older women, smoking, HPV-positive

D. All of the above

Active Learning

1. Review charts of patients with multiple risk factors. Determine whether your assessment matches the diagnosis and treatment notes.

2. Work with a partner to develop sample patient assessments that include multiple risk factors. Discuss the implications on oral health and treatment together.

3. Role-play with family, friends, or classmates. Have them challenge you by asking questions, providing limited information during the interview process, and discussing why you "need all this information from me."

4. Ask to shadow your dental hygienist. Plan to go in when he or she has a complicated case.

5. Look for cases and images on the Internet and textbooks that show examples of oral findings based on different risk factors. ■

REFERENCES

1. Douglass CW. Risk assessment and management of periodontal disease. *J Am Dent Assoc.* 2006;137(suppl):27S-32S.

2. Page RC, Beck JD. Risk assessment for periodontal diseases. *Int Dent J.* 1997;47(2):61-87.

3. Beck JD. Methods of assessing risk for periodontitis and developing multifactorial models. *J Periodontol.* 1994; 65(5 suppl):468-478.

4. Page R, Krall EA, Martin J, et al. Validity and accuracy of a risk calculator in predicting periodontal disease. *J Am Dent Assoc.* 2002;133(5):569-576.

5. Nunn ME. Understanding the etiology of periodontitis: an overview of periodontal risk factors. *Periodontol 2000.* 2003;32:11-23.

6. Pihlstrom BL. Periodontal risk assessment, diagnosis and treatment planning. *Periodontol 2000.* 2001;25:37-58.

7. Rivera-Hidalgo R. Smoking and periodontal disease. *Periodontol 2000.* 2003;32:50-58.

8. Grossi SG, Zambon JJ, Ho AW, et al. Assessment of risk for periodontal disease. I. Risk indicators for attachment loss. *J Periodontol.* 1994;65(3):260-267.

9. Grossi SB, Genco RJ. Machtei EE, et al. Assessment of risk for periodontal disease. II. Risk indicators for alveolar bone loss. *J Periodontol.* 1995;65(1):23-29.

10. Bergstrom J. Tobacco smoking and chronic destructive periodontal disease. *Odonotology.* 2004;92(1):1-8.

11. Tomar SL, Amsa S. Smoking attributable periodontitis in the United States: findings from NHANES III. *J Periodontol.* 2000;71(5):743-751.

12. American Academy of Periodontology Position Paper: tobacco use and the periodontal patient. *J Periodontol.* 1999;70(11):1419-1427.

13. Mavropoulus A, Aars H, Brodin P. Hyperaemic response to cigarette smoking in healthy gingiva. *J Clin Periodontol.* 2003;30(3):214-221.

14. Labriola A, Needleman I, Moles DR. Systematic review of the effect of smoking on nonsurgical periodontal therapy. *Periodontol 2000.* 2005;37:124-137.

15. Wan CP, Leung WK, Wong MC, et al. Effects of smoking on healing response to non-surgical periodontal therapy: a multilevel modeling analysis. *J Clin Periodontol.* 2009;36(3):229-239.

16. Heasman L, Stacey F, Preshaw PM, et al. The effect of smoking on periodontal treatment response: a review of clinical evidence. *J Clin Periodontol.* 2006;33(4):241-253.

17. Johnson GK, Hill M. Cigarette smoking and the periodontal patient. *J Periodontol.* 2004;75(2):196-209.

18. Heikkinen AM, Pajukanta R, Pitkäniemi J, et al. The effect of smoking on periodontal health of 15-16 year-olds. *J Periodontol.* 2008;79(11):2042-2047.

19. Albandar JM, Streckfus CF, Adesanya MR, Winn DM. Cigar, pipe, and cigarette smoking as risk factors for periodontal disease and tooth loss. *J Periodontol.* 2000;71(12):1874-1881.

20. Tomar SL, Winn DM. Chewing tobacco use and dental caries among U.S. men. *J Am Dent Assoc.* 1999;130(11):1601-1610.

21. American Cancer Society. Oral cavity and oropharyngeal cancer. http://www.cancer.org/Cancer/Oral CavityandOropharyngealCancer/DetailedGuide/oral-cavity-and-oropharyngeal-cancer-risk-factors. Accessed September 27, 2010.

22. Ezzo PJ, Cutler CW. Microorganisms as risk indicators for periodontal disease. *Periodontol 2000.* 2003;32:24-35.

23. Teles, RP, Haffajee AD, Socransky SS. Microbiological goals of periodontal therapy. *Periodontology.* 2000;42:180-218.

24. Mealey BL, Oates TW. Diabetes mellitus and periodontal diseases. *J Periodontol.* 2006;77(8):1289-1303.

25. Lalla E, Chang B, Lal S, et al. Periodontal changes in children and adolescents with diabetes. *Diabetes Care.* 2006;29(2):295-299.

26. Salvi GE, Collins JG, Yalda B, et al. Monocytic TNF-_ secretion patterns in IDDM patients with periodontal diseases. *J Clin Periodontol.* 1997;24(1):8-16.

27. Naguib G, Al-Mashat H, Desta T, Graves D. Diabetes prolongs the inflammatory response to a bacterial stimulus through cytokine dysregulation. *J Invest Dermotol.* 2004;123(1):87-92.

28. Salvi GE, Yalda B, Collins JG, et al. Inflammatory mediator response as a potential risk marker for periodontal diseases in insulin-dependent diabetes mellitus patients. *J Periodontol.* 1997;68(2):127-135.

29. Taylor GW, Burt BA, Becker MP, et al. Severe periodontitis and risk for poor glycemic control in patients with non-insulin-dependent diabetes mellitus. *J Periodontol.* 1996;67(10 suppl):1085-1093.

30. Saremi A, Nelson RG, Tulloch-Reid M, et al. Periodontal disease and mortality in type 2 diabetes mellitus. *Diabetes Care.* 2005;28(1):27-32.

31. Shultis WA, Weil EJ, Looker HC, et al. Effect of periodontitis on overt nephropathy and end-stage renal disease in type 2 diabetes. *Diabetes Care.* 2007;30(2):306-311.

32. Geurs NC. Osteoporosis and periodontal disease. *Periodontology 2000.* 2007;44:29-43.

33. Saito T, Shimozaki Y, Koga T, Tsuzuki M, Ohskima A. Relationship between upper body obesity and periodontitis. *J Dent Res.* 2001;80(7):1631-1636.

34. Al-Zahrani MA, Vissada NF, Borawskit EA. Obesity and periodontal disease in young, middle-aged, and older adults. *J Periodontol.* 2003;74(5):610-615.

35. Wood N, Johnson RB, Streckfus CF. Comparison of body composition and periodontal disease using nutritional assessment techniques: Third National Health and Nutrition Examination Survey (NHANES III). *J Clin Periodontol.* 2003;30(4):321-327.

36. Ciancio SB. Medications: a risk factor for periodontal disease diagnosis and treatment. *J Periodontol.* 2005;76 (11 suppl):2061-2065.

37. Spolarich AE. Managing the side effects of medications. *J Dent Hyg.* 2000;74(1):57-69.

38. Fox PC. Xerostomia: recognition and management. *Access.* 2008(special suppl):1-7.

39. Borrell LN, Beck JD, Heiss G. Socioeconomic disadvantage and periodontal disease: the Dental Atherosclerosis Risk in Communities Study. *Am J Public Health.* 2006;96(2):332-339.

40. Shiau HJ, Reynolds MA. Sex differences in destructive periodontal disease: a systematic review. *J Periodontol.* 2010;81(10):1379-1389.

41. American Cancer Society. Oral cancer. www.cancer.org/acs/groups/content/@nho/documents/document/oralcancerpdf.pdf. Accessed September 27, 2010.

42. American Cancer Society. Human papilloma virus (HPV), cancer, and HPV vaccines—frequently asked questions. http://www.cancer.org/cancer/cancercauses/othercarcinogens/infectiousagents/hpv/humanpapillomavirusandhpvvaccinesfaq/index. Accessed September 27, 2010.

43. American Cancer Society. Oral cavity and oropharyngeal cancer. http://www.cancer.org/Cancer/Oral CavityandOropharyngealCancer/DetailedGuide/oral-cavity-and-oropharyngeal-cancer-risk-factors. Accessed September 27, 2010.

44. D'Souza G, Kreimer AR, Viscidi R, et al. Case-control study of human papillomavirus and oropharyngeal cancer. *New Engl J Med.* 2007;356(19):1944-1956.

45. Offenbacher S, Beck JD, Jared HL, et al. Effects of periodontal therapy on rate of preterm delivery: a randomized controlled trial. *Obstet Gynecol.* 2009;114(3):551-559.

46. Michalowicz BS, Hodges JS, DiAngelis AJ, et al. Treatment of periodontal disease and the risk of preterm birth. *New Engl J Med.* 2006;355(18):1885-1894.

47. Mobley C, Marshall TA, Milgrom P, Coldwell SE. The contribution of dietary factors to dental caries and disparities in caries. *Acad Pediatr.* 2009;9(6):410-414.

48. Sohn W, Bart BA, Sowers MR. Carbonated soft drinks and dental caries in the primary dentition. *J Dent Res.* 2006;85(3):262-266.

49. Marshall TA, Eichenberger-Gilmore JM, Larson MA, Warren JJ, Levy SM. Comparison of the intakes of sugars by young children with and without dental caries experience. *J Am Dent Assoc.* 2007;138(1):39-46.

50. National Institute of Dental and Craniofacial Research. Dental caries (tooth decay) in children (age 2–11). NHANES 1999–2004. http://www.nidcr.nih.gov/Data Statistics/FindDataByTopic/DentalCaries/Dental CariesChildren2to11.htm. Accessed July 26, 2015.

51. Greenstein G, Hart TC. Clinical utility of a genetic susceptibility test for severe chronic periodontitis: a critical evaluation. *J Am Dent Assoc.* 2002;133(4):452-459.

52. Kornman KS, Crane A, Wang HY, et al. The interleukin-1 genotype as a severity factor in adult periodontal disease. *J Clin Periodontol.* 1997;24(1):72-77.

53. Armitage GC, Wu Y, Wang HY, et al. Low prevalence of a periodontitis-associated interleukin-1 composite genotype in individuals of Chinese heritage. *J Periodontol.* 2000;71(2):164-171.

54. Walker SJ, Van Dyke T, Rich S, et al. Genetic polymorphisms of the IL-1 alpha and IL-1 beta genes in African-American LJP patients and an African-American control population. *J Periodontol.* 2000;71(5):723-728.

55. American Dental Hygienists' Association. Standards for clinical dental hygiene practice. Adopted March 10, 2008. Chicago: American Dental Hygienists' Association. www.adha.org/resources-docs/7261_Standards_ Clinical_Practice.pdf. Accessed June 10, 2013.

56. Dental hygiene diagnosis: an American Dental Hygienists' Association position paper. http://www.adha. org/resources-docs/Diagnosis-Position-Paper.pdf. Accessed July 26, 2015.

57. Ask Advise Refer. Three minutes or less can save lives. http://www.askadviserefer.org. Accessed June 10, 2013.

58. American Academy of Periodontology. Gum disease symptoms. http://www.perio.org/consumer/4a.html#. Accessed June 10, 2013.

59. American Dental Association. Caries risk assessment form. http://www.ada.org/sections/professional Resources/pdfs/topic_caries_over6.pdf. Accessed February 20, 2014.

Part V

Diagnosis and Planning

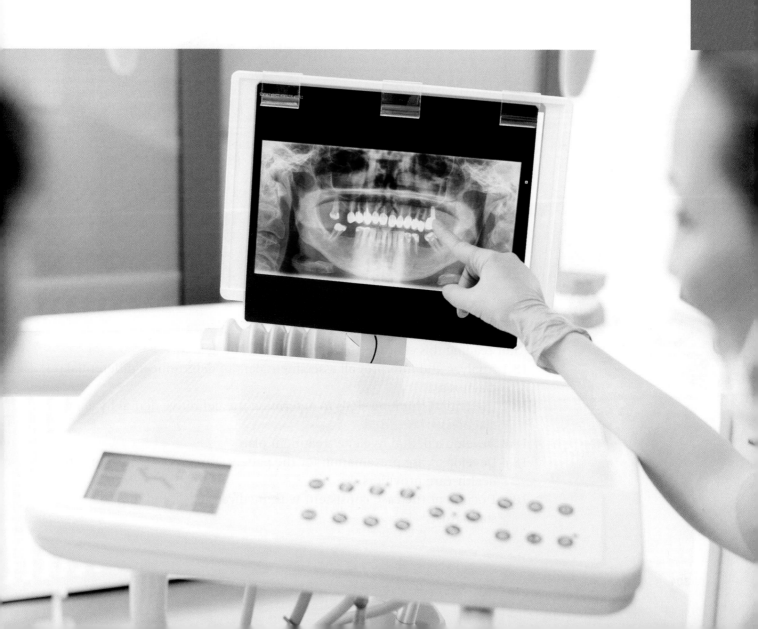

Chapter 18 | Dental Hygiene Diagnosis, Treatment Plan, Documentation, and Case Presentation

JoAnn R. Gurenlian, RDH, PhD • Deb Astroth, RDH, BS

KEY TERMS

battery
breach of contract
definitive diagnosis
differential diagnosis
expressed consent
implied consent
informed consent
informed refusal
treatment plan

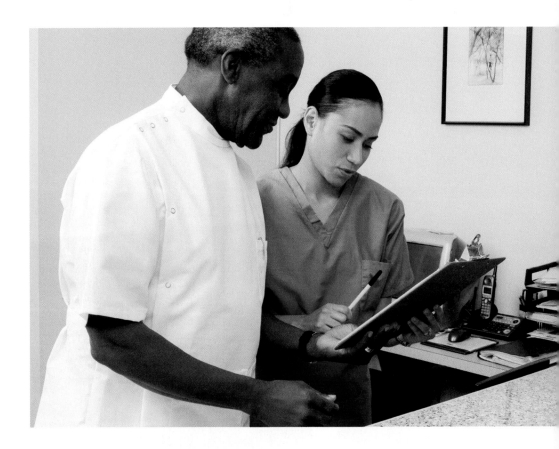

LEARNING OBJECTIVES

After reading this chapter, the student should be able to:

18.1 Analyze and interpret all assessment data to determine a differential diagnosis.

18.2 Use critical thinking skills to determine the definitive dental hygiene diagnosis.

18.3 Develop a dental hygiene treatment plan.

18.4 Develop a case presentation for the patient, caregiver, dentist, or other health-care providers.

18.5 Document the case consistent with medical, legal, and ethical standards.

KEY CONCEPTS

- Determining a dental hygiene diagnosis, formulating a treatment plan, and completely and accurately documenting all aspects of the dental hygiene process of care are elements of the standards for clinical dental hygiene practice.
- Identifying the goal of a case presentation, the intended audience, and the significant aspects to include are elements of both written and oral case presentations.

RELEVANCE TO CLINICAL PRACTICE

Formulating the dental hygiene diagnosis (DHDx) involves a process of clinical decision-making that takes into consideration the patient's health history, oral health needs and values, and findings from assessment procedures. The dental hygienist uses these resources to determine existing or potential health problems that require further intervention. These patient problems become the basis for creating a treatment plan. The **treatment plan** delineates the treatment interventions that the dental hygienist and the patient will implement. Use of a DHDx provides the basis for individualized treatment plans that will help each patient achieve optimum oral and general health.

DENTAL HYGIENE DIAGNOSIS

Diagnosis refers to the ability to recognize or identify a disease. It may be based on signs and symptoms, physical examination, interview with the patient or family, or both, and other pertinent health assessments. The dental hygienist is responsible for determining the DHDx and developing a treatment plan appropriate to the patient's needs.

Historical Perspective

From a historical perspective, the concept of the DHDx is relatively new. For years, dental hygienists were taught that formulating a DHDx was not within their scope of practice. Language used included the word *suspicious* for interpreting any clinical findings. For example, if a dental hygienist noted a large, black gaping hole on the occlusal surface of a tooth, he would state the tooth was "suspicious for a carious lesion." Only a dentist could determine the diagnosis for oral consideration.

In 1982, Miller[1] was the first person to discuss the concept of a DHDx, which sparked a lengthy discussion in the literature about the need to create diagnoses that were unique to the dental hygiene profession. Models for formulating a DHDx were promoted based on clinical decision-making and nursing diagnosis process and application.[2–4]

In 1985, the American Dental Hygienists' Association (ADHA) developed an approach to clinical practice through a model known as the dental hygiene process of care. This process of care comprised four steps: assessment, planning, implementation, and evaluation. This model was reflected in the publication *Applied Standards of Clinical Dental Hygiene Practice.*[5] The ADHA also adopted a definition for DHDx and supported its use of the DHDX as an integral approach to dental hygiene care. The standards were revised in 2008 to reflect changes in the development of the profession.

Current Clinical Practice Standards

Current clinical standards of practice are defined in the ADHA document entitled *Standards for Clinical Dental Hygiene Practice.*[6] These standards recognize the knowledge, skills, and professional scope of responsibility of dental hygienists with respect to oral health promotion and protection for individuals and groups. The expectations of these standards are that oral health will be improved through patient-centered comprehensive care. The current standards include six components of the dental hygiene process of care: assessment, diagnosis, planning, implementation, evaluation, and documentation as delineated in Figure 18-1.

Definition

As noted in the current standards, the *DHDx* is defined as "the identification of an existing or potential oral health problem that a dental hygienist is educationally qualified and licensed to treat."[6] Based on current findings from clinical assessments and/or the perceptions,

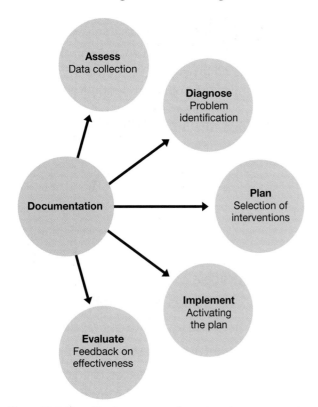

Figure 18-1. Dental hygiene process of care. (From the American Dental Hygienists' Association. *Standards for Clinical Dental Hygiene Practice.* March 10, 2008. Chicago, IL. 13 p, which was adapted from Wilkins, *Clinical Practice of the Dental Hygienist*, 2005.)

values, and beliefs of the patient, the DHDx may identify both existing and potential oral health problems. Further, the diagnosis points to conditions for which the dental hygienist can legally and educationally provide health care. This may include oral health education, debridement procedures, procedures designed to prevent oral diseases, as well as referrals to other health-care providers and re-evaluation procedures to determine the efficacy of treatment rendered and referral examinations conducted. For example, taking vital signs may reveal that the patient has hypertension and requires further evaluation. The dental hygienist may note hypertension as part of the medical component of the DHDx. Although the dental hygienist cannot diagnose hypertension or prescribe an antihypertensive medication, the dental hygienist is responsible for monitoring vital signs during subsequent appointments, encouraging adherence to medications prescribed by the patient's physician, noting any oral side effects of medications used, and referring the patient for further evaluation should blood pressure not improve once medication has been used.

The current standards recognize that the dental hygienist must be able to:

- Analyze and interpret all assessment data to evaluate clinical findings and formulate the DHDx.
- Determine patient needs that can be improved through the delivery of dental hygiene care.

- Incorporate the DHDx into the overall dental treatment plan.[6]

Purpose

The DHDx defines and specifies the types of problems presented by each patient, providing a bridge between the assessment phase of care and the development of the treatment plan. Once a diagnosis has been determined, the dental hygienist can develop a treatment plan that is both comprehensive in addressing all of the patient needs and is patient centered. Conducting this step in the standards of clinical practice helps the dental hygienist focus on factors and interventions that are necessary for each patient to achieve optimum oral and general health (see Application to Clinical Practice).

Diagnostic Terminology

Initially, when the DHDx models were presented, an attempt was made to create terminology in the form of diagnostic statements that were meaningful to the profession. Some of this terminology was based on that used for a nursing diagnosis. An example of this terminology comparing different models appears in Table 18-1. Although some authors of models of diagnosis prefer to maintain this approach, it has become

Application to Clinical Practice

With each patient who presents to clinical practice, challenges may exist in terms of oral health conditions. Some patients will present with specific problems they would like you to address as part of their chief complaint. Other patients will not have a high level of oral health awareness or may not notice any problems with their mouth. Using a variety of assessment tools, the dental hygienist will identify existing or potential problems that are unique to the patient. These problems become the basis for formulating a DHDx. Although most clinicians focus on periodontal problems or caries, patients may have other infections of the mouth, temporomandibular dysfunctions, among others, and systemic conditions (e.g., cardiovascular disease, diabetes mellitus, and arthritis). These findings are part of the DHDx that affects patient education practices and treatment plans. Creating a DHDx for each patient and informing them of these diagnoses helps the patient better understand her health status, interventions that can be accomplished within the dental/hygiene practice, as well as the rationale for referrals to other health-care professionals.

Also, as licensed health-care providers, dental hygienists are legally bound to adhere to the standards of care for the profession. If the DHDx is not identified and part of the patient record, the dental hygienist may be found negligent and held accountable if a lawsuit is pursued. ■

Table 18-1. ***Historic Comparison of Diagnostic Terminology***

Medical	Dental	Nursing	Dental Hygiene
Myocardial infarction	Periapical abscess	Injury, potential for	Knowledge deficit (specify)
Diabetes mellitus	Caries	Comfort, alternations in: pain	Noncompliance (specify)
Multiple sclerosis	Candidiasis	Infection, potential for	Fear, potential for
Rheumatoid arthritis	Chronic periodontitis	Skin integrity, impairment of	Potential for injury (specify)
Asthma	Hemangioma	Cardiac output, alterations in, decreased	Impairment of skin and mucous membrane integrity of the head and neck

clear that many health-care providers can share the same diagnostic terminology. How each practitioner incorporates this diagnosis into his treatment plan demonstrates the differences among professions. For example, a patient may present with a chief complaint of rheumatoid arthritis to a physician, nurse, dentist, and dental hygienist. The physician may prescribe an anti-inflammatory agent to alleviate pain. The nurse may evaluate the patient for the need for intermittent periods of rest and exercise. The dentist and dental hygienist may note that the patient has difficulty performing oral hygiene, resulting in gingivitis and caries. The dentist will treat the carious lesions restoratively, whereas the dental hygienist may treat the gingivitis, recommend oral care products that will assist in reducing bacteria and inflammation in the mouth and preventing caries, and recommend the use of adaptive devices for teeth and interdental cleansing at home. The health-care providers share the same diagnosis, but they use different approaches to care that are appropriate to their areas of expertise.

FORMULATING THE DENTAL HYGIENE DIAGNOSIS

Determining the DHDx involves correlating assessment information, the patient's perception of the problem and her complaints, and signs and symptoms, with known general and oral health conditions. In some cases, the condition or patient problem is readily identifiable, such as torus palatinus, an overgrowth of bone on the palate. In this case, the dental hygiene professional can document this torus as the **definitive diagnosis.** The definitive diagnosis represents the identification or determination of a disease, problem, or injury. When conditions have similar characteristics, signs, and symptoms, and a definitive diagnosis cannot be readily determined, the clinician identifies a **differential diagnosis** or listing in order of likelihood those conditions or diseases that may be producing the signs observed.

Arriving at a diagnosis requires the development of clinical reasoning, decision-making, and problem-solving skills. The process of diagnosis involves a standardized, systematic approach of summarizing assessment data into actual and potential problems, generating hypotheses as to the causes of these problems, performing further assessments if indicated, synthesizing information, and making a reasoned decision that represents the diagnosis. Becoming a dental hygiene diagnostician requires knowledge, attention to detail, active listening, critical thinking, and continuous self-directed learning to refine these skills.

Mueller-Joseph and Petersen[3] offered a system for categorizing information from the assessment process to ensure that key elements are included in the DHDx. These authors suggested classifying assessment data into 10 key areas as follows:

- Chief complaint—the patient's chief concern or reason he has attended the dental hygiene appointment
- General systemic—a comprehensive summary of the patient's general health, which may or may not influence dental hygiene treatment planning
- Dental history—data identified during restorative examination including caries, malformations, occlusal problems, stain, defective restorations, abrasion, erosion, attrition
- Oral habit—factors that influence oral findings including nail biting, chewing on lips and mucosa, chewing on other devices (e.g., pencils), and smoking
- Nutrition—dietary intake (proteins, carbohydrates, fats, sugars), calories, body mass index
- Hard tissue—lesions, swellings, nodules, asymmetry, change in color or texture, bleeding or suppuration, ulceration, pain or tenderness upon palpation
- Soft tissue—same as hard tissue
- Periodontal—inflammation, bone loss, loss of clinical attachment, bleeding, loss of papillae, fetid odor, pain, tooth loss, mobility, furcation involvement
- Oral hygiene—level of biofilm, calculus, and stain formation; brushing routine; other interdental cleaning activities
- Radiographic survey—radiolucencies, radio-opacities, impacted teeth, resorption, caries, calculus

For novice dental hygienists, it may be helpful to note a DHDx for each category as appropriate and identify what the cause might be for each condition (e.g., caries related to malposed teeth, diet high in sugar, and toothbrushing technique). Dental hygienists with more experience in pathology and periodontology may simply want to list the general health and oral health diagnoses as they are identified and then create a treatment plan related to each diagnosis.

Case Examples

Case A

Robert Patterson, a 49-year-old patient, presents with a chief complaint of dry mouth. He indicates that he has a recent history of depression and a long-standing history of bipolar disorder. His physician prescribed quetiapine (Seroquel) 300 mg daily, which may be used to treat both conditions.[7] The patient reports that his mouth has been very dry since he began taking this medicine and that it is interrupting his sleep because he is constantly drinking water and then has to go to the bathroom in the middle of the night. He is so tired he is having difficulty concentrating during the day and admits his home-care regimen has been reduced to brushing once per day. He no longer flosses or uses a mouthrinse as recommended by the dental hygienist. Based on this information alone, the DHDx would appear as:

DHDx: general health—bipolar disorder, depression, sleep disorder
Oral health—xerostomia related to medication used for mental health conditions
Nonadherence with home-care regimens

Case B

Maureen MacDougall is a 26-year-old patient who presents with a chief complaint of swelling of both lips of 2-day duration. Examination reveals diffuse swelling of the lips, maxillary greater than mandibular lip. The patient denies allergies to medications, products, and foods. She denies using any new oral health products. The patient denies difficulty breathing, speaking, or swallowing. The patient appears concerned about her appearance and is mystified by this onset of swelling. Further questioning reveals that the patient spent significant time over the previous weekend working in the yard helping her husband take down oak trees and clear brush from a recent storm.

DHDx: general health—noncontributory
Oral health—angioedema, possibly related to mild allergic response to oak trees

Case C

Samuel Stevenson is a 37-year-old patient who presents to your practice for his scheduled maintenance appointment with a chief complaint of oral ulcers. His medical history is significant for Crohn disease and allergies to penicillin, strawberries, and stings from wasps. The patient states that he noticed several small, but painful ulcers in his mouth over the last 3 days. The patient denies trauma to the oral cavity and denies ever having any oral health problems in the past. Clinical examination reveals three nonspecific ulcers of the hard palate and two on the left buccal mucosa that appear to be coalescing.

DHDx: general health—Crohn disease, allergies to penicillin, strawberries, wasp stings
Oral health—aphthous ulcers related to Crohn disease

TREATMENT PLAN

The dental hygiene treatment plan is based on the patient's health history, the assessment findings, and the dental hygiene diagnoses. It must also take into consideration the patient's goals, values, lifestyle, and current scientific evidence (see Evidence-Based Practice).[6] The *Standards for Clinical Dental Hygiene Practice* state that the dental hygienist must be able to:

- Identify, prioritize, and sequence dental hygiene interventions (e.g., education, treatment, and referral).
- Coordinate resources to facilitate comprehensive quality care (e.g., current technologies, pain management, adequate personnel, appropriate appointment sequencing, and time management).
- Collaborate with the dentist and other health/dental-care providers and community-based oral health programs (see Spotlight on Public Health).
- Present and document the dental hygiene treatment plan to the patient.
- Explain treatment rationale, risks, benefits, anticipated outcomes, treatment alternatives, and prognosis.
- Obtain and document informed consent and/or informed refusal.[6]

Evidence-Based Practice

With greater emphasis on providing evidence-based practice, dental hygienists can incorporate products and procedures as part of their treatment plan based on current scientific evidence. When patients inquire about the use of a particular toothpaste, mouthrinse, toothbrush, whitening procedure, or polishing procedure, use information from the most recent research to advise them. Informing patients about research findings can help them make treatment decisions, as well as product choices for themselves and their families. Using evidence-based practice provides another opportunity to better educate and inform patients about the latest interventions in oral health care. ■

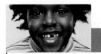

Spotlight on Public Health

Not only can dental hygienists formulate a DHDx and treatment plan for each patient, they can incorporate these same concepts when working in community settings. Families, employees of local businesses, and those with special medical conditions or disabilities would benefit from an oral health assessment, diagnosis, and comprehensive plan that includes education, provisions of oral care, and coordination of health services with other health-care providers. Referral and follow-through may be essential components incorporated to ensure that available resources are used. ■

Individualized dental hygiene treatment plans must consider not only the physical health of the patient but also the patient's goals for her oral health and her willingness to be an active participant in her care. The patient's nutrition history and lifestyle habits (exercise, tobacco use, alcohol consumption) are contributing factors that will impact the prognosis and final outcomes of treatment. The dental hygienist must be able to identify the patient's needs and determine whether the patient should be immediately referred or whether the patient would first benefit from dental hygiene interventions. An individual with uncontrolled diabetes, a patient with severe hypertension, and a patient with a painful tooth abscess are examples of patients who should be referred before most dental hygiene interventions.

The dental hygienist must acknowledge that dental hygiene interventions and referrals are integrated into the overall dental and/or health treatment plans for the patient. Most dental hygienists at some point in their careers, during the review of a patient's health history, have been asked, "Why do you need to know that?" Having full knowledge of the patient's physical and mental health may impact scheduling and sequencing of treatment. Some patients may do better with morning appointments because of physical mobility issues or perhaps they are better in the afternoon. There may be transportation issues that need to be taken into consideration. If the patient is going to be scheduled for anesthesia, he must be aware of the possible impact on his ability to speak or eat for a period after the procedure. Patients who are currently going through dialysis, chemotherapy, or radiation treatment should not be scheduled on the same days as those procedures or may need to delay treatment. Individuals with mental health problems may be able to tolerate procedures or interactions with people at certain times of the day or according to their medication schedules. Further information on working with patients with special needs is included in Part IV of this textbook.

Collaboration among the oral health providers and other health-care providers is essential for the patient and the providers (see Teamwork). Understanding among health-care providers that they can share the same diagnosis but intervene and treat according to their respective profession's scope of practice promotes an interdisciplinary and comprehensive approach to patient care. Within collaboration is the necessity to communicate effectively not only with the patient but also among the health-care providers. The dental hygienist is often the provider who initiates collaboration by contacting other providers either for consultation or referral. Consultations with dentists or specialists regarding oral health needs, or with physicians to confer regarding medications or current disease status, are a daily occurrence in today's dental hygiene practice.

Many varieties of forms are available for the treatment plan. Some use a checklist format, whereas others provide the practitioner the option to write her own plan. With advances in technology and federal mandates, many dental offices are going paperless and are using electronic health records. Computer-based patient record systems are commercially available; however, some have been found to have significant usability problems and steep learning curves.[8] Regardless of the format that is used, there seems to be agreement in the literature that the treatment plan should be based on current standards of evidence-based dental hygiene care and include:

- Patient profile or demographics
- Assessment findings
- Diagnosis and prognosis
- Goals and expected outcomes
- Treatment and treatment options
- Risks and benefits of treatment
- Referrals
- Evaluation strategies
- Maintenance schedule
- Financial implications
- Consent[3,4,9,10]

Teamwork

When formulating a DHDx and treatment plan, the dental hygiene practitioner does not work in isolation. This process involves collaborating with other dental specialists and health-care providers to identify a definitive diagnosis in some cases, to coordinate medical care needed, and to provide for the use of additional resources to improve the health of the patient. Working together with other specialists provides the patient with optimum results. Improving oral health is one way of helping to improve general health. ■

Assessment findings are thoroughly discussed in Part IV, Chapters 8 to 17. Data gathered during this phase are the foundation for the DHDx and the treatment plan. The treatment plan will parallel the findings from the assessment phase. This chapter focuses on the diagnosis and subsequent treatment plan. The diagnoses provide the treatment rationale. The patient's assessment findings (indices, intraoral photographs, radiographs, study models) are helpful visuals to provide further evidence for recommended treatment. The dental hygiene prognosis is a statement of the possible outcomes that can be expected from the dental hygiene interventions performed for that patient.[9]

Some authors have presented a three-prong approach to treatment plan development (patient profile, clinical evidence, case management),[11] whereas others have presented a phase approach.[10,12] A four-prong approach to each diagnosis, which includes prevention, therapy, maintenance, and referral, is presented in Table 18-2. Prevention identifies interventions to prevent further worsening or subsequent incidences of the problem. Therapy identifies all treatment interventions selected by the dental hygienist for the patient's diagnosis. Maintenance presents the recommendations for daily self-care, monitoring, and scheduled intervals for future dental hygiene care. Referrals would specify other health-care providers, as well as the areas of concern for consultation or referral, or both. When multiple diagnoses are present, it may be beneficial to complete all four areas of the treatment plan for each diagnosis and then address the prioritization and appointment sequencing to prepare a comprehensive dental hygiene treatment plan.

Treatment Options

The dental hygienist should offer treatment options in addition to the ideal treatment plan. Patients may have financial, time, or travel constraints that could impact their choice of plans. If the treatment plan is consistent with the patient's goals and the patient has had the opportunity to be an active participant in the development of the treatment plan, the patient is more likely to consent to the ideal treatment plan.

Risks and Benefits of Treatment

The risks and benefits of the proposed treatment should be explained to the patient. For example, a patient who receives quadrant debridement with anesthesia may experience the effects of the anesthesia for several hours after the procedure and have some initial gingival bleeding, subsequent recession, and/or root sensitivity. The benefits may include lack of daily gingival bleeding while brushing, reduction of gingival inflammation, and decreased root sensitivity.

Financial Implications

It is essential for patients to know and understand their financial responsibilities associated with their treatment. This is an integral part of the informed consent. Many patients who have dental insurance do not understand that the insurance contract between their employer and the insurance company specifies financial amounts for dental services provided, as well as frequency intervals within each calendar year. For example, Mrs. Jones's policy through her employer XYZ Company may allow for two prophylaxes at least 6 months apart and will pay $65.00 for each prophylaxis. They may also pay a specific amount for one dental examination a year and one set of four bitewing radiographs. Mrs. Jones is your patient and your fee is $75.00 for a prophylaxis. Mrs. Jones must be informed that her insurance coverage will cover $65.00 of your fee and she will be responsible for the remaining $10.00 for each prophylaxis during the year. The financial implications section of the treatment plan should specify the amount the insurance company is contracted to pay for the services (often referred to as the preauthorization) and the amount that the patient is responsible to pay.

Case Examples

Case A

Using the four-prong approach, the dental hygiene treatment plan for Robert Patterson, who was diagnosed earlier in this chapter, might look like this:

DHDx: bipolar disorder, depression, xerostomia related to medications for mental illness, nonadherence to home-care regimens

Prognosis: Robert is nonadherent with medications as reviewed and prescribed by his primary care provider. Robert is nonadherent with fluoride therapy, over-the-counter (OTC) salivary supplements, and has no signs of candidal infection. Robert is compliant with daily biofilm removal.

Appointment schedule: 1 1/2 hours prophylaxis; fluoride treatment; salivary testing; brushing, flossing, and rinsing instructions

Explain calendar to record compliance

Schedule 2-week follow-up for oral hygiene index and 3-month continuing care appointment

Table 18-2. A Four-Prong Approach to the Dental Hygiene Treatment Plan

Prevention	Treatment	Maintenance	Referral
Interventions to prevent further worsening or subsequent incidences of the problem or disease	Identify all treatment interventions selected by the dental hygienist appropriate to the patient's diagnosis	Interventions and recommendations for daily self-care, monitoring for the provider, and scheduled intervals for future dental hygiene care	Identify other health-care providers and the areas of concern that require consultation and referral

Prevention	Treatment	Maintenance	Referral
Provide fluoride therapy for caries prevention Perform CAMBRA to determine risk for disease	Evaluate for signs of candida infection and treat with antifungal medications	Home fluoride therapy	Refer to dentist if caries are present
Correlate with other diseases and medications to determine causative factors	Perform diagnostic salivary testing to determine risk level	Recommend use of OTC salivary supplements or prescription medications	Refer to primary care provider to review medications if determined to be cause of dry mouth symptoms
	Perform dental hygiene therapy	Schedule periodic re-evaluation appointments to monitor progress Have patient identify best time of day for follow-up appointments given mental health issues	
Discuss with patient when he performs oral hygiene, rationale for oral hygiene, and triggers to use to increase adherence	Discuss patient's perception of situation, reasons for nonadherence, when he is more amenable to perform daily regimen Modify home-care recommendations that patient will agree to perform	Give Robert calendar to record performance of oral hygiene regimen Schedule 2-week follow-up appointment to review adherence progress Make additional recommendations for improving home care as accepted by patient	

Treatment options: no fluoride treatment, no salivary testing

Risks of no treatment: caries, candidal infection, continuance of xerostomia

Fee: provide the patient with the amount that his dental insurance will cover and the amount for which he is responsible

Patient/Guardian Signature	Date
Provider	Date

Case B

Maureen MacDougall, 26-year-old patient with a chief complaint of swelling of both lips of 2-day duration.

DHDx: general health—no significant findings

Oral health—angioedema, possibly related to mild allergic response to oak trees

Prognosis: Elimination of all signs of maxillary and mandibular lip swelling. Maureen is compliant with referral to an allergist and calls office to report that oak tree allergy is confirmed, as well as allergy to poison oak and poison ivy. The allergist confirmed continued use of OTC antihistamine until all signs of lip swelling are eliminated.

Appointment schedule: 30 minutes
Review patient's medical/dental histories
Oral examination and further questioning
Recommend OTC antihistamine
Referral to an allergist
Advise patient to call with status report in 24 hours

Prevention	Treatment	Maintenance	Referral
Document patient's call and confirm allergies in patient's record	Recommend using an OTC antihistamine to see whether symptoms subside	Advise patient to call 24 hours after starting antihistamine to report status	Referral to an allergist for further evaluation and to determine definitive diagnosis

Treatment options: Do not recommend OTC antihistamine and see whether symptoms subside without intervention

Patient does not accept referral to allergist

Risks of no treatment: angioedema continues for several days

Angioedema is not related to oak trees and continues until causative agent is identified

Fee: provide the patient with the amount that her dental insurance will cover and the amount for which she is responsible

_____   _____
Patient/Guardian Signature   Date

_____   _____
Provider   Date

Case C

Samuel Stevenson is the 37-year-old patient who presents with a chief complaint of oral ulcers.

DHDx: general health—Crohn disease, allergies to penicillin, strawberries, and wasp stings

Oral health—aphthous ulcers related to Crohn disease

Prognosis: compliant with topical corticoid steroid application; compliant with referral to primary care physician; compliant with vitamin D supplement as recommended by physician

Appointment schedule: 1 hour

Review health history

Intraoral/extraoral examination

Review biofilm control methods

Supragingival and subgingival debridement

Selective polishing

Referral to primary care physician

Consultation with dentist regarding use of topical corticosteroids

Instruct patient on relationship of Crohn disease and vitamin D deficiency, nutritional counseling, and occasional aphthous ulcer appearances

Instruct patient to perform self oral examination

Treatment options: preprocedural antimicrobial mouthrinse (did not use because it might have irritated the ulcers)

Risks of no treatment: Failure to refer to primary care physician could result in the progression of coalescing ulcerations and nonrecognition of early signs of intestinal lesions that are associated with Crohn disease or diagnosis of another granulomatous disease

Fee: provide the patient with the amount that his dental insurance will cover and the amount for which he is responsible

_____   _____
Patient/Guardian Signature   Date

_____   _____
Provider   Date

CASE PRESENTATION

A case presentation may be developed for a variety of reasons.

- To acquaint the dentist with the dental hygiene treatment plan that is to be incorporated into the comprehensive dental treatment plan for a patient.
- To present the case to a patient and his or her caretaker.
- To present the case to another health-care provider to whom the patient is being referred for additional treatment (see Professionalism).
- To present the case (making sure confidentiality is not breached) during a staff meeting or a study club as a learning experience. Another way to share the case would be for publication in a newsletter or journal. In this final option, the publication may specify guidelines for submission of the case for publication.

The case presentation should cover all the areas that were previously identified as essential elements of the treatment plan. The dental hygiene case presentation should be presented to the patient and the individual

Prevention	Treatment	Maintenance	Referral
Instruct patient on the relationship between vitamin D deficiency and Crohn disease and the fact that occasional aphthous ulcers should be expected	Review health history Extraoral/intraoral examination Biofilm control review Supragingival and subgingival debridement Selective polishing	Schedule subsequent maintenance appointment	Referral to primary care physician for further evaluation of the current status of intestinal problems associated with Crohn disease and possible vitamin D deficiency
Instruct patient on self oral examinations to identify lesions and their relationship to other gastrointestinal problems associated with Crohn disease	Instruct patient on application and frequency of application of topical corticosteroids	Recommend periodic self oral examinations for lesions to aid in monitoring Crohn disease state	Consultation with dentist for prescription of topical corticosteroids

Professionalism

When dental hygienists are willing to discuss their DHDx and treatment plans, and provide case presentations to their dental colleagues and other health-care providers, they learn to work collaboratively with other members of health teams. Sharing this knowledge with physicians, nurses, therapists, public health officials, among others, increases the perception that dental hygienists can play a vital role as a member of a health-care team. Other providers will acknowledge the expertise of the dental hygienist, and all providers can learn from each other. Working with other colleagues to improve the health of the public is another way for dental hygienists to be stimulated to pursue lifelong learning. ■

who has the authority to grant consent if they are not the same person. The written documentation and the visual images such as charting, radiographs, study casts, intraoral photographs, and laboratory tests can help in explaining the patient's oral health status, recommended treatment, and expected outcomes. A concise presentation of the patient's assessment findings, the diagnosis and prognosis, the mutually developed goals for treatment, treatment options, risks and benefits of treatment, consequences of no treatment, evaluation strategies, referrals, and maintenance schedule would be appropriate to present. It is important to allow the patient to ask questions and to verify information with the patient to ensure that he or she has understood the explanations so that his or her consent is truly informed. Effective communication and active listening to the patient's questions, comments, and nonverbal cues will contribute to building trust between the dental hygiene provider and the patient, and the patient will feel more comfortable in making an informed consent.

CONSENT

Once the treatment plan has been presented, the dental hygienist must seek consent from the patient before proceeding with treatment. The patient's right to make decisions regarding his or her own health care is protected by state statute and case law. **Informed consent** means the patient has been informed by the practitioner of his or her health status, the risks and benefits of the treatment options available, the consequences of not receiving treatment, and all financial implications. The practitioner should not make promises or guarantees regarding treatment outcomes because each individual may respond differently to treatment.

Expressed consent may be given orally or written; however, if consent is stated on a signed and dated

document by both the patient and the practitioner it is difficult to dispute. Informed consent is validated when the document also includes treatment options, risks and benefits of treatment, and consequences of no treatment. **Implied consent** can be consent given by the patient's actions. For example, the patient arrives for his scheduled maintenance appointment and allows the dental hygienist to proceed with treatment.

Consent must be given by competent adults. In most states, an adult is defined as being 18 years of age. If the patient is still a minor, the consent must be obtained from the parent or legal guardian. The dental hygienist must determine who has the legal authority to consent to treatment for a minor or an incompetent individual. Elder individuals or terminally ill patients sometimes choose to grant other individuals the right to make decisions for them regarding their health care through use of a legal form referred to as a Durable Powers of Attorney for Health Care.

The treatment plan with a signed consent acts as an express contract between the patient and the professional. It is a written agreement that states the problems to be addressed, the services to be rendered, and the fees to be paid. The treatment plan should be signed, thereby giving consent, before any treatment is provided. If the treatment plan needs to be modified or additional treatment is needed, the plan should be revised and again signed and dated by both the patient and the practitioner. For example, if it is determined during treatment that the patient needs to be anesthetized to thoroughly debride a specific area of the mouth, or application of a fluoride varnish to decrease root sensitivity is indicated, this would constitute changes to the treatment plan that should be documented and signed. When a practitioner renders additional procedures without consent, the practitioner could be libel for **battery** if the patient chooses to take legal action. Examples of battery would be if the dental hygienist applied sealants without obtaining consent before placement or gave someone a fluoride treatment without consent. If a practitioner does not render the treatment in a reasonable time and within the standard of care, they can be libel for **breach of contract.**

Because patients have the right to make decisions regarding their health care, they may choose to refuse recommended treatment or referrals. This is referred to as **informed refusal** and should also be signed and dated in the patient's record. An example of this would be when a patient refuses a referral to a periodontist for periodontal treatment. See Chapter 2 for more information.

DOCUMENTATION

The current standards acknowledge that a dental hygienist has the following responsibilities:

- Document all components of the dental hygiene process of care.

- Objectively record all information and interactions between the patient and the practice (i.e., telephone calls, emergencies, prescriptions).
- Record legible, concise, and accurate information (i.e., dates and signatures, clinical information that subsequent providers can understand, ensure all components of the patient record are accurately labeled).
- Recognize ethical and legal responsibilities of record-keeping including guidelines outlined in state regulations and statutes.
- Ensure compliance with the federal Health Insurance Portability and Accountability Act (HIPAA).
- Respect and protect the confidentiality of patient information.

How the dental hygienist documents the patient's treatment plan and consent depends on the documentation options available in the work setting. Dental hygienists may be able to develop their own system or be able to give input into the record system being used (see Technology). The dental hygienist has an obligation as a licensee to practice according to the standard of care as discussed previously. Patient records are the first line of defense in any regulatory, civil, or criminal case. For records to be defensible, they must be accurate and legible. The dental hygienist may use acceptable abbreviations and initials; however, other health-care providers must be able to read and understand them. Also, the hygienist should be aware that patients may have access to their records. Anything that the health-care provider would not want read in a court of law or that one would not want the patient to see should not be put in the patient record.

Including the types of materials used, type and amounts of anesthesia, adverse reactions to treatment or medications, the postoperative instructions, and notations regarding treatment outcomes verifies the procedures and communications with the patient. In addition to recording all aspects of the dental hygiene process of care, the recording of all information and interactions with the patient is essential. Including entries regarding management of problems, the patient's questions and the answers provided, any unusual circumstances, and any secondary diagnoses and subsequent alterations to the treatment plan can be important. Post-treatment phone calls made

Technology

Technology has become a mainstay of health care. The creative dental hygiene professional can work with a company or alone designing a formal document for the practice that incorporates the DHDx and treatment plan. These forms can be computer generated, allowing the practitioner to print out a copy for each patient. Providing patients with a copy of the form and asking for their signature consenting to treatment is one means of increasing understanding of their oral health condition and may contribute to greater adherence to the treatment process. This process also provides a mechanism of proof that patients were properly informed of their oral health status and recommended treatment should a legal concern arise. ■

by the dental hygienist or other members of the staff, phone calls or correspondence between the dental hygienist and other health-care providers, third-party insurance submissions and receipts, and notations regarding frequently missed or broken appointments might be helpful in re-creating a scenario of treatment. All add to presenting a complete, accurate, and comprehensive reflection of the care, treatment, and management of the patient.

Computerized or electronic patient records can provide a convenient method of data entry and preservation. The U.S. courts have established the validity of using electronic health records.[13] The use of electronic records may contribute to increasing the legibility of records, provide easier and faster access to patient information, and contribute to increased collaboration among health-care providers in treating patients.

Regardless of the way that patient records are maintained, compliance with HIPAA was mandated for all dental practices on April 14, 2003. The act addresses rules for patient privacy, confidentiality, and security (see Chapter 2 for detailed information on HIPAA).[14,15]

Case Study

Mrs. Julie Ann Gordon, a 31-year-old woman, presents in the office as a new patient. She brings with her the completed medical/dental history that was mailed to her before her appointment. When he greets her, the dental hygienist notices that Mrs. Gordon is carrying a large water bottle. The forms that Mrs. Gordon completed indicate that her last oral health appointment was 4 years ago. She explains that at that time she had crowns placed on #6 to #8, #10, #11, and #22 to #27. After all that time in the dental chair, "The thought of going back was just too much." Mrs. Gordon is married and has a 7-year-old boy, Isaac, and a 5-year-old daughter, Isabel. She relates that she is very involved in her children's school activities and numerous charitable foundations.

Her medical history reveals common childhood illnesses of measles and chickenpox, hospitalizations for

Case Study—cont'd

both her children, and an appendectomy when she was 17 years old. She is 5′7″ tall, weight is listed as 115 pounds. Her blood pressure is 110/78 mm Hg RA, pulse is 76. She sees her gynecologist annually because she "never knows when she will have her menstrual cycle," but does not list a primary care physician. She is not taking any medications currently; however, she reports taking phenelzine sulfate (Nardil) for a few months about a year ago after her mother died. She takes a multivitamin, fish oil, and another multivitamin at night every day because she is "always on the run and I want to make sure I get what I need."

She scheduled this appointment because her teeth "really hurt when I drink or eat something cold or hot, it hurts when I chew, and I seem to always have a dry mouth."

Her extraoral and intraoral assessment reveals the following findings:

- The posterior teeth demonstrate severe erosion—significant in the mandible, extreme in the maxillary
- Posterior restorations appear to be "erupting"
- Generalized 1- to 3-mm recession in the posteriors
- Cervical decay in teeth #21, #28, and #29
- Tissue appears firm and fibrotic in posterior, although edematous around anterior crowns
- Bleeding upon probing in mandibular anteriors
- Light biofilm, patient reports brushing and flossing at least three times per day, uses floss and mouthrinse routinely

Radiographic assessment reveals interproximal decay on #5 mesial, #12 distal, and #13 mesial.

Case Study Exercises

1. Summarize the significant information from the assessment findings for Mrs. Gordon.
2. Determine the general and oral health dental hygiene diagnoses for Mrs. Gordon.
3. Create a treatment plan for Mrs. Gordon, including prevention, treatment, maintenance, and referral.
4. Based on this case and the treatment plan, are referrals warranted? If yes, explain why.
5. What parameters will be assessed at a re-evaluation appointment?
6. Before proceeding with treatment, the dental hygienist should:
   A. Present the dental hygiene treatment plan and obtain written consent.
   B. Present the patient with treatment options, the risks and benefits of treatment and no treatment, the financial implications for treatment, and obtain informed consent.
   C. Present the case to the dentist and obtain consent from the patient.
   D. Present the patient with treatment options, the benefits of treatment, the amount her insurance will cover, and obtain consent.

Review Questions

1. The dental hygiene diagnosis defines the type of problems presented by patients. This diagnosis bridges the gap between the assessment phase of care and the implementation phase of care.
   A. Both statements are true.
   B. Both statements are false.
   C. The first statement is true, but the second statement is false.
   D. The first statement is false, but the second statement is true.

2. The identification of a disease, problem, or injury is referred to as the:
   A. Differential diagnosis
   B. Conditional diagnosis
   C. Definitive diagnosis
   D. Proposed diagnosis
   E. Potential diagnosis

3. The dental hygiene treatment plan is based on the patient's health history, assessment findings, and dental hygiene diagnosis. It also includes the patient's goals, values, and lifestyle.
   A. Both statements are true.
   B. Both statements are false.
   C. The first statement is true, but the second statement is false.
   D. The first statement is false, but the second statement is true.

4. If challenged by a patient or other health-care provider about the process of care or procedures performed, the dental hygiene provider can refer to the guidelines for practice. This document is referred to as:
   A. *Standards for Clinical Dental Hygiene Practice*
   B. *Applied Standards for Dental Hygiene Practice*

C. *Applied Clinical Standards for Dental Hygiene Practice*

D. *Standards for Dental Hygiene Clinical Practice*

E. *Clinical Standards for Applied Dental Hygiene Practice*

5. All of the following are examples of cases that require referral before dental hygiene intervention EXCEPT:

A. Severe hypertension

B. Uncontrolled diabetes

C. Painful abscess with carious lesion

D. Generalized gingivitis

E. Uncontrolled hyperthyroidism

Active Learning

1. When conducting the case presentation for the patient, use graphics as visual prompts to assist the patient with understanding her oral health status. Such graphics may include use of an intraoral photograph, mirror for demonstrating on the patient, radiographs, health history form, and chartings of disease manifestations.

2. Engage the patient in a verbal interaction to discuss informed consent for the proposed dental hygiene treatment plan. Based on the patient's questions and tone of voice, evaluate how he is perceiving and understanding the information provided. Check for understanding by using active listening and questioning techniques.

3. After determining the DHDx for a given patient, use the four-prong approach to develop a dental hygiene treatment plan. Research the literature to identify support for the aspects included in the treatment plan. Use this research to provide evidence for the patient of the credibility of the treatment plan.

4. For any patient, practice providing sensory information regarding what treatment will be like for the patient. If you have planned to administer local anesthesia, describe for the patient what he will feel during and after the procedure. ■

REFERENCES

1. Miller SS. Dental hygiene diagnosis. *RDH*. 1982;2(4):46.

2. Gurenlian JR. Diagnostic decision making. In: Woodall IR, ed. *Comprehensive Dental Hygiene Care*. 4th ed. St. Louis, MO: Mosby; 1993:362-364.

3. Mueller-Joseph L, Petersen M. Dental hygiene process: diagnosis and treatment planning. Albany, NY: Delmar Publishers; 1995:1-16, 46-63.

4. Darby ML, Walsh MM. *Dental Hygiene Theory and Practice*. Philadelphia: W.B. Saunders; 1995.

5. American Dental Hygienists' Association. *Applied Standards of Clinical Dental Hygiene Practice*. Chicago: American Dental Hygienists' Association; 1985.

6. American Dental Hygienists' Association. *Standards for Clinical Dental Hygiene Practice*. Chicago: American Dental Hygienists' Association; 2008:8-9.

7. Wynn RL, Meiller TF, Crossley HL. *Drug Information Handbook for Dentistry*. 15th ed. Hudson, OH: Lexi-Comp; 2009.

8. Thyvalikakath TP, Monaco V, Thalmbuganipalle HB, et al. A usability evaluation of four commercial dental computer-based patient record systems. *J Am Dent Assoc*. 2008;139(12):1632-1642.

9. Wyche CJ. The dental hygiene treatment plan. In: Wilkins EM, ed. *Clinical Practice of the Dental Hygienist*. 10th ed. Philadelphia: Lippincott Williams & Wilkins; 2009:370-378.

10. Palleschi KM. Dental hygiene treatment plan and evaluation. In: Darby ML, Walsh MM, eds. *Dental Hygiene Theory and Practice*. 3rd ed. Philadelphia: W.B. Saunders; 2010:372-389.

11. Francis B. Case development, documentation, and presentation. In: Daniel SJ, Harfst SA, Wilder RS, eds. *Mosby's Dental Hygiene: Concepts, Cases, and Competencies*. 2nd ed. St. Louis, MO: Mosby; 2008:430-435.

12. Hodges KO. *Concepts in Nonsurgical Periodontal Therapy*. New York: Delmar; 1997:153-179.

13. Rhodes PR. The electronic record. In: Rose LF, Mealey BL, Genco RJ, Cohen DW, eds. *Periodontics, Medicine, Surgery, and Implants*. St. Louis, MO: Elsevier Mosby; 2004:163-171.

14. Health Insurance Portability and Accountability Act (HIPAA). http://www.hipaa.org. Accessed July 26, 2015.

15. HIPAA Administrative Simplification Statute and Rules. http://www.hhs.gov/ocr/privacy/hipaa/administrative/index.html. Accessed July 26, 2015.

Part VI

Treatment

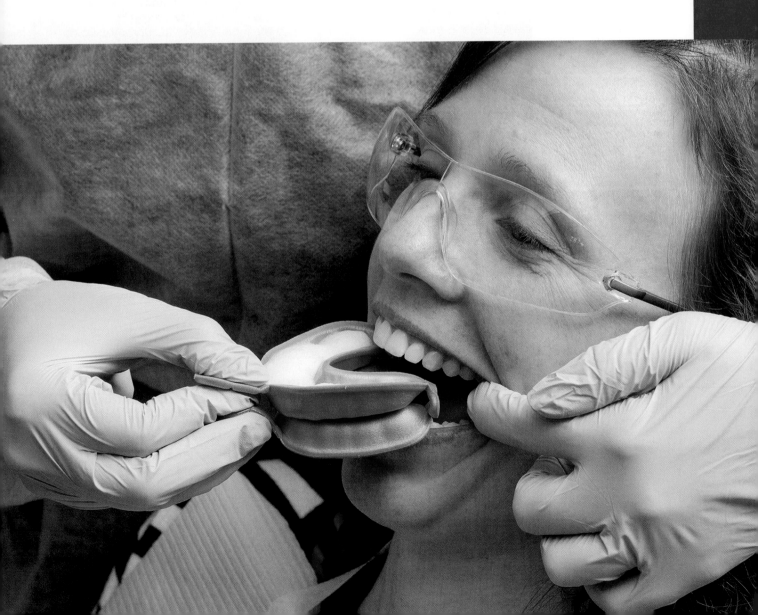

Chapter 19 | Devices

Carol A. Jahn, RDH, MS

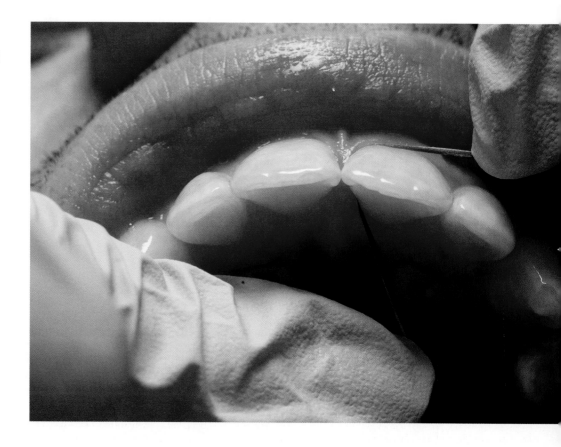

LEARNING OBJECTIVES

After reading this chapter, the student should be able to:

19.1 Discuss the role daily self-care plays in achieving and maintaining good oral health.

19.2 Explain the benefits and limitations of power and manual toothbrushes.

19.3 Compare and contrast the various types of interdental cleaning devices.

19.4 Recommend self-care devices to patients that are appropriate to their needs, interest, and ability.

19.5 Instruct a patient on how to use various types of self-care devices.

KEY CONCEPTS

• Tooth brushing is the primary and often only self-care habit utilized by most people.

• Interdental cleaning is needed by most patients to achieve good oral health.

• Successful recommendations include assessment of patient needs, ability, and interest, as well as instruction and education.

RELEVANCE TO CLINICAL PRACTICE

Daily self-care is critical to achieving and maintaining optimal oral health. The toothbrush is the most widely used self-care device, with 80% to 90% of people brushing one to two times per day.[1] Yet even the best-designed brushes cannot adequately clean between teeth, allowing for buildup of plaque biofilm. Most patients need some type of interdental cleaning. Compared with tooth brushing, only 10% to 30% of people use dental floss on a regular basis.[2]

The number and types of self-care options are larger today than ever. From manual and power toothbrushes to string floss, flossing aids/alternatives, interproximal brushes, toothpicks, and more for interdental cleaning, patients have a variety of choices (see Advancing Technologies). At the same time, the sheer volume of product offerings may confuse and overwhelm patients. One ideal product that can meet the needs of every patient does not exist. Dental hygienists play an important role in helping and motivating patients to find and use the product best suited for their unique situations. Table 19-1 shows how the recommendation of self-care devices fits into the dental hygiene process of care.

TOOTHBRUSHES

The first toothbrush is believed to have originated in China where early brushes had ox bone handles and hog bristles. It was not until the end of the 19th century that toothbrushes began to be used widely. In the late 1930s, toothbrushes started to be made with plastic handles and nylon bristles, making them affordable for everyone. The first "electric" toothbrush was introduced in the United States in the 1960s. Many of these early designs were not mechanically durable, so the life cycle was short lived.[1] Power brushes re-entered the U.S. market in the 1980s. Better designs, results of clinical research, and affordability have made them a mainstay in today's oral care marketplace.

Manual Toothbrushes

The **manual toothbrush** is still widely used by the majority of people in the United States.[3] The major advantage of a manual toothbrush over a power toothbrush is affordability. Other positive features of manual brushes include the wide variety of shapes, sizes, and configurations of both handles and heads (Fig. 19-1). This variety allows the user to find a design that personally provides him or her with the best brushing experience. These new brush-head configurations that feature various bristle heights, tufting, and angulation may enhance interproximal penetration and allow for greater coverage of the tooth surface when brushing.[4] Table 19-2 outlines the parts of a manual toothbrush.

The main disadvantage of the manual brush is that efficacy is dependent on the ability and technique of the user. The best-designed brush still needs to have correct placement in the mouth and an effective brushing motion.[4] Length of brushing time may also influence efficacy. Two minutes is the most commonly recommended brushing time; although data to substantiate this remain more anecdotal than evidence based. When the average person spends 1 minute brushing, he or she removes approximately 60% of the plaque biofilm present around teeth.[1]

Power Toothbrushes

Power toothbrushes have become increasingly popular since their reintroduction to the U.S. market in the

Advancing Technologies

Self-care products continue to evolve as manufacturers partner with patients and dental professionals to find devices that are pleasurable to use and make home plaque biofilm control easy. Staying current with what is new in the marketplace can be challenging. Continuing education courses, professional association meetings and trade shows, journal advertising and articles, corporate websites, and newsletters are just some of the ways that dental hygienists can stay on top of new products. Many companies offer free samples or discounted pricing on new products to entice dental professionals to try the product. Whether the product is free or discounted is generally dependent on the price point of the device. Manual products (e.g., toothbrushes and floss) are often offered as a free sample, whereas a power toothbrush or oral irrigator is more likely to be at a discounted price. ■

Table 19-1. *Self-care Devices and the Dental Hygiene Process of Care*

Process	Actions

Assessment	• Review and consider:
	  • Oral health status
	  • Past self-care practices/likes and dislikes
	  • Oral anatomy/embrasure size
	  • Manual dexterity
	  • Learning disabilities
	  • Economic status/product affordability
	  • Interest in the product

Dental hygiene diagnosis	• Analyze and interpret the assessment findings to determine what product(s) can best help the patient improve or maintain good oral health.
Planning	• Review the product choices with the patient. • Collaborate with the patient on the final choice including a discussion of rationale, risks, benefits, and anticipated outcomes from the product selection. • Set a goal for the frequency of product use. • Provide patient education on the selected product. • Identify how the patient will acquire the product (i.e., dispensed/purchased in the office or purchased through a traditional or online retailer).
Implementation	• Confirm the final choice and how it will be acquired. • Communicate with the patient within 1 to 2 weeks post appointment to verify that the product has been acquired and is being used. • Answer any questions the patient may have about using the product.
Evaluation	• At the next patient visit, use measurable assessment criteria (plaque control, bleeding, gingivitis) to evaluate the effectiveness of the product. • Communicate the findings to the patient. • Make any necessary adjustments and review product use. It may be necessary to switch products if the desired outcomes are not achieved.

late 1980s (Fig. 19-2). Market data indicate that approximately 30% of people use a power brush.[3] The major advantage of a power brush is that it simplifies the brushing process, thus reducing the effect that technique has on outcome. A power-brush user positions the bristles in the mouth, but brushing action and, in many cases, brushing length is predetermined due to the presence of a 2-minute timer. Power brushes have also been shown to need less force during brushing, which can be beneficial for patients at risk for abrasions and recession.[5] Power brushes have many different types of features that allow for selection based on personal preference. The most defining difference in power brushes relates to bristle design and motion, with oscillation and high-velocity sonic action the most popular. Oscillating designs are typically configured in a round head, whereas sonic action is most often found in a more traditionally shaped brush head. Power source is another factor. Some brushes are rechargeable, whereas others use replaceable batteries. Rechargeable brushes tend to have higher brush speeds and higher purchase prices than battery-operated brushes.

The major disadvantage of the power toothbrushes is cost. Some replaceable battery–operating models are quite inexpensive, but high-end oscillating and sonic models typically cost much more. Brush-head replacements are an additional expense. Another consideration is handle size. Power handles can vary in size and weight, which could be an issue for younger or older patients or people with disabilities.

The Scientific Evidence

Several literature reviews and one systemic review have evaluated the clinical outcomes (see Evidence-Based Practice) between power and manual toothbrushes.[6–9]

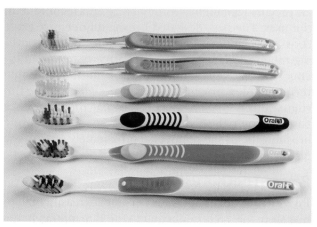

Figure 19-1. Manual toothbrushes.

Table 19-2. *Parts of a Manual Toothbrush*

Part	Design
Brush head	Working end that contains tufts of bristles or filaments
Brushing plane	Surface used for cleaning; may be flat, rippled, dome, multilevel, angled, or bilevel
Bristles/ Filaments	Generally nylon or synthetic; soft with end-rounded filaments
Stiffness	Bristles are generally identified as soft, medium, or hard based on the diameter, length, number, and angle of the filaments. Soft bristles are generally thinner and longer, whereas harder bristles are thicker and shorter; no standard exists among manufacturers, so can be variability of stiffness between brands
Handle	Part that is grasped during brushing; most are made from plastic or other polymers; various shapes; many ergonomically designed to aid in adapting the brush intraorally
Shank	Connects the head to the handle; generally the narrowest part of the brush

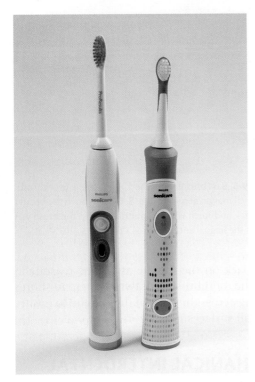

Figure 19-2. Power toothbrushes.

Powered toothbrushes reduce plaque and gingivitis more than manual toothbrushing in the short and long term. The clinical importance of these findings remains unclear. Observation of methodological guidelines and greater standardization of design would benefit both future trials and meta-analyses.[6] Other less-stringent

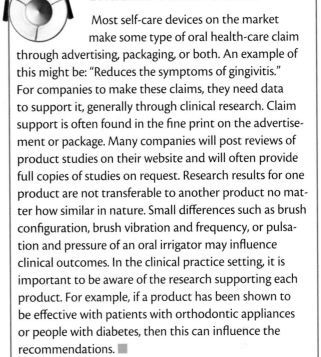

Evidence-Based Practice

Most self-care devices on the market make some type of oral health-care claim through advertising, packaging, or both. An example of this might be: "Reduces the symptoms of gingivitis." For companies to make these claims, they need data to support it, generally through clinical research. Claim support is often found in the fine print on the advertisement or package. Many companies will post reviews of product studies on their website and will often provide full copies of studies on request. Research results for one product are not transferable to another product no matter how similar in nature. Small differences such as brush configuration, brush vibration and frequency, or pulsation and pressure of an oral irrigator may influence clinical outcomes. In the clinical practice setting, it is important to be aware of the research supporting each product. For example, if a product has been shown to be effective with patients with orthodontic appliances or people with diabetes, then this can influence the recommendations. ■

literature reviews have found varying results.[7–9] A review that compared manual with sonic/ultrasonic brushes found that in patients with chronic gingivitis/periodontitis, sonic/ultrasonic brushes did not produce better results in removing plaque biofilm and reducing gingivitis than a manual brush.[7] Two reviews have observed better plaque biofilm removal but not better reductions in gingivitis for power versus manual toothbrushes.[8,9]

Many studies have compared one type of power toothbrush with another with varying outcomes.[5] Currently, it is generally accepted that there is no one type or brand of power toothbrush that has been demonstrated to be consistently significantly superior to other power brushes. For manual toothbrushes, a literature review of studies that compared a brush with a crisscross array of angled bristles with other types of manual and lower-end battery-powered toothbrushes found that the crisscross design generally removed significantly more plaque than the other types of brushes.[4] Given that the scientific evidence does not dictate one type of toothbrush over another, in the practice setting, clinical judgment and patient values will be equal determining factors in the type of brush that is recommended. It is wise to know the research on individual products so that the expected outcomes from using the product can be explained to the patient and reasonable goals set.

Brush Selection and Usage

Claydon[10] notes that the ideal toothbrush design removes plaque effectively, is safe on hard and soft tissues, and is user-friendly. The accepted industry standard is a toothbrush with soft bristles with end-rounded filaments generally no larger 0.23 mm in diameter. As a benchmark, most products should have been evaluated for safety and efficacy in at least one randomized clinical trial. The brush head should be appropriate to the size of the user's mouth and the handle suitable to the user's age and dexterity.[10] User-friendliness is one of the most important yet sometimes overlooked considerations. To be most effective, the patient has to like the toothbrush. If the product does not resonate with the patient, he or she may not use it or may use it with less frequency and duration. Other considerations for recommendation are outlined in Table 19-3.

The manual brushing technique used by most people is a horizontal scrubbing motion. Although many different techniques have been proposed, most research centers on plaque removal. There is little science that evaluates which technique is best for improving gingival health.[10] The **Bass brushing method,** demonstrated in Figure 19-3, is one of the most widely accepted methods because it targets the gingival margin. There are many other tooth-brushing methods and their indications for use are outlined in Table 19-4. When using a power brush, the patient should follow the technique recommended in the manufacturer's instruction guide.

Tongue brushing or cleansing is an additional component of complete mouth cleaning. The posterior dorsum of the tongue has an irregular surface that collects food particles and bacteria that cause a coating of the tongue. This area is a primary source of oral malodor or bad breath. Cleaning the dorsum of the tongue reduces oral malodor and contributes to overall oral cleanliness.

The tongue can be cleaned with a toothbrush or specialized tongue-cleaning device. To clean the tongue, the tongue should be extended so that the toothbrush or other device can access the dorsum. The toothbrush may be held vertically with the end of the head placed

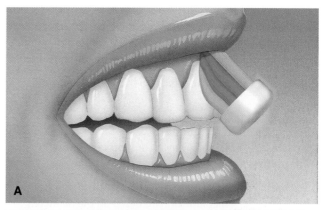

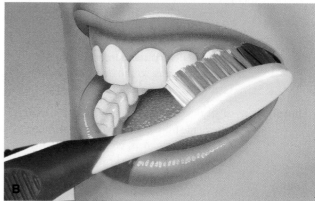

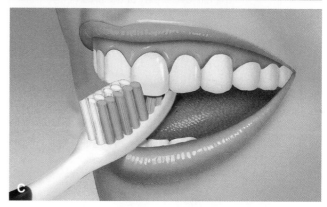

Figure 19-3. Bass brushing method. A, Place the toothbrush along the gingival margin at a 45° angle. B, Gently move the brush in a gentle back-and-forth vibrating motion. C, Tip the brush vertically to access the lingual anterior areas. Courtesy of Sunstar Americas, Inc.

as far back on the tongue as can be reasonably tolerated. The toothbrush is drawn forward in short strokes, working across the back of the tongue to ensure cleaning of all surfaces (Fig. 19-4).

MECHANICAL INTERDENTAL CLEANING

It is well established that most patients need some type of interdental cleaning tool in addition to tooth brushing for optimal oral health. The anatomy of the interdental area is not easily accessible by tooth brushing. The anatomy of the interdental area is an influencing factor in the type of interdental aid that is most appropriate for

Table 19-3. *Factors to Consider When Recommending Toothbrushes*

Factors	Considerations
Handle size	Shape and ergonomics of the handle Weight of handle Age and dexterity of the user
Brush-head size	Age and size of mouth of the user Brush-head configuration: round vs. traditional
Brush-head action	Oscillation vs. sonic
Bristle filaments	Round-ended nylon or polyester filaments No larger than 0.23 mm in diameter Thickness, stiffness, pattern of arrangement, density
Timer	2 minutes with 30-second signal to change quadrants the most common
Battery indicator	Helps user know when to recharge

Table 19-4. Tooth-Brushing Methods and Techniques

Method	Technique	Patient Selection
Bass/Sulcular brushing	• Filaments are directed at a 45° angle to the long axis of the tooth. • The brush head is gently vibrated back and forth with short strokes.	Any type
Stillman	• Brush is placed partly on gingiva and partly on cervical area. • Pressure is applied to blanch the tissue and handle rotates slightly.	Gingival massage and stimulation
Modified Stillman	• Same as Stillman plus a roll and vibrating brush stroke.	Exposed cervical and proximal surfaces Gingival massage
Charters	• Filaments are placed downward at a 45° angle toward the occlusal surface. • The filaments are flexed lightly and the brush is vibrated with a short back-and-forth motion.	Orthodontic appliances After periodontal surgery Fixed partial denture (bridge)
Rolling stroke	• Filaments are directly apical toward the teeth with the side of the brush on the attached gingiva. • The filaments are flexed and rolled slowly over the teeth.	Children In addition to the Bass, Charters, or Stillman methods

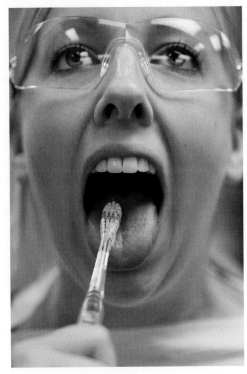

Figure 19-4. Cleaning the tongue.

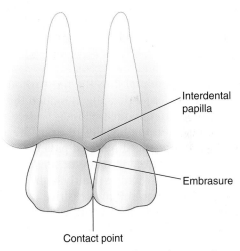

Figure 19-5. The gingival embrasure is the area between the teeth.

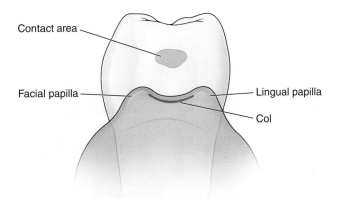

Figure 19-6. The col is a concave-shaped depression found directly under the contact point where the facial and lingual interdental papilla connect.

the patient. The area between the teeth is called the **gingival embrasure** (Fig. 19-5). In health, the interdental papilla fills the embrasure area and is narrowest at the contact and widest at the gingival margin. With attachment and bone loss, the embrasure widens and may be reduced in height or completely missing. The area where the facial and lingual interdental papilla connect is called the *col*. It is a concave-shaped depression found directly under the contact point (Fig. 19-6).

Because the epithelium in the col is thin, it can become inflamed more easily. With inflammation, the papilla swells and enlarges and the col becomes deeper. This is why most gingivitis starts in the col area.

The product dental professionals recommend most frequently for interdental cleaning is **dental floss.** Flossing is good practice for those with a normal embrasure; however, with bone and attachment loss, it may lose effectiveness. Flossing is often promoted as the gold standard for interdental care; research does not support this.[2] It is simply one tool. In terms of patient compliance with this recommendation, less than 30% of people use dental floss on a regular basis, and many who do use it are unable to master the technique to the extent that improves oral health.[2] In recent years, several different types of alternative products for interdental cleaning have become available. Many of these products, including floss holders, automated flossers, interdental brushes, picks, wooden sticks, and pulsating home irrigations (also called *oral irrigators, dental water jets,* or *water flossers*) have been shown to be viable, effective alternatives to dental floss (Fig. 19-7).[11] These products may be better for people with a reduced embrasure area. It is important to consider that flossing alternatives have sound science behind them and therefore provide patients with a tangible method for improving oral health.[11] Table 19-5 outlines the different products and indications for their use.

Dental Floss

Not only is string dental floss the most recommended method for interdental cleaning; it is often the first and only method recommended. Floss is widely available and affordable, and the benefits of using it are understood and acknowledged by most patients. It is available waxed or unwaxed in spools or single-use holders (Fig. 19-8). Flossing requires a fairly high level of manual dexterity and is technique sensitive to achieve improvements in oral health such as reductions in bleeding and/or gingivitis. Many patients simply cannot develop the skills necessary to adequately floss or may have tight contacts that are difficult to pass through. It

is accepted that floss reaches approximately 3 mm subgingivally, making it more appropriate for patients who are healthy or have gingivitis than for those with pockets 4 mm and deeper. The dental hygienist will need to determine on an individual basis whether flossing is the best method of interdental cleaning for the patient or whether a different device would be preferable. Procedure 19-1 demonstrates the proper use of dental floss.

A benchmark study by Graves et al[12] demonstrated the potential of effective flossing in reducing bleeding. Over a 2-week time frame, participants came to a research facility for supervised flossing while flossing on their own only on the weekends. At the conclusion of the study, the flossing group was nearly twice as effective as brushing alone in reducing bleeding (67% vs. 35%). In contrast, a systematic review comparing unsupervised tooth brushing and unsupervised flossing with tooth brushing alone found no significant benefit for plaque removal or gingivitis reduction with the addition of flossing. Of the studies reviewed, four demonstrated greater plaque biofilm removal and one better gingivitis reduction with the addition of floss.[2] This information does not mean that flossing cannot be effective. It does, however, demonstrate that many patients do not floss well enough or frequently enough to achieve a health benefit. Another systematic review on dental floss evaluated its ability to reduce interproximal caries. The investigators found that professional flossing on school days for 10 months reduced the caries risk by 40% in children with poor oral hygiene and no exposure to fluoride. Conversely, their data also showed that in the presence of fluoride, flossing did not reduce the incidence of caries in children. In addition, no studies were available that evaluated the effect of flossing and caries reduction in adults. The authors noted that there is no evidence that flossing is effective for caries reduction in the presence of topical fluorides.[13] Interestingly, the investigators of both systematic reviews reached similar conclusions—that the dental hygiene professional needs to determine on an individual basis whether high-quality flossing is an achievable goal and recommend accordingly rather than by routine.[2,13]

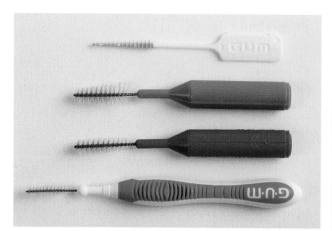
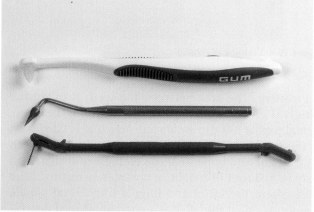

Figure 19-7. Interdental cleaning aids are an alternative to dental floss for improving oral health.

Table 19-5. Interdental Aids and Patient Considerations

Device	Patient Consideration/Applicability
Dental floss	• Healthy tissue or sulcus depth ≤3 mm • Good manual dexterity • Good contact easement
Dental floss holder	• Healthy tissue or sulcus depth ≤3 mm • Good contact easement
Interdental brushes	• Sufficient embrasure space needed • Exposed root surfaces • Difficulty getting floss through contact areas or maneuvering around teeth
Oral irrigator/ water flosser	• Unresolved gingivitis or bleeding • Orthodontic appliances • Implants • Deeper pockets • Difficulty with floss or other types of devices
Wood sticks	• Sufficient embrasure space needed • Exposed root surfaces • Difficulty getting floss through contact areas or maneuvering around teeth

Interdental Brushes

Interdental brushes are specially designed brushes with small nylon filaments twisted onto a stainless-steel wire. They may be round or conical and are available in a variety of widths to accommodate different embrasure sizes (see Fig. 19-5). The interdental brush is inserted from the buccal side of the mouth and gently moved

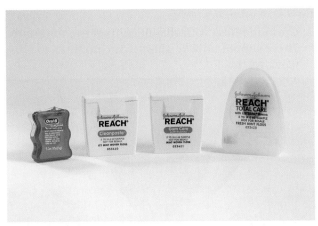

Figure 19-8. Dental floss is often recommended for interdental cleaning.

back and forth. Figure 19-9 demonstrates the placement of the interdental brush. The advantage of this product is that it is less technique-sensitive than string floss. For patients with bone or attachment loss, the interdental brush can help access and clean the concave col area.

To use an interdental brush, the product should fit snugly into the interdental space. If the size of the brush is too small, plaque biofilm removal may be diminished. Conversely, a size too large may result in discomfort or possibly trauma. The brush should never be forced through the embrasure space.

Systematic reviews comparing interdental brushes with floss found the interdental brush reduced interproximal bleeding and plaque significantly better than dental floss in patients with filled or open embrasures.[14,15] The interdental brush also removed more plaque biofilm than did dental floss. No difference was found between the devices on parameters of gingival

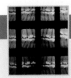

Procedure 19-1 Flossing

MATERIALS AND PREPARATION

Cut 18 inches of waxed or unwaxed dental floss. The type of floss chosen depends on how easy it is to get through the contact points. Waxed floss is preferable for tight contacts.

PREPROCEDURE

Tooth brushing may precede or follow flossing. There is no definitive evidence to suggest that time influences effectiveness.

Patient Education

Educate the patient on the use of the dental floss and how flossing benefits oral health.

PROCEDURE

1. Wrap the floss gently around the middle fingers, keeping about 4 to 6 inches between the middle fingers. Wrapping around the middle fingers keeps

the index fingers free to manipulate the floss around the tooth.

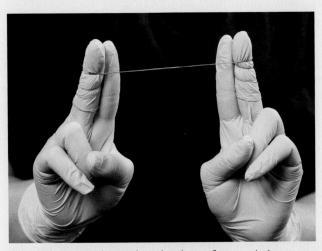

Step 1: Floss wrapped around two hands, two fingers pointing up.

2. Grasp the floss with the index fingers and thumb. There should now be about 1 inch of floss to work with.

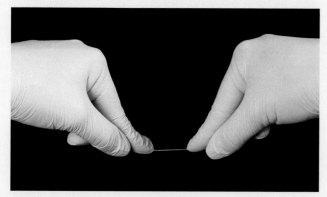

Step 2: Index fingers pressing down on floss.

3. Starting in the posterior area of either the upper or lower arch, gently glide the floss between the interdental contact area, being careful not to snap through the contact.

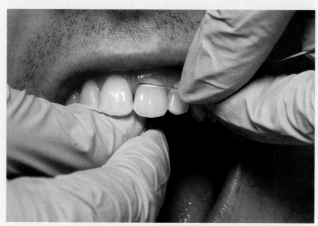

Step 3: Floss between two front teeth.

4. With the index finger, gently push on the floss to form a C-shape around one side of the tooth (buccal or lingual). With the floss in the C-position, gently guide the floss up and down the tooth from under the contact area, flexing slightly under the gingival margin three to four times.

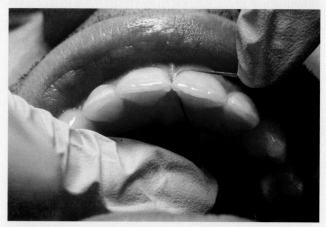

Step 4: Form a C-shape with floss.

5. Staying in the same interproximal area, push on the floss so that a C is formed on the opposing side and follow the same procedure. Once both sides have been cleansed, bring the floss back through the contact and proceed to the next interdental area.

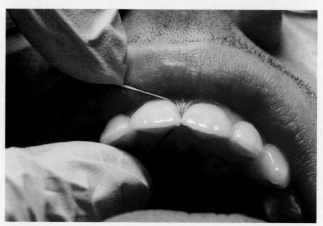

Step 5: Push and form a C on the opposing side.

6. Before proceeding through the next contact area, wind the used portion of the floss around one middle finger and unwind a clean section from the other finger.
7. Repeat steps 3 to 6 until all teeth have been flossed.
8. Dispose of floss in receptacle.

inflammation. When patient preference was evaluated, the subjects preferred the interdental brush over floss, citing it was easier to use.[15]

Wood Sticks

The **wood stick** is a triangular-shaped device traditionally made of soft wood such as balsa, bass, or birch. The wood stick is used by placing it from the buccal side between the teeth with the flat side down. A gentle back-and-forth, in-and-out motion is recommended. Figure 19-10 shows the proper placement of the wood stick. The wood stick may be moistened before use for comfort. Wood sticks are easy to use, portable, and disposable. Like interproximal brushes, there needs to be adequate embrasure space for placement, and the stick should never be forced. Wood sticks may also splinter with use and should be immediately discarded if this happens. In the last few years, plastic versions of the wood stick have entered the marketplace, with the advantage of this product that it will not splinter or lose shape when wet.

A systematic review compared wood sticks with dental floss. The data from this review found no differences in plaque biofilm removal between wood sticks and dental floss. For gingival inflammation scores, the wood stick was significantly better than dental floss.[16]

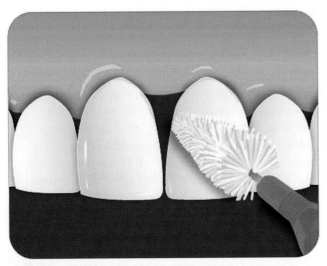

Figure 19-9. Placement of an interdental brush. Courtesy of Sunstar Americas, Inc.

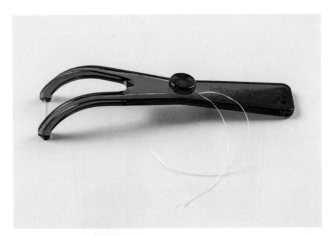

Figure 19-11. Floss holder.

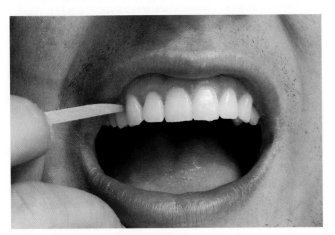

Figure 19-10. Placement of a wood stick.

Floss Holders, Automated Flossers, and Toothpicks

A variety of other types of mechanical interdental cleaners is also available, including floss holders, automated flossers, and toothpicks (Figs. 19-11 and 19-12). A report by the Canadian Dental Hygienists Association found select randomized trials supporting the safety, efficacy, and in some cases, patient preferences for these products. A 12-week trial comparing floss and a toothpick found no differences between the devices for the reduction of plaque biofilm and bleeding. Similar results were shown for floss-holding devices and automated flossers. The report further recommends that flossing should be recognized as having limitations, and dental hygienists should tailor oral hygiene education and instruction based on the patient and/or specific oral hygiene needs and preferences.[11]

PULSATING ORAL IRRIGATION

The pulsating **oral irrigator** was developed in 1962. Since that time, it has been known by several different

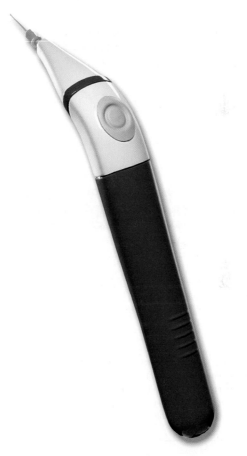

Figure 19-12. Waterpik Power Flosser. Courtesy of Water Pik, Inc.

names including dental water jet and, more recently, water flosser (Fig. 19-13). The oral irrigator works through pulsating lavage and a variable pressure setting. The most commonly available device has 1,200 pulsations per minute and a pressure range from 5 to 90 psi (Table 19-6). The advantage of the oral irrigator is that it is easy to use. The tip is held in place for approximately 3 seconds in the embrasure area before sweeping across the gingival margin to the next interproximal space (Fig. 19-14). Full-mouth irrigation can be accomplished in about 1 minute. The most common tip is made of hard plastic with a small opening (Fig. 19-15A).

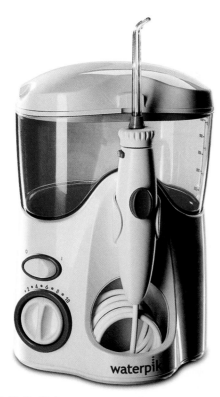

Figure 19-13. Oral irrigator. Courtesy of Water Pik, Inc.

Table 19-6. *Oral Irrigation Depth of Delivery*

Tip	Pocket Depth	Penetration
Classic jet tip	≤3 mm	71%
	4–7 mm	44%
	≥7 mm	68%
Site-specific tip	≤6 mm	90%
	≥7 mm	64%

Sources: Greenstein G. Research, Science, and Therapy Committee of the American Academy of Periodontology. Position paper: the role of supra- and subgingival irrigation in the treatment of periodontal diseases. *J. Periodontol.* 2005;76:2015-2027; and Jahn CA. The dental water jet: a historical review of the literature. *J. Dent. Hyg.* 2010;84(3):114-120.

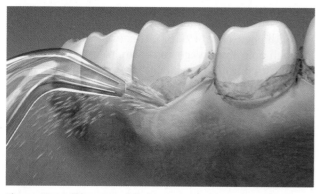

Figure 19-14. Placement of the jet tip. Courtesy of Water Pik, Inc.

Professionalism

You consider your office quite progressive as you offer a variety of different products to patients. You especially like the oral irrigator for periodontal maintenance patients. Recently, your dentist-employer received a phone call from a referring periodontist asking you to stop recommending irrigation because he believes it is not effective. You happen to know this periodontist's dental hygienist, so you ask her about it. She tells you that the hygienists in the practice recommend the product all the time but keep it from the doctor because they are aware that he is not favorable toward it. How could this situation be handled or improved? ■

It has been shown to deliver a solution approximately 50% the depth of the pocket.[17,18] In recent years, the tip has undergone several modifications. There is a tip with a soft rubber, latex-free conical configuration, which has been shown to enhance delivery into deeper periodontal pockets (Fig. 19-15B).[17,18] Two other tips feature bristle-type configurations for enhanced plaque biofilm removal. One has tapered bristles surrounding the tip opening (Fig. 19-15C), whereas the other features thin tufts projecting from the end of the tip (Fig. 19-15D). Other product modifications include cordless models, which allow for greater portability and use in the shower.

Compared with dental floss or other mechanical interdental aids, the oral irrigator has a higher initial investment price. Another limitation has been the dissemination of misinformation on the safety of the product. Some practitioners believe that the device can be damaging by driving bacteria into the pocket and furthering bone loss (see Professionalism). Scientific evidence seems to contradict this, concluding that the pulsating oral irrigator reduces subgingival bacteria up to 6 mm.[19]

The Scientific Evidence

The oral irrigator is one of the most evaluated self-care devices with a well-established body of evidence. Numerous randomized clinical trials have been conducted as systematic and literature reviews. Consistent reductions for bleeding and gingivitis are well established. A laboratory study found a 3-second application of pulsating water reduced plaque biofilm from treated areas (Fig. 19-16).[20] A single-use plaque study found that an oral irrigator added to manual tooth brushing reduced 29% more plaque than manual tooth brushing and flossing.[21] In addition, the large number of trials provides a documented profile on the safety of the product.[17,18,22] The oral irrigator has been studied and found safe and effective for people with crowns, bridges, implants, and orthodontic appliances, as well as for people with diabetes.[18]

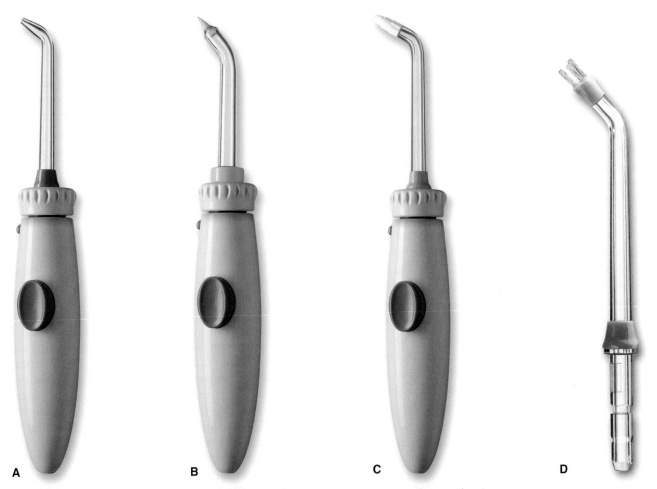

Figure 19-15. Water flosser tips. A, Classic jet tip. B, Pik Pocket tip. C, Orthodontic tip. D, Plaque Seeker tip. Courtesy of Water Pik, Inc.

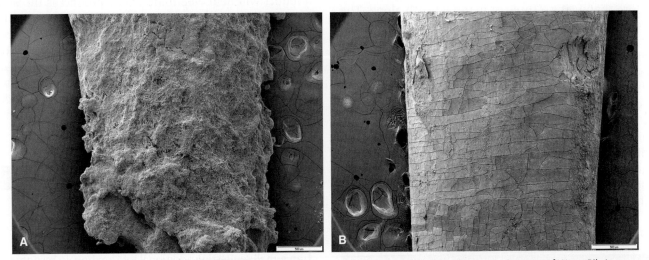

Figure 19-16. A, Before treatment with the oral irrigator. B, After a 3-second treatment with the oral irrigator. Courtesy of Water Pik, Inc.

The oral irrigator, now called a *water flosser,* has been found to be an effective alternative to string floss and superior to string dental floss in reducing gingival inflammation.[23–25] Plaque biofilm reduction was similar for all devices.[23,25] Adolescents with orthodontic appliances who used an irrigation tip with small tufted bristles surrounding the opening showed greater plaque removal than either brushing and

flossing via floss threader or tooth brushing alone.[24] When the oral irrigator was paired with a manual or power toothbrush and compared with traditional brushing and flossing, patients who added the oral irrigator had better reductions in bleeding, regardless of brush type. This finding indicates that even power toothbrush users may experience additional benefits from using a pulsating oral irrigator.[23] Patients who

Spotlight on Public Health

Each year since 2001, the West Suburban Dental Hygienists' Society (WSDHS) has participated in the Diabetes EXPO held in Chicago, Illinois. The EXPO is a free event sponsored by the American Diabetes Association, and its goal is to help people get expert information on preventing and managing diabetes and its complications. WSDHS is one of only a few groups that provide information on oral health. The dental hygienists from WSDHS bring different types of power and manual toothbrushes, and multiple types of interdental cleaning aids including dental floss, interproximal brushes, and a water flosser. Their main goal is to help people with diabetes understand the oral health implications and talk to them about how they can achieve and maintain good oral hygiene at home. Products are demonstrated on tooth models. WSDHS puts together goodie bags that contain a manual toothbrush, dental floss, coupons, and brochures on interdental aids and the water flosser. Approximately 10,000 people attended a recent EXPO, and WSDHS gave out more than 1,500 take-home bags. ■

added a water flosser to either sonic or manual tooth brushing reduced bleeding and gingivitis significantly more than using a sonic or manual brush alone. The combination of the water flosser and sonic toothbrush resulted in a 70% better reduction in bleeding and 52% better reduction in gingivitis; compared with manual tooth brushing, the water flosser was 159% better at reducing bleeding and 134% better at reducing gingivitis.[26]

Water and 0.12% chlorhexidine (CHX) are the agents most evaluated in an oral irrigator. CHX can be diluted because of the better interproximal and subgingival penetration of irrigation (Table 19-7). Water has been shown to be effective in numerous studies, although the addition of an antimicrobial does have the

potential to enhance effectiveness. One study that compared 0.6% irrigation, water irrigation, and 0.12% CHX rinsing found CHX irrigation superior to water irrigation but water irrigation superior to 0.12% CHX rinsing for reducing bleeding.[18] The oral irrigator will accommodate most types of agents. The one that is best for the patient depends on both oral health needs and patient preference.

PATIENT EDUCATION

Helping patients select the products that will meet their oral health needs and that they will use on a consistent basis is as much art as science (see Teamwork). Understanding the principles of evidence-based care (Chapter 6) as well as the development of good communication skills (Chapter 3) and behavioral change techniques (Chapter 4) will help to motivate patients to achieve optimal oral health. There is no one perfect device for all patients, nor is there any one device that "does it all." Suvan and D'Aiuto[27] capture this issue succinctly: "Best care for each patient rests neither in the clinician judgment nor scientific evidence but rather in the art of combining the two through interaction with the patient to find the best option for each individual."

It is the responsibility of the dental hygienist to help patients understand the importance of interdental cleaning. Taking into consideration oral anatomy, patient dexterity/physical limitations, and interest in using the product will help determine which product is the best choice for the patient. The hygienist should demonstrate the device to the patient. This can also help assist the patient in determining which product may work best for them. Whenever possible, it is important to provide the patient with a choice of devices, usually two to three. The ultimate goal is to collaborate with the patient as much

Table 19-7. *Commonly Used 0.12% Chlorhexidine Dilutions for Irrigation*	
Dilutions	**Preparation**
0.02%	1 part CHX to 5 parts water
0.04%	1 part CHX to 3 parts water
0.06%	1 part CHX to 1 part water
CHX, chlorhexidine.	

Teamwork

At a recent continuing education course, you learned about a new type of power toothbrush. In follow-up, you visit the company's website to learn more and send an e-mail requesting additional information. In response, you receive a phone call at the office from one of the company representatives who would like to make an appointment to stop by and tell you more about the new product. You talk with the other staff members including the doctor about the product, and everyone agrees that they would like to hear more. You schedule the representative to come in the following week. The doctor and other staff members thank you for taking the initiative. ■

as possible so he or she takes ownership of the product choice.

The patient's health is most important. In the past, manual brushing and flossing were the accepted methods for achieving oral health. Today, there are many options: power brushes, interdental brushes, wood sticks, floss holders, power flossers, and oral irrigators/water flossers.[7,8,12,16–18,21] Dental hygienists collaborate with patients to determine which products best meet each patient's needs (see Application to Clinical Practice).

Application to Clinical Practice

All patients who come in for a dental hygiene visit at the dental practice leave with a manual toothbrush and dental floss. Many times, this contradicts the self-care recommendations that you have just made. What changes can you make to better reflect that your actions support your recommendations? ■

Case Study

The dental hygienist is relatively new to the dental practice and is seeing most patients for the first time. Mrs. Rodriguez, a 68-year-old woman, is her next patient. Mrs. Rodriguez's medical history indicates overall good health except for osteoarthritis, for which she takes acetaminophen. She has been on maintenance therapy, alternating between the dental office and the periodontal office every 3 months. Her periodontal charting from the last visit indicates the return of some 5-mm periodontal pockets in posterior areas. The previous hygienist noted that she re-emphasized better flossing in those areas. Assessment confirms the presence of the pockets plus several new 4-mm pockets and general interproximal inflammation. In addition, there is significant plaque biofilm buildup along the gingival margin. Mrs. Rodriguez says that she is trying to floss but her arthritis makes it very difficult. She also reports challenges with her manual toothbrush.

Case Study Exercises

1. A history of osteoarthritis is likely to have an effect on:
   A. Salivary flow
   B. Ability to use dental floss
   C. Risk for oral cancer
   D. Tooth sensitivity
2. Based on the dental hygienist's assessment, what is the primary cause of Mrs. Rodriguez's increased pocket depth and inflammation?
   A. Systemic effect of osteoarthritis
   B. Medication use from osteoarthritis
   C. Inability to floss well enough to clean interproximally
   D. An undetermined systemic infection
3. What products might the dental hygienist recommend for Mrs. Rodriguez?
   A. Interdental brush
   B. Water flosser
   C. Power toothbrush
   D. Any of the above

Review Questions

1. Toothbrushes do not adequately clean the interproximal area. Most patients need some type of adjunctive interdental cleaning aid.
   A. The first statement is true. The second statement is false.
   B. The first statement is false. The second statement is true.
   C. Both statements are true.
   D. Both statements are false.

2. Which of the following best describes the major disadvantage of a manual toothbrush?
   A. Manual toothbrushes are affordable for most people.
   B. Toothbrush efficacy depends on the user's ability and technique.

   C. Novel brush-head configurations are available.
   D. Manual toothbrushes have a variety of handle designs.

3. What considerations should be taken into account when recommending a toothbrush?
   A. Manual dexterity
   B. Brush-head size in relation to the patient's mouth size
   C. Handle size
   D. All of the above

4. The Bass method of tooth brushing is the most widely accepted tooth brushing method because the bristles are placed toward the crown of the tooth.
   A. Both the statement and reason are correct and related.
   B. The statement and the reason are correct but NOT related.
   C. The statement is correct, but the reason is NOT.
   D. The statement is NOT correct, but the reason is correct.
   E. NEITHER the statement NOR the reason is correct.

5. Power toothbrushes are contraindicated in patients with recession or abrasion because they use more force than manual toothbrushes.
   A. Both the statement and reason are correct and related.
   B. The statement and reason are correct but NOT related.
   C. The statement is correct, but the reason is NOT.
   D. The statement is NOT correct, but the reason is correct.
   E. NEITHER the statement NOR the reason is correct.

Active Learning

1. Before recommending a manual toothbrush, use the brush in your own mouth at least twice.
2. Before recommending a power toothbrush, use the brush in your own mouth at least twice.
3. Try all the various types of interdental aids in your own mouth before recommending.
4. Try the oral irrigator in your own mouth at least twice before recommending.
5. Visit a local drug or mass retail store. Spend time in the oral care aisle and take note of the various product selections available.
6. Visit the exhibit floor of a trade show. Take time to visit the makers of various self-care devices. Ask about research, new products, and any support they have for dental recommenders. ■

REFERENCES

1. Van der Weijden GA, Timmerman MF, Danser MM, van der Velden U. The role of electric toothbrushes: advantages and limitations. In: Lang N, Attström R, Löe H, eds. *Proceedings of the European Workshop on Mechanical Plaque Control.* Chicago: Quintessence; 1998:138-155.
2. Berchier CE, Slots DE, Haps S, Van der Weijden GA. The efficacy of dental floss in addition to a toothbrush on plaque and parameters of gingival inflammation: a systematic review. *Int. J. Dent. Hyg.* 2008;6:265-279.
3. In house data, Fort Collins, CO: Water Pik; April 29, 2010.
4. Cugini M, Warren PR. The Oral-B CrossAction manual toothbrush: a 5-year literature review. *J Can Dent Assoc.* 2006;72(4):323.
5. Bowen D. An evidence-based review of power toothbrushes. *Compend. Contin. Educ. Oral Hyg.* 2002;9(1):3-16.
6. Yaacob M, Worthington HV, Deacon SA, Deery C, Walmsley A, Robinson PG, Glenny A. Powered versus manual toothbrushing for oral health. Cochrane Database of Systematic Reviews 2014, Issue 6. Art. No.: CD002281. DOI: 10.1002/14651858.CD0022. http://www.cochrane.org/CD002281/ORAL_poweredelectric-toothbrushes-compared-to-manual-toothbrushes-for-maintaining-oral-health. Accessed July 26, 2015.
7. Costa MR, Marcantonio RAC, Cirelli JA. Comparison of manual versus sonic and ultrasonic toothbrushes: a review. *Int. J. Dent. Hyg.* 2007;5(2):75-81.
8. Walmsley AD. The electric toothbrush: a review. *Br. Dent. J.* 1997;182(6):209-218.
9. Heasman PA, McCraken GI. Powered toothbrushes: a review of clinical trials. *J. Clin. Periodontol.* 1999; 26:407-410.
10. Claydon NC. Current concepts in toothbrushing and interdental cleaning. *Periodontology 2000.* 2008;48: 10-22.
11. Asadorian J. Canadian Dental Hygienists' Association Position Paper: flossing. *Can. J. Dent. Hyg.* 2006;40(3):1-10.
12. Graves RC, Disney JA, Stamm JW. Comparative effectiveness of flossing and brushing in reducing interproximal bleeding. *J. Periodontol.* 1989;60(5):243-247.
13. Hujoel PP, Cunha-Cruz DW, Bantling DW, Loesch WJ. Dental flossing and interproximal caries: a systematic review. *J. Dent. Res.* 2006;85(4):298-305.
14. Imai PH, Xiaoli Y, MacDonald D. Comparison of interdental brush to dental floss for reduction of clinical parameters of periodontal disease: a systematic review. *Can. J. Dent. Hyg.* 2012;46:63-78.
15. Slot DE, Dörfler CE, Van der Weijden GA. The efficacy of interdental brushes on plaque and parameters of gingival inflammation: a systematic review. *Int. J. Dent. Hyg.* 2008;6:253-264.
16. Hoenderdos NL, Slot DE, Paraskevas S, Van der Weijden GA. The efficacy of woodsticks on plaque and gingival inflammation: a systematic review. *Int. J. Dent. Hyg.* 2006;6:280-289.
17. Greenstein G; Research, Science, and Therapy Committee of the American Academy of Periodontology. Position paper: the role of supra- and subgingival irrigation in the treatment of periodontal diseases. *J. Periodontol.* 2005;76:2015-2027.
18. Jahn CA. The dental water jet: a historical review of the literature. *J. Dent. Hyg.* 2010;84(3):114-120.
19. Cobb CM, Rodgers RL, Killoy WJ. Ultrastructural examination of human periodontal pockets following the use of an oral irrigation device in vivo. *J. Periodontol.* 1988;59(3):155-163.
20. Goyal CR, Lyle DM, Qaquish JG, Schuller R. Evaluation of the plaque removal efficacy of a water flosser compared to string floss in adults after a single use. *J. Clin. Dent.* 2013;24:37-42.
21. Husseini A, Slot DE, Van der Weijden GA. The efficacy of oral irrigation in addition to a toothbrush on plaque and

the clinical parameters of periodontal inflammation: a systematic review. *Int. J. Dent. Hyg.* 2008;6:304-314.

22. Gorur A, Lyle DM, Schaudinn C, Costerton JW. Biofilm removal with a dental water jet. *Compend. Contin. Dent. Ed.* 2009;30(Spec Issue 1):1-6.

23. Barnes CM, Russell CM, Reinhardt RA, Payne JB, Lyle DM. Comparison of irrigation to floss as an adjunct to toothbrushing: effect on bleeding, gingivitis and supragingival plaque. *J. Clin. Dent.* 2005;16(3):71-77.

24. Sharma NC, Lyle M, Qaquish J, et al. The effect of a dental water jet with orthodontic tip on plaque and bleeding in adolescent patients with fixed orthodontic appliances. *Am. J. Orthod. Dentofacial Orthop.* 2008;133: 565-571.

25. Rosema NAM, Hennequin-Hoenderdos NL, Berchier CE, Slot DE, Lyle DM, van der weijden GA. The effect of different interdental cleaning devices on gingival bleeding. *J. Int. Acad. Periodontol.* 2011;13:2-10.

26. Goyal CR, Lyle DM, Qaquish JG, Schuller R. The addition of a water flosser to power toothbrushing: effect on bleeding, gingivitis, and plaque. *J. Clin. Dent.* 2012; 23:57-63.

27. Suvan JE, D'Aiuto F. Progressive, paralyzed, protected, perplexed? What are we doing? *Int. J. Dent. Hyg.* 2008; 6:251-252.

Chapter 20 | Dentifrices and Mouthrinses

Jennifer Pieren, RDH, MS

KEY TERMS

abrasives
active ingredients
antigingivitis agents
antimicrobial agents
antitartar agents
flavoring agents
humectants
inactive ingredients
preservatives
surfactants
thickening agents
xerostomia

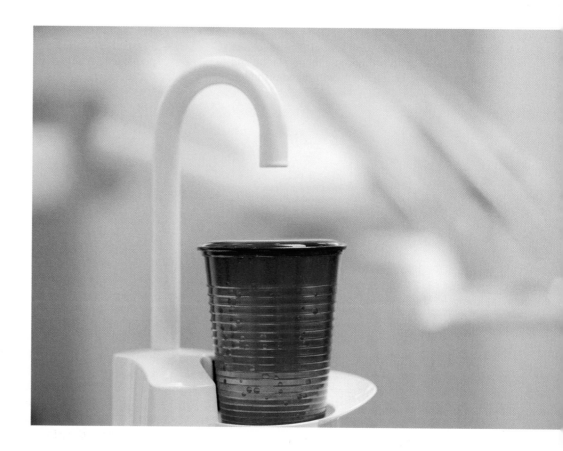

LEARNING OBJECTIVES

After reading this chapter, the student should be able to:

20.1 List and describe the basic ingredients of dentifrices and mouthrinses.

20.2 Select and recommend a dentifrice or mouthrinse for patients based on their needs.

20.3 Discuss the indications for use of different products based on their therapeutic ingredients.

20.4 Compare and contrast the active and inactive ingredients in dentifrices and mouthrinses.

20.5 Discuss potential adverse reactions for active and inactive ingredients in dentifrices and mouthrinses.

20.6 Identify key differences between prescription and over-the-counter dentifrices and mouthrinses.

20.7 Differentiate between the roles of the U.S. Food and Drug Administration and the American Dental Association in the regulation of dentifrices and mouthrinses.

KEY CONCEPTS

- Dentifrices and mouthrinses can be therapeutic adjuncts to brushing and flossing.
- An understanding of the different ingredients in dentifrices and mouthrinses can help the hygienist select the appropriate product to improve a patient's oral health.

RELEVANCE TO CLINICAL PRACTICE

Patients often ask their dental hygienist for information and advice regarding which toothpaste or mouthrinse would be the best choice for them. Substantial evidence supports the use of therapeutic dentifrices and/or mouthrinses as an adjunct to brushing and flossing. This chapter discusses common ingredients found in dentifrices and mouthrinses, and proper indications for their use. An understanding of the different ingredients in dentifrices and mouthrinses can help the dental hygienist recommend the appropriate product to improve a patient's oral health.

REGULATION AND CLASSIFICATION OF DENTIFRICES AND MOUTHRINSES

Dentifrices and mouthrinses are regulated by the U.S. Food and Drug Administration (FDA) in the United States. The FDA assures the safety and efficacy of products available to the public, and regulates both prescription and over-the-counter (OTC) drugs. Dentifrices and mouthrinses that are available without a prescription are considered OTC drugs, which are safe and effective for use by the general public without a physician's prescription.[1] The FDA classifies mouthrinses and toothpastes as therapeutic, cosmetic, or both. When toothpaste is classified as cosmetic, it is only required to meet safety guidelines and is not permitted to make claims of therapeutic value. When toothpastes are designated as therapeutic, they require extensive documented testing for efficacy and safety.[2] See Evidence-Based Practice.

Evidence-Based Practice

Patients commonly approach hygienists for advice on dentifrices, mouthrinses, or ingredients. With the assistance of today's technology, dental hygienists can research products and ingredients to evaluate their efficacy claims based on current evidence. When presented with these situations, consider the reliability, quantity, and quality of evidence, as well as your patients' needs (see Chapter 6 for more information). ■

DENTIFRICE

The primary job of a dentifrice, otherwise known as toothpaste, is to clean or remove plaque and debris from the teeth by enhancing the cleaning power of the toothbrush. Dentifrices are available as pastes, gels, and powders. Toothpastes, classified as cosmetic or therapeutic, are composed of inactive and active ingredients. **Inactive ingredients** help maintain the toothpaste's consistency to make it more palatable to the consumer. **Active ingredients** contribute to the therapeutic properties of the dentifrice.[3,4]

Inactive Ingredients in Dentifrices and Indications for Use

The common inactive ingredients found in toothpaste are:

- **Abrasives** and polishing agents (20%–60% of formulation): Aid in the removal of plaque/debris and stain. Examples include calcium carbonate, dehydrated silica gels, hydrated aluminum oxides, magnesium carbonate, phosphate salts, and silicates.[5] A variety of variables influence abrasiveness:
  - Particle size (grit)—larger particles increase wear on tooth surfaces.
  - Particle shape—irregularly shaped particles increase wear and abrasion on tooth surfaces. A smooth, round particle is less detrimental to the tooth.
  - Particle hardness—harder particles increase abrasion on tooth surfaces (for more information on particle hardness, see Mohs hardness scale, Chapter 29).

- pH level—higher acidity increases tooth surface mineral loss, particularly if dentin or cementum is exposed.
  - Glycerin—higher levels of glycerin increase abrasiveness on tooth surfaces because dissolution of insoluble materials is reduced.
  - Water—higher levels of water decrease abrasiveness on tooth surfaces because solution of soluble materials is increased.[6]
- **Surfactants** (1%–2% of formulation): Add foaming traits preferred by consumers. Surfactants reduce surface tension and suspend plaque and debris in an emulsion for easier removal during mechanical cleaning. Examples include sodium lauryl sulfate and sodium *N*-lauryl sarcosinate.
- **Humectants** (20%–40% of formulation): Prevent water loss from the preparation to prevent dehydration of the formulation. Although not their primary function, humectants can also contribute to the sweetness of the dentifrice. Examples include glycerol, propylene, glycol, and sorbitol.
- **Thickening agents**/binders (1%–2% of formulation): Stabilize dentifrice formulations and prevent separation of liquid and solid phases. These ingredients add bulk to the dentifrice. Examples include mineral colloids, natural gums, seaweed colloids, and synthetic cellulose.[3–5]
- **Flavoring agents,** sweeteners (up to 3% of formulation): Add flavors preferred by consumers. Flavoring agents should not promote tooth decay or contain sugar or any other ingredient that would promote tooth decay.[3,5,7] Examples include saccharin, xylitol, and other nonsugar sweeteners.[3,4]
- **Preservatives** (up to 3% of formulation): Preserve the toothpaste and prevent bacterial growth. Examples include alcohols, parabens, phenolics, and benzoates.[5,8,9]
- Dyes (up to 3% of formulation): Add colors to the product preferred by consumers. Examples include vegetable coloring.
- Fragrances (1%–1.5% of formulation): Add scents to the product and mask the taste, making the product more attractive to consumers. Examples include essential oils and menthol.[5]
- Water (15%–50% of formulation): Dissolves soluble particles and maintains the formulation.[6,10]

Active Ingredients in Dentifrices and Indications for Use

Most dentifrices are broadly classified and marketed to the public as agents for caries prevention, antitartar activity, whitening/cosmetic, antigingivitis/plaque formation reduction, or tooth sensitivity reduction. These ingredients typically constitute 1% to 2% of the dentifrice formulation[3,10]:

- Caries prevention: These toothpastes typically contain a form of fluoride (F) as the caries reduction agent. Other therapeutic ingredients can enhance fluoride uptake and aid in the remineralization process. Common active ingredients include fluoride, stannous fluoride, sodium fluoride, and sodium monofluorophosphate.[3,11,12]
- Antitartar/Reduction in calculus: These formulas inhibit calculus formation. It is generally thought that **antitartar agents** reduce crystal growth on the tooth surfaces. Common active ingredients include pyrophosphates, zinc citrate, chloride, triclosan, or stabilized stannous fluoride.[3,11,13]
- Cosmetic whitening: Cosmetic whitening can result from (a) mechanical removal of stain with abrasives; or (b) chemical breakdown of stain pigments with various compounds, such as hydrogen peroxide, papain, sodium citrate, or sodium tripolyphosphate.[3,11,14]
- Antigingivitis/Reduction in plaque formation: These formulas reduce the amount of supragingival biofilm and plaque accumulation. **Antigingivitis agents** are thought to be **antimicrobial agents** and reduce the pathogenicity of biofilm. Common active ingredients include triclosan (with vinyl methyl-ether maleic acid), zinc citrate, stannous fluoride, or a combination of essential oils.[3,11,15]
- Tooth sensitivity reduction: These formulations have been shown to desensitize enamel. These therapeutic ingredients work by decreasing nerve excitability or blocking dentinal tubules. Common active ingredients include arginine bicarbonate/calcium carbonate complex, potassium nitrate, or stabilized stannous fluoride.[3,11,16–18]

MOUTHRINSES

Mouthrinses can be used for a wide variety of reasons, including, with therapeutic ingredients, as adjunctive therapy to brushing and flossing (see Application to Clinical Practice). Some mouthrinses specifically aid the teeth by delivering fluoride. Others generally improve the total oral environment by reducing the overall bacteria. Like dentifrices, mouthrinses contain inactive and active ingredients and can be classified as either cosmetic or therapeutic.

Inactive Ingredients in Mouthrinses and Indications for Use

The common inactive ingredients found in mouthrinses are:

- Water: This is the main compound to stabilize other ingredients.
- Flavoring agents: Add flavors preferred by consumers. Flavoring agents should not promote tooth decay. Examples include saccharin, essential oils, and other nonsugar sweeteners.
- Humectants: Add body and prevent water loss from the preparation, inhibiting crystallization around the opening of the mouthrinse container. Examples include glycerin and sorbitol.[3]

Application to Clinical Practice

One of the most common questions asked of hygienists is whether the patient is using the right toothpaste or mouthrinse. Knowledge of the common therapeutic ingredients in dentifrices and mouthrinses, and indications for their use, will allow you to assist the patient in selecting a product that will best meet her needs. These interactions will also provide you with an opportunity to educate patients on the specific needs of their oral conditions.

For example, many patients today are focused on aesthetics, wanting white teeth. Not all of these patients will be ideal candidates for common whitening toothpastes, or they may have other conditions that need to be considered when suggesting products. In the case of a person with sensitive teeth who asks about using a toothpaste with whitening agents or abrasives, carefully consider each ingredient in the product. One solution may be to select a toothpaste with lower amounts of whitening agents that also contains a sensitivity ingredient such as potassium nitrate, fluoride, or both. ■

- Surfactants: Solubilize flavoring agent and provide foaming action preferred by consumers, remove oral debris, and have some limited antimicrobial properties. Examples include nonionic block copolymers, sodium lauryl sulfate (anionic), and cetyl pyridinium chloride (cationic).[3,19]
- Alcohol: Helps solubilize other ingredients. (Note: Although alcohol can denature bacterial cell walls, it serves as an inactive vehicle in most mouthrinses.)[3]

Active Ingredients in Mouthrinses and Indications for Use

Most mouthrinses are broadly classified and marketed to the public as agents for caries prevention, whitening/cosmetic, antigingivitis, oral malodor (halitosis), **xerostomia** (dryness of the mouth), cleaning/debridement, and topical pain relief.

- Caries prevention: These formulas typically contain a form of fluoride (F) as a caries reduction agent. When used, these mouthrinses have been found to enhance the fluoride uptake and aid in the remineralization process. Common active ingredients include sodium fluoride, stannous fluoride, and hydrogen fluoride.[3,20]
- Cosmetic whitening: These formulas are used to bleach teeth. The common active whitening ingredient is hydrogen peroxide 1.5% to 2%.[3,21]
- Antigingivitis: These formulations contain antimicrobial agents and ingredients that inhibit plaque formation. Common active ingredients include essential oils, chlorhexidine gluconate, and cetylpyridinium chloride.[3,22,23]
- Halitosis (oral malodor): These mouthrinses have agents that control growth of bacteria or deactivate volatile sulfur-containing compounds that are present due to the breakdown of amino acids. Common active ingredients include chlorhexidine, chlorine dioxide, cetylpyridinium chloride, and essential oils such as eucalyptol, menthol, thymol, and methyl salicylate. These mouthrinses can also include agents that inhibit odor-causing bacteria such as zinc salts, ketone, terpene, and ionone.[3,24,25]
- Xerostomia: These formulations reduce discomfort associated with dry mouth by coating the tissue or mimicking the feel of saliva in the mouth. Common active ingredients include salts, enzymes, cellulose derivatives, and/or animal mucins.[3,26]
- Cleaning/Debridement: The active ingredients in these formulas physically remove necrotic tissue and food particles. The common cleaning/debridement active ingredient is hydrogen peroxide (the bubbling action). (Note: These mouthrinses should not be used frequently or for extended periods when the active ingredient concentration is 3% or more, as they could damage oral tissues.)[3,19]

Advancing Technologies

Recently, the number of new products in the dental market has exploded. More and more therapeutic claims are being made, and dental professionals' original beliefs are being challenged. For example, most mouthrinses were once thought to just freshen breath. New evidence has suggested that some therapeutic ingredients in mouthrinses may add to the therapeutic benefit derived from brushing and flossing. Similar results have been found for essential oils, as they have been shown to offer therapeutic benefits in addition to brushing and flossing.[3,22]

However, not all studies have such positive results. Triclosan has been in the spotlight recently following studies suggesting that triclosan may alter hormone regulation in animals and contribute to making bacteria resistant to antibiotics. Although a wealth of information supports the benefit of triclosan in dentifrices, the "FDA is engaged in an ongoing scientific and regulatory review of this ingredient" in light of these studies.[28] So, as a professional, practitioners must not only be sure to evaluate each individual ingredient in the product before recommending it to patients, they must also stay up-to-date with the literature regarding safety and efficacy of the ingredients because the prevailing thoughts on the materials can change.[28] ■

- Topical pain relief: These mouthrinses contain topical local anesthetics to diminish pain. Common active ingredients include lidocaine, benzocaine/ butamben/ tetracaine hydrochloride, dyclonine hydrochloride, or low concentration phenol. Barrier mouthrinses also fit into this category. These formulas coat tissue ulcerations or soft tissue lesions to act as a physical barrier and reduce discomfort. Common active ingredients include hyaluronate, polyvinylpyrrolidone, and glycyrrhetinic acid.[3,26,27]

Discussion

All mouthrinses and dentifrices should be used as directed or prescribed with the indicated dose, duration, and frequency. For the maximum antiplaque or anticaries benefit, patients are generally recommended to rinse before going to bed without rinsing or drinking anything. Mouthrinses and dentifrices (OTC or prescription) should always be kept out of the reach of children.[3,29,30]

PRESCRIPTION PRODUCTS

The FDA defines a prescription drug as a product that requires a physician's authorization to purchase.[1] Prescription dental products usually include higher concentrations of active ingredients or can include other regulated drugs (see Professionalism). Prescription-strength mouthrinses and dentifrices have been found to be effective. Prescription-strength fluoride products have higher concentrations of fluoride. These products have been found to be very effective because higher levels of fluoride are generally directly related to increased reduction in caries. The maximum allowable fluoride in OTC dentifrices in the United States is 1,500 part per million (ppm). The maximum amount in mouthrinses is 230 ppm. Any product formulation containing more fluoride is only available by prescription.[4,30]

Professionalism

In addition to providing patient care, dental practices are also businesses. Often, OTC or prescription products are sold in the dental office for a profit. When you are hired, your office manager asks you to recommend only a certain brand of product that is sold in your office. You have knowledge of another product from a different brand that may provide a better therapeutic benefit for the patients in your office. Considering your role as a dental hygienist and your responsibility to your patient, what would you do? ▪

Teamwork

Working with other health-care professionals is imperative for comprehensive health care. Often patients have other systemic conditions or are undergoing treatments that can drastically affect their oral health. For example, the management of patients who are undergoing cancer treatment provides an excellent opportunity for collaborative treatment planning. Patients with cancer often experience varying degrees of oral mucositis, stomatitis, and xerostomia. Oncology teams often prescribe pain-relieving or compounded mouthrinses and encourage preventative dental services before, during, and after their treatment. Dental hygienists must work collaboratively with the other caregivers to develop a treatment plan to comprehensively treat the patient to ensure optimal healing and comfort. ▪

Products that contain chlorhexidine are only available by prescription. In addition, specialty mouthrinses can be prescribed in the form of compounded medicines for unique reasons. For example, a compounded mouthrinse may include many ingredients such as antihistamines, antifungals, topical anesthetics, and even antibiotics for pain relief. These mouthrinses can be prescribed by a dentist or other health-care professionals (see Teamwork).[25,27,31]

ADVERSE REACTIONS AND SPECIAL CONSIDERATIONS

Serious adverse reactions to dentifrices and mouthrinses have been reported as relatively low. Most reactions reported are contact-type reactions[3]:

- Gingival irritation or dental sensitivity: Some reactions from antitartar toothpastes have been reported in the forms of gingival irritation or dentinal sensitivity. Sodium laurel sulfate has also been reported as an irritant to some patients. Dentifrices are marketed without sodium laurel sulfate and antitartar ingredients in the event of a suspected reaction.
- Staining: Chlorhexidine, stannous fluoride, and cetylpyridium chloride have been associated with extrinsic staining. (Note: Chlorhexidine has also been associated with supragingival calculus formation over long-term use.)
- Chemical burning: Mouthrinses containing oxygenating agents have been associated with chemical burns of the oral mucosa, decalcification of the teeth, and black hairy tongue.[3]
- Fluorosis: When fluoride-containing products are used inappropriately or there is an increased accumulative exposure, the patient is at risk for fluorosis. Children

Spotlight on Public Health

The U.S. Department of Health and Human Services has proposed a new recommendation of 0.7 mg fluoride per liter of water to prevent dental caries, which is an increase over the original recommendation made in 1962. One of the reasons for the change is the increased access to and use of fluoridated dental products, including fluoridated mouthrinses and dentifrices. Children are at the highest risk for receiving more than optimal amounts of fluoride because of their inability to expectorate and rinse properly after using fluoridated products.[29] In addition, research has shown that parents are not always aware of the proper amount of toothpaste to use.[32] In response to these concerns, the CDC recommends that health professionals counsel patients on the appropriate amount and frequency of fluoridated dentifrice use[29] because these products remain an important method of reducing childhood caries. Information about the CDC's brush-up program and instructions to share with parents can be found at the CDC's website (brush-up campaign): http://www.cdc.gov/OralHealth/publications/resources/press_releases/brushup_pr.htm. Accessed July 26, 2015. ■

are especially at risk. Assessment and education on how to properly use fluoride is imperative (see Spotlight on Public Health).[3,30] Total fluoride exposure, especially of young children, should be evaluated carefully during the medical and dental history assessment and considered when planning interventions.

Table 20-1 contains additional special considerations for common active ingredients in dentifrices and mouthrinses.

When an adverse reaction is suspected from a toothpaste or mouthrinse ingredient, the patient should discontinue use and switch to a formula that does not have the suspected ingredient. Any patient who has a known sensitivity to an ingredient in a product should avoid using it. In addition, as discussed previously in this chapter, while the FDA assures the safety and efficacy of the products in the market, special consideration should be given to pregnant or pediatric patients when recommending products.

AMERICAN DENTAL ASSOCIATION SEAL OF ACCEPTANCE

The American Dental Association (ADA) Seal of Acceptance program is a voluntary program where a manufacturer can submit its product for review and acceptance by the ADA. The program requires that the product be cleared by the FDA and have ADA-mandated standardized testing. The manufacturer must submit a list of ingredients, indications, and claims. The manufacturer must also provide clinical trials and laboratory tests as required by the ADA seal guidelines to document the safety and efficacy of the product, as well as other criteria such as manufacturing processes. When the product is accepted, it may be marketed with the ADA Seal of Acceptance. Currently, only consumer products are eligible for the seal. Professional and prescription products are not eligible for consideration.[33]

Table 20-1. *Common Active Ingredients and Special Considerations*

Type	Common Ingredient	Efficacy	Special Considerations
Caries prevention	Fluoride Stannous fluoride Sodium fluoride Hydrogen fluoride Sodium monofluorophosphate	Effective in reducing caries[20]	Monitor pediatric patients to minimize amount of fluoride ingested Fluorosis[3]
Antitartar/ Reduction in calculus	Pyrophosphates Zinc citrate Triclosan Stabilized stannous fluoride	Significant reduction in calculus[3,8]	Minimal risk for dentinal hypersensitivity and/or tissue irritation[3]
Cosmetic whitening/ cleaning/ debridement	Hydrogen peroxide Papain Sodium citrate Sodium tripolyphosphate	A number of whitening toothpaste ingredients are effective at stain removal in laboratory studies, but evaluating clinical benefit has been problematic[3,8,14,20]	Possible burning sensation Abrasion Taste alteration Drying of mucosal membranes Enamel erosion Use cautiously in patients with low salivary flow or oral ulcerations[3]

Continued

Table 20-1. *Common Active Ingredients and Special Considerations—cont'd*

Type	Common Ingredient	Efficacy	Special Considerations
Antigingivitis/ Reduction in plaque formation	Triclosan (with vinyl methyl-ether maleic acid) Zinc citrate Stannous fluoride Chlorhexidine gluconate cetylpyridinium chloride Combination of essential oils	Significant reduction in biofilm formation and some reduction in gingivitis Triclosan with copolymer, zinc citrate, and stannous fluoride significantly improve plaque control and periodontal health[3,8,19]	Potential allergic reaction Burning sensation Bitter taste[3] Recent studies finding possible issues (hormone regulation and antibiotics resistance) with triclosan[28]
Tooth sensitivity reduction	Potassium nitrate Stabilized stannous fluoride	Potassium nitrate reduces sensitivity compared with regular fluoride toothpaste[3,8]	Potential allergic reaction[3]

Case Study

Sally is a 4 ½-year-old-girl brought in by her aunt for her annual prophylaxis. Upon examination, she has several new incipient carious lesions with minimal plaque. When asked about Sally's current oral hygiene habits, her aunt, who only babysits her after she gets home from preschool, is not sure how often Sally brushes or what kind of toothpaste is used. She is sure her sister buys "a great toothpaste" because it is from an organic health food store. Sally indicates that she brushes twice a day, swishes with a pink rinse, and takes her vitamins to stay strong and healthy. Sally also says she was just at her pediatrician last week for her school physical for the upcoming year.

Case Study Exercises

1. Who would be the best person to speak to before recommending any type of fluoride therapy for Sally?
   A. Speak to her primary caregiver to determine her total fluoride exposure.
   B. Contact her pediatrician to determine whether she is taking a supplement.
   C. Speak to her preschool teacher to determine whether she drinks city or well water while at school.
   D. Ask the person who brought her to the appointment.

2. What are the potential sources of fluoride for Sally?
   i. Water
   ii. Supplement
   iii. Toothpaste
   iv. Mouthrinse

   A. i and ii
   B. i, ii, and iii
   C. iii and iv
   D. All of the above
   E. None of the above

3. All of the following would be aspects to cover when educating Sally and her primary caregiver EXCEPT:
   A. Sally should be supervised when brushing.
   B. Sally can dispense as much fluoride toothpaste as she would like on her toothbrush.
   C. Toothpaste should be stored out of Sally's reach.
   D. Toothpastes and mouthrinses should only be used as directed.

4. All of the following are factors that should be considered when determining Sally's total fluoride exposure EXCEPT:
   A. How well Sally expectorates
   B. Where Sally lives
   C. What kinds of toothpastes and mouthrinses Sally use.
   D. Where Sally's mom buys her toothpaste

Review Questions

1. While performing a dental hygiene assessment, the dental hygienist notes that the patient has localized plaque-induced gingivitis, bleeding on probing, insufficient salivary function, abfractions, and generalized extrinsic staining. The patient indicates that she uses a whitening toothpaste, but it makes her "teeth hurt." What recommendations should the dental hygienist give this patient regarding her oral care?
   A. Tell the patient to discontinue using whitening products and advise her to use a toothpaste for sensitive teeth.
   B. Discuss the patient's clinical findings with her and help her select a toothpaste and mouthrinse that would best meet all of her needs.
   C. Recommend a product with triclosan, which has antigingivitis benefits, because treating the patient's gingivitis is the priority.
   D. Advise the patient to keep using her current products but to use them less often.

2. Inactive ingredients help maintain the toothpaste's consistency to make it more palatable to the consumer. Active ingredients contribute to the therapeutic properties of the dentifrice.
   A. Both statements are true.
   B. Both statements are false.
   C. The first statement is true; the second statement is false.
   D. The first statement is false; the second statement is true.

3. A patient asks if there is a more natural alternative to the OTC toothpastes that are on the market. He has been making his own toothpaste from a recipe he found online. He mixes baking soda, lemon water, and honey and brushes with it every night before bed. Based on this information, what should the dental hygienist be concerned about when conducting Sam's assessment?
   A. Caries risk
   B. Abrasion
   C. Erosion
   D. All of the above
   E. None of the above

4. Using the scenario from question 3, select the most appropriate points the dental hygienist should make during patient education.
   i. Recommend that the patient discontinue use of the current homemade dentifrice.
   ii. Review each ingredient of the homemade dentifrice and explain the concerns.
   iii. Ask the patient what he values for his oral health needs.
   iv. Review the patient's current needs and help him select a product.
   A. i and ii
   B. ii, iii, and iv
   C. i, iii, and iv
   D. All of the above
   E. None of the above

5. Chlorhexidine has been associated with extrinsic staining. Chlorhexidine used over a long period will result in a reduction of calculus formation.
   A. Both statements are true.
   B. Both statements are false.
   C. The first statement is true; the second statement is false.
   D. The first statement is false; the second statement is true.

Active Learning

1. Dispense different toothpastes onto a mixing pad. Observe the characteristics and properties of the toothpastes. Rub each toothpaste between your fingers. Is it gritty or smooth? Discuss the different ingredients and their purposes.
2. Brush with different toothpastes. What happens when you add water? Does it foam or not? What ingredients are present or missing?
3. Compare and contrast labels from different types of mouthrinses and toothpastes. Identify the different ingredients and their functions.
4. Rinse with different types of mouthrinses. What does the mouthrinse feel like? What is it doing (foaming, coating the tissues, etc.)?
5. Using written case studies with photos and radiographs, select appropriate mouthrinse and dentifrice options to meet the patient's needs. Discuss why these selections were made. Compare and contrast the options. ■

REFERENCES

1. U.S. Food and Drug Administration. Drugs, approvals & databases: Drugs@FDA glossary of terms. Silver Spring, MD: FDA. Updated February 2, 2012. http://www.fda.gov/Drugs/InformationOnDrugs/ucm079436.htm. Accessed October 23, 2012.

2. U.S. Food and Drug Administration. Guidance, compliance & regulatory information: is it a cosmetic, a drug, or both? Silver Spring, MD: FDA. Updated April 30, 2012. http://www.fda.gov/Cosmetics/GuidanceComplianceRegulatoryInformation/ucm074201.htm. Accessed October 23, 2012.

3. Mariotti AJ, Burrell KH. Mouthrinses and dentifrices. In: Ciancio SG, ed. *ADA/PDR Guide to Dental Therapeutics.* 5th ed. Montvale, NJ: ADA Publishing Division and Thomson PDR; 2009:305-321.

4. Collins FM. *Reflections on Dentifrice Ingredients, Benefits and Recommendations.* Tulsa, OK: Penn Well; 2009.

5. Lavoie F, Feeney N, McCallum L, Paquet M, Fortin Y, Nadeau D, et al. Evaluation of toothpastes and of the variables associated with the choice of a product. *Can J Dent Hyg.* 2007;41:42-56.

6. Darby ML, Walsh M. *Dental Hygiene: Theory and Practice.* 3rd ed. St. Louis, MO: Elsevier Health Sciences; 2010.

7. American Dental Association. Toothpaste. Chicago: ADA. http://www.ada.org/1322.aspx. Accessed January 3, 2013.

8. Davies R, Scully C, Preston AJ. Dentifrices—an update. *Med Oral Patol Oral Cir Bucal.* 2010;15(6):976-982.

9. Forward GC, James AH, Barnett P, Jackson RJ. Gum health product formulations: what is in them and why? *Periodontol 2000.* 1997;15:32-39.

10. Wilkins E. *Clinical Practice of the Dental Hygienist.* ed 11. Philadelphia: Lippincott Williams & Wilkins; 2013.

11. Sensabaugh C, Sagel ME. Stannous fluoride dentifrice with sodium hexametaphosphate: review of laboratory, clinical and practice-based data. *J Dent Hyg.* 2009; 83(2):70-78.

12. Walsh T, Worthington HV, Glenny AM, Appelbe P, Marinho VC, Shi X. Fluoride toothpastes of different concentrations for preventing dental caries in children and adolescents. *Cochrane Database Syst Rev.* 2010;(1): CD007868.

13. Netuveli GS, Sheiham A. A systematic review of the effectiveness of anticalculus dentifrices. *Oral Health Prev Dent.* 2004;2(1):49-58.

14. Joiner A. Whitening toothpastes: a review of the literature. *J Dent.* 2010;38(suppl 2):e17-e24.

15. Blinkhorn A, Bartold PM, Cullinan MP, Madden TE, Marshall RI, Raphael SL, Seymour GJ. Is there a role for triclosan/copolymer toothpaste in the management of periodontal disease? *Br Dent J.* 2009;207(3):117-125.

16. Parolia A, Kundabala M, Mohan M. Management of dentinal hypersensitivity: a review. *J Calif Dent Assoc.* 2011;39(3):167-179.

17. Li Y, Lee S, Zhang YP, Delgado E, DeVizio W, Mateo LR. Comparison of clinical efficacy of three toothpastes in reducing dentin hypersensitivity. *J Clin Dent.* 2011; 22(4):113-120.

18. West NX. Dentine hypersensitivity: preventive and therapeutic approaches to treatment. *Periodontol 2000.* 2008;48:31-41.

19. Moran JM. Home-use oral hygiene products: mouthrinses. *Periodontol 2000.* 2008;48:42-53.

20. Marinho VC. Cochrane reviews of randomized trials of fluoride therapies for preventing dental caries. *Eur Arch Paediatr Dent.* 2009;10(3):183-191.

21. Torres C, Perote L, Gutierrez N, Pucci C, Borges A. Efficacy of mouth rinses and toothpaste on tooth whitening. *Oper Dent.* 2013;38(1):57-62.

22. Gunsolley JC. Clinical efficacy of antimicrobial mouthrinses. *J Dent.* 2010;38(suppl 1):S6-S10.

23. Biesbrock AR, Bartizek RD, Gerlach RW, Terézhalmy GT. Oral hygiene regimens, plaque control, and gingival health: a two-month clinical trial with antimicrobial agents. *J Clin Dent.* 2007;18(4):101-105.

24. Armstrong BL, Sensat ML, Stoltenberg JL. Halitosis: a review of current literature. *J Dent Hyg.* 2010;84(2):65-74.

25. Fedorowicz Z, Aljufairi H, Nasser M, Outhouse TL, Pedrazzi V. Mouthrinses for the treatment of halitosis. *Cochrane Database Syst Rev.* 2008;(4):CD006701.

26. Napeñas JJ, Brennan MT, Fox PC. Diagnosis and treatment of xerostomia (dry mouth). *Odontology.* 2009; 97(2):76-83.

27. Scully C, Field EA, Randall C. Over-the-counter remedies for oral soreness. *Periodontol 2000.* 2008;48:76-84.

28. U.S. Food and Drug Administration. Triclosan: what consumers should know. Silver Spring, MD: FDA. Updated November 25, 2013. http://www.fda.gov/ForConsumers/ConsumerUpdates/ucm205999.htm. Accessed December 21, 2013.

29. Centers for Disease Control and Prevention. Community water fluoridation: questions and answers. Atlanta, GA: CDC. Updated October 22, 2012. http://www.cdc.gov/fluoridation/fact_sheets/cwf_qa.htm#6. Accessed December 21, 2012.

30. Centers for Disease Control and Prevention. Other fluoride products. Atlanta, GA: CDC. Updated January 6, 2011. http://www.cdc.gov/fluoridation/other.htm#5. Accessed December 21, 2012.

31. Wiseman M. The treatment of oral problems in the palliative patient. *J Can Dent Assoc.* 2006;72(5):453-458.

32. Wiener RC, Crout RJ, Wiener MA. Toothpaste use by children, oral hygiene, and nutritional education: an assessment of parental performance. *J Dent Hyg.* 2009; 83(3):141-145.

33. American Dental Association. Guidelines for earning the seal. Chicago: ADA. Updated 2011. http://www.ada.org/participationguidelines.aspx. Accessed January 3, 2013.

Chapter 21 | Cariology and Caries Management

Jacques Freudenthal, RDH, MHE

KEY TERMS

acidogenic bacteria

biofilm

buffer

caries

Caries Management by Risk Assessment (CAMBRA)

cariogenesis

cariogenic bacteria

cariology

carious lesion

cavity

confounder

coronal caries

demineralization

dental decay

determinants

early childhood caries (ECC)

hydroxyapatite

microorganism

pH

recurrent caries

remineralization

restoration

root caries

saliva

secondary caries

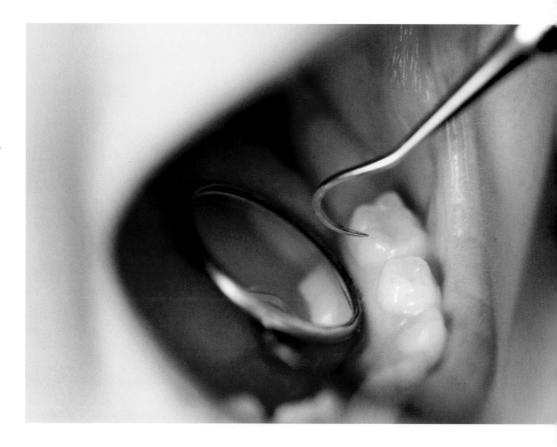

LEARNING OBJECTIVES

After reading this chapter, the student should be able to:

21.1 Discuss the most important distinctions among various terms used to describe the disease of mineralized structures.

21.2 Describe the multifactorial nature of the caries process.

21.3 Discuss the demineralization and remineralization processes and the importance of a balance between the two.

21.4 Explain the role fluoride and other preventive measures play in the remineralization process.

21.5 Describe how carious lesions are classified.

21.6 Discuss why early intervention using minimally invasive dentistry is critical to a therapeutic approach.

21.7 Identify the key elements of conducting a caries risk assessment.

21.8 Identify the specific primary risk factors and protective factors in the caries balance equation.

21.9 Explain how therapeutic recommendations differ among low-, moderate-, and high-risk status.

KEY CONCEPTS

- Caries is a multifactorial transmissible disease where cariogenic microorganisms interact in a dynamic relationship with factors that influence the disease process.
- The caries process can be reversed if it is identified in the early stages and protective factors are introduced.
- Fluoride is the primary therapeutic intervention in the prevention and control of caries.
- A caries risk assessment is essential in determining the level of risk and treatment protocols.
- A major paradigm shift to an interprofessional care model may help to identify, limit, and control oral diseases.

RELEVANCE TO CLINICAL PRACTICE

Current evidence reveals that the caries process exhibits a much more complex, multifactorial nature than was previously believed. Understanding the caries process has progressed from the early worm theory when barber surgeons hypothesized worms lived in the teeth and caused holes, to a research-based biological phenomenon.[1] Dental caries is a complex infectious disease process that afflicts 80% of the world's population. It is puzzling, though, how a largely preventable disease remains so prevalent.[1] New research is enhancing the understanding of the dynamic relationship among oral bacterial species, host dynamics, and measures that either promote or interfere with this disease process. Preventive regimens are key to minimizing caries risk and controlling the disease. Dental hygienists have expertise in designing and implementing preventive, oral, and nutritional education programs; they can effectively determine and recommend specific fluoride and nonfluoride caries preventive agents and recare intervals. Dental hygienists have the opportunity to take a leadership role in assisting patients to motivate themselves and in directing therapeutic care to decrease the burden of oral diseases and improve the quality of life for individuals and communities.

DEFINITIONS AND TERMINOLOGY

Many terms are used to describe the primary dental disease affecting the mineralized structures of the teeth: caries, dental caries, caries process, carious lesion, cavities, decay, and dental decay. Individuals, clinicians, educators, and researchers commonly use these terms interchangeably. No single definition exists and usage is not standardized. The definitions discussed in this section are based on a terminology used by professional associations and in the current literature.

Cariology is the study of dental caries and **cariogenesis,** the development of caries.[2] **Caries** is defined as a transmissible bacterial infectious disease process of the mineralized oral structures. The disease occurs on a continuum, resulting from repeated cycles of demineralization and remineralization over an extended period.[3] **Cavity** most accurately describes the end result of a localized chemical dissolution of the tooth structure caused by metabolic events taking place in the biofilms that cover the affected tooth surface(s) and denote a hole in the tooth.[4] In some cases, surgical treatment is required to remove the decayed tissue and restore function by preparing the tooth and placing a **restoration** to support the remaining tooth structure. If the decay has not reached the dentin, the lesion can most likely be remineralized. If the **carious lesion** progresses to involve the pulp, extensive treatment options, calcium hydroxide, endodontic therapy (root canal), or an extraction may be indicated. The term **dental decay** comes from the Latin words meaning "rottenness or decay," and it is commonly used interchangeably with the terms *cavity* and *cavitation*. A significant number of children and adults have teeth extracted because of extensive decay.

The most important distinction among the various terms is the stage they refer to along the continuum. Caries is a process that, if identified in the early stages, is reversible by remineralization of the affected area. Once cavitation or a break in the enamel occurs, remineralization is no longer feasible and restorative treatment is indicated. A shortfall of all of these common terms is that the definitions do not specify the extent of the lesion(s), whether the lesion is active or inactive, or the level of risk for the disease.

The terms *detection* and *diagnosis* are used regarding assessment of caries. Generally, clinicians detect a lesion(s) and diagnose disease(s).[5]

CAUSE OF THE INFECTION

Approximately 40 of the 700 to 800 identified species that inhabit the oral cavity have been implicated in the caries process, with new **microorganisms** identified every year.[6,7] Current science describes oral microorganisms in a dynamic **biofilm** with interrelated factors responsible for initiating the caries process. In the presence of fermentable carbohydrates (sucrose, glucose, fructose, and cooked starch), specific microorganisms produce organic acids (lactic, formic, acetic, and propionic) that are capable of dissolving the inorganic components (calcium and phosphate) from the enamel and dentin, resulting in a process called *demineralization*. The acid-producing microorganisms are referred to as **acidogenic** or **cariogenic** bacteria. A dynamic relationship exists among the cariogenic organisms, fermentable carbohydrates, saliva, and time.[8] The mere presence of cariogenic pathogens does not mean mineral loss will occur or cavitation will develop. However, cariogenic pathogens are essential for the process to occur, and active lesions have a strong association with dietary habits.[1]

The primary acidogenic microorganisms associated with the caries process include *Streptococcus mutans, Lactobacillus, Streptococcus sobrinus,* and *Actinomyces* species. The *Streptococcus* species, specifically *Mutans streptococci,* have been identified with early lesion development and primarily secrete lactic acid. *M. streptococci* are frequently dominant in early lesions. The *Lactobacillus* species increase in numbers, primarily on smooth surfaces in the later stages of lesion development where they thrive in a very low pH environment (3.0–3.5). Lactobacilli tend to suppress or displace other acidogenic bacteria because of the low pH and are one of the most acid tolerant of the cariogenic microorganisms.[9]

Microorganisms attach to the tooth via extracellular proteins called *extracellular polysaccharides* and *intracellular polysaccharides.* Extracellular polysaccharides promote greater bacterial adhesion and add mass to the biofilm. The extracellular polysaccharides produce the glue (glucans) that holds the microflora to the tooth, whereas intracellular polysaccharides serve as a storage reservoir for sucrose, enabling the bacteria to maintain a low level of acidity in the absence of fermentable polysaccharides. Sucrose is unique in that it is easily fermented compared with other starches and sugar alcohols.[9,10] Researchers now realize the early cause-and-effect diagrams of the caries process were oversimplified for such a complex disease process (Fig. 21-1).

A modified diagram keeps the major circles of the Venn diagram but includes additional factors that contribute to the caries process (Fig. 21-2). In the modified caries diagram, factors are labeled as determinants and confounders. The **determinants** are those factors that determine the outcome by interacting with each other and are located inside the circle. The **confounders** are those components not fully explained by the determinants alone such as knowledge, education, attitudes, behaviors, social class, and income.[10] The confounders are noted on the periphery and can also be referred to as risk indicators. The confounders may influence the risk assessment between individuals with similar determinant factors.[10]

The net loss or gain of minerals over time determines whether the process will result in repair of the tooth surface or cavitation. Because of the dynamic nature of the disease process, the patient must be assessed frequently to evaluate and monitor disease activity. Intervention at the earliest stages provides an opportunity to implement preventive strategies to reverse the manifestations of early disease.

Multifactorial Disease

The four primary factors implicated in the development of a carious lesion are: 1) a susceptible host tooth, 2)

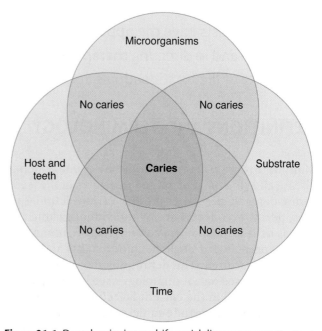

Figure 21-1. Dental caries is a multifactorial disease process. (Reprinted by permission from Macmillan Publishers Ltd: Yip K, Smales R. Oral diagnosis and treatment planning: part 2. Dental caries and assessment of risk. *British Dental Journal* 2012 Jul 28:213(2):fig 1.)

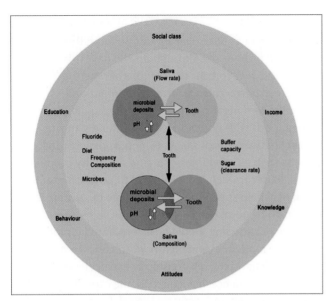

Figure 21-2. Determinants-confounders model in dental caries. (From Usha C, Sathyanarayanan R. Dental caries—a complete changeover (part I). *J Conserv Dent.* 2009 Apr-Jun;12(2):46-54. doi: 10.4103/0972-0707.55617. Copyright © Indian Journal of Conservative Dentistry.)

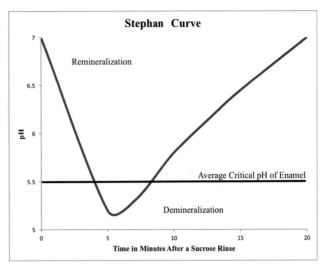

Figure 21-3. Stephan curve after a sucrose rinse.

acidogenic microorganisms, 3) available fermentable carbohydrate substrate, and 4) a sufficient period for these factors to occur. Many other risk factors and risk indicators are also involved in this complex process. Risk factors, including moderate or high cariogenic bacterial counts, visible biofilm, more than three between-meal snacks, and inadequate saliva flow, are the determinants of the disease. Risk indicators are factors or circumstances that are indirectly associated with the disease such as socioeconomic and epidemiological factors, education level, and special needs.[11]

The host factors with the greatest impact are the proportions and numbers of cariogenic bacteria, dietary habits, oral hygiene, and the quality and quantity of saliva. Caries as a disease process is not based solely on the presence of acidogenic pathogens and fermentable carbohydrates. The extent of the decline in pH and the length of time it takes to **buffer,** or bring the low **pH** to normal, are dependent on and influenced by an individual's quantity and quality of saliva, a process first reported by Stephan in the 1940s, which became known as the cornerstone for how the caries process works (Fig. 21-3).[12]

Refined carbohydrates have been widely implicated in the increased prevalence of caries. Frequent consumption of liquid or solid foods that cause the pH in the oral cavity to drop below the 5.5 threshold results in loss of minerals. It takes the saliva approximately 40 minutes to buffer the pH back to normal pH 7 after solid sugar or carbohydrate exposure and about 20 minutes for a liquid exposure. Studies have shown the low pH that results from bacterial metabolism is responsible for the loss of minerals.[13] See Evidence-Based Practice.

Saliva

Saliva, which is produced via the major salivary glands (parotid, submandibular, and sublingual), is an important

protective factor in the caries process. Saliva has the following functions:

- Lubricates the tissues of the mouth
- Aids in the clearance of food
- Secretes sodium bicarbonate, which buffers acids
- Initiates carbohydrate digestion
- Possesses antibacterial properties
- Serves as a reservoir for calcium, phosphate, and fluoride

A healthy flow rate increases saliva's buffering capability, dilutes the acids, and has adequate calcium and phosphate to foster remineralization. Multiple medications and radiation treatment can lead to a significant decrease in saliva quantity and quality. Xerostomia (dryness of the mouth) is a major risk factor in the caries process (Box 21-1). Chewing sugarless gums, candies, and lozenges can stimulate saliva flow for those with a dry mouth.

Demineralization/Remineralization Process

The caries process is a continuous cyclic process of demineralization and remineralization where an imbalance occurs. Under normal conditions, the pH of the oral cavity is close to a neutral pH and the saliva is saturated with calcium and phosphate ions to maintain this healthy environment. **Demineralization** (the loss of calcium and phosphate from the enamel surfaces of teeth) occurs when acid-producing *M. streptococci* and other cariogenic bacteria metabolize dietary fermentable carbohydrates. The acidic environment causes a decline in the pH in the oral cavity, which results in a loss of calcium and phosphate from the **hydroxyapatite** and fluorohydroxyapatite crystals of the enamel surfaces.[9,10]

The point at which demineralization occurs is dependent on the decline in pH and the length of time the teeth are exposed to the acidic environment. There is a point referred to as the "critical pH" in which the equilibrium shifts and demineralization occurs. Hydroxyapatite

Evidence-Based Practice

Two questions have been validated to help determine the frequency of consumption and, therefore, the oral exposure to a low pH environment[7]:

1. Do you drink liquids other than water more than two times daily between meals?
2. Do you snack daily between meals?

Dietary counseling for caries-prone individuals should include recommendations to limit sweetened between-meal snacks and drinks to reduce caries susceptibility. Refined sugars and fermentable carbohydrates comprise a large portion of most diets, making dramatic change difficult. It is the frequency of exposure rather than the amount consumed that results in more below-critical pH episodes during the day. Therefore, a healthier alternative is to consume sugars and carbohydrates with meals or just following mealtimes. If this is not possible, it is best to consume the food or beverage all at once over a short period rather than small bites or sips throughout the day. This approach strives to limit the amount of time the teeth are exposed to an acidic environment and allows the remineralization process to occur. Replacing refined foods with noncariogenic sweeteners and/or limiting between-meal snacks to noncariogenic food options such as vegetables, proteins, and dairy products should be recommended. Rinsing with water after a snack may help speed the buffering time of saliva and the return to normal pH.

Dietary counseling should be incorporated for individuals in the moderate- and high-risk categories to help them understand the relationship between dietary habits and caries experience. Inadequate home care allows the biofilm to mature and increases the risk for disease. Regular removal of the biofilm through thorough home care disrupts the biofilm so it does not mature and become pathogenic. ■

---

crystals begin to lose mineral content at a pH of 6.5 to 6.7, particularly in areas where the root surfaces are exposed. This shift occurs between 5.0 and 5.5 pH for fluorohydroxyapatite crystals.[9] Without intervention to halt the loss of minerals, the lesion may progress to exhibit a white spot lesion, which is the first "clinically visible sign" of the caries process. A white spot or opacity is a subsurface lesion and is considered a "manifestation" of the disease. With unimpeded progression, cavitation may result. Demineralization is considered an imbalance in the caries process.

Remineralization is the natural repair process where calcium and phosphate ions use fluoride as a catalyst to rebuild the crystalline structure histologically in the subsurface lesion. Remineralized crystals are more acid resistant due to fewer impurities and a lower carbonate content than the hydroxyapatite crystals. These new crystals are referred to as fluorapatite-like or fluorohydroxyapatite. The presence of low levels of calcium and phosphate, in conjunction with minimal amounts of fluoride, inhibits dissolution and enhances the remineralization process.

PREVENTIVE AND THERAPEUTIC THERAPIES

Topical fluorides are the primary intervention for the prevention and therapeutic control of caries. However, many other therapeutic therapies are available to augment the effects of fluoride in protecting the tooth surface. The widespread use of fluoride is responsible for the significant decline in the incidence of caries. The primary role of fluoride is to inhibit demineralization and enhance remineralization. Therapeutic fluoride is available in multiple forms and formulations including pastes, gels, foams, varnishes, mouthrinses, water, milk, and salt.

Fluoride Pastes, Gels, Foams, and Varnishes

Fluoride accumulates, is retained in the saliva and biofilm, and becomes available when an acid challenge occurs. After exposure to fluoride ions, an elevated concentration can be measured in the biofilm.[5] The concentration slowly diminishes over time and is greatly reduced after rinsing. To retain higher fluoride reservoirs, advise caries-prone individuals to spit out remaining toothpaste when brushing the teeth and avoid rinsing with water.

Box 21-1. *Measuring Saliva Flow*

- Stimulated saliva flow can be measured by the amount of saliva produced divided by the amount of time. Normal stimulated flow is 1 to 3 mL/min; less than 0.7 mL is considered low or salivary hypofunction.[7,54]
- A quick test for low salivary flow is to simply assess the floor of the mouth for dryness. Unstimulated saliva flow is measured by allowing saliva to pool in the floor of the mouth and is more predictable of caries risk than stimulated flow.[54]
- Another simple test can be conducted by observing the formation of saliva droplets on the mucosa of the inner lower lip for 1 minute. There should be multiple droplets forming with healthy salivary flow.[6] ■

The stannous fluoride ion has demonstrated the ability to both remineralize and interfere with bacterial activity. Fluoride varnish contains a 5% neutral sodium concentration in a resin base that is painted on the teeth to increase the contact time. The ADA Council on Scientific Affairs affirmed fluoride varnish is effective in preventing caries in the primary and permanent dentition, as well as in high-risk individuals if applied two or more times per year.[14] Professional gel and foam fluorides are available in acidulated phosphate and neutral sodium (NaF) formulations and must be applied for a full 4 minutes even though some are labeled as minute formulations. Single-dose varnish contains less fluoride and reduces the risk for ingestion compared with in-office gel and foam products.[14]

A systematic review confirmed toothpaste with a fluoride concentration of 1,000 parts per million (ppm) and higher demonstrates anticaries benefits in children and adolescents.[15] Adults may also benefit from this concentration. Higher-concentration fluoride products must be balanced with the risk for fluorosis for children younger than 5 or 6 years. Long-term evidence supports the use of mouthrinses that contain low concentrations (0.05% NaF) of fluoride as a daily rinse and 0.2% NaF for weekly use.[16,17] High-concentration (5,000 ppm) pastes and gels are recommended for those at high risk and are frequently distributed in the dental office for home use. These formulations contain 0.4% stannous fluoride or 1.1% neutral sodium fluoride and can be used in custom trays to increase contact time. They are formulated with and without abrasives. A formulation with an abrasive may increase compliance because it can serve as a substitute for toothpaste. Used as recommended and in conjunction with in-office fluoride applications, these formulations can be effective in promoting the remineralization process (Fig. 21-4).

Chlorhexidine Mouthrinses and Varnish

Mouthrinses that contain chlorhexidine (CHX) have shown degrees of effectiveness in caries prevention and control. Chlorhexidine is the most extensively studied agent that targets microorganisms in the biofilm associated with caries and periodontal diseases. Conflicting evidence exists regarding the effectiveness of CHX for the control of coronal caries despite showing temporary reductions in *M. streptococci* levels. An ADA expert panel concluded CHX did not show a statistically significant reduction in coronal caries.[18] A more recent study found CHX rinse demonstrated a significantly lower caries risk and suggested reduced caries increment.[19] Regarding varnish combining CHX with thymol, three randomized controlled trials showed efficacy against root caries.[18]

The **Caries Management by Risk Assessment (CAMBRA)** protocol recommends that individuals at high risk rinse with 10 mL CHX 0.12% for 1 minute daily for 1 week each month.[20] A 60-minute interval is recommended between the use of CHX and products that contain fluoride to enhance the effectiveness of both.

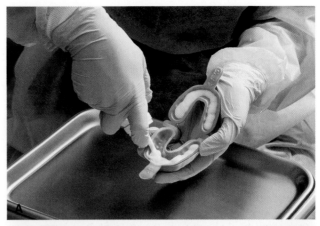

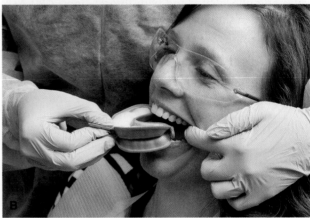

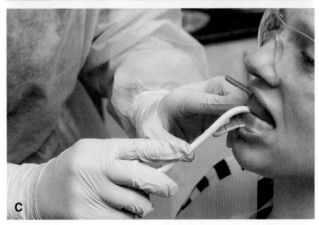

Figure 21-4. Fluoride application: (A) Fill tray with fluoride, (B) insert tray into patient's mouth, and (C) apply suction.

Use of a 40% CHX varnish has shown reduced incidence of root caries, but additional studies are needed to strengthen the evidence.[21] Ongoing research is needed to identify antibacterial and combination therapies that can inhibit cariogenic bacteria and enhance remineralization. Until new therapies are found, CHX may be the most effective antimicrobial for those at higher risk.[19]

Additional Measures

Additional measures used to combat caries in high-risk individuals include chewing gums, candies, lozenges, and pastes that contain casein phosphopeptide-amorphous calcium phosphate (CPP-ACP).

Casein Phosphopeptide–Amorphous Calcium Phosphate

CPP-ACP is incorporated into toothpastes, prophy pastes, and gels to facilitate deposition when exposed to calcium and phosphate in saliva. Developed from casein, a milk protein, CPP-ACP (Recaldent) binds to the tooth structure, allowing the ACP ions to penetrate and remineralize subsurface lesions. CPP-ACP is a milk-based product that is inorganic and highly soluble. It is created when dissolved calcium ions and phosphate ions react to form a noncrystalline insoluble salt. CPP-ACP speeds up the natural remineralization of demineralized enamel by coating the tooth with hydroxyapatite.[22,23] The calcium and phosphate bind with fluoride ions. CPP-ACP has also been shown to reduce white spot lesions on the enamel.[24]

Tricalcium Phosphate

Tricalcium phosphate (TCP) is a hybrid material created with a milling technique that fuses β-TCP and sodium lauryl sulfate or fumaric acid.[25] It was designed to increase the efficacy of fluoride remineralization. Products available with TCP include a 5,000 ppm sodium fluoride dentifrice and a 5% sodium fluoride varnish. A toothpaste with TCP was found to deliver more high-quality mineral above the surface and deep in the carious lesions, and provided superior surface and subsurface remineralization compared with a 5,000 ppm fluoride product alone.[26]

Calcium Sodium Phosphosilicate

Calcium sodium phosphosilicate (CSP) is a bioactive glass that has been available since the late 1960s to help regenerate bone. CSP reacts in an aqueous (or water) environment, and when exposed to saliva, ions of calcium, phosphate, and sodium are released. The sodium helps buffer the acid and then over time, the calcium and phosphate ions become accessible to support remineralization. CSP was initially established for the treatment of dentinal hypersensitivity.[27] In vitro and in situ studies propose that CSP can prevent dentin demineralization, remineralize root carious lesions, heal white spot lesions, and fill demineralized lesions.[28]

Xylitol

Much research has focused on the polyol sweetener xylitol because cariogenic bacteria are not able to effectively metabolize sugar alcohols and can influence a shift in the microflora.[29] Xylitol has been shown to reduce levels of *M. streptococci* in biofilm and saliva.[5] However, a minimum dose of xylitol is needed throughout the day (four times a day) to impact the *M. streptococci* counts. Xylitol varies in concentration and must contain at least 10% for therapeutic effectiveness.[5] Higher xylitol concentrations increase the cost and must be evaluated when recommending xylitol products.

Xylitol chewing gum marginally reduces the incidence of caries in children, and children with caries experience could also benefit from xylitol lozenges or hard candy, but there is not enough evidence to recommend xylitol syrup for children younger than 2 years or to recommend xylitol dentifrice.[18] There is also not enough evidence that xylitol, CHX, or calcium products given to mothers can reduce caries in children.[18]

Another therapeutic approach that may provide benefit includes fluoride-releasing dental materials. Dental sealants, glass ionomer cements, and resin composite materials are the most common fluoride-releasing materials currently used in dentistry. These materials have a synergistic effect when used with topical fluoride products and serve as a reservoir for fluoride. Fluoride rerelease is considered significant but is always lower than the release of fluoride when initially placed. Glass ionomers exhibit greater fluoride release and recharge abilities than resin-based materials.[30]

CLASSIFICATION OF CARIOUS LESIONS

Specific sites in the oral cavity are more susceptible to the caries process than others. The caries process may occur on the clinical crowns and root surfaces throughout the mouth. Caries may be classified by the type of caries or by one of the multiple classification systems for dental caries and restorations.

G.V. Black's Classification

Dr. G.V. Black developed a system of caries classification and nomenclature in the late 1800s that is still widely used today.[31] This classification system combines the surface type with the specific tooth surfaces, as well as the specific category of tooth (anterior vs. posterior), in a numerical order ranging from class I to class VI. For more information on G.V. Black's classification, see Chapter 12.

Classification Systems by Caries Type

In addition to classifying caries by the location, they are also classified by the type of caries: coronal, root caries, recurrent or secondary, and **early childhood caries (ECC).**

Coronal Caries

Coronal caries manifest in the enamel crystals covering the crown of the tooth occurring in pits and fissures, as well as on the smooth surfaces. Early signs of demineralization can be visible on a wet or dry tooth surface. Active enamel caries tend to appear chalky white with a matte or rough texture. Inactive caries tend to appear shiny with a smooth texture and may be white, yellow, brown, or black. A clean, shiny, smooth surface normally indicates an inactive lesion. Remineralization of the caries process requires an intact enamel surface. Light pressure using a blunt probe or the side of an explorer tip can be used to assess surface texture but not to assess for a "soft" spot. It can be challenging to determine whether a lesion will progress or remineralize; therefore, a risk assessment is necessary to help determine the proper course of treatment.[5]

Root Caries

Root caries occur below the cementoenamel junction by affecting the less mineralized cementum covering the root surfaces. Bacterial invasion and dissolution of cementum and dentin occur more rapidly than with enamel caries. Therefore, differentiating between active and inactive lesions helps determine the best approach to treatment. If the lesion is active, both preventive and surgical treatment may be indicated. A layer of biofilm covering the surface indicates activity of the lesion(s).[5] The surface may appear yellow or light brown with a texture that is either soft or leathery, or both. Inactive lesions tend to appear darker and may be dark brown or black.[5]

Root caries are commonly found in the elderly and those who have exposed root surfaces. Early detection of root caries is more challenging than coronal caries due to the increased rate of mineral loss and the lack of early clinical signs such as white spot lesions on enamel. A combination of visual and gentle tactile detection is recommended, as well as evaluation of the extent of involvement around the circumference of the root.[5]

Recurrent or Secondary Caries

Recurrent caries or secondary caries occur adjacent to existing restorations such as amalgam, composite, and crowns. Marginal integrity of restorations plays a significant role in the occurrence of recurrent caries. The decay occurs between the tooth surface and the margin of restorations. Both deficient and overhanging margins provide a nidus for bacteria to accumulate. Deficient margins allow microleakage under restorative materials, and excess or overhanging margins pose challenges to thoroughly remove food debris and biofilm and to remineralize these areas.

Recurrent caries are challenging to detect with both traditional methods (visual, tactile, radiographic) and new caries detection technologies. A cycle of re-restoring a tooth tends to increase in size and depth, sometimes leaving little natural tooth structure intact. Fifty to 60% of restorations are replaced because of secondary caries.[32] The preferred solution is to prevent the primary lesions from ever occurring and requiring a restoration. Variation and controversy exist in the literature as to the longevity of restorations based on specific teeth, clinician, type of material, size, age, sex, and cavity classification. Frequent recare may improve the longevity of restorations with early intervention where repair of the restoration, rather than replacement, is possible.

Early Childhood Caries

ECC is defined by the American Academy of Pediatric Dentistry (AAPD) as "the presence of one or more decayed, missing, or filled surfaces in any primary tooth in a child under the age of six."[33] Children in the age range of 12 to 30 months can exhibit a special pattern of caries that differs from that found in older children. The primary maxillary incisors and molars are the most susceptible to the caries process because the tongue and saliva provide some protection for the mandibular incisors. This pattern has been referred to in the past as "baby bottle tooth decay, bottle caries, and nursing caries." This severe form of caries is not limited to poor feeding habits but has a multifactorial cause, hence the change to ECC.[34,35]

Children are not born with the bacteria that initiate the caries process. Most children acquire the transmissible cariogenic microorganisms from their mothers or primary caregivers through sharing and tasting foods on a spoon or pacifier and intimate contact. This is referred to as vertical transmission. High counts of cariogenic microorganisms in mothers are associated with early colonization in their infants. Horizontal transmission may also occur between family members and other children.

Children with ECC tend to have a greater risk for new lesions in both the primary and the permanent dentitions. If the disease is extensive, it can become a family problem because of increased incidence of pain, diminished learning, hospitalization for treatment, and high economic costs. Young children exposed to frequent and prolonged use of a bottle with sugar-containing liquids and those who have low socioeconomic, minority, and immigrant status tend to have higher rates of disease.[36]

Dye et al. examined trends in oral health in the American population by comparing National Health and Nutrition Examination Survey (NHANES) data collected from 1988 to 1994 and 1999 to 2004. Although the oral health status of most of the U.S. population remained unchanged, the prevalence of dental decay in the primary dentition of preschool-aged children increased.[37] In 2009, similar NHANES data showed 24% of preschool-aged children from 2 to 5 years of age had a decay experience and 73% exhibited untreated

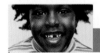

Spotlight on Public Health

Although the prevalence of dental caries has decreased over the past two decades, the prevalence has increased in the youngest and most vulnerable populations. Some communities experience a larger share of this burden than others. There appears to be a substantial disparity between racial and socioeconomic groups regarding access to oral and general health care. Caries is a complex multifactorial disease in itself; combined with the many complexities of community factors, it is even more challenging. Healthcare providers and public health officials must work together to design programs that will improve health care for all who live in our communities. Creative strategies that prevent diseases and lead to early diagnosis are needed. Public health policies that promote education, prevention, and access to care at an early age could positively impact both the personal and the financial burden on individuals, families, and governmental agencies. ■

Teamwork

Dentistry has traditionally been practiced as a separate entity from medicine. As more and more research confirms associations between oral health and systemic health, a need has emerged to move toward comprehensive health care that includes both dentistry and medicine. In 2003, the American Academy of Pediatrics recommended physicians play an integral role in children's oral health.[52] Oral health training tools such as the "Smiles for Life" curriculum[53] are tailored to healthcare professionals to provide quality information and improve identification of dental diseases and conditions. Medicine is in the beginning stages of integrating oral health training into medical professional education programs and residency training. Dental hygienists possess the skills needed to assist with this training. Interprofessional collaboration between dental and medical professionals may help lead to a better understanding of the complexity of oral diseases and the challenges of decreasing this burden on our population. A limited number of medical professionals are providing oral health screenings, assessments, and referrals, and applying preventive measures and anticipatory guidance at wellness visits. Comprehensive preventive care will be enhanced by the cooperation of all health professions in lowering the physical and financial burden of oral and systemic diseases by using a team approach. ■

Advancing Technologies

New technologies have provided advances in the healthcare field that have improved the quality of life for many citizens. Diagnostic technologies allow us to detect diseases earlier than ever before. The multifactorial nature of dental caries makes it unlikely that a single technology modality will have adequate sensitivity and specificity for the detection in all sites in the oral cavity. Future technologies capable of measuring caries activity would be a great leap forward and allow for earlier interventions. Advancing technologies may allow for a greater understanding of genetic and sex susceptibility to minimize destruction of oral tissues. For the present time, a combination of multiple diagnostic tools, techniques, and professional judgment is required for evidence-based quality care. ■

decay. A lack of access to and utilization of dental care is a significant concern in the preschool population (see Spotlight on Public Health and Teamwork).[38]

Awareness and preventive intervention in the first year of life may help improve the caries incidence over a person's life span. An increased awareness of this rampant disease by parents, teachers, and medical and dental providers could increase the utilization of dental care in pediatric populations.[37]

CARIES DETECTION METHODS

Traditional approaches to the detection of dental caries include visual, tactile, and radiographic methods. The most common method for detecting coronal carious lesions is by visual-tactile inspection. Research demonstrates a high ability to accurately identify sound tooth structure but a low ability to identify early lesion activity. The ability to measure activity is the goal of future caries detection methods (see Advancing Technologies).[5]

Visual Inspection

Visual inspection is an effective method to assess for changes in color and surface texture of coronal surfaces.

The International Caries Detection and Assessment System (ICDAS II) was developed by caries experts in Scotland in 2002 and updated in 2003. It is a visual system that provides a standardized method for diagnosing occlusal lesions.[20] This validated system measures degrees of lesion severity or depth and histological findings with a high degree of sensitivity and specificity for primary molars and permanent teeth.[5] The ICDAS system should be used with adjunctive diagnostic aids such as radiographs and caries detection tools that can monitor the nonsurgical or therapeutic treatment of early lesions.

Tactile Detection

Tactile detection of coronal lesions has traditionally involved using an explorer to assess for a soft area or stickiness. Scientific research encourages a major paradigm shift away from the traditional use of a sharp explorer to detect caries. Sharp explorers add little diagnostic value and can be detrimental if excess pressure is used, resulting in broken surface crystals from poking the lesion.[5,39]

Radiographic Detection

Radiographic detection is enhanced by using paralleling techniques for bitewing radiographs to detect interproximal lesions and root caries. Radiographs are most effective when comparisons can be made with previous films to identify progression or remineralization of lesions. Once the change in density is visible, the area is thought to be approximately 30% to 40% demineralized. Therefore, radiographically visible lesions are considered more advanced clinically than is visible on a radiograph. Occlusal caries are generally moderate or advanced lesions before they are radiographically visible. Radiographic sensitivity increases as lesions progress toward the dentin.

Emerging Technologies

Emerging technologies are being developed to identify and measure lesions in their earliest stages, something that traditional methods do not provide. Digital fiber-optic transillumination (DIFOTI), quantitative light-induced fluorescence (QFL), laser fluorescence, light-emitting diodes (LEDs), electrical caries monitor, and alternative current impedance spectroscopy (CarieScan) represent some of these new technologies.

Digital Fiber-Optic Transillumination

DIFOTI can be used to detect incipient and frank lesions, as well as fractures and recurrent caries. DIFOTI uses light to transilluminate and create a digital image where decay appears darker compared with the brighter healthy tooth structure. It has shown to be more sensitive in identifying lesions on the occlusal surfaces than interproximally and does not indicate depth of the lesions.[40,41]

Quantitative Light-Induced Fluorescence

QFL is an intraoral imaging system that uses specific wavelengths of light, creating a natural fluorescence of the teeth. Fluorescence decreases in areas of demineralization, resulting in a dark appearance compared with sound tooth structure. The QFL software measures the loss of fluorescence to monitor caries activity over time. Disadvantages include expense and a limitation to accurately distinguish among caries, stains, and developmental anomalies.[41]

Laser Fluorescence

Laser fluorescence detects changes in the density of tooth structure. The amount of fluorescence is related to the degree of demineralization allowing for longitudinal monitoring of caries and effectiveness of therapeutic measures. A limitation of this technology is the possibility of false-positive readings from the presence of biofilm, pastes, sealants, and other resin materials.[40]

Light-Emitting Diodes

LED devices are based on the reflection and reflectance of the emitted light. They are designed to detect changes in the optical translucency and opacity of the dental tissues. Additional studies are needed, as well as improvements in the ability of these devices to differentiate sound surfaces from enamel caries.[41]

Electrical Caries Monitor

Electrical caries monitor differentiates between sound enamel and carious lesions by measuring electrical resistance. This technology has the ability to monitor lesion progression and remineralization with a high degree of sensitivity and specificity.[42]

Alternative Current Impedance Spectroscopy

CarieScan's alternating current impedance spectroscopy uses electrical current to detect and quantify coronal caries in the early stages when therapeutic measures can be instituted to prevent disease progression. Color displays change to differentiate sound tooth structure from demineralized areas and advanced decay.[40]

A combination of multiple diagnostic tools and techniques, as well as professional judgment, is essential for the detection and treatment of caries in the earliest stages. These new technologies provide the opportunity to improve the oral health of patients through prevention, good disease management, and minimal intervention dentistry.

CARIES MANAGEMENT

No restorative material can sufficiently replace natural tooth structure in terms of longevity. New research encourages dental professionals to adopt more conservative approaches to prevent or treat carious lesions therapeutically in the earliest stages and preserve the natural tooth structure. Adhesive restorative materials allow for more conservative removal of tooth structure and are more conducive to repair versus replacement. A focus on patient-centered disease management rather than restorative surgical care is imperative to combat this complex multifactorial disease. A "minimally invasive" approach incorporates detecting, diagnosing, intercepting, and treating dental caries on a histological level using a therapeutic or medical model rather than a surgical model.[43] This means removing only the minimum amount of tooth structure and repairing, rather than replacing, restorations. Minimally invasive dentistry is more frequently referred to as minimal intervention dentistry. This concept is based on the patient's caries risk and the use of current therapies to prevent, control, and treat the disease. "Minimal intervention dentistry," "minimally invasive dentistry," or "preservative dentistry" is the approach to dentistry that should be practiced in the future.[44] However, this entails a philosophical change from what many practitioners learned in school and perform as clinicians to a philosophy of early intervention using minimal invasive dentistry.[45]

Dental Hygienist's Role in Caries Management

In a therapeutic treatment model, dental hygienists serve as preventive coordinators and monitor treatment outcomes. Successful outcomes frequently require dental hygienists to manage the infection, reduce risk factors, and motivate patients to be actively involved in all aspects of their disease through innovative preventive approaches and lifestyle changes. Identification of risk factors, risk indicators, and protective factors require patient engagement and open dialogue. Dental hygienists should review the medical history and evaluate both prescription and nonprescription drugs for oral side effects. Dry mouth can result as a side effect of systemic diseases (lupus, diabetes, cancers, thyroid disorders, etc.) and multiple medications. Not all factors can be altered, but strategies to treat the dry mouth can be incorporated into a daily routine (sugarless, mints or gum, frequent sips of water, products designed to treat dry mouth symptoms). Dental hygienists are educated to provide nutritional counseling regarding dietary habits and frequency of sweetened snacks as an essential aspect

Professionalism

The profession of dental hygiene is a growing and dynamic field. Dental hygienists are expanding their knowledge base by conducting research that adds to the body of dental hygiene evidence. Scientific research allows the profession to grow and provides exciting new findings that can be used to improve the health and quality of life for individuals and communities. Professional codes of conduct apply to both personal and professional behavior. With the explosion of social media, dental hygienists must be aware of the fine line between personal and professional demeanor. Competence, integrity, respect, and responsibility are all aspects of professionalism that must be upheld. ■

in the management of caries. Most lifestyle changes entail behavior modification, identification of motivating factors, and effective communication techniques that allow the patient to partner in determining strategies for the management of their disease status. This includes the determination of the continued care interval of 2, 3, 4, or 6 months. Generally, as caries risk increases, the frequency and intensity of preventive measures should correspond. Patients must understand the essential role they play in influencing the demineralization and remineralization process. This may be the most challenging aspect of caries management. Changing engrained dietary and lifestyle habits requires individuals to have a clear understanding of the disease process and an internal motivation to change behaviors. The traditional educational approach of persuasion and advice-giving has not proved sufficient to prevent oral diseases. Caries management requires much more than recommending that patients "brush," "floss," and "don't eat sugar."[44] Basic educational principles include: (a) individualizing the information, (b) active listening, (c) forming partnerships with patients,

(d) investigating the patient's values and long-term goals, (e) discussing pros and cons of making behavior changes, (f) respecting the patient's autonomy, and (g) providing support of individual choices (see Professionalism).[46] See Chapter 3 for information on motivational interviewing.

Risk Assessment

Managing caries risk involves conducting an assessment of caries risk. Risk assessment is the probability that an event or outcome will occur in the future.[47] This first step is important in determining the level of risk and treatment protocols.[48] Multiple studies show a history of caries is the single most reliable factor in identifying a future risk for caries activity.[49,50] Caries risk assessment (CRA) models have been developed to target both individual and community populations. Multiple versions are available for use in clinical practice and community settings.

Caries Management by Risk Assessment

CAMBRA is an evidence-based disease-management protocol designed for clinical practice. The conceptual model of CAMBRA is based on the caries balance where pathological factors (bacteria, limited quality and quantity of saliva, poor dietary habits) battle protective factors (healthy saliva, fluoride, sealants, antibacterials, probiotics, and a balanced diet). A group of caries experts developed two CRA forms and procedures to use in clinical settings.[47,50] One form is designed for children aged 0 to 5 years and the other for age 6 years through adult.[11] These one-page forms are easy to follow and can be used as part of the clinical examination procedures following the process of care model. Both forms identify disease indictors, risk factors, and protective factors. This information allows clinicians to determine whether the caries risk is balanced or imbalanced (Fig. 21-5).

If an imbalance is found, additional bacterial and salivary testing may be necessary to identify the level of risk (low, moderate, high, or extreme). The risk assessment determines the intensity and frequency of treatment and recare interval. Disease indicators include active decay (visible white spots, clinically or radiographic

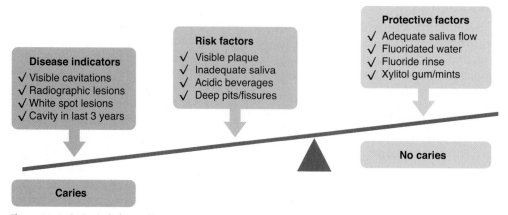

Figure 21-5. Caries imbalance diagram. (From Featherstone JB, Domejean-Orliaguet S, Jenson L. Caries risk assessment in practice for age 6 through adult. *J Calif Dent Assoc.* 2007 Oct;35(10):703-713. Reprinted with permission from The Journal of the California Dental Association.)

lesions, restorations placed in the past 3 years).[48,49] Risk factors of significance are heavy biofilm, frequent between-meal snacks, saliva-reducing medications, radiation therapy, deep pits and grooves, exposed roots, orthodontic appliances, and bedtime or continued use of a bottle with fluids other than water. Important protective factors include adequate saliva flow; living in a fluoridated community; regular exposure to fluoride multiple times a day through use of toothpastes, mouthrinses, professional-strength topicals, xylitol gum, or lozenges; and antimicrobial medicaments (Table 21-1). Individuals at low risk present with little or no history of white spot lesions, caries, restorations, or extractions. Moderate-risk patients have additional risk factors compared with low-risk patients. Low and moderate risk is based on the number of protective factors versus the number of risk factors. Those identified as high risk have continuing multiple risk factors or active lesions, or both. Those with cavitated lesions are automatically put in a high-risk category due to the strong predictive value of lesions requiring restorative

care in the past 3 years (Table 21-2).[11] The presence of any disease indicator and a dry mouth automatically puts individuals in an extreme risk category that requires aggressive management. Those with special needs may also fall into this risk level.[11] Individuals with special needs have varying levels of function that can impact their risk for oral diseases, including dental caries. Generally, the lower the level of function the more assistance is needed with home care because of dexterity and mental abilities. A team approach to professional oral care is essential to minimize oral diseases. Multiple medications frequently play a role in their risk for caries. The overall risk is determined by evaluating the number and severity of the disease indicators and risk factors using the caries balance model.[51] The mere presence of risk factors does not necessarily mean individuals have active disease or will in the future, but it is important to recommend a recare interval that is appropriate for their risk status. Generally speaking, the higher the risk the more frequent the recare (2–6 months) and intense the therapeutic recommendations.

Table 21-1. *Caries Risk Assessment Form—Children Aged 6 Years and Older/Adults*

Patient Name: _____ Chart #: _____ Date: _____
Assessment Date: _____ **Is this (please circle) baseline or recall?**

Disease Indicators (Any one "YES" signifies likely "High Risk" and to do a bacteria test**)	**YES = CIRCLE**	**YES = CIRCLE**	**YES = CIRCLE**
Visible cavities or radiographic penetration of the dentin	YES		
Radiographic approximal enamel lesions (note in dentin)	YES		
White spots on smooth surfaces	YES		
Restorations last 3 years	YES		
Risk Factors (Biological predisposing factors)		YES	
Mutans streptococci and *Lactobacillus* both medium or high (by culture**)		YES	
Visible heavy plaque on teeth		YES	
Frequent snack (>3× daily between meals)		YES	
Deep pits and fissures		YES	
Recreational drug use		YES	
Inadequate saliva flow by observation or measurement (**If measured, note the flow rate below)		YES	
Saliva-reducing factors (medications/radiation/systemic)		YES	
Exposed roots		YES	
Orthodontic appliances		YES	
Protective Factors			
Lives/work/school fluoridated community			YES
Fluoride toothpaste at least once daily			YES

Continued

Table 21-1. Caries Risk Assessment Form—Children Aged 6 Years and Older/Adults—cont'd

Disease Indicators (Any one "YES" signifies likely "High Risk" and to do a bacteria test**)	YES = CIRCLE	YES = CIRCLE	YES = CIRCLE
Fluoride toothpaste at least 2× daily			YES
Fluoride mouthrinse (0.05% NaF) daily			YES
5,000 ppm F fluoride toothpaste daily			YES
Fluoride varnish in last 6 months			YES
Office F topical in last 6 months			YES
Chlorhexidine prescribed/used 1 week each of last 6 months			YES
Xylitol gum/lozenges 4 × daily last 6 months			YES
Calcium and phosphate paste during last 6 months			YES
Adequate saliva flow (>1 mL/min stimulated)			YES

Bacteria/Saliva Test Results: *M. streptococci:*
Lactobacillus: **Flow Rate: mL/min. Date:**

VISUALIZE CARIES BALANCE
(Use circled indicators/factors above)
(EXTREME RISK = HIGH RISK + SEVERE SALIVARY GLAND HYPOFUNCTION)
CARIES RISK ASSESSMENT (CIRCLE): EXTREME HIGH MODERATE LOW
Doctor signature/#: _____ Date: _____

Source: Featherstone JB, Domejean-Orliaguet S, Jenson L. Caries risk assessment in practice for age 6 through adult. *J Calif Dent Assoc.* 2007;35(10):703-713.
  Reprinted with permission from The Journal of the California Dental Association.

Table 21-2. Caries Management by Risk Assessment: Clinical Guidelines for Patients Age 6 and Older

Risk Level###,***	Frequency of Radiographs	Frequency of Caries Recall Examinations	Saliva Test (Saliva Flow & Bacterial Culture)	Antibacterials Chlorhexidine Xylitol****	Fluoride	pH Control	Calcium Phosphate Topical Supplements	Sealants (Resin-Based or Glass Ionomer)
Low risk	Bitewing radiographs every 24–36 months	Every 6–12 months to re-evaluate caries risk	May be done as a baseline reference for new patients	Per saliva test if done	OTC fluoride-containing toothpaste twice daily, after breakfast and at bedtime. Optional: NaF varnish if excessive root exposure or sensitivity	Not required	Not required Optional: for excessive root exposure or sensitivity	Optional or as per ICDAS sealant protocol
Moderate risk	Bitewing radiographs every 18–24 months	Every 4–6 months to re-evaluate caries risk	May be done as a baseline reference for new patients or if there is suspicion of high bacterial challenge and to assess efficacy and patient cooperation	Per saliva test if done Xylitol (6–10 g/day) gum or candies. Two tabs of gum or two candies four times daily	OTC fluoride-containing toothpaste twice daily plus: 0.05% NaF rinse daily. Initially, 1–2 app of NaF varnish; 1 app at 4–6 month recall	Not required	Not required Optional: for excessive root exposure or sensitivity	As per ICDAS sealant protocol
High risk*	Bitewing radiographs every 6–18 months or until no cavitated lesions are evident	Every 3–4 months to re-evaluate caries risk and apply fluoride varnish	Saliva flow test and bacterial culture initially and at every caries recall appointment to assess efficacy and patient cooperation	Chlorhexidine gluconate 0.12% 10 mL rinse for 1 minute daily for 1 week each month. Xylitol (6–10 g/day) gum or candies. Two	1.1% NaF toothpaste twice daily instead of regular fluoride toothpaste. Optional: 0.2% NaF rinse daily (1 bottle), then OTC	Not required	Optional: Apply calcium/phosphate paste several times daily	As per ICDAS sealant protocol

Continued

Table 21-2. Caries Management by Risk Assessment: Clinical Guidelines for Patients Age 6 and Older—cont'd

Risk Level###,*,***	Frequency of Radiographs	Frequency of Caries Recall Examinations	Saliva Test (Saliva Flow & Bacterial Culture)	Antibacterials Chlorhexidine Xylitol****	Fluoride	pH Control	Calcium Phosphate Topical Supplements	Sealants (Resin-Based or Glass Ionomer)
				tabs of gum or two candies four times daily	0.05% NaF rinse 2× daily. Initially, 1–3 app of NaF varnish; 1 app at 3–4 month recall			As per ICDAS sealant protocol
Extreme risk** (High risk plus dry mouth or special needs)	Bitewing radiographs every 6 months or until no cavitated lesions are evident	Every 3 months to re-evaluate caries risk and apply fluoride varnish.	Saliva flow test and bacterial culture initially and at every caries recall appointment to assess efficacy and patient cooperation	Chlorhexidine 0.12% (preferably CHX in water-base rinse) 10 mL rinse for 1 minute daily for 1 week each month. Xylitol (6–10 g/day) gum or candies. Two tabs of gum or two candies four times daily	1.1% NaF toothpaste twice daily instead of regular fluoride toothpaste. OTC 0.05% NaF rinse when mouth feels dry, after snacking, breakfast, and lunch. Initially, 1–3 app NaF varnish; 1 app at 3 month recall.	Acid-neutralizing rinses as needed if mouth feels dry, after snacking, bedtime, and after breakfast. Baking soda gum as needed	Required: Apply calcium/phosphate paste twice daily	

*Patients with one (or more) cavitated lesion(s) are high-risk patients.

**Patients with one (or more) cavitated lesion(s) and severe hyposalivation are extreme-risk patients.

***All restorative work to be done with the minimally invasive philosophy in mind. Existing smooth surface lesions that do not penetrate the DEJ and are not cavitated should be treated chemically, not surgically. For extreme-risk patients, use holding care with glass ionomer materials until caries progression is controlled. Patients with appliances (RPDs, prosthodontics) require excellent oral hygiene together with intensive fluoride therapy, e.g., high fluoride toothpaste and fluoride varnish every 3 months. Where indicated, antibacterial therapy to be done in conjunction with restorative work.

###For all risk levels: Patients must maintain good oral hygiene and a diet low in frequency of fermentable carbohydrates.

****Xylitol is not good for pets (especially dogs).

DEJ, dentinoenamel junction; ICDAS, International Caries Detection and Assessment System; OTC, over-the-counter; RPDc removable partial denture.

Source: Adapted from Jenson L, Budenz AW, Featherstone J. Clinical protocols for caries management by risk assessment. J Calif Dent Assoc. 2007;35(10):714-723. Reprinted with permission from The Journal of California Dental Association.

Case Study

John and Sally are in their early thirties and have three children, ages 8, 6, and 4 years. They have had sporadic dental care the past few years because of lack of dental insurance. Kody, the 8-year-old, has composite restorations in both mandibular first molars and presents with generalized moderate biofilm. He states he forgot to brush that morning. The 6-year-old, Kyle, has no fillings or obvious decay, but he has white spot lesions and biofilm on the lingual surfaces of his mandibular molars. His first molars are fully erupted and he says he loves to brush his teeth. Klaire is 4 years old and this is her first visit to a dental office. She also likes to brush and lets her parents help when she brushes at night. John has class I restorations in all his posterior molars from when he was a teenager but no other evidence of new caries. Sally presents with little biofilm, remnants of sealant material in her second molars, and old class I amalgam restorations in her first molars with evidence of three interproximal lesions that require restorative care. She drinks multiple energy drinks a day to keep up with the three children and tends to snack between meals. She is not experiencing any sensitivity.

Case Study Exercises

1. Which family member has the highest risk for caries?
   A. John
   B. Sally
   C. Kody
   D. Kyle

2. Based on the case study, what is the caries risk status for Sally?
   A. Low risk
   B. Moderate risk
   C. High risk
   D. Extreme risk

3. What preventive recommendations would you recommend for the entire family?
   A. Use 1,000 ppm toothpaste two times daily.
   B. Place a reminder on the bathroom mirror to brush every morning and evening.
   C. Have fresh vegetables and cheese available for snacks.
   D. A and B
   E. A, B, and C

4. Which of the following specific measures would you NOT recommend for Sally?
   A. Reduce her energy drink consumption and/or drink it at mealtimes.
   B. Increase brushing to four times a day.
   C. Use prescription concentration fluoride (5,000 ppm) abrasive toothpaste.
   D. Choose gum and candies that contain xylitol.

5. What therapeutic recommendation(s) would you recommend for Kody and Kyle?
   A. Sealants on first molars
   B. Brushing twice a day for 2 minutes with 1,000 ppm toothpaste with parental supervision
   C. Fluoride mouthrinse once a day before bedtime
   D. A, B, and C
   E. None of the above

Review Questions

1. Which of the following plays the most important role in the remineralization process?
   A. Biofilm removal
   B. Limiting refined carbohydrates
   C. Fluoride
   D. Xylitol

2. Which of the following describes what occurs when the critical pH is reached?
   A. Demineralization occurs
   B. Remineralization occurs
   C. Neutral pH is reached
   D. Buffering occurs

3. What is the first clinical sign of demineralization?
   A. A dark spot in the pits and fissures
   B. A white spot lesion

   C. When a sealant is not retained
   D. Biofilm on the tooth surface

4. What is the single-most reliable factor in identifying a future risk for caries activity?
   A. Lack of community water fluoridation
   B. Poor dietary habits
   C. Low socioeconomic status
   D. Recent caries experience

5. Which of the following sugar alcohols has the greatest cariostatic effect?
   A. Sorbitol
   B. Mannitol
   C. Xylitol
   D. Glycol

Active Learning

1. Complete a 3-day diet diary. Record everything that you eat or drink during this period. Include at least one weekend day in the 3 days. Include all snacks, gum, candies, soft drinks, and so on. Circle and total all solid and liquid sugar/carbohydrate exposures in red. Multiply the number of solid exposures by 40 minutes and liquid exposures by 20 minutes (record as two different exposures if consumed 20 minutes apart). Add the solids and liquids to determine the total acid production for this period.

Form of Sugar	When Eaten	First Day	Second Day	Third Day
Liquid sugar	With meals			
(soda, sugar in coffee, etc.)	In between meals			
Solid sugar	With meals			
(cookie, cake, candy)	In between meals			

Grand total = _____ (sugar in liquid form)

Grand total = _____ (sugar in solid form)

_____ × 20 minutes = _____ ÷ 3 days = _____

Liquid Exposure   pH below   Acid Production   Daily liquid acid production

                              5.5

_____ × 40 minutes = _____ ÷ 3 days = _____

Solid Exposure   pH below   Acid Production   Daily solid acid production

                              5.5

Total daily acid production = _____ + _____ = _____

Liquid acid   Solid acid   Total time tooth is
production total   production total   exposed to acid daily
                                              (demineralization)

2. To demonstrate the amount of sugar in common beverages, place five glasses and five different sweetened beverages on a table. Have the class guess how many cubes of sugar are in each beverage (0.4 g sugar = 1 sugar cube). Have a different person come up and read each nutrition label. Add the number of corresponding sugar cubes to each glass. The person who guesses the closest to the total wins a prize (water bottle, pack of xylitol gum).

3. Eggshell Experiment: Obtain three jars or enough for each group and label each jar (1, 2, and 3). Place an unpeeled boiled egg in each jar. Pour in enough vinegar to cover the egg. Place a lid on the jar. Ask each group to record their observations each day. Remove the egg from the vinegar in jar 1 after the first day, remove the egg from jar 2 after the second day, and remove the last egg after the third day. Compare the groups' observations of changes that occurred to the eggshells. Relate how the eggshell is similar to the enamel on teeth and how enamel can break down from prolonged exposure to an acidic environment.

4. Stimulated saliva flow is easy to measure and can serve as an indicator of caries risk. Ask the patient to chew on paraffin wax and spit into a measuring vessel. The amount of saliva produced is measured in milliliters per minute. Normal flow is 1 to 3 mL/min, 0.7 to 1.0 mL/min is considered low, and less than 0.7 mL is very low. Discuss the results and make recommendations to maintain a healthy saliva flow or increase the flow if below normal.[8,47]

5. Choose three files of patients for whom you have completed comprehensive care. Remove identifying information. Review each patient's caries risk status and any recommendations you made to maintain or decrease their risk level. Share your findings with a classmate. Determine whether you accurately identified the risk level and whether there are additional therapeutic measures you could recommend. Evaluate recare interval and schedule an appointment if appropriate. ■

REFERENCES

1. Ruby JD, Cox, CF, Akimoto N. A review article. The caries phenomenon: a timeline from witchcraft and superstition to opinions of the 1500's to today's science. *Int J Dent.* 2010:1-10. doi:10.1155/2012/392730
2. Medical Dictionary for the Dental Professions. http://medical-dictionary.thefreedictionary.com/cariology. Accessed October 2, 2015.
3. Featherstone JD. Dental caries: a dynamic disease process. *Aust Dent J.* 2008;53(3):286-291.
4. Kawashita Y, Kitamura M, Saito T. Early childhood caries. *Int J Dent.* 2011:1-7. doi:10.1155/2011/725320
5. Rodrigues JA, Lussi A, Seemann. Prevention of crown and root caries in adults. *Periodontology 2000.* 2011;55:231-249.
6. Rosen B, Lamont RJ. Dental plaque formation. *Microbes Infect.* 2000;2:1599-1607.
7. Kutsch VK, Bowers RJ. *Balance. A Guide for Managing Dental Caries for Patients and Practitioners.* Tamarac, FL: Llumina Press; 2012.
8. Kleinberg I. A mixed-bacteria ecological approach to understanding the role of the oral bacteria in dental caries causation: an alternative to Streptococcus mutans and the specific-plaque hypothesis. *Crit Rev Oral Biol Med.* 2002;13(2):108-125.
9. Harris NO, Garcia-Godoy F, Nathe CN. *Primary Preventive Dentistry.* 7th ed. Cranbury, NJ: Pearson; 2009:29-45.
10. Carounanidy U, Sathyanarayanan R. Dental caries: a complete changeover (Part 1). *J Conserv Dent.* 2009; 12(2):46-54.
11. Featherstone JB, Domejean-Orliaguet S, Jenson L. Caries risk assessment in practice for age 6 through adult. *J Calif Dent Assoc.* 2007;35(10):703-713.
12. Stephan RM. Intraoral hydrogen ion concentrations associated with dental caries activity. *J Dent Res.* 1944; 23:257-266.
13. Marsh PD. Dental plaque as a biofilm and a microbial community—implications for health and disease. *BMC Oral Health.* 2006;6(suppl 1):S14.
14. American Dental Association Council on Scientific Affairs. Professionally applied topical fluoride: evidence-based clinical recommendations. *J Dent Educ.* 2007;71(3):393-402.
15. Walsh T, Worthington HV, Gleeny AM. Fluoride toothpastes of different concentrations for preventing dental caries in children and adolescents. *Cochrane Database Syst Rev.* 2010;(1):CD007868.
16. Featherstone JB. The science and practice of caries prevention. *J Calif Assoc.* 2000;13:887-899.
17. Marinho VC, Higgins JP, Sheiham A, Logan S. Combinations of topical fluoride (toothpastes, mouthrinses, gels, varnishes) versus single topical fluoride for preventing dental caries in children and adolescents. *Cochrane Database Syst Rev.* 2004;(1):CD002781.
18. Rethman M, Beltrán-Aguilar ED, Billings RJ, et al. Nonfluoride caries-preventive agents executive summary of evidence-based clinical recommendations. *J Am Dent Assoc.* 2011;142(9):1065-1071.
19. Featherstone JD, White JM, Hoover CI. A randomized clinical trial of anticaries therapies targeted according to risk assessment (caries management by risk assessment). *Caries Res.* 2012;46(2):118-129.
20. Jenson L, Budenz AW, Featherstone J. Clinical protocols for caries management by risk assessment. *J Calif Dent Assoc.* 2007;35(10):714-723.
21. Slot DE, Vaandrager NC, Loveren CV. The effect of chlorhexidine varnish on root caries: a systematic review. *Caries Res.* 2011;45:162-173.
22. Yengopal V, Mickenautsch S. Caries preventive effect of casein phosphopeptide-amorphous calcium phosphate (CPP-ACP): a meta-analysis. *Acta Odontol Scand.* 2009; 67(6):321-332.
23. Farooq I, Moheet IA, Imran Z, Farooq U. A review of novel dental caries preventive material: casein phosphopeptide–amorphous calcium phosphate (CPP–ACP) complex. *King Saud University J Dent Sci.* 2013;4:47-51.
24. Zhao J, Liu Y, Sun W and Zhang H. Amorphous calcium phosphate and its application in dentistry. *Chem Cent J.* 2011;5:40.
25. Karlinsey RL, Mackey AC, Walker ER, Frederick KE. Preparation, characterization, and in vitro efficacy of an acid-modified β-TCP material for dental hard-tissue remineralization. *Acta Biomater.* 2010;6:969-978.
26. Karlinsey RL, Mackey AC, Walker ER, et al. Remineralization potential of 5000 ppm fluoride dentifrices evaluated in a pH cycling model. *J Dent Oral Hyg.* 2010;2:1-6.
27. Andersson OH, Kangasniemi I. Calcium phosphate formation at the surface of bioactive glass in vitro. *J Biomed Mater Res.* 1991;25:1019-1030.
28. Burwell AK, Litkowski LJ, Greenspan DC. Calcium sodium phosphosilicate (NovaMin): remineralization potential. *Adv Dent Res.* 2009;21:35-39.
29. Maehara H, Iwami Y, Mayanagi H. Synergistic inhibition by combination of fluoride and xylitol on glycolysis by Mutant streptococci and its biochemical mechanism. *Caries Res.* 2005;39(6):521-528.
30. Dionysopoulos D, Koliniotou-Koumpia E, Helvatzoglou-Antoniades M, et al. Fluoride release and recharge abilities of contemporary fluoride-containing restorative materials and dental adhesives. *Dent Mater J.* 2013;32(2): 296-304.
31. Gladwin M, Bagby M. *Clinical Aspects of Dental Materials.* 4th ed. Philadelphia: Lippincott Williams & Wilkins; 2013.
32. Hicks J, Garcia-Godoy F, Donly K, Flaitz C. Fluoride-releasing restorative materials and secondary caries. *J Calif Dent Assoc.* 2003;31(3):229-245.
33. American Academy of Pediatric Dentistry. Reference manual. *Oral Health Policies.* 2011;34(6):50. http://www.aapd.org/media/Policies_Guidelines/P_ECC Classifications.pdf
34. American Academy of Pediatric Dentistry. Reference manual. *Oral Health Policies.* 2011;34(6). http://www.aapd.org/media/Policies_Guidelines/P_ECC Classifications.pdf
35. Institute of Medicine, Committee on an Oral Health Initiative. *Advancing Oral Health in America.* Published April 8, 2011. http://www.iom.edu/Reports/2011/Advancing-Oral-Health-in-America.aspx
36. Curzon MEJ, Preston AJ. Risk groups: nursing bottle caries/caries in the elderly. *Caries Res.* 2004;38 (suppl 1):24-33.
37. Dye BA, Tan S, Smith V. Trends in oral health status: United States, 1988–1994 and 1999–2004. National Center for Health Statistics. Vital Health Stat. 2007; 11(248).

38. Edelstein BL, Chinn CH. Update on disparities in oral health and access to dental care for America's children. *Acad Pediatr.* 2009;9(6):415-419.

39. *Diagnosis and Management of Dental Caries Throughout Life. NIH Consensus Statement.* 2001;18(1):1-30.

40. Amaechi BT. Emerging technologies for diagnosis of dental caries: the road so far. *J Appl Phys.* 2009;105:102047.

41. Rodriques JA, Hug I, Neuhaus KW, Lussi A. Light-emitting diode and laser fluorescence-based devices in detecting occlusal caries. *J Biomed Opt.* 2011;16(10):107003.

42. Rochlen G, Wolff, MS. Technological advances in caries diagnosis. *Dent Clin North Am.* 2011;55:441-452.

43. Rainey JT. Air abrasion: an emerging standard of care in conservative operative dentistry. *Dent Clin North Am.* 2002;46(2):185-209.

44. Young DA, Featherstone JB, Roth JR. Curing the silent epidemic: caries management in the 21st century and beyond. *J Calif Dent Assoc.* 2007;35(10):681-685.

45. Murdoch-Kinch CA, McLean ME. Minimally invasive dentistry. *J Am Dent Assoc.* 2003;134:87-95.

46. Freudenthal J. How to encourage change. *Dimens Dent Hyg.* 2010(9):60-65.

47. American Academy of Pediatric Dentistry. Guidelines for caries-risk assessment and management for infants, children, and adolescents. *Reference Manual.* Revised 2014. 32(6):101-108. http://www.aapd.org/media/Policies_Guidleines/G_CariesRiskAssessment.pdf

48. Ramos-Gomez FJ, Crall J, Gansky SA, et al. Caries risk assessment appropriate for the age 1 visit (infants and toddlers). *J Calif Dent Assoc.* 2007;35(10):687-702.

49. Doméjean-Orliaguet S, Gansky SA, Featherstone JB. Caries risk assessment in an educational environment. *J Dent Educ.* 2006;70(12):1346-1354.

50. Bader JD, Perin NA, Maupome' G, Rindal B, Rush WA. Validation of a simple approach to caries risk assessment. *J Public Health Dent.* 2005;65(2):76-81.

51. Doméjean-Orliaguet S, White, JM, Featherstone JB. Validation of the CDA CAMBRA Caries Risk Assessment—a six-year retrospective study. *J Calif Dent Assoc.* 2011; 39(10):709-714.

52. American Academy of Pediatrics. Oral health risk assessment timing and establishment of the dental home. *Pediatrics.* 2003;111:1113-1116.

53. Smile for Life, A National Oral Health Curriculum. www.smilesforlifeoralhealth.org. Accessed Oct 2, 2015.

54. Kutsch KV, Young DA. New directions in the etiology of dental caries disease. *J Calif Dent.* 2011;39:716-720.

Chapter 22 | Sealants

Rachel C. Kearney, RDH, MS

KEY TERMS

acid etching

autopolymerization

bisphenol A-glycidyl
    methacrylate
    (bis-GMA)

filled sealants

photopolymerization

polymerization

sealant

self-etching

unfilled sealants

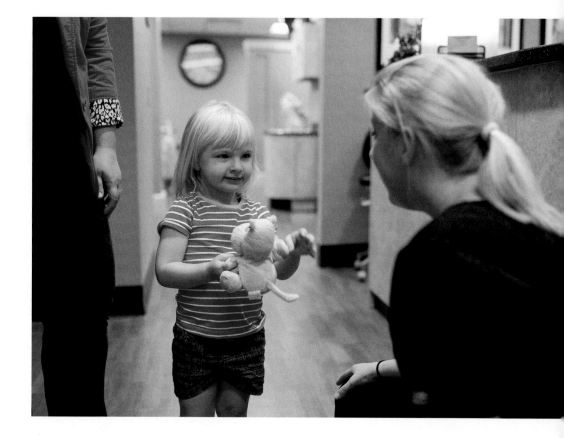

LEARNING OBJECTIVES

After reading this chapter, the student should be able to:

22.1 Discuss how sealants are part of an overall caries risk assessment and
    management protocol.

22.2 Outline the advantages and disadvantages of different types of sealants.

22.3 Successfully isolate a tooth in preparation for sealant placement.

22.4 Place a sealant and evaluate for retention.

22.5 Explain the sealant procedure to a patient.

KEY CONCEPTS

• Sealants are a primary way to prevent carious lesions in pits and fissures.

• Evaluation of sealants is a part of overall risk assessment.

• Proper technique and adherence to manufacturer's instructions are
  necessary for success in sealant placement.

RELEVANCE TO CLINICAL PRACTICE

Dental caries is the most common dental disease; it affects people of all ages. Five times more children have dental caries than asthma, hay fever, and chronic bronchitis combined. Eighty-five percent of adults have caries or have been treated for caries.[1] Caries is an infectious disease and, ironically, is preventable. Caries rates dropped drastically in the 1950s because of water fluoridation and increased use and awareness of the benefits of fluoride. Fluoride works best against smooth surface caries but does not always flow into the pits and fissures of teeth. It is well established that pit and fissure caries can be reduced by the placement of resin-based sealants. Studies show that reduction rates of caries range from 86% at 1 year to 58.6% at 4 years after placement.[2] It is crucial that dental hygienists be familiar with and skilled at the placement of dental sealants to effectively help their patients prevent oral disease.

WHAT ARE SEALANTS?

Definition

A dental **sealant** is a resin material that is placed into the pits and fissures of teeth at risk for caries. Sealants were first developed in the 1960s by Dr. Michael Buonocore and his colleagues at the Eastman Dental Center.[3] Over the last half century, sealants have advanced and improved and have become one of the primary ways of preventing pit and fissure caries.[4]

Composition

Dental sealants are composed of dimethacrylate monomers. These monomers may be **bisphenol A-glycidyl methacrylate (bis-GMA)** or urethane dimethacrylate. Types of sealants are classified by filler content, method of polymerization, color, and releasing properties (Table 22-1).

Fillers are added to sealants to increase the durability and make them more resistant to occlusal wear.[5] **Filled sealants** have silica and quartz particles added to increase strength and hardness. **Unfilled sealants** have less strength and hardness, but they usually do not require occlusal adjustment because occlusal forces will wear away any areas of the sealant that are high.

Sealants can be autopolymerized or photopolymerized. **Polymerization** is a chemical reaction in which monomers are linked to create a polymer.[6] In the case of dental sealants, polymerization refers to hardening. Materials for **autopolymerized**, or self-polymerized, sealants come in two parts, a catalyst and base, which must be mixed uniformly and placed quickly because polymerization starts as the materials combine. **Photopolymerized** sealants are polymerized by visible light. A curing light is used to harden the sealant once it has been placed into pits and fissures. The clinician is required to use proper safety glasses or shields when using a curing light because of its ultraviolet properties.

Sealants come in a variety of colors including opaque, tinted, and optically neutral. Tinted sealants have a slight color added to aid the application into the pits and fissures. Some tinted sealants turn white upon polymerization and aid in the application process. Tinted and opaque sealants make it easier for the clinician to see where the sealant has been placed and aid

Table 22-1. *Types of Sealants*			
Classification of Sealants			
Polymerization Method	**Filler Content**	**Color**	**Releasing**
Autopolymerized • Self-cured • Mixing two parts is required	Filled • Glass and quartz particles increase hardness and strength	Clear or optically neutral • Can be used in conjunction with caries detection devices	Fluoride releasing • Sealants that contain fluoride to increase caries resistance
Photopolymerized • Cured by light	Unfilled • Do not contain particles; less resistant to wear	Tinted • Aids in placement because of the contrast in color Opaque • Easy to evaluate for retention	Amorphous calcium phosphate releasing • Release calcium and phosphate ions to remineralize

in identifying sealant margins when assessing for retention at recall appointments. Optically neutral sealants allow for use with some caries detection devices.

Another option is to have a sealant that releases fluoride or amorphous calcium phosphate (ACP). Fluoride and ACP-releasing sealants have the potential to increase the resistance to caries and to remineralize incipient carious lesions. Fluoride has long been proved to aid in the prevention of caries.[1] ACP has shown potential to remineralize incipient carious lesions.[7,8] Currently, little research exists on using sealants as a vehicle to deliver ACP to pits and fissures, although there is great potential for this benefit (see Advancing Technologies).

How Sealants Work

Sealants work by creating a physical barrier between cariogenic bacteria and the susceptible pit and fissure surfaces of the tooth. For the sealant to bond to the tooth surface, acid-etching must be used to prepare the enamel surface. Etch is usually a 35% solution of phosphoric acid in a liquid or gel form. The **acid etch** creates a microscopic roughness on the enamel surface, which the sealant flows into; a mechanical bond is then created.[9] Etch is applied on the pits and fissures for 15 to 60 seconds (follow the manufacturer's instructions). Research shows that leaving acid etch in place for longer than 30 seconds does not increase the bond strength.[10,11]

INDICATIONS FOR SEALANTS

Risk Assessment

A proper risk assessment should be completed as part of the decision-making process for the placement of sealants (see Chapter 17). When the clinician determines that the patient is at risk for dental caries, sealants should be placed in the pits and fissures of potentially affected permanent teeth. Pit and fissure

Advancing Technologies

As with many dental products, dental sealants continue to improve as technology advances. Today, the market offers sealants that are colored to aid in visualization of placement; once polymerized, the sealant becomes white. Also available are sealants that are **self-etching.** Research has shown that these self-etching sealants have potential and would eliminate a step in the sealant procedure; however, retention rates associated with self-etching sealants have not been as high as those associated with etching with phosphoric acid and then rinsing.[9,10] ■

Spotlight on Public Health

The Columbus, Ohio, Department of Health has taken action to increase access to care and created a school-based dental sealant program. This program provides second and sixth graders in the Columbus Public Schools the opportunity to have dental sealants placed at their school. Schools that qualify for this program have a high concentration of low-income and minority students. Once the parents have given permission, students are screened, and dental hygienists and dental assistants place sealants on permanent teeth. The procedure is done at the school, during the school day, with portable dental equipment. Since 1986, more than 53,000 children have received more than 180,000 sealants. ■

sealants may also be placed on early carious lesions in children, adolescents, and young adults to decrease the progress of the lesion.[2] Assessments for caries include determining oral, medical, environmental, or behavioral risk factors (see Spotlight on Public Health). Oral risk factors may include history of caries or the presence of deep pits and fissures. An example of a medical risk factor would be a medication that causes xerostomia (dry mouth). Environmental risk factors are associated with the circumstances or surrounding in which the patient lives; for example, a patient who does not have access to optimally fluoridated drinking water is at risk for caries. Behavioral risk factors are primarily associated with oral hygiene habits. Poor oral hygiene and a highly cariogenic diet increase the likelihood of caries.[12]

Tooth Anatomy

Tooth anatomy is another factor to consider when creating a care plan that includes sealants. Debris and biofilm cannot be removed properly from pits and fissures with a toothbrush; therefore, there is a higher risk for caries in these areas. Pits and fissures on permanent teeth can be U-, V-, Y-, or Y2-shaped (Fig. 22-1).[13] Several types of pits and fissures may exist on the same tooth. Most commonly, sealants are placed on the occlusal surfaces of permanent molars and premolars. Anatomy of the lingual surfaces of the maxillary incisors should also be evaluated for sealant placement. Regardless of the location and shape of the fissures, sealants are an effective way to prevent caries in these areas.

Contraindications

Most patients will benefit from the placement of dental sealants, but there are contraindications to this procedure. Contraindications to sealant placement are:

- Allergies to any material in the sealant, as revealed by the medical history

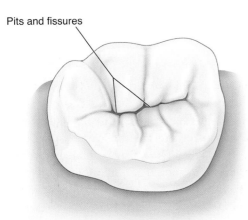

Figure 22-1. Pits and fissures have different shapes.

- Caries that extend into the dentin, which will not benefit from sealants the way incipient caries can; caries that extend into the dentin should be treated with restorative procedures
- Insufficient eruption; partial eruption can make it difficult to place sealant on all pits and fissures
- Coalesced, shallow, fused fissures; these flat fissures do not benefit from the placement of sealants
- Proximal caries; at this time sealants are not used to treat incipient proximal caries, but products are being developed to treat this area.

SEALANT PLACEMENT

Placement of pit and fissure sealants is a technique-sensitive procedure. Errors in sealant placement can lead to decreased retention and ineffectiveness of sealants. The most important principle of sealant placement is to maintain a dry field (see Application to Clinical Practice). Saliva contamination is a common reason for sealant failure. Patient behavior, age, salivary flow, and cooperation can all affect the placement of dental sealants.[14]

Ideally, sealants should be placed using a four-handed delivery technique. Four-handed delivery has

Application to Clinical Practice

You have decided to volunteer for Sealant Day, a day-long program run by your local dental hygiene society in conjunction with the local dental society. The event will take place in a school cafeteria. You have been put in charge of purchasing supplies for Sealant Day and you have discovered that patients will be seen in normal chairs and volunteers will be using flashlights instead of dental lights. You have some concerns about how you will maintain a dry field during sealant placement and what you will do if the sealant needs to be adjusted after evaluation. What are some of your ideas to solve these problems? ■

shown to increase the retention of sealants (see Teamwork).[7] Realistically, this is not always possible, so dental hygienists must be highly skilled in sealant placement both on their own and with an assistant.

Teamwork

Jill is waiting for her next patient to arrive; he is already 10 minutes late for his recall appointment, and he has a history of not showing up for his visits. While she is waiting she notices that another hygienist in the office, Beth, is trying to place sealants on a squirmy 6-year-old boy. No assistants are available to help at the moment, so you check at the desk to make sure your patient has not arrived; then you head into Beth's room to assist her with the sealants. Having an extra pair of hands makes it much easier to place the sealants in a dry field, and the two of you successfully finish all four sealants. Beth is grateful for your help and she says she will repay the favor if you ever need an extra hand. ■

Procedure 22-1   Sealant Placement

MATERIALS AND PREPARATION

Familiarity with the necessary materials and proper preparation for sealant placement is essential in utilizing time and resources. Being prepared for the procedure will eliminate stress and difficulty during the treatment.

Gather and organize the necessary materials before the patient's arrival.

Materials

Mirror. For indirect vision and retraction of the tongue
Explorer. To evaluate sealant retention

Air/water syringe tip. For rinsing and drying tooth surface during sealant placement
High-volume evacuation tip and/or saliva ejector. High-volume evacuation is preferred but can be difficult to handle if placing sealants without an assistant
Prophy brush on slow-speed handpiece. To clear the occlusal surface of debris before sealant placement
Cotton rolls and cotton-roll holders. Placed on the buccal and lingual sides of mandibular teeth and the buccal side of maxillary teeth being sealed
Dry angles. Triangular absorbent discs placed over the parotid duct to reduce salivary contamination

Sealant material. Many different options are available for sealant materials; always refer to manufacturer instructions before placing sealants

Acid etch. Usually, a 35% phosphoric acid etch in a liquid or gel; concentrations from 15%–50% are also used

Curing light (if appropriate). To set photopolymerized sealants

Floss. To ensure that interproximal areas have not been closed with sealant material

Articulating paper and holder. To evaluate the occlusion of the sealants

1.1% Neutral sodium fluoride and trays. To remineralize areas of enamel that were acid etched

Optional Items

Rubber dam. Provides the best isolation, but is not commonly used

Bite block. For patients who have difficulty keeping their mouths open

Toothbrush. Cleaning debris from the occlusal surface of teeth with a toothbrush is an accepted method of preparing a tooth for sealants

Pumice. Nonfluoridated pumice or nonfluoridated prophy paste can be used to prepare the teeth for sealants

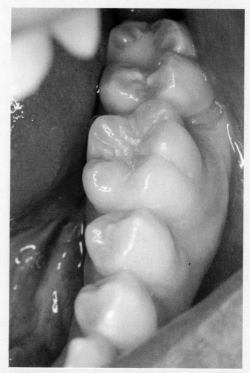

Tooth before sealant is placed.

PROCEDURE

1. *Prepare tooth.*
- There are many ways to prepare the tooth for sealant placement. Any of the following are acceptable methods for cleaning the surfaces of the pit and fissures:
  - Tooth brushing
  - Air abrasion
  - Prophy brush, with or without pumice
  - Explorer
  - Rinse any debris still in the area of sealant placement.

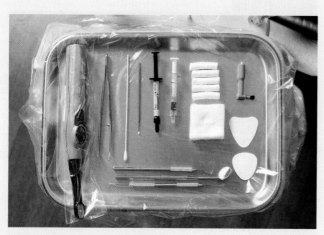

Materials needed to place sealants.

PREPROCEDURE

Patient Education

The patient, parent, or both must be educated on what a sealant is, how it will be applied, and the reason for sealant placement.

Informed Consent

Informed consent is required before placing sealants on all patients. Sealants are commonly applied on children's newly erupted teeth between the ages of 6 and 12 years. When treating the pediatric patients, it is essential to obtain consent from the parent or guardian before proceeding with treatment.

Selection of Teeth

- Based on the indications for sealants, identify which teeth are to be sealed.
- It is often helpful and time-efficient to work by quadrant.

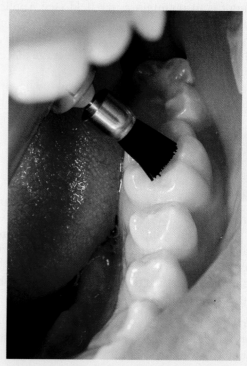

Prepare the tooth with a prophy brush.

2. *Isolate*.
- Isolation is an essential step in preventing contamination of sealants. Isolation should be completed by using cotton rolls and dry angles or, less commonly, by placing a rubber dam.
- Dry angles should be placed against the buccal mucosa to absorb salivary secretions from the parotid duct.
- Cotton rolls should be placed on the buccal and lingual sides of mandibular teeth to control salivary contamination.
- The maxillary teeth may require cotton rolls on the buccal side of the teeth to be sealed in the case of an active parotid gland.

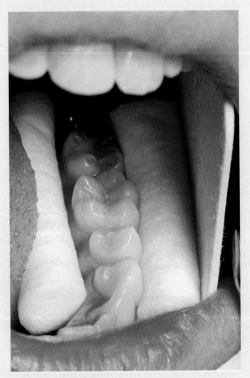

A properly isolated tooth.

3. *Dry tooth*.
- Dry the tooth with air from the air/water syringe.
- Ensure isolation is adequate and the tooth is completely dry.

4. *Apply acid etch*.
- Apply acid etch to pits and fissures for 15 to 30 seconds, or according to the manufacturer's directions.
- Rinse the tooth surface with water until free of etch (30–60 seconds).
- If high-volume evacuation is available, it should be used in this step to effectively and efficiently remove etch from tooth surface and minimize contact of etch with oral soft tissue.

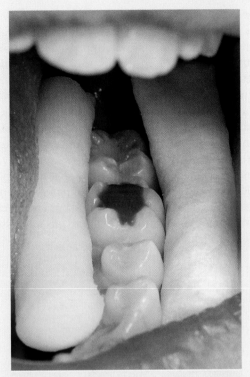

Etch on tooth.

5. *Dry tooth*.
- Evaluate isolation. If the area is not adequately isolated, re-isolate to prevent saliva contamination.
- Dry the tooth with air from the air/water syringe.
- Tooth may appear chalky white, but this is not essential to create proper adhesion.

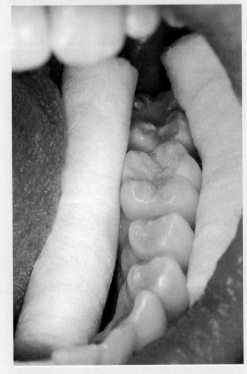

Chalky white etched tooth.

6. *Apply sealant.*
- Mix sealant material if autopolymerized.
- Using the sealant applicator, apply sealant to pit and fissures only. Be sure to apply sealant to buccal and lingual grooves, if indicated.
- If the sealant is photopolymerized, there is time to remove excess sealant material before curing. Once mixed, autopolymerized sealants begin to polymerize immediately, allowing little time to remove excess material.
- Some products come with a large application tip, which may distribute more sealant material than necessary. An explorer or microbrush is effective in distributing the sealant material into pits and fissures.

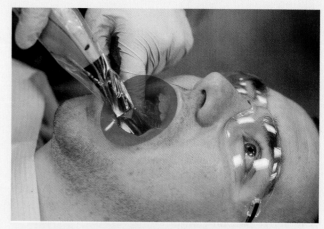

A curing light is used to cure the sealant.

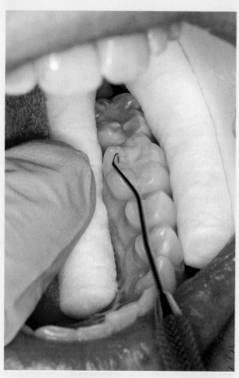

An explorer can be used to distribute the sealant.

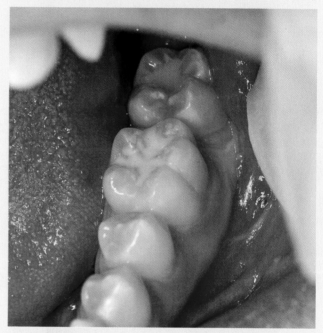

Cured sealant.

7. *Cure.*
- Autopolymerized sealants self-cure.
- Photopolymerized sealants need to be cured with a curing light.
  - Place the end of the curing light 5 to 10 mm above the newly placed sealant and turn on the light.
  - Be sure to use proper safety techniques with the curing light, which include proper safety glasses or shields for the clinician to block the light.

8. *Evaluate.*
- With the explorer, evaluate the sealant for air bubbles or voids. Also evaluate the margins for retention.
- If additional sealant material is needed, the area of placement should be re-etched.
- Occlusion should be evaluated with articulating paper on filled sealants only; unfilled sealants will adjust themselves. Specific attention should be paid to the articulation on the sealant itself. If occlusion is not correct, the sealant should be adjusted with a bur to allow for correct occlusion.

- Use floss to ensure that interproximal spaces were not closed with the sealant material. If interproximal spaces are closed, an appropriate bur or sandpaper strip may be used to remove the sealant material interproximally. The patient should be able to floss this area adequately.
9. *Remineralize.*
- Apply neutral sodium fluoride in a tray or fluoride varnish to remineralize areas on the teeth that were acid etched.

POSTPROCEDURE

After any dental procedure, the patient and, if the patient is a minor, the parent or guardian should be informed about the results of the procedure and given postprocedure instructions. The following issues should be discussed with the patient and parent or guardian after placing dental sealants:

- Evaluate how the patient tolerated the procedure.
- Chewing surface of the teeth may feel slightly different, but this sensation will diminish.
- Eating and drinking can resume after the specified time limit because of application of fluoride.
- The procedure is not likely to cause any discomfort postprocedurally.
- It is possible that the sealant might chip, but this is not an emergency.
- Proper oral hygiene should be reinforced.
- The sealant will be re-evaluated at each visit.

RETENTION AND REPLACEMENT

According to the research, sealants are retained on permanent molars at a rate of 76%. Most often sealant loss occurs soon after placement and is usually caused by poor technique in isolation (see Evidence-Based Practice).[5] At each recall visit, sealants should be evaluated by visual examination and with an explorer for retention and need of replacement. A sealant may come off completely or only partially. In either case, if this is noted on examination, the sealant should be redone. Sealants can be replaced without removing any retained sealant material. The area must be re-etched and isolated before placement to ensure proper retention.

DISCUSSION ISSUES

Bisphenol A and Estrogenicity

Patients have access to many resources through the media and internet sites. Often, a patient will read or hear about possible negative side effects associated with common procedures. One of the topics related to dental sealants is the potential for the sealant material to release bisphenol A (BPA). BPA has received publicity for its presence in plastic food containers and baby bottles. It has been established that low levels of BPA are released from unreacted monomers, such as those in a sealant. The concern is that BPA has a potential for estrogenicity, which has been reported to disrupt sperm production, prostate weight, and sexual differentiation and to alter mammary gland development in laboratory animals.[15]

Research has shown that these low levels of BPA are not detectable in saliva or the bloodstream 3 hours after sealant placement.[16,17] The U.S. Food and Drug Administration found that products on the market today are safe for use; therefore, the current protocol for use of sealants is appropriate and safe.[18] As a dental hygienist, it is important to be able to discuss the concerns that patients may have over certain procedures. Currently, the benefits of sealants outweigh the possible risk for exposure to BPA, although research continues on the potential risks of BPA exposure during sealant placement.

Sealants and Incipient Caries

Sealants can be successfully placed to prevent further progression of incipient caries. Originally, there was concern that the sealant would trap bacteria in the pit and the caries would proliferate. Currently, no findings substantiate this theory, and it has been found that sealants actually reduce the bacteria that cause decay, thus reducing the number of carious lesions.[2,19] It is also important to keep in mind that teeth with sealants have a lower rate of caries than teeth that are not sealed. When weighing the benefits of the sealant procedure, it is clear that areas of incipient caries can be sealed and may arrest the caries process. Researchers are also experimenting with sealing interproximal incipient caries.[20,21]

Evidence-Based Practice

Research shows that using good isolation and placement technique for sealants helps to increase the retention rate. If you notice that sealants are being lost soon after they are placed, or when patients come back for their recall visits the sealants are no longer present, it is time to evaluate your technique. Take deliberate notes on how isolation is done and what may be done to improve isolation. Also evaluate the manufacturer's directions and be sure to follow all instructions given. Maintaining a dry field is one of the most important steps in successful sealant placement, so spend some time evaluating your isolation technique and examine ways to improve your isolation. ■

Sealants continue to be part of an overall caries risk assessment and management protocol. Many types of sealants are available for use, so it is important to understand the basics behind each type of sealant. Choices should be made by clinicians after learning, using, and evaluating which product meets the needs of the patients and the clinician. When placing sealants, it is important to adhere to good techniques and follow manufacturers' instructions for placement to successfully place and retain the sealants.

Case Study

Jason, a 6 ½-year-old boy, tells his mother that he has a "sore spot" in the back of his mouth. His mother looks but cannot see anything. She calls the dental office to make an appointment to have Jason examined. The dental hygienist notes a mixed dentition during Jason's examination. Jason complains of a sore area posterior to the last molar in his mouth on the mandibular left. The hygienist also notes that Jason has had three restorations in the past year, and there is generalized moderate biofilm present.

Case Study Exercises

1. What primary teeth are likely to be completely erupted on the mandibular arch?
   A. A, B, C, H, I, J
   B. K, L, M, R, S, T
   C. K, L, M, N, O, P
   D. E, F, G, H, I, J

2. What permanent teeth are likely to be completely erupted on the mandibular arch?
   A. #21, #22, #23, #28, #29, #30
   B. #23, #24, #25, #26
   C. #18, #19, #20, #21
   D. #17, #18, #19, #30, #31, #32

3. The "sore area" on the gingiva posterior to the last primary molar is likely:
   A. An abscess
   B. Eruption of #30
   C. Eruption of #19
   D. Eruption of #3

4. Referring to question 3, Jason is at high risk for caries. The dental hygienist should recommend a dental sealant be applied immediately after full eruption.
   A. The first statement is true, but the second statement is false.
   B. The first statement is false, but the second statement is true.
   C. Both statements are true.
   D. Both statements are false.

5. Upon examination of the mandibular right, the dental hygienist notes the presence of tooth _____ immediately posterior to the last primary molar. What tooth is this?
   A. #19
   B. #31
   C. #18
   D. #30

Review Questions

1. Which of the following is the best indication for placing a dental sealant on a tooth?
   A. Caries that extend into the dentin
   B. Well-coalesced pits and fissures
   C. Not well-coalesced pits and fissures
   D. A child who cannot sit still

2. Which of the following descriptions best indicates the effectiveness of a pit and fissure sealant?
   A. Remineralizes the pit and fissures
   B. Creates a physical barrier from bacteria
   C. Prevents dental caries
   D. Allows dental caries to proliferate in fissures

3. What would you use to assess for excess sealant material on the occlusal surface?
   A. Articulating paper
   B. Dental floss
   C. A rubber dam
   D. Cotton-roll holders

4. What would you use to assess for excess sealant material in the proximal areas?
   A. Articulating paper
   B. Dental floss
   C. A rubber dam
   D. Cotton-roll holders

5. Acid-etched tooth enamel may appear:
   A. Dull and rough
   B. Dull and smooth
   C. Chalky white and opaque
   D. Smooth and reflective

Active Learning

1. Use an explorer on an extracted tooth (molars and premolars) to feel pits and fissures. Are they well-coalesced? If the answer is yes, there should be no "tug-back" areas.

2. Use an explorer on an extracted tooth (molars or premolars) with pits and fissures that are not well-coalesced. Use the explorer to feel the "tug back" of the area.

3. As you feel the "tug back'" in item 2, listen to the explorer as it pulls out of the sticky area.

4. Look at text pictures of pits and fissures under a microscope that demonstrate well-coalesced and poorly coalesced pits and fissures (Fig. 22-1).

5. Use visual aids (large model teeth), pictures, video, and radiographs to show examples of teeth that indicate the placement of sealants compared with teeth that do not need to be sealed. ■

REFERENCES

1. U.S. Department of Health and Human Services. *Oral Health in America: A Report of the Surgeon General.* Rockville, MD: U.S. Department of Health and Human Services, National Institute of Dental and Craniofacial Research, National Institutes of Health, 2000.

2. Beauchamp J, Caufield PW, Crall JJ, et al. Evidence-based clinical recommendations for the use of pit-and-fissure sealants. *J Am Dent Assoc.* 2008;139:257-268.

3. Handelman SL, Shey, Z. Michael Buonocore, and the Eastman Dental Center: a historic perspective on sealants. *J Dent Res.* 1996;75:529-534.

4. Ahovuo-Saloranta A, Hiiri A, Nordblad A, et al. Pit and fissure sealants for preventing dental decay in the permanent teeth of children and adolescents. *Cochrane Database Syst Rev.* 2008;(4):CD001830.

5. Powers JM, Wataha JC. *Dental Materials Properties and Manipulation.* 9th rev. ed. St. Louis, MO: Mosby Elsevier; 2008.

6. Gladwin M, Bagby M. *Clinical Aspects of Dental Materials Theory, Practice, and Cases.* 3rd rev. ed. Philadelphia: Lippincott Williams & Wilkins; 2009.

7. Llena C, Forner L, Baca P. Anticariogenicity of casein phosphopeptide-amorphous calcium phosphate: a review of the literature. *J Contemp Dent Pract.* 2009; 10(3):1-9.

8. Reynolds EC. Calcium phosphate-based remineralization systems: scientific evidence? *Aust Dent J.* 2008;53: 268-273.

9. Ferracane JL. *Materials in Dentistry Principles and Applications.* 2nd rev. ed. Philadelphia: Lippincott Williams & Wilkins; 2009.

10. Obeidi A, Liu P, Ramp LC, et al. Acid-etch interval and shear bond strength of Er, Cr:YSGG laser-prepared enamel and dentin. *Lasers Med Sci.* 2010;25(3): 363-369.

11. Reis AF, Aguiar FH, Pereira PN, Giannini M. Effects of surface texture and etching time on roughness and bond strength to ground enamel. *J Contemp Dent Pract.* 10;4:17-25.

12. Rethman J. Trends in preventive care: caries risk assessment and indications for sealants. *J Am Dent Assoc.* 2000;131:8-12.

13. Selecman JB, Owens BM, Johnson WW. Effect of preparation technique, fissure morphology, and material characteristics on the in vitro margin permeability and penetrability of pit and fissure sealants. *Pediatr Dent.* 2007;29:308-314.

14. Griffin SO, Jones K, Gray SK, et al. Exploring four-handed delivery and retention of resin-based sealants. *J Am Dent Assoc.* 2008;139:281-289.

15. Joskow R, Barr DB, Barr JR, Calafat AM, Needham LL, Rubin C. Exposure to bisphenol A from bis-glycidyl dimethacrylate-based dental sealants. *J Am Dent Assoc.* 2006;137:353-362.

16. Fung EY, Ewoldsen NO, St. Germain HA, et al. Pharmacokinetics of bisphenol a released from a dental sealant. *J Am Dent Assoc.* 2000;131:51-58.

17. Palanza P, Gioiosa L, vom Saal FS, Parmigiani S. Effects of developmental exposure to bisphenol A on brain and behavior in mice. *Environ Res.* 2008; 108:150-157.

18. American Dental Association. Statement on dental products and bisphenol a exposure. Published September 11, 2008. www.ada.org. Accessed May 15, 2009.

19. Amin HE. Clinical and antibacterial effectiveness of three different sealant materials. *J Dent Hyg.* 2008; 82:1-10.

20. Gomez SS, Basili CP, Emilson C. A 2-year clinical evaluation of sealed noncavitated aproximal posterior carious lesions in adolescents. *Clin Oral Invest.* 2005; 9:239-243.

21. Alkilzy M, Berndt C, Meller C, et al. Sealing of proximal surfaces with polyurethane tape: a two-year clinical and radiographic feasibility study. *J Adhes Dent.* 2009; 11(2):91-94.

Chapter 23 | Prostheses and Appliances

Catherine Draper, RDH, MS

KEY TERMS

abutment

appliance

Candida albicans

complete denture

denture

denture stomatitis

fixed bridge

implant

osseointegration

overdenture

peri-implantitis

peri-implant mucositis

permucosal seal

pontic

prosthesis

removable partial
   denture

titanium

ultrasonic cleaner

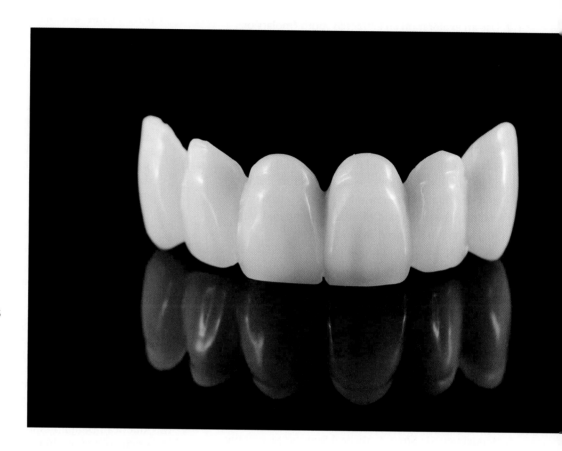

LEARNING OBJECTIVES

After reading this chapter, the student should be able to:

23.1 Describe the various ways missing teeth can be restored with fixed and removable prostheses.

23.2 Discuss the role dental implants play in replacing missing teeth.

23.3 Describe the various types of fixed and removable appliances used to influence the shape or function of the mouth and jaw.

23.4 Explain the importance of good oral hygiene, self-cleaning practices, and professional care for patients with prostheses and oral appliances.

23.5 Demonstrate appropriate self-care procedures for prostheses and oral appliances to a patient.

23.6 Discuss the necessary modifications in instrumentation for patients with implant-supported prostheses.

KEY CONCEPTS

• Missing teeth can be replaced with a variety of fixed and removable prostheses.

• Dental hygienists need to be familiar with all of the available treatment modalities for replacing missing teeth.

- Dental hygienists need to be familiar with the various types of fixed and removable oral appliances designed to influence the shape and function of the oral-facial structures.
- Prostheses and oral appliances require regular self-care and professional maintenance for optimal health and function.

RELEVANCE TO CLINICAL PRACTICE

The goal of modern dentistry is to restore individuals to optimal oral health in a predictable fashion regardless of oral disease, developmental defects, or injury to the oral and craniofacial system.[1] Millions of people in the United States alone experience dental caries, periodontal diseases, and anatomical defects such as cleft lip and palate. In 2004, more than 45% of adults in the United States, aged 65 years and older, were found to have six or more teeth missing.[2] Tooth loss caused by dental disease, congenital defects, and trauma affect an individual's ability to eat, swallow, and speak without discomfort, as well as her ability to maintain a healthy facial appearance. Malpositioned teeth and abnormal jaw relationships also influence an individual's ability to chew, eat, and speak, in addition to playing a role in the incidence of dental and periodontal infections and the individual's overall self-esteem. Oral disease caused by malignancies presents challenges in restoring function to the oral-facial structures. An estimated 30,000 cases of oral and pharyngeal cancers are diagnosed annually in the United States alone, creating a need for oral rehabilitation after surgical treatment.[3]

Dental hygienists must be well educated in the various treatment modalities and devices used in replacing missing oral structures, and they must recognize the various appliances that are designed to provide a therapeutic effect in the oral cavity. Dental hygienists must be able to educate patients regarding their treatment options and teach the appropriate self-care strategies. Dental hygienists must also be able to identify the materials used in oral prostheses and appliances, and apply the appropriate instrumentation principles for the professional care of these devices.

WHAT ARE ORAL APPLIANCES AND PROSTHESES?

Oral **appliances** are devices designed to provide a function or therapeutic effect in the mouth (Table 23-1). Appliances can be fixed, as in resin-bonded orthodontic bands and brackets, or removable, as in a removable retainer designed to maintain tooth position. **Prostheses** are artificial replacements of a missing body part (Table 23-2). An oral prosthesis can range from a **pontic** designed to replace a single missing tooth in a fixed bridge to complete **dentures** fabricated to replace all the teeth in the dentition. Oral-facial structures that are missing due to congenital defects such as a cleft palate or disease such as nasopharyngeal cancer can be replaced with an oral prostheses or obturator designed to close the defect.

ORAL APPLIANCES

Oral appliances, both fixed and removable, come in direct contact with the teeth and the oral tissues and require regular care and maintenance (Figures 23-1, 23-2, 23-3, and 23-4). Removable oral appliances serve a wide variety of functions ranging from custom-fitted fluoride trays and orthodontic retainers to full upper and lower dentures. Plaque biofilm forming on the appliance, as well as the adjacent tooth structures, can lead to inflammation, edema, gingival hyperplasia, enamel decalcification, and dental caries. Maintenance of optimal oral health is dependent on an individual's ability to clean the natural teeth and oral soft tissues, as well as the oral appliances. Patients must be familiar with the unique characteristics of their particular appliance and the materials it is made from to ensure its optimal function

Table 23-1. *Types of Oral Appliances*

Appliance	Function
Obturator	• Removable • Replaces a defect or opening created as the result of disease, trauma, or birth defect
Orthodontic appliance	• May be fixed or removed • Designed to influence the growth and/or position of the teeth and jaw structure
Orthodontic aligner	• Removable • Fabricated with the use of a computer-aided design system, sets of aligners are designed to fit over the biting surfaces of the maxillary and mandibular teeth; consecutive use of aligners repositions the teeth
Retaining appliance	• May be fixed or removable • Designed to hold the teeth in place after orthodontic therapy to stabilize the occlusion
Nightguard	• Removable • Worn while sleeping; designed to cover the occlusal and incisal surfaces of either the maxillary or the mandibular teeth to protect them from trauma caused by clenching or bruxing
Snore guard	• Removable • Designed to reposition the mandible to inhibit snoring
Splint	• May be fixed or removable • Designed to immobilize and stabilize the teeth while protecting them from occlusal forces • Can be worn day and night
Sports guard	• Removable • Designed to fit over the maxillary teeth and provide protection from possible trauma during athletic activities
Stent	• Removable • Designed to maintain or protect tissue such as in soft tissue grafting for periodontal defects; also used as a positioning guide in implant surgery

Table 23-2. *Types of Dental Prostheses*

Prosthesis	Function
Denture	• General term to describe an artificial substitute for missing natural teeth and the adjacent tissues
Complete (full) dentures	• Removable • Prosthesis that replaces an entire arch of missing teeth and the adjacent tissues • May replace the maxillary arch, mandibular arch, or both arches
Overdenture	• Removable or fixed • Complete denture supported by multiple dental implants
Removable partial denture	• Removable • Prosthesis designed to replace multiple missing teeth and the adjacent tissues
Fixed partial denture (bridge)	• Fixed • Prosthesis designed to replace one or more missing teeth • Bonded to the adjacent retained natural teeth or implant-supported restorations
Implant-supported crown	• Fixed • Prostheses to replace a single missing tooth attached by screw or bonding to an implant fixture

and to perform the appropriate self-care practices to maintain their oral health.

Dental Hygiene Considerations

Dental hygiene treatment considerations vary depending on the appliance. Control of the plaque biofilm and hard deposits on fixed and removable oral appliances is critical for maintaining oral health. Fixed orthodontic appliances, by the nature of their structure and position on the teeth, collect food debris and plaque biofilm (Fig. 23-5). Gingival inflammation, edema, and hyperplasia are common side effects of

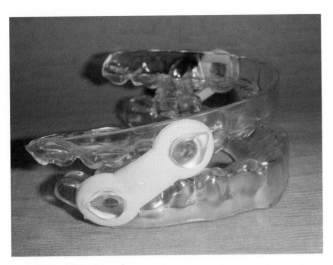

Figure 23-1. Snore guard.

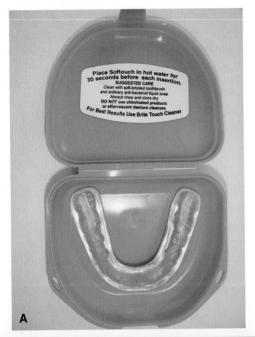

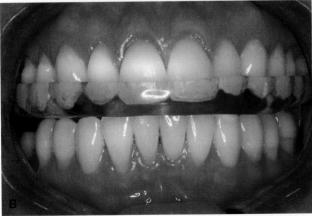

Figure 23-2. Nightguard in (A) storage case and (B) the mouth.

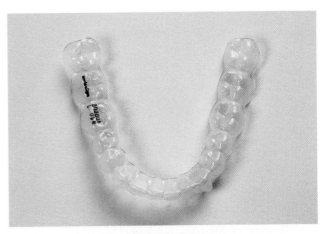

Figure 23-3. Removable orthodontic aligner.

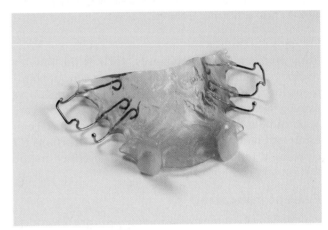

Figure 23-4. Hawley retainer.

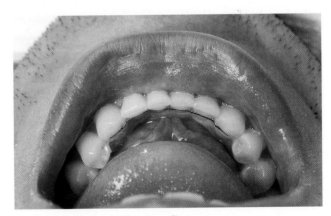

Figure 23-5. Fixed orthodontic appliance.

the plaque-retentive nature of orthodontic appliances. Patients undergoing orthodontic treatment may need more frequent continuing care intervals depending on their self-care abilities and overall periodontal health during active treatment.

Fixed appliances require thorough debridement at the continuing care appointment. Ultrasonic instrumentation or power scaling is an effective method of biofilm removal around fixed orthodontic appliances (Fig. 23-6). For detailed information on power scaling and ultrasonic instrumentation, see Chapters 25 and 26.

Fixed and removable appliances should be examined for irregular edges, broken or worn acrylic, bent or broken wires, as well as soft and hard deposits. Broken appliances need to be examined by the general dentist or orthodontist for evaluation and repair. Patients should

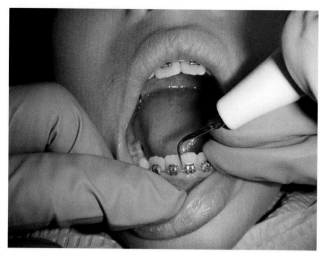

Figure 23-6. An ultrasonic scaler can be used to remove biofilm around a fixed orthodontic appliance.

bring any removable appliances, such as the Hawley retainer in Figure 23-4, to each dental hygiene appointment for regular maintenance. Removable appliances can be cleaned effectively at each continuing care appointment in a cleaning solution that has been immersed in an ultrasonic water bath. Instructions for cleaning a removable appliance are described in the section on dental prostheses.

Patient Education

Patient education regarding routine self-care is a critical component of the dental hygiene care plan for patients with oral appliances (see Teamwork 23-1).

Teamwork 23-1

Jill is a dental hygienist working in a busy general practice. Her patient Ms. Jones was in recently for her continuing care appointment. Jill and Dr. Smith identified a number of teeth that were exhibiting signs of attrition and occlusal wear. Ms. Jones admitted to being under stress at work and waking up with a sense of tightness in her temporomandibular joint. Jill and Dr. Smith discussed the protective benefits of a nightguard with Ms. Jones and took impressions during her dental hygiene appointment. Ms. Jones has an appointment today with Susie, one of the registered dental assistants in the practice, to pick up her nightguard. Susie will give Ms. Jones all the necessary patient education regarding adjusting to using a nightguard, daily cleaning of the appliance, and a reminder to bring the nightguard to each continuing care appointment for professional cleaning. Dr. Smith's practice has regular staff meetings and in-service training sessions so that all staff members are able to support each other and the patients they treat. ■

Key points should include:

- Oral appliances collect plaque biofilm and form calculus in the same manner as natural teeth.
- Plaque biofilm on an oral appliance can lead to oral infections.
- Follow the instructions of the oral health-care provider regarding the use of the specific oral appliance.
  - Some appliances such as an orthodontic aligner should be worn day and night with the exception of while eating.
  - Some appliances, such as nightguards and snore guards, are only worn while sleeping.
- Daily cleaning of the appliance is critical to maintaining oral health.
- Regular professional maintenance and cleaning will extend the life of the appliance.
  - Patients should be reminded to bring their appliances to their regular dental hygiene care appointments.

Although the number and type of removable oral appliances vary greatly, the basic principles of daily cleaning are similar. Daily self-care methods are discussed in the section Professional Prosthesis and Appliance Care.

Why Replace Missing Teeth?

The replacement of missing teeth is not a modern phenomenon. The first sets of dentures were crafted from animal or human bones as early as 700 BC. Seashells carved in the shape of teeth, precursors to modern dental implants, have been discovered in mandibles dating as far back as 600 AD. Individuals with tooth loss today have a number of predictable options for tooth replacement. Although teeth may be removed for orthodontic treatment or lack of function as in third molar extractions, there are risks involved in not replacing a functioning tooth. These risks include the migration of the opposing and adjacent teeth into the void created by the missing tooth and the loss of alveolar bone caused by lack of occlusal forces.

Understanding the Options for Tooth Replacement

It is important for patients to understand all of the options available for replacing their missing teeth so that they are able to make informed decisions regarding their treatment. After receiving information on the various treatment options, patients who decide to forgo treatment for replacing their missing tooth or teeth should complete and sign a statement of informed refusal. A written statement or agreement of informed refusal means that all of the various treatment options, risks, benefits, and alternatives have been explained and the patient is making an informed refusal of all treatment. The informed refusal process can be helpful in understanding a patient's reasons for not proceeding with treatment, such as cost, fear, or low value of oral health, while also protecting the practitioner from future misunderstandings with the patient regarding any consequences of not proceeding with treatment.

ORAL PROSTHESES

Fixed Partial Denture

A fixed partial denture is also commonly known as a **fixed bridge** (Fig. 23-7). This type of prosthesis is used to replace one or multiple missing teeth. Either natural teeth or dental **implants** can support a fixed bridge. The supporting teeth or implants are called retainers or **abutments.** The term *pontic* is used to describe the artificial tooth that has been fabricated to replace the missing natural tooth in a fixed or removable partial denture.

Types of Fixed Partial Dentures

Natural teeth serving as fixed bridge abutments are often prepared as full-coverage crowns to support the anticipated biting forces of the bridge. In some cases, though the abutment teeth are not prepared as full-coverage crowns and instead serve as supports for winglike extensions from the pontic. This type of fixed partial denture is also known as a Maryland bridge.

Fixed bridges are described in terms of the total number of teeth included in the prosthesis or units. Thus, a bridge that is designed to replace one missing tooth is called a *three-unit bridge* and a bridge designed to replace two missing teeth is called a *four-unit bridge*.

A fixed bridge is usually fabricated in the dental laboratory from a combination of metals and ceramics based on the prescription written by the restorative dentist. The exact combination of materials will depend on the number of units in the prosthesis, its location in the mouth, and the anticipated occlusal stresses.

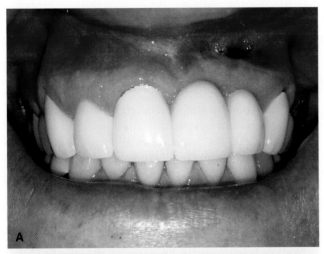

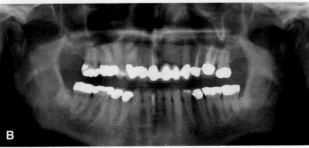

Figure 23-7. (A) Fixed bridge. (B) Radiograph of fixed bridge.

Dental Hygiene Care Considerations

Fixed bridges may be susceptible to problems depending on the complexity of the restoration, the materials used, and the oral health and hygiene of the patient. It is important for the dental hygienist to be aware of the following specific areas of a fixed bridge that require special attention during continuing care appointments.

- Abutment–pontic connection
  - May weaken because of occlusal forces
  - Examine for stress fractures
- Abutment teeth
  - Prone to trauma from occlusal forces
  - Check for mobility
- Restoration margins around the abutment teeth
  - Retain plaque biofilm
  - Increase the risk for recurrent caries and periodontal infections
  - Examine margins carefully with an explorer

Fixed bridge pontics that fit tightly against the alveolar ridge and oral mucosa can trap food debris and contribute to plaque biofilm retention. Chronic inflammation of the tissue beneath the pontic is a common finding in patients with fixed bridges. The anatomic configuration of the gingival surface of the fixed bridge pontic(s) can contribute to food debris and plaque biofilm retention. Chronic inflammation of the alveolar ridge tissue beneath the pontic is a common finding in patients with fixed bridges. This area should be thoroughly debrided at the continuing care appointment. An interdental cleaning device such as dental floss and a threader is very effective and also provides an opportunity for the dental hygienist to reinforce the patient's daily self-care technique when performed during the dental hygiene appointment. Care must be taken if rubber cup polishing is indicated for biofilm and stain removal. The dental hygienist should use a polishing agent that is appropriate for the materials used to fabricate the fixed bridge. See Chapter 29 for more information.

Patient Education

Patients must understand the anatomical features of their particular prosthesis and be able to practice the appropriate self-care techniques required to maintain it (Fig. 23-8).

Recommended Self-Care Practices

- Vigorously rinse with water or use an oral irrigator to remove oral debris before tooth brushing.
- Brush with a manual or power toothbrush and an appropriate fluoride dentifrice (see Chapters 19 and 20).
- Clean the interdental areas and under the missing teeth. A variety of devices and techniques are available for adapting to the surfaces of abutments and pontics, including:
  - Floss threading devices
  - Tufted floss with self threaders
  - Interdental brushes in varying widths and handle sizes

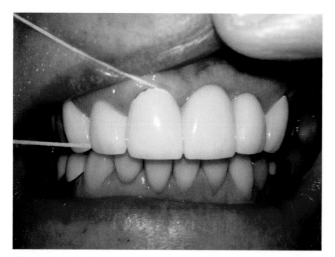

Figure 23-8. Flossing a fixed bridge.

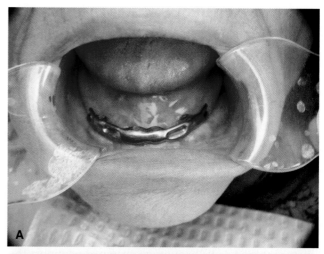

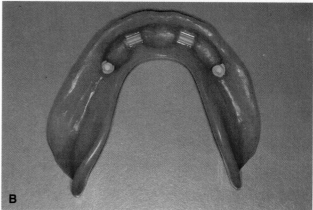

Figure 23-9. (A) Implant-supported lingual bar for overdenture. (B) Overdenture lingual view with attachments for implant-supported lingual bar.

- Interdental picks
- Oral irrigating devices

Removable Partial Dentures

The **removable partial denture** replaces multiple, but not all, teeth in an arch. Removable partial dentures are often fabricated with a metal framework and an acrylic base. The missing teeth are made of acrylic, porcelain, or metal and are mounted on the base. The prosthesis is fabricated to attach to the natural teeth via clasps, metal rests, or precision attachments. Some simple removable partial dentures are fabricated entirely from acrylic to replace one or more anterior teeth. These removable partial dentures are commonly referred to as *flippers,* named for the practice of flipping the appliance out on the tongue.

Complete Dentures

The **complete denture** is a removable prostheses fabricated to replace all of the teeth in a single arch or the entire dentition and the adjacent tissues. An **overdenture** is a type of complete denture that is supported by retained natural roots or dental implants rather than the alveolar ridge (Fig. 23-9). The retained roots or implants can provide greater support for the denture, improve biting forces, and decrease the resorption of the alveolar ridge.

Complete dentures consist of a denture base, often made of acrylic, and the teeth, which are made of acrylic, composite resin, or porcelain. The outer surface of the denture is a smooth, polished acrylic, whereas the inside impression surface that lies against the tissue does not have a smooth, polished finish. The inner surface may be treated with soft liners or tissue conditioners to improve the fit and comfort of the denture. Patients may also add adhesive materials to improve retention of the denture. Notably, the addition of liners and adhesives can increase the incidence of food debris and oral biofilm retention because of the challenges of effectively cleaning the inner surfaces of the prosthesis.[4]

Dental Hygiene Care Considerations

Complete dentures, removable partial dentures, abutment teeth, and the underlying tissues must be examined on a regular basis to check for optimal fit and maintenance of oral health. Abutment teeth often retain more biofilm and food debris because of the prosthetic attachment device, thus placing these key teeth at increased risk for dental caries and periodontal infections. Soft tissues covered by prostheses are susceptible to traumatic lesions and infections. Opportunistic fungal infections are a common problem with individuals with oral prostheses, particularly full dentures.[5] It is important for the dental hygienist to examine the prosthesis for any defects in the acrylic or the metal attachments. Broken or fractured attachments can alter the fit of the prosthesis and, in turn, affect the abutment teeth and the surrounding soft tissues. Wear patterns or flattened occlusal anatomy on the prosthesis may indicate abnormal bite forces and can precipitate a change in the underlying alveolar bone. Any abnormal findings with the prosthesis, the surrounding tissue, or teeth should be reported to the dentist for further care and treatment. Soft tissue responses are discussed further later in this chapter (see Complications Associated With Dental Prostheses and Appliances section).

Professional Prosthesis and Appliance Care

Professional cleaning of the removable prosthesis or appliance is an important component of the dental hygiene care plan. The rough, irregular surfaces on poorly maintained prostheses and appliances are conducive to bacterial and fungal growth.[6] Plaque biofilm, calculus, and stain formation will vary depending on the daily self-care practices of the individual patient. An **ultrasonic cleaner** is a device that transmits high-energy and high-frequency vibrations to a fluid-filled container to dislodge particles from immersed objects. The use of an ultrasonic cleaner is considered to be an effective method of cleaning soft and hard deposits off of removable prostheses and appliances. A cleaning and disinfectant solution can be used as the fluid for the ultrasonic device.

Although numerous commercial cleaning solutions are currently on the market for removable prostheses and appliances, research has shown that household products including bleach and vinegar can be equally effective provided that the product is appropriate for the material used in fabricating the prosthesis. Dentures fabricated without metal can be safely soaked in dilute sodium hypochlorite solutions, whereas a partial denture with metal claps will become corroded in a bleach solution over time (Table 23-3; also see Evidence-Based Practice 23-1).[7-10]

Evidence-Based Practice 23-1

A Cochrane review of randomized control trials comparing mechanical methods (brushing, ultrasonic cleaners) with a variety of chemical solutions found that there was a lack of evidence regarding the most effective method to clean a denture. The American College of Prosthodontists created a task force with the American Dental Association, the Academy of General Dentistry, the American Dental Hygienists' Association, and the National Association of Dental Laboratories to develop evidence-based guidelines for denture care. The guidelines include best practices for denture cleaning, denture care, and overall management of the patient with dentures ■

Source: Felton D, Cooper L, Duqum I, et al. Evidence-based guidelines for the care and maintenance of complete dentures: a publication of the American College of Prosthodontists. *J Am Dent Assoc.* 2011;142(suppl 1):1S-20S.

Table 23-3. *Household Products for Disinfecting Oral Appliances and Prostheses*

Product	Mode of Action	Disadvantages
Alkaline peroxide (combination of hydrogen peroxide and sodium bicarbonate)	• Oxygenating detergent • Antimicrobial	• May corrode metal • Removes only soft deposits
Sodium hypochloride (bleach)	• Dissolves biofilm and mucins • Antimicrobial	• Corrodes metal • Unpleasant odor and taste
Liquid hand soap	• Antimicrobial	
Vinegar	• Dissolves biofilm, mucins, and some hard deposits • Antimicrobial	• Corrodes metal

Procedure 23-1   Cleaning a Removable Prosthesis

MATERIALS AND PREPARATION

Familiarity with the necessary materials and proper preparation for cleaning a removable prosthesis is essential in utilizing time and resources. Being prepared for the procedure will eliminate stress and difficulty during the treatment.

Gather and organize the necessary materials before the patient's arrival.

Materials
Appropriate personal protective equipment (mask, gloves, eye protection)

Cup or small self-locking plastic bag laboratory	To transfer the prosthesis to the sink
Paper towels	To line the sink to protect the prosthesis
New or sterile toothbrush	To dislodge visible debris from the prosthesis
Label and pen	To label the plastic bag
Cleaning solution	Selection of a cleaning solution depends on whether the prosthesis or appliance contains metal; household products are effective cleaning solutions; commercial stain and tartar remover solutions may pose disposal issues because of their high acidity

Small beaker filled with water	To prevent the cleaning fluid from leaking into the ultrasonic solution
Hand instruments as needed	To scale residual calculus and stain on the outer surfaces of the prostheses

Preprocedure

PATIENT EDUCATION

Educate the patient about the ongoing need to keep the prosthesis clean. Provide the patient with a new brush to clean the prosthesis at each continuing care appointment to reinforce this teaching.

Procedure

1. *Remove the prosthesis.*
   - Ask the patient to remove the prosthesis.
   - Patients are often most comfortable with removing and inserting their own prosthesis.

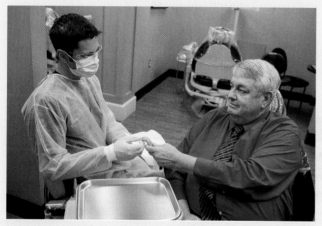

Patients are often most comfortable with removing and inserting their own prosthesis.

2. *Transfer to the dental laboratory.*
   - Place the prosthesis in a cup or small plastic bag and transfer the prosthesis to the dental laboratory.
3. *Clean the prosthesis.*
   - Place several paper towels in the bottom of the sink to protect the prosthesis in case it is dropped.
   - Use a new or sterile brush to dislodge any visible debris from the prosthesis or appliance.

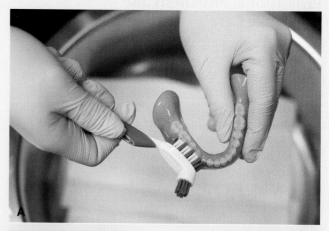

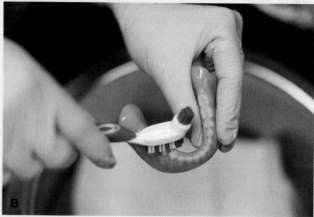

(A, B) Use a new or sterile brush to dislodge any visible debris from the prosthesis or appliance.

   - Label a self-locking plastic bag with the patient's name.
   - Carefully rinse the prosthesis or appliance.
   - Place the prosthesis or appliance in the self-locking plastic bag.
   - Select an appropriate cleaning solution.
   - Add the cleaning solution and close the bag.
   - Place the bag in a small beaker filled with water and immerse the beaker into an ultrasonic cleaner.

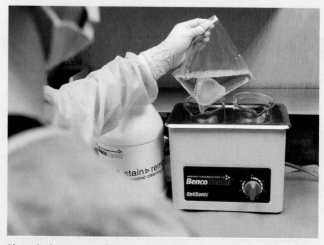

Place the bag in a small beaker filled with water and immerse the beaker into an ultrasonic cleaner.

- Process for 10 to 15 minutes. Processing time will vary depending on the ultrasonic unit and the quantity and hardness of the deposits.
- Remove the prosthesis or appliance from the bag and inspect it for residual deposits and stains.

4. *Utilize additional instrumentation.*
- Use hand instruments to scale residual calculus and stain on the outer surfaces only of the prostheses. Instrumentation on the impression side of the prosthesis may affect the fit.
- Polish any residual stains from the outer surfaces of the prosthesis with a fine-grit polishing agent.
- Hand instrumentation and rubber cup polishing can be completed in the operatory sink. Line the sink with paper towels to protect the prostheses in case it is dropped.

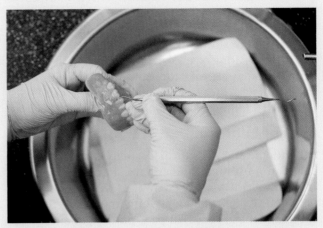

Use hand instruments to scale residual calculus and stain on the outer surfaces only of the prostheses. Instrumentation on the impression side of the prosthesis may affect the fit.

Postprocedure

- Return the clean prosthesis to the patient and have her insert it into her mouth. Ask the patient to confirm that the fit is comfortable.
- Reinforce that the prosthesis should be cleaned regularly.

COMPLICATIONS ASSOCIATED WITH DENTAL PROSTHESES AND APPLIANCES

Poorly fitting, damaged, or unhygienic prostheses put the underlying soft tissues at increased risk for erythema, edema, ulceration, hyperplasia, and infection. **Denture stomatitis** is the broad term given to the inflammation of the underlying soft issues that occurs as a result of mechanical, chemical, thermal, bacterial, viral, and allergic stimuli. ***Candida albicans,*** the most common fungus found in the mouth, often colonizes the irregular acrylic surfaces of the prosthesis and subsequently infects the underlying oral mucosa.[11] Although *C. albicans* is part of the normal microbial oral flora, an infection develops as the result of an overgrowth of the fungus. Persons who wear dentures are often more prone to candidiasis due to a number of cofactors including age, medication-induced xerostomia, diabetes, cardiovascular disease, immunosuppressive disorders, hormonal imbalances, and malnutrition.[12] Dry, cracked epithelium at the corners of the mouth can become colonized by *Staphylococcus aureus* and *C. albicans,* causing a condition known as angular cheilitis. Denture stomatitis and related candida infections, more commonly manifested in the maxilla, produce painful symptoms including burning and generalized tenderness.

Studies indicate that fungal infections in denture wearers and elderly adults have increased in prevalence

Spotlight on Public Health

Poor oral health has been observed in older populations around the world, especially affecting the lives of edentulous people. Findings from several studies indicate that denture stomatitis develops in 35% to 50% of persons who wear complete dentures and is most commonly found in elderly adults who live in nursing home facilities. A review of the causes and treatment of denture stomatitis stated that the 6-month incidence of denture stomatitis can be significantly reduced by educating nursing home caregivers about oral health care. Dental hygienists can play a vital role in providing education on denture care and hygiene for other allied health-care professionals and caregivers. Dental hygienists with alternative practice setting licenses, such as California's Registered Dental Hygienist in Alternative Practice, may also provide direct care to patients in nursing homes. ■

Sources: Frenkel H, Harvey I, Newcombe RG. Oral health care among nursing home residents in Avon. *Gerodontology.* 2000;17(1):33-38; Jainkittivong A, Aneksuk V, Langlais RP. Oral mucosal conditions in elderly dental patients. *Oral Dis.* 2002;8:218-223; and Sciubba JJ. Denture stomatitis. Medscape. Updated April 23, 2013. http://emedicine.medscape.com/article/1075994-overview. Accessed November 10, 2014.

(see Spotlight on Public Health). When allowed to progress, candidiasis may lead to more invasive systemic infection with serious complications.[13] Although there is currently no strong evidence linking oral malignancies to the wearing of an oral prosthesis, denture-related irritations may be cofactors in individuals with other risk factors for the development of oral cancer.[14] See Chapter 10 for more information.

Patient Education

Patient education is critical for anyone with a removable oral prosthesis. Studies have shown that edentulous patients have limited awareness of the need for prosthetic hygiene and long-term oral care.[15] Successful treatment depends, in part, on the patient's motivation to correctly use and maintain his prosthesis. The essential components of any education program for patients with a removable oral prosthesis include daily self-care techniques aimed at removing all loose debris and plaque biofilm, daily disinfection, and the importance of regular professional care. Patients also need to understand that wearing a denture or oral appliance increases their risk for fungal infections such as chronic candidiasis, because of the microscopically porous nature of the acrylic resin used to make the prosthesis.[7,11] Meticulous care of the denture is essential to reduce the risk for prosthesis-related infections. Mechanical cleaning and soaking in a disinfectant should be performed daily.[16]

Key points for patient education should include:

- Retention of food debris after eating can contribute to oral malodor.
- Removing the prosthesis and rinsing after eating will help remove excess food debris.
- Acrylic resins in oral prostheses harbor *C. albicans,* a common oral yeast.
- Soft tissues under an oral prosthesis that is not properly cleaned can become infected with *C. albicans.*
- A soft toothbrush should be used to gently brush the soft tissue, cheeks, and tongue.
- The soft tissues should be inspected regularly for any sore spots or changes.

Daily Prosthesis Care

- Clean and disinfect the prosthesis with a designated brush and a mild liquid soap.
- Place a small cloth in the sink to prevent breaking the prosthesis.
- Brush the outer and the inner surfaces.
- Rinse the prosthesis thoroughly with warm water. Hot water will distort the shape of the prosthesis.
- Avoid the use of toothpastes or abrasive cleaners. Abrasive particles scratch the acrylic resin and increase biofilm retention.
- Soak the prosthesis overnight in water or solution that is safe for overnight use (refer to Table 23-3). Soaking in very hot or boiling water can distort the prosthesis. Household products can be cost-effective cleaners and disinfectants. Care should be taken to

select a nonabrasive, noncorrosive product. Nightly removal of the prosthesis allows the soft tissue to "breathe" and helps prevent a candida infection.

Regular Dental Care

- Soft tissue examinations and oral cancer screenings should be performed on a regular basis.
- Prosthesis fit and overall function may change over time and need to be evaluated regularly.
  - Poor fit can lead to tissue trauma, accelerated bone loss, and difficulty eating and speaking.

DENTAL IMPLANTS

From an Unpredictable Art to Standard of Care

Historically, dental implants date at least as far back as the Egyptians; however, it was not until the 1950s, when Swedish medical researcher Per-Ingvar Brånemark described the phenomenon of osseointegration in a medical laboratory experiment, that modern implant science began to develop. **Osseointegration** is defined as the direct biological attachment of living bone to a **titanium** implant surface without any intervening soft tissue.[4] Although many different materials have been experimented with for implants, titanium alloy was found to be compatible with human tissues. Titanium alloy consists of the elementary substance of titanium along with traces of aluminum and vanadium.[17] Research over the past 50 years has transformed the discipline of implant dentistry from an unpredictable art to a well-grounded clinical science, improving the quality of life of individuals with varying degrees of tooth loss.[16] Brånemark's initial discovery has benefited the oral health of individuals around the world. The principles of osseointegration

Application to Clinical Practice

Julia is a recent dental hygiene graduate and is interviewing for her first position as a dental hygienist in a general practice. She found this practice through an internet employment advertisement and checked out the practice website before the interview. The website promotes services including full-mouth reconstruction and dental implants. Julia learned about dental implants during her rotation at the dental school affiliated with her program. Julia was also able to treat a patient in clinic who had undergone extensive dental treatment to reconstruct his dentition after losing a number of permanent teeth because of caries and periodontal disease. How should Julia prepare for her upcoming interview? What kind of questions should Julia ask the dentist regarding the restorative services that the practice offers? ■

also have a wide range of health applications ranging from orthopedic prosthetic limbs for amputees to osseointegrated hearing aids for individuals with severe hearing loss.[18]

Types of Dental Implants

There are three different types of dental implants: subperiosteal, transosteal, and endosteal. Each type has a specific use and function (Table 23-4). A defining characteristic among the three different types of dental implants is the way they integrate into the alveolar bone. Endosteal implant systems are the only implants that are placed *into* the alveolar bone of the mandible or maxilla. Early endosteal implants were blade shaped and could support multiple teeth. Modern endosteal implants mimic the length and width of a natural root. Screw-type endosteal implants are the most widely used implant systems in dentistry today and have demonstrated success rates of 96% or higher over a period of 20 years (Fig. 23-10).

Parts of an Endosteal Implant

The fixture, or body, is the portion of the implant that is screwed or tapped into the prepared bone. The fixture surface is often treated with a variety of materials and techniques ranging from hydroxyapatite coatings to sandblasted or acid-etched surfaces. Each implant manufacturer has its own unique patented finishing process designed to enhance osseointegration

Advancing Technologies 23-1

The implant manufacturing market is rapidly changing. Many new implant designs are being developed to meet the growing needs of consumers and dental professionals. In some cases, a tooth can be carefully extracted, an implant surgically placed in the extraction socket, and a temporary crown placed on the implant abutment in one appointment. This technique is called *immediate loading* or *provisionalization.* Occlusal contact with the opposing dentition will depend on the individual circumstances and the preferences of the surgeon. ■

(see Advancing Technologies 23-1). Special care must be taken not to scratch or gouge the surface of the implant fixture during instrumentation or self-care procedures.

The abutment serves as the connection between the fixture and the prosthesis, also called the *superstructure.* The abutment is often located subgingivally within the peri-implant crevice. Abutment design is dependent on the type of prosthesis that the implant or implants have been placed to support. Abutment configurations can range from straight and conical to angled or ball-shaped depending on the prosthesis.

Table 23-4. *Types of Dental Implants*

Design	Description	Use
Subperiosteal	• Titanium or Vitallium metal framework resting on the surface of the alveolar bone under the periosteum • Fabricated from impressions of the alveolar bone or from a computed tomography scan • Four posts emerge through the soft tissue from the metal framework • Not osseointegrated • Supported by fibro-osseous connective tissue interface	• Supports a complete overdenture • Indicated for individuals with narrow, atrophic alveolar ridges • Failure may be because of infection at the abutment site(s)
Transosteal	• Also known as a staple implant • Five- to seven-pin titanium or titanium alloy plate fitted to the inferior border of the mandible via an extraoral skin incision • Two or more terminal pins extend through the mandible to support an overdenture	• Only placed in the mandible • Indicated for individuals with an atrophic mandibular ridge or a deformed mandible • Increased probability of failure because of infection
Endosteal	• Titanium implants that are surgically placed within the bone of the mandible or maxilla • Also referred to as fixtures • Early forms were blade shaped • Current forms are cylindrical or screw shaped • Width and length vary depending on the anatomy of the tooth or teeth being replaced and the quantity and quality of the alveolar bone • May be designed with a very small diameter to serve as a transitional or mini implant • The most predictable and widely used dental implants	• May replace single or multiple teeth • May support a fixed or removable overdenture • May be designed to support a temporary prosthesis while osseointegration takes place • May provide a means for anchorage during orthodontic treatment

How a natural tooth attaches to bone   **How an implant attaches to bone**

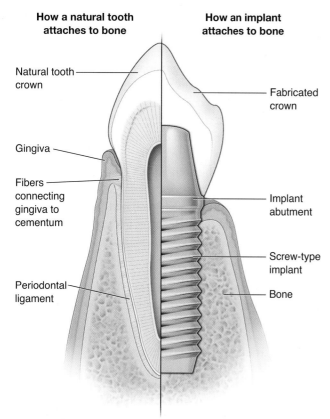

Natural tooth crown

Gingiva

Fibers connecting gingiva to cementum

Periodontal ligament

Fabricated crown

Implant abutment

Screw-type implant

Bone

Figure 23-10. Parts of the endosteal implant: the implant fixture, abutment, and superstructure or prosthesis.

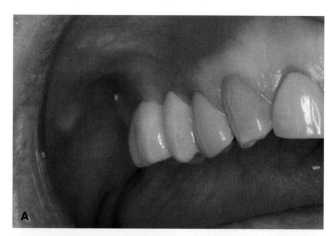

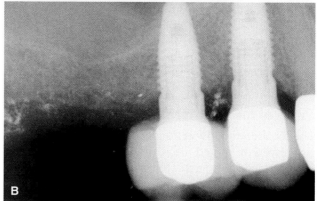

Figure 23-11. (A) Patient with implant-supported restorations. (B) Radiograph of implant-supported restorations.

Implant Restorations

An implant-supported prosthesis can vary from a single crown to fixed or removable dentures, depending on the restorative needs of the patient. Single-unit implant restorations provide patients with a predictable alternative treatment option to a fixed or removable bridge provided that the bone is adequate and there are no significant risk factors for successful implant placement. Improvements in surgical techniques and restorative materials can make it difficult to distinguish an implant-supported restoration from a natural tooth without an accompanying radiograph (Fig. 23-11).

Implant Prosthesis Retention Options

Implant restorations or prostheses may be either screw- or cement-retained, depending on the type of restoration, aesthetic concerns, and the preferences of the restoring dentist. Screw-retained restorations will have an access hole that is covered with a composite material. Some screw-retained prostheses necessitate periodic removal to facilitate cleaning around the implant abutments. Cement-retained restorations are bonded to the abutment in much the same fashion as a crown. In either system, it is possible for the restoration to become loose and need to be reconnected to the abutment.

Implant overdentures are dentures that are supported by implants rather than soft tissue. A variety of abutment systems exist ranging from two-unit ball-and-socket configurations to lingual bars supported by multiple implants. The overdenture may have plastic clips inserted into the lingual aspect of the prosthesis as part of an attachment system known as Hader bar and clips, named for the inventor of the process. These clips may need periodic replacement to maintain their function.

Implant–Bone–Soft Tissue Interfaces

Professional maintenance of dental implants requires an understanding of the bone and soft tissue interface with the implant. The osseointegrated implant demonstrates a direct contact between living bone and the implant surface without any intervening connective tissue. Unlike a natural tooth with a periodontal ligament attaching the tooth to the alveolar bone, the implant is integrated via the titanium–bone interface. Successful integration of the titanium fixture into the prepared implant site is influenced by a number of factors, particularly the quality and quantity of the patient's bone, as well as careful and aseptic surgical techniques (see Advancing Technologies 23-2).

Osseointegration requires an adequate amount of uninterrupted healing time for bone cells to integrate to the implant fixture. The average time for osseointegration ranges between 3 and 6 months, depending on the density of the bone. Typically, implants placed in the mandible integrate more quickly than in the maxilla. If connective tissue forms between the implant and the alveolar bone, osseointegration fails and the implant must be removed (Fig. 23-12).

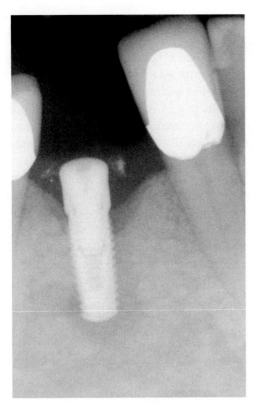

Figure 23-12. Radiograph of osseointegration failure.

Advancing Technologies 23-2

Advances in bone grafting techniques and imaging technologies have increased the number of individuals who successfully received dental implants. Bone can now be predictably augmented with grafts harvested from the patient (autogenous) or from other animal or acellular sources. Researchers are testing bone morphogenetic proteins, engineered from the cloning of the genes found in bone cells. Tissue engineering techniques open the possibilities for repairing severely damaged bone structures. Cone-beam computed tomography captures oral-maxillofacial images in three dimensions, enabling surgeons to effectively plan implant treatment. This is especially useful for patients with compromised bone or anatomical conditions that require special consideration. ■

The soft tissue interface formed with the implant fixture and abutment is called the *biological* or **permucosal seal.** This seal, formed by the junctional epithelium, creates a physiological barrier, protecting the implant–bone interface from the insults of bacterial plaque biofilm. The connective tissue adjacent to an implant is richer in collagen, contains fewer fibroblasts, and has a reduced blood supply compared with the gingival tissues that surround a natural tooth.[1] These biological differences help clarify why the peri-implant mucosa has a diminished capacity for self-repair in the presence of inflammation.

Peri-implant Disease

Peri-implant disease is the collective term given to the inflammatory reactions in the soft and hard tissues that surround dental implants. **Peri-implant mucositis** is the term used to describe the reversible, inflammatory reaction in the soft tissues that surround an implant, whereas **peri-implantitis** is an inflammatory reaction of the soft and hard tissues with a subsequent loss of supporting bone that surrounds an implant.[17] Bacterial plaque biofilm forms on the implant surfaces as soon as they are exposed in the oral cavity. The initial pellicle formation is similar to that on natural teeth.

Research supports the theory that the same periodontal bacterial flora of natural teeth colonize the peri-implant tissues, and that the progression of the disease process from gingivitis and periodontitis is similar.[19,20] Implants and their supporting tissues are described as ailing and failing depending on the extent of the inflammation.

Dental Hygiene Considerations

The dental hygienist works with the patient through all stages of implant treatment planning and maintenance.

Assessment

The first step in the continuing care appointment is the assessment of the peri-implant tissues, checking for the presence of visible plaque biofilm, calculus, and inflammation. The tissue that surrounds the implant should be evaluated for erythema, edema, changes in contour and consistency, as well as the presence of any suppuration around the sulcus (see Teamwork 23-2 and Box 23-1).

Teamwork 23-2

Successful dental implant therapy requires collaboration across the dental team. Specially trained general dentists, periodontists, and oral surgeons can surgically place implants. Dental laboratory technicians then precisely replicate the implant position to fabricate the restoration. Once the implant has osseointegrated, the general dentist or prosthodontist restores the implant. The dental hygienist works with the patient and the restorative dentist from the initial treatment planning to implant maintenance. The hygienist may be the first member of the dental team to note changes in the health of the peri-implant tissues. The surgeon who placed the implant often carries out treatment of an ailing or failing implant. Regular communication among the various team members is a key component of successful treatment. ■

Box 23-1. *Dental Hygiene Maintenance Procedures for Patients With Dental Implants*

The implant-supported restoration and surrounding soft tissue should be regularly evaluated for the following:
- Presence of plaque and calculus
- Color and texture of the peri-implant tissues
- Radiographic appearance of the implant and alveolar bone
- Mobility of the abutment or restoration
- Presence of exudate in the peri-implant sulci
- Salivary percolation or bubbling around the abutments resulting from pressure applied to the restoration
- Overall patient comfort and function
- Continuing care appointment schedule based on:
  - Prescription of the restorative dentist
  - General periodontal condition
  - Complexity of the implant restoration
  - Self-care abilities and motivation of the patient

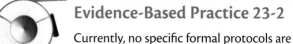

Evidence-Based Practice 23-2

Currently, no specific formal protocols are outlined in the professional literature for implant continuing care intervals. Some researchers recommend initiating a 3-month continuing care interval in the first year after implant placement. The interval can be extended later to 6 months in some cases, depending on the gingival health, oral hygiene status, and any additional risk factors. The hygienist, in consultation with the restorative dentist, should make an appropriate continuing care schedule based on the complexity of the implant restoration, the overall periodontal condition, and the patient's self-care abilities and motivation. ■

Implant mobility should be monitored at the continuing care appointment by gently tapping one side of the implant-supported prostheses with the tip of the mirror handle while placing the index finger of the opposite hand on the other side of the prosthesis. Movement of the restoration may indicate a failure in osseointegration or simply a loosening of the cement or screw-retained prosthesis. Loosened screws need to be tightened by the restorative dentist. In a screw-retained restoration, the integrity of the material used to seal the access hole should be monitored. Wear patterns may indicate the need for occlusal adjustment. Heavy occlusal forces contribute to a number of complications including the loosening or fracturing of abutment screws and implant failure.[21]

Radiographs should be taken during the continuing care appointment depending on the schedule determined in consultation with the restorative dentist (see Evidence-Based Practice 23-2). Radiographic interpretation has been shown to be a valuable measurement of an implant's success or failure. Patients are excellent sources of diagnostic information regarding the overall health of the implant. Pain or discomfort around the implant site may be the first indication of implant failure. Discomfort around the implant site may precede any radiographic changes.[22] All patients should be asked about the comfort of their dental implant(s) at each continuing care appointment.

Instrumentation

Thorough debridement of the bacterial biofilm and any hard deposits is as necessary for dental implants and their prostheses as it is for the natural dentition. Calculus that has formed on implant surfaces is softer and less tenacious than the calculus found on natural teeth

(Fig. 23-13). Supragingival calculus is more common than subgingival deposits.[21]

Instrument selection for dental hygiene care will depend on the position of the abutments and the prosthesis the implant system was designed to support. Scanning electron microscopic studies have shown that metal instrumentation produces scratching of the titanium implant abutment interface, causing greater plaque retention and inflammation of the peri-implant tissues.[23] Only instruments and other debridement devices made of materials designated to be safe for titanium surfaces should be used. A variety of plastic and graphite, as well as titanium and gold-tipped, hand instruments are available for implant instrumentation (Fig. 23-14). Instrument selection should be based on the abutment configuration and the implant-supported prosthesis that needs to be accessed for debridement.

Power instrumentation may be used when calculus and plaque need to be removed from the restoration and the abutment. Care should be taken that only power instruments with specially designed implant tips are used at low power and with ample irrigation.

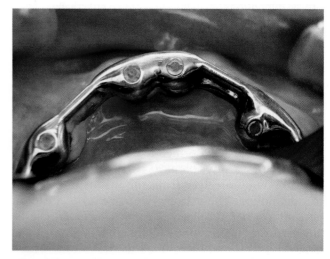

Figure 23-13. Implant with calculus formation.

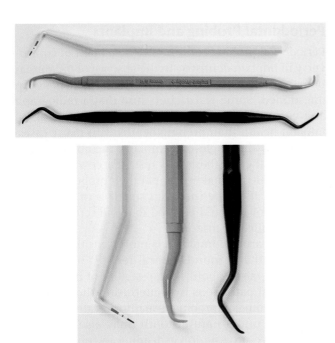

Figure 23-14. Instruments for use with dental implants.

Single-unit implant replacement crowns pose special challenges in accessing the supporting implant abutment. The circumference of the crown or base is often much wider than the abutment, making it difficult, if not impossible, to access the peri-implant crevice with an instrument. In these cases, it is necessary only to deplaque the crevice with an alternative plaque removal aid, such as floss (Fig. 23-15).

Implant fixture debridement may be necessary in the case of peri-implant disease. In a healthy implant, the threads or roughened surface of the implant fixture are below the biological seal and not visible. In the case of bone loss, the implant threads are exposed. The exposed areas may be deplaqued with a brush. If calculus is present, an appropriate hand or power instrument may be used.

In general, implant-supported restorations should only be polished when necessary for stain removal and

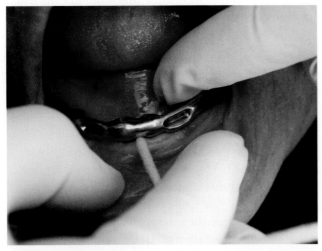

Figure 23-15. Floss used to debride a single-unit implant restoration.

to restore their luster. The polishing agent should be selected based on the restorative material used. Low-abrasive pastes, cleaning agents, and dentifrices can be used safely on implant restorations.[21] See Chapter 29 for more information.

Patient Education

Effective self-care strategies are crucial for the long-term health of the dental implant. Heavy plaque indices have been correlated to increased incidences of peri-implant mucositis.[24] The dental hygienist must evaluate the position of the implant prosthesis and abutments and their relationship to the soft tissue, and customize oral hygiene recommendations based on the patient's specific needs. Patient motivation and manual dexterity must also be considered when recommending oral hygiene devices. Research has demonstrated that when multiple oral hygiene devices are recommended, their use diminishes with the passage of time until only one device remains in use. Successful plaque control will be limited if the procedures require an inordinate amount of time, a high degree of manual dexterity, or a multitude of devices.

Patients need to understand the basic configuration of their particular implant restoration in order to learn effective plaque control techniques. Homecare devices must be safe for titanium implant surfaces and not cause trauma to the peri-implant mucosa. An interproximal cleaning device should be recommended in addition to a tooth brushing method in order to effectively clean the implant abutment. Numerous adjunctive devices are available ranging from flossing products specifically designed for implants to rubber tips, interproximal brushes, and oral irrigators.

The use of an antimicrobial solution, such as 0.12% chlorhexidine gluconate, may be a beneficial adjunct to mechanical plaque-removal devices. The chemotherapeutic agent can be applied locally to the peri-implant area by dipping the toothbrush, rubber tip, floss, or other plaque-control device into a small capful of the chlorhexidine gluconate before beginning the home care procedure. Chlorhexidine gluconate is also useful during the postsurgical healing phases when mechanical plaque removal may be contraindicated.[25] See Chapters 19 and 20 for more information.

Key points for patient education should include:

- The implant fixture mimics the root of the tooth.
- The abutment is like a post and connects the restoration to the implant.
- Implant restorations, like natural teeth, require daily maintenance to remain healthy.
- Implant restorations may become loose.
- Cements or screws may become loose.
- Implant fixtures may become infected.
- Any changes in the implant or restorations must be reported to the dentist.

Discussion Issues

Implants Versus Dentures

The use of dental implants to support a fixed or removable denture provides edentulous individuals with increased stability and improved occlusal forces compared with individuals with dentures supported by soft tissues. Alveolar bone needs stimulation to retain its shape and density. When teeth are lost, the occlusal forces decrease significantly. The average occlusal force in the molar region of a person with natural teeth averages between 150 and 250 pounds per square inch (psi), whereas the maximum occlusal forces of the edentulous individual are less than 50 psi. Individuals who have been wearing complete dentures for 15 years or longer may have occlusal forces as low as 5.6 psi, which significantly affects their ability to eat, chew, and speak.[1] The average edentulous patient can expect a 25% decrease in bone width and a 4-mm decrease in bone height in the first year following tooth loss. An ill-fitting, soft tissue–supported denture can accelerate this bone loss. Implant-supported prostheses have been shown to maintain the overall volume of alveolar bone as a result of the stimulation produced by the day-to-day function of the prosthesis (see Professionalism).

Professionalism

Oral implantology is a rapidly changing science. Attending continuing education programs sponsored by one of the professional organizations for dentists is a good way to learn more about this treatment option for tooth replacement. The International Congress of Oral Implantologists (ICOI) focuses on providing implant education to the entire dental team. The Association of Dental Implant Auxiliaries (ADIA) is a component of the ICOI and provides a variety of implant education and certification programs for dental hygienists, assistants, and office staff. Learn more about the ICOI and ADIA by visiting their website at: www.icoi.org. ▪

Periodontal Probing and Implants

Periodontal probing continues to be a point of controversy in implant dentistry. In the absence of inflammation, the benefit of probing peri-implant tissue has been questioned. Some researchers find that a radiograph and visual assessment are more reliable indicators of implant health than probing depths.[26] In many cases, particularly the single-unit implant, the anatomy and position of the prosthesis may restrict access to the peri-implant sulcus, making a parallel probe insertion impossible. If the peri-implant sulcus is to be probed, a plastic probe should be used to avoid scratching the titanium implant surface.

Probing around implants is more sensitive to force variations than around natural teeth.[19,27] Concerns have been raised about the possibility of introducing periodontal pathogens by penetrating the biological seal.[27] Bleeding on probing, usually indicative of active disease around a natural tooth, may also be caused by excessive probing forces leading to trauma to the biological seal around the implant fixture. A pressure-sensitive probe may be used to safeguard against excessive probing forces. Clinicians can expect to find that the gingival sulcus depth of a dental implant averages between 1.3 and 3.8 mm, compared with the average sulcus depth around a healthy natural tooth, which averages between 0.4 and 3 mm.[28] Probing is contraindicated in the first 3 months following the abutment connection to avoid disrupting the newly formed biological seal.[29,30]

SUMMARY

Many different devices can be placed in the oral cavity. All devices retain biofilm and have the potential of irritating oral tissues and leading to infection. Dental hygienists must be familiar with the various prostheses and appliances that can be used in the mouth and must be able to educate patients on their use and care. Dental hygienists must also be able to select the appropriate instruments and methods for professional care when handling prostheses and appliances.

Case Study

Mrs. Smith is 80 years old and recently moved to an assisted living facility near her daughter after her husband died. Mrs. Smith is in good general health for her age and is adjusting to her new living arrangement. Lately she has been complaining that she has a sore area under her upper partial denture that is making it difficult to eat. Mrs. Smith's daughter has called the dental office to have her mother seen for an examination. Mrs. Smith's health history indicates that she is currently taking a calcium channel blocker for high blood pressure and an antidepressant to help her sleep. It has been 2 years since Mrs. Smith had any regular dental hygiene care. When Mrs. Smith removes her partial denture, the hygienist sees that one of the clasps is broken and there are calculus deposits on #3 and #4. While making assessments, the dental hygienist notes that the palate is red and inflamed in a pattern that matches the metal framework of the partial

Case Study—cont'd

denture. When the hygienist asks Mrs. Smith how she cares for her partial denture, she replies that she brushes it like she does her natural teeth and rarely removes it.

Case Study Exercises

1. Which condition is most likely present on the palatal tissue of this patient?
   A. *C. albicans*
   B. Ulcerative stomatitis
   C. Denture stomatitis
   D. Squamous cell carcinoma

2. Mrs. Smith is at increased risk for dental caries and periodontal disease. Fluoride therapy has little effect in the dentitions of the elderly.
   A. The first statement is true, but the second statement is false.
   B. The first statement is false, but the second statement is true.
   C. Both statements are true.
   D. Both statements are false.

3. All of the following conditions could be considered contributory factors to Mrs. Smith's discomfort while eating EXCEPT:
   A. A poorly fitting partial denture
   B. Xerostomia

C. Hypertension
   D. Denture stomatitis

4. Patient education for Mrs. Smith should include all of the following points EXCEPT:
   A. The benefits of removing oral prosthesis for sleep
   B. The benefits of using toothpaste for cleaning the partial denture
   C. The regular use of prescription fluoride toothpaste
   D. The benefits of regular dental examinations

5. Xerostomia, maxillary prostheses, and poor diet can cause candida infections. A candida infection is the most likely cause of Mrs. Smith's pain when eating.
   A. The first statement is true, but the second statement is false.
   B. The first statement is false, but the second statement is true.
   C. Both statements are true.
   D. Both statements are false.

Review Questions

1. Which portion of the endosteal dental implant is surgically placed into the bone?
   A. Abutment
   B. Body or fixture
   C. Prosthesis
   D. Implant core

2. Plaque biofilm and calculus form only on natural teeth. Removable prostheses and appliances can increase an individual's risk for oral and systemic diseases.
   A. The first statement is true, but the second statement is false.
   B. The first statement is false, but the second statement is true.
   C. Both statements are true.
   D. Both statements are false.

3. Tooth loss can lead to all of the following complications EXCEPT:
   A. Drifting of the adjacent and opposing teeth into the missing space
   B. An atrophic alveolar ridge

C. Increased occlusal forces
   D. Difficulty in speaking

4. Acrylic denture material can become colonized with:
   A. Food debris
   B. Biofilm
   C. *C. albicans*
   D. Calculus

5. Which of the following best describes the reversible inflammatory process that can occur around a dental implant?
   A. Peri-implantitis
   B. Ischemia
   C. Necrosis
   D. Perimucositis

Active Learning

1. Use visual aids (typodont) to demonstrate how to floss under a fixed bridge versus a natural tooth.
2. Create a PowerPoint (5–10 slides) training presentation on the consequences of denture neglect for nursing home aides.
3. Go to the local pharmacy and check out the denture cleaning products. What are the various modes of action in each product? Describe how you will approach this topic with your patient.
4. Borrow a sample denture from the local dental laboratory. Close your eyes and feel the outer surface of the denture. Now run your fingers over the inner surfaces. How would you describe the surfaces?
5. Look at a diagram showing the cross section of a natural tooth. How does it compare with a dental implant? How do you think that the implant-supported tooth will feel versus the natural tooth when you check for mobility? ■

REFERENCES

1. Misch CE. *Contemporary Implant Dentistry.* 3rd rev. ed. St Louis, MO: Mosby; 2007.
2. Centers for Disease Control and Prevention. National Oral Health Surveillance System. http://www.cdc.gov/nohss/index.htm. Accessed February 21, 2010.
3. U.S. Department of Health and Human Services (HHS). *Oral Health in America: A Report of the Surgeon General.* Rockville, MD: HHS, National Institutes of Health, National Institute of Dental and Craniofacial Research; 2000.
4. Pereira-Cenci T, Del Bel Cury AA, Rodrigues-Garcia RC. In vitro Candida colonization on acrylic resins and denture liners: influence of surface free energy, roughness, saliva and adhering bacteria. *Int J Prosthodont.* 2007;20(3):308-310.
5. Pereira-Cenci T, Del Bel Cury AA, Crielaard W, Ten Cate JM. Development of candida associated denture stomatitis: new insights. *J Appl Oral Sci.* 2008;16(2):86-94.
6. Ramage G, Tomsett K, Wickes BL, Lopez-Ribot JL, Redding SW. Denture stomatitis: a role for Candida biofilms. *Oral Surg Oral Med Oral Pathol Oral Radiol Endod.* 2004;98(1):53-59.
7. Shay K. Denture hygiene: a review and update. *J Contemp Dent Pract.* 2000;1(2):28-41.
8. Pinto TM, Neves AC, Pereira MV, Cardoso AO. Vinegar as an antimicrobial agent for control of *Candida* spp. in complete denture wearers. *J Appl Oral Sci.* 2008;16(6):385-390.
9. Jagger R. Lack of evidence about the effectiveness of the different denture cleaning methods. *Evid Based Dent.* 2009;10(4):109.
10. de Souza RF, de Freitas O, Paranhos H, et al. Interventions for cleaning dentures in adults. *Cochrane Database Syst Rev.* 20097;(4):CD007395.
11. Gasparoto TH, Dionisio TJ, Oliveiria CE, et al. Isolation of Candida dubliniensis from denture wearers. *J Med Microbiol.* 2009;58:959-962.
12. Gonsalves WC, Wrightson AS, Henry RG. Common oral conditions in older persons. *Am Fam Physician.* 2008;78(7):845-852.
13. ten Cate JM, Klis FM, Pereira-Cenci T, et al. Molecular and cellular mechanisms that lead to candida biofilm formation. *J Dent Res.* 2009;88:105-115.
14. Stucken E, Weissman J, Spiegel JH. Oral cavity risk factors: experts opinions and literature support. *J Otolaryngol Head Neck Surg.* 2010;39(1):76-89.
15. de Castellucci BL, Ferreira MR, de Carvalho Calabrich CF, et al., Edentulous patient's knowledge of dental hygiene and care of prostheses. *Gerodontology.* 2008;25(2):99-106.
16. Jose A, Coco BJ, Milligan S, et al. Reducing the incidence of denture stomatitis: are denture cleaners sufficient? *J Prosthodont.* 2010;19(4):252-257. Accessed March 7, 2010.
17. Jalbout Z, Tabourian G. *Glossary of Implant Dentistry.* Upper Montclair, NJ: International Congress of Oral Implantologists; 2004.
18. Granstrom G. Craniofacial osseointegration. *Oral Dis.* 2007;13(3):261-269.
19. Heitz-Mayfienld LJ. Diagnosis and management of peri-implant diseases. *Aus Dent J.* 2008;53(1 suppl):S43-S48.
20. Quirynen M, Vogels R, Peeters W, et al. Dynamics of initial subgingival colonization of pristine periimplant pockets. *Clin Oral Implants Res.* 2006;17(1):25-37.
21. Humphrey S. Implant maintenance. *Dent Clin N Am.* 2006;50:463-478.
22. Lekholm U, von Steenberghe D, Herrmann I, et al. Osseointegrated implants in the treatment of partially edentulous jaws: a prospective 5 year multicenter study. *Int J Oral Malliofac Implants.* 1994;9:627-635.
23. Quirynen M, Bollen CM, Williams G, van Steenberghe D. Comparison of surface characteristics of six commercially pure titanium abutments. *Int J Oral Maxillofac Implants.* 1994;9:71-76.
24. Ferreira SD, Silva GL, Cortelli JR, et al. Prevalence and risk variables for peri-implant disease in Brazilian subjects. *J Clin Periodontol.* 2006;33(12):929-935.
25. Porras F, Anderson GB, Cafesse R, et al. Clinical response to 2 different therapeutic regimens to treat peri-implant mucositis. *J Periodontol.* 2002;73(10):1118-1125.
26. Deppe H, Wagenpfeil S, Donath K. Comparative value of attached measurements in implant dentistry. *Int J Oral Maxillofac Implants.* 2004;19(2):208-215.
27. Lindhe J, Meyle J. Peri-implant diseases: consensus report of the sixth European Workshop on Periodontology. *J Clin Periodontol.* 2008;35(suppl 8):282-285.
28. Mombelli A, Buser D, Lang NP, et al. Comparison of periodontal and peri-implant probing by depth force pattern analysis. *Clin Oral Implant Res.* 1997;8:448-454.
29. Bauman GR, Mills M, Rapley J, et al. Clinical parameters of evaluation during implant maintenance. *Int J Oral Maxillofac Implants.* 1992;7(2):220-227.
30. Greenstein G, Cavallaro J, Tarnow D. Dental implants in the periodontal patient. *Dent Clin N Am.* 2010;54:113-128.

Chapter 24 | Ergonomics

Juli Kagan, RDH, MEd

KEY TERMS

anteverted pelvis

dynamic sitting

ergonomics

magnification loupes

musculoskeletal disorders (MSD)

trigger points

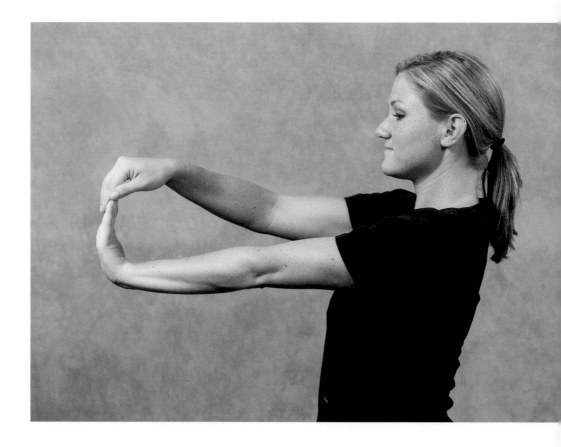

LEARNING OBJECTIVES

After reading this chapter, the student should be able to:

24.1 Define *musculoskeletal disorders*.

24.2 Define *ergonomics*.

24.3 State at least three common symptoms of musculoskeletal disorders.

24.4 Discuss the importance of an anteverted pelvis while performing clinical dental hygiene.

24.5 Describe at least two ways to open the pelvic angle while sitting.

24.6 Provide reasons to exercise while in the dental operatory.

24.7 Demonstrate one exercise each for the hands, neck, shoulders/upper trunk, back, and legs.

24.8 Explain why loupes and proper lighting are important for the dental hygienist.

24.9 List three aspects of instrument selection.

24.10 Explain four key concepts of instrumentation related to hand health.

KEY CONCEPTS

• Most musculoskeletal disorders (MSD) are insidious, but with applied knowledge about work environment (ergonomics), equipment adjustment, and patient and operator positioning, cumulative disorders can be minimized.

- Prevention of MSD occurs because risk factors are minimized or eliminated.
- An anteverted pelvis helps the body stay in a more upright position.
- Properly standing, sitting, and moving around the patient can help prevent musculoskeletal injuries.
- Chairside exercises, when done regularly and frequently, allow the clinician to work more comfortably and effectively.

RELEVANCE TO CLINICAL PRACTICE

Dental hygienists often complain about pain in their hands, arms, neck, shoulders, and upper and lower back. Clinically, these pains describe **musculoskeletal disorders (MSD).** These disorders are not the result of a single event but develop over time from the chronic use of repetitive, forceful, and awkward movements or postures at work or at home.[1] Affected areas include the soft tissues of the body, including nerves, tendons, and muscles. Symptoms may include pain, swelling, burning sensations, cramping, decreased range of motion, stiffness, muscle weakness, tingling, and numbness.

Studies regarding MSD among dental hygiene students are quite limited; however, musculoskeletal problems have become a significant issue for the profession of dentistry, including dental hygiene, and represent a significant burden. Factors that contribute to pain among dental professionals include poorly designed workstations, inadequate equipment, inappropriate work patterns, repetitive work, neck flexion, upper arm abduction, prolonged static postures, awkward positioning, and precise motions.[2] The key to preventing MSD is to minimize risk factors.

ERGONOMICS

Ergonomics is the scientific study of equipment design and workspaces focused on maximizing productivity by minimizing operator fatigue and discomfort. Examples of risk factors for operator fatigue and discomfort include:

- A poorly designed workstation including machinery that is illogically placed outside arm's reach
- Inadequate equipment such as dull instruments
- Ineffective and inefficient maneuvering around quadrants during instrumentation
- Inappropriate work patterns, such as contorting the body, not using indirect vision, and not following clock operator positioning
- Neck flexion and upper arm abduction caused by deviation from a neutral body position while working
- Prolonged static postures, especially when doing labor-intensive therapy, such as quadrant root planing

COMMON DENTAL MUSCULOSKELETAL DISORDERS

Three common MSD that dental hygienists experience are:

1. *Carpal tunnel syndrome:* Caused by compression of the median nerve in the carpal tunnel of the wrist. If not prevented, the hand may become "lazy" or "clumsy" with a loss in dexterity and strength. Treatments range from taking anti-inflammatory drugs to surgery.
2. *Rotator cuff problems or thoracic outlet syndrome:* Caused by swelling of the rotator cuff soft tissues of the shoulder and/or compressed nerves or blood supply passing to the arm. Both problems require worksite ergonomic interventions. Surgery should be a last resort for treatment.
3. *Myofascial pain syndrome:* Represents a range of symptoms that can present as a pain in the neck, shoulder,

and arm or back with possible trigger points. **Trigger points** are hyperirritable spots in the muscle that are associated with palpable nodules. The goal of treatment for this syndrome is to reduce pain and restore muscle function by strengthening and stretching muscles.

Prevention

Strategies for preventing MSDs include:

- Reducing the force of fingers while holding instruments
- Minimizing the load on the body when it is in one position for a prolonged period; that is, "taking the load off" by moving into a different position, even for a few moments simply to break the static cycle
- Improving posture
- Lessening vibrations from ultrasonics and handpieces
- Intentionally organizing the workplace setup for mindful musculoskeletal health
- Enhancing neutral postures whenever possible
- It is incumbent that the hygienist find a system of working in the mouth that is most efficient and effective to avert inappropriate work patterns

It is important to schedule a variety of procedures (e.g., sealants, root planing, radiographs, prophylaxis, and bleaching) throughout the day to avoid repetitive work patterning. It is ideal to avoid back-to-back repetitive prophylaxis appointments all day.

LOW-BACK PAIN

Clinical dental hygiene can be seen as an athletic event that requires tangible strength, physical endurance, and mental acuity. In the United States, approximately 85% of the population will experience a backache sometime in their life compared with an astounding 5% in other countries, where physical labor is part of the workday.[3] We live in a society that makes us move less, yet we were born to be active. Dental professionals practice in operatories where limited motion is emphasized and stabilization is stressed.

Low-back pain is a leading cause of occupational disability in dentistry. Studies show that low-back pain is frequently positively related to sitting duration. In fact, many experts believe that sitting is not a healthy position.[4,5] See Application to Clinical Practice 24-1.

People often think that sitting is a passive event, when, in fact, it is a very dynamic activity. Active sitting encourages the individual to move dynamically, because it is beneficial to the human body and can make some tasks easier to perform. The opposite of dynamic sitting is called *static sitting*, where the body is rigid, resulting in sustained mechanical tissue loading. Numerous problems occur when dangerous prolonged and unhealthy postures are sustained (Fig. 24-1). Table 24-1 lists common unhealthy working positions and solutions to prevent potential problems.

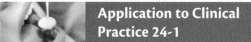

Application to Clinical Practice 24-1

It is possible for dental hygienists, as well as the entire dental profession, to practice pain-free for an entire career by understanding sound ergonomic principles and applying them on a consistent and routine basis. The International Ergonomics Association defines *ergonomics* as "the scientific discipline of interactions among humans and other elements that applies theory, principles, data, and methods to optimize human well-being and overall system performance." Applying ergonomics to the practice of dentistry could not only provide safety benefits, but a dental practice might also improve performance objectives through greater productivity.[29] ▪

ANTERIOR VERSION PELVIC POSITION

Terms such as *neutral sitting position, keeping the back straight,* and *keeping the head fairly straight* are ambiguous.[5] Attempting to hold these positions can be detrimental because the spine and its associated musculature are designed for motion. To improve posture and reduce muscle fatigue in a clinical environment:

- Position the patient so that your elbows are lower than your shoulders; keep your wrists even with or lower than the elbows.

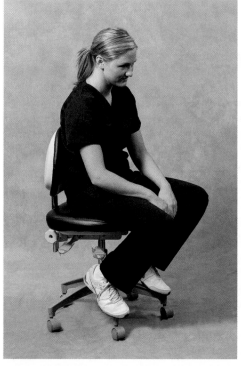

Figure 24-1. Poor posture can lead to musculoskeletal disorders.

Table 24-1. Unhealthy Working Postures and Solutions

Problem	Solution
Cervical (neck) rotation and laterally flexed	Maintain ears in line (above) with shoulders.
Arms abducted away from the body	Place arms by side near ribcage.
Arms in awkward forward position	Keep arms bent forward more than 20°.
Lumbar flexion (low back)	Preserve anterior version of pelvic girdle.
Trunk twisting	Use castors of a chair to turn.
Trunk laterally flexed	Align the trunk vertically.
Neck and upper and lower back are flexed	Entire spinal column is elongated.
Pelvis shifted in an oblique fashion	Sit on both sit bones (ischium) equally.
Wrists angled in different planes	Always align the wrist as if shaking a hand.
Patient chair is too high	Position yourself first; then move patient.
Feet close together or tucked under chair	Place feet flat and apart on the floor.

- Alternate between sitting and standing.
- Take breaks! Pausing even briefly and frequently can minimize fatigue and allow for muscle recovery (a term used in fitness), to reduce the risk for MSDs.
- Use properly fitted loupes to help with back, neck, and shoulder issues.
- Use properly fitted gloves and a more relaxed grip when holding instruments, whenever possible.
- Always work all body joints in a neutral position.
  - Neck: Keep it as vertical as possible and avoid tipping forward or to one side.
  - Shoulder: Keep shoulders horizontal and balanced on the chair. Avoid lifting, hunching, and sitting on one hip.
  - Spine: Lean from the waist in a "ready" position. Avoid a curved back.
  - Upper arm: Keep the upper arm parallel to the torso with the elbows at waist level and bent as if to shake someone's hand. Avoid greater than 20° abduction (arms flying away) from the body.
  - Forearm: Keep the forearm parallel to the floor and avoid closing it less than 60° to the upper arm.
  - Hand: Keep the thumb slightly higher than the little finger and keep the wrist aligned with the forearm. Avoid rotating the wrist or bending it up or down, as if the action resembled the crimping of a garden hose.

Dental hygienists sometimes use direct vision when indirect vision should be used. They also bend or twist to gain access to the oral cavity when changing the patient's position would allow easier access. The leaning, twisting, and reaching postures create imbalanced and overactive muscles. Ideally, when treating the mandibular arch, the patient should be positioned so that the chairback is lifted forward to bring the patient's occlusal plane as parallel to the floor as possible. When treating the maxillary arch, the chairback should be positioned as far back as possible so that the occlusal plane is perpendicular to the floor. Another consideration is to be sure the patient's head is as far back on the headrest as possible, because reaching or leaning over this additional space can lead to MSD that creep up over time. Practicing these adjustments is important, because many symptoms are not felt until after damage has been done.[6]

OPERATOR STOOL

The operator stool is important for preventing musculoskeletal injuries, because almost every syndrome or condition stems from improper seating. If the hips are offset, most other body parts are unbalanced. For example, when the pelvis is not centered in the middle of the chair and placed back into the seat/pan, one hip is commonly off center. If one hip is misaligned, then one hip is higher than the other. This translates to one side of the body being shorter and lower; this is often the right side for right-handed hygienists. Like a cascading effect, a lower right hip brings the right shoulder down, uneven with the left shoulder. Because the shoulder is lowered, the elbow must overcompensate and be lifted up to bring the arm up to a more stable parallel position. The lifted elbow contracts and fires up the deltoid and trapezius muscles, which fatigue quickly. If the elbow is not lifted enough, the wrist must flex to create parallelism of the instrument so that it can function most effectively. All of these conditions result from improper sitting positions.

For the left-handed hygienist, the left trunk will be shortened and lower than the right and the entire cascading effect occurs on that side. Think of the body's trunk as an accordion collapsed on one side. Now add twisting to the working side and it is easy to see how the spine is in an compromised position while working. Following this domino effect, it is easy to see how carpal tunnel syndrome, for example, is often not a problem that originates at the wrist, but rather begins at the seat. Most conditions of the body are due to improper alignment of the spine, shoulders, and hips.[7]

To avoid development of MSDs, the dental hygienist should sit up in the chair, with his or her buttocks at the back of the chair. When seated properly, the spine's natural curves should allow the head to be directly over the shoulders, which should be directly over the hips.

Most importantly, the coccyx, or tailbone, should be raised or even extended posteriorly to allow the pelvis to rotate forward, clockwise. The anterior spine of the hips (ilium) should be slightly forward of the sit bones (ischial tuberosities), so the hygienist can sit up with the tailbone (coccyx) back.

The goal of sitting is to maintain this pelvic and spinal alignment. Therefore, it is crucial to find or create a chair that places the pelvis in its anterior position *(anteversion)* in a supportive manner. This position reduces muscle strain and decreases intervertebral disk pressure. An **anteverted pelvis** facilitates healthy posture.[8] An elongated spine is integral to the health of the back, especially while seated.

With the thighs parallel to the floor, the hips are often at a 90° angle. In this position, the low back is frequently flattened (it loses its natural lumbar curve) and the pelvis rolls backward. This pelvic arrangement is a common cause of back pain. Conversely, when the pelvis is rotated too far anteriorly, the back muscles require constant contraction, expending tremendous energy.[9] This position is both unachievable and undesirable. Optimal or ideal sitting is between these two positions (Fig. 24-2).[10]

To sit in a neutral pelvic position:

1. Tilt the pelvis gently forward, placing your buttocks and base of the spine at an angle behind you with your behind, behind.
2. Stack the rest of the spine in a more or less straight line above the pelvis.
3. To prevent swaying, anchor the chest by engaging the internal oblique abdominal muscles just under the ribcage.[11]

An anteverted pelvis should not cause the low back to sway forward or become hyperextended. (Flexion would be the opposite effect.).

Another goal of any seated position is to keep the load on the spinal disks as low as possible by keeping the spine upright. The more an unsupported spine flexes the higher the disk load. Keeping the lower belly in and up almost always prevents this problem. To remember this action, create personal reminders. For example, every time you get an instrument off the tray, pull your lower belly in and up. Find personal ways to remind yourself that posture is less physical than it is mental.

Chair Options

One way to open the pelvis, helping to create anteversion, is to increase the chair height so that the angle of the hips opens to between 110° and 130°. This way the hips are slightly higher than the knees. The downward slant of the thighs also allows closer proximity to the patient. A saddle-shaped seat facilitates an opening of the hip angle and helps maintain the anteverted curve. Some stools are both saddle shaped and work in both active and passive positions. Alternating between the two active and passive positions is called **dynamic sitting,** where you alternate between half-standing and sitting (Figs. 24-3 and 24-4). In the active stance, the hygienist is literally in a "ready" position, like an athlete ready for action. This dynamic process is ideal because it keeps the hygienist moving throughout the day while working. In addition, sitting upright with the pelvis (ilia) forward and the hips open to about 110° in relation to the legs requires the least amount of

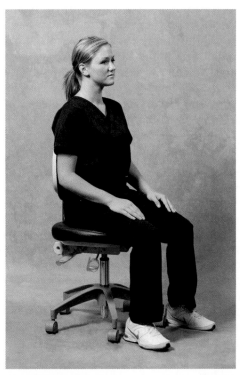

Figure 24-2. Optimal sitting position.

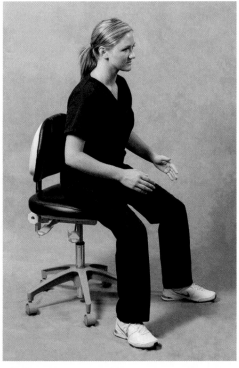

Figure 24-3. Dynamic active position.

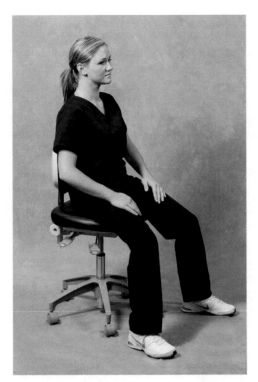

Figure 24-4. Dynamic passive position.

muscular effort to maintain the spinal curves and reduces disk pressure, which are factors in eliminating or reducing back pain.

TAKING A STAND

Sitting for long periods while leaning forward toward a patient, and performing repetitive motions such as scaling, builds the front of the body, making these muscles short and tight while the opposing back muscles overstretch, making them long and weak. More importantly, a slumped spine and upper body impairs the breathing mechanism by closing down the chest, lungs, and diaphragm. An excellent alternative to sitting while working is standing. Standing is a natural human posture and by itself poses no particular health hazard.[12]

Standing while performing clinical dental hygiene allows the large muscles of the legs and torso to contract and be active while providing a break for the vulnerable back and lumbar region (thereby transferring muscle activity and emphasis), improves circulation in the lower extremities, allows the upper body to be more relaxed, relieves stress on the intervertebral disks of the back to about 100 pounds,[13] promotes increased cardiovascular blood flow throughout the body,[14] allows for greater mobility around the patient chair, and provides more stability for the operator.

Another strategy to help prevent MSD is to move around the patient from *all* clock positions, including 1 and 2 o'clock for the right-handed practitioner (10 and 11 o'clock for the left-handed practitioner). Finally, attempt to schedule patients so that you alternate between

Application to Clinical Practice 24-2

Standing is the ideal position for treating the mandibular arch. During a periodontal maintenance or prophylaxis appointment, when both the maxillary and mandibular arches are treated, sit while treating the maxilla and stand for the mandible. Or stand for an entire quadrant of root debridement. ■

Application to Clinical Practice 24-3

Although it is important to keep moving around the patient, it is also important to be mindful of the neck while standing. Do not compromise the alignment of the neck structures just to stand. Be certain the patient chair is properly lifted to allow for sound standing principles. While working on the patient's mandibular arch/teeth, bring the headrest/backrest up so the patient's chin is as parallel to the floor as possible. Avoid compromising your neck and spine. DO NOT bend your back and crane your neck to get closer. If you are taller than average or your chair does not lift up high enough to counter this effect, standing may not be an alternative for you. The patient's size also may make a difference. Be mindful of both conditions. ■

long, difficult cases and short, easier cases.[15] See Application to Clinical Practice 24-2 and 24-3.

POSTURE

Tips to improve posture include:

- Develop the habit of checking your posture at specific times. For example, every time you begin a new quadrant during a prophylaxis or periodontal maintenance procedure, turn and stretch your trunk the opposite way you normally operate to counteract the contracted side. Or, whenever you are finished with hand instrumentation, open and close your fists four times.
- Change your position frequently. Stand to do the mandibular teeth and sit to do the maxillary teeth. Move around the patient and treat the mouth from both sides. Move equipment out of the way. Turn the entire chair from the base to gain access around 12 o'clock.
- Take care of your hips and bottom. Stretch the front of your hips (see the "Ill-E-O-So-As" exercise later in this chapter) and perform squats.

- Perform abdominal exercises with an extended spine. Do not pull on your neck or curl your spine while doing abdominal crunches. Keep the pelvis in a neutral position. Do not press the small of your back into the mat. Pilates or stabilizing exercises like the plank, balancing on your elbows while maintaining shoulder girdle stability, are best.
- Strengthen and elongate your back. Learn exercises that extend the back while standing, seated, on knees, or prone on elbows. These exercises often improve or eliminate back pain.
- Focus on the upper body. Learn exercises that strengthen the upper back and stretch the chest. A perfect exercise is holding 3-pound dumbbells with your arms at 90° and opening the elbows and closing the arms elbow to elbow, like you are closing and opening a book. The back action is more important than the front action. Stretch the chest (pectoralis muscles) and strengthen the upper back (upper and middle trapezius muscles).
- Vary your exercise regimen. Consider an elliptical machine for cardiovascular health or tennis for balance. Pilates emphasizes alignment and controlled movements of the spine, which can greatly improve posture. Yoga is superb for flexibility and reducing mental stress.
- Perfect your posture. Changing your *posture is more a mental phenomenon* than a physical occurrence. Imagine a helium balloon attached to the crown of your head rising up. Mind your body.
- Use magnification. When fit properly, **magnification loupes** improve visual perception and posture and provide precision with dental treatment. Dental hygienists who do not use magnification loupes often suffer from a multitude of musculoskeletal problems, which include back, neck, and shoulder injuries. These problems often occur because of the need to assume a shorter working distance to increase visual acuity.[14]

Loupes and Lighting

There are two types of loupes (magnification): through the lens and flip-up. Through the lens eyewear is individually customized to fit your eye width and other variables. Flip-ups hinge on top of a pair of safety glasses and can be heavy on the bridge of the nose. Like a purse or handbag worn over the shoulder, there are differences, both personally and functionally, between loupes. Many companies have a trial period. Take advantage of this opportunity and invest in loupes (Box 24-1). They will be an eye and back saver if fitted and used properly. Also, consider personal lighting. When properly selected and adjusted, lighting and magnification can support balanced musculoskeletal ergonomics. Conversely, improperly selected or poorly adjusted systems can contribute to, or may even create, unacceptable working postures.[15] See Advancing Technologies.

Overhead lighting should produce even, shadow-free, color-corrected illumination concentrated on the operating field.

Box 24-1. *Loupes*

- Custom eyewear can be expensive, but it is worth the price for a healthy body.
- There is a learning curve to using loupes, which can be challenging at first. Keep using them as long as they are fit perfectly for you until you are able to adjust to them.
- With increased magnification, your field size and brightness decrease.
- Loupes will greatly help you to see more clearly and effortlessly, thereby improving your clinical experience.
- Loupes can improve efficiency and effectiveness during clinical practice.
- Your posture can improve as long as your focal length and declination angle are correct.
- Magnification of 2.0 to 2.5 is often a good option for dental hygiene care. ■

 Advancing Technologies

In addition to magnification, consider using a headlight or headlamp to help illuminate the oral cavity. Being able to see more easily and clearly reduces stress to the musculoskeletal system. Headlights are lightweight and have a small, portable battery pack that fits in a uniform pocket. Sufficient lighting is a tool that is essential in preventing potential pain and compromising injury. When selecting a headlight, consider the adjustment of brightness, beam uniformity, and weight.[30] ■

HAND INSTRUMENTS

When using any instrument, the goal is to reduce force exertion while maintaining the hand/wrist in a neutral position; that is, there is no bend at the wrist and no hyperextension of the finger joints, particularly the thumb.

Selecting Instruments

When selecting an instrument, consider:

- Your intention for utilization
- Overall shape and size
- Handle shape and size
- The weight of the instrument (each hygienist may have a different preference)
- Whether the instrument feels balanced in your hand
- Maneuverability
- Ease of operation
- Ease of maintenance for both cutting edge and cleaning

When selecting hand instruments that will be held for a long period, look for larger-diameter, round, textured handles that are hollow or resin, because they are lighter and easier on the hand. Larger handles can be gripped with the pads of the fingers, thereby distributing the strain through a larger group of muscles.[16]

Color-coding may make instrument identification easier. Also consider different handle sizes and textures for probing, supragingival scaling (sickles), and universal instruments. Even subtle variation between instruments of various handle size can distribute muscle activity among hand and finger muscle groups, reducing fatigue.[17] Consider, for example, an instrument set up that has narrower and thinner handles for the probe and explorer, a round, metal handle that is serrated for universal use, and Gracey instruments with graphite handles. This arrangement allows you to select instruments with more efficiency and change handle diameter throughout the appointment, which will help prevent hand problems.

Keeping working edges sharp is key to decreasing hand stress. Instruments perform more effectively and efficiently when sharp. When an edge is dull, additional force is required to achieve the same result. Sharp instruments are vital for reducing excessive force during instrumentation, which is a risk for MSDs. No standard for an ergonomic instrument currently exists.

AUTOMATED INSTRUMENTS (HANDPIECES)

Handpieces should be as light as possible and well-balanced. Having a shorter hose length will help prevent drag and extra weight on the handpiece, thereby reducing extra stress on the hand and wrist. A pliable hose with a swivel mechanism in the barrel of the handpiece, which allows the instrument to rotate with minimal effort, is recommended.[18]

Additional Tips to Improve Posture

The following are additional recommendations to improve posture:

- *Consider arm support:* Free-motion elbow supports are a key component in reducing work-related MSD of the back, shoulders, and neck.[19] Make sure armrests are adjustable. Some armrests move as a clinician leans forward or back; others swing out of the way, and some remain fixed, according to a clinician's physical specifications.[20] Be aware that ergonomic chairs are designed to support weaknesses in the musculoskeletal system. However, nothing compares with a strong body at work.[21]
- *When in doubt, check it out:* Postural problems can have serious ramifications on an individual's life and livelihood. Consult a physical therapist, physiatrist, medical doctor, chiropractor, or other specialist when needed. Do not wait for symptoms to become aggravated; take action when symptoms begin.

- *Operatory/Workplace exercises:* Specific strength-training exercises are indicated for dental hygienists who are pain free. Most important are exercises that target the back and abdominal muscles, known as core-strengthening exercises. Stretching exercises may help prevent work-related MSD and break the cycle of discomfort-pain-muscle stiffness-injury-pain caused by awkward postures and continuous (isometric) or repetitive (isotonic) muscle contractions.[22] Other benefits of stretching may include increased flexibility, improved joint range of motion, improved circulation, enhanced posture, and stress relief.[23] Taking numerous breaks throughout the day to stretch is more important than stretching once a day during a major break, such as at lunchtime.[24,25]

Fitness Outside the Operatory

Keeping fit outside the workplace is equally, if not more important than exercising in the operatory. The key to preventing MSD is exercising consistently and routinely. For healthy adults, the latest guidelines from the American College of Sports Medicine and the American Heart Association suggest cardiovascular exercise at a moderate (30 min/day, 5 days a week) or vigorous intensity (20 min/day, 3 days a week). In addition to cardiovascular training, they advise including 8 to 10 strength-training exercises, working the back, shoulders, legs, hips, arms, and abdominals, and performing 8 to 12 repetitions of each, twice a week.[26]

Physical activity decreases pain, improves overall function, delays disability in joints, improves cardiovascular health, enhances glucose metabolism, boosts musculoskeletal health, improves psychological well-being, and keeps weight in check. A healthy weight reduces the stress on the ligaments and joints of the body.[27]

OPERATORY AND OFFICE EXERCISES

Navel In and Up

The most important of all exercises is the navel in and up exercise. Inhale and gently pull the navel toward the spine, then, more importantly, pull the navel *up* toward the ribs. Sit tall, with the shoulders relaxed and drawn down. Hold for about 5 to 10 seconds and release. Repeat 5 to10 times. Notice how the lift enhances spinal extension. This exercise can be done anytime throughout the day.

Hands

Most seasoned dental hygienists do not need to do hand-strengthening exercises because these muscles are often built up; however, it is important for students to do hand-strengthening exercises to manage instruments effectively. Squeezing and releasing a tennis ball is one example of a hand-strengthening exercise.

Open/Close

To perform this hand stretch spread the fingers as wide apart as possible. Then make a tight fist and release. This brings vital blood and circulation to the hands. Hold for 5 seconds and release. Hold for 10 seconds. Repeat five to eight times.

Wrist Flexor and Extensor Stretch

To perform a wrist flexor and extensor stretch, straighten the arm parallel to the floor. Bend the wrist so the fingers are pointing toward the floor. Gently press with the opposite hand, flexing your wrist, and try to bring the fingers closer to the inside of the wrist (Fig. 24-5). Making a fist while flexing greatly enhances this stretch. To counter the stretch, extend the fingers toward the ceiling. With the opposite hand, gently pull your palm and fingers toward you (Fig. 24-6). Repeat each exercise four to six times to relieve hand and wrist strain.

Neck Stretches

Stretching the neck improves range of movement and motion, a vital necessity for these most often overworked muscles of the dental professional. Stretching the neck will ease stiffness, reduce stress, and provide relief for recurring cervical muscle tension.

No

For the "no" exercise, turn your head to the right and then to the left, looking over each shoulder. Where your eyes go, your body will follow. Take your time to stretch your neck. Repeat four complete cycles.

Ear to Chest

The ear to chest exercise is especially beneficial on the opposite working side; for example, turning the head right for right-handed dental hygienists. Turn the head slightly to one side. Bring the ear to the chest (nipple) and exhale on the stretch. To stretch farther, place the hand on the side of the head and gently stabilize the head (Fig. 24-7). Keep the abdominals gently contracted and avoid lifting the shoulder or twisting the trunk. Reaching under a stool with the free hand, and pulling the shoulder down, will facilitate the stretch. Hold for 10 seconds. Return to the starting position very slowly and repeat two to three more times. Turn your head and repeat on the other side.

Shoulder Stretches

Dental professionals would be well-served to stretch and open the front chest muscles and strengthen the upper and middle back muscles.

Fingers Clasped and Arms Up to the Ceiling

An effective should exercise is to clasp your fingers in front of your chest and turn the palms outward (Fig. 24-8A). Inhale and lift the arms straight up to the ceiling, by the ears if possible (Fig. 24-8B). Hold for about 5 seconds and exhale as the arms descend

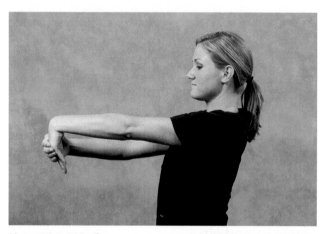

Figure 24-5. Wrist flex.

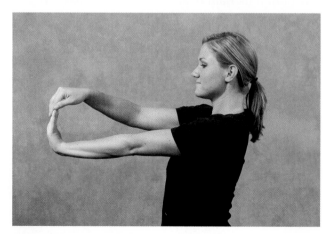

Figure 24-6. Wrist extend.

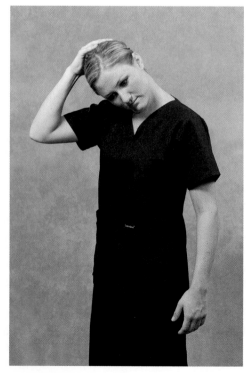

Figure 24-7. Ear to chest.

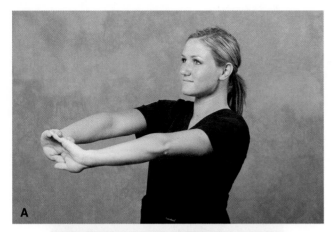

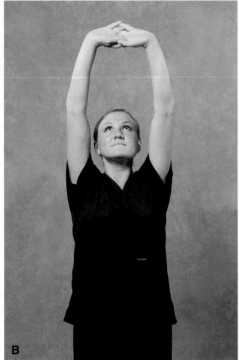

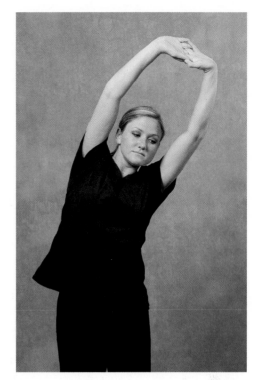

Figure 24-9. Lateral trunk stretch.

Figure 24-8. (A) Clasp fingers in front of chest and turn palms out. (B) Lift the arms up and stretch.

back down. Looking up enhances the stretch. Repeat four times. This is a great anytime stretch,

Set Your Shoulders Back

Sitting erect, take a full inhale and slowly exhale. As you breathe, lift the shoulders up, roll them around to the back, and place them down. Then allow the weight of the arms, behind your back, to depress the shoulder blades even farther. Keep your arms behind your back and lift your sternum up. Repeat five times. If there was one exercise to do all day—this is it!

Upper Body Stretches

Lateral Trunk Stretch (Variations: Arms Down or One Arm Overhead)

To perform a lateral trunk stretch, clasp the hands and lift them overhead. Sitting or standing tall with the abdominals slightly contracted, bend the trunk laterally to

one side (Fig. 24-9). Inhale on the lift and exhale on the lateral stretch. Hold for 5 seconds. Keep breathing. Stretch the opposite side. Repeat four times on each side.

Upper Trunk Extension

Sitting: Clasp your hands behind your head and sit tall. Slowly inhale and lift the sternum up and the upper back up and slightly backward to a point of maximal stretch. Look to the junction of the wall and ceiling or the ceiling itself. Keep your head in line with the spine, especially at the cervical vertebrae. Hold for 4 seconds. Return to the original position and repeat five times.

Standing: Place your hands on the back of your hips (at the iliac crest) and gently lift and extend the spine up and back. Inhale on the lift and exhale on the return. Hold for 5 seconds at the top. Tuck the tail slightly to avoid pinching the lower back. Repeat five times.

Note: This exercise may be contraindicated for people with disk or back problems. Consult a physician or therapist first.

Lateral Rotation/Spinal Rotation

To perform a lateral rotation/spinal rotation, sitting tall, open the knees and rotate the spine to one side and lift as you twist. For added stretch, use your hands on the chair backrest to deepen the twist. Keep your bottom stable, in the center of the chair (Fig. 24-10). Inhale on the twist and exhale on the release. Hold for 5 seconds on the twist. Repeat on the other side after five repetitions. Keep lifting the spine upward like a wine cork being lifted from its bottle.

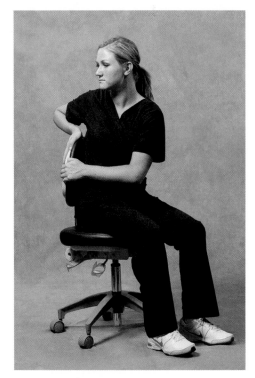

Figure 24-10. Spinal rotation.

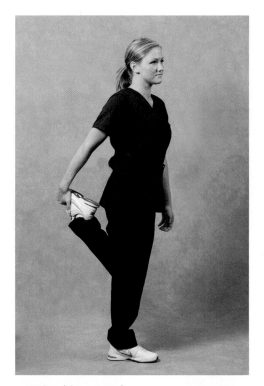

Figure 24-11. Quadriceps stretch.

For a further seated twist, cross one knee over the other and rotate laterally. Use the opposite hand to enhance the stretch.

On all rotations, where you look, your body will follow. Be mindful of your eye direction. Keep looking to the horizon or middle of a wall. Do not look up or down because that will twist the upper cervical spine unnecessarily.

Legs

Quadriceps Stretch

For a quadriceps stretch, bend one knee back and reach for the ankle with the same-side hand (Fig. 24-11). Hold the ankle. Place the opposite hand on a chairback or desk if necessary to maintain balance. Attempt to draw the knees together. To stretch the hip flexors, which are shortened and tight all day, gently pull the tail under in a counterclockwise rotation to bring the front hipbone backward. You should feel a terrific stretch at the top of the thigh, at the origin of the muscle. Hold for 5 to 10 seconds or two breath cycles. Repeat three times and then switch legs.

The "Ill-E-O-So-As" Stretch

The "Ill-E-O-So-As" stretch is the most important leg stretch. Standing at a wall or counter, place one foot about 2 feet away and the other foot about 4 feet away. Bend the front knee and press the back heel down in line with the hip (Fig. 24-12). For a deeper stretch, push the hips forward and counterclockwise, so the tail pulls under, without squeezing the gluteal (buttocks) muscles.

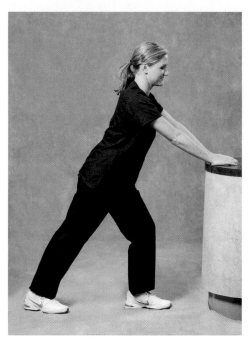

Figure 24-12. Ill-E-O-So-As stretch.

For an enhanced stretch, take the arm that is on the same side as the extended back leg straight up by the ear. Lift up and over to the opposite side. Hold for 5 to 10 seconds. Breathe. The stretch should be felt along the entire side of the body as well as inside the abdominal wall. Release and stretch two more times. Switch to the other side and repeat. Keep breathing.

SUMMARY

Prevention of work-related MSD is crucial. Most dental hygiene programs provide basic ergonomic education (patient/operator positioning and instrumentation), but additional education such as body mechanics or preventive exercises are generally unavailable or available only on a limited basis to dental hygiene students.

Integration of ergonomic education in dental hygiene curricula may help prevent MSDs in dental hygienists by enabling them to begin their dental hygiene careers with awareness of MSDs and good ergonomic work habits.[28] Incorporating numerous and frequent ergonomic principles and strategies into daily clinical practice will allow dental hygienists to have longer, more productive, healthier, and ultimately happier careers.

Case Study

The dental hygienist is working on her third patient of the day and has been debriding the lower left quadrant for an hour. Her back and neck are starting to bother her because she has been leaning to the right, creating a C curve in the side of her back, to see. The hygienist has only a few more teeth to complete the entire procedure and knows she can get to the end of the appointment without too much trouble. Her next appointment is a child; then she has an hour for lunch.

Case Study Exercises

1. What immediate changes could the hygienist make to improve her posture?
   A. Raise the chair and stand up to work.
   B. Have the patient reposition his head so it is down and away.
   C. Roll her shoulders up, around, and back.
   D. All of the above
2. What ergonomic equipment could the hygienist use to improve her visibility?
   A. Magnification/Loupes
   B. Headlamp
   C. Ergonomic stool
   D. All of the above

3. What trouble might the hygienist encounter if she continues working this way?
   A. Chronic backaches
   B. Shoulder pain
   C. Neck stiffness
   D. All of the above
4. What should the hygienist do during her lunch hour to help her be most productive in the afternoon?
   A. Rest in her operatory chair.
   B. Take a 20- to 30-minute brisk walk.
   C. Sit on the local park bench and read.
   D. Apply an ice pack to her neck.
5. What could the hygienist use in her operatory that would make it more ergonomic?
   A. A patient chair that allows the patient's head to be all the way at the back end
   B. An operatory chair with a flat, large seat pan so the hygienist's back could be flat against the backrest
   C. A tray of instruments that are set up on the counter to the right of the hygienist
   D. A computer that is set on a high shelf to the left of the hygienist, out of the patient's way

Review Questions

1. Applying sound ergonomic principles in a dental operatory could prevent most musculoskeletal disorders. Sitting during all procedures is one sound ergonomic suggestion.
   A. The first statement is true, but the second statement is false.
   B. The first statement is false, but the second statement is true.
   C. Both statements are true.
   D. Both statements are false.

2. To sit in an anteverted pelvic position:
   A. Sit up tall to place an arch in the back, roll the shoulders back, and stick out the coccyx.
   B. Tilt the pelvis forward slightly, lift the spine up, and slightly contract the muscles at the front upper ribs.
   C. Pull the tailbone under, pull the shoulders forward, and allow the navel to draw out.
   D. Sit tall, pull the navel in, and pull the shoulders back.

3. Benefits of stretching could include:
   A. Increased flexibility
   B. Increased range of motion
   C. Improved blood flow
   D. All of the above

4. An excellent postural exercise to do any time of day is:
   A. Navel in and up
   B. Wrist flexor and extensor
   C. Lateral trunk stretch
   D. Quadriceps stretch

5. One of the most important exercises for the seated professional is:
   A. Opening and closing the hands
   B. Seated lateral rotation/spinal twist
   C. "U" first
   D. The Ill-E-O-So-As stretch

Active Learning

1. Sit in a flat, noncontoured dental chair and tuck your tailbone under. Roll your shoulders forward while allowing your arms to hang down at your hips. Take a breath. How does it feel? Now, sit up, lift your chest, and inhale. How much difference do you sense between the two positions?

2. While seated, roll your pelvis forward so your back feels arched and your muscles are contracted. Hold this position for 10 full seconds. Then, curl your tailbone under and round your chest and shoulders forward. Hold this position for 10 full seconds. Find a point in between where you are balanced between the two positions and feel your sit bones underneath your bottom. Breathe. Note the change.

3. Facing an imaginary patient, see what happens when you create a cascading effect in your body by sitting on one sit bone (ischial tuberosity), allowing the bottom to literally "hang off" the chair edge. Lower your same-side shoulder down; lift your elbow up, crane your neck up, and twist it toward the imaginary patient. HOLD this position for 20 seconds. How does it feel? Now, sit balanced on both sit bones. Note the distinction.

4. Visit your local personal dental office and evaluate their chairs and other ergonomic equipment. Make notes. Take an active part in sitting, trying out loupes, viewing objects with a headlamp, or learning about any other products that help you in a clinical setting.

5. Review the seated exercises and perform three of your favorite. Commit to doing them, both in and out of the operatory. ■

REFERENCES

1. Hamann C, Werner R, Rhode N, Rogers P, Sullivan K. Upper extremity musculoskeletal disorders in dental hygiene: diagnosis and options for management. *Contemp Oral Hyg.* 2004;4:2-8.

2. Hayes M, Cockrell D, Smith D. A systematic review of musculoskeletal disorders among dental professionals. *Int J Dent Hyg.* 2009;7(3):159-165.

3. Volinn E. The epidemiology of low back pain in the rest of the world: a review of surveys in low- and middle-income countries. *Spine.* 1997;22(15):1747-1754.

4. Ahearn D. The 8 keys to selecting great seating for long-term health. *Dentistry Today.* 2005;24(9):128, 130-131.

5. Division of Occupational Health and Safety. Bethesda, MD: National Institutes of Health, Office of Research Services. http://dohs.ors.od.nih.gov/ergo_computers.htm. Accessed August 16, 2010.

6. Dylla J, Forrest J. Fit to sit: strategies to maximize function and minimize occupational pain. *J Mich Dent Assoc.* 2008;90(5):38-45.

7. Egoscue P. *Pain Free at Your PC.* New York: Bantam; 1999.

8. Gokhale E. *8 Steps to a Pain-Free Back.* Pendo Press; 2008:71-73.

9. Williams M, Hawley J, McKenzie R, van Wijmen P. A comparison of the effects of two sitting postures on back and referred pain. *Spine.* 1991;16(10):1185-1191.

10. Gokhale E. *8 Steps to a Pain-Free Back.* Pendo Press; 2008.

11. Gokhale E. Palo Alto, CA. August 2009. http://egwellness.com/get-your-behind-behind-you. Accessed July 14, 2010.

12. Working in standing/sitting positions. Hamilton, ON: Canadian Centre for Occupational Health and Safety. http://www.ccohs.ca/oshanswers/ergonomics/standing/sit_stand.html. Accessed March 10, 2010.

13. Nachemson A. The lumbar spine, an orthopaedic challenge. *Spine.* 1976;1(1):59-71.

14. Millar D. *Reinforced Periodontal Instrumentation and Ergonomics.* Philadelphia: Lippincott Williams & Wilkins; 2008:3-6.

15. Rucker LM, Beattie C, McGregor C. Declination angle and its role in selecting surgical telescopes. *J Am Dent Assoc.* 1999;130:1096-1100.

16. Martin J. Hand Tool Use and Design Principles (lecture). Dental Economics Summit 2000; American Dental Association; Chicago.

17. Oberg T, Karsznia A, Sandsjo L, et al. Workload, fatigue, and pause patterns in clinical dental hygiene. *J Dent Hyg.* 1995;69(5):223-229.

18. Pollack R. The ergo factor: the most common equipment and design flaws and how to avoid them. *Dentistry Today.* 1999:112-121.

19. American Dental Association. Chicago: Ergonomics for Dental Students. Updated 2008. http://www.ada.org/sections/educationandcareers/pdfs/ergonomics.pdf. Accessed August 18, 2010.

20. Osuna T. Elbow room. *RDH Maga*[...] [...]&TEMPLATE=/CM/HTMLDisplay.cfm&
21. Guignon A. Toxic or healthy seat [...] [...]764. Accessed August 17, 2010.
    2010;30(4). [...]*ody.* MindBody Publishing; Walnut
22. Kravitz L. The 25 most significa [...] [...]08.
    physical activity and exercise. [...] Assessment of ergonomic education
23. DaCosta B, Vieira E. Stretching [...] [...]rricula. *J Dent Educ.* 1998;62(6):
    musculoskeletal disorders: a s[...]
    Med. 2008;40(5):321-328. [...]Association. An introduction to
24. Choi S, Woletz T. Do stretchi[...] [...]actors, MSDs, approaches and
    work-related musculoskelet[...] [...]report of the Ergonomics and
    Environ Res. 2010;6(3). [...]rt Advisory Committee to Council on
25. Valachi B, Valachi K. Preve[...] [...]2004. www.http://rgpdental.com/pdfs/
    disorders in clinical dentis[...] [...]ics_paper(2).pdf
    134:1604-1612. [...]ng, positioning, and lighting. *Dimens Dent*
26. American College of Spor[...] [...]):36-37.
    http://www.acsm.org/AM[...]

Chapter 25 | Power Scaling

Michele Carr, RDH, MA

KEY TERMS

amplitude

cavitation

frequency

hertz (Hz)

lavage

magnetostrictive
  ultrasonic scaler

piezoelectric ultrasonic
  scaler

sonic scaler

ultrasonic scaler

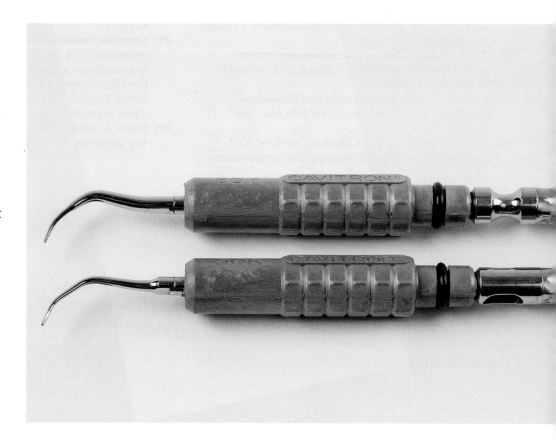

LEARNING OBJECTIVES

After reading this chapter, the student should be able to:

25.1 Discuss the principles and mechanisms of action for powered scaling devices.

25.2 Describe the types of power scaling devices that are available.

25.3 Understand and explain the advantages and disadvantages of power scaling compared with manual instrumentation.

25.4 Identify appropriate inserts/tips for use in a variety of clinical circumstances.

25.5 Describe the proper activation and care of ultrasonic inserts.

KEY CONCEPTS

• Power scaling can effectively treat a wide range of patient needs from maintaining oral health to treating patients with periodontal disease.

• Power scaling is an efficient and effective means for full-mouth debridement.

• Proper technique and tip selection is necessary for success in thorough debridement.

RELEVANCE TO CLINICAL PRACTICE

Power scaling has been used for periodontal procedures for more than 50 years and will continue to be used in the future. The evolution of power scaling devices and inserts has been tremendous. Due to current research findings regarding the pathogenesis of periodontal disease, power scaling can and should be used on nearly every patient undergoing periodontal debridement procedures, including routine visits for recare, periodontal maintenance, and periodontal therapy. New technology has allowed researchers to discover that bacterial plaque is sophisticated and exists as complex matrices called *biofilms*.[1] The only way to improve periodontal health is to remove or disrupt the biofilm.[2] This can be accomplished effectively with manual instrumentation or power scaling devices, but there are advantages when power scaling is used.

WHAT ARE POWER SCALING DEVICES?

Power scaling devices are electronically powered machines that create electrical currents that produce rapid vibrations of the instrument tip. These rapid vibrations remove calculus and debris and disrupt the biofilm.

TYPES OF POWER SCALING DEVICES

There are two general categories of power scaling devices: sonic scalers and ultrasonic scalers. **Sonic scalers** are connected to the dental unit's compressed air valve and are activated by the unit's foot control. **Ultrasonic scalers** have their own electronic generator and foot pedal, which attaches to the unit.

Mechanism of Action

Both sonic and ultrasonic devices, when activated, convert energy from the handpiece to produce vibrations at the tip.

Frequency

The number of times an instrument tip vibrates or cycles per second (cps) is referred to as the **frequency**. The **hertz (Hz)** is the unit of energy that measures the cps. Sonic scalers operate at a frequency of 3000 to 8000 cps.[3] Because of this low frequency, sonic scalers are not as effective as ultrasonic scaling devices.

Ultrasonic power scaling devices operate at a frequency between 18,000 and 50,000 cps depending on the type and manufacturer of the power scaling unit.[3] There are currently two types of ultrasonic scalers: magnetostrictive and piezoelectric (Figs. 25-1 and 25-2). **Magnetostrictive ultrasonic scalers** generate an elliptical, or figure-eight motion, whereas **piezoelectric**

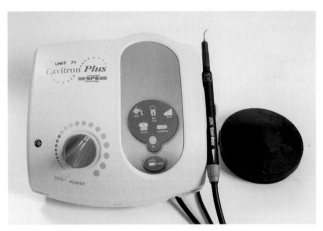

Figure 25-1. Magnetostrictive power scaling device.

ultrasonic scalers have a linear motion. Magnetostrictive units are available in 30K and 25K configurations and must use corresponding 30K or 25K tips, or inserts, made of a stack of metal strips or rods of ferromagnetic material. The tips are capable of being magnetized, resulting in an elliptical or figure-eight motion of the

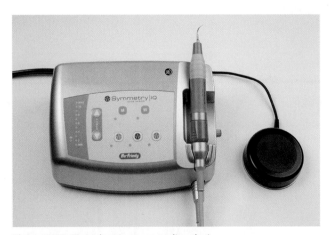

Figure 25-2. Piezoelectric power scaling device.

working end of the tip (Fig. 25-3). This type of motion allows the use of all sides of the working tip. Heat is generated when using magnetostrictive inserts; water is used as a cooling agent.

Piezoelectric units use tips that screw into a handpiece with a wrench-type device (Fig. 25-4). These tips alternate electrical currents applied to reactive crystals horizontally, resulting in a linear motion. Only the lateral sides of the working tip are activated. Little heat is generated when using these tips, minimizing the amount of water that is necessary. Piezoelectric units operate at a higher frequency than magnetostrictive units.

Amplitude

On both types of ultrasonic units, there is a power control and a water, or lavage, control feature. The power feature controls the **amplitude,** which is the distance the tip moves or the length of the stroke. Higher power delivers a longer, more powerful stroke, and low power delivers a shorter, less powerful stroke.

Lavage

The **lavage** (water) control feature adjusts the flow of water from the tip. Because water is used with power scaling devices, cavitation and acoustic microstreaming effects are created. Rapid movement of air bubbles from the tip of the insert, known as **cavitation,** creates shock waves that are responsible for bacterial cell death.[4] Acoustic microstreaming releases energy by the movements of small currents in the water.[5] Magnetostrictive and piezoelectric power scaling devices are equally effective in calculus removal.[6,7]

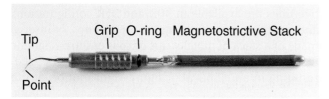

Figure 25-3. Parts of a magnetostrictive insert.

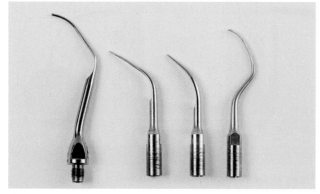

Figure 25-4. Piezoelectric tip.

Advantages of Power Scaling Devices

Although there is no difference in the effectiveness of power scaling and manual instrumentation, power scaling devices have significant advantages:

- Lavage, or irrigation, is the therapeutic washing of the periodontal pocket from the constant stream of water from the instrument tip. It improves vision by acting as a wash field and improves healing time by removing toxic bacterial by-products.
- Instrumentation time is reduced by one third compared with hand instrumentation.[8,9]
- Increased patient comfort results from less tissue distention.
- Operator ergonomics are improved because power scaling devices require less lateral pressure and less repetitive stress, and they are more efficient.
- Less root surface structure is removed.
- Tips do not need to be sharpened.

Disadvantages of Power Scaling Devices

Power scaling devices also have several disadvantages:

- Evacuation devices can be cumbersome.
- Patients may have increased sensitivity to the vibration of the tip or water flow, or both.

Indications for Use

Power scaling devices can be used for all types of periodontal debridement procedures, including deplaquing, supragingival and subgingival scaling, and root planing.

Contraindications

- Power scaling devices produce contaminated aerosols and should not be used on patients who have a predisposition to infection or a known communicable disease.
- Power scaling devices should be used with caution on patients with respiratory risk or those who are prone to gagging because of the flow of water.
- Patients who have older-model pacemakers should not be the recipients of power scaling from magnetostrictive units because their mechanism of action could interfere with the operation of the pacemaker. View the manufacturer's instructions.
- Power scaling should be avoided in areas of demineralization because it could cause further damage to weakened enamel areas. It should be used with caution

Application to Clinical Practice

Denise has just graduated from a dental hygiene program where students routinely used power scaling devices on their patients. She has accepted a position in a private dental practice and has discovered they do not use power scaling technology. Denise cannot imagine completing periodontal procedures without using ultrasonic instrumentation. She does not feel comfortable asking her new employer to purchase a power scaling unit because she does not want to appear demanding so early in her employment. Knowing the benefits that power scaling offers, should she ask her employer to purchase one for the office? Or should she purchase a unit herself after consulting with her employer? ■

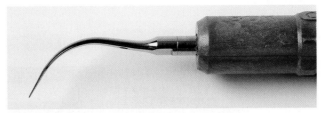

Figure 25-6. Periodontal or thin tip.

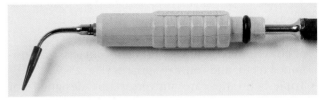

Figure 25-7. Implant tip.

around exposed root surfaces and primary teeth with large pulp chambers because these areas may be sensitive to the vibration of the tip or the heat generated.
- Power scaling devices should be used with caution around restorations to avoid damage to margins and surfaces. They should not be used around titanium implants unless a specialized implant tip is used.

Tip Types

Power scaling devices use a variety of tips and tip designs. There are two basic tip types:

- Standard or universal tips are comparatively bigger and bulkier tips used for moderate to heavy deposit removal. These tips can be used on any power setting (Fig. 25-5).
- Periodontal, or "slim," tips are approximately 40% thinner than universal tips and mimic a periodontal probe. Because these tips are thinner and longer, they provide better access to deeper periodontal pockets and are ideal for deplaquing inflamed, shallow pockets. Periodontal tips should be used on low-to-medium power (Fig. 25-6).

Specialty Tips

A variety of tips are available for specific tasks:

- Implant tips include a plastic cover that is placed over the metal tip to prevent damage to titanium implants (Fig. 25-7).
- Bladed tips are shaped like curets, thin in diameter, and designed for light to heavy supragingival deposits in shallow pockets.

- Diamond-coated tips are designed for enhanced access in periodontal pockets. They are used for light to medium deposit removal or for finishing.
- Swivel tips can be rolled between the hygienist's fingers to allow for better adaptation during instrumentation (Fig. 25-8).
- Illuminated tips provide light directly in the area of instrumentation. See Advancing Technologies.

Tip Designs

There are many types of ultrasonic tips. Choosing the correct tip for the type of treatment being provided will help maximize efficiency and help to safely treat patients with all levels of oral health.

- Straight tips are available in universal and slim types.
- Curved right and left tips are available in the slim design. They are most effective on interproximal surfaces

Advancing Technologies

Power scaling technology continues to evolve and improve. Ultrasonic scalers are superior to sonic scalers in their ability to break up bacterial biofilm, the cause of active disease. Ultrasonic tips are available in various lengths, shapes, thicknesses, and angulations, all of which are critical for ideal access and deposit removal. ■

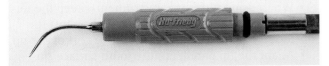

Figure 25-5. Standard or universal tip.

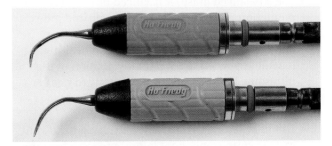

Figure 25-8. Swivel tip.

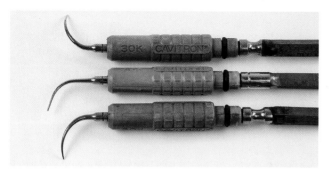

Figure 25-9. Curved right and left tips.

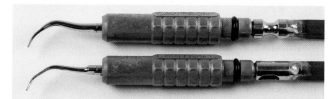

Figure 25-10. Triple bend tip.

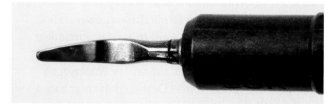

Figure 25-11. Beaver tail tip.

of posterior teeth, furcations, tight contacts, malpositioned teeth, and concave surfaces (Fig. 25-9).
- Triple-bend tips are universal tips designed for heavy-to-gross debridement (Fig. 25-10).
- Beaver tail tips are universal tips designed for heavy buccal and lingual deposits (Fig. 25-11).

Procedure 25-1 | Power Scaling

PREPARATION
- At the beginning of each day, flush the waterline to the power scaling device for 2 to 3 minutes to reduce bacterial contamination. Repeat for 20 to 30 seconds between patients.
- Before placing the power scaling insert into the handle on magnetostrictive units, fill the handpiece with water, lubricate the O-ring with water, and then firmly place the insert into the handpiece.
- Direct the patient to complete a 30-second preprocedural rinse with an antimicrobial solution to reduce the number of pathogens present in the aerosols.[10]
- Inform the patient that a power scaling device will be used for debridement.

Tip Selection
Tip selection is based on the following factors:
- Tissue health or disease
- Type, location, and amount of deposits
- Pocket depth and periodontal classification
- Root anatomy

PROCEDURE
1. *Position the patient*
   - Place the patient in a supine position.
2. *Grasp*
   - Use a balanced grasp. A balanced ultrasonic instrumentation grasp (between the thumb and index finger) aids to maximize ultrasonic technique and dental hygienist musculoskeletal health. It is achieved when the weight distribution of the ultrasonic handpiece feels heavy toward neither the front nor back of the instrument.
3. *Lateral pressure*
   - Use light lateral pressure. When using ultrasonic instruments, apply light lateral pressure for safe, effective calculus removal and patient comfort.

Pressure contrary to this is likely to lead to ineffective deposit removal (remaining calculus, remaining burnished calculus, or increased time for calculus removal) or possible root surface damage, or both. Use the same light lateral pressure (or less) when using an ultrasonic instrument to remove or disrupt bacteria and biofilm colonies.
   - Wrap the cord of the handpiece around the forearm or between the fingers of the dominant hand to reduce tension and torque.
4. *Fulcrums*
   - Extraoral and intraoral fulcrums can be used. Establish a fulcrum that will aid with the ideal adaptation of an ultrasonic insert to promote effective and safe deposit removal, minimize the risk for musculoskeletal disorders, and maximize patient comfort.
   - A fulcrum too close to the working surface may disrupt a balanced ultrasonic grasp and/or impinge on the hygienist's ability to achieve appropriate light lateral pressure because strength and leverage are not required for the removal of calculus with ultrasonic instruments. Therefore, alternate or advanced fulcrums may be used. Specifically, a cross arch and opposite arch fulcrum can provide improved access and adaptation while allowing for proper ultrasonic instrumentation grasp and lateral pressure. Basic extraoral fulcrums such as a chin-cup or knuckle-rest technique are also other options.
5. *Adaptation*
   - When using ultrasonic instruments, keep the terminal 2 to 3 mm of the tip adapted against the tooth at all times. This is the active part of the tip.
   - Adapt the tip parallel to the tooth surface close to 0° but no more than 15°. *The point of the tip should never be directed at the tooth surface.*

- Start at the lowest effective power setting to maximize patient comfort.
- Keep the tip moving at all times.
- Insert the tip subgingivally with the lateral surface of the tip against the tooth.
- Insert at the distal line angle and move toward the contact to instrument the distal surface (halfway across the interproximal surface).
- Reinsert the tip at the distal line angle and move across the buccal or lingual to the mesial line angle through to the mesial proximal surface.
- Use overlapping vertical, horizontal, and oblique brushlike strokes so that every millimeter of the tooth is instrumented.
- Use the same seating positions and sequence as manual instrumentation, and use indirect vision when necessary.

6. *Fluid evacuation*
- Use nondominant hand.
- High speed is preferred, with an assistant, to minimize aerosols.

- Saliva ejector can be used if working alone.
- Keep the evacuation device closest to the area of instrumentation.
- Deactivate the tip when necessary to allow complete evacuation.

7. *Evaluation*
- Evaluate the effectiveness of the procedure with the explorer.
- Reinstrument with the power device as necessary and determine the need for manual instrumentation.

POSTPROCEDURE

Following the procedure, discuss:
- How the patient tolerated the procedure
- Whether the patient experienced any tissue discomfort
- Proper oral hygiene

- Furcation tips are specifically designed for furcations. There is a 0.08-mm ball at the end of the tip to prevent gauging in the furcation area.

CARE AND MAINTENANCE OF EQUIPMENT

Power scaling tips should be evaluated for wear. As the tips of the inserts wear, scaling efficiency decreases.[11] Worn-out, broken, or bent ultrasonic scaling tips cannot effectively remove stain or calculus or disrupt biofilm. As a general rule, 1-mm tip wear results in approximately 25% loss of efficiency; 2-mm wear equates to a 50% loss of efficiency and should be replaced.

Standard autoclave bags provide a sterile environment; however, there is minimal protection if the bags are dropped or mishandled. Autoclavable instrument cassettes made from either metal or plastic are ideal storage units for magnetostrictive inserts, providing a secure environment for the stack and tip. Some piezo tips are housed in a protective carrier that also doubles as a tightening wrench, which can be sterilized in an autoclave bag. Autoclavable cassettes provide safe storage for ultrasonic insert tips.

Tips should be rinsed under water to remove gross debris before sterilization. Some manufacturers recommend not running ultrasonic tips through an ultrasonic cleaner because this may void the warranty. Always check manufacturer's recommendations for care and maintenance of equipment.

MICROULTRASONIC INSTRUMENTS

Microultrasonic instruments use smaller-diameter tips. These tips resemble the diameter of a periodontal probe and can be thinner. When used appropriately, microultrasonic tips cause less root surface damage and less excessive cementum removal, and provide better access to the base of the pocket and access to furcations.[12] Microultrasonic tips are thinner periodontal power scaling tips or specially designed ultrathin tips that are the manufacturer's response to clinician's demands for thinner tips. It is believed that

Teamwork

Wendy has decided to use power scaling on her patient who presents with heavy supragingival and subgingival calculus. As she is instrumenting she has to stop frequently because her patient is prone to gagging and the saliva ejector is not as effective as high-speed fluid evacuation. The patient has an active tongue and it is all she can do to retract the tongue, instrument, and use the saliva ejector. The dental assistant walks by and notices Wendy is struggling and offers to help with fluid evacuation using the high-speed suction. Wendy is able to complete the appointment with improved efficiency and patient comfort thanks to the help of the dental assistant. ■

these tips are more comfortable for the patient because there is less tissue distention. Ultrathin tips should be used only on low-to-medium power.

After clinical assessment and treatment planning, an armamentarium should be selected based on the needs of the patient. Power scaling is effective and efficient in treating a wide range of patients from healthy to periodontally involved. With improved units and tip designs, power scaling has the ability to improve dental hygiene and periodontal outcomes.

Case Study

A 37-year-old male patient presents to the dental office for a comprehensive examination and preventive prophylaxis. His chief complaint is that his gums bleed when he brushes his teeth and they are sore. It has been 12 years since his last dental visit. His medical history revealed exercise-induced asthma, and there were no contraindications to treatment. A full-mouth series of radiographs was taken and a comprehensive examination was performed, including an oral cancer screening, intraoral and extraoral examination, and restorative and periodontal charting. His clinical examination revealed red, inflamed, bulbous tissues in the presence of heavy supragingival and subgingival calculus. His probe depths ranged from 3 to 5 mm, his bleeding index was 78%, and his plaque score was 62%. His American Academy of Periodontology (AAP) classification was generalized, moderate adult periodontitis (AAP classification is discussed in Chapter 11).

Case Study Exercises

1. Which type of tip would be the best to begin initial periodontal therapy on this patient?
   A. Periodontal tip
   B. Universal tip
   C. Diamond-coated tip
   D. Furcation tip
2. Power scaling can be used for all types of periodontal debridement procedures. Power scaling devices are safe to use on existing restorations.
   A. The first statement is true, but the second statement is false.
   B. The first statement is false, but the second statement is true.
   C. Both statements are true.
   D. Both statements are false.
3. Before using power scaling on this patient, all of the following should be performed EXCEPT:
   A. Assess the patient's periodontium to determine the health of the tissue, type, and location of deposits and periodontal classification.
   B. Review the patient's medical history.
   C. Inform the patient that a power scaling device will be used.
   D. Have the patient complete a 60-second preprocedural rinse with an antimicrobial solution.
4. After initial debridement with power scaling is complete, what tip should be used to instrument this patient's deeper pocket depths?
   A. Beaver tail
   B. Triple-bend
   C. Slim
   D. Bladed
5. Power scaling should not used on this patient because he has a history of asthma.
   A. The statement is true, but the rationalization is false.
   B. The statement is false, but the rationalization is true.
   C. The statement and the rationalization are true.
   D. The statement and the rationalization are false.

Review Questions

1. The length of the stroke is controlled by the:
   A. Water setting
   B. Power setting
   C. cps setting
   D. Frequency setting

2. Piezoelectric tips have a (an) _____ movement whereas magnetostrictive inserts have a (an) _____ movement.
   A. Oblique; lateral
   B. Lateral; oblique
   C. Elliptical; linear
   D. Linear; elliptical

3. All of the following are advantages of power scaling devices EXCEPT:
   A. Tips/inserts need to be sharpened
   B. Cavitation
   C. Improved operator ergonomics
   D. Removes less root surface structure

4. The use of power scaling devices is contraindicated in all of the following cases EXCEPT:
   A. Patients who have older-model pacemakers
   B. Patients with controlled, mild asthma
   C. Patients who have a known communicable disease
   D. Patients who are prone to gagging

5. Standard or universal tips are designed for:
   A. Deplaquing shallow pockets
   B. Moderate-to-heavy deposit removal
   C. Finishing
   D. Implants

Active Learning

1. Activate the power scaling device and place the side of the tip on an area of heavy supragingival calculus such as the lingual of the mandibular anterior teeth. Watch the calculus being dislodged from the teeth.

2. As you prepare to use the power scaling device, listen to the high-pitched sound that is created. Raise and lower the power button and listen to the difference.

3. Before you activate the power scaling device, feel areas of calculus with the tip. Activate the device and begin calculus removal. Then feel the area with the tip again and note the difference.

4. Use visual aids such as pictures of dentitions with light, moderate, and heavy calculus to determine what tip diameter should be used according to the clinical circumstances. ■

REFERENCES

1. Overman P. Biofilm: a new view of plaque. *J Contemp Dent Pract.* 2000;1(3):18-29.
2. Sbordone L, Ramaglia L, Gulletta E, Iacono V. Recolonization of the subgingival microflora after scaling and root planing in human periodontitis. *J Periodontol.* 1990; 61(9):579-584.
3. Minsk L. The role of power scalers in periodontics. *Compend Contin Educ Dent.* 2005;26(2):128-132.
4. Bennett BL. Using power scaling to improve periodontal therapy outcomes. *Contemporary Oral Hygiene.* 2007; 7(6):14-21.
5. Walmsley DA. The possibility of pulsation. *Dimens Dent Hyg.* 2012;10(1):42-44.
6. Position Paper; sonic and ultrasonic scalers in periodontics. Research, Science and Therapy Committee of the American Academy of Periodontology. *J Periodontol.* 2000;71(11):1792-1801.
7. Oda S, Nitta H, Setoguchi T, et al. Current concepts and advances in manual and power-driven instrumentation. *Periodontol 2000.* 2004;36:45-58.
8. Hallmon WW, Rees TD. Local anti-infective therapy; mechanical and physical approaches. A systematic review. *Ann Periodontol.* 2003;8:99-114.
9. Tunkel J, Heinecke A, Flemming TF. A systemic review of efficiency of machine-driven and manual subgingival debridement in the treatment of chronic periodontitis. *J Clin Periodontol.* 2002;29(suppl):72-81.
10. Fine DH, Yip J, Furgang D, et al. Reducing bacteria in dental aerosols: pre-procedural use of antiseptic mouthrinse. *J Am Dent Assoc.* 1993;124(5):56-58.
11. Lea SC, Landini G, Wamsley AD. The effect of wear on ultrasonic scaler tip displacement amplitude. *J Clin Periodontol.* 2006;33(1):37-41.
12. Kwan JY. Enhanced periodontal debridement with the use of micro ultrasonic, periodontal endoscopy. *J. Calif Dent Assoc.* 2005;33(3):241-248.

Chapter 26 | Instrumentation Principles and Techniques

Ashlynn Le, RDH, MA

KEY TERMS

adaptation

angulation

curettage

digital motion activation

file

fulcrum

handle rolling

hoe

motion activation

pivoting

universal instruments

wrist motion activation

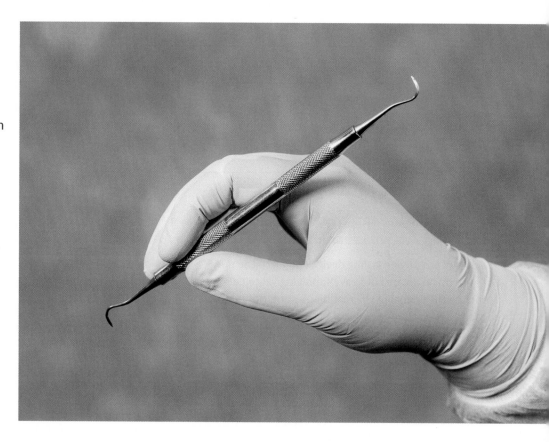

LEARNING OBJECTIVES

After reading this chapter, the student should be able to:

26.1 Use the modified pen grasp in practice.

26.2 Differentiate among the three parts of the working end of the curet and sickle scaler.

26.3 Adapt the working end of the anterior sickle scaler.

26.4 Demonstrate the process of inserting the working end of the sickle and curet into the sulcus or beneath the gingival margin.

26.5 Apply the appropriate working end of a universal curet to the distal surface of a mandibular posterior tooth.

26.6 Demonstrate the correct angulation of the instrument for the process of calculus removal.

26.7 Demonstrate wrist motion activation.

26.8 Demonstrate hand pivot and handle roll.

26.9 Use proper technique to stabilize the hand and instrument to perform an instrumentation stroke.

26.10 Use the correct techniques for instrument sharpening.

KEY CONCEPTS

- The major conventional methods for removing biofilm, calculus, and altered cementum are scaling and root planing.
- Risk evaluation includes the assessment of tissue healing patterns and pocket depth rates.
- The success of periodontal therapy is linked to the effectiveness of scaling and root planing.
- The success of treatment of patients with gingivitis and periodontitis in early stages depends on several factors, among them efficient patient education, recognition of the disease, and appropriate instrumentation.

RELEVANCE TO CLINICAL PRACTICE

Evidence-based care defines instrumentation for the processes of calculus and biofilm removal and ensures that treatment is optimum. Periodontal debridement (previously restricted to scaling and root planing) is essential to periodontal health for the following reasons:

1. It blocks the development of periodontal diseases through physical removal of biofilm and calculus deposits.
2. It creates a healthy environment that assists in keeping tissues intact and allows the gingival tissue to be restored, reducing and removing inflammation.
3. It contributes to better oral self-care by providing healing in those potentially disease-causing areas that patients cannot access themselves.[1]

This technique is also referred to as nonsurgical periodontal therapy. In general, it presupposes the removal of supragingival and subgingival deposits of calculus and biofilm. This procedure is technically challenging, and its efficiency is bound to the depth of the pocket, skill of the dental hygienist, anatomy of the root, time spent, and sharpness of instruments. Scaling and root surface debridement are normally conducted with the help of hand instruments and sonic or ultrasonic instruments. Traditional therapy is given during a series of appointments. Full-mouth disinfection may be used to reduce the risk of healing pockets being re-infected; the treatment is completed within 24 hours. However, systemic or local factors, as well as the technical aspect of the work, may restrict the effectiveness of this type of therapy. In this case, surgical approaches or adjunctive antimicrobials are used.[2]

The terms *scaling* and *root planing* were widely used in the past. *Scaling* is the removal of hard and soft deposits from the crown and root surfaces whereas *root planing* is defined as the removal of cementum and dentin that is impregnated with bacteria, endotoxins, and calculus.[3] The dental hygiene field uses the term *periodontal debridement*, because it presupposes preservation of cementum for a faster and more efficient healing process in patients. It also concentrates on the removal of calculus and bacteria biofilm from root and crown surfaces, but attempts to leave cementum intact. Because of the superficial association of endotoxin and cementum, it is unnecessary to remove the cementum, given the undesirable side effects such as pulpitis and hypersensitivity that may result from its removal.[4]

INSTRUMENT DESIGN

Periodontal instruments are available in single- and double-ended versions, depending on the number of working ends of an instrument. Double-ended instruments enhance the hygienist's workflow by allowing the use of either side of the instrument. When using a double-sided instrument, the hygienist does not have to stop and reach for another instrument.

Several combinations are possible for double-ended instruments:

- The working ends have almost equal functions, differing in size.
- The ends are right and left paired.
- The working ends are used for the same procedure but are different and have different applications.[5]

Paired double-ended instruments such as a curet are used more frequently than unpaired instruments such as an unpaired explorer (Fig. 26-1).

Handle

Handle design is essential to prevent cramping during extended periods of use, as well as musculoskeletal disorders caused by instrumentation. Use of #4 to #6 handles, which are large in diameter, is recommended to avoid musculoskeletal hand injuries.[6]

When selecting an instrument, the dental hygienist considers three characteristics of the handle:

- *Weight:* Hollow, lightweight handles increase tactile transfer and minimize fatigue.
- *Size, or diameter:* A handle that is too small lessens the hygienist's control over the instrument, leading to muscular fatigue. A handle that is large enough ensures maximum control and reduces cramps. However, a large handle may restrict the hygienist's movement in zones with limited access. It is advisable to have a set of instruments with several diameter options to accommodate all patients.
- *Texture:* The surface of the handle may be either knurled (have small ridges) or smooth. Knurled handles are preferred because they increase control over the instrument.[7]

Shank

The shank connects the handle to the working end and becomes narrower toward the working end. It may be angled to reach various areas in the patient's mouth. Shanks of dental instruments can be straight (having no angles), curved (or slightly bent), monoangle (one angle), binangle (two angles), and triple angle (three angles).[6] Most periodontal instruments are bent in at least one place, which gives the hygienist freedom to position the instrument against the tooth surface as necessary.

Simple shanks bend in one plane and are used for anterior teeth. Complex shanks bend in two planes and are used for both anterior and posterior teeth. Instruments, often with complex shanks, that are used in all areas of the mouth are referred to as **universal instruments.**[7] When examined from the front, a complex shank appears bent, whereas a simple shank appears straight (Fig. 26-2).

Shank Flexibility

Strength defines the flexibility of the shank and is one of the major characteristics of the shank. While performing instrumentation, dental hygienists apply varying degrees

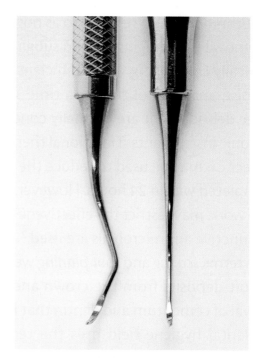

Figure 26-2. Complex shank (left); simple shank (right).

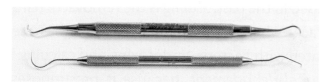

Figure 26-1. Paired, mirror image working ends (top) and unpaired, dissimilar working ends (bottom).

of pressure to achieve optimum contact with the tooth surface. The material and size of the shank determine its flexibility or strength. Shanks can be rigid, moderately flexible, or flexible.

Rigid shanks such as those found in sickle scalers are used to remove strongly attached calculus and deposits because they are thick and can endure the pressure necessary to remove heavy calculus. Their use is limited, though, because their rigidity restricts tactile conduction, reducing their effectiveness and complicating calculus detection.

Flexible shanks are thinner and, as their name suggests, bend when pressure is applied. Moderately flexible shanks provide better tactile contact, which enables successful detection and removal of moderately heavy subgingival deposits. Universal curets have a moderately flexible shank.

Flexible shanks are used primarily for the purpose of detecting and removing fine manifestations of subgingival calculus and deposits. Instruments with flexible shanks, such as explorers and some Gracey curets, provide the best tactile transfer to the hygienist.[7]

Extrarigid shanks, which are relatively new to instruments, are used when rigid instruments (curets) do not provide the most efficient scaling procedure for the patient. Their rigidity eliminates the possibility of the shank flexing while the hygienist is scaling heavy calculus. Curets with extrarigid shanks are designed especially for the initial stage of periodontal service for patients with heavy calculus.[8]

The Functional and Lower Shank

The functional shank covers the area from the working end of the instrument to the bend that is closest to the handle. The lower (terminal) shank is part of the functional shank and is the portion of the shank closest to the working end of the instrument (Fig. 26-3). The lower shank zone is crucial in the choice of working end, providing visual assistance, because the lower shank must be parallel to the instrumented surface.

Functional shanks can be long, short, or intermediate. Long functional shanks are used for instrumentation of the surfaces of teeth that are longer than 5 mm. Short functional shanks are designed for the removal of supragingival calculus deposits.[7]

Working End Design

The working end of the instrument may be a point, nib, blade, beak, or rounded end (Fig. 26-4). The working end determines the instrument's function. Some instruments are used to examine soft tissues or perform an initial assessment, whereas others are used for scaling. Design characteristics of the working end's face, back, cutting edges, and lateral surfaces contribute to its function. The *face* is the surface that separates two cutting edges, and the reverse side is called the *back* of the instrument (Fig. 26-5). Each side of the face is referred to as a *lateral surface,* and the *cutting edge,* a sharp one, is formed by the convergence of the two lateral surfaces.[7] There are other configurations; for example, the cutting edges of a curet form a surface called a *toe,* whereas the cutting edges on a sickle scaler converge to a point called a *tip.*

INSTRUMENT IDENTIFICATION

Instruments have similar functions but unique designs and numbers. The instrument's name normally reveals its designer or manufacturer. The manufacturer's number is carved or printed on the handle of the instrument (Fig. 26-6). It is used for ordering from databases or placement in the set of periodontal instruments. For example, Gracey curets are periodontal instruments named after Dr. Clayton H. Gracey, who designed them. Instrument shape, length, width, and other specifications

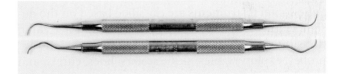

Figure 26-4. Universal instruments' working end designs.

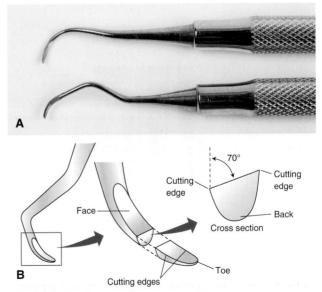

Figure 26-5. (A) Working ends. (B) Parts of the working end.

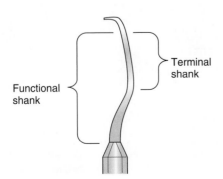

Figure 26-3. Terminal shank.

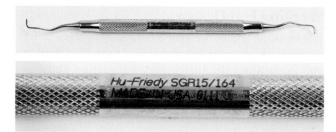

Figure 26-6. Gracey instrument handle.

may differ slightly among manufacturers, although the instruments may have identical design numbers. Some manufacturers color-code instruments to make them easy to identify.[8]

Working End Identification

Two numbers are stamped on the handles of double-ended instruments, one for each working end. The first Gracey series consisted of 14 single-ended and 7 double-ended instruments. Gracey's first double-ended instruments were labeled Gracey 3/4, Gracey 5/6, Gracey 11/12, and Gracey 13/14 (Fig. 26-7). The Gracey 15/16 and 17/18 are modified instruments created in response to dental hygienists' feedback. The Gracey 15/16, adapted from the 11/12, has a more acutely angled shank to facilitate access to the mesial surfaces of posterior teeth. The Gracey 17/18 is a modified 13/14 with a longer terminal shank and a shorter blade to enable easier access and adaptation to posterior distal surfaces, particularly molars.[8]

Instrument Classification

Periodontal instruments are classified based on the design features of the working ends. Hand-activated nonsurgical instruments are classified as follows: probes, explorers, files, sickle scalers, hoes, curets, and chisels.

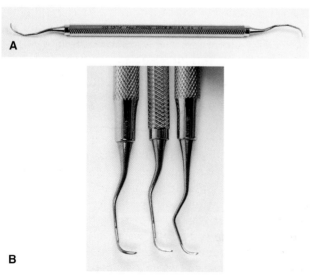

Figure 26-7. (A) Gracey 13/14 labeled on handle. (B) Gracey 3/4, 13/14, and 15/16 working ends.

INSTRUMENT ACTIVATION

Instrument activation is performed in several stages: adaptation, angulation, lateral pressure, and strokes. Using instruments for periodontal care is technically a combination of movements performed by the dental hygienist over the tooth surface to achieve the desired effect. These movements require skill and are performed according to a number of principles.

Grasp

In most cases, instruments are held with a modified pen grasp. In a modified pen grasp, the index finger and thumb hold the instrument handle. The middle finger is placed on the shank and the ring finger is used as a fulcrum (Fig. 26-8). A **fulcrum** is a finger that a hygienist uses to stabilize his or her hand when performing instrumentation and assessment. A well-established fulcrum guarantees stability, control, and injury prevention.[9]

Adaptation

Adaptation is the manner in which the working end of an instrument is positioned against the tooth surface. The focus is on making the working end of the instrument correspond with the contour of the surface. Correct adaptation must be done without damaging soft tissues and root surfaces. Adapting bladed instruments such as curets or pointed instruments like explorers is challenging because it is difficult to adapt them precisely.[10]

It is essential to keep the instrument in constant contact with the surface of the tooth. To achieve this, the hygienist adapts the tip to the contours of every surface and periodontal structures by rolling the instrument handle between the thumb and index finger. Every following stroke overlaps the previously finished one to guarantee that the hygienist covers the entire surface.[7]

The cutting edge of the working end has three conventional parts:

1. Leading third, most frequently used for instrumentation
2. Middle third
3. Heel third

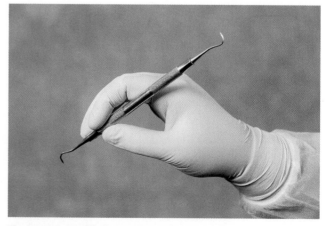

Figure 26-8. Modified pen grasp technique.

For example, the leading third of a curet is the toe of the working end, whereas the tip is the leading third of a sickle scaler.[10] Knowledge of dental and root anatomy is important for correct instrument adaptation. Longitudinal depressions are frequently found on proximal root surfaces. Depressions and multirooted tooth furcations are among the most challenging areas to instrument.

Angulation

Angulation describes the angle between the bladed instrument working end and the surface of the tooth. There are two guidelines to follow:

1. To insert the instrument beneath the gingival margin, the angle between the face and the tooth surface must be in the range of 0° to 40°.
2. To remove calculus, the angle must be 45° to 90°. The exact angle depends on the heaviness of calculus and its nature, the specificity of the procedure, and the state of the tissue during root planing or scaling. If the angle is smaller than necessary, the cutting edge will only burnish the calculus.[10] Curettage is done, however, at angles exceeding 90°. **Curettage** is the removal of the soft tissue in the periodontal pocket. This technique is not often used in the treatment of periodontal disease. Successful instrumentation is possible if the correct angulation is performed throughout the stroke.

The principles of adaptation and angulation are more important than they may seem at first. According to Pattison, working in accordance with them "can spell the difference between chronic, continuous infection and healing. Burnished calculus left behind from misunderstanding or misapplication of principles is not the harmless entity previously believed."[11]

Activation

Motion activation is the term that describes movements of the instrument to create a stroke on the surface of the tooth. There are two types of motion activation: wrist motion activation and digital motion activation.

Wrist motion activation is the rotating movement of the hand and wrist as one unit that allows the hygienist to apply additional power for the instrumentation stroke.[7] This type of activation is recommended for removing calculus with hand-activated instruments, because it causes less fatigue than using fingers only for instrumentation.

Digital motion activation is moving the periodontal instrument by flexing three fingers: thumb, index, and middle finger. The focus of this activation type is not strength, as it is applied by the machine, but flexibility.[7] Digital motion activation may be used with ultrasonic (power) instruments, periodontal probes, and explorers. It also applies to areas where access and freedom to maneuver are restricted. Using digital motion activation during scaling, however, can lead to muscle fatigue and repetitive stress injuries. Digital motion activation is less stable than wrist motion activation for scaling.

Tips for Digital Motion Activation

The following tips promote efficient digital motion activation:

1. Use a pencil for practice.
2. Grasp a pencil with a modified pen grasp (refer to Fig. 26-8) and take the starting position.
3. Perform the pull-push movements of the thumb, index, and middle fingers.
4. Direct the pencil tip away from the countertop toward your palm.
5. Restore the pencil to the initial position.
6. Do not apply power to the strokes.

Hand Pivot and Hand Roll as Parts of Activation

Pivoting is a joint swinging movement of the arm and hand conducted by balancing on the fulcrum finger.

Handle rolling (turning the handle of the instrument between the thumb and index finger to readapt the instrument to the surface of the next tooth) is a crucial adaptation technique, especially for root concavities and mesial line angles. For example, when using an explorer, the pivoting motion of the hand, wrist, and forearm pivot assists in achieving the proximal midline. Pivoting also advances instrument strokes on the proximal surfaces before the point of the tip crosses the midline. Hand rolling is performed with the help of either the thumb or the index finger.

Activation also comprises the rocking movement that extends the tip of the working end from epithelial attachment to the gingival margin. Strokes must be short, approximately 1 mm, and the hygienist should advance the instrument around the tooth. To keep it activated and adapted, the hygienist should continue rocking, rolling, and pivoting actions.[12]

Instrumentation Strokes

Removing subgingival calculus can be complicated. When working below the gingival margin, the hygienist cannot see the root surface or the deposits of calculus. In this situation, the hygienist has to use a systematic approach in performing the strokes for instrumentation. Only this pattern can result in complete coverage of the tooth surface and, therefore, successful instrumentation.

There are four types of strokes: placement stroke, exploratory or assessment stroke, scaling stroke, and root planing stroke (Table 26-1).[10] Placement stroke is performed to position the working end above the calculus or at the base of a pocket or sulcus. During the placement stroke, no pressure is applied. An exploratory stroke is a stroke with no pressure that is used to detect the location and depth of the calculus. A scaling stroke is used when activating the instrument for calculus removal. More pressure is applied to this stroke than any other type of stroke.

Table 26-1. Stroke Characteristics

	Assessment Stroke	Calculus Removal/Scaling Stroke	Root Planing Stroke
Purpose	• Evaluation of the tooth anatomy • Attachment level • Detection of calculus and biofilm	Calculus removal	Removal of residual calculus, biofilm
Instrument	Probes/explorers, curets	Sickle scalers, curets, files	Curets
Insertion		0°–40°	
Angulation	50°–70°	70°–80°	60°–70°
Lateral Pressure	Contact with the surface of the tooth, without pressure application	Moderate or firm	Light or moderate
Character	Fluid stroke; medium length	Powerful but short strokes	Light strokes of medium length
Direction		Vertical, oblique, horizontal	
Number of Strokes	Abundant, must cover the whole root surface	Limited; applied only to the necessary area	Abundant, must cover the whole root surface

Stroke Direction

Strokes are performed in the coronal direction, outward from the soft tissue sulcus base or pocket. Vertical, oblique, and horizontal strokes can be used to enable calculus removal in all areas.[10] Horizontal strokes performed with standard-blade curets are deemed highly effective if narrow deep pockets or tooth contours make the use of vertical or oblique strokes impossible. It may appear impossible using vertical strokes to insert and adapt the blade of a standard curet deep enough and avoid lacerating the tissue. Similarly, it may be unattainable to evade the creation of grooves in the root surface or traumatizing tissues using the toe of a conventional curet. Therefore, Reedy suggests "by directing the toe apically and using a series of carefully controlled, short, circumferential strokes, a standard curet blade can be better adapted to these convex and concave tooth surfaces."[13] There are two solutions:

1. Access to the problematic areas can be ensured through the use of mini-bladed and micro minibladed Gracey curets. These instruments may be adapted to the narrow contours in deep pockets or furcations. They may be applied with vertical strokes without injury to the tissue. Horizontal or oblique strokes may be used as well, but given the small size of the blade, the strokes cannot be inserted far subgingivally if the tissue is impossible to retract.
2. Standard universal or Gracey curets can be used in the areas with horizontal strokes. A series of short and highly controlled strokes are activated after inserting the blade toe into the deep pocket on a mesial or distal surface. The movement is directed from the lingual line angle to the facial line.

Horizontal strokes have three disadvantages:

1. They are potentially dangerous, which makes them difficult for beginners to perform. With the toe applied apically, the blade can damage soft tissues. This requires careful exploration of the pocket before activation of horizontal strokes.
2. These strokes are most often finger-flexing movements, which calls for a greater level of precision. At the same time, they are less powerful in comparison with wrist activation strokes. The stroke must be limited to 1 mm in restricted areas, but the tenacious calculus necessitates a combination of wrist motion and finger flexing. In this case, vertical or oblique strokes are more efficient.
3. Horizontal strokes are not always effective on heavy ledges because they are activated toward the most resistant dimension of the deposit, making this approach inappropriate in this case.

Regardless of the disadvantages, horizontal strokes are extremely useful for performing instrumentation in restricted areas and are a must for a skillful hygienist to master.[15]

Calculus Removal Stroke With Sickles

The working end of the sickle scaler arrives at a point at the tip; its cross section is triangular (Fig. 26-9). The blade is 90° angled to the lower shank and facing up. This shape allows access to the area linked to gingival embrasure and the narrow proximal contact. It also facilitates calculus removal. The instrument is considered the basic instrument for the removal of heavy supragingival calculus deposits, permitting better accessibility to the subgingival areas for curets.[3] When used

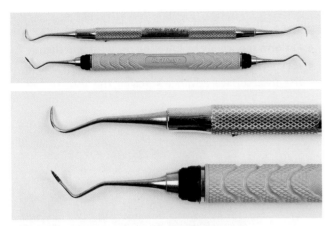

Figure 26-9. Anterior and posterior sickle scalers.

around the line angle, the sickle may lacerate tissues. Large calculus deposits can be removed in sections via short and precisely controlled strokes. Excellent knowledge of root morphology and work experience

give dental hygienists the ability to visualize the current position of the sickle to avoid laceration of soft tissues.[14]

Using the Anterior Sickle

Anterior sickles are designed for effective use in the anterior area. Straight blade, shank, and handle sickles are the most frequently used anterior sickles. There are also anterior curve sickles for scaling the anterior regions. The technique presupposes initiation of activation on the opposite side of the angle of the line, with the tip adapted while advancing into the interproximal surface. Apply lateral pressure on the pull stroke and insert the blade in the pocket while minding the tissue.[16,17] See Box 26-1.

Using the Posterior Sickle

Sickles with contra-angled shanks are used for adaptation to posterior teeth. These sickles may have straight or curved blades and are also referred to as Jacquettes.[7] See Box 26-2.

Box 26-1. *Using the Anterior Sickle Scaler*

1. Use the modified pen grasp for holding the instrument.
2. Set a finger on the incisal surface of a canine or mandibular left lateral.

4. Scale the facial surface away from the mandibular right, adapting the pointed tip to the surface. Use slight rocking movements to the patient's right.

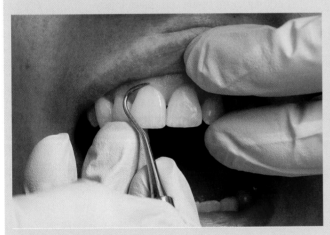

Position finger.

3. Start the insertion.

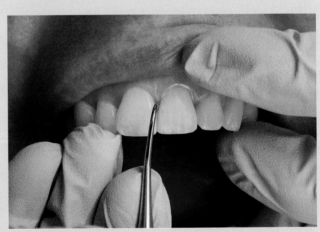

Scale away from the mandibular right.

5. Perform scaling on the distal surface.
6. Scale the mesial surface from behind, at the 12 o'clock position. ▮

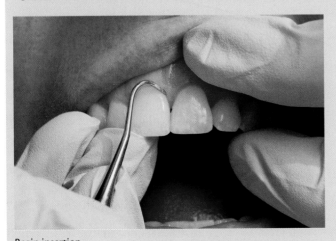

Begin insertion.

Box 26-2. *Using the Posterior Sickle Scaler*

1. Use the modified pen grasp for holding the instrument.
2. Set a finger on the occlusal surface of the mandibular right premolar.
3. Adapt the blade to the angle of the distal line of the mandibular right first molar. The lower shank must be maintained parallel to the scaling surface. Start the insertion of the cutting edge above the gingival margin in the case of supragingival calculus.

4. Perform the scaling by lowering the wrist and slightly rocking back on the fulcrum finger in the direction of the distal surface; advance in scaling the distal surface.

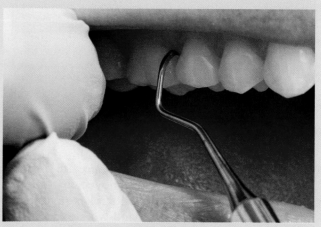
Scale in the direction of the distal surface.

5. Carry out adaptation of the second working end of the instrument to the mesial line angle of the mandibular right first molar. Adaptation should be done with care and precision to avoid movements that may cause tissue trauma or injury. ■

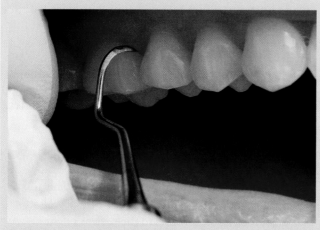
Adapt the blade.

Calculus Removal Stroke With Universal Curet

The working end of the universal curet is composed of two parallel cutting edges converging in a rounded toe. The blade face of the curet is positioned at a 90° angle to its shank, and both cutting edges are used for the calculus removal and debridement of the root surface. Standard universal curets normally have a bent working end; there is also an additional curve in the shank, which allows dual adaptation for both posterior and anterior teeth. Universal curets require accurate adaptation to ensure that the second edge does not traumatize tissue.[18] Universal curets can be used for the removal of subgingival and supragingival calculus and root planing. The angulation between the surface of the tooth and the blade must be 80° to 90° to achieve the lower shank parallelism. See Box 26-3.

Box 26-3. *Practicing Technique With Universal Curets*

1. Preparation and insertion:
   • Start insertion at a 0° angle, keeping the terminal shank to the tooth surface.
   • Carefully slide the working end below the gingival margin and on the facial surface of the root.
2. Preparation for a stroke:
   • Place the working end below the gingival margin. Slide the tip of the instrument down the margin, then slide the working end to the root until it reaches the calculus deposit.
   • Tilt the terminal shank closer to the tooth surface—the angulation between the face and the root must be 80°; the face of the curet should be positioned at a 90° angle to the terminal shank. Therefore, the curet

face and the shank should be tilted in the direction of the root surface for the correct angulation.
   • Lock on the toe third of the instrument.
3. Activate the calculus removal stroke:
   • Perform an instrumentation stroke directed from the tissue at the base of the pocket.
   • Maintain the toe third of the instrument and the facial surface locked.
   • Activate a short, biting stroke directed toward the deposit to remove a small bit of the deposit.
4. Cease the stroke with excellent precision, pressing the fulcrum finger to the occlusolingual tooth surface, pausing after each separate stroke. Relax fingers between the strokes. ■

Using the Universal Curet for the Anterior Region

Use of the instrument for the anterior teeth presupposes the division of the teeth in half at the midline, with the long axis becoming the initial point. All the surfaces that face the operator are subject to debridement with one working end of the instrument and the same cutting edge, whereas the opposite edge applies to the surfaces that face away from the operator.[18] See Box 26-4.

Using the Universal Curet for the Posterior Region

With the use of the universal curet for the posterior teeth, debridement must be started with the distal line angle, with one side of the blade advancing into the distal proximal surface. The opposite blade of the working end starts from the distal line angle into the mesial proximal surface through the lingual or facial aspect. The angulation maintained by the hygienist must be 70° to 80° by way of tilting the lower shank toward the surface of the tooth.[18] See Box 26-5.

TYPES OF INSTRUMENTS

Gracey Curets

In the 1930s, Dr. Clayton H. Gracey of the University of Michigan designed a series of innovative and adaptable curets capable of reaching the base of periodontal pockets.[19] Initially, Dr. Gracey and a blacksmith from Ann Arbor, Michigan, attempted to produce an instrument capable of reaching the surface of the tooth root inside the deep pocket without injuring the epithelial tissue of the oral cavity.[5] Eventually Dr. Gracey collaborated with Hugo Friedman, the founder of Hu-Friedy

---

Box 26-4. *Using the Universal Curet for the Anterior Region*

1. Use the modified pen grasp.
2. Set a finger on the incisal edge of the mandibular left lateral incisor.
3. Choose the necessary working end of the instrument and correct positioning.

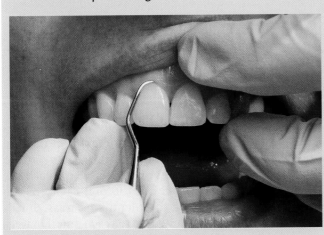

Position the working end of the universal curet.

4. Insert the blade in the subgingival direction at the midline point and activate a scaling stroke toward the mesial surface; move until the contact is reached and then withdraw the blade slowly.
5. Advance to the back position and then flip the instrument to choose the necessary working end.
6. Set a finger on the incisor edge of the mandibular right central incisor; then perform adaptation of the blade for the distal surface of the left central incisor.
7. Start the subgingival insertion of the instrument blade at the midline, keeping the toe faced toward the distal surface. Activate a stroke on the surface.
8. Assess the progress. ▪

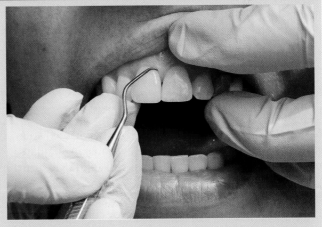

Insert the blade.

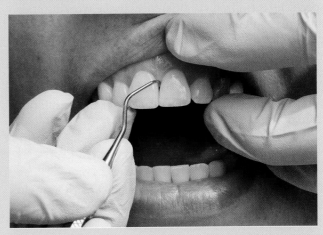

Activate a scaling stroke.

Box 26-5. *Using the Universal Curet for the Posterior Region*

1. Set a finger on the occlusal surfaces of the mandibular right premolars.
2. Choose the necessary working end, then insert the curet toward the periphery at the distal line angle maintaining 0° angulation.

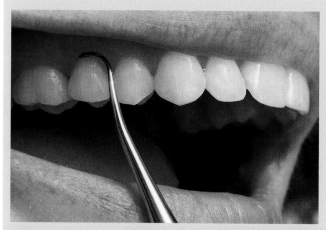

Insert the curet toward the periphery at the distal line angle.

3. Achieve appropriate angulation by raising the instrument handle and perform activation strokes in the direction of the distal surfaces using vertical upward and downward strokes. Having finished with the distal surface, approach the contact and then withdraw.

4. Using the same working end, flip the blade with the toe facing the mesial surface, then insert the toe third of the instrument at the distal line angle, maintaining 0° angulation to the pocket base.

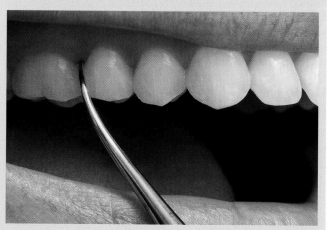

Insert the curet with the toe facing the mesial surface.

5. Set the necessary angulation to carry out strokes through the buccal surface.
6. Roll the instrument with the help of your thumb to adapt the cutting edge while scaling around the mesial line angle in the direction of the mesial surface. ■

Manufacturing Company, to create 14 single-ended area-specific curets.[8] Gracey curets are available in standard, miniature working end, extended shank, and rigid form.

Design

The primary difference between Gracey curets and other types of curets is that Gracey curets are area specific. This specificity is realized via differences in the working ends and utilization in certain regions of the oral cavity.[3] They can remove supragingival and subgingival calculus. Working ends of Gracey curets have only one cutting edge. In contrast with universal curets, Gracey curets have bends in the shank to facilitate access to the tooth surface, which contacts mechanically with the inferior third of the blade.[3] See Box 26-6.

Hoes

Design

The periodontal **hoe** is a large appliance with a single cutting edge created by the connection of the beveled toe and face of the razor blade. Its blade is bent at a 99° angle; the cutting edge is beveled at 45°.[10] Avoid traumatizing the epithelium tissue of the oral cavity with the back of the hoe blade when positioning the cutting edge at the junctional epithelium.

There are two types of hoes: single ended and double ended. Because the hoe is the paired appliance, the hygienist will need a set of four working ends to reach each of the four surfaces of the teeth: distal, buccal, mesial, and lingual. Hoes can be distinguished by their shank angulation, length, and size of the cutting edge.

Use

Long hoes with an angled bar are usually used to remove the calculus in the posterior regions of the oral cavity, because the length of their blade adapts badly to the proximal surfaces. Hoes are best used to reach the buccal and lingual surfaces of the oral cavity or the proximal regions next to the edentulous areas. Small-angled hoes are commonly used to reach anterior areas such as labial and lingual surfaces of the oral cavity. Because hoes are not adaptable and sensitive to touch, their subgingival utilization is permitted only in cases where the periodontal pocket is large and the tissue can be reflected away from the tooth easily. Force should not be used to insert a hoe subgingivally. See Box 26-7.

Files

Design

Files have numerous cutting edges.[19,20] A series of cutting edges are located on the base of the file. Each of the file's cutting edges is identical to the cutting edge of the hoe. The cutting edges are bent at a 90° to 105° angle toward the file's shank. The cutting edge's base, which can be round, oval, or rectangular, is situated on the shank's extension. Different kinds of shanks are

Box 26-6. *Technique for Using a Gracey Curet*

1. Hold the instrument in a modified pen grasp and ensure its cutting edge is parallel to the ground.
2. Choose the correct working end.
3. Arrange your fulcrum.
4. Position the lower shank of the instrument parallel to the surface of the tooth undergoing the treatment.
5. Smoothly insert the instrument subgingivally at the line angle.

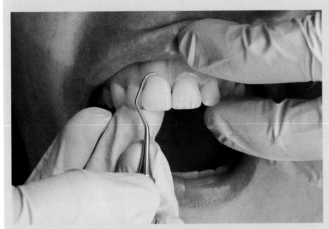

Insert the curet subgingivally at the line angle.

6. Adjust the lower third of the shank in relation to the tooth surface.

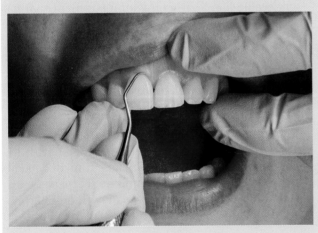

Adjust the lower third of the shank.

7. Move the stroke upward, to remove the subgingival calculus. ■

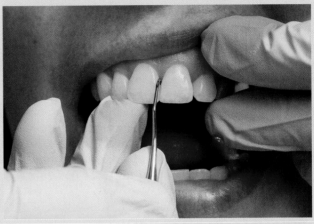

Move the stroke upward.

Box 26-7. *Technique for Using a Hoe*

- Carefully touch the tooth surface, moving the hoe vertically to ensure that the cutting edge of the instrument is located completely against the tooth. Moving the hoe in the indirect and horizontal manner can cause injury to the epithelium tissue of the oral cavity.
- The pull stroke can only be used while applying the hoe. Place the cutting edge of the hoe at a 90° angle toward the tooth surface. Ensure that the cutting edge of the hoe is located at a proper angle to the tooth surface before moving it in a pull-like manner. Otherwise, there is a possibility of the hoe's slipping, causing flattening and burnishing of calculus. There should be a double contact of the tooth surface and the hoe. Both the shank and the cutting edge of the hoe should contact the tooth surface to prevent the heavy deposits of calculus from breaking into small pieces. ■

useful in case of pocket depth or gingival margin atrophy. A file with a larger shank angulation is usually used to reach posterior teeth.[19]

Use

Files are used primarily to remove and break large, solid parts of calculus into smaller pieces. Files are not used in supragingival or subgingival areas with easily relocated tissue because of the length of their blade, their poor adaptability, and their lack of tactile sensitivity.

Files are similar to hoes in that they should not be used interproximally. They are much more appropriate for buccal and lingual surfaces, and for areas that are close to edentulous regions of the oral cavity. As with the hoes, the hygienist needs a set of four working ends to reach each of the four surfaces of the teeth.[19] See Box 26-8.

INSTRUMENT SHARPENING

Instruments are sharpened to generate a functionally sharp cutting edge and to safeguard the shape and contour of the appliance.[17] Sharp appliances improve palpable sensations, thus augmenting the efficiency of deposit elimination. Using sharp appliances also requires less force for removal of tooth biofilm and deposits. Dull instruments can burnish the calculus, which then is harder to remove. Moreover, the possibility of bacteria emerging, resulting in periodontal failure, is feasible if calculus residues remain in the tooth pocket. Newer metals are being developed that allow the cutting edge to maintain sharpness longer than traditional metals, thereby reducing the frequency of sharpening.

Differentiating a Sharpened Instrument From a Dull One

With use and autoclaving, the cutting edges of dental instruments gradually lose their sharpness and become

---

Box 26-8. *Technique for Using the File*

- Stabilize the file to verify its position.
- Locate the file's shank on the tooth and contact the tooth surface with the cutting edge.
- Activate the file in pull stroke manner.
- Because files and hoes are similar in configuration, use of a file is subject to the same restrictions as a hoe. The file must be moved extremely carefully to avoid injuring the epithelium tissue and the root surface with its straight cutting edge because of the lack of adaptability to bent surfaces of the tooth.[21]
- Files and hoes are not capable of eliminating all calculus beneath the tooth pocket because of the risk for relocation of the junctional epithelium. To avoid leaving calculus residues in the tooth pocket, use a curet to complete the removal of the tooth biofilm.[21]

---

rounded rather than angular. One of the best ways to estimate instrument sharpness is to draw the appliance lightly across an acrylic stick. A dull appliance will slide gently, whereas a sharp appliance will bite into the surface, leaving a light shaving trace.[17]

Sharpening Stones

Choosing the appropriate stone type for each instrument is of great importance. Sharpening stones are made from a variety of materials, from natural mineral to artificial stone with coarse abrasive crystals that appear to be even stronger than metallic stones.[19] The more abrasive sharpening stones with large crystals are used to sharpen the dullest instruments, whereas the finer sharpening stones with smaller abrasive crystals are used to sharpen slightly dull appliances. Instruments should be sharpened frequently to avoid having a very dull blade. Follow the manufacturer's instructions to obtain the best effect.

Principles of Sharpening

Keep the instrument's configuration in mind while sharpening it and adhere to the following principles:

- Sharpen instruments at the first sign of dullness. A dull instrument will not bite on the roof surface and the hygienist will need to apply amplified pressure for successful use, resulting in muscle fatigue.[17] Sharpening instruments regularly maximizes their serviceable life. Sharpening an instrument that has been allowed to become dull will require more force and utilization of a more abrasive sharpening stone. This can cause metal loss and reduce the life of the instrument.
- Choose the appropriate sharpening stone type according to the type of dental instrument (sickles, universal or Gracey curets) and the level of the instrument's dullness.
- Establish a proper angle between the sharpening stone and the cutting edge of the instrument depending on the type of instrument to be sharpened.
- Maintain a constant, firm grasp of both the sharpening stone and the instrument to be sharpened.

SHARPENING CURETS

Gracey Curets

The Gracey curet's blade is bent at a 70° to 80° angle between its front and lateral sides. The principles of Gracey curet sharpening are:

- Maintain a constant, firm grasp of the instrument to ensure that the face of its blade is parallel to the floor.
- Hold the sharpening stone perpendicular to the floor.
- The Gracey curet has only one cutting edge. Position the blade's face at a right angle to the sharpening stone, with the stone situated close to the cutting edge of the curet.

- Adjust the angle of the stone to be more obtuse on 10° to 20°. At this point, the angle of the blade's face toward the sharpening stone may be 100° to 110°.
- Make the sharpening stroke by shifting the instrument toward you, thus minimizing the development of a wire edge.[21] Start from the shank end of the curet's blade and move slowly to its curved toe.
- To maintain the exceptional curvature of the Gracey curet, track the instrument's contour while sharpening.
- To sharpen the curet blade's face, apply a cone-shaped sharpening stone toward the curet blade's face in a slight back-and-forth stroke manner. Perform no more than four to six strokes while sharpening the face of the blade.
- To estimate the sharpness of the appliance, use the acrylic stick test described earlier.

Universal Curets

To sharpen the universal curet appropriately, the curet's blade should be bent at a 70° to 80° angle between its front and lateral sides. Both cutting edges of the double-edged universal curets should be sharpened. When sharpening universal curets:

- Maintain a constant, firm grasp of the instrument to ensure that the face of its blade is parallel to the floor.
- Classify the appropriate angle for sharpening. Position the instrument so the blade's face is at a 100° to 110° angle toward the surface of the sharpening stone.
- Locate the side surface of the universal curet in such a way that the angle between the blade's face and the stone surface maintains the 90° value.
- Adjust the angle of the stone to be more obtuse on 10° to 20°. At this point, the angle of the blade's face toward the sharpening stone may be 100° to 110°.
- Start from the shank end of the curet's blade and move slowly to its curved toe. Make the sharpening

stroke by shifting the instrument toward you and constantly applying slight pressure.[18]
- To estimate the sharpness of the appliance, use the acrylic stick test. To protect the curet's toe from getting a cuspate look, sharpen the curet's blade completely, from its shank end to its toe. Sharpen all around the toe to maintain its sharp form.
- After finishing the first blade of the universal curet, move to the opposite end, and sharpen it using the same principles.

Sickles

The angle between the blade's face and the side surface of the sickle is similar to the curet's angle and equals 70° to 80°. To protect this angle, apply the sharpening stone toward the side surfaces of the sickle, the angulation of which should be equal to 100° to 110°.[17]

- Maintain a constant, firm grasp of the instrument and ensure that the face of its blade is parallel to the floor.
- Classify the appropriate angle for sharpening. Locate the sharpening stone in such a way that it has contact with the side surfaces of the sickle along its full length. The angle of the blade's face and the stone surface will be equal to 100° to 110°. For sickles with smooth side surfaces, try to preserve the angle size between 100° and 110°.
- Start from the shank end of the sickle's blade and move slowly to its toe. Make the sharpening stroke by shifting the instrument toward you, while constantly applying slight pressure to maintain the contact with the side surface of the blade.[17]
- To estimate the sharpness of the utilized appliance, use the acrylic stick test.
- After finishing the first blade of the sickle, move to the opposite end and sharpen it using the same principles.

Case Study

A dental hygienist decides to sharpen his instruments for the first time. He has a set of sickles, Gracey and universal curets, hoes, and files. He assembles the instruments and the appropriate sharpening stone for each instrument in his set, selects an instrument and sharpening stone, and begins the sharpening process.

Case Study Exercises

1. What is the best way for the dental hygienist to differentiate a sharpened instrument from a blunt instrument?
   A. Try it on his hand.
   B. Use it on the sheet of paper.
   C. Note time of its utilization.
   D. Use the acrylic stick.

2. What is the appropriate angle between the face of the blade and the stone while sharpening the Gracey curet?
   A. 70°
   B. 100°
   C. Right angle
   D. 80°

3. How should the hygienist rotate the sharpening stone to appropriately sharpen an instrument?
   A. Laterally
   B. By circular movement
   C. It should not be rotated
   D. In a seesaw manner

Case Study—cont'd

4. How should the hygienist sharpen the second universal curet's cutting edge?
   A. Like a Gracey curet's cutting edge
   B. In the same manner as the first cutting edge
   C. Like a sickle's cutting edge
   D. There is no need to sharpen it

5. The hygienist should position the sickle blade's face _____ to the floor while sharpening it.
   A. Parallel
   B. Perpendicular
   C. Bent 30°
   D. Bent 45°

Review Questions

1. The design number at the end of the instrument name identifies the:
   A. Working end
   B. Number of working edges
   C. Length of the handle
   D. Length of the shank

2. Three characteristics to consider when selecting an instrument handle are:
   A. Weight, diameter, and texture
   B. Weight, length, and diameter
   C. Length, diameter, and texture
   D. Weight, diameter, and length

3. Another term for a simple shank is:
   A. Straight shank
   B. Direct shank
   C. Round shank
   D. Rectangular shank

4. A complex shank:
   A. Is bent in two planes.
   B. Is not bent.
   C. Has a pointed end.
   D. Has multiple ends.

5. The universal curet has _____ working ends.
   A. 1
   B. 2
   C. 3
   D. 4

Active Learning

1. Working with a partner, take turns selecting an instrument and explaining its use.
2. Select an instrument and demonstrate how it is sharpened for the class. ■

REFERENCES

1. Sahayata VN, Patel VG. Evidence based periodontology. *J Dent Sci.* 2011;2(1):15-19. http://www.ddu.ac.in/academics/fds/wp-content/uploads/2010/12/4.Evidence-based-Periodontology.pdf. Accessed June 4, 2012.
2. American Dental Hygienists' Association. Standards for Clinical Dental Hygiene Practice. http://www.adha.org/downloads/adha_standards08.pdf. Published March 10, 2008. Accessed June 4, 2012.
3. O'Hehir TE. Debridement = scaling and root-planing plus. *RDH.* 1999;9(5). http://www.rdhmag.com/articles/print/volume-19/issue-5/columns/periodontics/debridement-scaling-and-root-planing-plus.html. Updated 2009. Accessed June 4, 2012.
4. Clerehugh V, Tugnait A, Genco R. *Periodontology at a Glance.* Hong Kong: Wiley-Blackwell; 2009.
5. Dibart S, Dietrich T. *Practical Periodontal Diagnosis and Treatment Planning.* Hong Kong: Wiley-Blackwell; 2010.
6. Donley T. Instrumentation for the Treatment of Periodontal Diseases. Chicago: American Dental Association Continuing Education Recognition Program; 2011. http://www.dentalhygieneexcellence.com/pdf/Instrumentation_for_treatment_of_perio_disease-Donley.pdf. Accessed June 5, 2012.
7. Phinney DJ, Halstead JH. *Delmar's Dental Assisting: A Comprehensive Approach.* 2nd ed. New York: Delmar Learning; 2003.
8. Profident. Hufriedy. http://www.profident.pl/oferta/hufriedy/pdf/Periodontal.pdf. Accessed June 5, 2012.
9. Millar D. *Reinforced Periodontal Instrumentation and Ergonomics for the Dental Care.* Philadelphia: Lippincott Williams & Wilkins; 2007.
10. Shalu B. *Periodontics Revisited.* New Delhi, India: Jaypee; 2012.
11. Pattison AM. Advancements in hand instruments. *Dimens Dent Hyg.* 2006;4(5):26, 28-29.
12. Millar D. Reinforced periodontal instrumentation and ergonomics. The best practice to ensure optimal performance and career longevity. *CDHA J.* 2009; 24(3):8-16.
13. Reddy S. *Essentials of Periodontology and Periodontics.* 2nd ed. New Delhi, India: Jaypee, 2008.
14. Matsuda SA. Anatomy of a stroke. *Dimens Dent Hyg.* 2008; 6(11):22-26.

15. Pattison AM. The horizontal stroke. Tips on technique. *Dimens Dent Hyg.* 2010;8(12):58.

16. Pattison AM. The secret use of sickle scalers. *Dimens Dent Hyg.* 2008;6(9):44, 46-47.

17. Registered Dental Hygienist Development. Anterior sickle. http://www.rdhdevelopment.com/. Updated 2009. Accessed June 7, 2012.

18. Scaramucci MK. The versatility of the universal curet. *Dimens Dent Hyg.* 2010;8(2):32, 36, 38.

19. Noble S, ed. *Clinical Textbook of Dental Hygiene and Therapy.* 2nd ed. Chichester, U.K.: John Wiley & Sons; 2012.

20. Bathla S. *Periodontics Revisited.* New Delhi, India: Jaypee Brothers, Medical Publishers; 2012.

21. Ireland R, ed. *Oxford Dictionary of Dentistry.* Oxford: Oxford University Press; 2010.

Chapter 27 | Nonsurgical and Surgical Periodontal Therapy

Ugo Covani, MD, DDS • Massimilliano Ricci, DDS, PhD

KEY TERMS

antimicrobial

debridement

junctional epithelium

laser

lipopolysaccharide (LPS)

modified Widman flap

open flap

osteoplasty

osteotomy

periodontal debridement

periodontal healing

periodontal surgery

perioscopy

regenerative technique

scaling and root planing
   (SRP)

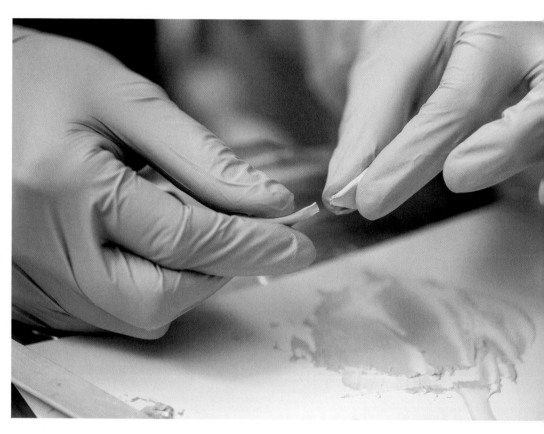

LEARNING OBJECTIVES

After reading this chapter, the student should be able to:

27.1 Explain the goals of nonsurgical and surgical periodontal therapy.

27.2 Outline biofilm formation.

27.3 Demonstrate the use of the perioscope.

27.4 Discuss how periodontal surgery is part of a periodontal rehabilitation protocol.

27.5 Indicate how the dental hygienist supports the periodontal patient in a surgical phase.

27.6 Explain surgical interventions to a patient.

KEY CONCEPTS

• Nonsurgical and surgical therapies may be necessary to control and treat periodontal diseases.

• Periodontal surgery is performed to treat severe periodontal pockets.

- Periodontal surgery follows an appropriate scaling and root planing (SRP) procedure, which is often sufficient to solve the majority of deep pockets.
- Periodontal healing is ideal when periodontal infection is completely eradicated. As a consequence, all surgical procedures have to be considered after periodontal treatment and followed by a dental hygienist.
- It is crucial that dental hygienists be familiar with periodontal surgical and nonsurgical procedures to effectively help their patients in attaining and maintaining periodontal health.

RELEVANCE TO CLINICAL PRACTICE

A number of types of periodontal diseases exist. Untreated periodontal disease can eventually lead to tooth loss and other health problems. Types of periodontal diseases include gingivitis, the mildest and only reversible form, aggressive periodontitis, chronic periodontitis, periodontitis as a manifestation of systemic disease, and necrotizing periodontal disease.[1]

The goal of periodontal therapy is to achieve successful periodontal regeneration. **Scaling and root planing (SRP),** sometimes referred to as **periodontal debridement,** can solve most periodontal problems, but it is often insufficient when a patient has deep pockets. Regenerative surgery is essential to regenerate a new periodontal apparatus and obtain satisfactory functional and aesthetic results.

Dental hygienists need to be familiar with periodontal surgical and nonsurgical procedures to effectively help their patients attain and maintain periodontal health. If in a general dental practice, and if all treatment measures fail, the patient should be referred to a periodontist. If periodontitis is detected as a manifestation of systemic disease, such as diabetes, the patient should also be referred to a physician.

ORAL–SYSTEMIC LINK

Links exist between periodontal diseases and systemic diseases and conditions. For example, patients with undiagnosed or poorly controlled type 1 (insulin-dependent) or type 2 (non–insulin-dependent) diabetes mellitus may be more susceptible to periodontal diseases than patients with well-controlled diabetes. Patients with poorly controlled diabetes should have a maintenance interval of about 3 months, shorter appointments, and appointments preferably in the morning. Drug-induced disorders, hematological disorders, and immune system conditions also affect treatment and prognosis.

NONSURGICAL THERAPY

Periodontal treatment includes the maintenance of the health, function, comfort, and aesthetics of all supporting structures and tissues in the mouth.[2] The goals of periodontal therapy are to preserve, improve, and maintain the natural dentition, dental implants, periodontium, and peri-implant tissues to achieve health, comfort, aesthetics, and function.[2] A healthy periodontal condition is described by the absence of inflammation, which may appear clinically as redness, swelling, suppuration, and bleeding on probing. A comprehensive periodontal examination and risk assessment should be performed, along with a diagnosis, prognosis, and treatment plan. Informed consent should be obtained, and all records documented.

Treatment of periodontal diseases should include patient education, management of oral–systemic interrelationships, and nonsurgical or surgical therapy. Adjunctive aids could include the use of lasers, the perioscope, chemotherapeutic agents, and occlusal therapy. All treatment should be evaluated and modified if necessary.

The goal of nonsurgical therapy is eliminating the causal agent of periodontal disease, bacterial plaque biofilm, and its associated factors. SRP reduces both gingival inflammation and probing depths, leading to a gain of clinical attachment in most periodontal patients.[3,4] SRP includes instrumentation of the crown and root surfaces of the teeth with hand, sonic, or ultrasonic instrumentation to remove plaque biofilm, calculus, and stains. The success rate of this treatment is assessed by re-established tissue health and patient compliance with an established maintenance regimen.

Success at the time of therapy is determined by visual and explorer evaluation of tooth surfaces. Use of the perioscope can be a helpful adjunct. Total calculus and plaque removal is impossible, especially at the base of deep pockets and furcations. Small, residual deposits do not appear to cause treatment failures. If areas remain unresponsive after scaling, rescale and add an **antimicrobial** agent such as tetracycline or doxycycline to the treatment to destroy or inhibit the growth of disease-causing microbes.

Biofilms are a complex community of microorganisms characterized by the excretion of an adhesive and protective extracellular matrix, microbe-to-microbe attachment, structural heterogeneity, genetic diversity, and complex community interactions.[5] A biofilm community comprises bacterial microcolonies, an extracellular slime layer, fluid channels, and a primitive communication system. Microorganisms experience major changes during their transition from planktonic (free-swimming) organisms to cells that are part of a complex community attached to a surface (Fig. 27-1). The initial goal of SRP was to create a glassy, hard, smooth surface by removing cementum or surface dentin, which is rough, impregnated with calculus, or contaminated with toxins or microorganisms. It was believed that endotoxins (**lipopolysaccharides [LPS]**) formed by gram-negative bacteria invaded the root structure and the diseased cementum should be removed. LPS, also known as lipoglycans, are large molecules that consist of a lipid and a polysaccharide joined by a covalent bond. LPS are found in the outer membrane of gram-negative bacteria, act as endotoxins, and elicit strong immune responses in animals. Current research indicates that toxins are superficially located on root surfaces and relatively easily removed.[6] Extensive root instrumentation is not required beyond the removal of calculus and plaque. Repeated removal of tooth structure is not a goal of periodontal therapy because it may result in thinned and sensitive root surfaces. Furthermore, removing the cementum hinders the regeneration potential of the site.

SRP is the definitive procedure designed for the removal of cementum and dentin that is rough or permeated, or both, by calculus or contaminated with toxins or microorganisms. Some soft tissue removal occurs. This procedure may be used as a treatment in some stages of periodontal disease or as part of presurgical procedures in others, or both. **Debridement** is a generalized term that signifies the removal of bacterial plaque biofilms and calculus deposits from crown or root surfaces, or both, and from within the pocket, without root surface removal. The terms are sometimes used interchangeably, and most studies are done using SRP.

Periodontal debridement and SRP may include hand or powered scalers or a combination of the two. The method of instrumentation does not determine success of treatment as much as the skills, knowledge, and expertise of the dental hygienist. According to research, both hand and powered instrumentation provided comparable clinical results in the treatment of periodontal disease.[7] Therefore, because both treatments are proven effective and safe, the choice of instrumentation is determined by the preference of the hygienist, patient, or both. Ultrasonic instruments combine the use of mechanical, irrigation, cavitation (the inward collapsing of bubbles of water), and acoustic streaming forces. Dental hygienists may prefer ultrasonic instrumentation because it increases efficiency, reduces time spent per tooth, and is physically less demanding for dental hygienists.

Hand instrumentation may be necessary because of contraindications for the patient or clinician. Contraindications include the use of ultrasonic instruments with unshielded pacemakers because the electromagnetic field generated by ultrasonic instruments can interfere with the functioning of some cardiac pacemakers.[8] However, ultrasonic instruments are safe to use with shielded pacemakers. Dentists and dental hygienists with an unshielded pacemaker should not operate ultrasonic scalers. Sonic scalers do not create an electromagnetic field and may be used as a substitute for ultrasonic instrumentation.

Periodontal healing after nonsurgical periodontal therapy occurs as repair of existing tissues rather than regeneration of tissues lost in the disease process. Periodontal pockets, alveolar bone, periodontal ligament, and epithelium will heal, inflammation will be resolved, long junctional epithelial attachment may occur, and gingival recession may result. Subgingival bacterial plaque biofilm will repopulate with younger, less pathogenic bacterial

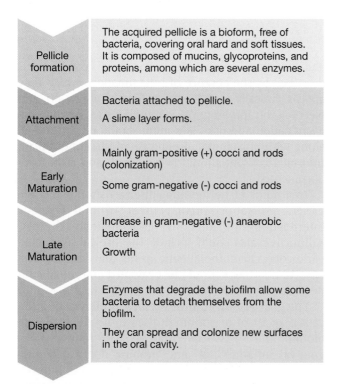

Pellicle formation	The acquired pellicle is a bioform, free of bacteria, covering oral hard and soft tissues. It is composed of mucins, glycoproteins, and proteins, among which are several enzymes.
Attachment	Bacteria attached to pellicle. A slime layer forms.
Early Maturation	Mainly gram-positive (+) cocci and rods (colonization). Some gram-negative (-) cocci and rods
Late Maturation	Increase in gram-negative (-) anaerobic bacteria. Growth
Dispersion	Enzymes that degrade the biofilm allow some bacteria to detach themselves from the biofilm. They can spread and colonize new surfaces in the oral cavity.

Figure 27-1. Stages of biofilm formation. (Sources: Hannig C, Hannig M, Attin T. Enzymes in the acquired enamel pellicle. *Eur J Oral Sci.* 2005;113(1):2-13; Marsh PD. Dental plaque as a microbial biofilm. *Caries Res.* 2004;38:204-211.

initially. Formation of new bone to replace lost bone, new connective tissue attachment to root surfaces, and new cementum on the root are not predictable outcomes of nonsurgical periodontal therapy. **Junctional epithelium** can be expected to take approximately 1 week to heal after debridement, whereas underlying connective tissue can take 4 weeks.

After SRP, the bacterial plaque shifts from the predominantly gram-negative flora found in periodontal disease to gram-positive bacteria. There is a decrease in motile forms, especially spirochetes, after treatment. The bacteria after nonsurgical periodontal therapy are much less pathogenic and similar to those present in health. In addition to being less destructive, bacteria also tend to repopulate in a specific order: *Streptococcus* and *Actinobacillus* species followed by *Veillonella, Bacteroides, Porphyromonas, Prevotella,* and *Fusobacterium* species, and finally *Capnocytophaga* species and spirochetes are the last to grow back.[9] The repopulation cycle may take as long as 6 months to complete, depending on the competency of the dental hygienist and patient plaque control. Repopulation also can occur in a shorter period, requiring a shorter maintenance interval.

Expected clinical responses include noticeable reduction in redness, inflammation, and bleeding. An easy way to remember this is the 3 C's: color, contour, and consistency. Generally, sites with deeper initial probe depths respond with greater improvements than shallower pockets. Pockets with initial depths of 4 to 6 mm tend to be reduced 1 to 2 mm, whereas initial pockets larger 7 mm show the greatest improvement of 1.5 to 3 mm.[10] Periodontal healing is greatest 3 to 6 weeks after nonsurgical periodontal therapy, but changes occur continually for up to 12 months after therapy. Probing to re-evaluate probe depths should not be done until at least 4 weeks after treatment.

Even clinically successful treatment has a great likelihood of pocket reinfection. Reinfection of periodontal pockets results from remaining biofilms, increased tolerance of microbes within a dense, mature biofilm to antibiotics, reservoirs of bacteria in calculus, and reservoirs of bacteria within the dentinal tubules of infected root surfaces and soft tissue.[5] A combination of SRP and locally delivered antimicrobials should be considered if nonsurgical therapy is the treatment of choice (Table 27-1). A meta-analysis indicated an overall significant reduction in pocket depth (PD) with adjunctive local antimicrobials versus SRP alone.[11]

Local Drug Delivery

Because periodontal diseases are a combination of bacteria, the immune response, self-care, and other factors, there are a variety of ways to manage the diseases. One critical element of therapy is to control the bacteria, conventionally done through mechanical debridement such as SRP. However, mechanical debridement alone may not remove the bacteria that have invaded hard or soft tissue, or are inaccessible in the furcations or other hard-to-reach areas.[12] Various locally delivered agents are used in the treatment of periodontal disease, including 10% doxycycline hycylate (Atridox), minocycline hydrochloride (Arestin), tetracycline hydrochloride (Periodontal Plus AB), and chlorhexidine gluconate (PerioChip). Local drug delivery, used with SRP, provides additional benefits in PD reduction compared with SRP alone.[12]

For an antimicrobial agent to be effective, the pathogen should be susceptible to the drug and not readily develop resistance for an adequate period. The periodontal pocket is a natural site for treatment with local sustained-release delivery systems, because it is easily accessible and gingival crevicular fluid provides an extraction medium for the drug.[13] Antimicrobial drugs, as site-specific dental formulations into the periodontal pocket, are a viable alternative to conventional periodontal therapy.[14]

Most locally delivered antibiotics and antimicrobials are delivered in a similar fashion. Procedure 27-1

Table 27-1. *Locally Delivered Antibiotics/Antimicrobials*

Antibiotics/ Antimicrobials	Active Ingredient	Polymer	Results of Studies
PerioChip	Chlorhexidine gluconate (2.5 mg)	Hydrolyzed gelatine	PerioChip plus SRP significantly reduced PD and increased CAL at 9 months compared with SRP alone.
Atridox	Doxycycline (10% or 50 mg)	Poly-DL-lactide	Treatment with Atridox alone produced improvements in PD and CAL at 9 months that were equivalent to SRP alone.
Arestin	Minocycline (1 mg)	Polyglycolide-co-DL-lactide	Subjects treated with Arestin plus SRP exhibited significantly greater PD reductions at 1, 3, 6, and 9 months versus SRP alone.

CAL, clinical attachment loss: PD, pocket depth; SRP, scaling and root planing.
Source: American Academy of Periodontology Statement on local delivery of sustained or controlled release antimicrobials as adjunctive therapy in the treatment of periodontitis (Academy report). *J Periodontol.* 2006;77:1458. http://www.joponline.org/doi/pdf/10.1902/jop.2006.068001. Accessed Oct 2, 2015.

Procedure 27-1 Placement of Minocycline Hydrochloride

MATERIALS AND PREPARATION

Familiarity with the necessary materials and proper preparation for antibiotic placement is essential in using time and resources. Being prepared for the procedure will eliminate stress and difficulty during the treatment.

Gather and organize the necessary materials before the patient's arrival.

Materials

Mirror	For indirect vision and retraction of the tongue
Explorer	To evaluate the teeth
Periodontal probe	To measure the periodontal pocket
Cotton pliers	Enables clinician to pick up small items and remove small items from the mouth They are also used to avoid contamination
High-volume evacuation tip and/or saliva ejector	High-volume evacuation is preferred but can be difficult to handle if placing antibiotic without an assistant
Minocycline hydrochloride cartridges	Contain the minocycline microspheres
Autoclavable stainless-steel handle	Holds the cartridge containing the minocycline microspheres

PREPROCEDURE

Patient Education

Educate the patient, parent, or both regarding what the antibiotic is, how it will be applied, and the reason for antibiotic placement. Antibiotics are indicated as an adjunct to SRP procedures for reduction of PD in patients with adult periodontitis. Antibiotics may be used as part of a periodontal maintenance program that includes good oral hygiene and SRP. Ask the patient about any known sensitivity or allergy to minocycline or any drug in the tetracycline family. Tetracycline class drugs are contraindicated for use in children and pregnant or nursing women because they may cause permanent discoloration of the teeth during tooth development.

Informed Consent

Informed consent is required before placing antibiotics on all patients. Antibiotics are commonly placed in periodontal pockets 5 mm or larger, along with SRP or periodontal maintenance.

Selection of Periodontal Pockets to Be Treated

• Identify the periodontal pockets that have been selected for antibiotic therapy.

PROCEDURE

1. *Syringe setup for placement of antibiotic*
   • Remove the cartridge from the tray.

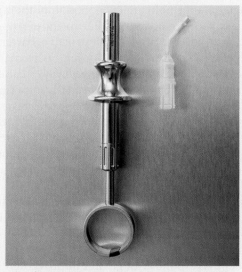

Remove the cartridge from the tray.

   • Insert the cartridge into the handle and twist until it locks into place.

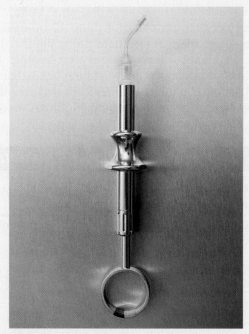

Insert the cartridge into the handle and twist until it locks into place.

   • Remove the tip cap before placing the antibiotic in the periodontal pocket.

2. *Placement of antibiotic*
- Place the cartridge tip into the periodontal pocket, parallel to the long axis of the tooth.

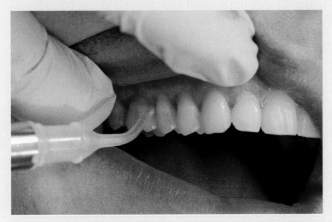

Place the cartridge tip into the periodontal pocket, parallel to the long axis of the tooth.

- Do not force the tip into the base of the pocket.
- Gently press the thumb ring to express the antibiotic powder while withdrawing the cartridge tip from the base of the pocket.
- If there is any resistance during delivery, withdraw the device farther.

- Once delivery is complete, retract the thumb ring and remove the cartridge.
- Appropriately discard the cartridge and sterilize the handle before reuse.

POSTPROCEDURE

Inform the patient (and parent or guardian if the patient is a minor) about the results of the procedure. Explain that one cartridge of the antibiotic was used to treat each pocket and note how many cartridges were placed. Discuss how the patient tolerated the procedure and reinforce proper oral hygiene. Provide the patient with postprocedure instructions, including:

- Resume brushing after 12 hours.
- Wait at least 10 days before using floss, toothpicks, or other devices to clean between the teeth and around treated areas.
- Avoid touching treated areas for 1 week except for routine brushing.
- Avoid eating hard, crunchy, or sticky foods for 1 week.
- Follow up with the dental hygienist and dentist by keeping scheduled appointments.

provides general instructions for placing minocycline hydrochloride. Always follow the manufacturer's instructions for a specific product.

Systemic Antibiotics

Most periodontal infections are dominated with anaerobic bacteria and will respond favorably to penicillin, amoxicillin, tetracycline, doxycycline metronidazole, and clindamycin or a combination of these antibiotics.[15] Although antibiotics are not routinely used for chronic periodontitis, they may enhance healing by reducing the bacterial load or eliminating specific pathogens for up to 6 months to 1 year. Like all other antimicrobial therapy, the effect is short-lived and may need to be repeated when symptoms of active disease, such as bleeding on probing and attachment loss, occur. More aggressive types of periodontitis require a combination of surgery and systemic antibiotics.

Lasers

The first **lasers** approved for dental/oral procedures were for soft tissue procedures such as gingivectomy, curettage, biopsy, and other procedures. Lasers used were the carbon dioxide lasers, Nd:YAG, argon, and diode lasers.[16] More recently, the Er:YAG has been approved for procedures on oral soft and hard tissues. The purported advantages of laser use are greater hemostasis, disinfection of the periodontal pocket, reduced use of anesthesia, and decreased healing time. In the case of a medically compromised patient, such as one taking anticoagulants, the use of a laser may be an advantage because of the reduced chance of bleeding. Disadvantages include the need for patient and clinician eyewear, cost, and size.

Meaningful comparison between various clinical studies or between laser and conventional therapy is difficult and probably impossible at the present time.[17] There are several reasons for this dilemma, such as different laser wavelengths; wide variations in laser parameters; insufficient reporting of parameters that, in turn, does not allow calculation of energy density; differences in experimental design, lack of proper controls, and differences in severity of disease and treatment protocols; and measurement of different clinical endpoints.

A need exists to develop an evidence-based approach to the use of lasers for the treatment of chronic periodontitis.[17] There is insufficient evidence to suggest that any specific wavelength of laser is superior to the traditional modalities of therapy. Evidence does suggest that use of the Nd:YAG or Er:YAG wavelengths for treatment of chronic periodontitis may be equivalent to SRP with respect to reduction in probing depth and subgingival bacterial populations. However, if gain in clinical attachment level is considered the gold standard for nonsurgical periodontal therapy, then the evidence supporting laser-mediated periodontal treatment over traditional therapy is minimal. Also, there is limited evidence suggesting that lasers used in an adjunctive capacity to SRP may provide some additional benefit.[18] Clinical application of lasers for the treatment of periodontal disease has continued to expand since their introduction for this purpose in the early 1990s but remains controversial.[19]

A number of state dental examining boards permit dental hygienists to use laser devices when used within their scope of practice and in adherence with state statutes. Laser use within the scope of dental hygiene practice as an adjunct device to SRP is most often cited, and training/education is necessary and should include a hands-on proficiency course provided by a recognized sponsor of continuing education (CE), in accordance with the current rules for CE for the state. Licensees using laser technology should maintain documentation of the satisfactory completion of the formal CE or training from programs that qualify for CE credits.[16] For information on states that allow hygienists to use lasers, and the authorizing rule, law, or policy that permits such use, visit the American Dental Hygienists' Association (ADHA) website or state boards of dentistry or dental hygiene.[20]

Perioscopy

Dental **perioscopy** is a nonsurgical procedure that is performed with a fiberoptic endoscope connected to a color high-definition monitor to diagnose and treat dental and periodontal diseases (Fig. 27-2).[21] A fiber with magnifying and illuminating capabilities is inserted into the endoscope sheath and then the endoscope explorer to provide detailed and highly magnified images of the diagnostic or treatment site, or both. Endoscope explorers are sterilizable dental instruments that hold the sheath/fiber complex, allowing for intraoral use. The explorers are configured to allow for subgingival viewing around each tooth. During periodontal instrumentation the explorer provides visual access for simultaneous ultrasonic instrumentation and subgingival viewing (Fig. 27-3).

The single-use disposable endoscope sheath provides a sterile intact barrier to pathogens, preventing any cross-contamination between the sheath and fiber and extending the life of the fiber. The sheath is also designed to deliver water irrigation to keep the endoscope lens free from debris. The 1.0-m length allows for full reach without touching the floor. The endoscope explorer shield is designed to hold the soft tissue away from the camera lens and along with water irrigation allows for video viewing of the subgingival environment.

Indications and Contraindications for Use of the Perioscope

Dental endoscopy (perioscopy) can be used for initial periodontal therapy, sites that have not responded to traditional nonsurgical debridement, maintenance patients with chronically inflamed or increasing pockets, residual pockets in maintenance patients who refuse surgical therapy and/or where surgery is contraindicated for medical or aesthetic reasons, and suspected subgingival pathology such as caries, root fractures, perforations, or resorption. As with all dental treatment, dental perioscopy should not be used on individuals with certain heart valve defects or artificial prosthesis without proper consultation with the patient's physician and possible antibiotic premedication.[22]

When initiating any nonsurgical periodontal therapy, clinicians (dental hygienists and dentists, as per state laws) must be aware of the treatment objectives, limitations of treatment (such as tooth anatomy, PD, and

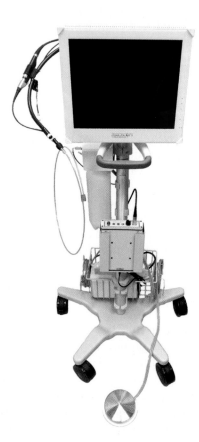

Figure 27-2. Perioscopy system with monitor. (Courtesy of John Y. Kwan, DDS, Perioscopy, Inc.)

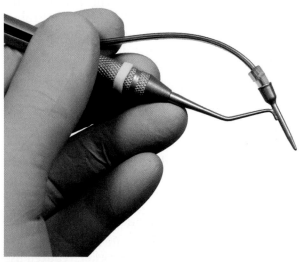

Figure 27-3. Endoscope explorer. (Courtesy of John Y. Kwan, DDS, Perioscopy, Inc.)

operator error), and whether treatment recommendations are in alignment with the severity of the disease. Treatment objectives include arresting the disease process, maintaining or regenerating periodontal/peri-implant support, and resolving or reducing periodontal/peri-implant inflammatory disease. Although dental endoscopy affords clinicians the opportunity to provide meticulous instrumentation, appropriate treatment recommendations should be based upon the level of disease to be treated and operator experience.

Factors that affect instrumentation in nonsurgical debridement include the amount of deposit; location of deposit; access for instruments such as narrow deep pockets, curved roots, close root proximity, overcontoured restorations, and the distal aspects of second or third molars; root morphology such as bifurcated and trifurcated teeth, concavities, line angles, depressions, and developmental grooves; anatomical considerations such as a small mouth, muscular tongue, tight cheeks, lips, and propensity for gagging; patient cooperation; and experience of the dental hygienist or dentist. Periodontal endoscopic debridement is difficult in patients with very inflamed pockets, abscesses, distal furcations of maxillary molars, narrow furcations and class III furcations, curved roots, close root proximity, and grossly overcontoured restorations.

Although mechanical debridement is essential in removing the bacterial bioburden from root surfaces, endoscopic debridement may also incorporate adjuncts. These can include systemic antibiotics, local delivery antibiotics, biologics (such as Emdogain and Gem 21S), lasers, and various chemical disinfection options.[23,24] Actively progressing periodontitis is virtually always associated with specific bacterial infections and often requires the adjunctive use of systemic antibiotic therapy.[4] By entering periodontal tissues and the periodontal pocket via serum, systemic antibiotics can affect organisms outside the reach of instruments or topical anti-infective chemotherapeutics. Systemic antibiotic therapy also has the potential to suppress periodontal pathogens residing on the tongue or other oral surfaces, thereby delaying subgingival recolonization of pathogens.[25] Because periodontal lesions often harbor a mixture of pathogenic bacteria, drug combination therapies have gained increasing importance and may even be required for eradication and prevention of periodontal infections by known periodontal pathogens that invade subepithelial periodontal tissue or colonize extradental domains from which they may translocate to periodontal sites.[25] Many dentists prescribe antibiotics empirically, based on clinical experience and/or the patient's medical history and sensitivity to the desired antibiotics. The rationale supporting this approach is that most pathogens are susceptible to the same antibiotics. Identification of specific bacteria is reserved for those situations where there is no or minimal clinical improvement after a course of systemic antibiotics or to ensure the elimination of the target bacteria.[26]

Using the Perioscopy System

The clinician (dental hygienist or dentist) places the endoscope fiber into a sterile sheath and then into the endoscope explorer. The fiber, sheath, explorer complex is then placed into the sulcus for subgingival viewing. When the dental endoscope is used subgingivally in a periodontal pocket, a loose film adhering to the tooth is frequently observed. This material is easily disturbed by the shield on the endoscope. During scaling of the subgingival root surface, this film loses adherence and is washed away by irrigation water flowing from the endoscope probe and is assumed to be biofilm.[27] Frequently, the gingival wall of a healthy sulcus is light pink, indicating health. In disease, islands of dark red blotch the pocket wall and may vary in color from a slight color change to deep red with an erythematous appearance, and may be discrete or diffuse.[27] In addition, these red areas have been shown to be primarily associated with calculus covered with biofilm, not biofilm alone, thus emphasizing the role of calculus in the pathophysiology of this chronic inflammatory periodontal disease.[27]

Periodontal endoscopy uses a two-handed technique: the endoscope in the nondominant hand (similar to holding a dental mirror) and the ultrasonic instrument in the dominant hand, moving together around the tooth while cleaning. Rarely, a "view, instrument, and view" technique is used when both the endoscope and the explorer are unable to simultaneously access the area being scaled. Beginning and finishing with one explorer in each segment before starting with another explorer is an integral part of the systematic approach to endoscopic debridement. This methodology is not unlike that taught for blind closed pocket instrumentation.

Ultrasonic powered instruments are the first choice with the periodontal endoscope. Typical ultrasonic inserts used are small and probelike. Endoscopically, they provide efficient root debridement, requiring only a small array of instruments. A full-mouth debridement typically requires only a straight probelike universal ultrasonic tip with an occasional need for curved or angled tips. These nonbladed ultrasonic tips are also less likely to remove healthy root structure. Just as most providers develop preferences and proficiencies with certain instruments, their use with the dental endoscope should prove useful. Efficiency is enhanced by fewer instrument changes and more instrument adaptation.

Diamond-coated ultrasonic instruments are used for advanced instrumentation in the removal of rough (globular) cementum, tenacious calculus, overhanging restorations, and subgingival enamel anomalies. Because of their cutting power, advanced skill is required in the use of diamond-coated ultrasonic tips. This is not only true with the cutting function, but to avoid damage to the explorer shield, sheath over the endoscope fiber, or the fiber itself.

Recommended training in dental endoscopy usually consists of an online video review, bench training, and patient hands-on training. This type of instruction is usually provided in-office and can also be provided as part of dental, dental hygiene, and periodontal clinical training. Most practitioners are confident performing the procedure after treating 20 to 30 patients.

Periodontal Surgery: An Overview

A variety of surgical techniques and procedures have been described in periodontology. Surgical procedures include gingivectomy, periodontal flaps, osseous (bone) contouring, bone grafts, and free gingival grafts.

Periodontal surgery aims to reduce PD and/or restore gingival contour to a state that can be maintained free of inflammation by the patient. In the past, a large number of surgical treatments to repair periodontal lesions have been proposed.[28] Before discussing the indications for periodontal surgery, a brief summary of periodontal healing is crucial.

Periodontal Healing: What Is the Key?

The American Academy of Periodontology defines periodontal regeneration as "the reproduction or reconstitution of a lost or injured part so that form and function of lost structures are restored. As a consequence, periodontal regeneration includes regeneration of alveolar bone, cementum, periodontal ligament and gingiva."[28] Although the famous experiments of Nyman, Karring, and colleagues[29] elucidated the concepts that govern periodontal regeneration, suggesting that only the cells of periodontal ligament have the capacity to regenerate the attachment, other authors indicated that various factors can contribute to the re-formation of attachment.

First, root surface conditions are critically important. Periodontal defects result from a gradual, variable destruction of the periodontium, which is due to the colonization of bacteria onto the root cementum.[30] Traditional root debridement, however, eliminates most bacteria and toxins, although many studies revealed that plaque and calculus remain in interadicular septa, lacunae, and surface concavities.[31] It is probable that this fact can jeopardize the normal healing process, contributing to the formation of junctional epithelium.

Furthermore, some types of root surfaces seem to be unfavorable for plasma absorption and clot stabilization.[32] In an animal study, Polson and Proye[33] extracted teeth, treated them with root planing, demineralized using citric acid, and placed them back into the sockets. They demonstrated that teeth reimplanted after SRP have different behaviors only compared with teeth replaced after root planing and demineralization of surfaces.[33] In fact, the demineralized root surface exhibits a fibrin linkage maturing into a connective attachment. This is a consequence of a more stable anchorage of the clot on this type of surface.[33] Moreover, it seems that the presence of residual antigenic material on the root surface could increase the number of neutrophil cells

in early phases of healing and, as a consequence, a bigger release of proteolytic enzymes, which, in turn, could delay maturation of the clot.[32]

The exact influence of the root surface is still unclear. It was shown that root surfaces clotted with heparin exhibited formation of an epithelial attachment, whereas at the control sites conditioned with saline, the epithelium was arrested at, or immediately apical to, the cementum–enamel junction.[30] In contrast, a reparation through a new attachment formation was observed when the surface was demineralized using citric acid or tetracycline.[34] Second, the adaption of the flap represents a factor of fundamental importance. The frail fibrin clot is crucial for the connective reparation, as shown in experimental models where the absence of a stable fibrin attachment led to a rapid epithelization of the defect.[35] As mentioned earlier, animal experiments indicate that the force necessary to detach the flap is hardly 200 grams after 3 days, increasing to 340 grams after 7 days.[29] As a consequence, these forces could easily compromise the clot stability.

The third factor involved is the morphology of the defect. As a matter of principle, the nature of defects is intimately related to the amount and disposition of the residual gingiva, the morphology of residual alveolar bone and periodontal ligament, and the particular anatomy of the tooth or teeth involved. Gingival units that exhibit a reduced width of keratinized tissue have been considered more susceptible to periodontal disease progression.[36] In contrast, the width of remaining attached gingiva is commonly not considered critical for the outcome of therapy.[37] Moreover, the position of individual teeth in the alveolar process may predispose them for suprabony, intrabony, and recession defects.[38] Root characteristics or variations such as bifurcations or trifurcations and root grooves appear to be particularly susceptible to disease progression.[39]

Morphology of the defect plays a key role also in the prediction of healing. This is related first to the amount of regenerative resources. For instance, the availability of regenerative resources is dramatically decreased in two- and one-wall intrabony defects. Second, the walls of the defect are able to protect the coagulum from mechanical forces; as a consequence, the stability of the clot is increased when the number of walls increases. In addition, it should be noted that for any periodontal defects, the amount and features of residual gingiva are critical for the achievement of a passive flap adaption and a primary wound closure.[40] All in all, these studies point out the crucial importance of the unimpeded absorption and of the adhesion and maturation of a stable fibrin clot for the formation of the connective tissue attachment over a long junctional epithelium. This concept should clearly be considered in all procedures of SRP or surgery.

What Is the Correct Approach in Periodontology?

Different approaches can be used to treat periodontal disease. Nonsurgical treatment versus surgical treatment, the choice of **regenerative techniques** versus resective techniques, and use of evidenced- and experienced-based therapy are all facets of evidence-based care.[41] Both nonsurgical and surgical approaches tend to reduce PD and increase attachment levels. However, an additional SRP treatment can often improve clinical attachment levels (CAL), reducing the need for surgical treatment.[42]

Clinicians agree that SRP results are better in the case of shallower pockets. After 3 years, the results of SRP and a surgical approach are indistinguishable. Topical antibiotic therapy in addition to SRP strongly increases a positive nonsurgical result.[43,44]

What Are the Indications to a Surgical Approach?

SRP is the best first step in treating periodontitis for several reasons:

- When pockets are due mainly to gingival hyperplasia, improvement in oral hygiene may result in resolution of inflammation and reduction in swelling, so surgery can be avoided.
- Reduction of probing depth may result from SRP.
- Reduction in inflammation means that hemorrhage at the surgery site is less of a problem.
- When pockets are shallow (< 5 mm), resolution after SRP may obviate the need for surgery.
- A surgical approach should be carefully evaluated, and clinicians should consider surgery only in patients who are able to maintain low plaque index levels and a reduced bleeding on probing index.
- Another requisite of a candidate for a surgical approach is the absence of severe systemic diseases, which could contraindicate any surgical therapy.

Before designating a patient to a surgical protocol, a series of parameters should be checked carefully. It is necessary to evaluate the probing depth after periodontal treatment considering that pockets greater than 5 mm have a worse prognosis than shallower pockets and also a higher probability of failure.[45] Moreover, the probability of success is linked to the severity of periodontitis, as well as tobacco use.[46]

What Is the Aim of a Surgical Approach?

Periodontal surgery aims to reduce PD and/or restore gingival contour to a state that can be maintained free of inflammation by the patient.[47] Surgical treatment includes a wide range of surgical techniques and procedures.

TYPES OF PERIODONTAL SURGERY

Gingivectomy
Indications

Indications for gingivectomy include:

- Gingival hyperplasia
- All conditions when probing depth is reduced but there are not changes in attachment levels

Technique

A probing evaluation indicates the depth and morphology of the pockets or tissues to be eliminated. Excess tissue to be removed is excised by an incision made at an angle of 45° to the long axis of the tooth, so that the blade impacts against the tooth slightly apical to the base of the pocket. Sterile swabs are used to control hemorrhage. Later a periodontal dressing may be placed to protect the wound area.

Flap Procedures

Flap procedures include a decontamination of root surface. They have different names according to the clinician who invented them. This approach should be considered as an adjunctive therapy. Flap procedures are essential in the presence of deep pockets because the mechanical control of plaque is difficult when a pocket is greater than 5 mm. This approach should induce a reduction of bleeding on probing, as well as a gain in attachment levels.[46] In contrast, the decrease of inflammation may result in a slight reduction of marginal gingiva.

The basic principles of flap design include:

- It should be wide enough to maintain adequate blood supply.
- It should be sufficiently large to expose possible bone defects.
- Incisions should allow movement of the flap without tension.
- Important vessels and nerves must be preserved.

Replaced Flap

This procedure, also known as **open flap** or **modified Widman flap,** involves suturing the flap in or near its original position.

Indications

The following are clinical indications for the need for open flap therapy:

- When access to the root and bone is desired, because it allows access to root and alveolar bone to enable removal of subgingival deposits and granulation tissue where pockets persist after hygiene phase therapy
- When pocket reduction is a goal, because it can reduce pockets and encourage a new epithelial and/or connective tissue reattachment at a more coronal level
- In osseous regenerative procedures, such as guided tissue regeneration (GTR)

Technique

The technique for completing open flap therapy is listed below.

- An intracrevicular incision is made around the necks of the teeth with the scalpel parallel to the long axis of the teeth. Care should be taken to preserve as much tissue as possible. (In the modified Widman flap, the pocket-lining epithelium is also excised via an inverse bevel incision).

- Vertical relieving incisions are required buccally if pockets are deep. Flaps should be sufficiently extensive to expose the marginal bone.
- Subgingival calculus deposits and granulation tissue are removed.
- The flaps are replaced with interrupted sutures, taking care to achieve approximation of wound edges interdentally where possible.

The aim of this intervention is to reduce PD and to facilitate oral hygiene maintenance.[45,48–50]

A modified approach involves additional bone remodeling. This intervention consists of a gingivectomy plus a modification of mucogingival morphology and then a remodeling of alveolar bone through **osteotomy** (removal of supporting bone) or **osteoplasty** (removal of nonsupporting bone to improve bone morphology). This resective approach could also involve dental tissue (root resection, tooth hemisection, and odontoplasty).

This last approach is ideal in case of increased gingival volume or bone volume, or when there are dental furcations. The result of this type of surgery is the complete resolution of the pocket, although a lengthening of the crown is often possible. In other words, this type of intervention tends to create a new periodontal attachment but in more apical position.

Repositioned Flap

With the repositioned flap treatment, the flap is repositioned apically, coronally, or laterally after surgery.

Indications

Indications for repositioned flap treatment include:

- To eliminate pockets by positioning the gingival tissue apically
- To increase the zone of keratinized gingivae
- To expose additional root for restorative procedures, that is, crown lengthening

Technique

Buccal and lingual/palatal flaps are raised using either intracrevicular or inverse bevel incisions.

- The flap is reflected and dissected from the alveolar process so that it is sufficiently mobile to enable repositioning.
- Any adherent granulation tissue or subgingival calculus deposits are removed.
- The flap is sutured in the desired position and may be held in position by the placement of a periodontal pack. Figures 27-4 and 27-5 show preparation and placement of a periodontal pack.

Regenerative Periodontal Surgery

GTR is defined by the American Academy of Periodontology as a procedure that attempts to regenerate lost periodontal structures through differential tissue responses.[28] This technique is ideal in cases of deep pockets (greater than 5 mm), and its results are more predictable if a greater number of residual walls of the defect are present.

GTR involves the use of resorbable or nonresorbable barriers (membranes) to exclude epithelial and connective tissue cells from the root surface during wound healing. It is believed to facilitate the regeneration of lost cementum, periodontal ligament, and alveolar bone. In theory, this technique should result in reconstructing the attachment apparatus rather than just root coverage. The membranes used during this procedure are most commonly made of materials such as expanded polytetrafluoroethylene (ePTFE), polyglactic acid, polylactic acid, and collagen.[51]

Other types of interventions include the placement of bone graft in the defects, root biomodification (regeneration using amelogenins), and the GTR technique, with the aim to reconstruct the periodontal defects and root furcations.[48,52–54]

Mucogingival surgery, which is considered a restorative surgery and includes connective and epithelial flaps, is limited to the restoration of original tissue architecture. It is not indicated in case of active periodontal infection.

Complications of Periodontal Surgery

Periodontal surgery almost invariably results in a degree of gingival recession, which has a number of consequences; for example:

- Increased exposure of the root surface may lead to dentine hypersensitivity.
- Increased tooth length may have implications for aesthetics in anterior teeth.
- Exposed root surface is more vulnerable to root caries.

Sutures and Periodontal Dressings

Some procedures require the placement of sutures. The goals of suturing are as follows: Provide adequate tension for wound closure but loose enough to prevent tissue ischemia and necrosis, maintain hemostasis, permit healing by primary intention, reduce postoperative pain, prevent bone exposure resulting in delayed healing and bone resorption, and permit proper flap position. There are different types of needles and suture materials. The nonresorbable category includes silk, polyester, nylon, and polytetrafluoroethylene (PTFE). Nonresorbable sutures must be removed. Resorbable sutures dissolve and include natural, plain gut, chromic gut, synthetic, and coated Vicryl.[55]

Periodontal dressings protect the wound after surgery. They also help to attain and preserve a close adaptation of the mucosal flap to the underlying bone and assist in providing patient comfort. A 0.12% chlorhexidine rinse is sometimes used as an antimicrobial for postoperative plaque control.

Comparative surgical studies have shown small differences between methods when evaluated over a few

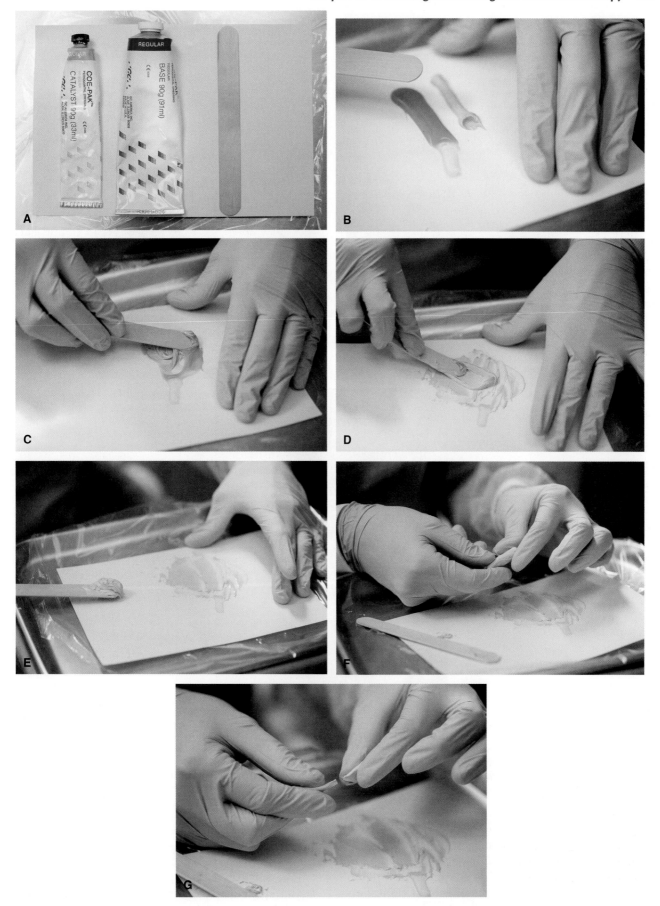

Figure 27-4. Preparing the surgical pack. (A) Assemble supplies: catalyst, base, and tongue depressor. (B) Dispense equal lines of the catalyst and base on paper. (C–E) Mix the base and catalyst with the wooden tongue depressor for several minutes. (F) Roll the paste into a cylinder. (G) Separate the cylinder into the appropriate size to cover the wound.

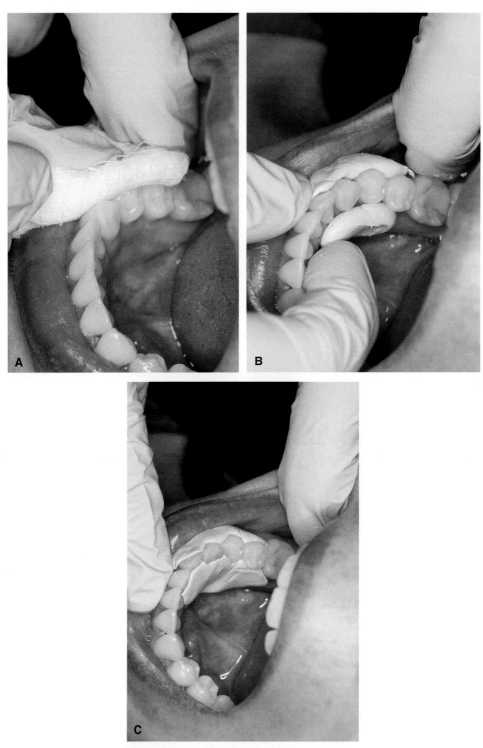

Figure 27-5. Placing the surgical pack. (A) Use cotton gauze to dry the area to be packed. (B) Place a strip of pack on the facial and lingual surfaces. (C) Gently apply pressure on the facial lingual surfaces to join the pack interproximally. Ensure that the pack does not interfere with occlusion.

years postsurgically. Results suggest that apical repositioning is more effective at reducing probing depth, replaced flaps (such as the modified Widman technique) offer slight advantages in terms of gain in clinical attachment, and procedures that involve extensive bone removal or exposure result in more bone loss and loss of attachment.[56]

DENTAL HYGIENE CONSIDERATIONS

Dental hygienists do not perform periodontal surgery, but they can contribute a great deal to the healing and health maintenance process. Patient education is vital to ensure that the patient is aware of the pros and cons of the surgical procedure and to ensure that self-care is optimal. Explaining the surgical procedures and why they are necessary will help answer anticipated questions and place the patient at ease. Instructions on tooth brushing, interdental cleaning, rinses if appropriate, and any other aids that will assist the patient should be demonstrated to the patient. The patient should then validate their understanding of the procedures by performing them for the dental hygienist. Frequent return visits for periodontal maintenance should be established to monitor health and self-care.

PERIODONTAL MAINTENANCE

When active periodontal therapy is complete, a recall and maintenance program is required. This allows the clinician to monitor plaque control and check for recurrent periodontal disease, often indicated by bleeding on probing. In general, recall intervals should initially be short (6–8 weeks) and then gradually extended provided the periodontium remains stable. The precise recall interval should be tailored to the patient's individual circumstances.

The American Academy of Periodontology has developed a parameter on periodontal maintenance.[57] Periodontal maintenance is an essential part of periodontal therapy for patients with a history of inflammatory periodontal diseases. It is most often performed by the dental hygienist. Patients should be informed of the disease process, therapeutic alternatives, potential complications, expected results, and their responsibility in treatment. Consequences of no treatment should be explained and documented. Failure to comply with a periodontal maintenance program may result in reactivation of the disease or progression of the disease process.

Case Study

A patient with diabetes arrives at the general dentist's office for his dental hygiene appointment. He takes insulin but is having difficulty controlling his blood sugar. The patient has gingival redness, swelling, suppuration, bleeding on probing, and two abscesses. Pocket depths are 6 to 8 mm.

Case Study Exercises

1. What is the diagnosis of the patient?
   A. Uncontrolled diabetes
   B. Controlled diabetes
   C. Periodontitis as a manifestation of systemic disease
   D. A and C
   E. B and C

2. Treatment would consist of all of the following EXCEPT:
   A. Preventive prophylaxis
   B. Referral to a periodontist
   C. Referral to a physician
   D. Treatment of acute infection

3. A dental hygienist in a periodontal office must care for this patient. The maintenance interval should be about 3 months, with shorter appointments, preferably in the morning.
   A. Both statements are true.
   B. Both statements are false.
   C. The first statement is true, but the second statement is false.
   D. The first statement is false, but the second statement is true.

Review Questions

1. The ultimate goal of periodontal surgery is to achieve successful periodontal regeneration. Scaling and root planing can solve most periodontal problems and is often sufficient when a patient has deep pockets.
   A. Both statements are true.
   B. Both statements are false.
   C. The first statement is true, but the second statement is false.
   D. The first statement is false, but the second statement is true.

2. Periodontal treatment includes the maintenance of the health, function, comfort, and aesthetics of all supporting structures and tissues in the mouth. Once periodontal disease has been diagnosed, SRP is the gold standard of nonsurgical periodontal therapy.
   A. Both statements are true.
   B. Both statements are false.
   C. The first statement is true, but the second statement is false.
   D. The first statement is false, but the second statement is true.

3. A comprehensive periodontal examination and risk assessment should be performed, along with a diagnosis, prognosis, and treatment plan. Informed consent should be obtained, and all records documented.
   A. Both the statement and the reason are correct and related.
   B. Both the statement and the reason are correct but are not related.
   C. The statement is correct, but the reason is not.
   D. The statement is not correct, but the reason is correct.
   E. Neither the statement nor the reason is correct.

4. Treatment of periodontal diseases should not include patient education, management of oral–systemic interrelationships, and nonsurgical or surgical therapy. The use of lasers, the perioscope, chemotherapeutic agents, and occlusal therapy are not a part of periodontal treatment.
   A. Both the statement and the reason are correct and related.

B. Both the statement and the reason are correct but are not related.
C. The statement is correct, but the reason is not.
D. The statement is not correct, but the reason is correct.
E. Neither the statement nor the reason is correct.

5. The goal of SRP is to create a glassy, hard, smooth surface with the removal of cementum or surface dentin that is rough, impregnated with calculus, or contaminated with toxins or microorganisms. Endotoxins (LPS) formed by gram-negative bacteria invade the root structure and this diseased cementum should be removed.
   A. Both the statement and the reason are correct and related.
   B. Both the statement and the reason are correct but are not related.
   C. The statement is correct, but the reason is not.
   D. The statement is not correct, but the reason is correct.
   E. Neither the statement nor the reason is correct.

Active Learning

1. Work in groups of four and prepare an oral presentation on the rationale between choosing nonsurgical and surgical therapy on a patient.
2. Prepare a PowerPoint presentation on the use of a periscope.
3. Create a decision tree for following the dental hygiene process of care with a new periodontal patient. ■

REFERENCES

1. Armitage GC. Development of a Classification system for periodontal diseases and conditions. *Ann Periodontol.* 1999;4(1):1-6.
2. Comprehensive periodontal therapy: a statement by the American Academy of Periodontology. *J Periodontol.* 2011;72:1790-1800. http://www.joponline.org/doi/pdf/10.1902/jop.2001.72.12.1790.
3. Kaldahl WB, Kalkwarf KL, Patil KD, Dyer JK, Bates RE Jr. Evaluation of four modalities of periodontal therapy. Mean probing depth, probing attachment level and recession changes. *J Periodontol.* 1988;59(12):783-793.
4. Ryan ME. Nonsurgical approaches for the treatment of periodontal diseases. *Dent Clin N Am.* 2005;49:611-636.
5. Cobb CM. Microbes, inflammation, scaling and root planing, and the periodontal condition. *J Dent Hyg.* 2008;82(suppl 3):4-9.
6. Corbet EF, Vaughan AJ, Kieser JB. The periodontally-involved root surface. *J Clin Periodontol.* 1993;20:402-410.
7. Ioannou I, Dimitriadis N, Papadimitriou K, Sakellari D, Vouros I, Konstantinidis. Hand instrumentation versus ultrasonic debridement in the treatment of chronic periodontitis: a randomized clinical and microbiological trial. *J Clin Periodontol.* 2009;36(2):132-141.
8. Rose LF, Mealey B, Minsk L, Cohen DW. Oral care for patients with cardiovascular disease and stroke. *J Am Dent Assoc.* 2002;133(suppl):37S-44S.
9. Perry D, Beemsterboer PL, Essex G. *Periodontology for the Dental Hygienist.* 4th ed. St. Louis, MO: Saunders; 2013.
10. Perry DA, Beemsterboer PL. *Periodontology for the Dental Hygienist.* Philadelphia, PA: Elsevier Science Health Science Division; 2007.
11. Hanes PJ, Purvis JP, Gunsolley JC. Local anti-infective therapy: pharmacological agents. A systematic review. *Ann Periodontol.* 2003;8:79-98.
12. Kalsi R, Vandana KL, Prakash S. Effect of local drug delivery in chronic periodontitis patients: a meta-analysis. *J Indian Soc Periodontol.* 2011;15(4):304-309.
13. Jorgens S. Efficient antimicrobial treatment in periodontal maintenance care. *J Am Dent Assoc.* 2000;131:1293-1304.
14. Nair SC, Anoop KR. Intraperiodontal pocket: an ideal route for local antimicrobial drug delivery. *J Adv Pharm Technol Res.* 2012;3(1):9-15.
15. Drisko C. The antimicrobial approach. *Dimens Dent Hyg.* February/March 2003. Available at: http://www.dimensionsofdentalhygiene.com/2003/02_February/03_March/Features/The_Antimicrobial_Approach.aspx. Accessed October 2, 2015.
16. Goldie M. Clinical application of lasers in dental hygiene. Dentistry IQ. *RDH eVillage Focus.* Published October 19, 2012. Available at: http://www.dentistryiq.com/articles/2012/10/clinical-application-of-lasers-in-dental-hygiene.html. Accessed: Oct 2, 2015.
17. Cobb CM. AAP-commissioned review. Lasers in periodontics: a review of the literature. *J Periodontol.* 2006;77(4):545-564.
18. Cobb CM. Lasers and periodontal therapy: the paradox of evidence vs. clinical perception. Maastricht,

the Netherlands: M(H)aastricht in Flow. September 28, 2012.

19. Workgroup to Develop Statement on Laser Use by Dental Professionals. American Academy of Periodontology Statement on the efficacy of lasers in the non-surgical treatment of inflammatory periodontal disease. *J Periodontol.* 2011;82(4):513-514. http://www.joponline.org/toc/jop/82/4.

20. American Dental Hygienists' Association website. http://www.adha.org.

21. Kwan JY. Perioscopy technology overview. Perioscopy Incorporated website. 2015. http://www.perioscopy-inc.com/perioscopy-technology.php. Accessed October 30, 2015.

22. Kwan JY, Workman PD. Micro ultrasonic endoscopic periodontal debridement: retrospective analysis of treatment with at least 1 year follow-up. Poster presented at American Academy of Periodontology Annual Session; 2009; Boston, MA. http://www.perioscopyinc.com/documents/aap_poster_boston_2009.pdf. Accessed Oct 2, 2015.

23. About Emdogain(tm). Straumann USA LLC website. http://www.straumann.us/en/home/recession/about-emdogain.html. Accessed October 2, 2015.

24. Osteohealth. Innovative Dental Solutions. Osteohealth Company. 2014. http://www.osteohealth.com/GEM21S.aspx. Accessed October 30, 2015.

25. Slots J, Ting MM. Systemic antibiotics in the treatment of periodontal disease. *Periodontol 2000.* 2002;28:106-176.

26. Serio FG, Serio CL. Systemic and local antibiotics and host modulation in periodontal therapy: where are we now? Part I. *Inside Dentistry.* 2006;2(2). Published by AEGIS Communications.

27. Wilson TG, Harrel SK, Nunn ME, Francis B, Webb K. The relationship between the presence of tooth-borne subgingival deposits and inflammation found with a dental endoscope. *J Periodontol.* 2008;79(11):2029-2035.

28. American Academy of Periodontology. *Glossary of periodontal terms.* 4th ed. Chicago, IL: American Academy of Periodontology; 2001. http://www.perio.org/sites/default/files/files/PDFs/Publications/GlossaryOfPeriodontalTerms2001Edition.pdf.

29. Nyman S, Gottlow J, Karring T, Lindhe J. The regenerative potential of the periodontal ligament. *J Clin Periodontol.* 1982;9:257-265.

30. Wikesjö UME, Claffey N, Egelberg J. Periodontal repair in dogs: effect of heparin treatment of the root surface. *J Clin Periodontol.* 1991;18:60-64.

31. Crespi R, Barone A, Covani U. Histologic evaluation of three methods of periodontal root surface treatment in humans. *J Periodontol.* 2005;76(3):476-481.

32. Polimeni G, Albandar JM, Wikesjo UME. Prognostic factors for alveolar re generation: effect of space provision. *J Clin Periodontol.* 2005;32:951-954.

33. Polson AM, Proye MF. Fibrin linkage: a precursor for new attachment. *J Periodontol.* 1983;54:141-147.

34. Kennedy JE, Bird WC, Palcanis KG, Dorfman HS. A longitudinal evaluation of varying widths of attached gingiva. *J Clin Periodontol.* 1985;12:667-675.

35. Wikesjö UME, Claffey N, Christersson LA, et al. Repair of periodontal furcation defects in beagle dogs following reconstructive surgery including root surface demineralization with tetracycline hydrochloride and topical fibronectin application. *J Clin Periodontol.* 1988;15:73-80.

36. Lang NP, Loe H. The relationship between the width of keratinized gingiva and gingival health. *J Periodontol.* 1972;43:623-627.

37. Tackas VJ. Root coverage techniques: a review. *J West SOC Periodont Periodont Abstr.* 1995;43:5-14.

38. Nielsen IM, Glavind L, Karring T. Interproximal periodontal intrabony defects. Prevalence, localization and etiological factors. *J Clin Periodontol.* 1980;7:187-198.

39. Leknes KN, Lie T, Selvig KA. Root grooves: a risk factor in periodontal attachment loss. *J Periodontol.* 1994;65:859-863.

40. Wikesjö UME, Selvig KA. Periodontal wound healing and regeneration. *Periodontol 2000.* 1999;19:21-39.

41. Caffesse RG. Resective procedures. American Academy of Periodontology. Proceedings of the World Workshop in Clinical Periodontics; Chicago, IL, 1989.

42. Caranza F. Glickman's Clinical Periodontology. 7th ed. Philadelphia, PA: WB Saunders Co.; 1990.

43. Morris ML. The unrepositioned muco-periosteal flap. *Periodontics.* 1965;3:147.

44. Stahl SS. Repair or regeneration following periodontal therapy? *J Clin Peridontol.* 1979;6:389-396.

45. Levine L. Periodontal flap surgery and the gingival fiber retention. *J Periodontol.* 1972;43:91-98.

46. Barrington EP. An overview of periodontal surgical procedure. *J Periodontol.* 1981;52:518.

47. Dedolph TH, Clark HB. A histological study of mucoperiosteal flap healing. *J Oral Surg.* 1958;16:367.

48. Caffesse RG, Ramfjord SP, Nasjleti CE. Reverse bevel periodontal flaps in monkeys. *J Periodontol.* 1968;39:219.

49. Ramfjord SP. Present status of the Modified Widman Flap procedure. *J Periodontol.* 1977;48:558.

50. Caffesse RG, Castelli WA, Nasjleti CE. Vascular response to modified Widman flap surgery in monkeys. *J Periodontol.* 1981;52:1.

51. Cortellini P, Clauser C, Prato GP. Histologic assessment of new attachment following the treatment of a human buccal recession by means of a guided tissue regeneration procedure. *J Periodontol.* 1993;64(5):387-391.

52. Becker W, Becker BE, Ochsenbein CO, et al. A longitudinal study comparing scaling, osseous surgery and modified Widman procedures. Results after one year. *J Periodontol.* 1987;59:351.

53. Ramfjord SP, Nissle RR. The Modified Widman Flap. *J Periodontol.* 1974;45:601.

54. Wirthlin MR. The current status of new attachment therapy. *J Periodontol.* 1981;52:529.

55. Silverstein LM. *Principles of Dental Suturing: The Complete Guide to Dental Closure.* Mahwah, NJ: Montage Media Corporation; 1999.

56. Palmer RM, Floyd PD. Periodontology: a clinical approach. 4. Periodontal surgery. *Br Dent J.* 1995;178(8):301-306.

57. American Academy of Periodontology. Parameter on periodontal maintenance. *J Periodontol.* 2000;71:849-850. http://www.joponline.org/doi/pdf/10.1902/jop.2000.71.5-S.849.

Chapter 28 | Management of Dentin Hypersensitivity

Lillian Caperila, RDH, MEd, and Ellen R. Guritzky, AAS, RDH, BS, MSJ

KEY TERMS

Brännström
  hydrodynamic theory

dentin tubules

iontophoresis

myelinated A-delta fiber

smear layer

Tomes fiber

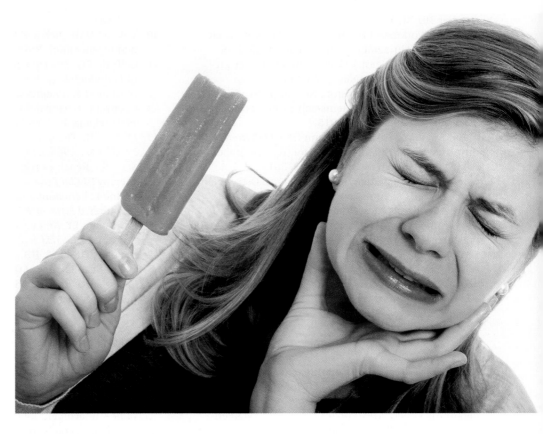

LEARNING OBJECTIVES

After reading this chapter, the student should be able to:

28.1 Describe dentin hypersensitivity and discuss the prevalence, cause, and symptoms.

28.2 Recognize by exclusion the cause associated with various entities of dentin hypersensitivity.

28.3 Identify the most common teeth affected by dentin hypersensitivity and predisposing factors that contribute to this condition.

28.4 Recognize transient and long-term occurrences of dentin hypersensitivity and recommendations for patient relief.

28.5 Discuss and compare preventive and therapeutic modalities in the treatment of dentin hypersensitivity.

28.6 Define the new and widely used generation of medicaments that support prevention and control of symptoms associated with hypersensitivity.

28.7 Develop an evidence-based approach to preventing dentin hypersensitivity in individualized patient cases.

KEY CONCEPTS

- Dentin hypersensitivity has been referred to as one of the most chronic and painful dental conditions that occurs often in the general population but is more prevalent in periodontal patients.
- Differential diagnosis of the cause of dentin hypersensitivity in conjunction with patient education ensures greater success in managing, preventing, and relieving symptoms of hypersensitivity.
- Evidence-based therapies are introducing a new generation of agents that enhance the combination of fluoride with calcium and phosphates in successfully treating chronic and painful symptoms while remineralizing tooth structure.

RELEVANCE TO CLINICAL PRACTICE

Dentin hypersensitivity is a common, chronic, and painful disorder experienced by a majority of the general population. Depending on its frequency and intensity of occurrence, patients may or may not report dentin hypersensitivity during routine dental visits. Dentin hypersensitivity may be transient or persistent and may cause difficulty in normal function on a daily basis.

Dental hygienists should be able to recognize symptoms of dentin hypersensitivity by completing a thorough dental history, examining clinical structures, and applying appropriate treatment modalities that resolve the associated symptoms. With the new diagnostic technologies and therapeutic medicaments available today, the dental hygienist is better equipped to identify and recommend treatment that can minimize or eliminate this dental disorder.

DEFINITION OF DENTIN HYPERSENSITIVITY

Dentin hypersensitivity is described as a sharp pain of limited duration that occurs at exposed dentin in response to a stimulus.[1,2] The stimulus may be caused through mechanical, chemical, thermal, evaporative, tactile, or osmotic provocation on the tooth surface. Dentin discomfort or pain resulting from known pathology or defect such as chipped or fractured teeth, cracked cusps, carious lesions, and/or leaky restorations would not be categorized as hypersensitivity.[2]

Dental Structures

It is necessary to review the associated dentin histology and the neural components that are responsible for the conduction of sensory stimuli perceived as pain within the tooth to understand the nature of dentin hypersensitivity. Enamel is the most highly calcified and hardest tissue in the body. Dentin is a tubular, branched structure that connects the pulp to the enamel–dentin junction.

Dentin is 70% inorganic material, 18% organic material, and 12% water. Healthy dentin is covered by enamel in the clinical crown and by cementum in the anatomical root portion of the tooth (Fig. 28-1). The dentin tubules are filled with fluid and are important to hydraulically transfer and relieve stresses on the tooth. The dentin is composed of thousands of small channels known as **dentin tubules,** which contain odontoblastic processes, or **Tomes fibers,** bathed by tissue fluids and minerals.

Mature dentin is mainly inorganic tissue that consists of many dentin tubules that extend from the dentino-enamel junction in the crown area or the dentino-cemental junction in the root area to the outer wall of the pulp. After the maturation of dentin, the cell bodies of the odontoblasts remain in the pulp along its outer wall and inside the tooth. The Tomes fiber and odontoblast within each of the dentin tubules communicate with the pulp. Dentinal fluid surrounds the cell membrane of the odontoblast from the cell body in the pulp.

Three types of sensory nerve fibers are found in the pulpal side of the dentin tubules: A-delta fibers, A-beta fibers, and C-fibers. Stimulation of any of these fibers

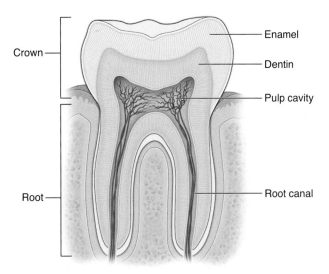

Figure 28-1. Tooth structure.

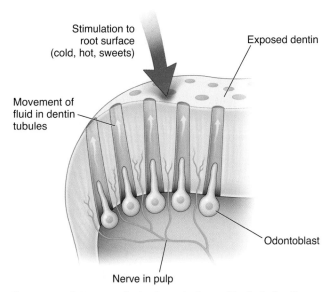

Figure 28-2. Brännström hydrodynamic theory. Physical stimuli applied to exposed dentin causes fluid movement in the dentin tubules. The fluid movement stimulates nerve receptors sensitive to pressure, which the patient perceives as a sharp pain.

will be felt as tooth pain, but more specifically, each of these types of nerve fibers elicits variances in pain sensation and its source of stimulation.

The **myelinated A-delta fibers** elicit a well-localized, sharp pain considered responsible for dentin hypersensitivity. A-beta fibers also produce sharp pain of short duration, but they are more responsive to electrical stimulation. C-fibers are unmyelinated and produce a dull, nonlocalized, aching pain that is felt with direct pulpal stimulation. Consequently, depending on the activation of certain nerve fibers, pain is felt in different ways.

CAUSATIVE AND PREDISPOSING FACTORS

Brännström hydrodynamic theory, developed in the 1960s, is the most widely accepted theory regarding the cause of dentin sensitivity. According to the hydrodynamic theory, when physical stimuli such as cold or heat are applied to exposed dentin, fluids in the tubules are disturbed. The stimulation produces an outward flow of tubular fluid through capillary actions. While the dentin tubules are open and exposed to the oral environment, the A-delta fibers surrounding the odontoblasts are stimulated. The fluid movement stimulates nerve receptors sensitive to pressure, which the patient perceives as a sharp pain (Fig. 28-2).[3]

No matter which form of stimulus is applied to the exposed dentin surface area, the patient will perceive this stimulus in the pulpal region as a painful reaction. In addition to the type of stimuli exposed to the tooth surface, the number of dentin tubules present at the surface also affects dentin hypersensitivity. The likelihood that a patient will experience dentin hypersensitivity is directly proportionate to the number of exposed dentin tubules.

When evaluating a patient, the dental hygienist identifies all known predisposing factors that create exposed dentin tubules (Box 28-1). Dentin may become exposed to the oral environment through parafunctional habits, periodontal implications, enamel wear or erosion, and anatomical abnormalities. The **smear layer,** a thin layer of organic debris that develops on the tooth surface after procedures such as root planing or cutting with a dental bur, covers the tubules and provides relief from dentin sensitivity.

Conducting a thorough medical, dental, and social history with the patient can be very helpful in the identification of environmental or predisposing factors that contribute to or exacerbate dentin sensitivity. Even if patients do not report chronic sensitivity, their initial interview may provide pertinent information that is useful at a later time during treatment. Predisposing factors may be clinical signs of gingival recession, anatomical anomalies on the teeth surfaces, dietary and lifestyle habits (such as sucking on lemons, drinking through a straw, brushing vigorously, or using home whitening agents), or a history of restorative and periodontal therapy.

PREVALANCE OF DENTIN HYPERSENSITIVITY

In the general practice population, the reported prevalence rate of dentin hypersensitivity may vary between 4% and 74%.[4,5] These disproportionate numbers may be explained by the methods used to collect these data and how the noted sensitivity is defined in the survey. Although there may be high numbers of documented

Box 28-1. *Predisposing Factors That Create Exposed Dentin Tubules*

Parafunctional Oral Habits
- Excessive toothbrush patterns or hard-bristle toothbrush
- Poor oral hygiene directly affects the gingival inflammatory response, which can result in gingival recession and dentin exposure
- Grinding and attrition to the teeth expose dentin surfaces
- Abrasion of root surfaces with excessive picking by fingernails, toothpicks, or similar objects of habit

Periodontal
- Gingival recession may be caused by acute or chronic periodontal inflammation, anatomical defects, or abrasion created by incorrect tooth brushing or parafunctional oral habits
- Exposed dentin surface as a result of repositioned gingival tissues during periodontal flap surgery procedures
- Extensive tooth and root instrumentation that removes excessive cementum and exposes underlying dentin surfaces
- Use of smokeless tobacco, causing severe gingival recession related to the quid, a noxious chemical in this product
- Occlusal forces in conjunction with periodontal disease activity may directly lead to further gingival recession and dentin exposure

Enamel Loss
- Erosive dissolution of extrinsic enamel by habitual ingestion of acidic foods or drinks with pH less than 5.5
- Patients who experience intrinsic erosion of enamel or cementum as a result of chronic acidic exposure during episodes of regurgitation related to bulimia or gastroesophageal reflux disease
- Brushing teeth immediately after ingestion of acidic foods and drinks damaged the enamel
- Ineffective plaque control may contribute to enamel demineralization, further leading to sensitivity

Anatomical Abnormalities
- Thin labial alveolar bone or the occurrence of a fenestration on the labial plate may contribute to gingival recession
- Malpositioned teeth may create thin, alveolar bone and consequently lead to gingival recession
- In approximately 10% of cases, dentin may become exposed when enamel and cementum do not meet at the cementoenamel junction (This does not necessarily indicate sensitivity but can be a predisposing factor.)

Frenum attachment and associated fibers attached closer to the gingival margin may create gingival recession during masticatory functions. ■

---

cases of sensitivity, there is a smaller population that has been accurately diagnosed as having cervical dentin hypersensitivity according to set diagnostic criteria.[6] Error in documented cases of sensitivity may be due to patients who choose not to seek treatment because they do not perceive this as a severe oral health problem. Conclusively, it appears that the incidence rate of hypersensitivity in most populations ranges between 10% and 30% of the general population,[7] while one study estimated a 73% to 98% prevalence rate in periodontal patients.[8] Dental hygienists who treat patients with periodontal disease should expect a higher prevalence of dentin hypersensitivity.

Other factors associated with prevalence of dentin hypersensitivity show that female individuals have a slightly higher occurrence over male individuals. Although the difference is not statistically significant, the most accepted explanation is due to better attention to oral hygiene habits, which may lead to greater incidence of sensitivity related to fastidious and greater frequency of oral care habits especially on buccal surfaces.[9,10]

Reports of dentin hypersensitivity may range from teenaged cases through adults 70+ years of age. The peak age period is between 30 and 40 years and slowly diminishes over the age of 40 years as changes in the dentin are responsible for decreasing the dentin exposure. The formation of reparative or tertiary dentin associated with attrition, abrasion, caries, or restorative procedures will obliterate the opening of dentin tubules, further reducing symptoms of sensitivity to stimuli. This may explain a diminished sense of pain associated with exposed dentin with older patients who have signs of chronic tooth wear as reparative dentin forms in reaction to chronic wear and attrition of normal occlusal function.[11] Dental visits that include regular topical fluoride and home-applied fluoride toothpaste will build a protective layer on exposed dentin and cementum that further contribute to decreasing sensitivity of the dentin in the adult population.

In order of frequency, the teeth most commonly affected by dentin hypersensitivity are: canines and first premolars, incisors, second premolars, and molars. The anatomical architecture of the alveolar bone and thin gingival tissue in the buccal aspects of these teeth predisposes the dentin to greater exposure and sensitivity.[6,9] Studies that record data related to dentin sensitivity had a negative correlation to plaque scores in those sites. This demonstrates that it is not the bacterial plaque as a chief factor but the improper plaque-removal techniques that contribute to abrasion and gingival recession, further leading to greater occurrence of sensitivity. Patients who demonstrate right-handed dominance during brushing techniques will eventually produce greater severity of dentin abrasion on the left side of their mouth and elicit sensitivity on those sites more often than the right side.

Dentin hypersensitivity may be described as "transient" when it occurs during or shortly after a procedure that is often correlated with exposed or compromised dentin or enamel integrity. Sensitivity most often occurs in periodontal patients, and symptoms may persist for a longer period or until the exposed dentin surfaces are protected with permanent restorations or gingival coverage of the root surfaces. Mild or transient episodes of hypersensitivity may also be associated with recent placement of restorations, teeth bleaching (in-office or take-home tray wear), or a recent periodontal scaling and/or root planing procedure. These symptoms are more likely to dissipate with a professional desensitization treatment followed by daily home-applied dentifrices containing ingredients to depolarize neural transmission or tubular occlusion of dentin surfaces. Nonetheless, professional recommendations may consider a "pretreatment" in using a fluoride-based gel worn in a tray for approximately 2 weeks before teeth bleaching or a 5000 ppm sodium fluoride dentifrice at home before an extensive scaling and root planing procedure. Fluorides will be more effective in pretreatment phase rather than the use of a potassium salt for post-treatment relief.[12]

DENTAL HYGIENE DIAGNOSIS OF DENTIN HYPERSENSITIVITY

Dentin hypersensitivity is diagnosed by a process of exclusion. It is recognized and treated successfully following a process of eliminating known pathological causes. Signs and symptoms related to pathological conditions such as dental caries, pulpal trauma or damage, chipped or fractured teeth, and/or fractured, marginal leakage, or failing restorations are not considered or managed as dentin hypersensitivity from dentin exposure.[13]

The basic erosive wear examination (BEWE) was developed to offer a scoring system and diagnostic tool for the management of erosive tooth wear. The BEWE is a partial scoring system recording of the most severely affected surface in a sextant. The cumulative score guides treatment planning for the condition. The four-level score grades the appearance or severity of wear on the teeth from no surface loss (0), initial loss of enamel surface texture (1), distinct defect, hard tissue loss (dentin) less than 50% of the surface area (2), or hard tissue loss more than 50% of the surface area (3). Differentiating between lesions restricted to enamel and dentin can be difficult, particularly in the cervical area. Buccal/facial, occlusal, and lingual/palatal surfaces are examined, and the highest score is recorded. BEWE scores are:

0 = No erosive tooth wear
1 = Initial loss of surface texture
2 = Hard tissue loss less than 50% of surface area
3 = Hard tissue loss more than 50% of surface area

Scores of 2 and 3 will have dentin involvement. The result of the BEWE is not only a measure of the severity of the condition but also a guide for management.[14]

Dentin is naturally sensitive because of its close functional relationship with the dental pulp. However, because of enamel and cementum coverage in a normal, healthy tooth anatomy, the dentin does not exhibit sensations upon direct stimulus. A microscopic examination of dentin reveals numerous and wider dentin tubules present when there is known reported sensitivity of this dental tissue. These observations are consistent and support the hypothesis of the Brännström hydrodynamic theory.[11]

More than 90% of all known sites of dentin hypersensitivity are found at the cervical margins of buccal or labial surfaces of the teeth. The hypersensitivity develops in two phases. First, a *localized lesion* develops as a result of exposure of the dentin either by gingival recession or loss of enamel surface. When tooth brushing abrades enamel structure, it happens as a secondary process following the apical recession of the gingival margin. Second, the *initiation of the lesion* occurs when the smear layer is lost and opens access directly to the dentin tubules. During this stage of the process, enamel erosion becomes the significant cause of the loss of this protective layer, leaving dentin tubules vulnerable for the communication of stimuli from the dentin surface to the reactive pulp.[5,13]

When a patient presents with a complaint or symptoms of sensitivity, it is helpful for the dental hygienist to follow the steps in Box 28-2 to establish a conclusive diagnosis of dentin hypersensitivity.

MANAGEMENT OF DENTIN HYPERSENSITIVITY

A wide selection of treatment options are available in dentistry today to manage dentin hypersensitivity. They are categorized as either chemical or physical agents based on their mode of action to minimize symptoms and provide patient relief. Depending on the cause of the sensitivity and the patient's pain threshold, the success of a chosen therapy may be determined by whether the source of discomfort comes from exposed dentin tubules or neural transmission related to the fluid conduction occurring within the tubules.

Transient hypersensitivity may occur immediately after a dental procedure such as periodontal instrumentation, periodontal surgery, extensive restorations, and tooth-whitening procedures. The dental hygienist should anticipate this possibility and recommend home-applied desensitizing agents to reduce the symptoms as a preventive approach. If patient-applied agents do not bring relief, it may be necessary to have the patient return to administer a professionally applied medicament with both analgesic and blocking properties for the sensitive sites.

Box 28-2. *Screening for Dentin Hypersensitivity*

Patient Information (subjective data)
- Do you currently experience tooth sensitivity?
- When does this occur? (identification of stimulus)
- Duration of the pain?
- Occurs how often?
- Contributing diet or lifestyle habits?
  - This includes identification of acidic foods or liquids consumed daily.

Clinical Criteria (observed during examination)
- Gingival recession
- Toothbrush abrasion
- Presence of cervical plaque
- Sites of tooth demineralization
- Loss of enamel or cementum
- Exposed areas of dentin/cementum
- Malpositioned teeth (related to gingival position and recession)
- Abfraction

- Gingival position related to past periodontal procedures
- Signs of cusp grinding, bruxism, clenching habits
- History of recent teeth bleaching or periodontal instrumentation
- Recently placed restorations
- Abnormal flow or presence of saliva to prevent demineralization

Radiographic Criteria
- Identification of caries or pulpal infection eliminates preliminary diagnosis of dentin hypersensitivity
- Identification of radiolucency at cervical areas may implicate possible erosion, abrasion, or abfraction until clinical examination confirms these findings to rule out caries
- No radiolucent areas found under present restorations

Treatment Options

Two major groups of treatment options are used to treat dentin hypersensitivity: those that plug/block and occlude dentin tubules, and those that interrupt the transmission of neural impulses. Table 28-1 lists desensitizing agents and their mode of action directed at either nerve impulses or tubular occlusion.[15]

In using an agent that contains potassium nitrate, the mode of action relies on elevating the potassium ion concentration within the dentin tubules and creates a state of hyperpolarization of the nerves. This reduces nerve excitation and causes them to become insensitive to any further stimulation for a short duration.

The selection of a blocking agent or tubule obtundent to occlude or plug the dentin tubules is recommended when the clinical examination reveals dentin exposed to the oral environment and accompanied by symptoms of pain or discomfort when any form of stimuli provokes a reaction by the patient. This is the most common explanation and treatment used in dental care for the symptoms reported at a patient visit. An extensive selection of therapeutic products can be

Table 28-1. *Desensitizing Agents and Their Mode of Action*

Classification of Desensitization Agents	Mode of Action	Process
Nerve hyperpolarization	Potassium nitrate	Interrupt nerve impulse conduction
Tubule obtundents	Fluorides Oxalates Calcium compounds Sodium citrate Strontium chloride	Precipitate calcium fluoride or other compounds to block exposed or open tubules
Protein precipitants	Strontium chloride Silver nitrate Formaldehyde Glutaraldehyde	Block tubules and narrow tubule diameter by coagulation of proteins and amino acids
Calcium phosphate technology	Amorphous calcium phosphate Casein phosphopeptides/amorphous Calcium phosphate Calcium sodium phosphosilicate Arginine calcium carbonate	Calcium phosphate diffusion and salivary availability to replace lost minerals and occlude tubules

applied by a dental professional in-office, as well as products the patient can use daily at home. Best success in relieving painful symptoms is achieved with repeated applications that follow any disturbance of the smear layer that forms on tooth surfaces during routine tooth-brushing patterns.[15]

A third category of treatment known as **protein precipitants** demonstrates a coagulation of proteins within the dentin tubule lumen, consequently decreasing the tubular diameter and interrupting the nerve transmission and fluid flow to the pulp.

Since the late 1990s, a new category of desensitization agents, calcium phosphate technology, has emerged. These agents suggest that both occlusion of the tubules and replenishment of lost minerals in the tooth structure reduce sensitivity and restore the health of enamel and dentin. Calcium and phosphates are replaced with compounds including fluoride, calcium, phosphate, and carbonate. In addition to penetrating tooth surfaces, the compounds saturate the salivary with fluoride and minerals that can remain available to infiltrate structures that are compromised by abrasion and demineralization.

Delivery Modes

There are three modes of desensitization treatment delivery: home-applied agents, professionally applied agents, and professionally prescribed home-applied agents. Products that require a prescription for use at home by the patient are subject to regulatory guidelines and must be supervised by a dental professional.

Treatment and Patient Education Plan

In developing a treatment plan following the diagnosis of dentin hypersensitivity, it is essential to identify all behavioral risks and contributory factors before the delivery of any selected agent. A patient education plan should include the following steps: (a) observe tooth-brushing techniques in all affected sites to revise the direction, force, and pressure; (b) replace the patient's toothbrush with a "soft" nylon bristled brush or instruct the patient in using a soft brush attachment for power-driven toothbrushes; and (c) discuss the patient's daily eating habits and advise him or her to avoid consuming highly acidic foods and drinks to excess or high frequency.

When the patient education plan has addressed all contributory factors for dentin hypersensitivity, it is important to document current symptoms, duration, and stimuli that provoke a painful response and to create a well-thought-out therapy plan to address these factors.

The dental hygienist and patient formulate a preventive approach. Once the patient has been instructed to improve brushing and flossing techniques, avoid acidic foods, and maintain a regular dental appointment, the dental hygienist should also identify any contributory factors that may initiate or perpetuate clinical symptoms of sensitivity. A list of preventive recommendations for

dentin hypersensitivity for patients and professionals is provided in Box 28-3.[8]

To date, there is no single treatment for dentin hypersensitivity. Recommended treatments may depend on the recognized cause or individual's threshold to pain. When considering therapeutic management of the symptoms, it is best to select the most conservative and least expensive treatment. Suggesting a home-applied dentifrice remains the first choice of care followed up with a 2- to 4-week post-treatment evaluation to assess resolution of painful symptoms and comfort to the patient during normal function. If this approach proves unsuccessful, then a professionally applied product or prescription for home-applied products may be the next step in proper care.[15]

At this point in the decision-making process, and with no success in home-applied therapy, it becomes necessary for the clinician to implement an in-office therapy that combines tubular occlusion and analgesic comfort. Following this procedure, patient education should be reviewed to ensure that the patient is not creating an abrasive action that may remove the effects produced by the professional treatment. This includes a "soft-bristle" toothbrush and observation of the patient's technique in applying a desensitizing dentifrice to follow at home. Some electric toothbrushes offer a mode for people with sensitive teeth. Placing a lot of pressure when teeth are being cleaned can be detrimental and aggravate dentin hypersensitivity. Some power brush models have pressure sensors that will indicate to the patient via a beep or light that too much

---

Box 28-3. *Preventive Recommendations for Dentin Hypersensitivity*

Suggestions for Patients
- Avoid medium- to hard-bristle toothbrushes.
- Avoid brushing teeth immediately after consumption of acidic foods or liquids.
- Avoid excessive pressure during brushing, especially at the cervical region of teeth.
- Avoid picking or scratching at the gingival margin or misuse of toothpicks/dental aids.
- Rinse mouth with neutral water after consumption of acidic snacks or liquids.

Suggestions for Professionals
- Avoid excessive instrumentation of root surfaces during periodontal scaling and root planing procedures, especially at cervical sites.
- Follow criteria for "selective polishing" when possible; rotary polishing with abrasive agents should be avoided on exposed dentin surfaces.
- Recommend conservative steps in whitening teeth: use lower-strength peroxides, limit wear time of products, and avoid contact with gingiva to minimize irritation. ■

pressure is being applied. The best results occur when patients do not rinse immediately after brushing with these products.

The need for another post-treatment evaluation in 2 to 3 weeks will offer the option of another series of professional application or the need to restore the tooth with a surgical restoration or adhesive protection for permanent relief and normal oral function.

Procedure 28-1 provides a step-by-step process for assembling the supplies and performing a desensitization procedure to manage a patient's symptoms of dentin sensitivity.

HOME-APPLIED TREATMENT OPTIONS

Over-the-counter products for relief of dentin sensitivity usually contain a potassium salt such as potassium nitrate, potassium chloride, or potassium citrate. Remineralizing toothpastes contain sodium fluoride and calcium phosphate salts.

Since the start of this decade, several clinical trials were published that compare the use of potassium-containing dentifrices. Potassium nitrate decreases the excitability of the intradental nerves by altering the membrane potential.[15–18] Select studies demonstrated better results in reducing sensitivity when using 5% potassium nitrate or 3.75% potassium chloride compared with baseline or negative controls. Other products using combinations of potassium nitrate and 0.454% stannous fluoride in a silica base or potassium nitrate and 0.243% sodium fluoride in a silica base reduce mild symptoms of discomfort with frequent use.[19,20]

Instruct patients to use these products twice daily and avoid rinsing immediately after their application to avoid diluting the paste and active ingredients and reducing their efficacy. Desensitization products are most successful when applied consistently with a soft-bristle toothbrush.

Additional desensitizing agents marketed as rinses and gels may contain active ingredients of sodium fluoride, sodium silicofluoride, and stannous fluoride. Because these ingredients are designed to form a calcium-fluoride compound that serves to reduce the radius of the tubule and occlude the opening to these pathways in dentin, they are suggested for long-term use for best results.[15]

Potassium nitrate-containing pastes or gels are recommended for immediate treatment of mild to severe sensitivity; chronic, long-term relief is best achieved with continual use of fluoride-containing products to support layered applications to seal off exposed dentin surfaces.[15]

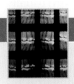

Procedure 28-1   Application of a Desensitizing Agent

MATERIALS
Mirror
Cotton rolls, dry angle, or mouth retractor
Air/water syringe
Locking pliers
2 × 2-inch gauze square
Cotton-tip applicators or cotton pellet with locking pliers
Dappen dish
Anesthetic syringe and local anesthesia (local anesthesia may be necessary if the patient experiences discomfort during debridement and application of the agent)

PREPROCEDURE
Patient Education
Review symptoms and site location with the patient. Explain how the desensitizing agent will be applied, the reason for its application, and post-treatment expectations.

PROCEDURE
1. Gather and organize materials before the patient's arrival.
2. Remove all superficial debris and plaque from the tooth surface. If the patient experiences discomfort during debridement, administer local anesthesia, then continue.
3. Isolate the specific site(s) to be treated with cotton rolls or dry angles.
4. Blot the site with dry gauze square.
5. Review specific manufacturer's instructions for agent application.
   - If liquid or gel agent is used, apply with tips or pellet applicator.
   - If varnish is used, apply with brush applicator supplied.
6. Apply very light air to site to assess need for second application.
7. Discard all disposable materials and sterilize reusable supplies.
8. Document the procedure by date, tooth identification, BEWE, and process used in patient chart/file.
9. Recommend a desensitization dentifrice to be used twice daily with soft-bristle toothbrush.
10. Schedule a postprocedure evaluation or telephone call to assess success of professional treatment.
    - If symptoms persist, schedule a second visit to reapply in-office desensitizing agent.
    - Document this information by date and patient's response.

PROFESSIONAL TREATMENT OPTIONS

Desensitizing agents recommended to patients for home use are typically easy to purchase and apply with a toothbrush. When relief is not attained in a reasonable amount of time following the use of desensitizing dentifrices, the dental professional will offer alternative procedures that require an office visit.

Professionally applied or prescribed agents may include one of the following: fluorides (as gels, rinses, or topical varnish), precipitants (oxalates, calcium-phosphate compounds, calcium hydroxide), primers that contain hydroxyethyl methacrylate (5% glutaraldehyde), or polymerizing agents (glass ionomer cements, adhesive resin primers). Other procedures that involve ancillary equipment include iontophoresis, lasers, or the placement of a permanent restoration.

When a selected fluoride agent is considered for use, it may be one of the following categories: sodium fluoride, stannous fluoride, or hydrogen fluoride. The mechanism of action of the fluorides is primarily to decrease the permeability of the dentin, possibly by precipitation of insoluble calcium fluoride within its tubules.[13] Professionally applied fluoride agents are more potent than those applied at home. Furthermore, the percentage of fluoride ion concentration varies with the classification and vehicle of delivery.

Sodium fluoride varnish is gaining increased acceptance in treating localized sites of sensitivity. Fluoride varnish is classified as a device with approved U.S. Food and Drug Administration claims to treat desensitization and application as a cavity liner. Using a varnish agent allows ease in application, provides quick drying on tooth surface, and sustains a high concentration of fluoride ions into the exposed dentin surface, as well as continued fluoride concentration in salivary components. Topical fluoride varnishes are less likely to be removed after application because of their intact precipitate compared with gels or solutions that naturally rinse away immediately after application.[21,22]

Potassium Nitrate

Potassium nitrate (1%–15% solutions; 5%, 10% in gels) is also used in professional applications in an aqueous solution or an adhesive gel. It reduces nerve excitability by blocking repolarization of nerve endings.

Potassium Oxalates

Potassium oxalates (3% potassium oxalate or 6.8% ferric oxalate) reduce dentin permeability and occlude tubules, but they have been more successful in laboratory studies than in clinical studies. Although some reported studies show success in alleviating sensitivity, many studies proved to be unclear because of the nature of experimental designs.[23]

Calcium Compounds

Calcium compounds (amorphous calcium phosphate (ACP), calcium hydroxide, casein phosphopeptides-amorphous calcium phosphate (CPP-ACP), and calcium sodium phosphosilicate and, more recently added, an arginine bicarbonate complex) are all specific compound formulations that primarily work to deliver calcium and phosphates that create a precipitate and facilitate the occlusion of open dentin tubules. Theoretically, the end result is not a new approach to reducing sensitivity, but with the latest generation of ACP-driven technologies, there is an added benefit of restoring the lost components of inorganic minerals in both the enamel and dentin structure. Consequently, by replacing denatured dentin, the goals of reducing sensitivity may be attained by the formation of fluorapatite and greater success in tubular occlusion.[24,25]

Adhesives and Resins

Adhesives and resins (primers, sealants, etch and primer adhesives, oxalic acid and resins, varnishes) are a class of agents that provide longer-lasting relief for sensitivity because of their properties of adhesion and permanent placement on exposed dentin structures. Upon re-evaluation following reports of little success in the initial trial of home-applied desensitizing toothpastes, a clinician may consider selecting a product in this category in the next step of resolving symptoms of hypersensitivity. The primers, sealants, and adhesives are usually a two-step process using an initial primer step of acid etch to prepare the tooth surface for better retention of the polymers and resins.[26] This group of agents demonstrates a sustained adherence to prepared dentin compared with home-applied pastes. Most fluoride-based varnishes do not require a primer and may be included in both categories of adhesive or fluoride therapies to diminish patient discomfort by their concentration of active ingredient and stability in placement.

Miscellaneous Procedures

Miscellaneous procedures (iontophoresis, lasers, and permanent restorations) include a variety of alternative procedures that are considered when the symptoms persist and more permanent options must be explored. **Iontophoresis** is the application of a mild electrical current to a dentifrice when it is applied to the teeth to increase its effectiveness. Iontophoresis is not commonly used because it involves special equipment. The mechanism of action is occluding the dentinal tubules by the diffusion of fluoride ions into dentin tissue. This action occurs because of the electromagnetic property of negatively charged fluoride and electrodes reacting to the ions in hydroxyapatite, which results in occlusion of the tubules.[27]

Laser Therapy

Laser therapy is an application that is used in a wide variety of dental procedures as technology replaces traditional equipment and clinical therapies. The target action in using lasers is to precipitate plasma proteins and seal off dentin tubules for immediate relief. Some options for laser therapy include neodymium:yttrium-aluminum-garnet (Nd:YAG) laser, the erbium YAG (Er:YAG) laser, and gallium-aluminum-arsenide low-level lasers. If a dental practice invests in laser equipment to serve in alternative procedures, then it makes good sense to use lasers for treating hypersensitivity because its results show great promise.[28,29]

Restorative or Periodontal Plastic Procedures

Restorative or periodontal plastic procedures are the most aggressive procedures performed to minimize or eliminate dentin hypersensitivity caused by exposed root surfaces that has not dissipated after several weeks of home-applied desensitization agents. The first choice of restorative material is resin composite or glass ionomer, which sustains adequate root coverage and is placed most often at the cervical aspect of the root. Depending on the extent of the sensitive lesion, the tooth or teeth may be restored with veneers or full-coverage precious or semiprecious crowns.

After a definitive examination that correlates exposed cervical dentin as an inevitable soft tissue healing response related to nonsurgical instrumentation or surgical pocket elimination, or both, it is necessary for the clinician to be prepared to treat transient or chronic root hypersensitivity. Exposed root surfaces associated with severe localized gingival recession caused by inflammation or parafunctional oral habits may require connective tissue graft procedures to achieve coronal reattachment and coverage of the root surface.

Generalized root exposure created from a periodontal surgical pocket elimination procedure may present generalized patterns of tooth and root sensitivity as a result of rapid dentin exposure to the oral environment. Because this does not afford the dentin time to establish a natural smear layer containing salivary fluorides, calcium, phosphorous, or proteins, it becomes necessary to begin a regimen of daily application of a home-applied desensitizing dentifrice (potassium nitrates) for quicker relief if sensitivity is imminent. More often, a clinician will prescribe a 1.1% sodium fluoride gel to be used at home twice daily to increase the available fluoride of 5,000 ppm with intent to build a protective layer to reduce generalized sensitivity.

In some cases where sensitivity is thought to be associated with abfraction caused by excessive occlusal forces, some dental clinicians will recommend that the patient undergo a complete occlusal adjustment to reduce these factors initially and re-evaluate results over a 4- to 6-week post-treatment period.

Case Study

During routine care at the dental office, a 35-year-old patient indicates that she has been experiencing transient sharp pain when she drinks hot and cold beverages. She asks what is causing the pain and what she can do to avoid it.

Case Study Exercises

1. Each of the following habits may cause dentin hypersensitivity EXCEPT:
   A. Grinding the teeth
   B. Using whitening products
   C. Using excessive force when brushing the teeth
   D. Consuming foods and beverages with a high sugar content

2. To prevent dentin hypersensitivity, the patient should brush her teeth immediately after consuming acidic foods and beverages. To avoid dentin hypersensitivity, the patient should use a soft-bristle toothbrush.
   A. The first statement is true, but the second statement is false.
   B. The first statement is false, but the second statement is true.
   C. Both statements are true.
   D. Both statements are false.

3. After unsuccessful home-applied treatments, a professional-strength desensitizing agent is applied in the dental office. Which of the following instructions should the dental hygienist give the patient for home care?
   A. Using a soft toothbrush, brush the teeth twice a day with a desensitizing dentifrice.
   B. Rinse the mouth with desensitizing rinse three times a day instead of brushing for the first 2 days after treatment.
   C. Avoid using any dentifrice the day of treatment, then resume normal brushing the day after treatment.

Review Questions

1. Which teeth typically have the highest incidence of dentin hypersensitivity?
   A. Anterior and lateral
   B. Lateral and canine
   C. Canine and premolar
   D. Premolar and molar

2. There can be as many as _____ dentinal tubules in a square meter of dentin.
   A. 10,000
   B. 20,000
   C. 30,000
   D. 40,000

3. What is the layer of collagen and calcified material that cannot be brushed off but yet blocks the dentinal tubules?
   A. Amelogenic layer
   B. Calcium calcified layer
   C. Isotropic layer
   D. Smear layer

4. How much time does it take dietary acids to cause marked openings of tubules?
   A. 1–2 minutes
   B. 2–3 minutes
   C. 2–3 seconds
   D. 3–4 seconds

5. The hydrodynamic theory is a currently accepted theory that fluid movement creates pressure on nerve endings within the dentinal tubule. Excessive tooth brushing may predispose a patient to dentin hypersensitivity.
   A. Both statements are true.
   B. Both statements are false.
   C. The first statement is true, but the second statement is false.
   D. The first statement is false, but the second statement is true.

Active Learning

1. Conduct an internet search for professionally applied and take-home therapies for tooth sensitivity related to general root exposure and sensitivity. Prepare a brief presentation for the class explaining how you conducted the search, how each product works, and how they differ from each other.
2. Working with a partner, take turns being patient and dental hygienist and apply desensitizing agent. ▪

REFERENCES

1. Addy M. Dentine hypersensitivity: definition, prevalence distribution and etiology. Edited in Orchardson R & Gillam D. *J Am Dent Assoc.* 2006;137:990-998.
2. Canadian Advisory Board on Dentin Hypersensitivity. Consensus-based recommendations for the diagnosis and management of dentin hypersensitivity. *J Can Dent Assoc.* 2003;69:221-226.
3. Strassler HE, Serio FG. Dentinal hypersensitivity: etiology, diagnosis, and management. American Dental Association Continuing Education Recognition Provider. http://www.ineedce.com/courses/2057/pdf/1103cei_sensitivity_rev1.pdf. Published November 2009. Accessed November 18, 2014.
4. Rees JS, Addy M. A cross-sectional study of dentin hypersensitivity. *J Clin Periodontol.* 2002;29:997-1003.
5. Orchardson R, Collins WJN. Clinical features of hypersensitive teeth. *Br Dent J.* 1987;162:253-256.
6. Fischer C, Fischer RG, Wennberg A. Prevalence and distribution of cervical dentine hypersensitivity in a population in Rio de Janiero, Brazil. *J Dent.* 1992; 20:227-276.
7. Barthold PM. Dentinal hypersensitivity: a review. *Australian Dent J.* 2006;51(3):212-218.
8. Drisko CH. Dentin hypersensitivity—dental hygiene and periodontal considerations. *Int Dent J.* 2002; 52:385.
9. Flynn J, Galloway R, Orchardson R. The incidence of "hypersensitive" teeth in the west of Scotland. *J Dent.* 1985;13:230-236.
10. Addy M, Mostafa P, Newcombe RG. Dentine hypersensitivity: the distribution of recession, sensitivity and plaque. *J Dent.* 1987;15:242-248.
11. Absi EG, Addy M, Adams D. Dentine hypersensitivity: a study of the patency of dentinal tubules in sensitive and non-sensitive cervical dentine. *J Clin Periodontol.* 1987;14:280-284.
12. Tilliss T. Addressing the pain of dentinal hypersensitivity. *Dimens Dent Hyg.* 2010;8(4):46-50.
13. Al-Sabbagh M, Andreana S, Ciancio SG. Dentinal hypersensitivity: review of aetiology, differential diagnosis, prevalence, and mechanism. *J Int Acad Periodontol.* 2004;6:8-12.
14. Bartlett D, Ganss C, Lussi A. Basic erosive wear examination (BEWE): a new scoring system for scientific and clinical needs. *Clin Oral Investig.* 2008;12(suppl 1):65-68. http://www.ncbi.nlm.nih.gov/pmc/articles/PMC2238785/#!po=6.25000. Accessed November 18, 2014.
15. Orchardson R, Gillam DG. Managing dentin hypersensitivity. *J Am Dent Assoc.* 2006;137:990-98.
16. Swift EJ. Treating the twinge. *Dimens Dent Hyg.* 2006; 4:24, 26.

17. Peacock JM, Orchardson R. Effects of potassium ions on action potential conduction in A- and C- fibers of rat spinal nerves. *J Dent Res.* 1995;74:634-641.

18. Markowitz K, Bilotto G, Kim S. Decreasing intradental nerve activity in the cat with potassium and divalent cations. *Arch Oral Biol.* 1991;36(1):1-17.

19. Poulsen S, Errboe M, Hougaard O, Worthington HW. Potassium nitrate toothpaste for dentine hypersensitivity (Cochrane Review) In: The Cochrane Library. Oxford, U.K.: Update Software; 2005;1.

20. Schiff T, Zhang YP, DeVizio W, et al. A randomized clinical trial of the desensitizing efficacy of three dentifrices. *Compend Contin Educ Dent.* 2000;21(suppl 27):4-10.

21. Stadecker W. Effectively treating dental hypersensitivity. *Dentistry Today.* 2011;14:36. http://www.dentistrytoday. com/component/content/article/132-pain-management/ 4343-effectively-treating-dental-hypersensitivity. Accessed November 18, 2014.

22. Petersson LG. The role of fluoride in the preventive management of dentin hypersensitivity and root caries. *Clin Oral Invest.* DOI: 10.1007/s00784-012-0916-9. http://link.springer.com/article/10.1007%2Fs00784- 012-0916-9#page-2.

23. Pillon FL, Romani IG, Schmidt ER. Effect of a 3% potassium oxalate topical application on dentinal hypersensitivity after subgingival scaling and root planing. *J Periodontol.* 2004;75:1461-4.

24. Schiff T, Mateo LR, Delgado E, Cummins D, Zhang YP, DeVizio W. Clinical efficacy in reducing dentin hypersensitivity of a dentifrice containing 8.0% arginine, calcium carbonate, and 1450 ppm fluoride compared to a dentifrice containing 8% strontium acetate and 1040 ppm fluoride under consumer usage conditions before and after switch-over. *J Clin Dent.* 2011; 22(4):128-138.

25. Petrou I, Heu R, Stranick M, et al. A breakthrough therapy for dentin hypersensitivity: how dental products containing 8% arginine and calcium carbonate work to deliver effective relief of sensitive teeth. *J Clin Dent.* 2009;20(1):23-31.

26. Prati C, Cervellati F, Sanasi V, Montebugnoli L. Treatment of cervical dentin sensitivity with resin adhesives: 4 week evaluation. *Am J Dent.* 2001;14:378-382.

27. Singal P, Gupta R, Pandit N. 2% sodium fluoride Iontophoresis compared to commercially-available desensitizing agent. *J Periodontol.* 2005;76:351-357.

28. Sgolastra F, Petrucci A, Severino M, Gatto R, Monaco A. Lasers for the treatment of dentin hypersensitivity: a meta-analysis. *J Dent Res.* 2013;92(6):492-499.

29. Benetti AR, Franco EB, Franco EJ, Pereira JC. Laser therapy for dentin hypersensitivity: a critical appraisal. *J Oral Laser Applications.* 2004;4:271-278. http:// jola.quintessenz.de/jola0404_s271.pdf. Accessed July 28, 2014.

Chapter 29 | Polishing

Aubreé Chismark, MSDH, RDH

KEY TERMS

abrasion

air polishing

extrinsic stain

feldspar

grit

intrinsic stain

manual polishing

Mohs scale of hardness

polishing

power polishing

prophy paste

remineralization

selective polishing

therapeutic polishing

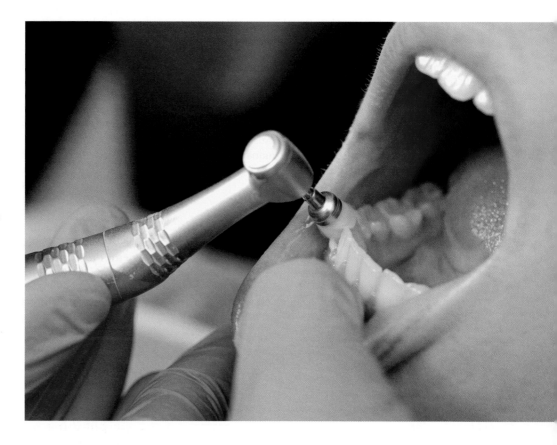

LEARNING OBJECTIVES

After reading this chapter, the student should be able to:

29.1 Explain selective polishing to patients.

29.2 List the indications and contraindications of manual, power, and air polishing.

29.3 Apply the technique of manual, power, or air polishing in the clinical setting.

29.4 Describe the armamentarium needed for each polishing procedure.

29.5 Select a prophy paste or air-polishing powder based on the patients' needs.

KEY CONCEPTS

• Polishing is a technique used to remove extrinsic stain from the enamel surface.

• Evaluating the need for polishing is based on the needs of each patient.

• Selecting the appropriate polishing technique is necessary based on the patient's health history.

RELEVANCE TO CLINICAL PRACTICE

Polishing is a technique that is used on most patients toward the end of a dental hygiene appointment. Different types of polishing methods include manual, power, and air polishing. The purpose of polishing is to remove extrinsic stains that cannot be removed with hand or ultrasonic instruments from enamel surfaces or before sealant placement. Many patients feel the most important part of their hygiene visit is when they have their teeth polished because they "feel smooth and appear shiny and white." It has been suggested that untrained clinicians should not perform polishing because the outer surface of the enamel layer, which contains fluoride, may be removed, and damage to restorative materials including amalgams, composites, and porcelain may occur.[1]

The dentist and dental hygienist are the most qualified clinicians in the dental office to make the decision as to when a patient should receive polishing during an oral prophylaxis appointment.[1] Therefore, learning the types of polishing methods used during a dental hygiene appointment and knowing when to incorporate them is important when assessing a patient. In this chapter, we discuss the different polishing methods, indications, contraindications, and armamentarium used for each procedure.

STAINS

Extrinsic Stains

Stains that are formed on the outer surface of enamel within biofilm and are caused by external factors that can be removed with hand instruments and polishing are called **extrinsic stains.** Hand or ultrasonic instruments should be used first to remove as much stain as possible before polishing. Causes of extrinsic stains include but are not limited to the following: smoking, coffee, tea, dark fruit juices, red wine, chlorhexidine, and stannous fluoride. These stains appear as brownish or black. Black line stain, which is commonly seen on the maxillary posterior lingual surfaces, is caused by poor oral hygiene habits. Green stain is commonly seen in children and also forms because of poor oral hygiene habits. For more information on stains, see Chapter 13.

Intrinsic Stains

Stains that are formed on the inner surface of enamel and cannot be removed with hand instruments, ultrasonic instruments, or polishing are called **intrinsic stains.** Causes of intrinsic stain while the teeth are forming include excessive fluoride ingestion (fluorosis) and intake of tetracycline. Fluorosis appears white-to-brown in color, and tetracycline causes the enamel to appear gray.[2] Intrinsic staining can also occur after tooth development because of trauma, amalgam restorations, and smoking.

POLISHING

Selective Polishing

Selective polishing, which is polishing of specific teeth that present with only extrinsic stains, is used to reduce damage to the enamel, cementum, and dentin. Most dental hygienists continue to polish all of the teeth regardless of the presence of stain. It is important to educate patients on the reasons why their teeth may or may not be polished during an oral prophylaxis procedure. Treatment planning for polishing should be based on caries risk, abrasion, erosion, exposed dentin, stain, and types of restorations present.[3]

In a recent study to examine the abrasiveness of polishing on the enamel surface, extracted teeth were polished on the buccal surfaces 150 times for 5 seconds to replicate 75 years of semiannual polishing. Results showed that a lifetime of routine polishing has minimal effect, if any, on enamel thickness.[4] Evidence-based decision-making supported by evaluation of scientific literature, in addition to clinical expertise, is in the best interest of the patient and is also required of dental hygienists. [5]

Abrasive Agents

Abrasion is the removal of a surface by means of friction, and **prophy paste** is used during manual or power polishing to remove extrinsic stain from the enamel surface. Prophy pastes contain abrasive agents, and manufacturers determine their ability to increase surface roughness according to abrasive grit levels.[6] These pastes are prepared as extra-fine, fine, medium, and course grit. Prophy pastes should be chosen based on evidence and the needs of the patient.[3,6] The type of prophy paste used is determined by the amount of stain present after hand and ultrasonic instrumentation. The higher the amount of stain present on the enamel surface, the more abrasive the paste that should be used. The more abrasive a prophy paste is, the larger the **grit** size, leading to effective stain removal and possibly more abrasion. Pumice and glycerin are the most common ingredients found in prophy pastes. The mineral **feldspar** is a cleaning agent that is low in abrasives and is available in powder form. It can be mixed with water or sodium fluoride to polish the teeth.[3] Feldspar can be used on enamel and restorations because it will not abrade the surfaces.[3]

The higher the speed used with manual or power polishing, the amount of pressure used, and the quantity of particles applied to the tooth surface will affect the degree of abrasion. Using a slower speed, lighter pressure, and a wet prophy paste is recommended to reduce the rate of frictional heat produced. Using these skills when polishing will reduce the degree of abrasion and prevent injury to the pulp.

Finishing Strips

Finishing strips, which are made of plastic or linen, can be used to remove stain from interproximal surfaces when necessary. These strips come in different widths and grit sizes, including an abrasive and a smooth side. The finishing strip used is chosen based on grit size, which is dependent on the amount of stain present. The abrasive side should be used against the enamel surface using a back-and-forth motion until the stain is removed. The last step is to floss the area to ensure all abrasive materials have been removed from the interproximal surface.

Mohs Hardness Value

Mohs scale of harness is a scale that compares the hardness value of ingredients found in prophy pastes with enamel, dentin, and cementum. According to Mohs hardness value, enamel is 5.0 and dentin is 3.0 to 4.0. The values listed for abrasive agents found in prophy pastes range from 0.4 to 9.3, with potassium at 0.4 and boron at 9.3.[3] The Mohs hardness value for pumice is 6.0, which is the most common abrasive agent used in prophy paste.[7] Manufacturers usually do not disclose the amount of ingredients found in prophy pastes;[3] therefore, it is important to choose a paste based on the amount of stain present (see Table 29-1).

Therapeutic Polishing

Therapeutic polishing involves using a prophy paste that includes ingredients that have been added for remineralization and to reduce hypersensitivity (see Teamwork). Fluoride was the first ingredient to be added to prophy paste, although it does not have the

Table 29-1. Mohs Hardness Value of Dental Tissues and Abrasive Agents Used in Prophy Pastes and Air-Polishing Powders

	MHV
Dental Tissue	
Dentin	3.0–4.0 (3)
Enamel	5.0 (3)
Abrasives	
Potassium	0.4 (3)
Glycine	2.0 (15)
Calcium carbonate	2.5 (15)
Sodium bicarbonate	2.5 (7)
Aluminum trihydroxide	4.0 (15)
Calcium phosphosilicate (Sylc)	4.0+ (15)
Pumice	6.0 (7)
Boron	9.3 (3)

MHV, Mohs hardness value.

same effectiveness as professionally applied fluoride.[8] **Remineralization** is the process in which minerals and fluoride are deposited into demineralized areas of the enamel. Ingredients that have been added for remineralization and to reduce high caries risk include calcium, phosphate, and fluoride. Ingredients added to reduce hypersensitivity include arginine-calcium carbonate and calcium sodium phosphosilicate.[8] More research is needed to determine how effective therapeutic prophy pastes are in promoting remineralization and reducing hypersensitivity for dental hygienists to make evidence-based decisions.[8]

Teamwork

Dental hygienists can collaborate with various health-care professionals to improve oral hygiene behaviors. For example, Registered Dental Hygienists in Advanced Practice (RDHAP) go into nursing homes and treat patients. Although nurses cannot selectively polish teeth, it is a good opportunity for dental hygienists to teach them the proper techniques of brushing and flossing when caring for their patients, as well as how to appropriately care for partial and full dentures. ■

Polishing Restorations

Maintaining the integrity of restorative materials when polishing is essential. Aesthetic restorative materials used in dentistry include composite and porcelain, with composite being the most commonly used aesthetic material. Because composite has a lower Mohs hardness number than enamel, polishing these restorations with prophy paste can increase surface roughness, which allows bacteria to be retained.[9] Porcelain is used for crowns and veneers, has the greatest translucency, can be glazed or polished, and is the hardest restorative material when it comes to aesthetics.[9] If the brand of the aesthetic restoration is known, follow the manufacturer's instructions for polishing. Otherwise, a cleaning agent that contains feldspar and rubber cup polishing can be used on all restorative materials without causing damage (see Evidence-Based Practice).[9]

Manual Polishing

Manual polishing is a technique performed by using a Porte polisher, which has an orangewood tip attached to a contra-angle. Due to advancing technologies, dental hygienists do not commonly perform manual polishing. Some hygienists, however, may use it to apply desensitizing products. See Table 29-2 and Procedures 29-1 and 29-2.

Table 29-2. *Manual Polishing*

Indications	Contraindications	Armamentarium
Extrinsic stain Application of desensitizing agents	Exposed root surfaces Exposed dentin and cementum Caries Demineralization Individuals with an adverse reaction to prophy paste or desensitizing agent	All personal protective equipment (PPE) for the dental hygienist and safety glasses for the patient Mirror Contra-angle Orangewood tip Air/water syringe Saliva ejector High-volume evacuator Prophy paste Floss Gauze

Procedure 29-1 Manual Polishing Extrinsic Stain Removal

MATERIALS AND PREPARATION

Gather and organize the necessary items before the patient arrives.

Materials

All personal protective equipment (PPE)	To protect the patient and clinician from aerosols and spatter
Mirror	For indirect vision and retraction
Contra-angle	To hold the orangewood tip in place
Orangewood tip	For stain removal
Air/water syringe	To rinse and dry the teeth
Saliva ejector	To remove excess saliva and prophy paste
High-volume evacuator	To remove excess saliva and prophy paste; to reduce aerosols and spatter
Prophy paste	For stain removal
Floss	To remove prophy paste from interproximal surfaces
Gauze	To wipe the orangewood tip of excess saliva
Petroleum jelly	To prevent cracking or drying of the lips

Preprocedure

REVIEW MEDICAL HISTORY

Review the medical history to determine whether any contraindications to manual polishing exist (Table 29-3).

Table 29-3. Medical Contraindications to Polishing

Manual Polishing	Power Polishing	Air Polishing
Individuals with an adverse reaction to prophy paste or desensitizing agent	Individuals with a communicable disease Individuals with upper respiratory disease Individuals who are immunocompromised Individuals with an adverse reaction to prophy paste	Individuals with a communicable disease Individuals with upper respiratory disease Individuals who are immunocompromised Individuals with sodium restrictions[26] Individuals wearing contact lenses[26] Individuals with an adverse reaction to air-polishing powder

PATIENT EDUCATION
The patient must understand the reason for treatment and how the procedure will be done.

SELECTION OF TEETH
The selection of the teeth to be polished will be based on the need for extrinsic stain removal.

Procedure
1. *Prepare.*
   - Insert the orangewood tip into the contra-angle.
   - Use a mirror for indirect vision or retraction.
   - Insert the saliva ejector or high-volume evacuator into the patient's mouth.
2. *Apply.*
   - Apply infection-control barriers to equipment as necessary.
   - Apply petroleum jelly to patient's lips to prevent cracking or drying.
   - Add prophy paste to the tip and spread evenly over two to three teeth.
   - Starting at the cervical third, apply the tip to the tooth with light-to-moderate pressure and use a vertical stroke starting at the distal and moving toward the mesial; apply the tip to the middle third with light-to-moderate pressure using a vertical stroke moving from distal to mesial; apply the tip to the incisal third with light-to-moderate pressure using a vertical stroke moving from distal to mesial.
   - As you continue to polish, wipe the tip with gauze to remove excess saliva.
3. *Rinse.*
   - Rinse the teeth with water using the air/water syringe and saliva ejector or high-volume evacuator.
4. *Evaluate.*
   - Re-evaluate the surfaces polished to ensure all stain has been removed.
   - Use a finishing strip to remove stain from interproximal surfaces if necessary.
5. *Floss.*
   - Floss all teeth to remove paste from the interproximal surfaces.

Postprocedure
- After any dental procedure the patient and, if the patient is a minor, the parent or guardian should be informed about the results of the procedure and given postprocedure instructions.
- Discard the orangewood tip and sterilize the contra-angle handpiece for each patient.
- Document the procedure in the patient's chart.

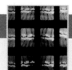

Procedure 29-2 Desensitizing With Porte Polisher

MATERIALS AND PREPARATION
Gather and organize the necessary items before the patient's arrival.

Materials

All PPE	To protect the patient and hygienist from aerosols and spatter
Mirror	For indirect vision and retraction
Contra-angle	To hold the orangewood tip in place
Orangewood tip	To apply desensitizing agent
Air/water syringe	To dry the teeth
Saliva ejector	To remove excess saliva and desensitizing agent
High-volume evacuator	To remove excess saliva and desensitizing agent; to reduce aerosols and spatter
Desensitizing agent	To reduce sensitivity
Gauze	To wipe the orangewood tip of excess saliva or to dry the teeth
Petroleum jelly	To prevent cracking or drying of the lips

Preprocedure
REVIEW MEDICAL HISTORY
Review the medical history to determine whether any contraindications to applying desensitizing agent exist (refer to Table 29-3).

PATIENT EDUCATION

The patient must understand the reason for treatment and how the procedure will be done.

SELECTION OF TEETH

The selection of the teeth to be desensitized will be based on the need for sensitivity reduction.

Procedure

1. *Prepare.*
   - Insert the orangewood tip into the contra-angle.
   - Use a mirror for indirect vision or retraction.
   - Dry the tooth surface with air or gauze.
   - Insert the saliva ejector or high-volume evacuator into the patient's mouth.
2. *Apply.*
   - Apply infection-control barriers to equipment as necessary.
   - Apply petroleum jelly to patient's lips to prevent cracking or drying.
   - Add desensitizing agent to the tip and spread evenly over the sensitive surface using a circular motion and light pressure.
   - Allow the surface to dry. Do not rinse with water.
3. *Evaluate.*
   - Re-evaluate the surfaces to ensure the areas have been thoroughly covered with the desensitizing agent.

Postprocedure

- After any dental procedure the patient and, if the patient is a minor, the parent or guardian should be informed about the results of the procedure and given postprocedure instructions.
- Discard the orangewood tip and sterilize the contra-angle handpiece for each patient.
- Document the procedure in the patient's chart.

Power Polishing

Power polishing is used with a slow-speed hand-piece, disposable prophy angle or prophy brush, and prophy paste (Fig. 29-1, Table 29-4, Advancing Technologies, and Procedure 29-3). Power polishing is recommended for individuals with extrinsic stains and is used to prepare the tooth surface before sealant placement. A prophy angle can be used on the facial, lingual, and occlusal surfaces of the teeth, whereas a prophy brush should be used on the occlusal surfaces only. Polishing with extra-fine or fine prophy paste is suggested for light-to-moderate stain; medium to coarse prophy paste can be used for heavy stain removal.

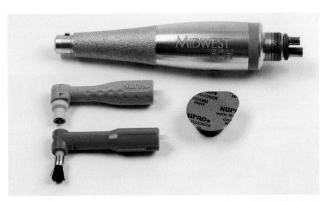

Figure 29-1. Handpiece, prophy brush, prophy angle, and prophy paste.

 Advancing Technologies

Improving technology is important especially for ergonomic purposes. Slow-speed handpieces are now made to be lighter and with a wider diameter to reduce hand fatigue, while some handpieces are even cordless and come with a wireless rheostat (Fig. 29-2). ■

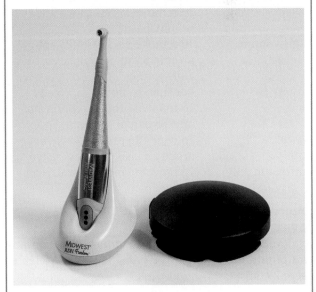

Figure 29-2. Cordless handpiece with wireless rheostat.

Table 29-4. *Power Polishing*

Indications	Contraindications	Armamentarium
Extrinsic stain	Exposed root surfaces	All personal protective equipment for the dental
Before sealant placement	Exposed dentin and cementum	hygienist and safety glasses for the patient
	Caries	Mirror
	Demineralization	Slow-speed handpiece
	Amalgam restorations	Disposable prophy angle
	Composite restorations	Air/water syringe
	Porcelain or gold crowns	Saliva ejector
	Individuals with a communicable disease	High-volume evacuator
	Individuals with an adverse reaction to	Prophy paste
	prophy paste	Floss
		Gauze

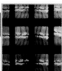

Procedure 29-3 | Power Polishing

MATERIALS AND PREPARATION

Gather and organize the necessary items before the patient's arrival.

Materials

All PPE	To protect the patient and clinician from aerosols and spatter
Mirror	For indirect vision and retraction
Slow-speed handpiece	To hold the prophy angle in place
Disposable prophy angle	For stain removal
Air/water syringe	To rinse and dry the teeth
Saliva ejector	To remove excess saliva and prophy paste
High-volume evacuator	To remove excess saliva and prophy paste; to reduce aerosols and spatter
Prophy paste	For stain removal
Floss	To remove prophy paste from interproximal surfaces
Gauze	To wipe the prophy angle or prophy brush of excess saliva
Petroleum jelly	To prevent cracking or drying of the lips

Preprocedure

REVIEW MEDICAL HISTORY

Review the medical history to determine whether any contraindications to power polishing exist (refer to Table 29-3).

PATIENT EDUCATION

The patient must understand the reason for treatment and how the procedure will be done.

Selection of Teeth

Selection of the teeth to be polished is based on the need for extrinsic stain removal.

Procedure

1. *Prepare.*
   - Place a disposable prophy angle onto a slow-speed handpiece.

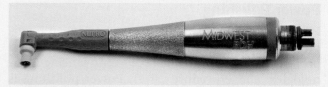

Prophy angle attached to handpiece.

   - Align the prophy angle with the guide pin and lock into place.
   - To ensure the prophy angle is locked into place, step on the rheostat and operate the prophy angle outside the mouth.
   - Insert the saliva ejector or high-volume evacuator into the patient's mouth.
2. *Apply.*
   - Apply infection-control barriers to equipment as necessary.
   - Apply petroleum jelly to patient's lips to prevent cracking or drying.

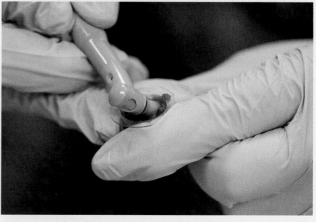

Apply prophy paste to cup.

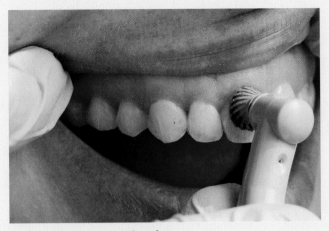

Apply prophy paste to tooth surface.

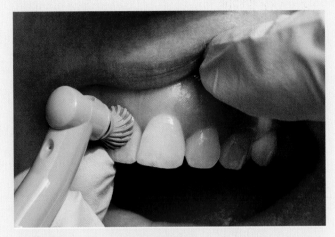

Apply prophy paste to the buccal surface.

- Apply a modified pen grasp onto the slow-speed handpiece and establish a fulcrum.
- Apply a small amount of prophy paste to the prophy cup and spread the paste evenly over the facial surfaces of two to three teeth.
- Starting at the distal surface of the tooth, press the prophy angle enough so that it flares into the interproximal surface.

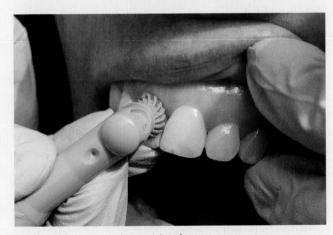

Apply prophy paste to the mesial surface.

- Polish two to three teeth at a time, making sure the enamel surface is covered with prophy paste at all times to avoid overheating the teeth.
- Polish the occlusal surfaces with a prophy brush.

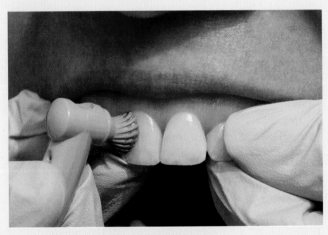

Apply prophy paste to the distal surface.

- Step on the rheostat and polish each tooth starting with the cervical third, the middle third, and then the incisal third at a low speed of 1,500 to 3,000 rpm.[10]
- Lift the prophy cup off the tooth, apply to the direct facial of the tooth, lift the prophy cup off the tooth, then apply to the mesial surface of the tooth, pressing so the prophy cup flares into the interproximal surface. Continue polishing the middle third and then incisal third of the tooth.

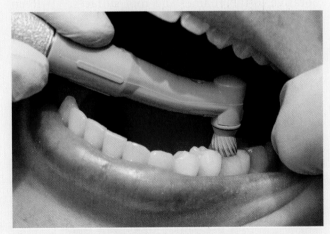

Apply prophy paste to the occlusal surface.

- A saliva ejector or gauze can be used to remove excess saliva from the prophy cup or prophy brush.
3. *Rinse.*
   - Rinse the teeth with water using the air/water syringe and saliva ejector or high-volume evacuator.
4. *Evaluate.*
   - Re-evaluate the surfaces polished to ensure all stain has been removed.
   - Use a finishing strip to remove stain from interproximal surfaces if necessary.
5. *Floss.*
   - Floss all teeth when finished to remove paste from the interproximal surfaces.

Postprocedure

- After any dental procedure the patient and, if the patient is a minor, the parent or guardian should be informed about the results of the procedure and given postprocedure instructions.
- Discard the prophy angle and sterilize the slow-speed handpiece for each patient.
- Document the procedure in the patient's chart.

Air Polishing

Air polishing was introduced in the 1980s and uses compressed air, water, and sodium bicarbonate powder (Fig. 29-3). Air polishing is helpful for heavy extrinsic stain removal, plaque removal from orthodontic appliances, and to remove bacteria in occlusal fissures before sealant placement (Table 29-5).[11,12] Direct air polishing of sealants is not recommended because it may damage the seal coating.[13] Powder emission rates vary among different brands of air-polishing devices depending on the amount of powder present in the chamber. It is important to follow the manufacturer's instructions and refill the powder chamber to the suggested level to ensure safety and effectiveness.[14]

Air-Polishing Powders

Most air-polishing powders contain sodium bicarbonate, which has a Mohs hardness value of 2.5.[7] This powder is used for heavy stain removal and may be abrasive to the enamel and root surfaces.[15,16] Even though the Mohs hardness value is relatively low, it is abrasive when used on composites, glass ionomers, and gold.[17–19] Sodium bicarbonate also reduces the dentin bond strength of resin composites.[20] Avoid polishing exposed dentin and cementum because sodium

bicarbonate can cause a loss of structure when sprayed directly on those areas for a continuous amount of time.[21]

Low-abrasive powders are less abrasive to root cementum and dentin and are effective in plaque removal.[16] Glycine has a Mohs hardness value of 2.0 and can be used for light stain removal.[15] Glycine causes minimal damage to cementum, dentin, and gingival

Table 29-5. *Air Polishing*

Indications	Contraindications	Armamentarium
Extrinsic stain	Exposed root surfaces	All personal protective equipment for the dental hygienist and safety glasses for the patient
Orthodontic appliances	Exposed dentin and cementum	
Before sealant placement	Caries	
	Demineralization	Mirror
	Amalgam restorations	Face shield
	Composite restorations	Hair bonnet for the dental hygienist
	Porcelain or gold crowns	Air/water syringe
	Severe gingival inflammation[26]	Saliva ejector
	Individuals with a communicable disease	High-volume evacuator
	Individuals with upper respiratory disease	Handpiece
	Individuals with sodium restrictions[26]	Insert
	Individuals wearing contact lenses[26]	Air-polishing powder
	Individuals with an adverse reaction to air-polishing powder	Floss
		Gauze
		Petroleum jelly

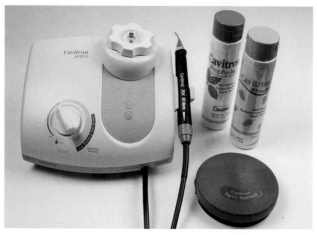

Figure 29-3. Prophy jet and prophy powder.

epithelium and is less abrasive on composites than is sodium bicarbonate.[18,19,22,23] Calcium carbonate has a Mohs hardness value of 2.5 and is an effective alternative to sodium bicarbonate, especially for patients on a sodium-restricted diet.[15] Calcium phosphosilicate (Sylc) has a Mohs hardness value of 4+ and is used to desensitize root surfaces.[15]

An alternative air-polishing agent that contains aluminum trihydroxide has a Mohs hardness value of 4.0. This powder is abrasive and is commonly used for air abrasion techniques.[15] Avoid air polishing with aluminum trihydroxide on luting cements, resin composites, glass ionomers, and cast restorations.[17] See Procedure 29-4.

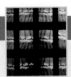

Procedure 29-4 Air Polishing

MATERIALS AND PREPARATION

Gather and organize the necessary items before the patient's arrival.

Materials

All PPE	To protect the patient and clinician from aerosols and spatter
Mirror	For indirect vision and retraction
Air/water syringe	To rinse and dry the teeth
Saliva ejector	To remove excess saliva and air-polishing powder
High-volume evacuator	To remove excess saliva; to reduce aerosols and spatter
Handpiece	To hold the insert in place
Insert	For air-polishing powder and water delivery
Air-polishing powder	For stain removal
Floss	To remove air-polishing powder from interproximal surfaces
Gauze	To wipe the insert of excess saliva
Petroleum jelly	To prevent cracking or drying of the lips

Preprocedure

REVIEW MEDICAL HISTORY

Review the medical history to determine whether any contraindications to air polishing exist (refer to Table 29-3).

PATIENT EDUCATION

The patient must understand the reason for treatment and how the procedure will be done.

SELECTION OF TEETH

Selection of the teeth to be air polished is based on the need for extrinsic stain removal.

Procedure

1. *Prepare.*
   - Turn on the air-polishing unit.
   - Step on the foot pedal and, holding the handpiece over a sink, flush with water for 2 minutes at the beginning of the day and 30 seconds between patients.
   - Turn off the unit and fill the powder chamber with appropriate air-polishing powder until it reaches the top of the center tube.
   - Set the powder and lavage flow according to the amount of stain present: clockwise for heavy stain and counterclockwise for lighter stain.
   - Place the insert into the handpiece.
   - Turn on the unit, hold the handpiece over a sink, and step on the foot pedal to ensure the water and powder flow evenly out of the insert.
   - Insert the high-volume evacuator into the patient's mouth.

2. *Apply.*
   - Apply infection-control barriers to equipment as necessary.
   - Apply petroleum jelly to patient's lips to prevent cracking or drying.
   - Apply a modified pen grasp onto the handpiece and establish a fulcrum.
   - In the anterior region, use your hand and the patient's lip to contain aerosols; in the posterior region, use the patient's cheek to contain aerosols in addition to high-volume evacuation.
   - Aim the air-polishing insert at the middle third of the tooth, holding the tip 3 to 4 mm away from the tooth surface.
   - Use a circular motion and avoid aiming the tip at the gingival margin.
   - Polish two to three teeth at a time, rinsing the patient's mouth frequently with water by depressing the foot pedal halfway.
   - Angle the tip 60° for anterior teeth, 80° for buccal and lingual surfaces of posterior teeth, and 90° for occlusal surfaces.

3. *Rinse.*
   - Rinse the teeth with water using the air/water syringe and saliva ejector or high-volume evacuator.
   - Have patient rinse and expectorate at the sink.

4. *Evaluate.*
   - Re-evaluate the surfaces polished to ensure all stain has been removed.
   - Use a finishing strip to remove stain from interproximal surfaces if necessary.

5. *Floss.*
   - Floss all teeth when finished to remove air-polishing powder from the interproximal surfaces.

Postprocedure
- After any dental procedure the patient and, if the patient is a minor, the parent or guardian should be informed about the results of the procedure and given postprocedure instructions.

- Remove the insert and sterilize.
- Flush the handpiece for 30 seconds, then sterilize.
- Follow manufacturer's instructions for daily and weekly maintenance.[24,25]
- Document the procedure in the patient's chart.

Case Study

Emily Smith is a healthy 37-year-old female who is a sales representative and travels 3 weeks out of each month. Emily takes an oral contraceptive and multivitamin daily, and high blood pressure runs in her family. Emily drinks one to two glasses of wine 5 days a week, drinks coffee every morning, and drinks green tea throughout the day. The vital signs taken at her dental visit today are: blood pressure 130/90, pulse 70, respirations 12. Emily is unhappy with the appearance of her teeth. She presents with light-to-moderate stain on her maxillary and mandibular anterior teeth on both the facial and lingual surfaces. She is also concerned about the dark shadows surrounding the amalgams on teeth #29 and #30.

Case Study Exercises

1. According to Emily's health history, all of the following instruments can be used to remove the stain from the maxillary and mandibular anterior teeth EXCEPT:
   A. Power polishing
   B. Air polishing
   C. Hand instruments
   D. Manual polishing

2. Which of the following techniques would be the best option to remove Emily's extrinsic stain?
   A. Selective polishing
   B. Air polishing
   C. Power polishing
   D. Manual polishing

3. The dark shadows surrounding the amalgams on teeth #29 and #30 are examples of extrinsic stain. Replacing the amalgams with composite may improve the aesthetic appearance of #29 and #30.
   A. The first statement is true, but the second statement is false.
   B. The first statement is false, but the second statement is true.
   C. Both statements are true.
   D. Both statements are false.

4. The stains on the maxillary and mandibular anterior teeth were most likely caused by all of the following EXCEPT:
   A. Coffee
   B. Wine
   C. Oral contraceptive
   D. Tea

5. Hand instruments should be used first to remove stain from the maxillary and mandibular anterior teeth. Air polishing is a technique that can be used to remove the shadows surrounding teeth #29 and #30.
   A. The first statement is true, but the second statement is false.
   B. The first statement is false, but the second statement is true.
   C. Both statements are true.
   D. Both statements are false.

Review Questions

1. Which of the following is a common abrasive ingredient found in prophy paste?
   A. Sodium bicarbonate
   B. Feldspar
   C. Fluoride
   D. Pumice

2. Therapeutic polishing can be used for all of the following EXCEPT?
   A. Remineralization
   B. To reduce hypersensitivity
   C. To remove stain
   D. To reduce caries

3. Contraindications to air polishing include all of the following EXCEPT:
   A. Before sealant placement
   B. Amalgams
   C. Sodium-restricted diet
   D. Exposed root surfaces

4. Power polishing includes all of the following EXCEPT:
   A. Prophy paste
   B. Sodium bicarbonate powder
   C. Slow-speed handpiece
   D. Prophy angle

5. Which of the following can cause intrinsic stain?
   A. Tetracycline
   B. Chlorhexidine
   C. Tea
   D. Coffee

Active Learning

1. Use intraoral photos to show examples of extrinsic stain and specify which polishing technique(s) would be used.
2. Using a slow-speed handpiece, step on the rheostat, bringing the speed to a consistent 1,500 to 3,000 rpm, close your eyes, and listen to the speed that should be used when power polishing.
3. After setting up the air-polishing unit, hold the tip over a sink and depress the foot pedal halfway to see the flow of water only. Next, step all the way on the foot pedal to see the water and powder combination.
4. Use intraoral photos to show examples of intrinsic versus extrinsic stain. ▪

REFERENCES

1. American Dental Hygienists' Association. Position on the oral prophylaxis. American Dental Hygienists' Association. https://www.adha.org/resources-docs/7115_Prophylaxis_Postion_Paper.pdf. Approved April 29, 1998. Accessed November 24, 2013.
2. Harris NO, García-Godoy F, Nielsen Nathe C. *Primary Preventive Dentistry.* 8th ed. Upper Saddle River, NJ: Pearson; 2013:145.
3. Barnes CM. The science of polishing. *Dimens Dent Hyg.* 2009;7(11):18-20, 22.
4. Pence SD, Chambers DA, van Tets IG, Wolf RC, Pfeiffer DC. Repetitive coronal polishing yields minimal enamel loss. *J Dent Hyg.* 2011;85(4):348-357.
5. Forrest JL, Miller SA, Overman PR, Newman MG. *Evidence-Based Decision Making: A Translational Guide for Dental Professionals.* Philadelphia, PA: Lippincott Williams & Wilkins; 2008:7.
6. Avey KD, DeBiase CB, Gladwin MA, Kao EC, Bagby MD. Development of a standardized abrasive scale: an analysis of commercial prophylaxis pastes. *J Dent Hyg.* 2006;80(1):1.
7. Barnes CM. An in-depth look at air polishing. *Dimens Dent Hyg.* 2010;8(3):32, 34-36, 40.
8. Barnes CM. The evolution of prophy paste. *Dimens Dent Hyg.* 2011;9(3): 50, 52.
9. Barnes CM. Polishing esthetic restorative materials. *Dimens Dent Hyg.* 2010;8(1):24, 26-28.
10. KERR TotalCare: Perfect Pearl Disposable Prophy Angle IFU. http://www.totalcareprotects.com/education/documents/category/manual-ifu. Published 2012. Accessed April 14, 2012.
11. Gerbo LR, Barnes CM, Leinfelder KF. Applications of the air-powder polisher in clinical orthodontics. *Am J Orthod Dentofacial Orthop.* 1993;103:71-73.
12. Brocklehurst PR, Joshi RI, Norheast SE. The effect of airpolishing occlusal surfaces on the penetration of fissures by a sealant. *Int J Paediatr Dent.* 1992;2:157-162.
13. Engel S, Jost-Brinkmann PG, Spors CK, Mohammadian S, Müller-Hartwich R. Abrasive effect of air-powder polishing on smooth-surface sealants. *J Orofac Orthop.* 2009;70:363-370.
14. Petersilka GJ, Schenck U, Flemmig TF. Powder emission rates of four air polishing devices. *J Clin Periodontol.* 2002;29:694-698.
15. Lennemann T. Air polishing: overview. *Can J Dent Hyg.* 2011;45(3):145-148.
16. Petersilka GJ, Bell M, Mehl A, Hickel R, Flemmig TF. Root defects following air polishing. An in vitro study on the effects of working parameters. *J Clin Periodontol.* 2003;30:165-170.
17. Johnson W, Barnes CM, Covey DA. The effects of a commercial aluminum airpolishing powder on dental restorative materials. *J Prosthodont.* 2004;13(3):166-172.
18. Giacomelli L, Salerno M, Derchi G, Genovesi A, Paganin PP, Covani U. Effect of air polishing with glycine and bicarbonate powders on a nanocomposite used in dental restorations: an in vitro study. *Int J Periodontics Restorative Dent.* 2011;31(5):e51-e56.
19. Salerno M, Giacomelli L, Derchi G, Patra N, Diaspro A. Atomic force microscopy in vitro study of surface roughness and fractal character of a dental restoration composite after air-polishing. *Biomed Eng Online.* 2010; 9:59. http://www.biomedical-engineering-online.com/content/9/1/59. Accessed December 3, 2011.
20. Frankenberger R, Lohbauer U, Tay FR, Taschner M, Nikolaenko SA. The effect of different air-polishing powders on dentin bonding. *J Adhes Dent.* 2007;9:381-389.
21. Galloway SE, Pashley DH. Rate of removal of root structure by the use of the prophyjet device. *J Periodontal.* 1986;58(7):464-469.
22. Tada K, Kakuta K, Ogura H, Sato S. Effect of particle diameter on air polishing of dentin surfaces. *Odontology.* 2010;98:31-36.
23. Petersilka G, Faggion CM, Stratmann U, et al. Effect of glycine powder air-polishing on the gingiva. *J Clin Periodontol.* 2008;35:324-332.
24. Dentsply Professional Cavitron(tm) PROPHY-JET® Air Polishing Prophylaxis System, Directions for Use Section 8: Techniques for Use; 8.6 Proper Angulation of the Air Polishing Insert without JetShield(tm), page 11. Available from: https://www.dentsply.com/content/dam/dentsply/pim/manufacturer/Preventive/Air_Polishing_Units/Table_Top_Units/Cavitron_Prophy_Jet/Cavitron-Prophy-Jet-Cavitron-Prophy-Jet-TapOn-8qta9aj-en-de-fr-it-es-1402. Accessed Oct 8, 2015. Dentsply Professional York, PA.

25. Dentsply Professional Cavitron(tm) PROPHY-JET® Air Polishing Prophylaxis System, Directions for Use Section 3: Precautions; 3.2 Precautions for Air Polishing Procedures, page 3. Available from: https://www.dentsply.com/content/dam/dentsply/pim/manufacturer/Preventive/Air_Polishing_Units/Table_Top_Units/Cavitron_Prophy_Jet/Cavitron-Prophy-Jet-Cavitron-Prophy-Jet-TapOn-8qta9aj-en-de-fr-it-es-1402. Accessed Oct 8, 2015. Dentsply Professional York, PA.

26. Dentsply Professional Cavitron(tm) PROPHY-JET® Air Polishing Prophylaxis System, Directions for Use Section 8: Techniques for Use; 8.5 Performing Air Polishing procedures without JetShield(tm), page 10. Available from: https://www.dentsply.com/content/dam/dentsply/pim/manufacturer/Preventive/Air_Polishing_Units/Table_Top_Units/Cavitron_Prophy_Jet/Cavitron-Prophy-Jet-Cavitron-Prophy-Jet-TapOn-8qta9aj-en-de-fr-it-es-1402. Accessed Oct 8, 2015. Dentsply Professional York, PA.

Chapter 30 | Esthetics

Nicole Giesey, RDH, BSDH, MSPTE • Ruthie Palich, RDH, BSAS, MHHS • Mechee Thomas, RDH, BSAS, MSPTE

KEY TERMS

calcium peroxide

carbamide peroxide

composite veneer

computer-aided design/computer-aided manufacturing (CAD/CAM)

crown

digital impression

direct restoration

external whitening

hydrogen peroxide

indirect restoration

inlay

internal whitening

onlay

over-the-counter (OTC) whitening

porcelain veneer

professional whitening

sodium perborate

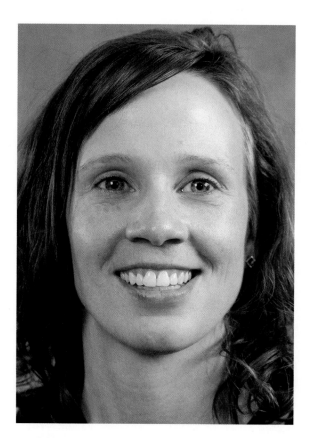

LEARNING OBJECTIVES

After reading this chapter, the student should be able to:

30.1 Discuss various esthetic options to present to the patient.

30.2 Discuss the advantages and disadvantages of esthetic restorations.

30.3 Discuss clinical and homecare techniques of esthetic restorations.

30.4 Explain CAD/CAM technology versus traditional methods of manufacturing.

30.5 Explain the difference between professional and over-the-counter whitening methods.

30.6 Explain mechanism of action, side effects, and contraindications of whitening methods.

30.7 Outline available delivery methods and products for whitening.

30.8 Explain whitening procedures and post-treatment care to the patient.

30.9 Discuss whitening outcomes on various types of enamel.

30.10 Discuss ethical and safety considerations with regard to esthetic dentistry.

30.11 Explain treatment planning considerations for the esthetic patient.

KEY CONCEPTS

- Esthetic dentistry has grown significantly and has changed how dentistry is performed today.
- There are two types of esthetic restorations: direct and indirect.
- CAD/CAM technology has changed the method of fabrication for certain esthetic restorations.
- Dental hygienists play an important role in preserving and maintaining esthetic restorations.
- There are two styles of tooth whitening: professional, which includes in-office and take-home methods, and over the counter.
- Whitening outcomes vary on different types of enamel.
- It is the dental hygienist's role to assist in managing the esthetic patient in all aspects of dental hygiene care, from treatment planning to maintenance.

RELEVANCE TO CLINICAL PRACTICE

Over the past 20 years, the focus on cosmetic dentistry has grown tremendously. Society's belief that a whiter, brighter smile equates with health and physical attractiveness has led to increased interest in elective cosmetic dental procedures. As a result, the use of tooth-colored or esthetic restorative materials and tooth whitening procedures are now very common in today's dental office.

The role of the dental hygienist in presenting esthetic treatment options and maintaining the patient is crucial. The hygienist has the unique opportunity to converse with and treat patients at regular intervals. Thus, the dental hygienist must be well informed about current esthetic treatment options and how they are incorporated in treatment planning, professional maintenance procedures, and patient education.

In this chapter, various esthetic restorative choices are discussed, including composites, crowns, veneers, inlays, and onlays. In addition, a comprehensive review of tooth whitening is presented. This chapter also focuses on dental hygiene considerations for in-office treatment, as well as at-home maintenance of the esthetic patient. Because dental hygienists play a central role in educating and maintaining esthetic patients, hygienists need to be well versed and confident in their knowledge of esthetic dentistry.

WHAT ARE ESTHETIC RESTORATIONS?

There are two styles of esthetic restorations: indirect and direct. **Indirect restorations**, which include crowns, inlays, onlays, and veneers, are fabricated outside of the mouth, usually in a dental laboratory. Indirect restorations are customized for a precise fit in the mouth. They are strong, long lasting, and provide very attractive results. Indirect restorations also tend to be more costly than direct restorations because of the length and number of appointments required, use of materials, and laboratory fees.

Direct restorations involve placing a soft, malleable filling material, such as a composite, directly onto the tooth. A direct restoration sets quickly, is relatively inexpensive, and can be done in a single procedure. However, direct restorations are not as strong as indirect restorations and are not recommended for large restorations. The materials used most commonly for esthetic restorations are composites, porcelain, and glass-ionomer cements.[1]

INDIRECT ESTHETIC RESTORATIONS

Inlay and Onlay

When a tooth is to be restored with an intracoronal restoration, such as an amalgam or a composite, but the dentist feels the decay or fracture compromises the integrity of the tooth and its ability to withstand occlusal forces, an **inlay** may be indicated. An inlay restores the occlusal surface without including the cusp of a posterior tooth.[2] If the decay or fracture involves the cusp or cusps of a tooth, and enough healthy tooth structure remains, an **onlay** may be a viable choice for restoration.[2] Inlays and onlays are indirect restorations that are precisely fitted to a cavity in a tooth and permanently cemented into place. These restorations are similar to a crown in that the tooth is prepared, an impression is taken, a temporary restoration is made, and the impression is sent to a dental laboratory for fabrication. Once completed, the inlay or onlay is placed into the preparation and seated with permanent cement.

The advantages of an inlay or onlay include superior resistance to occlusal forces, excellent marginal integrity, and exceptional interproximal contouring.[3] As well, compared with a full-coverage crown, an onlay allows for a more conservative restoration that still provides strength and protection for a compromised tooth.[3] In the past, inlays and onlays were usually fabricated from gold. However, with the emphasis on esthetics in many cases, inlays and onlays can be fabricated from indirect composite and porcelain and are virtually undetectable from outside the mouth.

Crown

The most common indirect esthetic restoration for both anterior and posterior teeth is a full-coverage crown.[3] A **crown**, sometimes referred to as a cap, is a restoration made to completely cover a tooth and improve the function and esthetics of the tooth. Crowns are generally indicated for several reasons. Perhaps the most frequently seen situation where a crown is needed is when a large restoration compromises the ongoing health and function of a tooth. When a large portion of a tooth is lost due to decay and is replaced by a restoration, the structural integrity of the tooth is greatly compromised and the tooth is at greater risk for fracture. Therefore, a full-coverage crown is an ideal choice to strengthen and protect a fragile tooth.[3]

A tooth that has undergone endodontic treatment, or root canal therapy, generally requires a crown. During root canal therapy, a small opening is made on the occlusal or lingual surface to access the pulp chamber within the tooth. The nerve and blood supply are then cut off from the tooth and the pulp chamber and root canals are cleaned, shaped, and filled to prevent further infection. This tooth is now considered nonvital. Consequently, the tooth structure becomes very brittle and may darken over time. Thus in most situations, it is recommended that posterior teeth are crowned after endodontic therapy. Anterior teeth, on the other hand, are exposed to considerably less occlusal force than are posterior teeth; therefore, a crown may not be necessary. In many cases, an endodontically treated anterior tooth can be successfully restored with a direct restoration, such as a composite. Over time, however, teeth that have had root canal therapy tend to darken or discolor. For anterior teeth, this discoloration becomes an esthetic issue, and a crown or a veneer (discussed later in the chapter) may be desired simply to preserve an acceptable appearance.

A crown may be recommended when a veneer is not an acceptable option because of the patient's occlusion, existing restorations or decay, fractures, a history of bruxism, or an edge-to-edge bite.[3] When these conditions are problematic for veneer placement, a crown is an excellent option to change the shape, color, and size of a tooth and provide a strong, long-lasting restoration.

Materials

From an esthetic standpoint, a porcelain-fused-to-metal (PFM) crown or all-ceramic crown is the best choice for an attractive smile. PFM crowns have a metal shell on which a **porcelain veneer** or covering is placed. The metal shell provides strength for the tooth, and the porcelain covering gives the crown a tooth-like appearance. However, PFM crowns only have porcelain showing on the areas of the crown that are visible in the mouth, with the remaining surfaces being metal. The metal margins can cause a dark appearance near the gingival margin that may be undesirable to the patient. If this is a concern, an all-ceramic crown can be recommended.

All-ceramic crowns, which are restorations without a metal shell, are ideal for esthetic restoration. There is no metal margin, and therefore no dark shadowing occurs. This feature is especially desirable for an anterior tooth because it closely mimics natural tooth color.[3] There are different types and brands of all-ceramic crowns, including leucite reinforced, porcelain fused to alumina, and zirconium.[2] The dentist usually decides on the type and brand of crown.

Traditional Crowning Process

The traditional process of crowning a tooth requires two appointments. During the first appointment, the tooth is prepared for an impression by removing approximately 1 to 2 mm of tooth structure from all five tooth surfaces of the tooth. Then, an impression is taken of the tooth to be crowned, as well as the surrounding teeth, using special impression materials. Typically, an impression of the opposing arch is also taken to ensure the new crown will not affect the patient's occlusion. A temporary crown is fabricated for the prepared tooth and is cemented using temporary cement. The impression of the crown preparation and the model of the opposing arch are then sent to a dental laboratory for the crown to be manufactured. The process generally takes 1 to 2 weeks for the laboratory to fabricate the crown and return it to the office to be permanently seated in the patient's mouth.

Computer-Aided Design/Computer-Aided Manufacturing Restorations

With the development of **computer-aided design/computer-aided manufacturing (CAD/CAM)** technology, dentistry's approach to crown preparation and manufacturing has changed significantly. Although many offices do not have this technology on-site, growing numbers of dentists are investing in CAD/CAM systems. Therefore, it is important that dental hygienists have a basic knowledge of this technology. CAD/CAM systems offer dental professionals an efficient, reliable, and precise method for fabricating crowns, inlays, onlays, and veneers and other esthetic dental restorations in the office while the patient waits.[4] CAD/CAM technology uses a scanner to obtain an image of a prepared tooth called a **digital impression** (Fig. 30-1). Special software then designs a replacement part for the missing portion of the tooth. The design is sent to a milling machine, where the restoration is carved out of a solid block of material, such as composite resin or ceramic (Fig. 30-2).[4] The finished restoration is then permanently cemented onto the prepared tooth. This process eliminates the need for a temporary crown and an additional visit by the patient.

Advantages and Disadvantages of Computer-Aided Design/Computer-Aided Manufacturing

As with any technology, there are advantages and disadvantages to CAD/CAM systems. The most notable advantage is that this technology allows the patient to have a customized restoration done in one appointment. The need for multiple appointments, temporary restorations, and additional anesthetic is eliminated. As

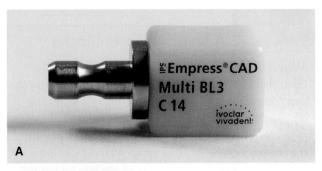
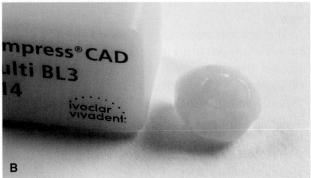

Figure 30-2. (A) Porcelain block before milling. (B) CAD/CAM crown.

a result, less chair time is required, less material is used, and less manipulation of the tooth occurs. Also, CAD/CAM affords clinicians complete control over the artistic aspects of crown fabrication, such as shade, staining, and glazing.[4]

Arguably, the biggest disadvantage of an in-office CAD/CAM system is the cost, which can be $100,000 or more, with additional costs for materials, maintenance, and software upgrades.[4] As well, specialized training that may or may not be included with the purchase price is needed for the dentist and dental staff who operate the system. Also, not all restorative cases can be completed in this manner. For instance, when a tooth is fractured subgingivally, the optical scanner may not be able to capture the margin adequately because of the surrounding gingiva. Therefore, the dentist may choose to crown the tooth using the traditional method.[4]

Although CAD/CAM technology may not be the right choice for every office, it is imperative that dental professionals have a basic understanding of the technology.

Porcelain Veneer

Porcelain veneers are thin pieces of porcelain used to re-create the natural look of teeth and provide strength and resilience comparable to natural tooth enamel. A porcelain veneer, often referred to as an indirect veneer, is prepped in the mouth.[5] An impression is taken and sent to the laboratory for the fabrication. If a veneer is not made chairside and an impression needs to be taken and sent to the laboratory to make the veneer, it is considered indirect.[6] A direct veneer is made directly chairside and is usually composed of composite material. **Composite veneers** are referred to as direct veneers. Indications for a veneer (either direct or indirect) include slight misalignment of teeth, discoloration

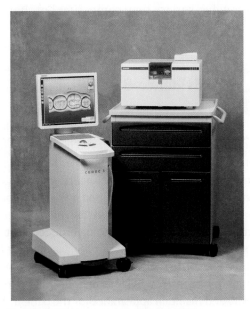

Figure 30-1. CAD/CAM computer milling machine.

Advancing Technologies

Many technologies are currently advancing within the dental field. Because esthetic dentistry is in such demand, new technology in this branch of dentistry is increasing rapidly. Digital radiography, 3-D computer-assisted tomography (CAT) scanning, and digital photography are the newest technology for imaging. All three capture digital images in the format of computer files for instant viewing.

The intraoral camera is a wand-like device with a small camera on the end to use inside the mouth to capture pictures. These pictures can be used for patient education, insurance claims, and before-and-after comparisons of dental work. The CAD/CAM system incorporates 3D imaging by scanning the area and sending the information to a milling machine to fabricate a restoration according to the specifications determined from the digitally scanned images.

Shade matching is always challenging, and new technology can lend a hand. VITA Easyshade® Advance 4.03D shade matching for multicolor enamel matching is a digital shade matcher that reads the tooth and displays a shade. Laser prepping, air abrasion to prep caries, and laser therapy for esthetic gingivectomy have also become popular. These methods are very conservative as compared with the older methods that are available.

Wand anesthesia allows patients to relax and receive anesthesia without the feeling of a shot. This advanced technology is especially helpful for nervous patients. Finally, digital video disc (DVD) glasses that patients can wear during in-office whitening or long appointments allow patients to relax the neck and watch a movie without strain during treatment. ■

of teeth, and to perfect the look of teeth.[7] Composite veneers are made chairside using a composite material. Composites are a mixture of glass filler particles and polymerizable (either self- or light-activated) resin.[5] They are esthetically not as polished as porcelain, but achieve their purpose when done correctly. Staining at the margins can occur more frequently than with porcelain veneers. Porcelain is a stronger material than composite.[7]

A porcelain veneer is a cosmetic procedure and is not usually covered under an insurance plan. The patient usually pays 100% for a veneer. Sometimes when a direct or composite veneer is completed it is coded as a four + surface composite and is covered by insurance according to the policy's restorative coverage. There are Current Dental Terminology (CDT) codes for porcelain veneers, direct composite veneers, and anterior composite restorations covering four or more surfaces. Each code has a unique description, and it is up to the dentist to determine which treatment will be used.

DIRECT ESTHETIC RESTORATIONS

Composites

Composite restorations are now the most popular restorations used in a dental office for both anterior and posterior restorations. Composites are used as fillings and as a cosmetic intervention, as with the veneers discussed previously. Composite fillings are completed chairside and come in a variety of shades. The dental assistant and dentist evaluate the shade using the shade guide. As stated previously, composites are a mixture of glass filler particles and polymerizable (either self- or light-activated) resin.[5] When polished and placed correctly, they can be difficult to detect.

Composites can be microfilled, hybrid, nanofilled, packable, flowable, or small particle.[7] Small-particle composites are nearly obsolete and may only be seen in older patients. The other types of composites are much more common, and it can be difficult to distinguish among them. Most composite materials can be polished with a rubber polisher followed by the composite polishing paste recommended by the composite manufacturer or a paste specifically designed for composite polishing done by dental hygienists. Hybrid composites should be polished with aluminum oxide paste and a water-filled rubber polishing cup.[1] It is contraindicated to use air powder polishing (prophy jet) and ultrasonic devices on composite restorations, as well as medium- or coarse-grit prophy paste, because these will cause severe scratching and compromise the integrity of the composite.

Glass Ionomer

Glass-ionomer restorations are not as commonly used as composites because they are esthetically inferior to composite materials. However, because glass-ionomer material is fluoride releasing, there are certain situations where it is still indicated.[1] Glass-ionomer restorations have a rougher surface than composites but should still be polished using slow speed and light pressure with a

Evidence-Based Practice

Research shows that using a medium- or coarse-grit prophy paste on esthetic restorations is contraindicated.[1] If you notice that your patient's esthetic restorations seem to be retaining more staining, you may want to evaluate your polishing procedure. Surface roughness caused by medium- or coarse-grit prophy paste can cause staining to adhere to esthetic restorations. Use of polishing products that are recommended by the manufacturer or that are safe for all esthetic materials is advised. Employing the appropriate polishing regimen on esthetic materials can increase longevity and maintain appearance for the patient. ■

product safe for glass-ionomer surfaces. Glass-ionomer restorations should always be lubricated with petroleum jelly or water before polishing.[1] As with composites, ultrasonic instrumentation and medium- and coarse-grit prophy pastes are contraindicated on glass ionomer.

Dental Hygiene Considerations for Esthetic Restorations

Dental hygienists share the responsibility of maintaining the integrity of restorations with the patient. Dental hygienists must be able to identify esthetic restorations to determine appropriate treatment during a routine recall appointment. Because most esthetic restorations are virtually unrecognizable, ample time is needed for a thorough examination. Dental hygienists should utilize the explorer, mouth mirror, compressed air, current charting, and radiographs to aid in determining where restorations exist. Magnification using loupes or an intraoral camera is also extremely helpful. Once the restorations are detected, the dental hygienist can decide how to proceed.

Dental hygienists must be prepared to modify the routine recall appointment and armamentarium to accommodate the esthetic patient. For example, when scaling teeth with existing restorations, it is recommended that scaling near the restoration be done in a lateral direction so as not pull on or damage the margin.[8] Not all restorations adapt cleanly against the tooth. Faulty and leaky margins can cause snagging of instruments that could result in accidentally pulling or chipping the restoration. Also, bulky margins will leave a ledge of material that can create difficulty when scaling. Care needs to be taken when scaling restorative margins to ensure that plaque removal is done gently so as not to damage the restoration.

Using a sonic or ultrasonic device directly on a restored surface is not advised because these instruments can scratch the surface and loosen the restorations. It is acceptable to use ultrasonic instrumentation with thin precision inserts on low-power apical to the restoration margin.[7]

Understanding the significance of proper polishing is essential for the dental hygienist. Basic knowledge of polishing agents is also important. Prophylaxis polishing pastes generally come in either powders or flours that are mixed with water or mouthrinse, or commercially prepared polishing agents, or prophy pastes, available from dental manufacturers. Commercially prepared pastes come in coarse, medium, and fine grits. Using a standard medium- or coarse-grit prophy paste on every patient is unacceptable. When a patient has esthetic restorations present, taking into consideration the type of material and the needs of the patient is very important for successful maintenance. Dental hygienists should not overlook the specific requirements of each patient and his or her esthetic restorations. For example, polishing porcelain restorations requires the dental hygienist to consider whether the porcelain is glazed or unglazed. Glazed porcelain is smoother and

more stain resistant than unglazed porcelain, but can still require occasional polishing to remove staining and restore a smooth surface. Glazed porcelain can be polished with a diamond paste (used dry) and a Robinson brush.[1] If the diamond paste comes in different grit sizes, it should be used according to the manufacturer's instructions. Conversely, the surface of unglazed porcelain is usually rougher and attracts more stain. If unglazed porcelain is rough, it should be smoothed before polishing, using dry diamond paste and a Robinson brush.[1] If there is staining present, diamond paste used with a rubber polishing cup is helpful.[1] Only those products safe for porcelain surfaces should be applied, and following the manufacturer's instructions is always recommended. In addition, caution should be used with ultrasonic instrumentation because it can fracture porcelain, alter margins, and loosen the restoration. Also, if the restoration is done poorly, the margins may have overhangs on them. When scaling around the margins, be careful not to pull on the restoration.

Patient Education for Esthetic Restorations

The dental hygienist's role in maintaining esthetic restorations includes patient education. Providing the instruction patients need to preserve the quality and appearance of their restorations is a key component of the esthetic recall appointment. Recommend that patients brush two to three times per day with a soft-bristle toothbrush using gentle sulcular brushing. Instruct patients to use the least abrasive toothpaste available to prevent damage to esthetic restorations.[1] Encourage patients to floss at least once daily and to use interdental cleaning aids such as superfloss, interdental brushes, toothpicks, and triangular wooden tips according to gingival embrasures. Advise patients to avoid using mouthrinses with high alcohol content, which can soften and stain esthetic materials.[9] To prevent staining, encourage patients to reduce or avoid consumption of coffee (hot or cold), tea (hot or cold), red wine, blueberries, dark cherries, dark colas, grape juice, blue-colored mouthrinses, and tobacco products.[9]

Dental hygienists are in an excellent position to evaluate a patient's oral habits for potential problems. Individualize instructions for patients with a history of clenching or grinding, nail biting, ice chewing, excessive "picking" at restorations, and other detrimental behaviors.

When biofilm removal is complete, the dental hygienist should consider which type of fluoride is safe for the patient's restorations. A fluoride varnish is ideal. Acidulated phosphate fluoride (APF) should not be used on patients with esthetic restorations due to the etching of margins. APF can also cause breakdown of filler particles in composites.[10] APF fluorides are ideal for patients with no resin restorations or fixed orthodontic appliances. Neutral sodium fluoride is ideal for patients with resins, crowns and bridge, implants, sealants and orthodontic fixed appliances. Proper gingival brushing needs to be addressed with all patients, especially those with faulty fillings. Recommendation of good floss such as a polytetrafluoroethylene (Teflon) dental floss, rather than a thread-type floss that may shred, will help alleviate some frustration patients may have when flossing. Overhanging margins may make floss shred or tear.

Esthetic restorations will not change color with whitening. Advise patients with esthetic restorations who want to whiten their teeth that their composite fillings will not change color. This is very important if they have large anterior restorations.

TOOTH WHITENING

The dental hygienist is an important source of information on many topics. Factors to consider when discussing a patient's whitening goals are the different methods available, materials, ingredients, and mechanism of action.

Before starting a whitening treatment, the dentist and dental hygienist should perform a thorough comprehensive oral examination. The examination should include a review of the patient's medical and dental history, oral hygiene assessment, visual/tactile oral cancer screening, comprehensive periodontal and caries assessment, and assessment of the condition of existing restorations and hypersensitivity areas. Tooth discolorations may need treatments other than whitening. An examination will identify which teeth are healthy and candidates for whitening. Some tooth discolorations caused by pathology include decay, abscessed teeth, color and/or leakage of existing restorations, internal root resorption, and other diseases. Whitening would only mask these types of pathology.

After determining that the patient is a candidate for whitening, obtain the patient's current tooth shade, take intraoral pictures, and document the findings.

External Methods

External whitening products (applied to the tooth's surface) are available in over-the-counter and professional strengths.

Over-the-Counter Products

Whitening mouthrinses, strips, and toothpastes can be purchased without consulting a dentist. **Over-the-counter (OTC) whitening** products are very weak in strength as compared with professional-strength whitening given at the office. Their main ingredient is hydrogen peroxide in a weakened concentration.[11]

Take-Home Professional Whitening Methods

Professional whitening strips and gels for use in trays can be given to the patient to apply at home (Fig. 30-3). Although they are similar to the over-the-counter methods, professional whitening methods have a much higher concentration of ingredients. They achieve the whitening goal faster due to their increased

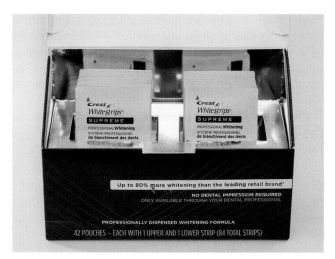

Figure 30-3. Professional whitening strips.

concentration. The dentist prescribes the appropriate-strength gel for each patient.

Prefilled and custom trays are available. Prefilled trays are dispensed to patients with the manufacturer's instructions on usage. Custom trays are fabricated in the dental office. The hygienist or dental assistant takes alginate impressions of the patient's teeth. Dental stone is poured into the impressions to make models of the teeth. A vacuum is used to heat and press down a clear square sheet of plastic over the model to make a tray. The plastic is suctioned with the vacuum press to the model to ensure a perfect fit. The plastic is trimmed, and rough edges are buffed out so the tray does not cut or rub the patient. The edges can be heated over a Bunsen burner to make a smooth lip.

When the tray is ready to be delivered to the patient, a short appointment is made. This appointment will achieve delivery and fitting of the trays. Demonstrate gel insertion into trays so that the patient is confident doing it at home. It is important to take a baseline shade using the Vita shade guide or technology (Fig. 30-4).

The dentist prescribes the appropriate-strength gel for the individual patient. Two common ingredients used in professional-strength whitening products are carbamide peroxide and hydrogen peroxide. The strengths in each differ by percentage due to the fact that carbamide peroxide breaks down into hydrogen

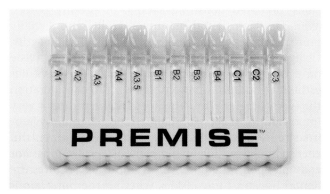

Figure 30-4. Vita shade guide.

peroxide. Therefore, a whitening product containing 10% carbamide peroxide yields approximately 3.5% hydrogen peroxide.[12] Tooth whitening gel products can range from 10% to 40% in strength, containing either carbamide peroxide or hydrogen peroxide concentrations.

Patient education instructions are very similar to those in the OTC methods, but in this case the patients have already had an examination to ensure dental caries are not present. Other than product usage, patient education on how to keep the trays clean and safe should be discussed. The trays can be rinsed and brushed with a clean, soft toothbrush. They can be stored in a special box that is given to the patient upon delivery of the trays. A fluoride varnish may be applied before whitening to protect against sensitivity. Fluoride application may be covered by the patient's insurance plan, the patient may elect to pay for it, or the dentist may include it in the cost for whitening.

Patient education regarding good hygiene measures such as a specific tooth-brushing technique tailored to the individual patient and flossing, with demonstration of both methods, would be discussed during patient education. A prescription-strength sensitivity-control toothpaste is typically recommended for use.[13] An extra-soft toothbrush is ideal during whitening to prevent toothbrush abrasion of enamel. Patients should also be scheduled for a follow-up procedure to see if their whitening goals have been met and address any issues they may have. A fluoride varnish can be reapplied at this appointment as well.

In-Office Professional Whitening

Depending on state law, either the dentist or the hygienist can perform in-office professional whitening. Refer to your state's laws and regulations before performing any task. The in-office whitening is completed by blocking all of the patient's tissue with a gingival block and curing light. Proper isolation of all tissue is necessary to ensure no tissue is exposed during the treatment. After all cheek retractors are in place and isolation of tissue is complete, a proper suction and application is ready. Follow the manufacturer's instructions. Typically, gel is placed on the teeth and a light is used to incorporate the material into the enamel (Fig. 30-5). After this application is complete, it is usually repeated as directed. It is best to remove the bulk of the material first through surgical suction.

One product uses the light within a mouthpiece and allows the patient to complete this procedure at home. It is available in both over-the-counter and professional strengths.

Internal

Internal whitening, placing a whitening agent to the interior of the tooth, is recommended for teeth that are nonvital. Internal whitening may be performed or recommended because internal tooth resorption has occurred from trauma causing discoloration from loss of

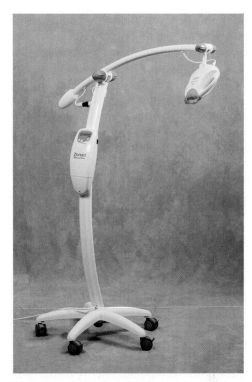

Figure 30-5. Light-emitting diode (LED) whitening machine.

tooth substance.[14] Internal whitening is only performed by a dentist in a dental office.

Method, Materials, Ingredients, Mechanism of Action

Internal whitening involves placing a cotton-soaked pellet of 35% hydrogen peroxide into a pulp chamber and placing a heat probe at a higher temperature than that used for vital teeth.[15] This is called the "walking bleach" technique. Whitening agents used for internal whitening include **carbamide peroxide**, **hydrogen peroxide**, **sodium perborate**, and **calcium peroxide**.[12] The whitening agent ranges from 10% to 35% strength. Studies show that 35% carbamide peroxide and 35% hydrogen peroxide are equally effective in internal whitening procedures and are more effective than sodium perborate.[16] This procedure can only be performed on a tooth that has had root canal therapy. It can be performed the same day a root canal is performed and sealed, or a tooth can be reopened to apply the bleaching agent.

Another approach to internal whitening is to place an amount of whitening agent inside the root-canaled tooth followed by a cotton pellet and a temporary filling. The patient is then released from the office and scheduled to return a few days later to add more whitening agent inside the tooth as many times as needed to achieve desired lightening of the tooth.[14] It is up to the dentist to determine whether or not the patient is a candidate for internal whitening and thus recommend which procedure is best. It is prudent to recommend that the patient whiten adjacent teeth by external methods to ensure maximum whitening potential and uniformity throughout the dentition. Before beginning any whitening treatment, external or internal, a shade guide should be used to compare pre- and post-treatment shades.

Once the tooth has reached the desired shade, a permanent filling is placed. The final shade results will be evident 2 weeks after whitening completion. A potentially negative outcome of this procedure is the possibility of internal or external root resorption if some has not already occurred, especially if there has been trauma to the tooth.[14] If the outcome is not what the patient expected or desired, restorative options should be explored further, such as post and core with either an all-ceramic crown or PFM crown.

Dental Hygiene Considerations

It is important that either the dentist or dental hygienist educates the patient on the condition of his or her mouth and what the likely outcomes would be if internal whitening were performed. It is also important that the clinician understands the patient's expectations of treatment and explains realistic outcomes. Typically, a tooth requiring internal whitening is a root-canaled tooth that cannot be whitened with external whitening methods. A successfully obturated and sealed root canal is required to prevent the whitening agent from reaching periapical tissue.

Patient Education for Maintenance

Internal whitening usually lasts longer than external whitening; however, there is no time frame in which a tooth should be retreated with internal whitening because it depends on the individual patient. At routine cleaning appointments the dental hygienist should use a shade guide to assess the treated tooth's shade and plan for whitening retreatment when appropriate. The role of the dental hygienist is to professionally remove extrinsic staining, calculus, and plaque at re-care visits and discourage the consumption of certain foods and beverages that can cause staining. An oral hygiene assessment and education should be performed as well so that patients understand their role in optimizing their whitening potential. OTC whitening products and re-touch-ups with professional procedures will prolong the treatment. Patients who actively engage in whitening may show improvement in their overall oral hygiene and be more likely to keep their re-care appointments.

INDICATIONS AND CONTRAINDICATIONS FOR WHITENING

Before recommending whitening options to patients, the dentist and dental hygienist should perform a comprehensive oral examination to assess for indications and contraindications for whitening (Box 30-1). The examination should include a review of the patient's

Box 30-1. *Contraindications for Whitening*
• Women who are pregnant or lactating
• Patient undergoing active orthodontic treatment
• Children (age is up to the dentist's discretion)
• Patient with active periodontal disease
• Patient with restorative needs
• Patient with allergy to bleaching ingredients
• Patient with dental restorations that cover the facial surface of the tooth
• Exposed root surfaces
• Xerostomia
• History of dental hypersensitivity[15,17]

medical and dental history, an oral hygiene assessment, a visual/tactile oral cancer screening, and a comprehensive periodontal and caries assessment. The condition of existing restorations and hypersensitivity areas should be assessed. Tooth discolorations may need treatments other than whitening. An examination will identify which teeth are healthy and candidates for whitening. The best candidates for whitening are those with generalized yellowing of natural teeth. Some tooth discolorations caused by pathology include decay, abscessed teeth, color and/or leakage of existing restorations, internal root resorption, and other diseases. Whitening performed on any of these types of pathology would only mask the problem. Ultimately it is the dentist who determines whether whitening is an appropriate course of treatment.

SIDE EFFECTS OF WHITENING

The most common side effects of whitening are tooth sensitivity and gingival irritation. Demineralization has also been reported due to the overuse of whitening products, especially if active decay is present already. Side effects found in those patients who choose bleaching methods at their own discretion include changes to existing dental restoratives. Due to the variability in concentration among OTC and professional whitening systems, dental materials are greatly affected if the patient attempts to apply bleaching agents to restorations.

Tooth sensitivity is temporary and often referred to as reversible pulpitis or Brainstorm's hydrodynamic theory.[17] Tooth sensitivity results from the whitening agent or other external factor entering through the enamel and dentin tubules and causing a sensation in the pulp. A higher peroxide concentration results in greater likelihood of tooth sensitivity. Patients who experience sensitivity in general should be cautioned before whitening that the procedure could exacerbate the sensitivity. Advising the patient of this side effect will enable the patient to make a fully informed decision and prevent unexpected discomfort.

Desensitizing agents are commonly recommended in conjunction with whitening treatments. Products that contain fluoride, potassium nitrate, and amorphous calcium phosphate are available in gels, pastes, and mouthrinses. They can be applied through brushing, rinsing, and finger or tray application. To prevent the incidence of sensitivity, it is recommended that patients use the desensitizing agent before, during, and after whitening treatment.

Desensitizing agents can be applied in whitening trays for 10 to 30 minutes before or after applying the whitening agent. Lower concentrations of the desensitizing agents can be found over the counter; however, the higher concentrations must be prescribed or dispensed by a dentist. It is recommended that patients brush with a desensitizing toothpaste for 2 weeks before whitening.

Some whitening agents contain desensitizing ingredients to reduce tooth sensitivity. The dental hygienist should read the manufacturer's instructions completely to accurately educate the patient on the use of specific whitening products and additional product recommendations.

Gingival irritation results from the tissue being exposed to a whitening agent. Most commonly this occurs when ill-fitted or overfilled trays cause the whitening agent to overflow onto the gingiva, tongue, or other mucosal tissues. Blanching or whitening of the tissues can occur, but it is only temporary. To prevent gingival irritation, an effective barrier should be applied to the tissue before the whitening agent is applied for in office procedures. The dental hygienist should educate the patient regarding proper use of the whitening agent and materials for at-home use before dispensing them.

Whitening products and procedures may produce unwanted side effects on dental restorations, including porcelain restorations, glass-ionomer cement, composite material, and amalgam restorations. Applying a bleaching agent at any level of concentration, especially higher concentrations, can cause undesirable results such as increased roughness, cracking, decreased hardness, greater staining susceptibility, microleakage, and material washout.[17] Whitening products and procedures should be individualized based on the presence of restorations. They are generally not recommended for restorations because the risks outweigh the benefits.

WHITENING OUTCOMES ON VARIOUS TYPES OF ENAMEL CONDITIONS

Tobacco Use

Patients who smoke or chew tobacco typically exhibit extrinsic nicotine staining and generalized yellowing of the teeth. Whitening treatments can improve the color of the patient's teeth, but it may take 1 to 3 months of consistent whitening applications to reach maximum results. Factors that influence whitening outcomes include the amount, type, duration, and frequency of use of the tobacco product and the individual's oral hygiene regimen. If discolorations remain around existing restorations after whitening treatments, replacement of the restorations should be recommended. Successful whitening may motivate patients to cease using tobacco to maintain an esthetic smile.

Tetracycline Stains

It is difficult to achieve successful whitening results with tetracycline-stained teeth. This type of staining occurs when a pregnant mother ingests an antibiotic from the tetracycline family (doxycycline, oxytetracycline, minocycline, chlortetracycline, demeclocycline) during tooth formation. Adults who take a minocycline medication for a long duration can also exhibit this type of staining.[14] Stains range in color from gray to blue, brown, or yellow. Brown and yellow stains are most responsive to whitening treatment; gray and blue stains are least responsive. To achieve maximum results with tetracycline staining, whitening treatments of a longer duration, perhaps up to a year, may be required. The patient should be advised that treatment will be lengthy and more costly, and will require more effort on the patient's part. Prolonged whitening applications also present a higher likelihood for sensitivity.

Dental Fluorosis

Dental fluorosis occurs when excessive fluoride is absorbed during the enamel formation process, resulting in demineralization. This can cause brown and yellow staining, white flecks, and white spots or striations. The level of severity depends on the amount and duration of fluoride intake.[18] Whitening may not eliminate the discolorations but it will lighten the enamel around the discoloration, making it more uniform. When a satisfactory outcome is not achieved with whitening treatments, an alternative option should be explored and selected, such as the possibility of porcelain veneers, composite restorations, all-ceramic crowns, or PFM crowns.

Hypocalcification

Demineralization is a stage of the dental care process in which calcium and phosphorous minerals are removed from the tooth structure by acidogenic bacteria. Remineralization occurs when these minerals are added back to the tooth from fluoride in food, beverages, or products, resulting in the appearance of a white spot. When remineralization forms a hypocalcified area and causes an undesirable appearance of "white spots," patients may choose a whitening product to correct the problem. However, without proper education and product recommendation, whitening agents applied to hypocalcified areas will only enhance the whiteness and make the lesions more noticeable. An attempt to whiten teeth with localized hypocalcification areas can show improvement within 1 year of treatment if used in conjunction with amorphous calcium phosphate (ACP) products. ACP products promote tooth remineralization and reduce bleaching-induced sensitivity (see Chapter 21 for additional information on ACP). For generalized areas, however, bonding with composite resin or porcelain veneers is more likely to produce a pleasing result.[5]

Combination Therapy

Combination therapy with whitening and microabrasion may be recommended to produce a more esthetic and uniform result. Microabrasion "entails using a slow running handpiece with pumice composed of a mild form of hydrochloric acid that can remove microns of enamel."[5] One or more treatments may be required to remove or lighten darker stains.

PATIENT EDUCATION FOR POST-WHITENING CARE

Patient education is a primary responsibility of dental hygienists. The importance of regular re-care visits following whitening treatments should be stressed. Professional cleanings and routine examinations will prolong the integrity of dental restorations and whitening treatments, although the effects of whitening procedures are not permanent. Assess shade changes at re-care visits and recommend whitening retreatment when appropriate. Advise patients to reduce or avoid consumption of foods and beverages that cause stains, such as coffee, tea, red wine, blueberries, dark cherries, dark colas, grape juice, and tobacco products.[9] Recommend OTC and professional products as needed, and provide instruction for oral hygiene homecare.

PROFESSIONALISM AND ESTHETIC DENTISTRY

Ethical and Safety Considerations

It is prudent to ask patients to sign an informed consent before the beginning of any whitening or restorative procedure. The consent should describe the procedure, alternative treatment options, cost, risks, and potential complications or side effects that could occur with treatment. Signature of the consent form indicates that the patient fully understands the procedure and consents to treatment. The dentist decides on an appropriate age limit for performing specific procedures. However, legally, a patient under the age of 18 requires a guardian's consent before treatment.

Research shows that carbamide peroxide does not cause further need for root canal therapy, internal or external resorption, extreme or permanent sensitivity, or harmful effects on tooth structure when used for whitening procedures. It should be recommended and should never be abused. Research also failed to show any effects of the highest concentrations of hydrogen peroxide for tooth whitening procedures on enamel and dentin in regard to erosion, abrasion, reduced surface hardness, wear resistance, or changes to morphology.[19]

Presenting a Treatment Plan

Once the patient has undergone a thorough intra-/extra-oral examination of the soft and hard tissues and a treatment plan has been presented for restorative needs, the next step after the appropriate professional cleaning is whether or not esthetic treatment is a concern or priority for the patient. Usually within the first 15 minutes of the appointment the patient shares his or her chief complaint(s) and concerns (Fig. 30-6). It is the hygienist's role to answer any questions the patient has about various procedures the dentist recommended or discussed. It is not the hygienist's role to diagnose decay, disease, cancer, or any other condition. Dentists highly value a hygienist who is competent and confident in explaining and discussing esthetic procedures with patients. Esthetic procedures should be presented in a noninsulting and nonjudgmental manner. Telling patients they would look better with whiter teeth or with veneers insinuates that they do not look good now.[14] One approach would be to include this as a question on the medical dental history as an option of whether or not patients desire whiter, straighter teeth. Or the hygienist can ask the patient, "Is there anything about your smile you are unhappy with or wish you

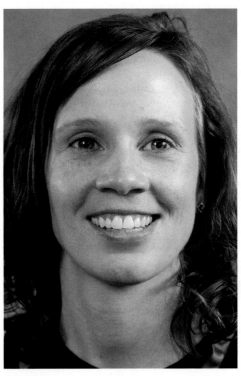

Figure 30-6. Many patients ask about cosmetic dentistry to achieve an esthetically pleasing smile.

could change?" This allows patients to reflect on their appearance in a nonjudgmental way. Another option is to place brochures or pamphlets throughout the office about procedures that are offered, such as veneers, crowns, whitening, amalgam filling replacement, and so forth. Intraoral pictures with an intraoral camera are a useful tool when presenting treatment plans and showing patients exactly what their teeth look like. This is an effective tool to use when recommending esthetic restorations, along with supplemental tools such as tooth models and pictures.

Dr. Van Haywood has done extensive research on whitening and published books and articles with a plethora of information and treatment planning recommendations. He developed an approach for recommending whitening to a patient.[14] He recommends that an individual's teeth color should match the color of the whites of his or her eyes. If the patient's teeth are darker than the whites of the eyes, whitening treatment will likely improve the patient's tooth color shade. Conversely, it can be distracting if a patient's teeth are whiter than the whites of the eyes. It is important that the whitening option be discussed before any restorative treatment, especially anterior esthetic procedures. Ultimately, realistic patient expectations are essential to patient satisfaction with esthetic treatment. The hygienist's role is to educate the patient on which teeth will or will not likely respond to whitening treatment and discuss other treatment options.

Case Study

A 64-year-old woman presents at the dental office for a routine cleaning. She has no medical conditions and is very excited about her granddaughter's upcoming wedding. She wants to look like a movie star when she smiles for the wedding. She esthetically has teeth of a shade D2 and she has a diastema (space) between #8 and #9. She tried a whitening rinse with no result. She is also a smoker and heavy coffee drinker.

Case Study Exercises

1. The patient is a smoker and a heavy coffee drinker. Determine how well her teeth will respond to professional whitening treatment.
   A. Very responsive
   B. Moderately responsive
   C. Least responsive
   D. Somewhere between A and B

2. The dentist may recommend either full crowns or porcelain veneers as esthetic treatment to close the diastema between #8 and #9. The dentist would plan for whitening treatment before starting esthetic restorative treatment.
   A. The first statement is true. The second statement is false.
   B. The first statement is false. The second statement is true.
   C. Both statements are true.
   D. Both statements are false.

3. Rank in order the steps you would recommend the patient take in optimizing whitening potential.
   A. ____Patient begins using sensitivity control toothpastes, either over-the-counter or prescription strength.
   B. ____Complete prophy.
   C. ____Recommend that the patient reduce stain-causing food, beverages, and habits.
   D. ____Obtain a current full-mouth radiograph (FMX) and complete examination by the dentist.
   E. ____Complete restorative treatment to treat any infection or decay present.
   F. ____Patient begins the recommended whitening treatment.
   G. ____Complete esthetic restorative treatment.

4. What type of prophy paste would you recommend for this patient if she follows through with esthetic treatment?
   A. Fine-grit prophy paste
   B. Medium-grit prophy paste
   C. Coarse-grit prophy paste

5. Which of the following should be obtained from the patient before treatment?
   A. Consent form for whitening treatment
   B. Consent form for esthetic treatment
   C. Neither A nor B is necessary as long as you get verbal consent.
   D. Both A and B are necessary.

Review Questions

1. Which of the following is one way to detect esthetic restorations?
   A. Using compressed air through air/water syringe
   B. Polishing with a fine-grit prophy paste
   C. Using fluoride treatment with neutral sodium
   D. Obtaining a thorough health history

2. When considering homecare for a patient with esthetic restorations, the hygienist should NOT recommend which of the following?
   A. Sulcular brushing with a soft-bristle brush
   B. Using an alcohol-based mouthrinse one to two times daily
   C. Avoiding coffee, red wine, and dark colas
   D. Using the least abrasive toothpaste available

3. Which of the following is NOT an esthetic restorative material?
   A. Porcelain
   B. Amalgam
   C. Composite
   D. Glass ionomer

4. An onlay is different from an inlay in that
   A. an onlay contains amalgam.
   B. an onlay involves a cusp or cusps of the tooth.
   C. an inlay is fabricated chairside.
   D. none of these—they are the same.

5. Which of the following is NOT an advantage of a crown?
   A. Strength
   B. Longevity
   C. Esthetics
   D. Cost

Active Learning

1. Use an explorer on an extracted tooth that has a tooth-colored restoration. How does the surface of the restoration feel versus the enamel?

2. Use pictures, videos, and radiographs to show examples of teeth that have been restored with esthetic restorations, such as composites, veneers, PFM crowns, and ceramic crowns.

3. Show text pictures of composite restorative material that has been scratched by polishing with a coarse-grit prophy paste.

4. Using an extracted tooth with a tooth-colored restoration, scratch the surface of the enamel and the restoration with an explorer. Are there any scratch marks present on the restoration? Do these surfaces sound differently when scratched? ▪

REFERENCES

1. Barnes C. Polishing esthetic restorative materials. *Dimens Dent Hyg.* 2010;8(1): 24, 26-28.
2. Parashar VP, Kortkar H, Cook A. The balance between function and esthetics. *Dimens Dent Hyg.* 2010; 8(11):54-59.
3. Radz GM. Indirect posterior restorations: a look at the current state of the industry. *Dent Econ.* 2012;102(7). Available from: http://www.dentaleconomics.com/ articles/print/volume-102/issue-7/features/indirect-posterior-restorations-a-look-at-the-current-state-of-the-industry.html.
4. Trost L, Stines S, Burt L. Making informed decisions about incorporating CAD/CAM system into dental practice. *J Am Dent Assoc.* 2006;137(9 suppl):32S-36S.
5. American Academy of Cosmetic Dentistry. Porcelain veneers. 2011. Available from: http://www.aacd. com/index.php?module=cms&page=574.
6. Noble WH, Gupta S, Vallee J, Schulze K. Advances in all-ceramic restorations. *Dimens Dent Hyg.* 2012; 10(5):60-63.
7. Calley, K. Maintaining the beauty and longevity of esthetic restorations. *Dimens Dent Hyg.* 2009;7(6): 38-41.
8. Goldstein RE. Behind a beautiful smile. *Dimens Dent Hyg.* 2003;1(7):14-16, 18.
9. Goldstein, RE, Garber DA, Schwartz CG, Goldstein, GE. Patient maintenance of esthetic restorations. *J Am Dent Assoc.* 1992;123:61-67.
10. Hosoya Y, Shiraishi T, Puppin-Rontani RM, Powers JM. Effect of acidulated phosphate fluoride gel application on surface roughness, gloss, and colour of different type resin composites. 2011;39(10):700-6. doi:10. 1016/j.jdent.2011.08.002.
11. Proctor and Gamble. Crest 3D white. 2013. Available from: http://www.3dwhite.com.
12. ADA Council on Scientific Affairs. Tooth whitening/ bleaching: treatment considerations for dentists and their patients. 2009. Available from: http://www.ada. org/sections/about/pdfs/HOD_whitening_rpt.pdf.
13. Colgate-Palmolive Company. Dental-indications for use. 2012. Available from: http://www.colgateprofessional. com/dental-indications/dentin-hypersensitivity.
14. Haywood V. *Tooth whitening: indications and outcomes of nightguard vital bleaching.* Hanover Park: Quintessence Publishing Co., Inc; 2007.
15. Woodall, Irene, et al. *Comprehensive dental hygiene care.* St. Louis: Mosby; 1989. 650 p.

16. Kim MY, Lum SOY, Poh RSC, Lee GP, Lim KC. An in vitro comparison of bleaching efficacy of 35% carbamide peroxide with established intracoronal bleaching agents. *Int Endod J.* 2004;37(7):438-488.

17. Nagelberg R. Professional whitening services: prioritizing and implementing success. ADA CERP. 2013; 1-15.

18. Mittal N, Jain J. A conservative approach for management of flurorosed anterior teeth. *Indian J Dent.* 2012;3(2):118-121.

19. Suliman, M. An overview of bleaching technique: 1. history, chemistry, and safety and legal aspects. *Dent Update.* 2004;31:608-616.

Part VII

Anxiety and Pain Management

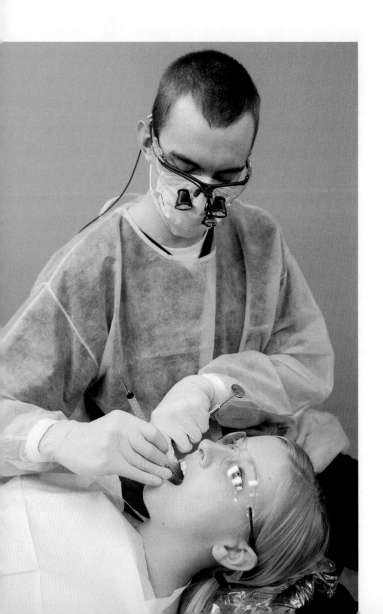

Chapter 31 | Dental Fear and Anxiety Management

Jackie Foskett, RDH, BA, CH

KEY TERMS

dental anxiety
dental fear
dental phobia
iatrosedation
relaxation response
stress response

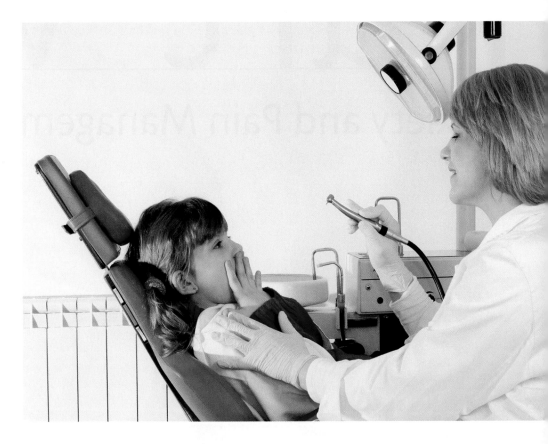

LEARNING OBJECTIVES

After reading this chapter, the student should be able to:

31.1 Distinguish between dental fear, anxiety, and phobia.
31.2 Identify the causes of dental anxiety and fear, and discuss their effects on patients and the dental team.
31.3 Explain the stress response.
31.4 Assess a patient's degree of fear or anxiety, and plan and implement cognitive and behavioral strategies to reduce dental anxiety and discomfort.
31.5 Apply behavioral strategies to manage anxious children.

KEY CONCEPTS

• Dental fear, dental anxiety, and dental phobia are related, yet distinct.
• Dental fear and anxiety affect people's oral and general health and well-being, lower their pain threshold and pain tolerance, and affect dental hygiene care.
• It is important for the dental hygienist to know the symptoms of the stress response and how to help patients who experience it.

- Establishing a dental fear management program that utilizes assessment tools, communication, and cognitive and behavioral tools is beneficial for patients and clinicians.
- Pharmacological agents provide a role in managing fearful dental patients. Although prescribing and administering them is out of the scope of practice of dental hygienists, they can be part of the dental team's comprehensive dental fear management plan.
- Pain control management is an important aspect of any dental fear management program.
- Managing children who are afraid of dentistry requires different skills than those used for adults.

RELEVANCE TO CLINICAL PRACTICE

Dental fear and dental anxiety are still prevalent among the general population, despite current pain relief measures and dental professionals' awareness of the problem.[1] According to numerous dental fear surveys, between 10% and 20% of adults in the United States avoid seeking regular dental treatment due to extreme dental fear.[2] The prevalence of dental fear has not changed significantly since the 1950s.[2,3] Additionally, various dental fear assessments show that 45% of patients report having moderate dental fear while obtaining oral health care.[4] The problems associated with dental anxiety and fear not only affect the oral health and treatment of a large percentage of the population, but they can also affect the dental clinician's ability to adequately treat his or her patients.[4]

The dental hygienist, being the dental team's prevention specialist and the team member who often spends the most time with patients, has the opportunity to positively affect patients' oral health care by effectively minimizing and managing fear and pain appropriately. Planning and managing patients' dental fears, anxiety, and pain will naturally result in a less stressful work environment for the dental hygienist as well.

DEFINITIONS

Dental anxiety, fear, and phobia are related, yet distinctive, terms that are often used interchangeably, especially by patients. All of these states produce similar physiological and cognitive responses in the body. **Dental fear** is described as a reaction to a known danger, stimulus, or an immediate threat. This uncomfortable reaction can be mental, emotional, or physical.[5] The sight of dental instruments, for example, can be an immediate threat to a dentally fearful patient. This threat may produce such physiological changes as tachycardia, profuse perspiration, and hyperventilation, along with numerous other physical, mental, and emotional states associated with the "fight-or-flight" syndrome, or stress response. This patient may literally feel like running from the circumstances! This phenomenon is short lived, as the responses subside once the threat is no longer present.

Dental anxiety is a nonspecific, ambiguous feeling of unease. It is anticipatory in nature, as there is no immediate threat and the source of the future threat is unknown. The dentally anxious patient will feel apprehensive, have negative thoughts, and imagine that negative experiences will occur about an upcoming dental appointment.[6] The major distinction between dental fear and dental anxiety is the immediacy of the threat or stimulus.

Significant fear, to the degree of being excessive, irrational, and persistent in response to either the presence of the threat or stimulus or the anticipation of that threat, is **dental phobia**. Fearful or anxious patients often will refer to themselves as being dental phobic.

What distinguishes a true dental phobic patient from the anxious or fearful patient is the intensity of the fear of the threat. A dental phobic patient will avoid the situation. This is the patient who does not seek regular oral health care and is generally only seen for emergency visits. A patient with dental phobia who does present in the dental office will be extremely fearful and exhibit poor coping skills. This perpetuates a negative cycle of imprinting the phobia further in the patient's mind. Referral to a mental health professional may likely be needed to proceed with any further dental care (see Professionalism).

THE EFFECTS OF DENTAL ANXIETY

The effects of dental fear or anxiety reach far. As stated previously, between 10% and 20% of the adult population avoids regular dental care. This can result in social embarrassment, poor self-esteem, and even, in extreme cases, personality changes.[7] When dental care is avoided due to extreme fear, people will often endure pain as long as possible until it exceeds the pain they had anticipated at a dental office. Even patients who are not extremely fearful, but who fall into the category of moderately anxious or fearful, will often cancel appointments, delay treatment, or wait longer than recommended for their dental hygiene preventative care appointment. The consequences of delayed dental care can be detrimental to the patient's oral and systemic health.

Avoidance and delay of treatment produces more treatment, increased costs, and, very often, more pain. What could have been a small restoration for minor decay now requires a more costly crown. Longer delays may now result in endodontic treatment of the tooth, another anxiety-producing event, and a more costly one.

Periodontal conditions are likely to be more severe, too. This results in more extensive treatment such as scaling and root planing, the use of local anesthetics delivered by the dreaded "needle," more visits, and often an additional referral to a periodontist. The cost of care keeps adding up.

The ultimate cost, however, is the "vicious cycle of dental fear," as termed and studied by Armfield et al (Fig. 31-1).[1] Their research validated previous theories and research on how dental fear contributes to avoidance of dental care, leading to more dental problems, which, in turn, most often results in negative dental experiences, which exacerbates the original dental fear.[1] The effects of the vicious cycle of dental fear reinforce the need for all dental professionals to establish a comprehensive dental anxiety and pain management program.

Children who are fearful of the dental profession are set up to become caught in this vicious cycle of dental fear if their fear is not managed immediately. Managing the dentally fearful child requires a different set of tools and behaviors that all dental professionals should know. Children represent the future, and their oral health is vital to a thriving community.

Finally, it is important to understand how the effects of dental fear extend to all dental professionals as well. In the article "Stress, Fear and the Well Dental Office," the author states, "A daily caseload ranging from patients in intense pain to routine care with underlying fear/anxiety can cause wear and tear on the psyche of dentists and the entire office team. Over time, symptoms of this stress become more noticeable."[6] It requires additional energy, focus, and time to treat fearful patients, which, when not properly managed with an anxiety and pain control plan, can cause distress and burnout for the dental hygienist and other oral health-care practitioners.

Onset and Etiology of Dental Fear and Anxiety

For many years, dental anxiety had been regarded as originating in childhood and persisting into later life.[8] Locker et al found, instead, that only 50% of the dentally anxious participants reported that their dental fear began in childhood, 22% reported that it began

Professionalism

Treating dentally fearful patients requires the dental hygienist to be professional at all times. Exhibiting confidence, along with compassion for the patient's problem, shows the patient that he or she is in good hands and helps to establish the rapport so essential to the patient's success. Being a professional also includes identifying and referring patients whose psychological problems may require skills beyond the average practitioner's ability to treat the patient successfully. ■

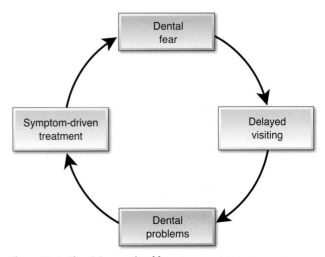

Figure 31-1. The vicious cycle of fear. (From Armfield JM, Stewart JF, Spencer AJ. The vicious cycle of dental fear: exploring the interplay between oral health, service utilization and dental fear. *BioMed Central Ltd.* 2007. doi:10.1186/1472-6831-7-1.)

in adolescence, and 27% reported adult-onset of dental anxiety.[8] Understanding this is crucial to the dental hygienist and other dental staff to ensure that all patients, not just children, are given the care and attention for preventing or reducing dental anxiety.

Dental fear and anxiety can be learned through a variety of experiences, regardless of age of onset. Children generally learn to be dentally fearful either by a direct unpleasant or traumatic dental experience or through vicarious learning.[8] Vicarious learning of dental fear results when other people, such as role models, peers, and/or society, influence an individual before he or she actually has the experience. An example of vicarious learning of dental fear would be when a child, who has never been to a dental office, observes, consciously and unconsciously, his or her parent being nervous when talking about an upcoming dental appointment and concludes that there is something to fear when going to the dentist. Another child might hear negative stories of one or more dental experiences dramatized over and over again by a dentally fearful parent, with the result that the child forms the belief that "bad" things happen when at the dentist. Both of these children may well exhibit fearful physiological and behavioral responses at their first dental visits, even though they did not have a direct adverse personal experience themselves.

The most-cited cause of dental fear comes from a *direct* personal experience as a result of a past traumatic or unpleasant dental episode occurring in childhood.[8] This classical direct conditioning model, wherein a stimulus such as pain produces the fear response, results in expectations of painful future treatments and can have lasting consequences, perpetuating the vicious cycle of dental fear. It is interesting to note from various studies how adolescent and adult onset of dental anxiety is linked more closely to personality traits and the overall anxiety of the individual than to simply a response to a stimulus.[8,9]

In addition to direct conditioning (painful or unpleasant experience provoking the fear response) and vicarious learning (learning fear from another's experience), dental fear and dental anxiety can be associated with personality traits and general psychological behaviors of individuals. For example, studies on general anxiety have shown that people who are generally anxious will tend to engage in negative or catastrophizing thinking. These same anxious people are shown to have three times as many negative thoughts as patients with low anxiety.[9] This type of thinking will reinforce any previous negative dental experience, and produce negative anticipation of any future dental care.

Fear of pain, perception, loss of control, perceived danger, unpredictability, disgustingness, and embarrassment may contribute to dental fear.

Fear of Pain

Numerous research studies define fear of pain as a key component of dental fear. Bradley et al found that individuals anticipating a painful stimulus showed greater heightened physiological responses, such as accelerated heart rate and changes in skin conductance, than when actually experiencing the uncomfortable stimulus.[10] Participants with high dental fear reported the anticipation of the uncomfortable stimulus to be more unpleasant than participants with low dental fear. Additionally, patients with high dental fear rated a mildly uncomfortable stimulus as being more uncomfortable than did those with low dental fear.[10,11] It can be inferred that pain threshold and pain tolerance are lowered whenever fear or anxiety is present. According to Milgrom et al, this has been clinically and experimentally established.[5] Commonly reported fear of pain includes pain associated with receiving an injection and drilling of teeth. Even noninvasive procedures, such as prophylaxis, can be seen as painful, and therefore feared.

Perception

Armfield et al propose that not all dental fear is acquired from experience, but rather through cognitive means. Their study Cognitive Vulnerability and Dental Fear found that a person's *perception* of a stimulus or situation is at the core of dental fear.[12] Perceptions of uncontrollability, unpredictability, dangerousness, and disgustingness are the specific elements that create powerful feelings of vulnerability. The Cognitive Vulnerability Model (Fig. 31-2) describes how exposure to dental stimuli or situations provokes an individual's particular schema, or system, of vulnerability, creating a series of emotional, behavioral, and physiological reactions.

Uncontrollability. Uncontrollability is often described by patients as feeling helpless or experiencing loss of control. Being in a supine position in the dental chair makes many fearful dental patients feel vulnerable and as if they have no control. Holding the mouth open for the dentist or hygienist to apply instruments adds to the perception of being helpless and having no control. These feelings are exacerbated by the perception of the dental office as a dangerous place.

Dangerousness. The dentally fearful patient worries that he or she will be harmed, something unpleasant will happen, and he or she will be uncomfortable at the dental office, whether or not discomfort has actually occurred in the past.[12]

Unpredictability. There has been little research into the role of unpredictability in relation to dental fear.[12] It makes sense that such an association would exist, as dental patients cannot view what is happening in their own mouths and are, for the most part, unable to anticipate when pain might occur.[12] If the hygienist or dentist fails to adequately explain the procedure, it is likely that the patient will also find the treatment process to be unpredictable, adding to his or her fear.

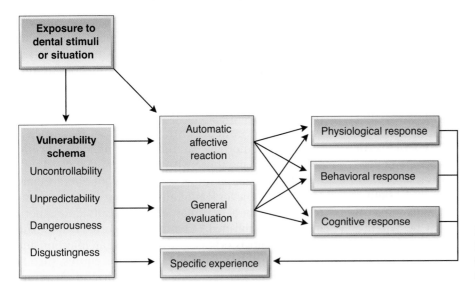

Figure 31-2. The Cognitive Vulnerability Model. (From Armfield JM, Slade GD, Spencer AJ. Cognitive vulnerability and dental fear. *BMC Oral Health.* 2008;8[2]. doi:10.1186/1472-6831-8-2.)

Disgustingness. This characteristic of the Cognitive Vulnerability Model was not examined in the Armfield et al study, nor has there been much research regarding the role of disgust in dental fear. However, there is some evidence that perception of disgustingness may be related to odors in the dental environment and fear of contamination with germs and disease.[12] There also seem to be generalized feelings of disgust related to blood, saliva, and peering into the mouth among the general population, which may be relevant to dental fear. Most dental professionals have probably heard negative comments about their profession related to this idea, such as "How can you work in someone's mouth? That is disgusting." Certainly, this is an area that needs more investigation. Even though it may not be as significant of a factor in dental fear as uncontrollability, dangerousness, and unpredictability, it behooves the dental hygienist and other members of the dental team to know it could be a perception factor involved in dental fear.

Embarrassment. Patients often cite embarrassment in surveys on dental fear as a reason to fear going to the dentist. A patient who has long neglected his or her oral health may feel embarrassed by or ashamed of that neglect and might fear being ridiculed or lectured.[1] Many people consider their mouths to be a very intimate aspect of their bodies, and having someone peering into their mouths can make them feel very vulnerable. This embarrassment and vulnerability can overlap with feelings of perceived helplessness and loss of control.[1]

The causes of dental fear and dental anxiety are many and complex. They include direct negative experiences, vicarious learning experiences, and cognitive and behavioral responses unique to each individual. The dental hygienist, being a key member of the dental team, can use this information to alleviate dental fear for his or her patients to support them in breaking the cycle of dental fear (see Spotlight on Public Health).

STRESS RESPONSE: THE SYMPATHETIC AND PARASYMPATHETIC NERVOUS SYSTEMS IN ACTION

The **stress response** is what happens to the body when fear is evoked. *Stress*, as defined by Hans Seyle, is a physical, emotional, psychological, and behavioral response to a particular situation or stressor.[13] Anything that is perceived by an individual as a threat to his or her well-being, whether real or imagined, causes what is often referred to as the fight-or-flight syndrome. For example,

Spotlight on Public Health

Although the literature is filled with research studies on dental fear and anxiety, its causes, and potential remedies, there is little information available on how this is being addressed as a public health concern. With the national emphasis on containing overall health-care costs, it would make sense to include dental health care in the equation. With the knowledge that dental fear leads to avoidance of care, which most often leads to more extensive and expensive treatments, it is imperative that dental fear and anxiety be recognized as a public health problem. Dental hygienists, taking the role as preventive care specialists, can position themselves as leaders in educating the public on how they can have a positive dental experience and avoid costly treatments. ■

in the dental office, if a patient perceives a threat, such as fear of pain, the stress response is immediately activated. It starts off in the hypothalamus of the brain, turning on the sympathetic division of the nervous system. In essence, it is turning on an alarm system, and preparing the body to fight, flee, or even freeze, another form of protection.[14]

The sympathetic nervous system is responsible for releasing the various stress hormones, including adrenaline and cortisol. These chemicals work to increase focus and concentration, and to speed reaction time. Heart rate increases and blood pressure rises, and the blood vessels constrict in the skin and other less vital organs of the body and dilate in the large muscles in the body, such as the legs and arms, to support the body in surviving.

After the removal of the threat, the parasympathetic system takes over to restore homeostasis to the body. Blood pressure decreases, blood vessels open to allow increased blood flow throughout the body, and neurotransmitters, such as endorphins, are released to replace the stress chemicals.[15]

It is important for the dental hygienist to understand the implications of the stress response when treating all patients, as any procedure could become stressful for a patient at any given moment due to perceived stressors or fear-evoking stimuli. When fear is present, there is more overall tension in the muscles (part of the stress response), resulting in more discomfort and fear of more pain to come. This produces feelings of vulnerability and the perception of unpredictability of what will happen next, along with feelings of uncontrollability, which instills more fear and heightens the stress response, which continues to cycle further into the chain of dental fear, if not immediately managed.[12] Observing patients' behaviors, in addition to gathering information from a verbal and physical assessment, will assist the hygienist in being prepared to manage patients' dental fear and stress response (Box 31-1).

MANAGEMENT PROGRAM

Evidence has shown that the cycle of dental fear perpetuates itself and has not changed significantly in the last 50 years.[1,2,3] Considering the number of people who avoid oral health care due to dental fear, anxiety, or phobia, having an articulated dental anxiety and pain control management program is extremely important.

A viable dental anxiety and pain control management program offers various benefits to the clinical practice:

- *Identification of dentally fearful patients* who are accessing regular dental care, yet are dentally fearful or anxious, to manage their oral health care appropriately.
- *Identification of the more highly dentally fearful patient* who is in the vicious cycle of dental fear, to help break that cycle and provide the oral care on a regular basis.

Box 31-1. *Observations for Signs of Stress and Anxiety in Patients*

Anxious Behaviors in Waiting Area
- Fidgeting
- Pacing
- Startled reactions
- Deep sighs/rapid breathing
- Rapid head movements
- Frequent changing of positions
- Nervously talking
- Statements of fear of dentists
- Negative statements about dentists

Anxious/Fearful Behaviors in Dental Treatment Chair
- Quiet demeanor; no talking
- Tense facial muscles
- Hands gripping chair
- Sweaty palms
- Perspiration on upper lip
- Rapid breathing
- Holding breath

- *Patient compliance:* When patients' fears are appropriately addressed and managed, the vicious cycle of dental fear can be broken and patients' oral health can be maximized.
- *Patient retention:* A viable dental anxiety and pain control plan builds rapport between the patient and oral health-care provider, which in turn keeps the patient coming back and referring friends and family as well.
- *Less stress* for the dental hygienist and other dental team members—having tools to help patients have a more comfortable experience, and perform oral care procedures with more ease—means that the hygienist and other dental staff feel more satisfied in their chosen field and less likely to experience burnout.
- *Promotes more positive associations with dental care:* As patients' fear concerns are addressed, pain is managed, and their overall experience in the dental office becomes easier, the negative associations can be reduced and be replaced with more positive ones.

Components of a Dental Fear and Anxiety Management Program

Assessment

Assessment sets the groundwork for the dental hygienist in understanding an individual's degree of anxiety or fear. It provides a means to plan the best course of action for any patient's unique needs. Several components and tools are used for a thorough assessment of dental anxiety and dental fear:[16]

- *Health and dental history questionnaires:* Health history questionnaires can provide pertinent information, such as past and present mental and other health conditions that could indicate emotional stresses. A questionnaire should also provide a list of current medications. The use of medications, such as antidepressants or drugs for anxiety, or even chronic use of pain relievers, can alert the hygienist to emotional or behavioral issues that could affect how the patient perceives his or her treatment.

- Most dental history questionnaires lack sufficient questions regarding patients' past dental experiences or their feelings about dental care. What questions they do have are generally too broad for the hygienist and dental team to effectively learn about their patients' past negative dental experiences or dental fears. A separate comprehensive dental history questionnaire is necessary. In addition to questions regarding current dental problems, oral homecare habits, and cosmetic desires, a comprehensive dental history questionnaire would include questions specific to dental anxiety. Questions can be designed to elicit a direct response on the form and to be conducive to further dialogue during a verbal interview, when the hygienist will be sure to approach all questions in a sensitive manner (Box 31-2).
- *Assessment surveys:* Assessment surveys are tools to identify levels of dental fear. There are various widely used tools for assessing dental anxiety and fear, such as Corah' Dental Anxiety Scale; Corah's Dental Anxiety Scale, Revised; the Modified Dental Anxiety Scale; and the Dental Fear Survey.
  - *Corah's Dental Anxiety Scale (DAS).* This tool is widely used and quite easy to administer. It consists of four brief multiple-choice questions pertaining to various dental treatment scenarios. Answers to the four questions are rated from 1 to 5, with scores ranging from 4 (no anxiety) to 20 (severe anxiety). Scores of 13 or 14 are indicative of moderate anxiety; those of 15 or higher indicate a highly anxious, fearful, or even phobic patient.[13]
  - *Corah's Dental Anxiety Scale-Revised (DAS-R).* In this assessment, the same four questions as used in the original DAS are revised to eliminate gender-specific terminology. The tool includes dental hygienists, in addition to dentists, as oral health-care providers (Fig. 31-3).[17]
  - *Modified Dental Anxiety Scale (MDAS).* This scale contains five questions with answers ranging from "not anxious" to "extremely anxious." The minimum score is 5, and the maximum is 25. According to Humphris, the author of the MDAS, evidence suggests that the mere completion of the questionnaire can significantly reduce anxiety in the practice setting.[18] A scoring value of 19 or greater indicates high dental anxiety. Although the assessment is based on the original DAS, the language of the questions is a bit different and the answers all contain the word *anxious* in them (Fig. 31-4).[18,19]
  - *Dental Fear Survey (DFS).* The DFS contains 20 items for the patient to rate from 1 to 5, with 5 being high intensity. These items relate to three areas of dental fear: avoidance of dental care due to fear, physiological responses (e.g., tensing of muscles during treatment), and fear of specific objects and/or situations in the dental environment (e.g., seeing or hearing the drill). A patient with a score of 75 or higher is considered to be highly dentally fearful. According to Heaton et al,[2] the DFS is highly reliable in predicting the dental fear of patients during dental treatment.[20]
  - *Dental Beliefs Survey.* This survey, developed by Smith et al in 1984, is designed to be complementary to the DFS, but focuses on a patient's *perceptions* of how the dental professional affects, or contributes to, the problem of the patient's dental fear.[21,22] It investigates three significant areas of concern: professionalism, or ethics; communication; and lack of control.[22] Some examples of questions are the following: *I have had dentists say one thing and do another (ethical); I feel uncomfortable asking questions (communication); Once I am in the chair, I feel helpless (lack of control).* This survey seems to be most beneficial for patients who have generalized anxiety or those who are distrustful, and would likely be used only after having procured that information from other assessments.

Interview Process

The verbal interview process is an integral component of a comprehensive dental anxiety and pain control management program. During the interview process, rapport can be built between the dental hygienist or other dental professional and the patient. One of the main objectives in conducting a verbal interview is to demonstrate to the patient the concern that the professional feels about

---

> ### Box 31-2. *Sample Questions for Dental History or Verbal Interview*
>
> 1. When was your last dental visit?
> 2. What was that dental visit for?
> 3. Have you had any unpleasant dental experiences in the past?
> 4. May I ask what happened when you had an unpleasant experience?
> 5. How do you generally feel when you know you have a dental appointment? Fine? Nervous? Extremely anxious?
> 6. Can you help me understand what is it about the dental office that is upsetting to you?
> 7. Did your parents have a positive attitude about going to the dentist?
> 8. Have you been satisfied with your previous dental care providers? If not, what was the cause of your dissatisfaction?
> 9. Is there any particular dental procedure that causes you the most anxiety?
> 10. What can I do to make your visit here today as comfortable as possible for you?

Corah's Dental Anxiety Scale, Revised (DAS-R)

Name _____   Date _____

Norman Corah's Dental Questionnaire

1.   If you had to go to the dentist tomorrow for a check-up, how would you feel about it?

   a. I would look forward to it as a reasonably enjoyable experience.
   b. I wouldn't care one way or another.
   c. I would be a little uneasy about it.
   d. I would be afraid that it would be unpleasant and painful.
   e. I would be very frightened of what the dentist would do.

2.   When you are waiting in the dentist's office for your turn in the chair, how do you feel?

   a. Relaxed.
   b. A little uneasy
   c. Tense.
   d. Anxious.
   e. So anxious that I sometimes break out in a sweat or almost feel physically sick.

3.   When you are in the dentist's chair waiting while the dentist gets the drill ready to begin working on your teeth, how do you feel?

   a. Relaxed.
   b. A little uneasy.
   c. Tense.
   d. Anxious.
   e. So anxious that I sometimes break out in a sweat or almost feel physically sick.

4.   Imagine you are in the dentist's chair to have your teeth cleaned. While you are waiting and the dentist or hygenist is getting out the instruments that will be used to scrape you teeth around the gums, how do you feel?

   a. Relaxed.
   b. A little uneasy.
   c. Tense.
   d. Anxious.
   e. So anxious that I sometimes break out in a sweat or almost feel physically sick.

Scoring the Dental Anxiety Scale, Revised (DAS-R)
(this information is not printed on the form that patients see)
a = 1, b = 2, c = 3, d = 4, e = 5   Total possible = 20

Anxiety rating:

9 - 12 = moderate anxiety but have specific stressors that should be discussed and
   managed

13 - 14 = high anxiety

15 - 20 = severe anxiety (or phobia). May be manageable with the Dental Concerns Assessment but
   might require the help of a mental health therapist.

Figure 31-3. Corah's Dental Anxiety Scale, Revised (DAS-R). (From Ronis RL, Hanson CH, Antonakos CL. Equivalence of the original and revised dental anxiety scales. *JDH.* 1995;Nov-Dec: 69. Reprinted with permission.)

the patient's concerns.[22] Effective two-way communication is a key aspect of establishing a positive relationship and helps build the trust that an anxious patient needs to feel. Evidence has shown how the behavior and demeanor of the dental professional greatly influence the perception a patient will have of his or her experience.[6,22] A calm, confident, and reassuring manner goes a long way in conveying to the patient that he or she is being taking seriously, and can even influence the patient's experience on that visit. The dental hygienist needs to be respectful, show concern, and never embarrass the patient, and needs to carefully choose words

Can you tell us how anxious you get, if at all, with your dental visit?
Please indicate by inserting X in the appropriate box.

1.   If you went to your dentist for **treatment tomorrow**, how would you feel?

Not   Slightly   Fairly   Very   Extremely
anxious ☐   anxious ☐   anxious ☐   anxious ☐   anxious ☐

2.   If you were sitting in the **waiting room** (waiting for treatment), how would you feel?

Not   Slightly   Fairly   Very   Extremely
anxious ☐   anxious ☐   anxious ☐   anxious ☐   anxious ☐

3.   If you were about to have a **tooth drilled**, how would you feel?

Not   Slightly   Fairly   Very   Extremely
anxious ☐   anxious ☐   anxious ☐   anxious ☐   anxious ☐

4.   If you were about to have your **teeth scaled and polished**, how would you feel?

Not   Slightly   Fairly   Very   Extremely
anxious ☐   anxious ☐   anxious ☐   anxious ☐   anxious ☐

5.   If you were about to have a **local anesthetic injection** in your gum, above an
upper back tooth, how would you feel?

Not   Slightly   Fairly   Very   Extremely
anxious ☐   anxious ☐   anxious ☐   anxious ☐   anxious ☐

Instructions for scoring (remove the section below for use with patients)

The Modified Dental Anxiety Scale. Each item scored as follows:

Not anxious   =   1
Slightly anxious   =   2
Fairly anxious   =   3
Very anxious   =   4
Extremely anxious   =   5

Total score is a sum of all five items, ranging from 5 to 25. A score of 19 or above indicates
a highly dentally anxious patient, possibly dentally phobic.

Figure 31-4. The Modified Dental Anxiety Scale (MDAS). (From Humphris GM, Morrison T, Lindsay SJE. The Modified Dental Anxiety Scale: validation and United Kingdom norms. *Comm Dent Health.* 1995;12:143-150. Available from http://www.biomedcentral.com/1472-6831/13/29; BMC Oral Health 2013, 13:29. doi:10.1186/1472-6831-13-29)

that encourage the patient to express his or her concerns, worries, doubts, and fears. The tone of the professional's voice is equally important. If the hygienist's tone conveys belittlement, criticism, or disbelief at what the patient is communicating, it will produce a negative impression, no matter what words are being said (see Box 31-1).[22] The verbal interview can be conducted before or after the patient has completed one of the dental fear surveys. Conducting the interview after the DFS allows the dental hygienist to have access to the answers the patient reported on the DFS. That information will assist the hygienist in sensitively asking the appropriate questions to discover more about the circumstances of the patient's fear and how to effectively proceed with treatment. See Application to Clinical Practice.

Summing Up the Need for Assessments

Most research has shown that dental professionals recognize anxious patients, yet many feel ill-equipped to effectively deal with dental anxiety.[22] They also feel anxious themselves when working on anxious patients, and are dubious about discussing fear with their patients for fear of making it worse.[22] Yet research has shown that patients actually feel relieved when asked about and being able to express their fears and anxiety about dental care.[23] In light of that evidence, it seems prudent for the dental hygienist to take a proactive stance and to proceed in using the various assessment tools available to provide the best experience possible for the patient, helping to break the vicious cycle of dental fear.

Application to Clinical Practice

A new patient in the waiting area is looking very nervous. She has already seen the dentist at a previous appointment, so you look in her records to learn more about her. The notes from the dentist and dental assistant indicate that they did not use a formal dental fears assessment survey when they initially saw her due to time constraints. The notes indicated that the patient reported to the dentist that she has had moderate to severe dental anxiety for as long as she can remember. She has not had her teeth cleaned in at least 5 years because she has been afraid to step into a dental office. She has some toothaches, which caused her to seek help. The dentist did some triage and palliative care using nitrous oxide and local anesthetic. He wants her to have a complete periodontal assessment before he continues further. What are some things you would do to make her dental hygiene care appointment as comfortable as possible? ■

Teamwork

Addressing patients' dental fear and anxiety requires the participation of the entire dental team. Having a comprehensive dental fear management program will ensure that each team member understands his or her role in helping identify these patients. Effective communication within the team assures that appropriate management tools and techniques can be implemented.

For example, when the fearful patient is being relaxed by the hygienist, other staff members are cognizant of the patient's needs and the procedure, making sure they are being quieter and nondisruptive in the operatory.

Teamwork may also include referring a patient to an appropriate health-care professional or other professional, such as a psychologist, a biofeedback specialist, or hypnotherapist, when the management of that patient is out of the scope of the dental team's practice.

Teamwork is an essential component of managing dental fear, not only for the patient, but for the dental team as well. ■

Cognitive and Behavioral Management

A comprehensive dental anxiety and pain control management program must go beyond the initial written and verbal assessments, which determine the degree of dental anxiety; it must provide tools for managing the cognitive (mental/psychological) and behavioral aspects of the patient. Research has shown how a wide variety of cognitive and behavioral strategies can effectively reduce dental anxiety and reduce patients' discomfort.[23]

Environment and Staff

A key element in managing patients' fear and anxiety starts with providing a comfortable dental environment. When walking through the door to a dental office, the patient must feel welcomed and acknowledged, not only by a positive attitude from the front desk staff, but from the physical surroundings as well. Relaxing furniture, warm colors, and soft, soothing music can provide an atmosphere of comfort, ease, and safety, setting positive expectations right from the beginning. Feelings of helplessness, of being out of control, and of not having their needs attended to are some of the concerns anxious patients express in self-reports on dental anxiety.[22] To convey an attitude of concern for the patient, it is important for the front desk staff to inform patients, especially the dentally anxious ones, if there is any delay in the schedule, instead of keeping them waiting, wondering when they will be seen, and reinforcing those beliefs (see Teamwork).

In the treatment areas, to ensure that dentally anxious or fearful patients do not see fearful stimuli such as dental instruments, it is best to cover instruments with the patient napkin or keep them out of sight until the patient is reclined and the hygienist is ready to use them. The environment needs to look professional and comfortable at the same time. Medicinal smells need to be reduced or eliminated through optimal ventilation or aromatherapy. Ensuring that the environment is as quiet as possible, free from the high-pitched sound of dental handpieces and other patients' negative comments or sounds of pain, will enhance feelings of comfort for these patients. Some anxious patients can be concerned about infection control issues; therefore the treatment room needs to be viewed as clean, with the appropriate barrier protections for the patient to observe, while at the same time not appearing too medicinal. The dental hygienist, as a pivotal member of the dental team, should dress professionally and avoid the all-white institutional look, which can promote white-coat syndrome. These are examples of **iatrosedation**, defined as "the act of making calm by the doctor's [dental hygienist's] behavior." These types of verbal and nonverbal communications (behaviors) can positively influence patients' responses in the dental office. An attitude of confidence, caring, and concern by the hygienist goes a long way in helping to allay dental fears (Box 31-3).[24]

Communication and Rapport

As already alluded to in various sections of this chapter, positive communication is one of the most important aspects when treating a dentally fearful or anxious patient.[22] Positive communication is not just dependent on the words thoughtfully chosen by the dental hygienist; it also provides a platform for the patient to feel comfortable to express fears without being ridiculed, dismissed, or embarrassed. Positive communication leads to good rapport, which establishes a trusting relationship between the patient and hygienist. Trust provides a foundation to support the patient in feeling less anxious or fearful. Good communication and rapport-building skills should be practiced by all staff members, beginning with the front desk and extending to all team members in the back treatment rooms.

Listed here are some strategies for positive communication and rapport building:

- Exude a warm and caring demeanor when greeting and escorting the patient back to the treatment room.
- Be genuine and engaged when inquiring about how the patient is feeling. Maintain eye contact, which builds rapport.
- Explain the treatment plan for the appointment and what will occur. Inquire if the patient has any questions about the procedure. This addresses the concern that some fearful patients have about not knowing what is going on and the perceived loss of control, and also takes away any surprise elements.[12,22,25]
- Obtain the patient's permission to start. Granting this permission allows the patient to feel some control over the circumstances, shows respect for his or her fear of loss of control, and provides a positive experience to help form more positive expectations going forward.
- Communicate how the patient can participate by stopping the procedure; for example, tell the patient, "If at any time you need me to stop, simply raise your hand, and I will stop." The patient may test this protocol several times to be certain that the hygienist will be true to his or her word before the patient can feel safe enough to relax and allow the treatment to continue.[22,25]
- Keep asking how the patient is doing as the oral care procedure proceeds. This shows that the dental hygienist is caring and respectful of the patient's comfort and is not just hurrying to get the procedure done.
- Choose words to help direct the focus to a positive outcome.[22] Telling the patient "There may be some discomfort when I scale this area" produces less anxious anticipation than saying, "This is probably going

to be painful." "I am going to numb that area for you so you can be comfortable" is more positively phrased and produces less anxiety than "I am going to give you a shot."
- Set up positive expectations for the future. Communicate to the patient how well he or she did during the procedure. Communicate that the patient can expect the same attention to his or her needs at each oral care visit. If there was a procedure done, such as scaling and root planing, use language that encourages the patient to expect a positive result and minimal discomfort. Statements such as, "The procedure went very well today. I expect your gums to heal normally. Most patients experience very little discomfort, and I imagine this will be the case for you as well. You can take a mild analgesic such as ibuprofen, if you would like, and rinse with warm salt water, and that should be fine. You may call the office if you should experience anything different, but I am not expecting that you will need to" work well to set up positive expectations for healing and comfort. The research in the arena of positive expectations or beliefs is promising in helping health-care professionals understand more about the power of the placebo effect. Bruce Lipton, PhD, author of *Biology of Belief,* defines the placebo effect as when the mind, through positive suggestions, improves health.[26] The dental hygienist and dental team should help their fearful patients have thoughts and expectations toward healing and health to assist further in breaking the vicious cycle of dental fear.[22]

Cognitive and Behavioral Management Techniques

At the Dental Fears Research Clinic at the University of Washington in Seattle, Dr. Peter Milgrom and his team use a wide variety of cognitive and behavioral techniques to reduce their patients' fears and anxiety, assist them in coping with the procedures, and manage their pain. These techniques work very well in a specialized clinic, and have also provided an immense amount of research to assist the general practitioner in treating fearful dental patients. However, for the general practice clinician, it is not feasible to know how to use all of the techniques, as some require specialized training. It is important, though, for the dental hygienist to learn about various techniques that are available and which ones can be utilized most easily and successfully to help anxious and fearful patients.

Distraction. Distraction shifts the patient's attention from the dental procedure to something else. Milgrom et al rank it as one of the easiest coping strategies and the one most familiar to dental professionals.[22] Many studies have shown it to be an effective means to lessen anxiety for mildly to moderately anxious dental patients. In one study by Frere et al, audiovisual (AV) glasses (AV glasses are worn by patients, allowing them to watch and hear either TV shows or movies) were used during the dental prophylaxis procedure. The results were positive for patients who were *not* highly anxious. They reported reduced anxiety and pain, although some of them did report missing the interaction with the clinician.[27] The highly anxious patients did not receive any benefits with this distraction, and, in fact, some reported that it interfered with their own coping mechanisms. The use of an assessment tool, including a verbal interview, can assist the hygienist in learning what can help the patient.

Other types of distraction include conversation, television, use of headsets or CD players with music, audio books, or guided relaxation, all self-selected by patients (see Advancing Technologies). Another type of distraction, especially good for those patients who have a tendency to gag, is to have the patient raise one leg when taking radiographs. This changes the focus from the radiograph in their mouths to the leg being lifted from the chair. Because the brain can only truly focus on one thing at a time, it is an effective distraction method. Children can be distracted by conversations about something special to them.

Things to note when considering distraction to help reduce anxiety include the following:

- Distraction works best on mildly to moderately anxious patients.
- Patients may still need a rest break.
- It works best for short-duration procedures.
- It may not be effective for patients being administered local anesthetics.

Modeling. Modeling is a behavior strategy that works well with children, because they are natural observers and learn behaviors through watching others. When modeling is used, the fearful child views someone else, usually a peer or an older sibling, undergoing a procedure. The child can watch a live demonstration or a video. The observation provides information about the procedure and the appropriate behavior during the procedure.[28] This experience is nearly identical to vicarious learning, one of the causes of dental fear in children, only now the method is used purposefully for producing a positive outcome for the child. Studies have shown that when fearful and disruptive children were shown videos of other children doing well and receiving praise for their behavior, the fearful/disruptive children had significant reductions in their negative behaviors. They had learned the appropriate coping skills to use during their own procedures by watching the successful performance of the observed children.[28]

Modeling can be accomplished in the private setting by having a younger child watch an appropriately behaved older sibling having oral health-care provided.

Tell–Show–Do. Tell–Show–Do is a procedure that is also very successful with children, although adults can benefit as well. Milgrom uses this technique at his dental fears clinic.[22] It is especially useful for teaching patients about new sensations. It provides information and uses demonstration before proceeding with a procedure. An example might be showing the patient how an instrument will touch the teeth and the gums on a model, after first telling the patient what will be happening. The next step is to tell the patient that the same thing is now going to happen to his or her own teeth. The procedure is then performed while keeping the patient informed throughout and also allowing the patient to interact. Sometimes having the patient hold a mirror is useful too, as it can create a disassociation from the fear and the patient can actually see what is happening. It is important to continue to keep the patient informed as to how long the procedure will take and how far it has already progressed; this helps to reduce the patient's anxiety.[22,28]

Relaxation Techniques

Relaxation techniques elicit the **relaxation response,** a term coined by Herbert Benson, MD.[29,30] The relaxation response, the opposite of the stress response, activates the parasympathetic nervous system, bringing the body back from the rigors of the fight-or-flight phenomena. Various biochemicals assist in the process, and the heart and respiratory rates decrease, blood pressure is lowered, and muscle tension is decreased. This physiological relaxation allows the mind to relax as well. It seems that it is not possible to have physical relaxation and an anxious mind at the same time, because the brain cannot process those two feelings simultaneously. The body and mind work together, so if the body is relaxed, the mind becomes relaxed. This works both

Advancing Technologies

With the increasing use of personal electronic devices, it is now easier than ever for patients to download various apps to their smartphones or mp3 devices that support them in having a more comfortable dental experience. Patients can easily listen to music of their choice on their own devices, or the dental team can suggest an application suitable for them to use. There are apps for everything from guided relaxation to audio books, all designed to help distract the patient from the environment and make them feel more comfortable.

Another popular use of technology for the dentally fearful patient is movie eyeglasses. This technology allows patients to enjoy a movie of their choice, distracting them from the visual triggers that cause them to feel fearful. ▪

ways: If the mind is calm, the body releases muscle tension and relaxes. Relaxed patients experience less physical and mental discomfort during dental care.[22] Relaxation techniques include focused breathing exercises, muscle relaxation, and guided imagery, or a combination of any or all of these. It is important before implementing any relaxation technique to explain to the patient how relaxation diminishes discomfort and how it will help him or her to manage the anxiety. This would also be the ideal time to inquire if the patient uses any special coping techniques in other stressful situations, so as not to add any additional stress by asking the patient to learn something new. Asking the patient's permission to guide him or her in the relaxation process is essential. Box 31-4 provides a sample script for preparing the patient for a guided relaxation exercise.

Focused Breathing. One of the easiest techniques for dental hygienists to teach and for patients to learn is focused breathing. When a patient is anxious or fearful, he or she often breathes in short, shallow breaths or sometimes even holds his or her breath. Inefficient breathing results in oxygen-poor blood circulating in the body, which, in turn, adds to the cycle of physical tension, more stress, and poor coping skills.[22] The hygienist can help patients elicit the relaxation response by teaching them the coping skill of focused deep breathing. Focused deep breathing allows more oxygen to flow to the brain and muscles, and brings a sense of calm. This technique can demonstrate to the patient how he or she can use inner resources to manage the anxiety. The dental hygienist can model the technique, breathing along with the patient, providing a benefit for both the patient and the professional. Box 31-5 gives instructions on how to guide patients in focused breathing.

Progressive Muscle Relaxation. Progressive muscle relaxation, originally devised in 1938 by Edmund Jacobsen, a physician and researcher of muscle physiology, is a systematic technique to help people relax; it is easy to learn and is effective.[22,31] This type of relaxation starts with slow tensing of individual muscle groups for 5 to 7 seconds, followed by release of the tension and relaxation of the same set of muscles for 20 to 30 seconds. The tension–relaxation process progresses from the lower to upper body, eliciting more and more relaxation along the way. The dental hygienist guides the patient through the process while bringing the patient's attention to the difference between a tense and a relaxed muscle. Relaxed muscles help the mind, in turn, to relax, which reduces anxiety. Box 31-6 provides instructions.

Box 31-4. *Preparing the Patient for Guided Relaxation*

The dental hygienist should explain to the patient each relaxation technique that is offered and obtain permission from the patient to begin.

Enrolling language:

"I would like to help you feel better during this procedure by using some guided relaxation [or guided imagery, or guided focused breathing]. Would you like me to help you with that?

"These guided techniques can help your muscles relax and help your mind focus on pleasant, calming thoughts of your choice. When your muscles are relaxed, tension cannot be present. When your mind is focused on something pleasant, your body will respond by feeling more relaxed and calm. When you feel more relaxed, the sensations of the procedure feel more comfortable.

"With your permission, we can begin. Please know that you will be in control at all times and can signal me to stop, if you would like. I think you will find that this [these] technique[s] will work very well for you.

"Would you like to go on a 'mental vacation,' or simply allow all of the muscles in your body to feel relaxed as you focus on them one by one? We can do both, if you would like, and even start with focusing on your breathing first. What would you like to try?" ▪

Box 31-5. *Guided Focused Breathing*

Explain to the patient how being tense causes shallow breathing, which causes tense muscles, which cause more discomfort. When deeper breathing is practiced, more oxygen flows into the muscles, allowing them to relax, release, and let go. Be sure to obtain the patient's permission to begin (see Box 31-4).

1. Simply bring your attention to your breathing.
2. Perhaps you would like to bring your hands to rest on your abdomen so you can feel how your abdomen rises and falls when you inhale and then exhale. Right...
3. Take a good deep breath first and then release it. The body relaxes more each time you exhale.
4. Now all you have to do is keep your focus on your breathing and notice how you feel when you do. Whenever you find your mind wanting to focus somewhere else, you can simply remember to bring your attention back to your breathing and your hands on your abdomen.
5. I will keep reminding you periodically, if that is okay with you.
6. Whenever you need my attention, you can simply signal me by raising one of your hands and I will stop what I am doing and give you my full attention. ▪

Box 31-6. *Guided Progressive Muscle Relaxation*

Explain to the patient how consciously tensing the muscles and then relaxing them allows the patient to feel the difference between tension and relaxation. As the patient continues to do this, the body begins to relax. This technique can be combined with and follow focused breathing. Use a soft, soothing, and calm voice. Be sure to obtain the patient's permission to begin (see Box 31-4).

"We will begin by making sure that you are as comfortable as you can be in the dental chair. Uncross your legs and place your arms somewhere that feels best for you. Do whatever you need to do to get yourself comfortable. Good. Now, we are going to start with your hands. Clench your hands into a fist...tighten them...for a count of five—1, 2, 3, feel the tension?...4, 5. Good. Now release the tension and relax your fists and hands...notice how loose and relaxed they feel? Good. Now, do the same with your arms and up to your shoulders and neck...bring your shoulders up to your ears...tighten them—1, 2, 3, 4, 5...feel the tension...now...just let them go and relax them...do you feel the relaxation, the looseness, the softness? Good. Now, bring your attention down to your feet and legs...curl your toes, tighten your calves...just enough to feel some tension...do you feel it? Good. Now, let go and relax your toes, feet, and calves. Nice and relaxed now. Feel how much looser they are? Good, you are doing great. Now...tighten the upper legs and your buttocks and feel the tension—1, 2, 3, 4, 5. Good, now let go. Notice how loose they feel? Good. Bring your attention to your face and jaw...just scrunch your face and clench your jaw—1, 2, 3, 4, 5...and now let go...feel all the tension drain right out of your face...as your jaw opens slightly...and you feel your whole body sinking in to the chair...feeling loose and relaxed...allowing your entire body to stay relaxed, with your mouth open now...a natural position for your relaxed face....as we continue on....you did a great job at relaxing your body, a great job at helping yourself feel more comfortable."

Guided Relaxation. Guided relaxation differs from progressive relaxation in that it does not incorporate the alternating tensing and relaxing of the muscles. Instead, it focuses the mind to assist the body in relaxing the muscles. The hygienist can guide the patient to relax all of the various muscle groups by simply asking him or her to focus attention on the area and giving the patient suggestions of relaxation. Usually, guided relaxation is used in combination with focused deep breathing. The process can begin with having the patient focus on inhaling and exhaling deeply, then, after a few focused breaths, having the patient focus on the muscles relaxing. Relaxation is a natural response of the body, and, if the patient has given permission to be guided for the benefit of reducing anxiety, he or she should start to feel some relief in a very short time.

It can be helpful for the hygienist to practice using the slow and soft tone of voice that is best for this technique by recording a script first and listening to it to experience the guided relaxation firsthand, and to learn how to guide others in this technique. Alternatively, purchasing a prerecorded commercial relaxation CD and listening to it repeatedly will also provide the opportunity to experience guided relaxation while learning how to become comfortable in applying it with patients. Box 31-7 offers a sample of brief guided relaxation combined with guided imagery.

Guided Imagery. Guided imagery is similar to both guided relaxation and distraction because it is a guided method, usually incorporating relaxation, and it distracts the mind from the outer circumstances, instead focusing the patient on his or her own inner world. It is like a directed daydream or a mental vacation that utilizes the imagination of the patient.[22,31,32] In this technique, the hygienist guides the patient in focusing on a scenario the patient has chosen. The dental hygienist supports the patient's focus and daydream by verbally cueing him or her with mental images and other sensory details. Filling in such details as colors, sounds, and even textures keeps the imagination engaged while allowing the patient a pleasant inner experience away from the experience of the dental hygiene care. Using a soft, slow voice enhances the pleasantness of the experience for the patient. To begin using guided imagery, the dental hygienist asks if the patient has a favorite vacation spot or where the patient would go to relax. Guided imagery can follow the focused breathing technique and then some guided relaxation, or the patient can simply be invited to close the eyes (for better focus and to block out any fear-inducing stimuli) and simply be guided to that special place. Upon completing the dental hygiene care, the hygienist can suggest to the patient that he or she use this technique at any time to experience relaxation and a mental vacation (see Box 31-7).

Focused Attention. Focused attention, as discussed by Milgrom et al in *Treating Fearful Dental Patients,* has been shown in various studies to influence the experience of pain by increasing pain tolerance.[22] It incorporates the distraction technique because attention is focused on something other than the dental care. An example of focused attention could be when a patient focuses on a problem he or she is mentally engaged in solving, keeping the focus on the problem instead of the dental

Box 31-7. *Guided Relaxation Combined with Guided Imagery*

Explain to the patient that using the imagination can help relax the body and the mind, and help him or her feel more comfortable and at ease while on a "mental vacation." This technique can be combined with and follow focused breathing. Use a soft, soothing, and calm voice. Ask where the patient would like to go on vacation or somewhere to relax fully. Be sure to obtain the patient's permission to begin (see Box 31-4).

"We will begin by making sure that you are as comfortable as you can be in the dental chair. Uncross your legs and place your arms somewhere that feels best for you. Do whatever you need to do to get yourself comfortable. As we begin, you may find it easier to focus when you close your eyes...or, if you want to wait until you are absolutely ready to close your eyes, you can do that as well; it is your choice. Good...now focus for a few moments on your breathing...take a good deep breath; right...and let it out slowly...good. Do that a couple of more times...and each time you inhale, you might imagine you are inhaling relaxation, and every time you exhale, you are allowing relaxation to drift down over your entire body. You are doing great. Now...as you relax more and more with each and every breath, your imagination becomes more fluid... it is easier to imagine now that a wonderful wave of relaxation is starting from your head all the way down to your toes, relaxing every single muscle as this wave of relaxation passes through your body...allowing you to sink deeper into the chair...deeper into relaxation...good...now imagine that place you said you would like to be. Allow yourself to be there fully in your mind, focusing on the colors you may notice there...noticing the feel of the air on your skin...as you notice if there are any pleasant aromas you can smell...or perhaps you may hear some sounds...or you may simply hear the sound of silence. Notice, especially, how good it feels to be in this special place today...notice how calm, comfortable, and serene you feel being here. This is a place you can go to in your imagination anytime you wish to take a wonderful relaxing mental vacation. You can go to this place or any other place you chose every time you come in to the dental office. In fact, you may find it so much easier next time, even as you step into the door to the office, how much more comfortable you are...and when you sit in the dental chair, you find it is so much better as you just naturally go to your wonderful vacation spot and relax and enjoy the experience."

When it is time to end the dental care procedure, you can then say, "In a few moments, we will be all done...you have done such a great job...and, when you are ready, you can simply open your eyes, stretch your arms and legs, and come back to an alert state, feeling good, refreshed, and ready for the rest of your day." ■

care. Another example may be when someone mentally recites a prayer or a phrase (mantra) over and over again. Focused attention could also be used to direct the patient's attention to his or her body, focusing, for example, on a hand resting on the arm of the chair, or otherwise focusing attention on keeping a particular body area relaxed. For example, the dental hygienist could guide the patient to focus on his or her hand or hands being loose and relaxed while resting comfortably on his or her lap or the arm of the chair.[22] Because this technique is internally generated, it might be best used with patients already accustomed to practicing this strategy in other areas of their lives. Focused attention could be combined with focused breathing, and guided relaxation and guided imagery.

Hypnosis. Hypnosis is a natural focused state of mind. It has been described as being an inner ultrafocused and alert state in which the cognitive mind is less active and more relaxed. As the analytical and logical mind becomes more relaxed, it allows the individual to be more open to suggestions. During this state, the individual is more aware of his or her inner world of senses and imagery, which can be enhanced to provide comfort and pleasure, and aid in controlling anxiety.[33–38] Although practicing formal hypnosis requires specialized training, it is prudent for the dental hygienist to understand that when fearful patients are relaxed through guided relaxation and/or guided imagery, and focused attention, they are essentially in a focused state of mind that allows them to be naturally more open to suggestions. For example, most people have experienced the phenomena of being so absorbed in a book or movie that they feel they are part of it. When there is a tense or scary event in the book or movie, it will provoke the same physiological responses as if it were happening for real. This is a natural hypnotic state, and people go in and out of it on a regular basis during the day. Understanding of this natural state, even without formal training, should give the hygienist incentive to use words (suggestion) that help the patient have a positive experience. This makes it equally important *not* to use words that imply failure or might provoke anticipation of pain to occur during or after the procedure. This is called the nocebo effect, which is the opposite of the placebo effect (Box 31-8).

When the dental care provider is not trained in using hypnosis, the patient should be referred to a qualified hypnotherapist, who can assist the patient in overcoming dental fear and anxiety, and teach the patient self-hypnosis to use for future dental appointments. Unfortunately, the word *hypnosis* still provokes images of people quacking like ducks or engaging in some other stage hypnosis behavior, feeding into the misconception of being controlled by the hypnotist. These misconceptions and myths are unfounded and require the dental hygienist to be knowledgeable about hypnosis

Box 31-8. *Definition of the Nocebo Effect*

The opposite of the placebo effect (in which the mind, through positive suggestion or perception, thinks that a medicine or treatment that is otherwise ineffective will improve health), the *nocebo effect* is when the mind perceives negative suggestions about a treatment or medicine, and that perception negatively affects health and well-being.[26] ■

to convince the patient of its usefulness for him or her when indicated.

Some of the advantages of hypnosis that can benefit both the patient and the dental care clinician are as follows:

- *Decreased anxiety*: The dental care provider is able to treat the patient effectively, without involving sedation drugs and exposing the patient to their side effects.
- *Pain management*: The patient can learn to elicit mild to profound analgesia for operative and postoperative procedures, reducing the need for pain medications.[39]
- *Control of bleeding and salivation*: The autonomic nervous system can be influenced with hypnotic suggestions and imagery, which eases the clinician's care during treatment and assists in the patient's healing (with less bleeding).
- *Reduced healing time*: Hypnosis can help the body's healing responses through suggestions of a quick recovery, and suggestions pertaining to how the healing response works (e.g., "all the cells that assist in healing are making their way to the area that was worked on today, doing what the body knows how to naturally do so well").
- *Control of gagging*: Suggestions are used that work with the autonomic nervous system to effect change in this response. This results in the patient no longer needing to feel embarrassed, reducing the anxiety that would have accompanied the anticipation of gagging.
- *Control of bruxism and other habits such as thumb sucking and tongue thrusting*: These unconscious behaviors respond very well to hypnotic suggestions and therapeutic hypnotherapy.
- *Smoking cessation*: Hypnosis has been shown to be effective in helping people to stop smoking, providing additional benefit to a patient's oral and overall health. Referral to a hypnotherapist specializing in smoking cessation is optimal.

Biofeedback. Biofeedback measures a patient's physiological responses using electronic equipment. The information is then converted into visual, auditory, and/or other types of feedback signals, informing the patient of his or her own physiological state. The patient's awareness of these responses teaches him or her how to voluntarily control them. Stress responses, such as an accelerated heart rate and elevated blood pressure, can be brought to the patient's attention through biofeedback, enabling the patient to monitor and control bodily functions that the patient previously thought it was not possible to control.[22] Biofeedback has been used successfully for stress-related medical conditions, such as tension headaches, muscle pains, irritable bowel syndrome, and insomnia. It has also been used successfully to treat myofascial pain, teeth clenching, and bruxism, along with dental fear.[22] Biofeedback requires specialized equipment and training. It is out of the scope of practice for a dental hygienist, and therefore the patient must be referred to a biofeedback specialist.

Systemic Desensitization. Systemic desensitization is a process that gradually exposes a patient to a hierarchy of fearful stimuli while the patient is in a relaxed state.[22] Although it is similar to Tell–Show–Do, the important difference is that the patient is in a relaxed state while being exposed to the fearful stimuli. Because the desensitization starts with the least fearful stimuli and substitutes relaxation instead of fear, the patient learns to feel calm as he or she gradually progresses through the hierarchy to the original fearful stimulus. This can be done first through rehearsals or practice using the imagination and then in the real setting with the real stimuli.[22] Box 31-9 provides a sample of a simple systematic desensitization procedure.

Use of Pharmacological Agents

Although prescribing pharmacological drugs is out of the scope of practice for dental hygienists, they are part of the dental team and will want to be informed to help in planning a course of action for the fearful patient. Milgrom et al[22] state the importance of not only assessing which drug might be best, but also that the dental professional must communicate to the patient that there are alternative options to heavy sedation. Heavy sedation takes away a patient's coping skills, resulting in the same "out-of-control" feelings that dominate many patients' fears. It is important to use behavioral therapies in combination with any appropriate sedation to ensure behavior predictability, efficient treatment, and patient safety during dental care.[22]

Pain Control Management

Pain control management is an important aspect of dental hygiene care for the dentally anxious patient. As previously discussed, unpleasant experiences, whether direct or indirect, and physical pain are the major causes of dental fear and anxiety.[22] Because anxiety and fear result in lower pain tolerance, it behooves the dental hygienist to remember this when considering pain control support. Along with behavioral and cognitive approaches, the use of topical and

> **Box 31-9. *Example of a Simple Systematic Desensitization for Scaling Teeth***
>
> Patient thinks about having teeth cleaned with "those" instruments
> *Hygienist instructs patient to take a deep breath and focus on breathing and relaxing*
> Patient feels a scaler on a finger or fingernail
> *Hygienist instructs patient to take a deep breath and focus on breathing and relaxing*
> Patient watches a video of someone getting their teeth cleaned
> *Hygienist instructs patient to take a deep breath and focus on breathing and relaxing*
> Patient watches in a mirror while the hygienist positions the scaler in the mouth
> *Hygienist instructs patient to take a deep breath and focus on breathing and relaxing*
> Patient watches in a mirror as the hygienist rubs the scaler against the tooth
> *Hygienist instructs patient to take a deep breath and focus on breathing and relaxing*
> Hygienist places the instrument in the sulcus and against the tooth surface
> *Hygienist instructs patient to take a deep breath and focus on breathing and relaxing*
> Hygienist scales the tooth
> *Hygienist instructs patient to take a deep breath and focus on breathing and relaxing*
> Hygienist scales a quadrant
> *Hygienist instructs patient to take a deep breath and focus on breathing and relaxing*
> Hygienist scales the entire dentition
> *Hygienist instructs patient to take a deep breath and focus on breathing and relaxing*

local anesthetic drugs can be instrumental in having patients experience a pain-free dental appointment.[22] Experiencing a pain-free dental appointment will go a long way in helping the dentally anxious patient break the vicious cycle of dental fear (see Chapter 33 for thorough coverage of local anesthetics).[1,22] Reducing dentinal hypersensitivity is another means to reduce unpleasantness and discomfort during the dental hygiene appointment. There are many products available for this problem, and the dental hygienist should be familiar with their applications to make the patient more comfortable during his or her appointment (see Chapter 28). Finally, the use of nitrous oxide, although not the panacea for all dentally anxious patients, is a viable asset in managing pain (see Chapter 32).

CONSIDERATION AND MANAGEMENT OF THE ANXIOUS CHILD

When treating children, it is important for the dental team to remember that many dentally fearful people associate their fear of dentistry with a negative childhood experience, and a good, or poor, experience can set the foundation for future dental care. The hygienist must actively create a safe environment that provides for a positive experience and helps form a positive attitude for the child's future dental experiences. Patience and knowledge of developmental factors are considerations for the entire dental team when treating children, and help to build trust and cooperation. Prevention is easier than treatment.[22]

When treating the already fearful child, keep in mind that strategies that are successful for adults do not always work well for children. Children under the age of 5 years cannot follow long, detailed explanations, although modeling and the Tell–Show–Do technique have been shown to be effective. Fearful children are especially prone to feeling anxious in situations they perceive as being out of their control, or when feeling trapped and thus vulnerable. It is important to give them a sense of some control or participation. An example is to let them hold the saliva ejector or to ask them to raise their hand if they feel any discomfort. Milgrom et al propose that when children perceive that they have some control, they exhibit less fear.[22] Simple choices such as "Would you like to start here or here?" give children a sense of control. Of course, the hygienist must always follow through with the child's choice to keep building rapport. Complimenting children on how well they are doing ("you are doing a great job keeping your mouth open"; "thank you for holding Mr. Thirsty (the saliva ejector); you are a big help") in age-appropriate language provides incentive for cooperative behavior. Keeping children informed as to how much longer the procedure will take communicates respect and concern. Milgrom et al also promote teaching age-appropriate relaxation techniques for children to acquire coping skills. Showing children a limp and loose doll and asking them to imagine being as loose and limp as that doll can help them begin to learn to relax tense muscles.[22]

SUMMARY

Understanding how dental fear can affect a patient's oral health for a lifetime should provide the dental hygienist with a mind-set that focuses on creating a thoughtful, caring, and concerned dental care environment for the patient. Learning and applying the various cognitive and behavioral techniques that effectively reduce anxiety, promote relaxation, and give patients better coping skills are the building blocks for that environment. It is imperative for dental hygienists to keep building and improving that environment not only to help break the vicious cycle of dental fear for patients, but also to contribute to their own health and well-being and thrive as practitioners in dental care.

Case Study

A dental hygienist who is new to the office is seeing a patient of record for the first time. She has reviewed the patient's record and noticed a few notes about how nervous the patient tends to be during the dental hygiene appointment and how it was difficult to work on the patient due to her tenseness. There is a very old dental fears assessment survey in the patient's chart, which has not been updated for 5 years. This outdated dental fears assessment did not indicate that the patient was fearful of dental procedures.

Curious about the patient's recent propensity to be anxious during her dental hygiene care appointments, the dental hygienist decides to reassess the patient via a verbal interview process. With the patient sitting up, she asks the following questions:

Dental Hygienist: "Before we begin, I'd like to tell you that I want to help you have a comfortable experience today.

Patient: Okay. What can you do?

Dental Hygienist: I've seen some notations in your chart that you seem to be very nervous about having your teeth cleaned, which started about a year and a half ago. May I ask you some questions about that?

Patient: Yes, go ahead.

Dental Hygienist: Has anything changed in your life or here in the dental office that now has you feeling nervous?

Patient: I'm glad you asked, because I was afraid to say anything. I don't want to be a bad patient, so I just try to steel myself every time I come in.

Dental Hygienist: Can you tell me what happened to make you nervous?

Patient: The last time I was having a filling done on my lower right back tooth, I started to feel some pain, as if the anesthetic wasn't working very well. It wasn't terrible, but I tried to let the dentist know and he was busy talking to the assistant and wasn't paying any attention. I kept thinking he'd notice how tense I was, but he didn't. I kept thinking it might keep getting worse and worse, and I felt scared. It didn't get worse, but I felt anxious the whole time. I didn't say anything to him, as I thought perhaps I was just being a baby. Now, it seems every time I'm in the dental chair, my body just tenses right up. I never used to be this way.

Dental Hygienist: I'm so sorry that happened to you. I want you to know that you can tell us if anything is not working for you. You simply can raise your hand to signal us to stop. I will let the doctor know what happened, and I'm sure he will make sure that doesn't happen again. Meanwhile, let's focus on how we can make today's visit the best for you. Would that work for you?

Patient: Yes, I'd love that. I don't like feeling this tense and afraid.

Dental Hygienist: I understand completely. I'd like to use a guided relaxation and guided imagery process with you. Studies have shown how relaxing physically helps us perceive sensations in our bodies in a much more positive manner. Additionally, when you use your imagination to go to a "happy place," or some place that is very pleasant to you, your mind acts as if it's real, and your brain produces those feel-good hormones you've probably heard of, called endorphins. Those endorphins further support your body in feeling good, and you can take a mini-vacation in your mind and feel good the whole time, just like you do when you are on vacation enjoying yourself. How does that sound?

Patient: If it works, it'll be good. Let's give it a try.

Dental Hygienist: Okay. First, begin by bringing all your attention and focus to your breathing.

The dental hygienist continues by instructing the patient in using focused breathing, guiding her in relaxing her body, and using guided imagery to create that wonderful mini-vacation in the mind for the patient.

Throughout the appointment, as the dental hygienist is working, she reminds the patient of her special place and how great she is doing. At the end of the appointment, she reminds the patient how relaxed she was during this time in the dental chair and how the patient can go to her "happy place" in her mind any time she comes into the dental office. The dental hygienist also comments on how relaxed the patient's face looks as the she is coming back to the seated position in the chair.

As the patient leaves, she tells the dental hygienist that this was the most relaxing time she's ever had in the dental office and that she will remember this experience. The front office employee has heard what has happened and also comments on how relaxed the patient looks. The patient leaves feeling very good.

Case Study—cont'd

Case Study Exercises

1. After reading the patient's record, what else could the dental hygienist do to be sure the patient's dental fears were being addressed?
   A. Think to herself: "Oh no, this is going to be unpleasant."
   B. Apply topical anesthetic without telling the patient what she is doing and why.
   C. Have the front desk staff give the patient a new dental fears assessment form to complete when the patient comes in.
   D. Complete a new dental fears assessment form with the patient at the same time as the verbal interview.

2. The hygienist was demonstrating what type of behavior when she addressed the patient's anxiousness?
   A. Rapport
   B. Distraction
   C. Good communication skills
   D. Focused attention
   E. Both rapport and good communication skills

3. The hygienist chose not to use topical anesthetic for the prophylactic procedure. What was she teaching the patient?
   A. That the hygienist is in control
   B. Good coping skills for the future
   C. That relaxation provides comfort
   D. That the patient's fear does not matter to her
   E. Both good coping skills for the future and that relaxation provides comfort

4. Which statement would most likely be true?
   A. The hygienist was stressed out the whole time she was with the patient and relieved when the patient finally left.
   B. The hygienist felt calm and comfortable and enjoyed working on this patient.
   C. The patient was pretending to be relaxed to please the hygienist.

5. Guided relaxation and guided imagery are difficult to learn and should not be used by anyone not trained in cognitive behavior, such as a counselor or psychotherapist.
   A. True
   B. False

Review Questions

1. According to various dental fears surveys, how prevalent is dental fear among the general population?
   A. 5–10%
   B. 40–45%
   C. 10–20%
   D. 30–40%

2. Although planning and managing patients' dental fears and anxiety can be useful for the dental hygienist, it is time consuming and not likely to change the patient's experience in the dental environment. Using one or more of the various dental fear assessment tools to help manage patients' dental fears and anxiety may require extra time and may embarrass the patient, causing more stress for both dental hygienist and patient.
   A. Statement 1 is true.
   B. Statement 2 is true.
   C. Both statements are false.

3. Dental fear
   A. is less problematic now than it used to be.
   B. is defined as a reaction to a threat or a known danger.
   C. is a nonspecific feeling of unease.
   D. produces the fight-or-flight syndrome.
   E. is defined as a reaction to a threat or a known danger and produces the fight-or-flight syndrome.

4. Which of the following is NOT a possible result of dental anxiety?
   A. Social embarrassment
   B. Poor self-esteem
   C. Timely treatment
   D. More costly dental treatment

5. Avoidance and delay of treatment results in more treatment, increased costs, and, very often, more pain. Periodontal and endodontic treatments do not generally have a major effect on the dentally fearful patient.
   A. Both statements are true.
   B. Both statements are false.
   C. The first statement is true, but the second is false.
   D. The first statement is false, but the second is true.

Active Learning

1. Working in teams of two students, take turns being patient and dental hygienist. Choose one or two of the following scripts to practice (the enrolling language in Box 31-4 can be used as a lead-in to any of the others)
   a. Guided Focused Breathing (Box 31-5)
   b. Guided Muscle Progressive Relaxation (Box 31-6)
   c. Guided Relaxation Combined with Guided Imagery (Box 31-7)

   The patient pretends to be tense and anxious by breathing shallowly and clenching the hands or gripping the chair. The patient listens and notices the tone of the hygienist's voice while also paying attention to how those words are affecting her or his body. The hygienist reads the script(s) while observing how the patient is responding to the words and tone of voice.

   Switch roles and, when complete, record all observations and what was learned through playing the role of patient and hygienist.

2. Working in teams of two students, take turns being patient and dental hygienist. Follow the instructions in Box 31-9 describing desensitization for scaling teeth. If a video of a patient's teeth being scaled is not available, move to the next instruction. After the first patient has completed the desensitizing process, the hygienist asks the patient to describe the experience. The hygienist documents the patient's comments. Repeat the process by switching roles. ■

REFERENCES

1. Armfield JM, Stewart JF, Spencer AJ. The vicious cycle of dental fear: exploring the interplay between oral health, service utilization and dental fear. *BioMed Central Ltd*. 2007. doi:10.1186/1472-6831-7-1.
2. Heaton L, Carlson C, Smith TA, Baer RA, de Leeuw R. Predicting anxiety during dental treatment using patients' self-reports: less is more. *J Am Dent Assoc*. 2007;138;188-195.
3. Smith TA, Heaton LJ. Fear of dental care: are we making any progress? *J Am Dent Assoc*. 2003;134(8):1101-1108.
4. Binkley CJ, Gregg RG, Liem EB, Sessler DI. Genetic variations associated with red hair color and fear of dental pain, anxiety regarding dental care and avoidance of dental care. *J Am Dent Assoc*. 2009;140:896-905.
5. Milgrom P, Kleinknecht R, Weinstein P, Getz T. *Treating fearful dental patients: a patient management handbook*. Seattle, WA: Behavioral Dental Publications; 1985.
6. Kamin, V. Fear, stress, and the well dental office. *Northwest Dent*. 2006;85(2):10-18.
7. Moore R, Bordsgaard I, Rosenberg N. The contribution of embarrassment to phobic dental anxiety: a qualitative research study. *BMC Psychiatry*. 2004;4:10. doi:10.1186/1471-244X-4-10.
8. Locker D, et al. Age of onset of dental anxiety. *JDR*. 1999; 78(3):790-796.
9. Rowe, MM. Dental fear: comparisons between younger and older adults. *Am J Health Stud*. 2005;20(3/4): 219-224.
10. Bradley MM, Silakowski T, Lang PJ. Fear of pain and defensive activation. *Pain*. 2008;137(1):156–163. doi:10.1016/j.pain.2007.08.027.
11. Van Wijk AJ, Hoogstraten J. Experience with dental pain and fear of dental pain. *JDR*. 2005;84(10): 947-950. doi:10.1177/154405910508401014.
12. Armfield JM, Slade GD, Spencer AJ. Cognitive vulnerability and dental fear. *BMC Oral Health*. 2008;8(2). doi: 10.1186/1472-6831-8-2.
13. Corah NL. Development of a dental anxiety scale. *J Dent Res*. 1969;48:596.
14. Biology Reference. Stress response. Available from: http://www.biologyreference.com/Se-T/Stress-Response.html.
15. Wikipedia. Stress (biology). Available from: http://en.wikipedia.org/wiki/Stress_%28biology%29.
16. Newton JT, Buck DJ. Anxiety and pain measures in dentistry: a guide to their quality and application. *J Am Dent Assoc*. 2000;131(10):1449-1457.
17. Ronis RL, Hanson CH, Antonakos CL. Equivalence of the original and revised dental anxiety scales. *J Dent Hyg*. 1995;69:270-272.
18. Humphris GM, Dyer TA, Robinson PG. The Modified Dental Anxiety Scale: UK general public population norms in 2008 with further psychometrics and effects of age. *BMC Oral Health*. 2009;9:20. Available from: http://www.biomedcentral.com/1472-6831/9/20.
19. Humphris GM, Morrison T, Lindsay SJ. The Modified Dental Anxiety Scale: validation and United Kingdom norms. *Comm Dent Health*. 1995;12:143.
20. Kleinknecht RA, Klepac RK, Alexander LD. Origins and characteristics of fear of dentistry. *J Am Dent Assoc*. 1973; 86(4):842-848.
21. Smith TA, Weinstein P, Milgrom P, Getz T. An evaluation of an institution-based dental fears clinic. *J Dent Res*. 1984;63:272.
22. Milgrom P, Weinstein, P, Heaton, L. *Treating fearful dental patients; a patient management handbook*. 3rd ed. Seattle, WA: Dental Behavioral Resources; 2009.
23. Daily YM, Humphris GM, Lennon MA. Reducing patients' state anxiety in general dental practice: a randomized controlled trial. *JDR*. 2002;81:319-322.
24. Wikipedia. White coat hypertension. Available from: https://en.wikipedia.org/wiki/White_coat_hypertension.
25. Harp H, et al. A patient's perspective on how hygienists can decrease patient anxiety. *J Dent Hyg*. 2000;74(4):322.
26. Lipton B. *Biology of belief*. 2005. Hay House, Inc. Carlsbad, CA.
27. Frere CL, et al. Effects of audiovisual distraction during dental prophylaxis. *J Am Dent Assoc*. 2000;132:1031-1038.
28. Do C. Applying the social learning theory to children with dental anxiety. *J Cont Dent Prac*. 2004;5(1):1-8.
29. Benson H. *The relaxation response*. New York, NY: Avon; 1975.
30. Smith L. *Of mind and body*. New York, NY: Henry Holt and Co, Inc.; 1997.
31. Rossman M. *Guided imagery for self healing*. Tiburon, CA: Kramer; 2000.
32. Naparstek B. *Staying well with guided imagery*. New York, NY: Warner; 1994.
33. Alladin A. *Hypnotherapy explained*. United Kingdom: Radcliffe; 2008.

34. Fross G. *Handbook of hypnotic techniques: with special reference to dentistry*. Tampa, FL: Florida Hypnosis Center; 1988.

35. Grindler J, Bandler R. *Trance-formations neuro-linguistic programming and the structure of hypnosis*. Boulder, CO: Real People Press; 1981.

36. Hadley J, Staudacher C. *Hypnosis for change*. New York, NY: MJF Books; 1996.

37. GSC Home Study Courses. *567: Hypnosis in dentistry-implications and risks*. Sacramento, CA: GSC Home Study Courses; 2006.

38. Elman D. *Hypnotherapy*. Ventura, CA: Westwood Publishing; 1983.

39. Montgomery CH, DuHamel KN, Redd WH. A meta-analysis of hypnotically induced analgesia: how effective is hypnosis? *Int J Clin Exp Hypn*. 2000;48(2):138-153.

Chapter 32 | Nitrous Oxide/ Oxygen Sedation

Ann Brunick, RDH, MS

KEY TERMS

analgesia

anesthesia

anxiolytic

biohazard

conscious sedation

tidal volume

titration

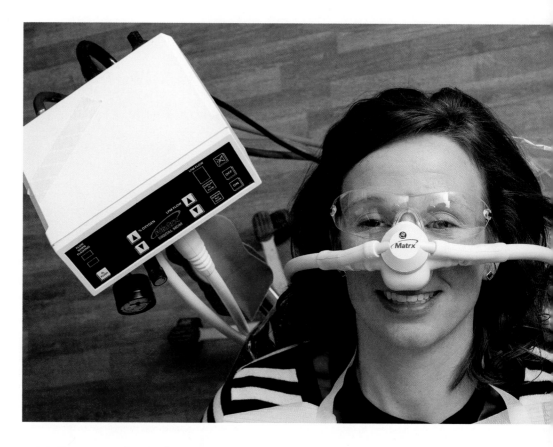

LEARNING OBJECTIVES

After reading this chapter, the student should be able to:

32.1 Explain the advantages and disadvantages of using nitrous oxide/ oxygen sedation as compared with other methods.

32.2 Discuss indications and contraindications of the use of nitrous oxide/oxygen sedation.

32.3 Identify the physical, chemical, and pharmacokinetic properties of nitrous oxide and oxygen.

32.4 Discuss the principles of respiration physiology, individual biovariability, and drug titration.

32.5 Recognize the armamentarium used to administer nitrous oxide/oxygen sedation.

32.6 State the importance of informed consent and preoperative patient assessment.

32.7 Describe the appropriation administration technique for nitrous oxide/oxygen sedation.

32.8 Identify the signs and symptoms of appropriate sedation.

32.9 Describe the procedure for recovery assessment, documentation, and patient dismissal.

32.10 Explain the importance of minimizing nitrous oxide exposure to the operator and office personnel.

32.11 Describe current recommendations for the prudent, ethical, and legal use of nitrous oxide/oxygen sedation for pain and anxiety management.

KEY CONCEPTS

- Nitrous oxide/oxygen sedation is an effective method for managing a patient's pain and anxiety.
- The titration method of administration is the current standard for clinical practice.
- Minimizing exposure to trace gas is important for all members of the health-care team.

RELEVANCE TO CLINICAL PRACTICE

There are many reasons why an individual may need pharmacological assistance during a dental appointment. Unfortunately, patients often present with pain and/or anxiety. Depending on their life circumstances, patients may wait to seek care until their pain is intolerable. And for those with any level of medical/dental anxiety, even the process of seeking care is a traumatic experience. Dental professionals may be called upon to treat both a patient's disease and his or her pain and anxiety. However, professionals have many options to assist these patients. Using nitrous oxide/oxygen sedation appropriately can result in a patient who is relaxed, comfortable, and able to tolerate many types of procedures.

INTRODUCTION

Nitrous oxide is a drug with a long history of use as an agent to ease pain and minimize anxiety. It first appeared in the late 1700s and was enthusiastically touted by a dentist, Dr. Horace Wells, in the mid-1800s. He used the drug routinely for extracting teeth. This advent of pharmacological intervention revolutionized how surgical procedures were completed and provided a segue for other agents and general **anesthesia**.[1]

Significant progress was made regarding the development and use of general anesthetics. Ether and chloroform were introduced. However, the acceptance and use of nitrous oxide expanded across the country and internationally, especially in the dental community. It was also determined that oxygenating the blood was important, thus the suggestion that oxygen be administered concomitantly with nitrous oxide. The extensive use of nitrous oxide and oxygen without incident established a safety record that continues until this day.

The modern-day world of pharmacology is astounding. Professionals struggle to stay current with the continuous outpouring of new medications. Reactions, side effects, and interactions with other drugs are reminders for constant vigilance and oversight of every patient. Nitrous oxide has several advantages in this respect. For the extent of its history, there has never been a documented case of a nitrous oxide allergy. It is nonirritating to mucosal tissues and it has very few interactions with other body systems. It can be used on most individuals and works well with a range of ages, abilities and disabilities, and other health/disease situations.[2]

Conscious sedation and ambulatory health care work very well together. Same-day procedures and outpatient clinics/facilities offer options to patients that are less expensive and less time intrusive. Oral, intravenous (IV), and nitrous oxide/oxygen sedation are common ways to assist those procedures that do not require general anesthesia. Dental procedures, traditionally done in an ambulatory setting, are currently being done with any or a combination of these methods. It is important to note that nitrous oxide can be used in combination with other drugs; however, diligent monitoring of the patient is required in any situation involving polypharmacy.

INDICATIONS

Nitrous oxide/oxygen sedation is primarily used to reduce pain and alleviate fear and anxiety. It can be used alone or in careful combination with other agents. **Analgesia** and/or pain modulation can be accomplished using nitrous oxide and oxygen. As with any other drug, individual biovariability can enhance or limit the extent of effect. Individuals differ in their perceptions of, reactions to, and tolerance of pain. Individuals also vary in how they perceive, react to, and tolerate pain within themselves on different occasions. Many factors influence the interpretation of pain at any given time. Pain is often accompanied by fear and anxiety. Anxiety often presents as a nervous preoccupation with having an unpleasant or worrisome experience; it is a symptom of an apprehensive, or uneasy, feeling about a situation or event. Fear is a response to a perceived threat; it is a distressing sensation in response to something specific. People can name their fears and will say, for example, "I am afraid of needles, spiders, heights." Fear will provoke a physiological response in many cases. It is common to see perspiration, increased heart rate and respiration, cool and clammy skin, and/or shaking. People may shed tears, faint, clutch the arms of a bed or chair, refuse to cooperate, be silent, or talk obsessively. In these cases, nitrous oxide and oxygen can promote calmness and tolerance. It assists patients in coping with the situation at hand. As an **anxiolytic**, it encourages relaxation and comfort. Patients who are phobic and present irrational reactions to and behavior in a specific situation are likely to need additional pharmacological or behavioral intervention. General anesthesia may be the best option in these cases.

Pain, anxiety, and/or fear can also induce systemic stress. Being able to calm an individual by reducing situational hypertension and tachycardia could prevent an untoward emergency situation such as myocardial infarction or stroke. Similarly, it is important to keep stress levels low in a person with asthma so as to ward off an attack. Patients who are calm and relaxed will be more cooperative, which leads to safe and effective care.

In addition, nitrous oxide and oxygen will suppress a hyperactive oral gag reflex. To maximize success of dental procedures such as radiographs, impressions, and rubber dam placement in individuals with this sensitivity, it is recommended to use nitrous oxide/oxygen sedation.

Spotlight on Public Health

Many disciplines in addition to dentistry use N_2O/O_2 sedation because of its many advantages. More U.S. hospitals are incorporating its use within their emergency rooms to assist patients with anxiety-provoking and/or painful situations. ■

CONTRAINDICATIONS

What makes the use of nitrous oxide/oxygen sedation appealing and useful is that there are very few relative contraindications. There are situations in which postponement of a procedure is recommended or medical consultation is advised; however, the majority of contraindications are relatively uncommon. Contraindications are outlined as follows:

- Pregnancy: As with any drug, it is recommended to avoid administration in the first trimester. It has been historically recommended that dental procedures be performed during the second trimester; however, before use of nitrous oxide and oxygen (N_2O/O_2) in either the second or third trimester, the patient's physician or obstetrician/gynecologist should be consulted and options should be discussed.

- History of or current drug/substance abuse: It is recommended to refrain from treating any person who presents for treatment who is high, inebriated, or in any way under the influence of drugs or substances that are not appropriately prescribed. Also, it would be appropriate to evaluate individuals with a history of substance abuse or who are recovering from addictions because nitrous oxide has euphoric effects.

- Inability to communicate: Persons who are not mentally able to comprehend the intent and details of the procedure, or who are unable to communicate the drug effects to the dental hygienist, are not candidates for N_2O/O_2 sedation. Careful assessment of each patient is critical in this instance. Professional discretion should be used with any patients who have cognitive difficulties, varying stages of Alzheimer's disease, autism spectrum disorder, or language barriers.

- Problematic situations due to gas expansion: Nitrous oxide is a gas with expansive pharmacokinetic properties. Several health conditions and medical procedures are affected when nitrous oxide is introduced. Medical consultation with attending physicians is recommended if the patient has had recent tympanic membrane surgery (i.e., replacement/repair of the eardrum), bowel impaction or specific intestinal/colon distention concerns, ocular surgery in which perfluoropropane or sulfur hexafluoride was implanted in the eye, pneumothorax, or cystic fibrosis.[2]

- Bleomycin sulfate therapy: Patients who are receiving bleomycin sulfate as a cancer treatment should not be given N_2O/O_2 sedation because of potential problems with the oxygen administration and the propensity for pulmonary fibrosis.[3]

- Other chronic obstructive pulmonary disease (COPD) conditions: Patients with chronic bronchitis, emphysema, or other debilitating respiratory diseases should not be treated with N_2O/O_2 sedation until an attending physician is consulted. Once again, the administration of oxygen may be of concern rather than the nitrous oxide. The increased oxygen may interfere with the hypoxic respiratory drive of these individuals.

- Psychoses and other mental illness: It is advised to avoid using N_2O/O_2 sedation on individuals with conditions that warrant treatment with psychotropic drugs or antidepressants, or who are ill and are not being treated (e.g., bipolar disorder, schizophrenia). Untoward complications can present themselves in certain individuals. Careful consideration of each individual situation is advised, and a conservative approach is recommended.
- Upper respiratory condition/sinus infection: Conditions that affect nasal and bronchial airflow will result in inadequate sedation due to the inability of the gas to be inspired and moved through the respiratory system. Often, this situation is resolved with the postponement of the appointment until the infection clears.

GAS PROPERTIES

Nitrous oxide is a tightly bound molecule of nitrogen and oxygen that does not separate in the body. It is a naturally occurring gas in the atmosphere but is also easily manufactured for specific use. The manufacturing process is simple; the raw ingredient ammonium nitrate is heated, thus producing nitrous oxide, water, and a few impurities. It is nonflammable by nature; however, it supports combustion and possible explosion in the presence of flame or high temperature and pressure. Its molecular weight is 44 and its specific gravity is 1.53, which indicates that it is heavier than air. And, because of its boiling point of 53°C (127°F), its liquid form will vaporize into a gas at room temperature. Nitrous oxide is stored as a liquid in cylinders and pressurized at 750 psi. A full cylinder will primarily be liquid with minimal vapor, and the dial indicator will not drop as the gas is being used until there is very little liquid left in the cylinder. The cylinder will be cool to the touch during use due to the vaporization of the gas as the liquid contacts the ambient air. In the United States, cylinders filled with nitrous oxide are color-coded blue.

Oxygen comprises 21% of the earth's atmosphere and is of significant proportion in the human body and water. It, too, is combustible, so it is important that neither oxygen nor nitrous oxide come in contact with a hydrocarbon source such as a grease or lubricant. Oxygen is compressed as a gas into cylinders at 2,000 psi. Unlike nitrous oxide, it can be monitored on the dial as it is being used. The dial drops accordingly, so there is never a question as to the amount left in a cylinder. It is typical to use approximately 2.5 times as much oxygen as nitrous oxide during sedation. In the United States, cylinders filled with oxygen are color-coded green.

Nitrous oxide is considered a relatively insoluble drug, which means only minimal amounts are dissolved in blood and barriers to the brain are easily crossed. This is advantageous clinically because the onset of sedation and subsequent recovery occur quickly. In addition, nitrous oxide has a much greater partial pressure gradient than nitrogen (air). This makes nitrous oxide very expansive in nature. Because of this, nitrous oxide will replace any nitrogen molecule. Physiologically, this replacement results in nitrous oxide filling any air space in the body. This will result in either an increase in volume or pressure depending on where the air is located. If the space has rigid confines, such as bone or cartilage, the result will be added pressure. If the space is within nonrigid boundaries, additional volume will be noted. This property is the reason for some of the situations in which nitrous oxide use is contraindicated.[2]

RESPIRATORY PHYSIOLOGY

The fast onset of action because of the pharmacokinetic properties of nitrous oxide is mirrored in recovery. Nitrous oxide quickly diffuses out of the blood and back into the lungs to exit the same way it entered. The advantage of this is that the drug is not metabolized in the liver like other drugs. People with compromised liver function, hepatitis, or any other condition affecting the liver are not of concern with nitrous oxide/oxygen administration. The literature has historically identified concern with the rapid exodus of nitrous oxide within the respiratory system in that oxygen saturation levels were shown to decrease during the time when the nitrous oxide flow was terminated. The phenomenon of "diffusion hypoxia" was cited as problematic and leading to hypoxic (decrease in oxygen) conditions. There was concern that a patient's physiology would be negatively affected during this time; however, recent and current literature has not shown support for any significant oxygen desaturation, or any clinical ramifications.[4] It is regarded as a "best practice" to postoperatively oxygenate the patient to avoid lethargy, headache, or nausea. It is typical to administer a minimum of 3 to 5 minutes of 100% oxygen postoperatively for the patient's comfort. And it is certainly appropriate to continue this postoperative oxygenation for as much time as is necessary until the patient feels he or she is recovered.[5]

The volume of gas inspired into an individual's lungs, or **tidal volume**, is important to know because this will determine the amount of flow necessary to maintain patient comfort during respiration through the nasal hood and achieve sedation. Obviously, if there is inadequate flow to the patient, he or she will experience a "suffocating" feeling, whereas too much flow will likely leak out of the hood and blow across the patient's face and be wasted. To determine the correct amount of nitrous oxide and oxygen flow to give the patient, it is necessary to assess his or her minute volume. The lung capacity of an average adult is approximately 500 mL. If this amount is multiplied by an average minute respiratory rate of 12 to 16, the result is approximately 6 to 7 liters per minute (L/min).[6] An average minute volume for a child is approximately 3 to 5 L/min. A patient's minute volume changes as the person ages; however, minute volume is not likely to change between frequent appointments. Once minute volume is established, it should remain constant throughout a sedation experience.

ARMAMENTARIUM

N₂O/O₂ sedation can be delivered from either a centralized or a portable system. A centralized system pipes gas to operatories, and the large tanks are housed away from the treatment area (Figs. 32-1 and 32-2).

A portable unit is similar to a rolling cart that can be transported from place to place; smaller tanks are attached directly to the self-contained unit (Fig. 32-3).

Each system utilizes cylinder safety features to avoid gas flow from the wrong line. Both systems incorporate regulators, which decrease the pressure of the gas from the tank to a level tolerable by human physiology. Both systems also utilize the same hoses and gas mechanism. Use of a centralized system is more economical but requires new construction or significant remodeling of a facility. A portable system may be preferable when

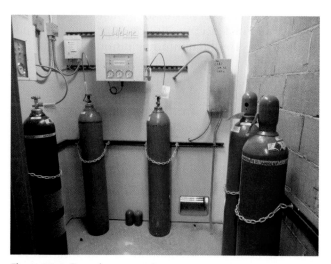

Figure 32-1. Central system tank room.

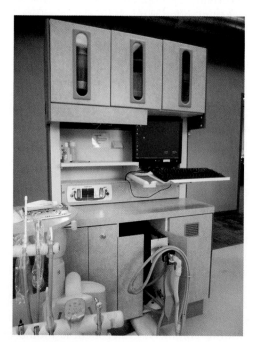

Figure 32-2. Central system operatory.

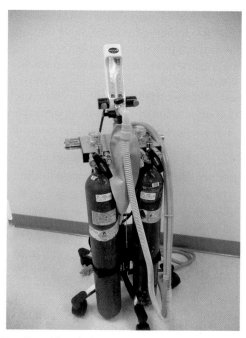

Figure 32-3. Portable sedation unit.

N₂O/O₂ sedation is used less frequently (see Application to Clinical Practice 32-1).

A major piece of equipment needed is the flowmeter. Both nitrous oxide and oxygen flow into the flowmeter, where they can be mixed and adjusted; the combination of gases then flows through tubing to the patient. There are many variations of the flowmeter; however, the amount of gas being delivered is visible on the face of the machine. Dials, knobs, and/or levers are used to adjust the flow of gases during use, depending on the type of flowmeter. Some units have glass tubes with silver balls that float within when gas is being administered, whereas others have flashing light-emitting-diode (LED) displays (Fig. 32-4).

There are several safety features available. All currently manufactured units are designed to ensure a minimal delivery of 30% oxygen, and some have features

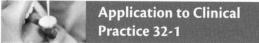

Application to Clinical Practice 32-1

The dentist for whom you work does not have a central nitrous oxide/oxygen system in the office. He indicates that he did not use this type of sedation much in dental school and does not think it is necessary. You feel very comfortable with the procedure because N₂O/O₂ sedation was taught to clinical competency in your dental hygiene educational program. You think it would assist you with many of your patients who are anxious and "afraid of the needle." How would you approach your employer about the addition of a portable unit for your operatory? What would you describe as the advantages of having this available for your patients? ■

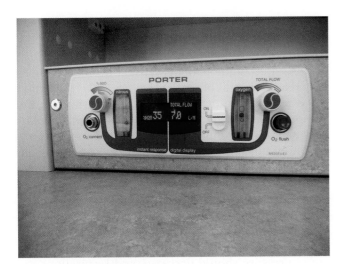

Figure 32-4. Digital flowmeter.

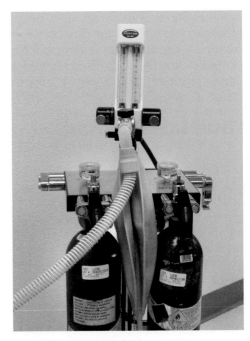

Figure 32-6. Collapsing reservoir bag.

such as audible alarms or locks. Each unit must have an oxygen fail-safe system; this system prevents the inadvertent flow of 100% nitrous oxide if the oxygen source is depleted. Sedation units are also advantageous in an emergency situation because oxygen can be obtained immediately, without having to leave an operatory.

A 2- to 3-liter reservoir bag attaches to the flowmeter and offers additional gas to the patient if necessary, and allows for visualization of the patient's inspiration and exhalation. Typically, the bag is kept two-thirds full during the procedure. The reservoir bag is used to confirm the appropriate amount of gas flow to the patient. If the bag collapses, there is an insufficient amount of gas to the patient; conversely, if the bag overinflates, there is an excessive and unnecessary amount of gas flow (Figs. 32-5 and 32-6).

Continuous monitoring of the reservoir bag is an important part of the administration procedure. Again, tidal volume should remain consistent throughout the procedure.

Gas reaches the patient through hoses attached to the flowmeter; a nasal hood, which is fitted over the patient's nose, is connected to the ends of the hoses. The hoses and nasal hood *must* have the ability to scavenge the exhaled gas from the patient, which means that one or two hoses extract the used gas from the patient and one end of the conduction tubing is connected to an evacuation system (Fig. 32-7).

Failure to utilize equipment with these capabilities is practicing below the standard set by the U.S. Occupational Safety and Health Administration (OSHA).[7] Operating without scavenging capability could affect the health of office personnel and/or place the office in legal jeopardy.

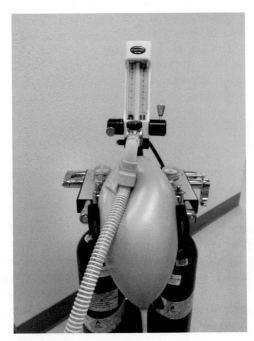

Figure 32-5. Overinflating reservoir bag.

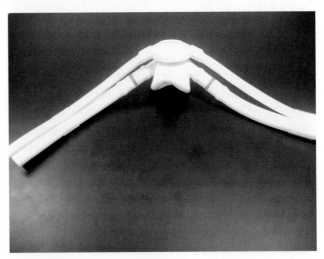

Figure 32-7. Scavenging nasal hood.

The nasal hood must fit snugly over the patient's nose so that gas does not leak into the nearby airspace. There are several size and scent options among manufacturers. Many are for single-patient use, whereas others can be sterilized. Most items are latex-free.

SEDATION EXPECTATIONS

N_2O/O_2 sedation is a safe and effective method for helping patients relax and be comfortable in a situation in which they have pain, fear, anxiety, or a sensitive oral gag reflex. When administered appropriately, the end result of N_2O/O_2 sedation is a pleasant, nonthreatening, productive appointment. It is important to note that not all patients react the same when given a drug, nor does the same patient react the same way to that drug on different occasions. Therefore, it is unacceptable to administer a percentage of nitrous oxide based on the amount given at a previous appointment or at an arbitrary, prearranged level. Each sedation experience must be considered individually.[2]

The method of administration for N_2O/O_2 sedation is titration. **Titration** involves administering a drug in incremental doses over a period of time until a desired endpoint is reached. This technique maximizes patient comfort, uncovers any possible idiosyncratic reactions early in the treatment, and delivers only the necessary amount of drug needed for the specific situation. Currently, this technique is considered the standard of care for N_2O/O_2 sedation (see Application to Clinical Practice 32-2).

The goal of N_2O/O_2 sedation is to help the patient relax and be comfortable. The titration method of administration works well to achieve this goal. By administering increments of nitrous oxide over a period of time, the patient can feel its effects gradually without concern. Signs and symptoms of sedation vary among individuals. It is important to inform the patient of what to expect, but also indicate that not all patients experience the same sensations. Ideally, anything the patient feels that is comfortable should not be alarming. For example, some patients sense a heavy feeling as they relax, whereas others feel lighter. N_2O/O_2 sedation is vasodilating, so patients may show flushing in the face or neck; they should feel comfortably warm. A tingling sensation around the mouth and at extremities is common, but not always apparent. As patients relax, the operator should notice that their body language changes and becomes less rigid. Shoulders may drop, hands loosen, and brows unfurl. Eye movement and blink rate should slow, with a possible glazed look; smiles should come easily (Fig. 32-8).

Physiologically, the patient's heart rate should slow, blood pressure should decrease, and respirations are likely to deepen and lessen. In ideal N_2O/O_2 sedation, the patient is always aware of his or her surroundings and knows what is being done. The patient is able to participate in conversation and respond to operator directions. Most important, the patient has control of his or her cough and gag reflex.

Signs and symptoms of appropriate sedation disappear when too much nitrous oxide is administered. Oversedation can occur because the operator is administering the drug too quickly, the dose of drug is too great, or a combination of both. In these cases, the patient is now uncomfortable. Patients experience many signs and symptoms of discomfort. Patients may feel dizzy, nauseous, lightheaded, or faint. They may suddenly feel hot or experience an intense tingling throughout the entire body. These sensations are likely to alarm the patient, thereby replacing the relaxed feeling with one of distress. In other cases, oversedated patients may not be able to keep their eyes or their mouths open. They may slur their words or not make sense while attempting to talk. Patients may dream, hallucinate, show signs of agitation, and/or display combative behavior; patients may vomit or become unconscious. Vomiting is significant during sedation in that it could result in aspiration of stomach contents due to the fact that the cough/gag reflex is not as actively engaged. This poses a life-threatening situation.

Application to Clinical Practice 32-2

You have recently begun working in a fast-paced dental office. It is the philosophy of the dentist to administer 50% nitrous oxide and 50% oxygen from the onset when using N_2O/O_2 sedation. When you have complied with this directive, several of your patients have experienced nausea and vomited or have complained of headaches and dizziness. The majority of them indicate that they do not want to be sedated again because of their bad reactions. You understand and feel comfortable using the titration technique, and know that this is the recommended administration technique. How could you handle this situation with the dentist? ■

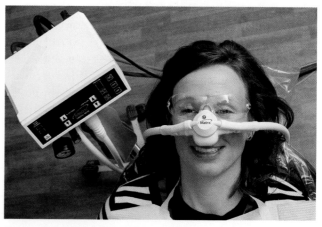

Figure 32-8. Appropriate N_2O/O_2 sedation.

For any sedation, the American Society of Anesthesiologists (ASA) recommends that patients avoid liquid and light food for a minimum of 2 to 6 hours, respectively, before sedation, with longer periods for heavy meals or fried/fatty foods.[8]

Ethical and Legal Responsibilities

It is the operator's ethical and legal duty to diligently monitor the patient during any sedation. It is unacceptable to leave the patient alone at any time (see Teamwork). Anyone administering N_2O/O_2 sedation must be certified in cardiopulmonary respiration (CPR) and be knowledgeable about and capable of handling an emergency situation. The ASA recommends that any nonanesthesiologist be responsible for the intended level of sedation and the next higher sedation level. This requires the operator to make sure an educated decision has been made based on careful preoperative assessment measures about whether the patient is a good candidate for N_2O/O_2 sedation.[8]

PREOPERATIVE ASSESSMENT

Assessment of risk is a critical preoperative procedure. A current medical history must be reviewed for each patient before N_2O/O_2 sedation. It should be determined that there are no relative contraindications, and if anything is questioned, consultation with an appropriate medical provider should be obtained. There should be a legitimate purpose for the use of N_2O/O_2 sedation that is related to a recognized indication. It is not ethically appropriate to administer this drug to a patient who requests it as a way to unwind after a stressful workday.

Blood pressure values, pulse, and respiration rates are vital signs that are recommended preoperatively and postoperatively when administering nitrous oxide and oxygen (Fig. 32-9). If the concentration of

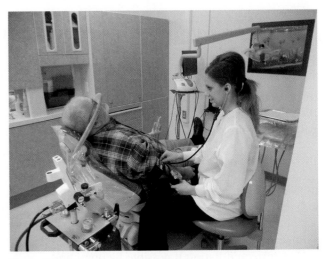

Figure 32-9. Postoperative assessment.

nitrous oxide is 50% or greater, it is recommended to obtain intraoperative vital signs as well. Use of a pulse oximeter to measure arterial blood oxygenation is also recommended with concentrations at 50% or above. It is important to note the patency of the airway. Patients should be able to breathe easily without obstruction. Typically, airway assessment involves ensuring no previous problems with sedation have been encountered, checking for clear passages, and evaluating the extent of the oropharyngeal opening. Again, it is important that the person administering the drug be proficient in management of airway obstruction and be diligent in monitoring the patient for signs of hypoxia. Emergency equipment such as positive-pressure ventilation, high-volume suction, oropharyngeal airway inserts, and other appropriate emergency medications must be available when sedation is administered.[8]

INFORMED CONSENT

Before any procedure, informed consent must be obtained from the patient. The patient must understand the intent and purpose of the procedure. The patient must also know what to expect and how to tell the operator if he or she senses anything uncomfortable or distressing. Risks associated with the procedure should be communicated to the patient, along with what to expect if this type of sedation is not used. Patients should always be given options for alternative methods of assistance. It is critical to make sure patients have had the opportunity to ask questions and have them answered to their satisfaction. It is prudent to have a separate consent form for N_2O/O_2 sedation and to obtain a written signature before each sedation experience. Parents/guardians are responsible for relaying informed consent for any child under age 18, unless there are specific legal circumstances. Procedure 32-1 details the steps for administering nitrous oxide/oxygen.

Teamwork

Your patient has postponed dental treatment because of her fear of the dental office. She had several bad experiences as a child and is now a fearful adult patient. She is in need of a full mouth series of radiographs and is worried about her gag reflex. You have communicated the benefits of using N_2O/O_2 sedation and obtained her informed consent. The radiographs are taken with little or no trouble and she is relaxed, comfortable, and ready to get her teeth cleaned. You know you cannot leave her alone while she is being sedated, so you ask another hygienist to assist as you process the radiographs. She willingly obliges, knowing that the patient's safety is always important. ■

Procedure 32-1 Nitrous Oxide/Oxygen Administration

The technique for administering N_2O/O_2 sedation is straightforward. There are steps to be completed before contact with the patient, in the sedation experience with the patient, and after the patient is dismissed.[2]

PREOPERATIVE PREPARATION

Steps to be completed before patient contact are as follows:

- Secure tanks to portable unit if applicable.
- Open tanks.
- Ensure suction adequacy and operation.
- Maximize ventilation if possible by opening doors/windows to outside.
- Turn on unit if applicable.
- Visually inspect reservoir bag, conduction tubing, and nasal hood apparatus for leaks or tears; assemble and connect to unit.
- Drape with transparent bag if this is desired method of disinfection.

PROCEDURE INITIATION

Steps to be completed with the patient are as follows:

- Review patient's health history.
- Obtain informed consent.
- Take preoperative vital signs; record on sedation record.
- Establish minute volume.
  - Set oxygen flow at approximately 6 to 7 L/min (4–5 L/min for child); use minute volume if known from previous visit.
  - Fit nasal hood on patient, securing the strap behind the headrest.
  - Fill reservoir bag two-thirds full if not already filled.
  - Adjust L/min if bag overinflates (decrease O_2) or collapses (add O_2).

Nitrous Oxide Titration

- For a machine with two independent controls, it is necessary to manually keep the minute volume constant. For example, as nitrous oxide is added, it will be necessary to decrease the oxygen so as to maintain the established volume.
- Some machines automatically maintain the minute volume; therefore, it is not necessary to adjust the level of oxygen as the nitrous oxide is introduced.
- As mentioned, there are many variations of flowmeters. Some machines display the percentage of nitrous oxide being delivered. In this case, there is no need for calculation. Some machines display the amount of oxygen being delivered; subtraction from 100 is necessary to determine the percentage of nitrous oxide. Some machines have balls within tubes that float when gas is flowing. The tubes are marked 1 to 10, with short hash marks between whole numbers. The sum of the two numbers at the level of both floating balls equals the total liters

flow per minute. This sum should equal the minute volume established at the beginning of the procedure. It is important to note that these numbers *do not* correspond with the percentage of gas being delivered. Instead, the actual percentage of N_2O is calculated by dividing the N_2O L/min by the total liters per minute.

It is important to be very familiar with the flowmeter being used.

- Begin by adding approximately 10% to 20% nitrous oxide. Wait for a short period of time (i.e., 1–3 minutes) before administering additional nitrous oxide increments. Increments of 5% to 10% are appropriate. As signs and symptoms appear, wait longer between doses; the peak action of each dose is likely within 3 to 5 minutes. Gauge the frequency of intervals according to how the patient is reacting.

Patient Monitoring

- Continuous careful monitoring of the patient is required while performing the required procedures.
- N_2O/O_2 sedation works well for those patients who are anxious about needles and receiving local anesthesia. The combination of N_2O, O_2, and a local anesthetic can promote a successful dental experience.
- If the patient becomes uncomfortable at any time, it is important to determine the extent of the discomfort. If he or she indicates that a lesser amount is desired, the operator should decrease the amount of nitrous oxide being delivered. Tell the patient what has been done and that the effects will lessen within a very short time. If the patient is extremely distressed, combative, or agitated, it is necessary to completely remove all nitrous oxide and ensure the patient that only oxygen is being delivered. In this situation, also tell the patient that the effects will soon disappear and that he or she will begin to feel normal within a very short time. Calm reassurance by the operator will assist the patient in these situations.
- Never leave the patient alone during N_2O/O_2 sedation.

RECOVERY/PATIENT DISMISSAL

- At the point at which the majority of the intense procedure has been completed, it is necessary to terminate the nitrous oxide flow and deliver 100% oxygen to the patient.
- A minimum of 5 minutes of 100% postoperative oxygen is recommended before the assessment of recovery. These 5 minutes can be completed while the operator is finishing a procedure and not necessarily at the end of the appointment.
- At the end of the 5 minutes, it is necessary to evaluate the recovery of the patient. Without taking off

the nasal hood, set the patient upright and obtain postoperative vital signs. Values should be within 10 mm/Hg for blood pressure readings compared with the preoperative values. The postoperative pulse rate should also be within 10 beats per minute and respirations within 5 compared with those taken preoperatively. If the numbers are not within these ranges, administer 100% oxygen for another 5 minutes, and take them again.[2]

- Once vital signs are completed, it is then appropriate to ask the patient how he or she is feeling. Ask about any of the following: dizziness, lethargy, nausea, lightheadedness, grogginess, or headache. If the patient answers affirmative to any, administer 100% oxygen for another 5 minutes, and ask the patient again.
- Postoperative oxygen can be given in 5-minute increments for as long as it takes for the patient to feel normal and ready to leave.
- The operator has the ethical and legal responsibility to determine when the patient may be dismissed. Although unlikely, it is possible the operator could recommend that the patient be discharged to an escort and not dismissed on his or her own accord.

DISINFECTION AND STERILIZATION

Disinfection and sterilization of the equipment is the step that follows dismissal of the patient. Draping the unit with a clear bag decreases the amount of surface disinfection necessary for the flowmeter and the reservoir bag. It is not necessary to disinfect the inside of the reservoir bag because it is not exposed to exhaled gas. The conduction tubing and the nasal hood are exposed to the operating environment. Wipe the hoses with a surface disinfectant and dispose of the nasal hood unless it is sterilizable. Most newly manufactured, latex-free nasal hoods are designed for single-patient use and are not sterilizable; they can be disposed of.

DOCUMENTATION

Documentation of any procedure is critical in all aspects of health care, and it is especially important when administering a drug. Documenting all aspects of N_2O/O_2 sedation is both ethically and legally required. And, each state's medical and/or dental practice act may require specific documentation. It is wise to consult the laws and rules of the state(s) in which the dental hygienist is licensed.

Information from a sedation experience should be recorded with other procedural information occurring at an appointment. A reason for using N_2O/O_2 sedation should be listed along with all preoperative vital sign values. Once the patient's tidal volume has been established, it should be recorded. This is the one value that can be referred to at a subsequent appointment. Once the procedure has been completed, postoperative vital signs are recorded, as is the amount of time and the peak percentage at which nitrous oxide was administered. Recovery is documented by recording the number of minutes that postoperative 100% oxygen was delivered and any subjective comments made by the patient. As always, if there are any specific comments or adverse conditions associated with the procedure, it is important to record as much information as possible at the time because it is not prudent to add comments at a later date. It is recommended that the person administering the drug should be the person to both dismiss the patient and document the procedure. A general rule is to sign or initial any entry made in a patient's record. An operator's signature or initials should also be consistent between every patient record.

MINIMIZING TRACE GAS

Repeated exposure to high levels of nitrous oxide, whether intentional or unintentional, can have negative biological effects. No health-care provider should be using nitrous oxide for recreational use. Neurological impairment such as decreased dexterity and numbness in the extremities has been reported by those who abuse nitrous oxide. This may or may not result in permanent injury.

Chronic exposure to high levels of trace nitrous oxide gas can be hazardous because of the inactivation of a vitamin B_{12}–dependent enzyme, methionine synthase. This enzyme is necessary for major physiological functions involving DNA, bone marrow, and cellular reproduction. For this reason, all health-care providers using N_2O/O_2 sedation should continuously monitor all equipment for leaks to ensure their minimal exposure.

In 1977, the National Institute for Occupational Safety and Health (NIOSH) and the American Conference of Governmental Industrial Hygienists (ACGIH) set exposure limits for personnel working with nitrous oxide. These recommendations have not been updated since their initial invocation and are enforceable during any office inspection. The limit that was set for a dental office setting is not to exceed 50 ppm.[9]

Minimizing the amount of trace gas contamination should be a priority for any dental setting using N_2O/O_2 sedation, which requires first determining the extent of nitrous oxide contamination. A measuring device that uses infrared spectrophotometry can be utilized to detect trace gas in ambient air. In addition, personal monitoring devices or badges can track nitrous oxide exposure over time with absorbent material.

It is recommended to establish and follow a protocol that is designed to keep **biohazard** risk and personnel exposure as low as possible. Manufacturers recommend

Advancing Technologies

N_2O/O_2 sedation equipment continues to improve in design, delivery mechanisms, and safety features; new products are well tested. Research is ongoing relative to biohazard concerns of practitioners who work with nitrous oxide, and safety is one of the highest priorities for manufacturing companies. ■

that flowmeters be calibrated every 2 years; tank connections, conduction tubing, and reservoir bags should be frequently checked for leaks. The adequacy of the vacuum should be determined at each patient visit, and it is vital that the patient knows to minimize talking and to inhale through his or her nose. Any air exchange that allows nitrous oxide to vent outside is beneficial, whether it is from a built-in system or an open window or door. As previously stated, it is mandatory that all nasal hoods have scavenging capabilities, which means that there are one or two hoses that carry exhaled gas from the patient through the suction to be vented outside.[10]

The health and safety of any health-care provider exposed to nitrous oxide is always important. Routine assessment of the effectiveness of scavenging protocols is a necessary part of nitrous oxide/oxygen sedation. Operators must be knowledgeable and vigilant about the extent of their exposure and follow best-practice protocols for minimizing trace gas.

RECOMMENDATIONS FOR BEST PRACTICES

Codified laws and rules vary between states as to the requirements for the administration of N_2O/O_2 sedation. Licensing agencies enforce the parameters of practice to ensure best practices are provided for the public, whose care they protect. Varying levels of supervision

exist, and it is likely that a dental hygienist must have the direct supervision of a dentist to administer this type of sedation. It is important to be educated on the laws and rules under which a professional is governed in any state.

Informed consent is critical to proper patient care. Make sure the patient is knowledgeable about the intent of the drug, associated risks, alternative sedation methods, and cost, and has had the opportunity to ask any questions. Effective communication with patients is a key aspect of successful outcomes. Written consent by the patient or parent/guardian for every sedation experience is prudent practice.

Ethical practice requires that professionals use good judgment in all patient care decisions. Nitrous oxide and oxygen should be administered for an appropriate reason, such as reducing pain and alleviating anxiety or suppressing a hyperactive gag reflex. It should not be administered for patients who do not need it, just as other drugs should not be prescribed for illegitimate reasons. Patients should also not dictate the amount of nitrous oxide they desire or expect to be delivered.

Standards of care have been established for the safe and efficacious delivery of N_2O/O_2 sedation. The titration technique of administration is the recommended practice, along with the use of updated scavenging equipment and protocols. Practitioners should stay abreast of emerging technologies and refresh their knowledge with continuing education.

SUMMARY

Nitrous oxide and oxygen have been used safely and effectively for well over 150 years as a conscious sedation method. Its professional use began in the field of dentistry, and it continues to be widely used in general and specialty dental practices. It has been adopted and accepted into a myriad of other health disciplines, with its use continually expanding. It is used worldwide and can be used on many individuals because of its limited interaction with body systems and negative reactions. With best practices in place, N_2O/O_2 sedation can promote a positive experience for both patient and operator.

Case Study

Your next patient, Jeremy, is a 28-year-old male. Finances were tight when he was growing up, and his parents did not have any type of insurance for him and his two sisters. He has been working at various jobs since high school, mostly in construction. He got his commercial driver's license (CDL) and has been driving a truck for a company that transports lumber to worksites. Jeremy has not had a history of regular dental care but has visited a local community dental center on occasion. He never liked going to the dentist because he always had to have big fillings or a tooth pulled. The sound of the drill or the "thing that polishes your teeth" really bothers him. He knows he needs to make an appointment; he just keeps putting it off.

Case Study Exercises

1. It is important to acknowledge Jeremy's anxiety and empathetically communicate that it is good that he came to this appointment. Verbalize how you think

Case Study—cont'd

N_2O/O_2 sedation can help him, and cite the advantages it has when it is combined with local anesthesia.

2. Jeremy has never had N_2O/O_2 sedation before. He trusts you when you say it will help him become relaxed and comfortable; however, he wants to know what to expect. What will you tell him?

3. As you finish your procedure with Jeremy, you administer 100% postoperative oxygen for 5 minutes. You take his postoperative vital signs and he says he still feels "groggy" and is not quite ready to go. What is your next step?

Review Questions

1. The person responsible for assessing the adequacy of patient recovery following N_2O/O_2 sedation is the
   A. patient.
   B. person administering the drug.
   C. person monitoring the patient.

2. N_2O/O_2 has significant negative effects on the _____ system.
   A. hepatic
   B. endocrine
   C. genitourinary
   D. renal system.
   E. None of these is correct.

3. The reduction of pressure from the cylinder to an appropriate level for patient inhalation is accomplished by the
   A. nasal hood.
   B. nonrebreathing valve.
   C. regulator.
   D. oxygen flush valve.

4. The dentist who has posthumously been recognized as the "Father of Anesthesia" due to his clinical use of nitrous oxide is
   A. Humphry Davy.
   B. Joseph Priestley.
   C. Gardner Quincy Colton.
   D. Horace Wells.

5. All of the following are relative contraindications of N_2O/O_2 EXCEPT which one?
   A. Hypersensitive gag reflex
   B. Severely claustrophobic patients
   C. Current upper respiratory infection
   D. First trimester of pregnancy
   E. Alcohol intoxication or drug use

Active Learning

1. Look at pictures of people's faces and body language, especially those in an uncomfortable situation, and try to determine their level of pain or anxiety/fear. Often the presence of pain can be seen in the pallor of the skin; anxiety or fear can be seen in the tenseness of the shoulders, hands, or neck.

2. Review the administration technique steps in sequence. Visualize the order and how you want the patient to respond. Anticipate what problems could occur and how you will handle the situation.

3. Working with a partner, practice your patient assessment skills. Perform the procedure for taking blood pressure, pulse rate, and respiration. Know the classifications and associated values for normal, prehypertension, and Stages 1 and 2 hypertension. ■

REFERENCES

1. Chancellor JW. Dr. Wells' impact on dentistry and medicine. *J Am Dent Assoc.* 1994;125:1585.
2. Clark M, Brunick, A. *Handbook of nitrous oxide and oxygen sedation.* St. Louis, MO: Mosby/Elsevier; 2008.
3. Fleming P, Walker PO, Priest JR. Bleomycin therapy: a contraindication to the use of nitrous oxide-oxygen psychosedation in the dental office. *Pediatr Dent.* 1988; 10(4):345.
4. Jeske AH, et al. Noninvasive assessment of diffusion hypoxia following administration of nitrous oxide analgesia. *Anesth Prog.* 2004;51(1):10.
5. Lampe GH et al. Postoperative hypoxemia after nonabdominal surgery: a frequent event not caused by nitrous oxide. *Anesth Analg.* 1990;71:597.
6. George R, Light R, Matthay M, Matthay, R. eds. *Chest medicine: essentials of pulmonary and critical care medicine.* 5th ed. Philadelphia, PA: Lippincott Williams & Wilkins; 2005.
7. McGlothlin JD, Crounch KG, Mickelsen RI. *Control of nitrous oxide in dental operatories.* DHHS No (NIOSH) 94-129. Cincinnati, OH: U.S. Department of Health

and Human Services, Public Health Service, Centers for Disease Control and Prevention, National Institute for Occupational Safety and Health, Division of Physical Sciences and Engineering, Engineering Control Technology Branch; 1994.

8. ASA Task Force. Practice guidelines for sedation and analgesia by non-anesthesiologists. *Anesthesiology.* 2002;96(4):1004.

9. Bruce DL, Bach MJ. *Trace effects of anesthetic gases on behavioral performance of operating room personnel.* HEW publication No (NIOSH) 76-169. Cincinnati, OH: US Department of Health, Education, and Welfare; 1976.

10. ADA Council on Scientific Affairs, ADA Council on Dental Practice. Nitrous oxide in the dental office. *J Am Dent Assoc.* 1997;128:364.

Chapter 33 | Local Anesthesia

Gwen Grosso, RDH, MS • L. Teal Mercer, RDH, MPH

KEY TERMS

absolute contraindication
acid–base balance (pH)
afferent nerve
amides
depolarize
efferent nerve
ester
infiltration
ischemia
isotonic
local anesthesia
lumen
negative aspiration
nerve block
pharmacokinetics
positive aspiration
relative contraindication
trismus
vasoconstrictor

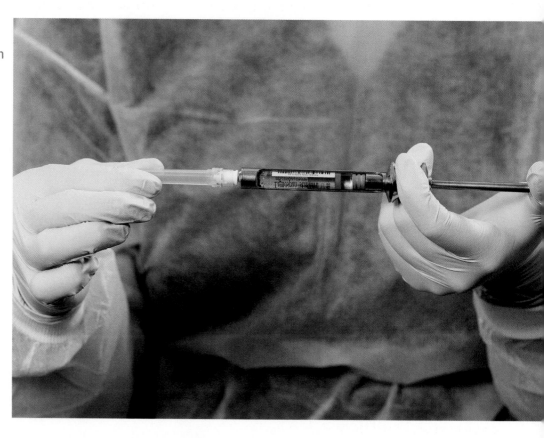

LEARNING OBJECTIVES

After reading this chapter, the student should be able to:

33.1 Articulate the importance of adequate pain control as a prelude to providing quality dental care.

33.2 Describe the physiological mechanism of nerve conduction.

33.3 Explain how local anesthetics prevent nerve transmission.

33.4 Identify and describe the pharmacology of the commonly used local anesthetic agents and vasoconstrictors.

33.5 Recognize disease conditions and medications that may alter or contraindicate the use of local anesthetic agents and/or vasoconstrictors.

33.6 Recognize signs and symptoms of local and systemic complications associated with the administration of local anesthetic agents.

33.7 Explain why local anesthetics may not be as effective in an area of injury (infection).

33.8 Describe the neuroanatomy of the trigeminal nerve.

33.9 Identify the armamentarium for local anesthesia.

33.10 Describe the techniques for administration of local anesthesia.

33.11 Identify the anatomical landmarks associated with administration for the following injections: ASA, MSA, PSA, IO, GP, NP, Gow-Gates and IA nerve block, buccal, mental, and incisive.

33.12 Identify which nerve, teeth, and soft tissue structures are anesthetized with each of the preceding injections.

KEY CONCEPTS

- Local anesthetics play an invaluable role in the provision of the dental hygiene process of care.
- **Local anesthesia** is defined as a temporary loss of sensation in a specific area of the body without loss of consciousness.
- Two major classes of injectable local anesthetics exist: **esters** and **amides.**

RELEVANCE TO CLINICAL PRACTICE

Local anesthetics play an invaluable role in the provision of the dental hygiene process of care. Studies indicate that 10% to 20% of the U.S. population experiences moderate to high levels of dental anxiety. This fear prohibits regular dental visits, resulting in poor oral health.[1] The dental office is unique in that patients often avoid the office because of the fear of pain associated with treatment, yet pain often brings patients to the dental office. Pain is a response that protects the body from harm. Many individuals who are fearful of dentistry worry about receiving oral injections.[2] Patient comfort enables the clinician to provide comprehensive care while reducing anxiety and increasing patient compliance.

LOCAL ANESTHESIA

Local anesthesia is defined as a temporary loss of sensation in a specific area of the body without loss of consciousness. **Infiltration** anesthesia is an injection that supplies anesthesia to an area near or adjacent to the area to be treated, generally an area of a few centimeters (Fig. 33-1). **Nerve block** anesthesia is achieved when an anesthetic solution is deposited near a nerve trunk or nerve plexus (Fig. 33-2). A nerve block provides anesthesia to multiple teeth. The clinical effects of both the infiltration and nerve block are a reversible blockage of peripheral nerve conduction (see Application to Clinical Practice).

Nerve Conduction

The dental neural plexus is a complex network of nerves supplying the teeth and the supporting structures.

Trigeminal Nerve

The trigeminal nerve (5th cranial nerve), the largest cranial nerve, provides the sensory innervation for the teeth, tongue, bone, and soft tissue of the oral cavity. The trigeminal nerve also provides the motor root for the mandibular nerve. The trigeminal nerve is divided into three branches: the ophthalmic, maxillary, and mandibular nerves (Fig. 33-3).

Ophthalmic Nerve. The ophthalmic nerve (V1) is the smallest division of the trigeminal nerve and is an afferent nerve, a nerve that carries information from the periphery of the body to the central nervous system (CNS). The ophthalmic nerve provides sensory information from the

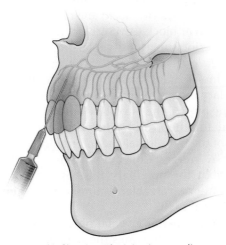

Figure 33-1. Local infiltration. The injection supplies anesthesia to the area to be treated.

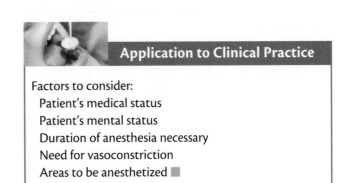

Application to Clinical Practice

Factors to consider:
   Patient's medical status
   Patient's mental status
   Duration of anesthesia necessary
   Need for vasoconstriction
   Areas to be anesthetized ■

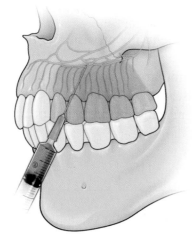

Figure 33-2. Nerve block. The anesthetic is deposited near a nerve trunk or nerve plexus at a distance from the area to be treated.

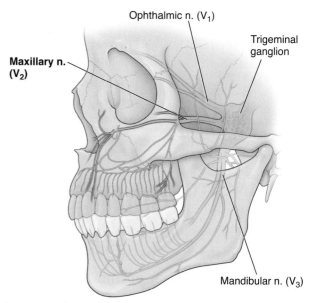

Figure 33-4. The maxillary nerve has fewer variations and less density of the maxillary and palatal bones than the mandibular nerve.

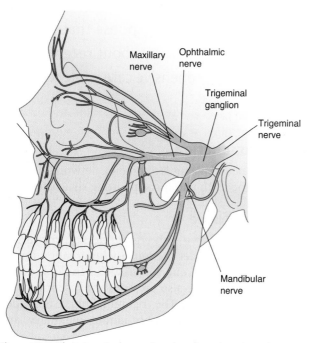

Figure 33-3. The trigeminal nerve has three branches: the ophthalmic, maxillary, and mandibular nerves.

eyeball, conjunctiva, cornea, orbit, forehead, and the ethmoid and frontal sinuses. Sensory information is carried from three main branches—the nasociliary nerve, frontal nerve, and lacrimal nerve—toward the brain by traveling through the superior orbital fissure of the sphenoid bone.

Maxillary Nerve. The maxillary nerve (V_2) enters the skull through the foramen rotundum of the sphenoid bone and branches off into four regions: the cranium, the pterygopalatine fossa, the infraorbital, and the face (Fig. 33-4). This afferent nerve provides sensory information from the maxilla, maxillary sinuses, palate, nasal cavity, and nasopharynx.

The nasopalatine nerve (NP) is a branch of the pterygopalatine nerve. This nerve crosses the roof of

the nasal cavity and ultimately enters the incisive canal and continues through the incisive foramen. The nasopalatine nerve innervates the palatal mucosa of the premaxilla area.

The greater palatine nerve (GP) is another branch of the pterygopalatine nerve. The GP innervates the posterior hard palate and posterior lingual gingiva before entering the greater palatine foramen. The lesser palatine nerve innervates the soft palate and palatine tonsils before traveling through the lesser palatine foramen in the palatine bone.

Local anesthesia for the maxillary division of the trigeminal nerve is more often successful than for the mandibular division because the maxillary division has fewer variations and less density of the maxillary and palatal bones (Fig. 33-4). The most common maxillary injections include the infiltration of the posterior superior alveolar (PSA), middle superior alveolar (MSA), anterior superior alveolar (ASA), greater palatine (GP), and nasopalatine (NP). Less common injections include the infraorbital block (IO block) and the anterior middle superior alveolar block (AMSA block).

The posterior superior alveolar nerve (PSA) is an afferent nerve that innervates the maxillary sinus, maxillary molars, periodontium, and buccal mucosa of the maxillary molars. Nerve branches of the PSA originate in the pulp of the maxillary molars, exit through the apical foramen, and join with the PSA nerve branches of the interdental and interradicular branches of the PSA nerve. Collectively, these PSA nerve branches exit the maxillary tuberosity through the posterior superior alveolar foramina before entering the infraorbital canal.

The middle superior alveolar nerve (MSA) is an afferent nerve that innervates the maxillary premolars and, often, the mesiobuccal root of the maxillary first molar, along with the periodontium and buccal mucosa of these areas. The nerve branches of the MSA start in the pulpal tissue of the maxillary premolars and first molar. The nerve branches exit through the apical foramen, join with the interradicular and interdental branches, travel along the lateral wall of the maxillary sinus, and then enter the infraorbital canal. The MSA is not always present. When absent, innervation is provided by the PSA and anterior superior alveolar nerve (ASA).

The ASA is an afferent nerve that innervates the maxillary canine, lateral, and central incisor teeth, along with the periodontium and buccal mucosa of these areas. The nerve branches of the ASA originate in the pulpal tissue of these maxillary teeth, exit through the apical foramen, travel along the anterior wall of the maxillary sinus, and then join with the interdental branches before entering the infraorbital canal.

Mandibular Nerve. The mandibular nerve (V$_3$) enters the skull through the foramen ovale of the sphenoid bone (Fig. 33-5). It is the largest of the three trigeminal divisions, and provides both afferent and efferent nerve branches. **Efferent nerve** branches carry impulses away from the CNS to the periphery of the body. Nerve blocks are more common when anesthetizing the mandible due to the density of the bone. The most common mandibular injections include the inferior alveolar block (IA), buccal block, mental block, and incisive block. The Gow-Gates block (GG) is effective, although not as commonly used.

The sensory branches of the mandibular nerve innervate the skin of the temporal region, cheeks, lower lip, and lower part of the face; mucous membrane of the cheek; anterior two-thirds of the tongue; mandibular teeth; mandibular bone; temporomandibular joint; and parotid gland. The motor branch of the mandibular nerve innervates the masticatory muscles, mylohyoid muscles, and anterior belly of the digastric muscle. The mandibular nerve passes through the foramen ovale of the sphenoid bone to enter the skull.

The buccal nerve, or long buccal nerve, a branch of the mandibular nerve, is an afferent nerve that innervates the skin of the cheek, buccal mucosa, and buccal gingiva of the mandibular molars. The buccal nerve begins in the skin of the cheek, retromolar triangle, and gingival tissue of the mandibular molars. The nerve crosses the anterior border of the ramus at the level of the occlusal plane and travels between the two heads of the lateral pterygoid muscle before reaching the external surface of the masseter muscle.

The lingual nerve is an afferent nerve that innervates the body of the tongue, the floor of the mouth, and the lingual gingiva of the mandibular teeth. The lingual nerve travels from the sides of the tongue to the base of the tongue, where it then travels superiorly and just medial to the inferior alveolar nerve.

The inferior alveolar nerve (IA) is an afferent nerve that provides pulpal innervation of the mandibular teeth and the periodontium of these teeth. It is derived from the merging of the mental and incisive nerves. Once these two nerves merge, the IA nerve joins the intradental, interradicular, and apical nerves of the mandibular posterior teeth. The IA travels through the mandibular canal until it exits the mandibular foramen on the medial surface of the ramus. The IA then runs posterior and lateral to the lingual nerve and ultimately passes through the foramen ovale of the sphenoid bone.

The mental nerve is an afferent nerve that innervates the chin, lower lip, and labial mucosa of the anterior teeth and premolars. Once leaving these tissues, the mental nerve travels through the mental foramen and joins with the inferior alveolar nerve.

The incisive nerve is an afferent nerve that provides pulpal innervation to the mandibular premolars and anterior teeth. The incisive nerve starts in the pulpal tissue of these teeth, and then exits the apical foramen before joining up with the mental nerve and forming the inferior alveolar nerve.

Nerve impulses are electrical in nature and occur when a stimulus is applied to a resting or polarized nerve. The nerve in this resting state has a large number of sodium ions (Na$^+$) on the outside and a large number of potassium ions (K$^+$) on the inside. Upon stimulation, the exterior of the nerve cell allows an influx of sodium ions to cross the cell membrane, which causes the sensation of pain. Calcium ions (Ca^{++}) that are present in the cell membrane assist the sodium into the cell, beginning the first step in nerve depolarization.

The goal of local anesthetics is to decrease or block the sensation of pain by decreasing the amount of

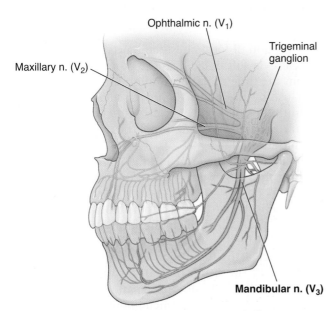

Ophthalmic n. (V$_1$)

Trigeminal ganglion

Maxillary n. (V$_2$)

Mandibular n. (V$_3$)

Figure 33-5. The mandibular nerve has afferent and efferent nerve branches. Because of the mandible's bone density, nerve blocks are commonly used to anesthetize this region.

Advancing Technologies

WAND

The CompuDent and Single Tooth Anesthesia (STA) System are commonly referred to as the Wand. This is a single-use, disposable needle and microtube that deliver a slow, steady, and precise volume of anesthesia. The increased comfort of the injection is attributed to the controlled rate of anesthetic delivery.

SAFETY SYRINGES

In an attempt to minimize accidental needle sticks, "safety" syringes were introduced. These are disposable, sterile, single-use needle/syringe systems that enable the needle to be sheathed by the syringe to prevent accidental injury. Two products currently available are the UltraSafety Plus XL and the Hypo Safety Syringe. ■

Table 33-1. Esters and Amides

	Esters	Amides
Metabolism	In plasma	In liver
Molecular chain	Oxygen	Nitrogen
Generic name	One "i"; e.g., tetracaine	Two "i's"; e.g., mepivacaine
Allergenicity	Highly allergic	Unknown to cause sensitivity

Spotlight on Public Health

Although local anesthesia is permitted in most states, each state has a unique dental hygiene practice act. Dental hygienists are responsible for knowing the requirements particular to their practice site. For example, some states permit hygienists to deliver local anesthesia with direct supervision, whereas some states require general supervision.

Local anesthesia requirements may be further delineated when hygienists work in public health facilities. When local anesthesia is permitted with general supervision or unsupervised, dental hygienists have the autonomy to provide adequate pain control while increasing access to care. ■

---

sodium ions (Na+) able to penetrate the cell membrane.[3] Local anesthetics attach themselves to receptors in the nerve membrane and block the conduction of nerve impulses by decreasing the permeability of the nerve membrane, possibly by attaching to the calcium ions. A reduction of the passage of sodium ions will **depolarize** the membrane, resulting in a less excitable state and causing a loss of sensation.

Local anesthesia is the main modality for the reduction of dental pain (see Advancing Technologies). Ideally local anesthetic agents should have the following qualities:

- Potency
- Reversible
- Absence of local reactions
- Absence of systemic reactions
- Absence of allergic reactions
- Rapid onset
- Satisfactory duration
- Low cost
- Long shelf-life
- Easily metabolized and excreted

Amide and Ester Agents

Two major classes of injectable local anesthetics exist: **esters** and **amides** (Table 33-1). Their chemical arrangement allows the drugs to diffuse through extracellular fluid and attach themselves to receptors in the nerve membrane.[4] Novocaine (procaine), the first dental anesthetic, was an ester. Novocaine is no longer available for dental injections due to its high incidence of allergic reactions. However, patients commonly refer to a dental injection as "getting novocaine." Currently, there are various local anesthetic drugs available for dental use (see Spotlight on Public Health).

Pharmacokinetics

Pharmacokinetics is the study of the action of drugs within the body, including the mechanisms of absorption, distribution, metabolism, and excretion.[3]

- Absorption of local anesthetics occurs in the bloodstream via soft tissue. It is the progression of a drug from the time of administration until it is available for use by the body. Highly vascular areas rapidly absorb the anesthetic. Local anesthetics used in dentistry have vasodilating properties resulting in systemic absorption.
- Distribution of the local anesthetics is the process by which the drug is delivered to the tissues and fluids of the body.
- Metabolism, also referred to as biotransformation, is the process by which the local anesthetic drug is transformed from an active drug to an inactive substance. This reduces or eliminates the possible toxicity of the drug. Biotransformation of amides occurs in the liver due to hepatic enzymes. Esters are primarily biotransformed in the blood or plasma by cholinesterase.
- Excretion of local anesthetic drugs is accomplished primarily by the kidneys through the passage of urine.

Factors That Affect Absorption

Local anesthetics are absorbed into the bloodstream via soft tissues. The **acid–base balance**, also referred to as the **pH** of the environment, can determine the rate of absorption. The concept of pH refers to the acid–base balance within intracellular and extracellular fluids. The goal of the body is to maintain an acid–base balance or homeostatic environment. Acids have a higher hydrogen ion concentration and want to give up hydrogen ions. Bases have a lower hydrogen ion concentration and can accept hydrogen ions.

pH is measured on a scale from 0 to 14. The lower the number, the more acidic is the solution; conversely, the higher the number, the more basic is the solution. A pH of 7 is considered neutral. The anesthetic in the dental cartridge is a weak base with a pH of 4.5.

The homeostatic mechanisms of the pH maintain the pH of blood at approximately 7.4 pH. If an infection is present, the pH is decreased to an acidic 6.5. This acidic environment reduces the ability of the anesthetic to be effective. An area of infection may also be difficult to anesthetize completely due to increased vascularity and dilution of the anesthetic drug due to the inflammation.

Vasoconstrictors

Local anesthetics, by their chemical makeup, have vasodilating properties. The addition of a **vasoconstrictor** such as epinephrine causes the **lumen,** or diameter, of the blood vessel to narrow, thus decreasing blood flow. Vasoconstrictors are always expressed as a ratio, 1 gram of solute in 1,000 mL of solution. Epinephrine and levonordefrin are common vasoconstrictors. Common concentrations of epinephrine used in dentistry are 1:100,000 and 1:200,000. The systemic effects are heart related and cause an increase in blood pressure, heart rate, and oxygen demand. Levonordefrin (Neo-Cobefrin) is a synthetic form of epinephrine that is added to mepivacaine at a concentration of 1:20,000. Levonordefrin is one-fifth as potent as epinephrine and therefore has less systemic effect on the heart muscle. The risks and benefits of adding a vasoconstrictor to an anesthetic agent are listed in Table 33-2.

Patients prescribed tricyclic antidepressants are at a greater risk for development of dysrhythmias with epinephrine administration; therefore its dose should be minimal. The administration of either levonordefrin or norepinephrine is absolutely contraindicated in patients taking tricyclic antidepressants. Patients being treated with nonselective beta blockers are at increased risk for elevation of blood pressure accompanied by reflex bradycardia. Monitoring of blood pressure is essential; according to Malamed, patients with blood pressure readings greater than 200 mm Hg/115 mm Hg should not undergo elective dental treatment.[5] Table 33-3 lists common tricyclic antidepressants, and Table 33-4 lists common nonselective beta blockers.

Duration of Action

Local anesthetics can be classified by their duration of action:

- Short-pulpal anesthesia: approximately 30 minutes
- Intermediate-pulpal anesthesia: approximately 60 minutes
- Long-pulpal anesthesia: approximately 90 minutes

Table 33-5 summarizes common local anesthetics.

Dosage

The maximum recommended dose (MRD) is the maximum quantity of a drug that can be safely administered.[6] This information is provided with the product insert. However, the following information is also required: patient's medical status, weight, and age.

To determine the MRD, multiply the patient's weight by 2 mg/lb, then divide the result by the 36 mg that the cartridge contains. For a patient weighing

Table 33-3. *Common Tricyclic Antidepressants*

Generic Name	Trade Name
Amitriptyline	Elavil
Clomipramine	Anafranil
Imipramine	Tofranil

Table 33-2. *Benefits and Risks of Vasoconstrictors*

Benefits	Risks
Slow absorption to surrounding tissue	Potential for local **ischemia**
Decrease systemic toxicity	Systemic interaction
Prolong duration of the anesthetic agent	Potential adverse effects in patients who are taking beta blockers or antidepressant drugs

Table 33-4. *Common Nonselective Beta Blockers*

Generic Name	Trade Name
Nadolol	Corgard
Timolol	Blocadren
Pindolol	Visken
Penbutolol	Levatol
Propranolol	Inderal

Table 33-5. Local Anesthetic Agents

Generic Name	2 % lidocaine HCL	2% lidocaine w/epi	3% mepivacaine plain	2% mepivacaine w/levonordefrin	Prilocaine	4% Articaine HCL	Bupivacaine
Trade Name	Xylocaine	Xylocaine w/epi, Octocaine	Carbocaine Polocaine	Carbocaine Polocaine	Citanest Forte	Septocaine	Marcaine
Vasoconstrictor	NO	YES	NO	YES	YES	YES	
Vasoconstrictor concentration	N/A	1:100,000	N/A	1:20,000	1:200,000	1:100,000 1:200,000	
Duration	Short	Intermediate	Short	Intermediate	Long	Intermediate	
Pulpal	5–10 min	60 min	20–40 min 20 min via infiltration 40-min block	60 min	60–90 min	60–75 min	
Soft tissue	60–120 min	3–5 hours	2–3 hours	3–5 hours	3–8 hours	3–6 hours	

N/A = not applicable.

Note: Always review patient's medical history and follow manufacturer guidelines regarding maximum recommended dosage.

80 lb receiving 2% Lidocaine HCL and epinephrine 1:100,000:

$$80 \text{ lb} \times 2 \text{ mg/lb} = 160$$

$$160/36 \text{ mg} = 4.4 \text{ cartridges}$$

Cardiac Considerations

The dose for patients with ischemic heart disease is 2 carpules of lidocaine with 100,000 of epinephrine.

Topical Anesthesia

Topical anesthesia is used for short-duration pain management of the gingiva and mucous membranes (see Teamwork). Dental hygienists may use topical anesthesia in the following situations:[7]

• To minimize patient discomfort during instrumentation
• Before administration of local anesthesia
• To minimize a patient's gag reflex
• Before removing sutures

Topical anesthetic is applied to the surface of the mucous membrane and acts on the terminal nerve endings. Topical anesthetic is only effective on 2 to 3 mm of surface tissue and does not contain vasoconstrictors; therefore, it is effective for only a short period of time.

Common types of topical anesthetic are outlined in Table 33-6.

Oraqix topical anesthetic is 2.5% lidocaine and 2.5% prilocaine. Oraqix is unique because it is designed to be applied into the periodontal pocket. Oraqix has thermosetting properties, which means it becomes a gel when exposed to heat. Oraqix has a 30-second onset time and a duration of 20 to 30 minutes. Oraqix is indicated for pain management during diagnostic or treatment procedures such as probing or scaling and root planing. See Procedure 33-1 for details about Oraqix application and Procedure 33-2 for local anesthesia application.

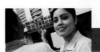

Teamwork

Teamwork is essential to a professional atmosphere. Dental hygienists can administer local anesthesia to their patients for scaling and root debridement and restorative care. This allows the dentist to spend his or her time providing services that a dental hygienist cannot provide. ▧

Table 33-6. *Topical Anesthetics*				
Brand Name	**How Supplied**	**Concentration**	**Onset**	**Duration**
Benzocaine	Gel	20%	1–2 min	5–15 min
	Liquid	20%	30 sec	10–20 min
Cetacaine	Spray	2% tetracaine 14% benzocaine	30 sec	30–60 min
Lidocaine	Ointment	5%	1–2 min	5–15 min
Oraqix	Liquid that turns to gel at body temperature	2.5% lidocaine 2.5% prilocaine	30 sec	20–30 min

Procedure 33-1 Oraqix Application

MATERIALS

Oraqix dispenser (2 parts: dispenser and barrel)
Oraqix carpule
Oraqix blunt-tipped applicator

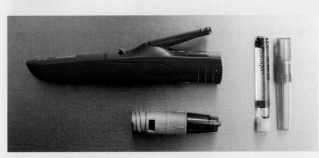

Oraqix application materials.

1. Place Oraqix cartridge in the dispenser.

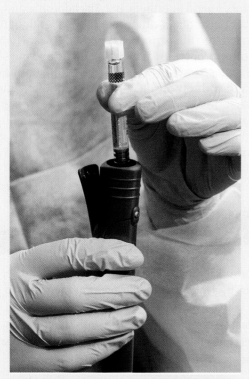

Place Oraqix cartridge in the dispenser.

   a. Ensure that the internal-ratchet mechanism is reset by pressing the reset mechanism.
2. Place the barrel onto the dispenser and twist into place.

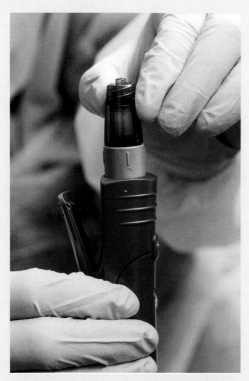

Place barrel onto dispenser and twist into place.

3. Place the blunt-tipped applicator onto the dispenser. Twist into place.

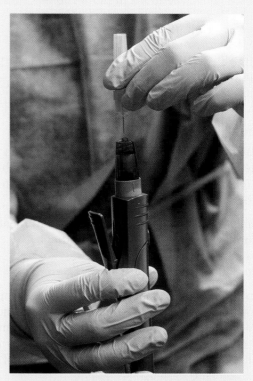

Place the blunt-tipped applicator onto the dispenser. Twist into place.

4. Take the cover off of the blunt-tipped applicator.
5. Place the blunt-tipped applicator into the periodontal pocket.

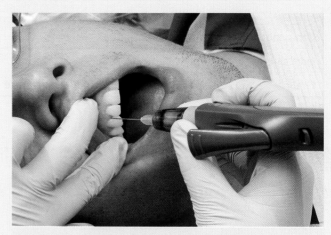

Place the blunt-tipped applicator into the periodontal pocket.

   a. Move to the base of the pocket, like a probe.
   b. Apply gel at the base of the pocket.
6. Oraqix has an onset time of 30 seconds and lasts for a duration of 20 to 30 minutes.

Procedure 33-2 Local Anesthesia Application

MATERIALS AND PREPARATION

Familiarity with the necessary materials and proper preparation for applying local anesthesia is essential in utilizing time and resources. Being prepared for the procedure will eliminate stress and difficulty during the treatment.

Gather and organize the necessary materials before the patient's arrival.

Materials

Syringe	Autoclavable, lightweight, and capable of providing effective aspirations.
Needle	Stainless steel, disposable, 25- or 27-gauge needle. The term *gauge* refers to the diameter of the needle opening, or lumen; the higher the gauge number, the smaller the diameter of the lumen. Long needle is approximately 32 mm; short needle is approximately 20 mm.

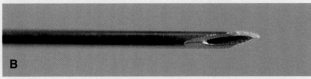

A. Parts of the needle. B. Beveled needle.

Cartridge	Prefilled 1.8 mL; store at room temperature, away from light. The cartridge contains the local anesthetic drug and may also include a vasoconstrictor. If a vasoconstrictor is added, the cartridge will also contain sodium bisulfite as a preservative. Sodium chloride is also added to make the solution **isotonic**.
Topical anesthetic	Decreases the discomfort of needle penetration. Topical anesthesia utilized before dental injections is usually in gel form. The topical

anesthetic is absorbed through the mucous membrane and is effective on surface tissue (2–3 mm). A minimal quantity is applied to the site for approximately 1 minute. Consult manufacturer recommendations.

Applicator sticks	For application of topical and pressure anesthesia. Due to the possibility of breakage, sterilizing cotton swabs is not recommended when using them for pressure techniques.
Cotton gauze	For tissue preparation and retraction.
Hemostat	To assist in the unlikely occurrence of needle breakage.
Sharps container	For safe disposal of sharps in compliance with regulations of the Occupational Safety and Health Administration (OSHA).

PREPROCEDURE

Preparation

Review the patient's medical history to determine whether there are any contradictions to treatment. Assess the need for anesthesia by reviewing the treatment plan. The anesthetic utilized will be determined by the medical history and treatment indicated.

PROCEDURE

1. *Assemble the syringe*

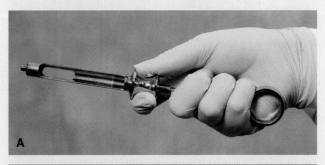

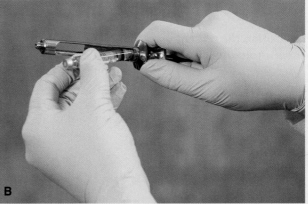

PSA nerve supraperiosteal/infiltration. A. Retract the piston to allow the cartridge to slide onto the barrel. B. Insert the cartridge with the rubber stopper toward the piston.

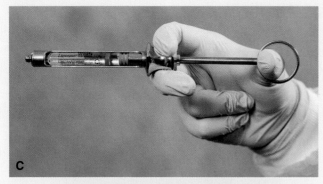

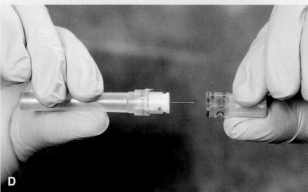

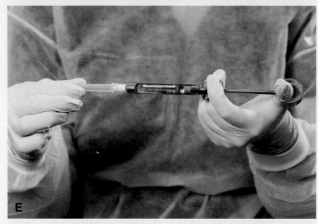

C. Release tension on the piston and confirm that the cartridge is fully seated. D. Gently turn the cap on the needle to break the seal and open the needle. E. Screw the needle securely onto the needle adapter.

- Orient the needle so the bevel will be toward the patient's bone during the injection.
- Test the syringe assembly.

2. Position the patient

Have the patient rinse with an antimicrobial rinse. Place the patient in a supine position for the injection procedure. The clinician is seated to have a better view of the anatomical landmarks. This is comfortable for the clinician and is helpful in case the patient faints (syncope).

3. Prepare tissue

- Wipe the injection site with a clean 2 × 2 gauze.
- Apply a small amount of topical anesthetic. Wait 1 to 2 minutes and then wipe off the excess topical solution. If administering a palatal injection, consider the use of a cotton-tipped applicator for pressure anesthesia.
- Retract the patient's lip or cheek for easier access to and better visibility of the injection site. Hold the soft tissue taut between two fingers. Keep the syringe out of the patient's sight.

4. Inject and aspirate

- Insert the needle with the bevel placed toward the bone into the injection site. The local anesthetic solution drip can be seen from the beveled side. For an anesthetic solution to be effective and safe, it must not be delivered directly into a blood vessel. Before depositing any anesthetic solution, and throughout the injection, aspirate by holding the needle steady at the appropriate deposition site and creating negative pressure within the cartridge. When using a standard harpoon-style syringe, gently pull the thumb back against the ring. Generally, 1 to 2 mm is all that is needed.
- A **negative aspiration** occurs when no blood is visible in the cartridge. The syringe should then be rotated a quarter turn and the aspiration repeated to prevent a false positive.
- A **positive aspiration** occurs when blood is seen flowing into the cartridge. At this point the needle needs to be withdrawn. Both the needle and the cartridge may need to be replaced to determine the result of subsequent aspirations.

5. Rate of application

- Slowly deposit the anesthetic solution to reduce the risk of overdose, decrease complications, and increase patient comfort. Although the rate of approximately 2 minutes for the deposition of 1.8 mL is considered safe and comfortable, Malamed suggests that "a more realistic time span in a clinical situation...is 60 seconds for a full 1.8 mL cartridge."[3]

6. Recap the needle

- Carefully withdraw the needle after completing the injection and recap the needle.
- OSHA regulations require that needles be recapped using the one-handed "scoop" technique or a mechanical device to hold the needle sheath. Check state practice laws for additional requirements; for example, Ohio state law requires the use of a card prop.

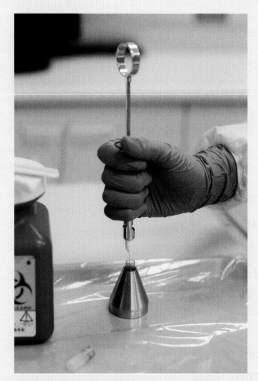

One-handed scoop recapping technique with weighted cap holder.

- Needles should never be bent. This will increase the possibility of injury to the patient or clinician.
- After needles are recapped and removed from the syringe, they must be placed into an appropriate sharps container. Sharps containers should be readily accessible.

POSTPROCEDURE

Treatment Entry and Legal Documentation

Record the date of visit, medical status, reason for using the anesthetic, and topical and local anesthetic agents used in the patient's chart. Indicate if a vasoconstrictor is used, and record the concentration level. Include the injection sites, needle(s) used, result of aspirations, total volume administered, effect of anesthesia (profound), duration if unusual, patient acceptance, any adverse reaction, and instructions provided.

TREATMENT ENTRY EXAMPLE

12/13/xx Update Med hx, no contraindications to treatment or anesthesia. Blood pressure 122/78. 5% benzocaine used as topical before injections. Scaled UR buccal quadrant with 1 carpule of 2% lidocaine 1:100,000. Injected PSA, MSA, ASA, all negative aspirations. Patient reported profound anesthesia and no complications were noted.

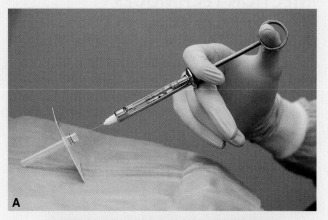

A

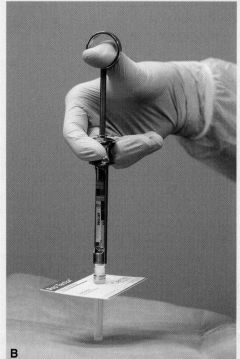

B

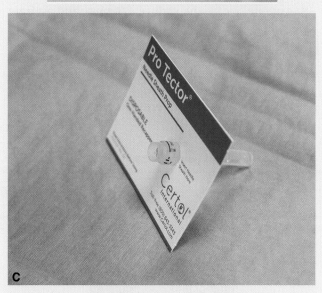

C

One-handed scoop recapping technique with a card prop.

INJECTION TECHNIQUES

Posterior Superior Alveolar Nerve Block

The posterior superior alveolar (PSA) nerve block provides pulpal anesthesia for the maxillary third, second, and first molars and associated buccal soft tissue (Fig. 33-6). The mesiobuccal root of the first molar is not anesthetized.

Needle

• 25- or 27-gauge short needle

Landmarks

• Height of the mucobuccal fold
• Maxillary tuberosity
• Zygomatic process of the maxilla

Procedure

1. Prepare tissue.
2. Orient bevel of needle toward bone.
3. Patient is in a supine position, with the head turned slightly toward the clinician. Patient's mouth is partially open, pulled toward the injection side. For left PSA nerve block, a right-handed clinician should sit at the 10 o'clock position facing the patient. For a right PSA nerve block, a right-handed clinician should sit at the 8 o'clock position facing the patient.
4. Retract and pull tissue taut.
5. Insert needle into the height of the mucobuccal fold (over 2nd molar).
6. Hold the syringe parallel with the long axis of the tooth.
7. Advance needle upward at a 45° angle, inward at a 45° angle, and backward at a 45° angle until the needle has been advanced approximately 16 mm.
8. Aspirate, rotate the syringe 1/4 turn, and aspirate again.
9. If both aspirations are negative, slowly deposit approximately 0.9 mL over 30 to 60 seconds. Aspirate several times during the procedure.
10. Slowly withdraw the syringe.
11. Recap the needle as directed in Procedure 33-2.

12. Wait 3 to 5 minutes to determine the quality of anesthesia, and assess the patient for any complications.
13. Document the type of injection, negative aspiration, the type of anesthetic used, the number of cartridges delivered, and any complications.

Infiltration for Posterior Superior Alveolar, Middle Superior Alveolar, and Anterior Superior Alveolar Blocks

Posterior superior alveolar (PSA), middle superior alveolar (MSA), and anterior superior alveolar (ASA) blocks provide small areas of pulpal and soft tissue anesthesia (Fig. 33-7).

Needle

• 25- or 27-gauge short needle

Landmarks

• Height of the mucobuccal fold
• Maxillary tuberosity
• Zygomatic process of the maxilla

Procedure

1. Prepare tissue.
2. Orient bevel of needle toward bone.
3. Patient's mouth is partially open, pulled toward the injection side. Patient is in the supine or semisupine position. To administer an ASA nerve block on the right, a right-handed clinician sits at a 10 o'clock position facing the patient. For the left ASA nerve block, a right-handed clinician sits at the 8 or 9 o'clock position facing the patient.
4. Retract and pull tissue taut.
5. Insert needle into the height of the mucobuccal fold over the target area. For example:
   • PSA: Over distal buccal root of 2nd molar providing pulpal anesthesia for Mx 3rd, 2nd, and 1st molars and associated buccal soft tissue (excluding the mesial buccal root of the maxillary 1st molar)
   • MSA: Over 2nd premolar (anterior to zygomatic) providing pulpal anesthesia for the Mx 1st and 2nd premolar and associated buccal soft tissue
   • ASA: Over canine/lateral incisor providing pulpal anesthesia for canine, lateral, and central incisors and associated soft tissue

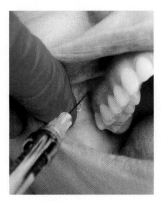

Figure 33-6. PSA nerve block.

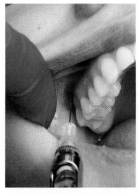

Figure 33-7. PSA nerve supraperiosteal/infiltration.

6. Hold the syringe parallel with the long axis of the tooth.
7. Advance the needle until the bevel is at or above the apical region of the target tooth.
8. Aspirate two times.
9. If both aspirations are negative, slowly deposit approximately 0.6 mL over 30 seconds. Do not allow the tissue to swell, or balloon, a sign that the anesthetic was deposited too quickly.
10. Slowly withdraw the syringe.
11. Recap the needle as directed in Procedure 33-2.
12. Wait 3 to 5 minutes to determine the quality of anesthesia and assess the patient for any complications.
13. Document the type of injection, negative aspiration, the type of anesthetic used, the number of cartridges delivered, and any complications

Infraorbital Nerve Block

The infraorbital (IO) nerve block anesthetizes the ASA, MSA, and IO nerves (Fig. 33-8).

Needle

- 25-gauge long needle

Landmarks

- Height of the mucobuccal fold
- Infraorbital notch
- Infraorbital foramen

Procedure

1. Prepare tissue.
2. Locate infraorbital foramen. Palpate the infraorbital foramen and hold your finger over it.
3. Orient bevel of needle toward bone.
4. Retract the tissue.
5. Insert needle into the height of the mucobuccal fold over the first premolar.
6. Hold the syringe parallel with the long axis of the tooth.
7. Advance the needle until the bevel gently contacts bone.
8. Aspirate.
9. If aspiration is negative, slowly deposit approximately 0.9 mL to 1.2 mL over 30 to 40 seconds. Maintain pressure with your finger over the infraorbital foramen

throughout the injection and for 1 minute after the injection.
10. Slowly withdraw the syringe.
11. Recap the needle as directed in Procedure 33-2.
12. Wait 3 to 5 minutes to determine the quality of anesthesia and assess the patient for any complications.
13. Document the type of injection, negative aspiration, the type of anesthetic used, the number of cartridges delivered, and any complications.

Greater Palatine Block

Used for pain control during periodontal procedures, the greater palatine (GP) block anesthetizes the posterior portion of the hard palate (Fig. 33-9).

Needle

- 27-gauge short needle

Landmarks

- Greater palatine foramen
- Junction of the maxillary alveolar process and the palatine bone
- Maxillary 1st and 2nd molar

Procedure

1. Patient is supine with mouth open wide, neck extended, and head turned to right or left, depending on injection site. For the right greater palatine nerve block, a right-handed clinician sits at an 8 o'clock position directly facing the patient. For the left greater palatine nerve block, a right-handed operator sits at an 11 o'clock position directly facing the patient.
2. Injection site is about 2 mm anterior to greater palatine foramen. Using a cotton swab, palpate posteriorly from the maxillary 1st molar along the alveolar process and palatine bone. The swab will "fall" into the depression created by the greater palatine foramen, which is usually distal to the maxillary 2nd molar.
3. Prepare tissue.
4. Advance the syringe from the opposite side of the mouth at a right angle to the palate.
5. Apply pressure for at least 30 seconds at the area of the foramen with a cotton swab in the left hand. Note ischemia (blanching) at injection site.

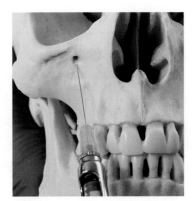

Figure 33-8. IO nerve block.

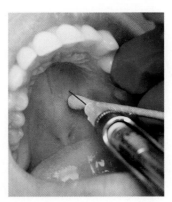

Figure 33-9. GP block.

6. Direct the needle in from the opposite side of the mouth.
7. Gently place the bevel against the ischemic tissue.
8. Apply enough pressure to bow the needle slightly.
9. Deposit a small amount of anesthesia.
10. Straighten the needle and penetrate the mucosa.
11. Continue to deposit small amounts of anesthesia throughout the procedure.
12. Insert needle about 2 to 5 mm.
13. Aspirate. If aspiration is negative, slowly deposit 0.45 to 0.6 mL of anesthetic (1/4–1/3 cartridge).
14. Slowly withdraw the syringe.
15. Recap the needle as directed in Procedure 33-2.
16. Wait 3 to 5 minutes to determine the quality of anesthesia and assess the patient for any complications.
17. Document the type of injection, negative aspiration, the type of anesthetic used, the number of cartridges delivered, and any complications.

Nasopalatine Nerve Block

The nasopalatine (NP) nerve block anesthetizes the anterior portion of the hard palate, from mesial of right first premolar to mesial of left first premolar (Fig. 33-10).

Patient should open wide, extend neck, and turn head right or left (to increase visibility).

Needle

• 25- or 27-gauge short needle

Landmarks

• Incisive papilla

Procedure

1. Position patient in a supine position with neck extended, head turned right or left to increase visibility, and mouth open wide.
2. Prepare tissue.
3. Apply pressure to the side of the incisive papilla with swab in left hand (if right handed). Incisive papilla should be ischemic (blanched).
4. Place bevel against ischemic tissue. Do not insert the needle directly into the incisive papilla.
5. Apply enough pressure to bow needle.
6. Deposit a small amount of anesthetic.
7. Straighten the needle and penetrate tissue.

8. Deposit small amounts of anesthesia while advancing needle. Depth of penetration is less than 4 mm.
9. Aspirate. If aspiration is negative, deposit slowly (15–30 seconds) 0.45 mL (1/4 cartridge) of anesthetic.
10. Slowly withdraw the syringe.
11. Recap needle as directed in Procedure 33-2.
12. Wait 3 to 5 minutes to determine the quality of anesthesia and assess the patient for any complications.
13. Document the type of injection, negative aspiration, the type of anesthetic used, the number of cartridges delivered, and any complications.

Inferior Alveolar Nerve Block

Often referred to as the *mandibular nerve block*, the inferior alveolar (IA) nerve block anesthetizes mandibular teeth to midline and buccal soft tissue anterior to the mandibular first molar (Fig. 33-11). The lingual nerve is commonly anesthetized at this time, anesthetizing the lingual soft tissue, floor of the mouth, and anterior two-thirds of the tongue.

Needle

• 25-gauge long needle

Landmarks

• Coronoid notch
• Pterygomandibular raphe
• Occlusal plane of mandibular posterior teeth

Procedure

1. Position patient in supine position with neck extended, head turned right or left to increase visibility, and mouth open wide.
2. Height of Injection
   • Palpate coronoid notch, and stretch tissue laterally.
   • Imagine a line running posterior from your finger (or thumb) to the deepest part of the pterygomandibular raphe. This line should be parallel to the occlusal plane of the mandibular teeth.
3. Insertion
   • Buccal mucosa on the medial side of the ramus, 6 to 10 mm above the mandibular occlusal plane, almost at the deepest recess of the pterygomandibular raphe. The needle approaches from the opposite labial commissure.

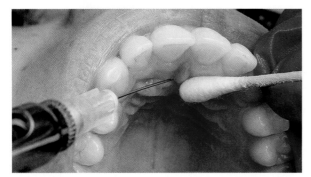

Figure 33-10. NP block.

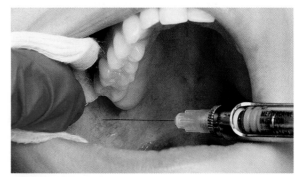

Figure 33-11. IA block.

- The long needle is inserted into the pterygo-mandibular space until it contacts bone, an average depth of 20 to 25 mm (proximally 3/4 of long needle).
- When bone is contacted, withdraw about 1 mm.
- Aspirate. If aspiration is negative, slowly deposit 1.5 mL of anesthesia over 60 seconds.
- Slowly withdraw needle.
- Recap needle as directed in Procedure 33-2.
- Sit patient up.
- Wait 3 to 5 minutes to determine the quality of anesthesia and assess the patient for any complications.
- Document the type of injection, negative aspiration, the type of anesthetic used, the number of cartridges delivered, and any complications.

Gow-Gates

The Gow-Gates (GG) mandibular block anesthetizes the inferior alveolar, mental, incisive, lingual, mylohyoid, and auriculotemporal nerves. The buccal nerve is anesthetized 75% of the time.

Landmarks

- Corners of the mouth
- Lower border of the tragus
- Mesiolingual cusp of the maxillary second molar

Procedure

1. Prepare tissue.
2. Locate the lower border of the tragus and corner of the mouth. Place thumb on the coronoid notch. Retract tissue.
3. Insert needle just distal to the maxillary second molar. The needle approaches from the opposite labial commissure. The needle should be parallel with the angle between the labial commissure and the lower border of the tragus notch.
4. Penetrate tissue until the needle contacts the neck of the condyle, usually 25 mm.
5. Withdraw the needle 1 mm, and aspirate. If negative aspiration, slowly deposit 1.8 mL of anesthetic solution over 60 to 90 seconds.
6. Slowly withdraw the needle.
7. Recap needle as directed in Procedure 33-2.
8. Direct the patient keep his or her mouth open for 1 to 2 minutes.
9. Return the patient to a seated position.
10. Wait 5 minutes to determine the quality of anesthesia and assess the patient for any complications.
11. Document the type of injection, negative aspiration, the type of anesthetic used, the number of cartridges delivered, and any complications.

Buccal Nerve Block

The buccal (B) nerve block anesthetizes the buccal soft tissue of mandibular molars (Fig. 33-12).

Needle

- 25- or 27-gauge long or short needle

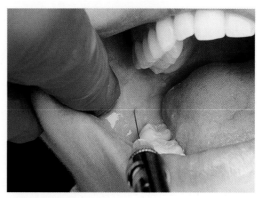

Figure 33-12. Buccal nerve block.

Landmarks

- Mandibular molars
- Coronoid notch

Procedure

1. Position patient in the supine position with neck extended, head turned right or left to increase visibility, and mouth open wide. Prepare tissue.
2. Orient bevel of needle toward the bone. Pull the buccal soft tissue laterally. Syringe is parallel to occlusal surface.
3. Insert needle distal and buccal to the terminal molar on the anterior border of the ramus.
4. Penetrate tissue until it contacts bone, usually 1 to 2 mm.
5. Aspirate. If negative aspiration, slowly deposit 0.3 mL over 10 seconds.
6. Slowly withdraw the syringe.
7. Recap needle as directed in Procedure 33-2.
8. Wait 3 to 5 minutes to determine the quality of anesthesia and assess the patient for any complications.
9. Document the type of injection, negative aspiration, the type of anesthetic used, the number of cartridges delivered, and any complications.

Mental/Incisive (M/I) Nerve Block

The mental nerve innervates the buccal mucosa anterior to the mental foramen to the midline and the lower lip and chin to midline. The incisive nerve innervates the pulpal tissue of the premolars, canines, and incisors. The lingual soft tissue is not anesthetized with this injection (Fig. 33-13).

Needle

- 25- or 27-gauge short needle

Landmarks

- Mandibular premolars
- Mucobuccal fold

Procedure

1. Prepare tissue.
2. Orient bevel of needle toward bone. Retract and pull tissue taut. Direct patient to close mouth partially to increase access, and locate the mental foramen.

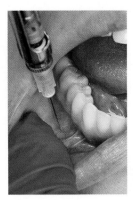

Figure 33-13. Mental/incisive nerve block.

3. Insert needle into the mucous membrane, at the canine or first premolar. Advance the needle toward the mental foramen to a depth of 5 to 6 mm.
4. Aspirate.
   - Positive aspiration occurs 5.7% of the time.
   - If negative aspiration, deposit 0.6 mL (1/3 cartridge) over 20 seconds.
5. Slowly withdraw the syringe.
6. Recap needle as directed in Procedure 33-2.
7. Wait 3 to 5 minutes to determine the quality of anesthesia and assess the patient for any complications.
8. Document the type of injection, negative aspiration, the type of anesthetic used, the number of cartridges delivered, and any complications.

Tables 33-7 and 33-8 summarize information about maxillary and mandibular injection sites.

ADVERSE SYSTEMIC REACTIONS

Systemic reactions to local anesthesia usually are a result of an excessive amount of the local anesthetic agent. The possible causes of an elevated blood level or drug overdose are related to administration of an excessive amount of anesthetic agent.[8] This may be based on the patient's medical status, rapid absorption into the circulatory system due to the rate of injection, or an intravascular injection that may have been prevented by utilizing a proper aspirating technique.

Adverse reactions may also occur if the patient has reduced kidney or liver function, which would affect the metabolism and/or excretion of the drug. With significant renal dysfunction, the body metabolizes all drugs more slowly, increasing the risk of overdose. Medical consult is advised; limit doses of all drugs depending on severity.[1]

Adjust dosage of drugs metabolized by the kidneys when glomerular filtration rate (GFR) is less than 60.[9] However, local anesthetic dosage adjustment is generally not required. Patients receiving hemodialysis should avoid dental care on the day of hemodialysis.

An allergic reaction, a rare occurrence with amide anesthetic agents, could be caused by the sodium bisulfite added as a preservative. Symptoms of an allergic reaction can be mild (rash) to severe (anaphylaxis).

MEDICAL CONDITIONS

Malignant Hyperthermia

Malignant hyperthermia is a genetically transmitted syndrome. According to Malamud, although malignant hyperthermia was previously considered an **absolute contraindication** for the use of amide local anesthetics, it is now believed to be a **relative contraindication** to the use of amides.[3] Medical consultation is necessary before treating a patient with this condition.

Methemoglobinemia

Methemoglobinemia is a condition that occurs due to conversion of a hemoglobin molecule into a molecule that has less ability to carry oxygen. Prilocaine and articaine should be avoided in patients with methemoglobinemia.[10]

Tables 33-9 and 33-10 outline the signs and symptoms associated with moderate to high blood levels of anesthesia.

ADVERSE LOCAL REACTIONS

Proper injection techniques are imperative to reduce the potential for adverse complications such as hematoma, paresthesia, trismus, needle breakage, epithelial desquamation, and postinjection lesions.

Hematoma

Hematoma is the result of puncturing a blood vessel during an injection. The PSA injection is a common site for a hematoma due to the close proximity of the pterygoid plexus to the PSA deposition site. Apply pressure and ice to the area to minimize swelling and bleeding. Once the hematoma has stabilized, instruct the patient to apply ice intermittently for 6 hours and avoid aspirin. Also advise the patient that temporary discoloration of the skin is likely. Although a hematoma is not always preventable, proper injection techniques (e.g., depth of penetration) and knowledge of anatomy can minimize the occurrence.[11]

Paresthesia

Paresthesia is the result of trauma to the nerve during the administration of local anesthesia. Pressure from edema, high drug concentrations, or vasoconstrictors and their preservatives may also play a role in paresthesia.[11] The patient will report a feeling of numbness and tingling. This will most often affect the lingual nerve following an inferior alveolar injection. To reduce the incidence of paresthesia, always deposit anesthetic solutions slowly. If paresthesia does occur, reassure the patient that it is generally temporary. Schedule an

Table 33-7. Maxillary Injection Sites

	Posterior Superior Alveolar (PSA) Block	Middle Superior Alveolar (MSA) (infiltration)	Anterior Superior Alveolar (ASA) (infiltration)	Infra-Orbital (IO) Block	Greater Palatine (GP)	Nasopalatine (NP)	Supraperiosteal
Injection Site	Height of mucobuccal fold over the 2nd molar	Height of mucobuccal fold over the 2nd premolar	Height of mucobuccal fold over the canine	Height of mucobuccal fold over first premolar	Soft tissue just anterior to the greater palatine foramen	Incisive foramen, beneath the incisive papilla	Depth of mucobuccal fold over the apex of the targeted tooth
Nerves anesthetized	Posterior superior alveolar	Middle superior alveolar	Anterior superior alveolar	Anterior and middle superior alveolar	Greater palatine	Nasopalatine	Large terminal branches
Gauge	25 or 27 gauge	25 or 27 gauge	25 or 27 gauge	25 gauge	25 or 27 gauge	25 or 27 gauge	25 or 27 gauge
Needle Length	Short needle (20 mm)	Short needle (20 mm)	Short needle (20 mm)	Long needle (32 mm)	Short needle (20 mm)	Short needle (20 mm)	Short needle
Depth	16 mm	Less than 5 mm	Less than 5 mm	16 mm (until bone is contacted)	Until bone is contacted (3–6 mm)	3–6 mm	Less than 5 mm
Volume	0.9–1.8 mL	0.6–0.9 mL	0.6–0.9 mL	0.9–1.2 mL	0.45 mL	0.45 mL	0.6 mL
Operator position	8 or 9 o'clock	8 or 9 o'clock	8 or 9 o'clock	10 o'clock	R: 8 or 9 o'clock L: 11 o'clock	8 or 9 o'clock	8 or 9 o'clock

Table 33-8. Mandibular Injection Sites

Injection Site	Inferior Alveolar (IA)	Gow-Gates (GG)	Buccal (B)	Mental/Incisive (M/I)
Teeth anesthetized	Mandibular teeth to midline	Mandibular teeth to midline	Soft tissue buccal to mandibular molars	M: Buccal soft tissue anterior to mental foramen to midline, skin of lower lip I: pulpal fibers of the premolars, canine, and incisive teeth
Nerves anesthetized	IA: Inferior alveolar, incisive, mental Li: Lingual	IA: Mental, incisive, lingual, mylohyoid, and auriculotemporal B: 75% of the time	Buccal nerve	M: Mental nerve I: Incisive nerve
Gauge	25-gauge needle	25-gauge needle	25- or 27-gauge needle	25- or 27-gauge needle
Needle length	Long needle (32 mm)	Long needle	Long or short needle	Short needle
Depth	Approx. 20–25 mm	25–27 mm	1–4 mm	5–6 mm
Volume	0.9–1.8 mL	1.8 mL	0.3–0.45 mL	0.45–0.9 mL
Operator Position	8 or 9 o'clock	8 or 10 o'clock	8 or 9 o'clock	8 or 9 o'clock or 11 o'clock

Table 33-9. Elevated Levels of Local Anesthesia

	Signs	Symptoms	Treatment
Moderate blood levels	Central nervous system (CNS): excitation, apprehension, talkativeness, confusion, nervousness, slurred speech Cardiovascular system (CVS): elevated blood pressure, heart rate, and respiratory rate	Lightheadedness, restlessness, dizziness, headache, blurred vision, disorientation	Monitor vitals; administer oxygen Time—drug will begin to metabolize
High blood levels	CNS: tonic-clonic seizures, CNS depression CVS: reduced blood pressure, heart rate, and respiratory rate	Loss of consciousness	Summon emergency medical assistance, basic life support

Table 33-10. Elevated Levels of Vasoconstrictor (Heart Related)

Signs	Symptoms	Treatment
Elevated systolic pressure, increased heart rate	Tension, restlessness, perspiration, palpitations, respiratory difficulty	Monitor vitals; administer oxygen

appointment to evaluate, and document all interactions. Record in detail the extent of the paresthesia. Refer the patient to the appropriate specialist.

Trismus

Trismus is the limited ability to open the jaw or discomfort of the jaw caused by muscle spasms due to contact with the medial pterygoid muscle during an injection.[12] Avoidance of multiple injections and use of nontraumatic techniques can minimize this occurrence.

Needle Breakage

Needle breakage is almost always avoidable. To avoid needle breakage:

- Never insert a needle to its hub or bend it.
- Select the needle based on the injection; for example, a 25-gauge needle is appropriate when an injection requires a significant depth.

If a needle does break, remain calm. Instruct the patient not to move. If the needle is visible, use cotton pliers or a hemostat to remove it. If the needle is no longer visible, the site where the needle has penetrated the mucosa should be marked with a permanent marker. The dental hygienist and/or dentist will contact a maxillofacial surgeon for immediate consultation. The maxillofacial surgeon will try to retrieve the broken dental needle under general anesthesia. Record the incident in the patient's chart.

Epithelial Desquamation

Epithelial desquamation (sloughing of tissue) may occur due to prolonged application of topical anesthesia. Follow manufacturer recommendations when applying topical anesthetics. Patients experiencing epithelial desquamation may require analgesics to minimize the discomfort.

Postinjection Lesions

Ulcerations/lesions may occur after an intraoral injection. Latent lesions may develop after manipulation of the oral tissues. Topical analgesics may be necessary to relieve discomfort. Lesions usually resolve within 7 to 14 days.

Case Study

Mr. Brian Jones is a 32-year-old man with a history of mental illness. He is a social drinker and smokes approximately three packs of cigarettes per week. His last prophylaxis appointment was 4 years ago. He presents with 4 to 5 mm pockets, bleeding upon probing, and generalized fibrotic tissue. He also is treated for migraines. His blood pressure is 124/92. He is taking the following medications: Effexor, Paxil, Pamelor, Elavil, and Tenormin.

Case Study Exercises

1. The patient will need to be anesthetized for quadrant scaling. Considering his medical history, what factors should be taken into consideration?
   A. Drug interactions
   B. Patient's age
   C. History of migraines
   D. Blood pressure
2. Because quadrant scaling is to be performed on the mandibular left, which injections will be necessary?
   A. PSA
   B. MSA
   C. IO
   D. IA, buccal, mental
3. Shortly after anesthetizing Mr. Jones with 2% lidocaine with 1:100,000 epinephrine, he appears nervous and indicates that his heart is racing. What has caused these reactions?
   A. Lidocaine
   B. Epinephrine
   C. Allergic reaction
   D. Anxiety
4. How should the hygienist manage these clinical symptoms?
   A. Monitor vitals
   B. Remain with patient
   C. Have oxygen available
   D. All of the above

Review Questions

1. What is the standard volume in a dental local anesthetic carpule?
   A. 1.55 mL
   B. 1.8 mL
   C. 0.18 mL
   D. 18 mL

2. What would typically cause trismus following the delivery of a local anesthetic?
   A. Injecting into a blood vessel
   B. Contacting the lingual nerve
   C. Multiple injections in the same area
   D. Local anesthetic deposited into the parotid gland

3. Which of the following nerves exits the skull through the foramen ovale?
   A. Facial nerve
   B. Ophthalmic nerve
   C. Maxillary nerve
   D. Mandibular nerve
   E. Glossopharyngeal nerve

4. What is the function of the sodium chloride contained in an anesthetic solution?
   A. Makes the solution isotonic
   B. Acts as a preservative
   C. Vasoconstriction
   D. Sterile water

5. The technique for obtaining pulpal anesthesia by depositing local anesthesia close to the nerve endings is called
   A. block injection
   B. infiltration injection
   C. posterior superior alveolar nerve block
   D. block injection or infiltration injection
   E. block injection or posterior superior alveolar nerve block

---

Active Learning

1. Note the label on the cartridge with the product name and expiration date. Pull back on the thumb ring with the tip of the thumb. Insert the cartridge with the rubber stopper toward the harpoon and the diaphragm toward the needle opening. Is the harpoon engaged into the rubber stopper?

2. Once you have ensured that the harpoon is engaged into the rubber stopper, remove the safety cap from the short needle. Screw the needle into the syringe. With the palm up, be sure that the large window faces the operator. The index finger and middle fingers should be on either side of spool or winged grip of the syringe and the thumb properly engaged in the thumb ring. Test the thump grasp and harpoon engagement by pulling back on the thumb ring. This creates a negative pressure that enables the clinician to aspirate. Remove the needle sheath and express several drops of solution from the needle. Aspirate red juice from a small cup. Observe the color through the cartridge window.

3. Practice recapping the needle using a needle-stick protector. Now practice recapping using the scoop technique. Which method was easier for you to accomplish by yourself while maintaining safe protocol? ■

REFERENCES

1. Prajer R, Grosso G. Quelling the anxiety: Strategies for treating patients with anxiety disorders. *Dim Den Hyg.* 2005;3(6):40-41.
2. Milgrom P, Coldwell SE, Getz T, et al. Four dimensions of fear of dental injections. *J Am Dent Assoc.* 1997;128: 756-766.
3. Turley S. *Understanding pharmacology for health professionals.* 4th ed. Upper Saddle River, NJ: Pearson; 2010. p. 449.
4. Yagiela J, Dowd F. *Pharmacology and therapeutics for dentistry.* 6th ed. St. Louis, MO: Elsevier Mosby; 2010. p. 939.
5. Malamed ST. *Handbook of local anesthesia.* 6th ed. St. Louis, Mo: Elsevier Mosby; 2012. p. 399.
6. Bassett K, DiMarco A, Naughton D. *Local anesthesia for dental professionals.* 2nd ed. Upper Saddle River, NJ: Pearson; 2014. p. 402.
7. Becker D, Dionne R, Phero J. *Management of pain and anxiety in the dental office.* Philadelphia, PA: Saunders; 2002. p. 418.
8. Haveles E. *Applied pharmacology for the dental hygienist.* 6th ed. Maryland Heights, MO: Mosby Elsevier: 2011; p. 382.
9. Moini J. *Focus on pharmacology essentials for health professionals.* 2nd ed. Upper Saddle River, NJ: Pearson; 2012. p. 730.
10. Pickett F, Terezhalmy G. *Basic principles of pharmacology with dental hygiene applications.* Philadelphia, PA: Lippincott Williams and Wilkins; 2009. p. 328.
11. Prajer R, Grosso G. *DH notes dental hygienist's chairside pocket guide.* Philadelphia, PA: F. A. Davis; 2011. p. 223.
12. Tortora G, Grabowski S. *Principles of anatomy and physiology.* 8th ed. New York, NY: Wiley; 2002. p. 985.

Part VIII

Evaluation

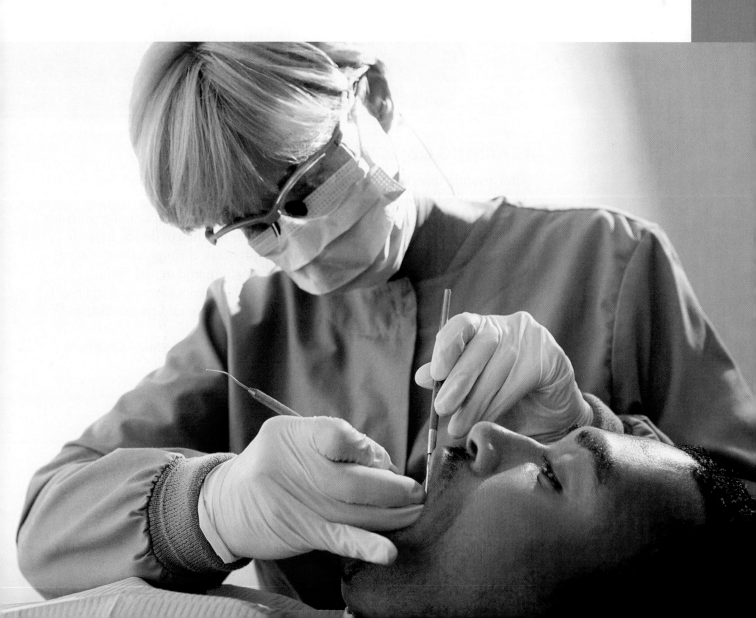

Chapter 34 | Evaluation

Ann O'Kelley Wetmore, RDH, BSDH, MSDH

KEY TERMS

evaluation

evidence-based decision
    making

formative evaluation

outcome measurements

patient advocacy

prognosis

quality assurance

referral

summative evaluation

supervised neglect

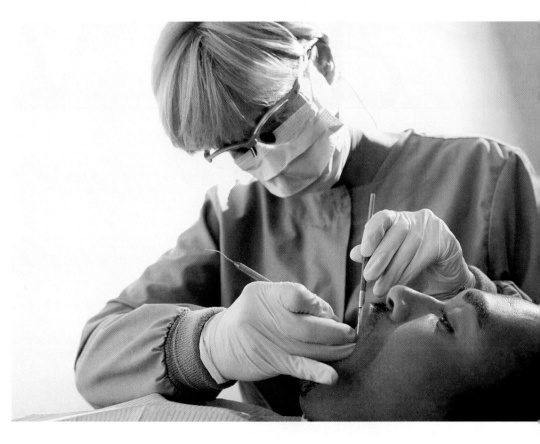

LEARNING OBJECTIVES

After reading this chapter, the student should be able to:

34.1 Describe the taxonomy of the evaluation process.

34.2 Choose the appropriate assessment mechanism to evaluate the outcome of dental hygiene care for all scopes of the practice of dental hygiene.

34.3 Demonstrate the attributes of patient advocacy through effective communication and collaboration with the patient and dental team.

34.4 Formulate an evidence-based, ethical, and legal decision-making process to evaluate the outcome of dental hygiene care in clinical practice and programs.

34.5 Analyze results of treatment implementation to determine prognosis of dental hygiene therapy.

34.6 Recognize the difference between diagnosis and prognosis.

34.7 Identify the criteria for referring a patient to dental specialists.

34.8 Identify the principles of risk management and quality assurance.

KEY CONCEPTS

- Clinical measurements and indices are used for evaluating treatment outcomes.
- Diagnosis determines the disease, and prognosis refers to the prediction for whether or not the patient will heal from that disease.

- Guidelines from dental specialty professions and practice acts provide criteria for referrals to dental specialists.
- Effective communication with patients and other health-care providers is important in evaluation of the dental hygiene process of care.
- Use of evidence-based decision making assures positive treatment outcomes.

RELEVANCE TO CLINICAL PRACTICE

Mueller-Joseph and Peterson identified evaluation as the fifth phase of the Assessment, Diagnosis, Planning, Implementation, Evaluation, and Documentation (ADPIED) dental hygiene process of care.[1] In 2008, the American Dental Hygienists" Association (ADHA) published the Standards for Clinical Dental Hygiene Practice that recognized the ADPIED as a "critical thinking model of the process of care."[2] Evaluation is the final step in providing comprehensive care for the patient. Subsequently, evaluation is the concluding phase of the clinical reasoning process.

WHAT IS EVALUATION?

According to Merriam-Webster, evaluation is the process "to determine the significance, worth, or condition of, usually by careful appraisal and study."[3] **Evaluation** is the measurement of the outcomes of dental hygiene treatment. Criteria must be measurable either qualitatively or quantitatively. Measurement tools should be reliable and valid. A reliable tool yields the same results every time.[4] A valid tool measures what it is supposed to measure.[4] Additionally, the dental hygienist is legally, ethically, and morally bound to use an evidence-based method of evaluation. Throughout ADPIED, the clinician uses the decision-making process.

The ADHA Clinical Standards of Practice identifies evaluation as a threefold process in which the clinician uses measurable criteria, communication skills, and collaboration with other professionals to complete the evaluation phase of the ADPIED dental hygiene process of care.[2] The dental hygienist:

1. Uses assessment criteria to evaluate the **measurable outcomes** of dental hygiene care (e.g., probing, plaque control, bleeding points, retention of sealants, etc.).
2. Demonstrates **patient advocacy** by communicating the outcomes of dental hygiene care to the patient, dentist, and other health-care and dental care providers.
3. Collaborates to determine the need for additional diagnostics, treatment, **referral**, education, and continuing care based on treatment outcomes and self-care behaviors.

Although evaluation was initially identified as the final step in the ADPIED dental hygiene process of care, evaluation is actually an ongoing process embedded in the provision of comprehensive dental hygiene care. For example, the clinician evaluates the assessment data, evaluates the diagnosis, evaluates the appropriateness of the treatment plan, evaluates the results of implementation, and, finally, evaluates the results of comprehensive care. This chapter discusses the evaluation process, both formative and summative, as it relates to the final phase of providing comprehensive care.

Taxonomy of Evaluation

The evaluation process is either formative, an ongoing process, or summative, a results process.[5,6] The clinician utilizes both formative and summative evaluation to determine the effectiveness of care. Table 34-1 provides a taxonomy of formative and summative evaluation in the ADPIED process of care.

Evaluation Tools

Evaluation tools must be measurable and reliable; to that end, the clinician should use evidence-based evaluation tools. Tools used during the assessment phase for gathering data to aid in diagnosing and planning are considered reliable because they will be used to measure the same criteria in the evaluation phase.[4] Armamentarium for the assessment and evaluation phase of ADPIED includes a clean mouth mirror; an explorer to detect hard and soft deposits; an explorer to detect caries; a probe that delineates not more than 2 mm between hashing, such as the UNC 15; sterile gauze; and disclosing solution. A hand mirror and intraoral camera are helpful for the patient to observe findings and will aid the clinician in demonstrating and discussing findings. The clinician may find the use of loupes and a personal headlight useful in gathering assessment and evaluation data.

Table 34-1. Formative and Summative Evaluation in the ADPIED Dental Hygiene Process of Care

ADPIED	Formative			Summative		
	Strategies/Tools		Role of Clinician	Strategies/Tools		Role of Clinician
Assessment	Evaluation of histories at each appointment	Patient feedback. Communication skills and cultural sensitivity	Listen to patient feedback and adapt therapy according to patient's expressed needs	Initial evaluation of effect on therapy based on patient histories. Evaluation of effect of therapy on the patient histories	Patient feedback. Comparison of pre- and post-therapy assessments. Communication skills and cultural sensitivity	Document and communicate expected and real outcomes
	Evaluation and comparison of clinical findings at each appointment in a multi-appointment therapy program	Dental hygiene armamentarium, clinical examination, indices, patient feedback	Listen to patient feedback and adapt therapy according to patient's expressed needs	Evaluation of clinical findings to determine outcomes of therapy	Use of intraoral and extraoral photographs to compare tissue changes. Use of software to compare periodontal changes	Document and communicate evaluation findings to the patient
	Evaluation of vital signs at each appointment.	Equipment for measuring the four vital signs: blood pressure, pulse, respiration, and temperature	Take and record vital signs to determine possible therapy adaptations and/or need for referral. Document and communicate evaluation findings to the patient	Initial evaluation of vital signs to determine the effect on therapy. Weight and height may also be noted. Evaluation of effect of therapy on the vital signs of the patient	Equipment for measuring the four vital signs: blood pressure, pulse, respiration, and temperature.	Take and record vital signs to determine possible therapy adaptations and/or need for referral. Document and communicate evaluation findings to the patient
	Evaluations of radiographs at re-care appointments	Equipment for taking radiographs and processing, either manually or digitally	Use evidence-based method to determine frequency and type of radiographs. Document and communicate radiographic findings to the patient	Initial evaluation of radiographs	Equipment for taking radiographs and processing, either manually or digitally	Use evidence-based method to determine frequency and type of radiographs. Document and communicate radiographic findings to the patient
Diagnosis	Evaluations of assessment data at re-care appointments to confirm or adjust initial periodontal diagnosis	Communication skills and cultural sensitivity. Armamentarium for assessment procedures, and feedback from patient histories	Use evidence-based decision-making process to determine the periodontal diagnosis of the patient. Use evidence based decision-making process to determine caries risk of the patient	Evaluation of initial assessment data to form a periodontal diagnosis	Communication skills and cultural sensitivity. Armamentarium for assessment procedures, and feedback from patient histories	Use evidence-based decision-making process to determine the periodontal diagnosis of the patient. Use evidence-based decision-making process to determine caries risk of the patient

	Evaluation of assessment data at re-care appointments to determine caries risk of the patient Evaluations by comparison of previous and current assessment data at re-care appointments to determine the presence of and/or risk of oral pathology	Communication skills and cultural sensitivity Armamentarium for assessment procedures, and feedback from patient histories Armamentarium for assessment procedures, and feedback from patient histories	Document and communicate diagnosis to the patient Use evidence-based decision-making process to determine caries risk of the patient Document and communicate caries risk to the patient Use evidence-based decision-making process to determine the risk and/or presence of oral pathology Document and communicate to the patient the risk and/or presence of oral pathology	Initial evaluation of assessment data to determine caries risk of the patient Evaluation of initial assessment data to determine the presence of and/or risk of oral pathology	Communication skills and cultural sensitivity Armamentarium for assessment procedures, and feedback from patient histories Armamentarium for assessment procedures, and feedback from patient histories	Document and communicate diagnosis to the patient Use evidence-based decision-making process to determine caries risk of the patient Document and communicate caries risk to the patient Use evidence-based decision-making process to determine the risk and/or presence of oral pathology. Document and communicate to the patient the risk and/or presence of oral pathology.
Plan	Ongoing evaluation of all patient data to assure a needs-based treatment plan	Skills in listening, communication, goal setting, motivational interviewing, and anticipatory guidance Cultural sensitivity	Document and communicate any adjustments in the treatment plan based on patient feedback	Evaluation of all patient data and current research to assure needs-based and evidence-based treatment plan	Skills in listening, communication, goal setting, motivational interviewing, and anticipatory guidance Cultural sensitivity	Document and communicate to the patient the treatment plan and obtain informed consent
Implementation	Ongoing evaluation of removal of hard and soft deposits	Appropriate instruments to achieve maximum tactile sense and detect deposits	Evaluate for effective removal of deposits Inform patient of findings	Evaluation of nonsurgical therapy after 4–6 weeks to determine future therapies: re-care, referral, maintenance	Appropriate instruments to achieve maximum tactile sense and detect deposits Periodontal probe calibrated within 1 mm or an electronic probe	Summarize findings and discuss future therapy needs with the patient

Continued

Table 34-1. Formative and Summative Evaluation in the ADPIED Dental Hygiene Process of Care—cont'd

ADPIED	Formative		Summative	
	Strategies/Tools	Role of Clinician	Strategies/Tools	Role of Clinician
Ongoing evaluation of the effectiveness of pain control measures	Communication skills and cultural sensitivity	Use patient feedback, both verbal and nonverbal, to evaluate effectiveness of pain control measures	Evaluation of the effectiveness of pain control measures and a summary of what methods were the most effective; Communication skills and cultural sensitivity	Summarize effective pain control measures and document for future reference; Communicate with future practitioners a summation of effective pain control measures
Ongoing evaluation of pathologies	Communication skills and cultural sensitivity; Knowledge of evidence-based diagnostic tools available	Use appropriate diagnostic tools; Refer to specialist for differential diagnosis	Biopsy to determine pathology; Communication skills and cultural sensitivity	Communicate with patient and specialist regarding referral and results of the referral.
Ongoing evaluation of caries risk assessment	Communication skills and cultural sensitivity; CAMBRA; Radiographs; Clinical examination of the dentition	Describe the etiology of caries; Use CAMBRA to decide on remineralization therapies; Document findings, therapy recommendations, and patient compliance	An evaluation resulting in a diagnosis of active caries; Communication skills and cultural sensitivity; CAMBRA; Radiographs; Clinical examination of the dentition	Document caries findings; Provide education to patient on caries etiology and risk
Ongoing evaluation of the self-care of the patient	Communication skills and cultural sensitivity; Plaque indices	Provide feedback and make self-care adjustment recommendations accordingly	Evaluation of current self-care regimen before referral to a specialist; Communication skills and cultural sensitivity	Document current self-care regimen and results
Ongoing evaluation of the soft tissues	Intraoral photographs; Hand mirror	Demonstrate findings to the patient and document any changes	Evaluation of soft tissues at the completion of therapy; Plaque indices; Intraoral photographs; Hand mirror	Demonstrate findings to the patient and document the presence of healing

Evaluation	Ongoing evaluation of goals and therapy	Communication skills and cultural sensitivity Human Needs Model of Care Risk factors	Use the data gathered from formative evaluations to make therapy modifications or refer the patient for therapies at any time during the dental hygiene process of care	Develop a prognosis and recommend future care	Communication skills and cultural sensitivity Risk factors Comparison of pre- and postclinical findings		Using the data gathered from summative evaluations, refer the patient for therapies at the completion of the ADPIED process Use outcomes measures to determine future care needs
	Evaluation of the clinician	Communication skills and cultural sensitivity Self-assessment Reflective learning Critical thinking Evidence-based decision making Patient feedback	Use all available resources to maintain quality assurance	Evaluation of the clinician	Communication skills and cultural sensitivity Self-assessment Reflective learning Critical thinking Evidence-based decision making Patient feedback		Use all available resources to maintain quality assurance
Documentation	Legal and ethical obligation for accurate documentation	Paper Electronic patient record	Document all findings, therapies, and data gathered	Legal and ethical obligation for accurate documentation	Paper Electronic patient record	Document all findings, therapies, and data gathered Communicate with specialist all findings	

Indices that quantify plaque, such as the O'Leary plaque score and Plaque Assessment Scoring System (PASS), are commonly used in clinical practice.[7,8] Although there are other indices for measuring self-care and disease progression, they are mostly used in clinical research. See Chapter 14, Indices, for more information on indices.

A paper- or computer-based charting system is used to document all assessment and evaluation data. When comparing data, consistency and calibration are important; therefore all clinicians should be proficient in the use of both systems.

Evidence-Based Decision Making

In addition to the armamentarium used in evaluation, the clinician utilizes critical thinking skills and scientific evidence in **evidence-based decision making** about patient care (see Chapter 6, Evidence-Based Care, for more information on evidence-based care and decision making).[2,9] Evaluation is the process of determining the results and the outcomes of the provision of comprehensive care. The clinician is bound ethically, morally, and legally to use current scientific evidence and standards of care when ascertaining the effects of care. The ADHA Standards for Clinical Dental Hygiene Practice is a benchmark for the clinician for evaluation in the practice of dental hygiene.[2] This chapter provides the clinician with additional resources and guidelines for evaluating the dental hygiene process of care.

Evaluation of Assessment Data

During the assessment phase of the dental hygiene process of care, the clinician evaluates the data gathered from the patient by taking histories, completing a clinical examination, and exposing radiographs.

Patient Histories

A thorough medical and dental history is completed for each patient, along with biographical data. The clinician also evaluates the socioeconomic status of the patient. Communication skills are crucial in conducting the interview with the patient and reviewing the patient's history. It is important to observe the patient for any nonverbal communication that may be indicative of the patient's psychological state. For example, a patient with sweat on the brow or upper lip may be anxious.

A summative evaluation of the patient's history aids in determining a diagnosis and plan. **Formative evaluation** is accomplished by reviewing the patient's history at each appointment during the treatment series and assessing any changes. For example, a patient being treated for hypertension may report a change in antihypertensive medication from nifedipine (Procardia, Adalat, Nifediac) to lisinopril (Prinivil, Zestril). Upon assessment, the clinician may note positive changes in the gingival status due to the drug change and periodontal therapies.

Vital Signs

Taking and recording patient vital signs at each appointment is an example of a continuing formative evaluation of the patient's status. A **summative evaluation** may be made by comparing vital signs taken at the initial appointment with vital signs taken at the evaluation appointment. For example, a patient demonstrates a slightly elevated blood pressure at the initial appointment and the clinician initiates a conversation about the etiology of hypertension, determining that the patient is a heavy user of sodium chloride. The clinician provides nutritional counseling on the dangers of excess salt, makes recommendations for decreasing sodium in the diet, and asks the patient to set a goal for reducing salt consumption by 50%. Upon review of patient goals at the final appointment, it is determined that the patient has cut his salt consumption. A summative evaluation notes a decrease in blood pressure from his initial to final appointment.

Clinical Examination

An extraoral and intraoral examination is completed. The clinician evaluates the findings and the patient's history to determine a differential diagnosis of any potential pathology. Formative evaluation is ongoing with each visit when the clinician continues to evaluate extraoral and intraoral tissues. An example of a summative evaluation is a biopsy to determine pathology.

At the initial visit and all subsequent initial visits in a series of appointments, the clinician will complete a dental chart, sometimes called an odontogram, of the existing and needed restorations and any deviations in the dentition. Additionally, a periodontal chart noting probe depths, bleeding points, suppuration, clinical attachment level, mobility, furcations, and any mucogingival defects will be recorded. A description of the soft tissue response is documented at each appointment to determine the progress of wound healing and is formative in nature. A summative evaluation is done when the clinician compares the soft tissue response pre- and post-therapy. Photographs of the tissue and/or intraoral digital photographs are valuable tools for determining the tissue response to therapy. Odontogram and periodontal chartings are compared pre- and post-therapy to quantify a summative evaluation of therapy.

A plaque index such as the O'Leary Plaque Record or PASS should be used to quantify plaque and determine a self-care regimen. This particular measurement may be used as a formative evaluation tool to provide data to the clinician and the patient on the effectiveness of the patient's self-care. The use of disclosing solution and a plaque index not only quantifies the amount and area of the plaque but also provides a qualitative visual tool for patients to see where their self-care needs improvement. This information will help the clinician to adjust self-care recommendations and personalize the self-care goals and plan. Plaque indices and other dental indices used to evaluate the patient's self-care may be used as summative evaluation tool to determine a diagnosis and subsequent plan, or after completion of therapy to determine outcomes of treatment in the dental hygiene process of care. See Advancing Technologies.

Radiographic Examination

Radiographs are a valuable tool to ascertain information that cannot be gathered by visual examination. A summative evaluation is completed after every radiographic series to determine pathology. Radiographs are rarely used to determine the outcomes of therapy; exceptions include the endodontist and orthodontist, who rely on radiographs for establishing a successful outcome. In most cases, radiographs are used in the re-care and maintenance phase as an evaluation of previous care.

Evaluation of Diagnosis

After thorough and complete gathering of assessment data, the clinician uses critical thinking skills to evaluate the findings and make a clinical judgment regarding the diagnosis. Furthermore, the clinician must inform the patient of the diagnosis and provide a justification for the diagnosis.[10] Documentation of this communication is crucial in risk management.

Advancing Technologies

Computer-based dental practice management software is used to document financial data and maintain electronic patient records. These electronic-based programs allow digital transfer of radiographs and patient records via e-mail attachments to referring specialists. E-mail is an efficient system for communicating with referring specialties and patients. Computer-based periodontal and dental charts provide a visual display for chairside use. For example, during the evaluation phase of care, the clinician may use a computer-generated graph of pre- and post-therapy periodontal chartings to visually demonstrate areas of change. This is an excellent visual tool for patient education during the evaluation phase of therapy. Patient education software programs allow the clinician to use graphics and audio and video media to educate the patient on disease, prevention, treatment procedures, and self-care strategies. Software designed for risk assessment provides patients with a record of their risks, diagnosis, and suggested treatment modulators. In the future, cloud computing and apps may present the clinician with new ways of tracking patient self-care or providing handheld oral health education information. Indeed, patients could be in charge of maintaining their personal health information in an electronic format. Emerging technology may present the clinician with more opportunities to stay connected and access knowledge from Web 2.0. ■

Periodontal Diagnosis

Figure 34-1 demonstrates the dynamic aspects of a periodontal diagnosis and how risk factors, poor self-care, systemic disease, and tobacco use can influence a diagnosis of health versus disease. The current guidelines from the American Association of Periodontology provide the clinician with an evidence-based method of diagnosing and classifying periodontal disease (see Chapter 35, Maintenance, for more information).

Caries Diagnosis

Oral health is also evaluated by the condition of the dentition. Caries Management by Risk Assessment (CAMBRA) is a tool used to evaluate a patient's caries risk and provide diagnostic criteria. An evaluation for caries is a summative process. The clinician uses clinical assessment findings, risk factors, and radiographs to evaluate the dentition for the presence of or potential for caries. Figure 34-2 illustrates the etiology of caries. See Chapter 21, Cariology and Caries Management, for more detailed information on caries detection and CAMBRA.

Oral Pathology

Clinical findings, radiographs, and risk factors are evaluated by the clinician to discern whether abnormal findings are pathological or benign. Screening methods for oral pathologies include in-chair brush cytology and use of light sources and dyes to help the clinician with chairside differential diagnoses. Other noninvasive diagnostic tools in the future may include use of nanoparticles and light to discern normal and abnormal tissues. Currently the ultimate method of determining pathology is a surgical incision biopsy evaluated by an oral and maxillofacial pathologist. See Chapter 10, Extraoral and Intraoral Examination, and Chapter 17, Risk Assessment, for detailed information on assessing for oral pathology.

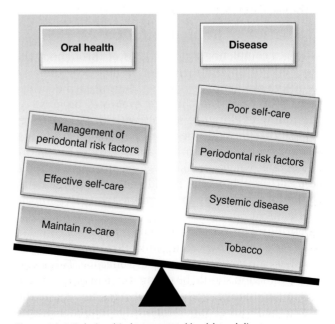

Figure 34-1. Relationship between oral health and disease.

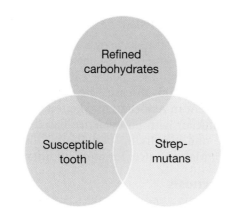

Figure 34-2. Etiology of caries.

Evaluation of Plan

The use of evidence in itself is another formative evaluation method. The clinician evaluates current studies on diagnosis and therapy to determine the best treatment plan for the patient. The clinician then presents the plan to the patient using patient informed consent (PARQ):

P = procedure planned
A = alternatives or recommendations
R = risks: "what if I do or do not proceed?"
Q = questions: are there any unanswered questions?

The benefits of PARQ in obtaining informed consent include employment of a legal-risk-management strategy and the opportunity for the patient to evaluate the treatment plan. By explaining the procedures in the plan and the alternatives or recommendations, followed by the patient asking questions, the clinician allows the patient to be the decision maker. Use of PARQ helps the clinician to avoid making assumptions about the patient's needs or wants. Additionally, utilization of PARQ allows the clinician to evaluate the patient's response to the treatment presented and make clinical judgments that maintain the standard of care.

Evaluation of Implementation

Whether completing a prophylaxis or throughout the sequence of appointments for nonsurgical therapy, formative evaluation is ongoing. During each debridement procedure, the clinician evaluates progress by alternating exploratory strokes with working strokes using a curette. With the use of powered instruments, an experienced clinician may adjust strokes to explore for deposits. For greater tactile sense, an explorer should be used throughout the debridement and at the completion of the therapy to determine the success of the debridement.

During all implementation procedures, the clinician must use effective communication to determine whether pain control measures are effective. This formative evaluation should be documented in order to provide a summative evaluation of pain control at the end of the series of appointments for reference during future treatment. When the patient is referred to other health-care providers, the referring clinician should communicate this summative evaluation of pain control to assure the best potential outcome for the patient's pain management.

Any previously noted potential pathologies should be followed during the course of therapy and evaluated at each appointment, and recommendations should be made accordingly. Appropriate referrals and/or use of other diagnostic tools can and should be implemented at the initial appointment or at any time in the sequence of appointments to achieve a differential or definitive diagnosis. The clinician must communicate the importance of diagnosis and/or continued evaluation by the patient for differences in the noted lesion. A method of self-evaluation for oral pathologies should be demonstrated to all patients so that they can continue to evaluate oral lesions for changes that may indicate a pathological condition.

The standard of care is for the periodontium of the patient to be stable before restorative therapies. If the patient is experiencing pain due to caries, the clinician will adjust the sequence of appointments in the implementation phase. Palliative restorative therapy should be implemented to alleviate pain and then periodontal therapy may be continued.

At each subsequent appointment, soft tissue changes in the previously treated areas are evaluated for healing and delayed wound healing. Changes in the color, texture, and form of the soft tissues should be noted. Delayed healing may be a sign of residual subgingival deposits that the clinician should address. In addition, the self-care of the patient should be evaluated and adjustments made to the self-care regimen. Indices such as the O'Leary plaque record and PASS provide documentation of the effectiveness of patient self-care.[7,8] To ensure that the patient understands the value of self-care, it is important to reiterate any self-care or postoperative instructions to ensure patient understanding. Self-care learning is facilitated through repetition, a well-known learning technique, when the clinician discusses the importance of self-care at each appointment. Another benefit of a multi-appointment sequence for nonsurgical therapy is that the clinician has an opportunity to develop a positive patient–provider relationship. Patient compliance is crucial to successful treatment outcomes and better **prognosis**, a prediction for whether or not the patient's disease will heal.[11,12]

Evaluation of Care

Care is evaluated both formatively and summatively. Table 34-1 describes the formative process of evaluation in the ADPIED dental hygiene process of care. At the completion of therapy, a summative evaluation of the periodontal status of a patient along with assessments will determine the prognosis and the future care for the patient.[13] The clinician and patient determine whether the treatment goals and outcomes of therapy have been met using a twofold process that is both qualitative and quantitative. Qualitative evaluations are more subjective; however, it is important for the clinician to evaluate care in this manner to validate the patient's feelings. Good rapport with a patient leads to compliance. Quantitative evaluations are linked to prognosis and real or predicted outcomes. Results of evaluating care will determine the prognoses and the need for termination of therapy, re-care schedule, maintenance, and/or referral.

Qualitative Evaluation

Research demonstrates that patients feel vulnerable during treatment; therefore effective communication between the patient and clinician is important so that the patient feels in control of the situation.[14] The clinician should constantly evaluate the patient's verbal and nonverbal cues to determine whether the patient understands all processes needed to provide comprehensive care. The clinician should avoid making assumptions about the patient's knowledge of oral health. The clinician must strive to educate the patient on oral health using current research and excellent communication skills. An educated patient can then make an informed decision about care. Effectively communicating formative and summative evaluation results with the patient, good rapport, and accurate documentation are recognized techniques for risk management.[15] See Chapter 3, Communication Skills, for more information on communication strategies.

The clinician must be culturally competent during the evaluation of care.[2,16] The clinician must understand the learning process and determine where the patient is on the learning process continuum.[3,17] Open-ended questions about current self-care, the patient's knowledge level of oral health, and long-term oral health goals will help the clinician evaluate the patient's understanding of treatment and self-care needs.[17] See Chapter 3, Communication Skills, for detailed information about communication strategies and communicating with a diverse clientele.

The Human Needs Conceptual Model provides a framework for clinicians as they evaluate patient care.[18] This model is a holistic approach that identifies the individual needs of the patient. The following eight human needs are evaluated throughout the dental hygiene process of care:[18]

1. Protection from health risks: This is the need to avoid medical contraindications during care. A thorough medical history, taking of vital signs, and modifying care appropriately will meet this human need.
2. Freedom from stress: This is the need to feel safe, free of fear, and emotionally comfortable throughout care. This need is related to cultural competence, nurturing, education, and pain management.
3. Wholesome facial image: This need is met when the clinician is aware of the patient's facial features and makes recommendations to improve esthetics and function with cultural competence and sensitivity.
4. Skin and mucous membrane integrity of head and neck: To meet this need, the clinician provides comprehensive care in order to maintain and improve the patient's head and neck, including self-care education, periodontal and nutritional care, and screening and referrals for oral cancer.
5. Biologically sound dentition: This need is met through evaluation for caries, caries preventive strategies, and restorative care.
6. Conceptualization and problem-solving: The need to be informed and educated is met using language and cultural competence.
7. Freedom from head and neck pain: Use of pain control measures ensures that this need is met.
8. Responsibility for oral health: This need is met through providing patient education and allowing patients to make decisions about their own health.

The clinician may use this model to evaluate comprehensive care as opposed to the completion of tasks or procedures.[18]

Quantitative Evaluation of Treatment Outcomes and Prognosis

Quantitative data determine the effectiveness of the implementation of the treatment plan. This may be referred to as the treatment outcomes. Additionally, evaluating risk factors is important in the plan and evaluation phase of dental care.[19] During the evaluation phase, the clinician identifies risk factors that may suggest "disease onset and/or progression, defined as a deteriorating risk profile."[19] The clinician uses decision-making skills in evaluating assessment and/or outcome data, and individual risk assessment.[13]

In addition to evaluating treatment outcomes, the clinician uses summative evaluation data to determine a prognosis. Prognosis is a prediction as to the progress, course, and outcome of a disease.[3] Periodontal prognosis has been identified as the "expected longevity of teeth with or without periodontal therapy."[20] Prognosis may differ when discussing individual teeth as opposed to the entire dentition.

Upon completion of nonsurgical therapy, the patient should be advised to return for a reevaluation procedure. The American Academy of Periodontology defines reevaluation as the "assessment of a patient's periodontal status and risk profile after therapy to be used as a basis for subsequent patient management."[13] The clinician should evaluate the following aspects during the clinical reevaluation procedure:

Gingival wound healing: Observe and document the areas of soft tissue inflammation. Plaque control and systemic conditions may influence results even after completion of nonsurgical therapy.[21] Inform and demonstrate findings to the patient.

Plaque: Complete a plaque index such as the O'Leary Plaque Record or PASS and compare it with previous scores. Explain the findings to the patient. The patient's ability to remove bacterial pathogens effectively is a factor in determining a good or poor prognosis for arresting disease.[21,22]

Bleeding: A complete recording of all areas that bleed upon probing should be noted. A reduction in the amount of bleeding upon probing indicates subgingival wound healing and possible reattachment of the junctional epithelium.[23] Conversely, the clinician should use bleeding on probing as an indication that there are residual subgingival deposits or other systemic factors delaying or impeding wound healing. Any observed suppuration indicates active infection in the site and is noted for further evaluation.[19] Patient compliance with plaque control is related to reduced plaque and bleeding on probing.[12]

Attachment: A complete periodontal examination, including probe depths, site of the gingival margin, and any mucogingival defects, should be completed and documented. The clinical attachment level should be calculated to determine the loss or regain of attachment. Research suggests that clinical attachment loss is significant in determining the prognosis of an individual tooth.[20,24,25] "Increasingly severe attachment level" is consistent as a risk for tooth loss, with or without respect to any other tooth conditions.[26]

Furcation: The severity of furcation involvement is directly related to the criteria for referral to a specialist.[13] Teeth with furcation involvement have a poorer prognosis because of loss of attachment and bone height.[27, 28] The clinician must explore the furcations with a furcation probe, such as the Nabors probe, and document all furcations on the periodontal chart. Note that the furcations may increase compared with the initial assessment due to the removal of subgingival deposits during nonsurgical therapy. Oral self-care measures should be adjusted in order to reduce the biofilm in the furcation.

Mobility: The presence of mobility is a risk factor for a poor prognosis. Tooth mobility related to bone loss has a poorer prognosis than tooth mobility related to inflammation or trauma.[29] Note that there may be an increase in tooth mobility compared with the initial assessment due to the removal of hard deposits that "held" the tooth in the socket. An occlusal analysis should be performed to determine the presence of occlusal trauma, believed by some to be a contributing factor to periodontal disease.[30,31]

Research demonstrates that there are many risk factors for periodontal disease. The clinician evaluates if there are other risk factors, such as systemic disease, that may influence the outcomes of care. Evaluate the patient for the following risk factors:

Use of tobacco: Smoking is directly related to periodontal disease and is a major risk factor.[27,28] Patients who continue to smoke have a worse prognosis than patients who do not smoke or who quit.[20] The clinician should reinforce the importance of quitting tobacco and encourage patients to comply with a tobacco cessation program.[32] Ongoing evaluation of compliance is important because of the potential for relapse.[32] The clinician must educate the patient and document patient progress toward tobacco cessation.

See Chapter 4, Health Education and Promotion, for information on helping patients with tobacco cessation.

Nutrition: Having the patient complete a food diary for assessment and guidance and for comparison with the initial food diary is an effective evaluation tool.[33] Nutritional counseling goals should be reviewed and discussed. Goals that have been met should be praised, followed by a discussion of future nutritional goals.[33,34] Nutritional risk factors related to poor prognosis include lack of calcium and vitamin C.[35,36]

Age, gender, and heredity: Classic studies demonstrate that the risk of chronic periodontal disease and the potential for a good prognosis are directly related to getting older. There is no conclusive evidence to suggest one gender is more at risk for periodontal disease than the other; however, some literature suggests that women have a greater potential for periodontal disease than men due to hormonal influences.[37,38] Heredity is a risk factor; the clinician should evaluate risk by questioning the patient about the current dentition of his or her parents and whether one or both parents have a history of periodontal disease.

Systemic factors: Emerging research demonstrates that numerous diseases and conditions affect the overall prognosis for the dentition. The clinician must constantly evaluate the patient's current health status. Diseases and conditions that have a positive correlation with a poor prognosis for maintaining a healthy periodontium include diabetes, immunodeficiency states, neutrophil disorders, osteoporosis, and stress.[21,27,28,38–43]

Referrals

A critical part of the evaluation process is referral. Using the data gathered from either formative or summative evaluations, the clinician may choose to refer the patient for therapies at any time during the dental hygiene process of care. Although it is sometimes difficult to "let the patient go," the clinician is bound morally, ethically, and legally to refer a patient when it is determined that the scope of care required is beyond that of the practitioner. Good patient–clinician communication and appropriate referrals prevent **supervised neglect**, "a case in which a patient is regularly examined and shows signs of a disease or other medical problems but is not informed of its presence or progress."[44] Principles of referral are based on guidelines from dental specialties and practice acts (Table 34-2).

Practitioners should establish relationships with all dental specialists and other health-care providers, for example a registered dietitian, a physician, and an acupuncturist. Communication with the clinicians, patients, and specialists should be open. An open dialogue using e-mail, phone, or letters leads to a relationship of mutual respect. Established methods of sharing data must be adhered to and agreed to by both the referring practitioner and the specialist (see Teamwork).

Table 34-2. *Specialist, Specialty, and Referral Guidelines*

Specialist	Specialties Approved by the American Dental Association (ADA)	Referral Guidelines
Endodontist	Endodontics: The branch of dentistry concerned with the morphology, physiology, and pathology of the human dental pulp and periradicular tissues. Its study and practice encompass the basic and clinical sciences, including biology of the normal pulp and the etiology, diagnosis, prevention, and treatment of diseases and injuries of the pulp and associated periradicular conditions. (Adopted by ADA, December 1983)	AAE Endodontic Case Difficulty Assessment Form and Guidelines, available from American Association of Endodontics website, http://www.aae.org/
Oral and Maxillofacial Pathologist	Oral and maxillofacial pathology: Oral pathology is the specialty of dentistry and discipline of pathology that deals with the nature, identification, and management of diseases affecting the oral and maxillofacial regions. It is a science that investigates the causes, processes, and effects of these diseases. The practice of oral pathology includes research and diagnosis of diseases using clinical, radiographic, microscopic, biochemical, or other examinations. (Adopted by ADA, May 1991)	Submission Policy on Excised Tissue, available from the American Academy of Oral & Maxillofacial Pathology website, http://www.aaomp.org/
Oral and Maxillofacial Radiologist	Oral and maxillofacial radiology: The specialty of dentistry and discipline of radiology concerned with the production and interpretation of images and data produced by all modalities of radiant energy that are used for the diagnosis and management of diseases, disorders, and conditions of the oral and maxillofacial region. (Adopted by ADA, April 2001)	To locate an oral and maxillofacial radiologist, see the Academy of Oral & Maxillofacial Pathology website, http://www.aaomr.org/
Oral and Maxillofacial Surgeon	Oral and maxillofacial surgery: The specialty of dentistry that includes the diagnosis and surgical and adjunctive treatment of diseases, injuries, and defects involving both the functional and esthetic aspects of the hard and soft tissues of the oral and maxillofacial region. (Adopted by ADA, October 1990)	See the American Association of Oral and Maxillofacial Surgeons website, http://www.aaoms.org/
Orthodontist	Orthodontics and dentofacial orthopedics: The dental specialty that includes the diagnosis, prevention, interception, and correction of malocclusion, and neuromuscular and skeletal abnormalities of the developing or mature orofacial structures. (Adopted by ADA, April 2003)	The American Association of Orthodontists provides guidelines for referral at http://www.aaomembers.org/press/HealthCareProfessionals/index.cfm
Pedodontist	Pediatric dentistry: An age-defined specialty that provides both primary and comprehensive preventive and therapeutic oral health care for infants and children through adolescence, including those with special health-care needs. (Adopted by ADA, 1995)	Guideline on Periodicity of Examination, Preventive Dental Services, Anticipatory Guidance/Counseling, and Oral Treatment for Infants, Children, and Adolescents available from the American Association of Pediatric Dentistry, http://www.aapd.org/
Periodontist	Periodontics: Specialty of dentistry that encompasses the prevention, diagnosis, and treatment of diseases of the supporting and surrounding tissues of the teeth or their substitutes and the maintenance of the health, function, and esthetics of these structures and tissues. (Adopted by ADA, December 1992)	Guidelines for the Referral of Periodontal Patients available from the American Academy of Periodontology, http://www.perio.org (These guidelines are also found in Chapter 35, Maintenance, of this text.)

Continued

Table 34-2. *Specialist, Specialty, and Referral Guidelines—cont'd*

Specialist	Specialties Approved by the American Dental Association (ADA)	Referral Guidelines
Prosthodontist	Prosthodontics: The dental specialty pertaining to the diagnosis, treatment planning, rehabilitation, and maintenance of the oral function, comfort, appearance, and health of patients with clinical conditions associated with missing or deficient teeth and/or oral and maxillofacial tissues using biocompatible substitutes. (Adopted by ADA, April 2003)	Prosthodontic Diagnostic Index available from the American College of Prosthodontists website, http://www.prosthodontics.org/
Implantologist*	*Currently there is no approved implantology specialty. Implants are part of the curriculum for periodontology, oral and maxillofacial surgery, and prosthodontology.	
Other Professional Specialists		
Physician	A person educated, clinically experienced, and licensed to practice medicine as usually distinguished from surgery	American Medical Association, http://www.ama-assn.org/
Endocrinologist	Physician who specializes in the diagnosis and treatment of conditions affecting the endocrine system such as diabetes	American Association of Clinical Endocrinologists, http://www.aace.com/org/
Cardiologist	Physician who specializes in the structure and function and disorders of the heart	American College of Cardiology, http://www.cardiosource.org/
Registered Dietitian	A food and nutrition expert who has met academic and professional requirements, including: • Earned a bachelor's degree with coursework approved by the ADA's Commission on Accreditation for Dietetics Education • Completed an accredited, supervised practice program at a health-care facility, community agency, or foodservice corporation • Passed a national examination administered by the Commission on Dietetic Registration • Completes continuing professional educational requirements to maintain registration	American Dietetic Association, http://www.eatright.org/

Teamwork

Given the oral–systemic connection, interdisciplinary care benefits the patient, the oral health-care providers, and the medical and dental specialists. Practitioners who choose to provide interdiscipliary care must give their time, trust, support, and commitment to maximize the potential for successful interdisciplinary patient care. The initial care provider (either a generalist or specialist) builds the relationship and then in turn refers the patient to a competent health-care provider or providers, and the trust is transferred. Trust and confidence among the care providers facilitates the professional relationship needed to provide interdisciplinary care. Leadership and teamwork are crucial for successful treatment co-therapy; one caregiver, usually the initial care provider, must be the point of contact for the patient to avoid fragmented multi-disciplinary care. The key element to maintaining working relationships among all providers of care is communication. A communication protocol needs to be established and followed by all providers in order to meet all of the needs of providers and patients. The treatment plan and the decision-making process are ongoing and shared to best serve the needs of the patient. An added benefit is that the care providers share knowledge and skills, therefore learning from each other and promoting lifelong learning.[51] ■

The clinician may find that keeping a registry of contact information is useful. This registry can be created in hard copy with a list of providers under each category or electronically through a contact list sorted by category. In addition, business cards and referral forms, either electronic or paper, are useful in providing the patient with a referral.

Documentation of the referral in the patient record is crucial to track patient progress and risk management. Sometimes the patient will refuse the recommendation of the clinician for referral. In this case, the clinician should objectively document the conversation between the clinician and patient in the patient record. It is important to note that the clinician should continue to recommend a referral to the patient at all subsequent visits until the reason for the referral is resolved. Additionally, the patient record should note any patient visits to a specialist or health-care provider. An example is when a patient is referred to a periodontist upon completion of the evaluation of nonsurgical periodontal therapy because of a bony defect distal to the second molar resulting from a third molar extraction. The patient accepts the referral as noted in the patient record. When the patient returns for a re-care visit, the dental hygienist, upon reviewing the patient record, notices that the patient saw the periodontist; however, he declined to have treatment to manage the defect. The dental hygienist must use communication skills to verify why the patient chose not to have the treatment and to educate the patient about the benefits of correcting the defect. Upon evaluation of this conversation, the clinician may choose to refer to another specialist or encourage the patient to continue with the planned therapy by the first periodontist. The clinician should document carefully the conversation with the patient and complete the established office protocol for a referral, including another referral to the original periodontist or another periodontist depending on feedback from the patient.

Referral to another care provider when needed is essential, as is consultation during therapy to obtain another health-care professional's opinion. Medical consults, especially for medically complex patients, are an essential part of the evaluation process of care.[45] Collaborative interactions with other health-care providers assure a positive outcome for the patient. Additionally, the clinician benefits through gaining knowledge that adds to lifelong learning.

Evaluating the care of the patient and making decisions on the future care for the patient is integral to the evaluation phase of the ADPIED process of care. In addition to meeting the needs of the patient, the clinician must assess his or her personal performance as well the profession's standards of care. Quality assurance is a professional responsibility of both the individual practitioner and the profession.

Professionalism and Quality Assurance

It is importance for the clinician to identify patient needs and make recommendations based on need and standard of care. The clinician must use effective communication skills to inform the patient of the benefits of oral health and all treatments, including alternate therapies.[46] When the clinician educates the patient in an effective manner, patients are able to understand the relationship between health and disease.[14,14,46] This new knowledge helps the patient make and accept treatment choices that are appropriate and be compliant with treatment recommendations.[14,46] When a patient chooses an evidence-based therapy, the likelihood of legal action is decreased.[46] Ultimately, effective patient education and communication contribute to the health of the patient.[14,46,46]

Quality communication and rapport between the patient and clinician and excellent documentation are the expected standard of care.[15,46] In addition, communication and documentation are crucial in risk management.[15]

Evaluation is more than just a part of the ADPIED process of care; it is also part of the clinician's responsibility to assure quality in practice. Self-assessment and peer review are strategies to promote **quality assurance**.[47,48] Within health care, quality assurance refers to "systematic monitoring and evaluation of the various aspects of a project, service, or facility to ensure that standards of quality are being met."[3] Dental practices should implement mechanisms and systems to evaluate quality assurance. These processes may include random chart or electronic record audits, patient satisfaction surveys, monitoring of sterilization and infection control systems, radiation safety, licensure verification of all personnel, and utilization of standards of care.

The clinician has a professional obligation to the philosophy of a self-regulating profession to empower its registrants to be responsible and accountable for their practices. Continuous quality improvement is beneficial for dental hygienists, the dental hygiene profession, and the public it serves.[49,50]

SUMMARY

Evaluation is an ongoing, formative process in the ADPIED dental hygiene process of care and is the fifth and summative process in providing evidence-based comprehensive care.[1,2] The clinician uses critical thinking skills to form a clinical judgment about the future care of the patient based on patient feedback, clinical findings, and risk factors.[2] Future care options may include completion of care and determination of re-care interval, the maintenance phase of periodontal therapy, and/or referral to additional providers or specialists for additional therapies.

Case Study

Mr. Tang is a 36-year-old male of Asian descent. He is currently employed in finance and is studying for his securities license. He reports a pollen allergy and takes allergy injections as needed.

Mr. Tang has been smoking for about 20 years and currently smokes one pack of cigarettes per day. Mr. Tang reported that he had quit smoking for almost a year and then went back to it after his girlfriend broke up with him. Mr. Tang set a goal to try to quit smoking.

Mr. Tang has not had adequate dental treatment in the past; his sister is a dental student, which is why he is seeking periodontal therapy. Previous therapy includes "quick cleanings" at a dental clinic and some minor restorative work by his sister.

A nutritional diary completed by Mr. Tang for one weekend day and analysis by the clinician with the patient revealed shortages in the following food groups: protein, vegetables and fruits, and dairy. Grains were met, although mostly with white rice or Asian noodles. Mr. Tang does not have a refined sugar habit other than in coffee. Even though he does not show clinical signs of being prone to caries, the clinician encouraged him to try sugar substitutes or drink coffee black. The clinician recognized that the patient does not eat breakfast. The clinician informed Mr. Tang about the need for protein, especially for healing, and the importance of breakfast. Mr. Tang set a goal to eat breakfast and increase dairy and protein intake.

Mr. Tang has chronic moderate to severe periodontal disease, as evidenced by his clinical attachment loss, probe depths, mobility, furcation involvement, bleeding, and radiographic bone loss, both horizontal and vertical. He relates that his parents lost their teeth.

Case Study Exercises

1. During the evaluation phase of Mr. Tang's therapy, all of the following risk factors are contributing to the patient's prognosis EXCEPT which one?
   A. Loss of attachment
   B. Nutritional status
   C. Occlusion
   D Oral self-care
   E. Smoking

2. Mr. Tang states that he has noticed loose teeth since the completion of nonsurgical therapy. The clinician should take which action?
   A. Evaluate the mobile teeth for replacement with implants.
   B. Inform the patient that they are loose because the supragingival calculus was holding them in his mouth.
   C. Inform the patient to eat a soft diet and avoid chewing on the mobile teeth.
   D. Perform an occlusal equilibration.
   E. Refer the patient to a periodontist.

3. Mr. Tang completed nonsurgical therapy. At the reevaluation appointment, he still has probe depths greater than 5 millimeters and has purulent exudates in the distolingual area of tooth 12. Which practitioner is the best choice for a referral?
   A. Endodontist
   B. Implantologist
   C. Oral maxillofacial surgeon
   D. Periodontist
   E. Physician

4. Mr. Tang has set two goals for the improvement of his personal health. Because Mr. Tang made the goals, the clinician does not have to evaluate these goals.
   A. Both statements are true.
   B. Both statements are false.
   C. The first statement is true, but the second statement is false.
   D. The first statement is false, but the second statement is true.

5. Mr. Tang's overall prognosis is good. Mr. Tang had nonsurgical therapy and does not need to see a periodontist.
   A. Both statements are true.
   B. Both statements are false.
   C. The first statement is true, but the second statement is false.
   D. The first statement is false, but the second statement is true.

Review Questions

1. When does the evaluation process begin?
   A. At the reevaluation appointment
   B. At comparison between pre- and post-therapy probe depths
   C. At review of the patient's histories
   D. During the referral process

2. How should the evaluation methods and tools be determined?
   A. Based on assessment methods
   B. Based on diagnostic methods
   C. Based on the plan
   D. Based on implementation methods
   E. All of these choices are correct.

3. Examples of summative evaluation include all of the following *except* which one?
   A. Evaluation of medical history
   B. Evaluation of dental history
   C. Careful subgingival exploration during implementation
   D. Pre- and post-therapy comparison of periodontal findings
   E. Diagnosis of radiographic findings

4. Monitoring a patient's pain during nonsurgical therapy is an example of a formative evaluation of care. A summative evaluation of the effectiveness of pain control measures should be documented in the patient record.
   A. Both statements are true.
   B. Both statements are false.
   C. The first statement is true, but the second statement is false.
   D. The first statement is false, but the second statement is true.

5. It is a dental hygienist's legal and ethical responsibility to
   A. assess and determine patient oral health.
   B. document patient information.
   C. evaluate therapy to determine further treatments.
   D. plan and implement patient care.
   E. All of these choices are correct.

Active Learning

1. Create a podcast detailing the main concepts of the chapter.
2. Contact a dental office or clinic and ask how staff members implement evaluation methods. ▤

REFERENCES

1. Mueller-Joseph L, Peterson M. *Dental hygiene process: diagnosis and care planning*. Albany, NY: Delmar; 1995. p. 178.
2. American Dental Hygienists' Association. Standards for clinical dental hygiene practice. *Access*. 2008;5(3):3-15.
3. Merriam-Webster Online Dictionary. Evaluation and quality assurance. 2010. Available from: http://www.merriam-webster.com/netdict/evaluation.
4. Darby ML, Bowen D. *Research methods for oral health professions*. St. Louis, MO: Mosby; 1980. p. 208.
5. Scriven M. *The methodology of evaluation*. Lafayette, IN: Purdue University; 1966.
6. Taras M. Assessment—summative and formative—some theoretical reflections. *Brit J Educ Stud*. 2005;53(4):466-478.
7. Butler BL, Morison O, Low SB. An accurate, time-efficient method to assess plaque accumulation. *J Am Dent Assoc*. 1996;127(12):1763, 1766; quiz 1784-1785.
8. O'Leary TJ, Drake RB, Naylor JE. The plaque control record. *J Periodontol*. 1972;43(1):38.
9. American Dental Hygienists' Association. Dental hygiene diagnosis: An American Dental Hygienists' Association position paper. 2010. Available from: http://www.adha.org/resources-docs/Diagnosis-Position-Paper.pdf.
10. Gurenlian JR. Dental hygiene diagnosis revisited. *Access*. 2001;15(7):34.
11. Chace RS, Low SB. Survival characteristics of periodontally-involved teeth: A 40-year study. *J Periodontol*. 1993;64(8):701-705.
12. Miyamoto T, Kumagai T, Jones JA, Van Dyke TE, Nunn ME. Compliance as a prognostic indicator: Retrospective study of 505 patients treated and maintained for 15 years. *J Periodontol*. 2006;77(2):223-232.
13. American Academy of Periodontology. Guidelines for the management of patients with periodontal diseases. *J Periodontol*. 2006;77(9):1607-1611.
14. Stenman J, Hallberg U, Wennström JL, Abrahamsson KH. Patients' attitudes towards oral health and experiences of periodontal treatment: A qualitative interview study. *Oral Health Prev Dent*. 2009;7(4):393-401.
15. Dym H. Risk management techniques for the general dentist and specialist. *Dent Clin North Am*. 2008;52(3):563.
16. Fitch P. Cultural competence and dental hygiene care delivery: Integrating cultural care into the dental hygiene process of care. *J Dent Hyg*. 2004;78(1):11-21.
17. Hodges, KO. *Concepts of non-surgical periodontal therapy*. 1998.
18. Darby ML, Walsh MM. Application of the human needs conceptual model to dental hygiene practice. *J Dent Hyg*. 2000;74(3):230-237.
19. American Academy of Periodontology. Guidelines for periodontal therapy. *J Periodontol*. 2001;72:1624-1628.

20. Schonfeld SE. The art and science of periodontal prognosis. *Calif Dent Assoc J.* 2008:175-179.

21. American Academy of Periodontology. Epidemiology of periodontal diseases. *J Periodontol.* 2005;76:1406-1419.

22. Dzink JL, Tanner AC, Haffajee AD, Socransky SS. Gram negative species associated with active destructive periodontal lesions. *J Clin Periodontol.* 1985;12(8): 648-659.

23. Lang NP, Joss A, Orsanic T, Gusberti FA, Siegrist BE. Bleeding on probing. A predictor for the progression of periodontal disease? *J Clin Periodontol.* 1986;13(6): 590-596.

24. McGuire MK, Nunn ME. Prognosis versus actual outcome. II. The effectiveness of clinical parameters in developing an accurate prognosis. *J Periodontol.* 1996; 67(7):658-665.

25. McGuire MK, Nunn ME. Prognosis versus actual outcome. III. The effectiveness of clinical parameters in accurately predicting tooth survival. *J Periodontol.* 1996; 67(7):666-674.

26. Gilbert GH, Shelton BJ, Chavers LS, Bradford, Edward H. Predicting tooth loss during a population-based study: Role of attachment level in the presence of other dental conditions. *J Periodontol.* 2002;73(12):1427-1436.

27. Grossi SG, Genco RJ, Machtei EE, Ho AW, Koch G, Dunford R, Zambon JJ, Hausmann E. Assessment of risk for periodontal disease. II. Risk indicators for alveolar bone loss. *J Periodontol.* 1995;66(1):23-29.

28. Grossi SG, Zambon JJ, Ho AW, Koch G, Dunford RG, Machtei EE, Norderyd OM, Genco RJ. Assessment of risk for periodontal disease. I. Risk indicators for attachment loss. *J Periodontol.* 1994;65(3):260-267.

29. Newman, MG, Takei, HH, Klokkevold, PR. *Carranza's clinical periodontology.* 10th ed. Carranza FA, editor. St. Louis, MO: Saunders Elsevier; 2006. p. 1286.

30. Fu JH, Yap AU. Occlusion and periodontal disease-where is the link? *Singapore Dent J* [Internet]. 2007; 29(1):22-23.

31. Bhola M, Cabanilla L, Kolhatkar S. Dental occlusion and periodontal disease: What is the real relationship? *J Calif Dent Assoc.* 2008;36(12):924-930.

32. American Dental Hygienists' Association. Ask. Advise. Refer. Available from: http://www.askadviserefer.org/.

33. Palmer, CA. *Diet and nutrition in oral health.* Upper Saddle River, NJ: Pearson Prentice Hall; 2007. p. 496.

34. Stegeman, CA, Ratliff, JR. *The dental hygienist's guide to nutritional care.* 3rd ed. St. Louis, MO: Saunder Elsevier; 2010. p. 441.

35. Nishida M, Grossi SG, Dunford RG, Ho AW, Trevisan M, Genco RJ. Dietary vitamin C and the risk for periodontal disease. *J Periodontol.* 2000;71(8):1215-1223.

36. Nishida M, Grossi SG, Dunford RG, Ho AW, Trevisan M, Genco RJ. Calcium and the risk for periodontal disease. *J Periodontol.* 2000;71(7):1057-1066.

37. Tezal M, Wactawski-Wende J, Grossi SG, Ho AW, Dunford R, Genco RJ. The relationship between bone mineral density and periodontitis in postmenopausal women. *J Periodontol.* 2000;71(9):1492-1498.

38. Genco RJ. Current view of risk factors for periodontal diseases. *J Periodontol.* 1996;67(suppl 10):1041-1049.

39. Genco RJ. Periodontal disease and association with diabetes mellitus and diabetes: Clinical implications. *J Dent Hyg.* 2009;83(4):186-187.

40. Genco RJ. Pharmaceuticals and periodontal diseases. *J Am Dent Assoc.* 1994;125(suppl):11S-19S.

41. Genco RJ, Glurich I, Haraszthy V, Zambon J, DeNardin E. Overview of risk factors for periodontal disease and implications for diabetes and cardiovascular disease. *Compend Contin Educ Dent.* 2001;22(2):21-23.

42. Genco RJ, Ho AW, Grossi SG, Dunford RG, Tedesco LA. Relationship of stress, distress and inadequate coping behaviors to periodontal disease. *J Periodontol.* 1999; 70(7):711-723.

43. Genco RJ, Ho AW, Kopman J, Grossi SG, Dunford RG, Tedesco LA. Models to evaluate the role of stress in periodontal disease. *Ann Periodontol.* 1998;3(1): 288-302.

44. Mosby. *Mosby's dental dictionary.* 2nd ed. St. Louis, MO: Elsevier; 2008. p. 816.

45. Brown RS, Farquharson AA, Plash TM. Medical consultations for medically complex dental patients. *J Calif Dent Assoc.* 2007;35(5):343-349.

46. Schultz C. Making standard of caring part of the standard of care. *J Calif Dent Assoc.* 2009;37(9):639-645.

47. DeVore L, Fried JL, Dailey J, Qori CG. Dental hygiene self-assessment: A key to quality care. *J Dent Hyg.* 2000; 74(4):271-279.

48. Forrest JL. Quality assurance concepts and skill development: Results of a national study. *J Dent Hyg.* 1995; 69(3):114-121.

49. Imai P. From quality assurance to continuous quality improvement: Why dental hygiene needs to change— continuous quality improvement ideas from the nursing profession. *Can J Dent Hyg.* 2006;40(3):126.

50. Bilawka E, Craig BJ. Quality assurance and dental hygiene. *Int J Dent Hyg.* 2003;1(4):218-222.

51. West JD, O'Connor RV, Cook DH. The interdisciplinary referral. *Dent Today* [Internet]. 2002;21(11):98-105. Available from: http://ezproxy.library.ewu.edu:2048/ login?url=http://search.ebscohost.com.ezproxy.library.ewu.edu/login.aspx?direct=true&db=cmedm&AN =12483934&site=ehost-live&scope=site

Chapter 35 | Maintenance

Lisa Bilich, RDH, BS, MEd

KEY TERMS

implant maintenance
informed consent
informed refusal
maintenance
periodontal maintenance
   (PM)
prophylaxis
self-efficacy

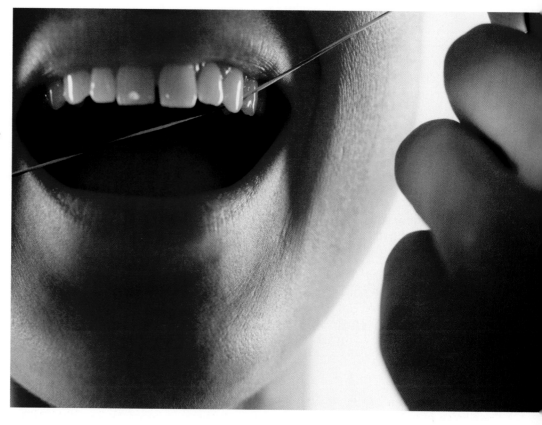

LEARNING OBJECTIVES

After reading this chapter, the student should be able to:

35.1 Evaluate the roles of the dental hygienist, dental team, and patient in maintaining dentition.

35.2 Relate concepts of evaluation to the maintenance phase of dental hygiene therapy.

35.3 Identify contributing factors and signs of the recurrence of dental diseases.

35.4 Make evidence-based decisions regarding medicaments and adjunct treatments for patients in the maintenance phase.

KEY CONCEPTS

• Determine the criteria for a maintenance care plan, including proper continuing care intervals based on the patients' risk assessment.

• Oral maintenance is an important part of overall health.

• Dental implants, when present, are an important part of the maintenance care plan and may require therapy adjustments.

• The maintenance appointment may include locally delivered antimicrobials, depending on the patient's oral risk assessment and periodontal findings.

RELEVANCE TO CLINICAL PRACTICE

Oral health maintenance is an important part of the dental hygiene treatment plan. It is the means for the patient to maintain healthy tissue and dentition free of disease. The hygienist is the preventive specialist in the dental practice. **Maintenance** is an ongoing treatment that occurs either after active therapy or as a routine prophylaxis. The hygienist collects assessment data, provides a dental hygiene diagnosis based on assessment data, implements appropriate therapy, evaluates treatment outcomes, and documents outcomes of therapy.

WHAT IS ORAL HEALTH?

Definition

The definition of oral health has expanded beyond just teeth. The National Institute of Dental and Craniofacial Research has defined *oral health* as:

> being free of chronic oral-facial pain conditions, oral and pharyngeal (throat) cancers, oral soft tissue lesions, birth defects such as cleft lip and palate, and scores of other diseases and disorders that affect the oral, dental, and craniofacial tissues, collectively known as the *craniofacial complex.*[1]

Oral Health Versus Systemic Health

Oral health cannot be separated from systemic health. Hygienists are charged with maintaining the health of each patient under their care. Hygienists are in a position to monitor the oral health of the patient and understand the risk factors associated with diseases in the oral cavity. Caries and periodontal disease are considered chronic diseases that will need to be monitored by the dental professional. The dentist, hygienist, and patient must work together to maintain health in the oral cavity (Fig. 35-1).

CRITERIA FOR DETERMINING A MAINTENANCE CARE PLAN

There is no way of predicting which patient will exhibit periodontal breakdown or when it will occur. Risk factors are important in determining the care plan for patients. A risk factor is not causative but increases the likelihood of the patient developing the disease. It is known that the increase of plaque and calculus has a negative influence on the periodontium. Smoking has been linked to a twofold increase in disease progression, making the use of tobacco one of the most significant factors in determining the type of care and frequency.[2] The hygienist will use the assessment data to formulate the plan for the type and frequency of care.

ASSESSMENT

To accurately assess the current periodontal condition of the patient, the standard protocol for a maintenance appointment is as follows:[3]

1. Update of medical and dental histories
2. Intraoral and extraoral examination
3. Full dental charting
4. Oral risk assessment
5. Update/review of appropriate radiographs
6. Full periodontal charting
7. Evaluation of deposits
8. Review of patient's homecare

Medical and Dental History

It is important to ask patients about changes in their medical conditions since the last appointment. Asking targeted questions about specific conditions and/or medications is necessary to find essential information that may alter treatment, affect maintenance ability, or identify a potential medical emergency. Taking of vital signs must be included during the appointment. The hygienist may be one of the first health-care workers to identify a medical concern with a patient through the recording of vital signs. Vital signs included in the

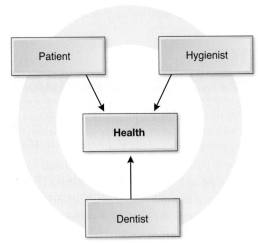

Figure 35-1. The dentist, dental hygienist, and patient work together to ensure the patient's oral health.

assessment are weight, height, blood pressure, pulse, respiratory rate, and temperature.[4] It is necessary to contact the patient's physician regarding certain conditions, such as heart surgery, joint replacement, myocardial infarction, stroke, or uncontrolled diabetes.[5]

The dental history will include the chief concern, what brought the patient into the office. The clinician must address the patient's needs as part of individualized care (see Application to Clinical Practice). Also included in this assessment is any treatment the patient may have had since the last appointment with the dental hygienist. If restorative care has been provided, it is necessary to ask the patient if there are any concerns with the treatment outcomes.[6]

Intraoral and Extraoral Examination

The hygienist often spends more time with the patient than do other dental professionals. It is important to note any risk factors for oral cancer and any changes in the skin of the head and neck or the oral mucosa. The conversation with the patient during the intraoral and extraoral examination has to tie in risk factors for oral and pharyngeal cancer if risk factors are noted on the medical history form. Risk factors for oral cancer include tobacco use, alcohol use, gender, sunlight exposure, poor nutrition, human papilloma virus (HPV), immune suppression, and lichen planus. It is estimated that 8 out of 10 oral cancers could be prevented by refraining from tobacco and alcohol use.[7]

Radiographs and Dental Charting

Bitewing radiographs are used not only for the detection of caries but also to monitor bone level, quality of interproximal bone, furcation involvement, and calculus deposits. The frequency of radiographs should be based on individual patients' clinical signs and symptoms of disease activity. Intraoral photographs may be necessary to support radiographs in the presence of periodontal disease. Vertical bitewing radiographs are the standard of care for patients who have had a history of bone loss. The vertical bitewings will show more of the crestal alveolar bone. An updated full mouth series of radiographs may be needed periodically. Clinical

Application to Clinical Practice

Conversations with the patient during the medical review can include the importance of oral health to overall health. Explaining the higher risk of cardiovascular disease to patients with periodontal disease and high blood pressure will help them make informed decisions regarding dental hygiene treatment. Specific, targeted questions about chronic diseases the patient presents with will help you start to understand the beliefs and values of the patient. ■

judgment must be used and based on individual patient risks for caries and periodontal disease.[8] A panoramic radiograph may also be useful as a supplement for the detection of osteoporosis.[9]

The dental chart needs to be updated to denote any caries present or new restorations from the last appointment. Radiographs and visual examination can be used to update this examination. Any defective restorations and/or margins also need to be noted because these conditions may be a risk factor for periodontal disease. Caries risk can alter the maintenance plan and will be taken into consideration in developing a maintenance plan.

Oral Risk Assessment

Oral risk assessment is part of the maintenance plan and can affect the patient's optimum periodontal maintenance schedule. A risk assessment includes identifying factors that will increase the risk that the patient will develop a disease such as caries, periodontal disease, or oral/pharyngeal cancer in the oral cavity. The following sections discuss factors that will affect the patients' periodontal health and can affect individual intervals of care.

Compliance with Maintenance Schedule

The prognosis for patients who maintain a regular periodontal maintenance schedule is better than that for patients who are irregular about their care. The number of teeth lost by noncompliant patients is approximately five times greater than that for patients who are compliant.[10] There are many potential reasons these patients have increased risk of attachment loss. Calculus and plaque are two factors that have been shown to have a higher risk of continual disease progression (Fig. 35-2).[2]

It has been estimated that approximately 52% of patients will maintain a regular maintenance schedule after 5 years.[11] After 10 years the rate drops to 37%.[10] Research has shown that self-efficacy is a major factor in patients' maintenance of their appointment schedule and their homecare regimen. Self-efficacy as it pertains to dentistry is how patients feel about their ability to improve their health. This becomes critical in a chronic disease, such as periodontal disease, that patients cannot monitor easily.

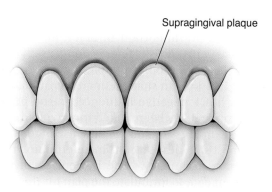

Supragingival plaque

Figure 35-2. Supragingival plaque with associated inflammation.

The dental hygienist can help the patient increase self-efficacy through behavior modification. Patient behavior modification can include setting goals with patients and not for patients. The goals must be reasonable and attainable. Another tactic to raise self-efficacy is to determine the appropriate homecare aid for the patient that can easily be incorporated into the existing oral hygiene routine. The dental hygienist should introduce one aid at a time and not overwhelm the patient with too many aids or tasks. Defining the role the patient must take in the disease process will help the patient to realize the importance of compliance.[12] See Chapter 4, Health Education and Promotion, for in-depth coverage of strategies to help patients improve their health.

Dental insurance has also shown to have an effect on patient compliance. If treatment is covered, the patient may be more likely to accept the treatment.[13] Communication with the patient needs to include the benefits and limitations of insurance. Dental insurance was never meant to be all inclusive of dental treatment; it is seen more as a way to defray costs. Each plan is dictated by the employer, the plan, and the premium. Maximum benefits have not significantly changed in 40 years. The patient will most likely have to pay out of pocket for optimum oral health.[14]

Smoking

Smoking is one of the most significant risk factors for periodontal disease. Half of the cases of periodontitis can be attributed to smoking. Smoking has an effect on immune response and healing rates and will affect the rate of progression and the effects of treatment. Clinically the hygienist can expect to see deeper pockets, greater attachment loss, and more calculus. Smoking masks bleeding, which means that bleeding on probing is not an accurate indicator of disease.[15]

A tobacco cessation program should be adopted by the hygienist. Research has shown that after quitting tobacco, a patient has the same risk of attachment loss as a patient who has never smoked.[15] Barriers to tobacco cessation counseling have been identified as:

- Lack of time by hygienist to counsel
- Lack of confidence of the hygienist to counsel patient on tobacco cessation
- Lack of insurance reimbursement
- The hygienists' perception that referring to a helpline is not personal enough to meet the needs of tobacco cessation

Hygienists have the skills to conduct a successful tobacco cessation program. They educate patients on oral health, patients trust them, and follow-up is routine in the dental office (see Teamwork).[16] Refer to Chapter 4, Health Education and Promotion, for information on tobacco cessation strategies.

Diabetes

Patients with uncontrolled diabetes are 2 to 3 times more likely to have periodontal disease than patients

Teamwork

The office manager greets the next hygiene patient. While the patient is waiting for the hygienist, the office manager starts a conversation with him about his recent attempt to quit smoking. He is excited to report that he has not had a cigarette in 2 days. The dentist overhears the remark and congratulates the patient on his success. The hygienist greets the patient in the waiting room with, "I hear you are working hard on quitting—that is great to hear!" He then continues the conversation in the treatment room, asking the patient if there is anything else he can do to help support the patient with his decision. As the appointment ends, the hygienist hands the patient an extra toothbrush for making an effort to quit smoking. ■

without diabetes. Patients with active periodontal disease may also have a hard time controlling their glycemic level. People with type 1 or type 2 diabetes will also have a greater risk of gingival hyperplasia, aggressive periodontitis, and periodontal abscesses.[17]

Treatment modifications for the diabetic patient include taking blood pressure at each appointment because diabetes is a risk factor for cardiovascular disease. A consultation with the patient's physician may be necessary if any complications have taken place. Make sure to update the medical history with special attention to medications, the current A1C levels, and most recent blood sugar reading. A1C is the measure of the level of glucose levels within the last 12 weeks and is considered a more accurate test of control than blood sugar reading.[17] During the intraoral examination, monitor the patient for xerostomia, burning mouth syndrome, enlarged parotid gland, and fruity smell on the breath. A thorough periodontal examination is necessary to monitor for active periodontal disease and detect periodontal abscesses. Morning is usually the best time for an appointment for the diabetic patient, when blood glucose is more likely to be stable; ask if the patient has had breakfast and what the patient ate for breakfast.[17]

Nonmodifiable Factors

Some factors cannot be modified but have an effect on periodontal disease. As the patient ages, more attachment loss is seen. This may be due to the patient being exposed to other risk factors for a longer period of time, such as periods of poor homecare routines or stress. The progression does slow down, with aggressive periodontitis rarely seen in the patient over age 50. Males are more likely to show disease progression than women.[10] All of these factors need to be taken into consideration as the dental hygienist and dentist recommend an ideal maintenance interval to maintain optimum oral health.

PERIODONTAL CHARTING

A full periodontal chart should be assessed at each appointment. This charting should include pocket depths, recession, furcation involvement, exudates, mobility, and bleeding on probing. Due to the random bursts of activity that can occur in periodontal disease, it is important to complete a full periodontal charting to recognize early signs of occurrence or reoccurrence of disease (Fig. 35-3).[18] It is useful to compare previous charts and discuss the results with the patient. Patient participation is necessary for optimal results in treatment.

Bleeding on probing cannot be the only determining factor of disease progression (Fig. 35-4). Smoking will reduce bleeding, but there can still be disease activity. Medications can increase the chance of bleeding with no disease progression present. The dental hygienist must take into consideration all clinical parameters when determining disease activity (see Advancing Technologies).[14]

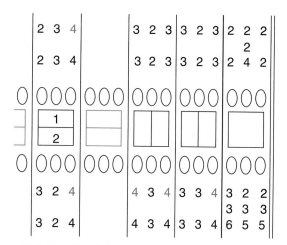

Figure 35-3. Periodontal chart showing attachment loss with furcation involvement.

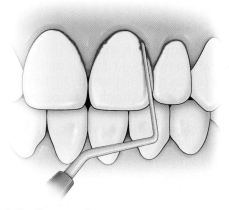

Figure 35-4. Bleeding on probing.

Advancing Technologies

The use of a computer-based charting program can help the dental hygienist explain the disease progression to the patient. The use of comparison graphs gives the clinician visual documentation of treatment outcomes and the need for future treatment (Fig. 35-6). ■

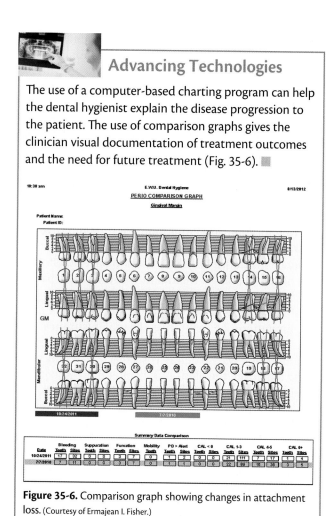

Figure 35-6. Comparison graph showing changes in attachment loss. (Courtesy of Ermajean I. Fisher.)

EVALUATION OF DEPOSITS

Plaque has been identified as a major etiological factor in periodontal disease and therefore needs to be assessed at each periodontal maintenance appointment.[19] Plaque will initiate inflammation, which is seen clinically as gingivitis. Gingivitis does not necessarily progress to periodontitis, although it is known that chronic inflammation is a risk factor for loss of attachment. The Plaque Control Record developed by O'Leary, Drake, and Naylor is a common index used to evaluate plaque. Plaque will be evaluated on all four surfaces of teeth present. Disclosing solution can be used to help the patient see the plaque.[20]

Calculus is also a risk factor for progression of attachment loss and is important to note.[21] Careful exploration with an explorer like the ODU 11/12 and examination of recent radiographs will assist the clinician in determining the amount of hard deposits. Air from the air/water syringe is beneficial in determining supragingival calculus. Gingival condition can be a guide if there are subgingival deposits. Inflammation can be a clue that there is either subgingival plaque or calculus.

HOMECARE

A systematic review of the literature has shown that homecare plus professional care is the ideal combination to reduce the chance of continual loss of attachment.[22] A patient seen by the oral health-care provider on a regular basis can be closely monitored for areas that are difficult for the person to reach with homecare aids. Use of a disclosing agent will benefit the patient by allowing the patient to physically see where plaque has been missed with brushing and/or interdental cleaning. It should be emphasized that supragingival plaque is an important etiological factor in the progression of periodontal disease and needs to be adequately controlled.[19]

DENTAL HYGIENE DIAGNOSIS

Dental hygiene diagnosis is defined by the American Dental Hygienists' Association (ADHA) as: "the identification of an existing or potential oral health problem that a dental hygienist is educationally qualified and licensed to treat."[23] Dental hygienists work with dentists and other health-care providers to provide optimum oral health to all patients. The dental hygiene diagnosis analyzes the assessment data to arrive at a risk assessment on which to base a treatment plan for dental hygiene therapy and a prevention plan.[24]

The interpretation of the assessment data will help identify patient needs. Identification of individual needs will help optimize dental hygiene care. The dental hygiene diagnosis does not focus just on the disease state but also on the reason for the problem. As it relates to maintenance, the dental hygienist will need to assess the data to determine whether the patient is presenting in health or will need active therapy.[24]

An example of a dental hygiene diagnosis is as follows: A patient who is taking a calcium channel blocker comes to the practice for an examination. During the intraoral examination, the dental hygienist notices generalized large, rolled margins. The dental hygiene diagnosis of this would be possible gingival hyperplasia due to the calcium channel blocker. The treatment would be referral to a physician for possible medication change.

DENTAL HYGIENE TREATMENT PLAN

The dental hygienist must prioritize dental hygiene treatment within the scope of his or her practice. The dentist and dental hygienist will collaborate to determine a comprehensive treatment plan for optimum oral health for the patient. The clinician will analyze the assessment data and provide evidence-based care based on that data. The hygienist will include all treatment that may be initiated, such as pain management, caries control, and polishing.[23]

When analyzing the assessment data, the clinician must determine whether active disease is present. Signs of disease may be seen clinically as an increase in probing depths from attachment loss of gingival inflammation, radiographic evidence of alveolar bone loss greater than that in previous radiographs, or bleeding on probing with no risks associated with increased bleeding. If there is active disease, the dental hygienist then needs to determine the extent of disease; that is, whether it is localized or generalized. Interpretation and evaluation of these data will help determine whether the patient needs to have active therapy or if a maintenance appointment is appropriate (Fig. 35-5).

Informed Consent

The hygienist has the ethical and legal obligation to inform the patient of the current disease state based on assessment data gathered and treatment options for the condition present, which is considered **informed consent**. The informed consent must be discussed and signed before treatment begins. The informed consent must contain:

1. Reason for treatment
2. Risks and benefits of treatment
3. Risks of not accepting treatment
4. Time to ask questions
5. Adequate time to accept/decline treatment without coercion

It is important to note that the treatment needs to be explained in patient-friendly terms so the patient can thoroughly understand all information before a true informed consent can be ascertained. Treatment costs should be included with this consent so that the patient knows what to expect. Alternative treatments should be included with this consent. Patients who

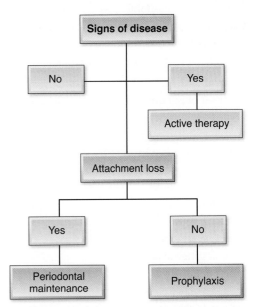

Figure 35-5. Decision tree showing how to assess for the correct dental hygiene treatment.

refuse treatment should sign an **informed refusal**. The signed refusal should include a statement stating that the patient understands the risk of not accepting treatment and that the condition has been thoroughly explained but the patient refuses treatment at this time.[25]

Referrals are an important part of informed consent. Effective periodontal maintenance requires the patient, the hygienist, the general dentist, and the specialist to collaborate for the patient's optimum oral health. The dentist and hygienist need to discuss which patients can be maintained in the general dentist office and which will need to see a periodontist (Box 35-1). Some patients may alternate between the general dentist office and the periodontist. It is the role of the hygienist to inform the periodontist's office of the condition of the patient when he or she comes to the general practice. Cooperation among the practices will benefit the patient.[3]

Maintenance Therapies

After informed consent has been attained, individualized treatment based on assessments and risk factors can be implemented. This phase will not only include dental hygiene therapy, but also therapies based on the current risk factors, including treatment for hypersensitivity, caries control, nutritional counseling, and oral hygiene instruction.

Debridement

If a patient presents with few or no signs of disease, the appropriate implementation is the prevention of

---

Box 35-1. *Recommendations for Referral to a Periodontist*

Level 3: Patients Who Should Be Treated by a Periodontist

Any patient with:
- Severe chronic periodontitis
- Furcation involvement
- Vertical/angular bony defect(s)
- Aggressive periodontitis (formerly known as juvenile, early-onset, or rapidly progressive periodontitis)
- Periodontal abscess and other acute periodontal conditions
- Significant root surface exposure and/or progressive gingival recession
- Peri-implant disease
- Any patient with periodontal diseases, regardless of severity, whom the referring dentist prefers not to treat

Level 2: Patients Who Would Likely Benefit From Comanagement by the Referring Dentist and the Periodontist

Any patient with periodontitis who demonstrates at reevaluation or any dental examination one or more of the following risk factors/indicators* known to contribute to the progression of periodontal diseases:

Periodontal Risk Factors/Indicators
- Early onset of periodontal diseases (before the age of 35 years)
- Unresolved inflammation at any site (e.g., bleeding upon probing, pus, and/or redness)
- Pocket depths greater than 5 mm
- Vertical bone defects
- Radiographic evidence of progressive bone loss
- Progressive tooth mobility
- Progressive attachment loss
- Anatomic gingival deformities

- Exposed root surfaces
- A deteriorating risk profile

Medical or Behavioral Risk Factors/Indicators
- Smoking/tobacco use
- Diabetes
- Osteoporosis/osteopenia
- Drug-induced gingival conditions (e.g., phenytoins, calcium channel blockers, immunosuppressants, and long-term systemic steroids)
- Compromised immune system, either acquired or drug induced
- A deteriorating risk profile
- It should be noted that a combination of two or more of these risk factors/indicators may make even slight to moderate periodontitis particularly difficult to manage (e.g., a patient under 35 years of age who smokes).

Level 1: Patients Who May Benefit from Comanagement by the Referring Dentist and the Periodontist

Any patient with periodontal inflammation/infection and the following systemic conditions:
- Diabetes
- Pregnancy
- Cardiovascular disease
- Chronic respiratory disease

Any patient who is a candidate for the following therapies who might be exposed to risk from periodontal infection, including but not limited to the following treatments:
- Cancer therapy
- Cardiovascular surgery
- Joint-replacement surgery
- Organ transplantation

*It should be noted that a combination of two or more of these risk factors/indicators may make even slight to moderate periodontitis particularly difficult to manage (e.g., a patient under 35 years of age who smokes).

From Guidelines for the Management of Patients with Periodontal Diseases, by the American Academy of Periodontology (AAP), 2006, 727, pp. 1607-1611. Reprinted with permission.

periodontal disease. Clinically the patient may have localized slight recession, localized slight inflammation, or tight and healthy tissue. The appropriate treatment is **prophylaxis.** Care provided would include removal of plaque, staining, and calculus to prevent irritation of the tissues and the initiation of periodontal disease. The appropriate insurance code would be 01110.[14] The key ideas are that there is no disease present and little or no attachment loss.

The patient who had active therapy in the past is more at risk for periodontal breakdown as exhibited through attachment loss. Clinically this patient may have slight to moderate periodontitis, one or more risk factors for periodontitis, and/or localized areas demonstrating active disease. The appropriate treatment for this patient is **periodontal maintenance (PM).** Care provided would include removal of plaque, staining, and calculus to prevent further loss of attachment. Periodontal maintenance goes beyond prophylaxis in the need for site-specific scaling and root planing in areas that have shown disease progression and/or signs of inflammation. The appropriate insurance code would be 04910.[14] Periodontal maintenance has been referred to as continuing care or supportive periodontal care. The American Academy of Periodontics (AAP) has deemed *periodontal maintenance* as the accepted term.[26] See Professionalism.

Polishing

Polishing can be an important part of the maintenance appointment. Polishing can help remove plaque and staining above the gumline. It is not necessary to polish all surfaces of the teeth, and the hygienist needs to determine the necessity of polishing. Air powder polish can also be used on patients with heavy stains. Air powder polisher is contraindicated for use on crowns, cementum, implants, and the patient on a sodium-restricted diet.[27] Refer to Chapter 29, Polishing, for complete information on polishing.

Professionalism

The hygienist is seeing a patient today for her regular 3-month periodontal maintenance. The patient is recently divorced and has already called the front office to tell the receptionist that she cannot afford any "x-rays" and only wants the minimal treatment today. She wants to keep her appointment, though, because she realizes how important her teeth are to her health. When the hygienist finishes the assessments, she informs the patient she will need to revisit nonsurgical periodontal therapy (NSPT) due to active disease. The patient says she will not receive NSPT and in fact only wants a basic cleaning. What are the hygienist's ethical obligations? ■

Newly exposed cementum due to healing may cause the patient sensitivity. The dental hygienist will have to decide if a desensitizing product is enough for the patient. Local anesthesia may be necessary to make the patient comfortable enough to complete dental hygiene therapy. Topical anesthesia may be adequate if only the tissue is involved. Part of clinical decision making is choosing the appropriate product to use to adequately complete the maintenance appointment. Refer to Chapter 28, Hypersensitivity, for product suggestions.

Special Care for the Implant

Dental implants are becoming more common and are being used to replace missing teeth. Some of these teeth may have been lost due to periodontitis. This is important because the risk factors for periodontal disease remain the same and will affect the implant. The main considerations with implants are that the lack of periodontal ligament and the weak fiber attachment with some epithelial attachment. The implant is held in place with osseointegration, a tight interface between the implant and surrounding bone. This puts the implant at higher risk for attachment loss called *peri-implantitis.*[28]

During the maintenance appointment, the dental hygienist should look for signs of a failing implant. The signs to look for are as follows:[28]

- Gingival inflammation
- Increased pockets
- Mobility
- Radiolucencies associated with the implant
- Bone loss around the implant

Evaluation of the implant must be done at every maintenance appointment. Metal instruments can compromise the surface of the implant, so a plastic probe should be used to measure pocket depths. An increase of probing depth of 0.5 mm to 1.0 mm in the first year after an implant is placed is considered normal. An increase of 0.6 mm to 0.8 mm every year is within normal limits. Probing healthy tissue around an implant that exhibits no signs of inflammation is controversial. It is believed that too much force with probing can compromise the epithelial attachment.[29] Radiographs will be taken of the implant on the same schedule as that for the natural teeth; the one difference is that a periapical will need to be taken because the bitewing will not show the apices of the implant.[29]

During the maintenance appointment, the dental hygienist will use special instruments for **implant maintenance** that will not scratch the surface of the implant. Plastic, graphite, or gold-tipped hand instruments can be used. Special ultrasonic tips designed for use with implants can also be used. Calculus will be loosely attached to the implant due to the titanium surface. Removal should only require light pressure. Optimum homecare needs to be reinforced at each appointment due to the susceptibility of the implant to attachment loss. Any signs of attachment loss need to be brought to the attention of the dentist and may require a referral to a periodontist (see Box 35-1).[29]

For an implant that is showing signs of inflammation, the hygienist should take the following steps:[28]

- Review and emphasize homecare with the patient.
- Debride the area with appropriate instruments.
- Perform subgingival irrigation with chlorhexidine to reduce subgingival flora.
- Possibly use a locally delivered antimicrobial with a prescription from the dentist.

The dentist may want to prescribe a systemic antibiotic such as amoxicillin or another appropriate medication if there are signs of inflammation and attachment loss.[28]

The implementation phase needs to include any caries-reducing treatment, including fluoride (see Evidence-Based Practice). The hygienist needs to evaluate the patient's caries risk based on risk assessment. Risk factors for decay include xerostomia, root exposure, active decay, and low fluoride use. Patients with moderate or high risk of caries should receive either gel or varnish fluoride. The evidence shows that patients at moderate

Evidence-Based Practice

- Amorphous calcium phosphate (ACP) polishing paste can benefit a patient with demineralization because it can help deposit calcium and phosphate into the tooth structure. The addition of fluoride can help increase the uptake.[31]
- A new product on the market, a calcium sodium phosphosilicate bioactive glass, sold under the trade name NovaMin, has been shown to promote remineralization when combined with fluoride. This product works even in the absence of saliva. It seems to be especially beneficial for root surfaces.[32] ■

risk for caries should receive treatment every 6 months, and those at high risk for caries should receive treatment every 3 to 6 months.[30]

Locally Delivered Antimicrobials

During the implementation stage, the hygienist may find areas that are not responding to treatment. If there are isolated areas that are demonstrating active disease, the hygienist may choose to use a locally delivered antimicrobial (Table 35-1). It is important to note that the dentist must prescribe this treatment before it is delivered. Debridement must be completed before an adjunct is delivered. The advantage of a locally delivered antimicrobial is that the clinician does not have to rely on patient compliance, as is the case with take-home products.

Some guidelines on when to use this treatment are as follows:[14]

- Pocket equal to or greater than 5 mm
- Bleeding on probing without any systemic medication effects
- Pockets not responding to treatment
- Implant showing signs of failure
- Poor surgical candidates

Continuing Care Intervals

Patients who have demonstrated a chronic disease and present with risk factors will benefit from professional care (see Spotlight on Public Health). Research has shown that patients with periodontitis have more attachment loss than periodontally healthy patients over time, even with a maintenance schedule. Patients with higher levels of subgingival plaque have demonstrated a greater loss of attachment.[33] Evidence has shown that the 3-month interval is appropriate for at least the first year of PM. This treatment plan will help the hygienist monitor the patient for signs of disease, remove deposits that the patient cannot or will not remove, assess implant health, and review homecare routines.[3]

Table 35-1. *Locally Delivered Antibiotics/Antimicrobials*

Medication	Days Medication Is Effective	Contraindications	Special Notes
Chlorhexidine Chip 2.5 mg PerioChip ®	7–10 Bacterial suppression up to 11 weeks	Pockets less than 5 mm	Can be used on pregnant patients
10% doxycycline gel Atridox®	7 Bacterial suppression up to 6 months	Allergy to doxycycline Pregnancy Patients with developing teeth	Smokers respond better to combination of scaling and root planing (SRP) and minocycline than SRP alone
Minocycline Hydrochloride 1 mg Arestin®	21	Allergy to doxycycline Pregnancy Patients with developing teeth	Smokers and diabetics respond better in combination with SRP than SRP alone

Spotlight on Public Health

The dental hygienist is an important part of overall health. The dental hygienist can deliver care in hospitals, long-term care facilities, and community-based clinics to help maintain oral health, which will maintain overall health. The dental hygienist is the key to prevention of disease and maintenance of oral health. An example of the dental hygienist helping maintain health is a school-based sealant program. The risk of decay is reduced, which will help maintain tooth structure. ■

The interval for care needs to be tailored to the individual patient. A more medically compromised patient who has many risk factors may benefit from a 2-month PM. The patient who has little attachment loss, practices good homecare, and does not demonstrate continual attachment loss may be able to have a maintenance appointment every 4 to 6 months. Continual evaluation of the tissue, attachment, and risk factors at each appointment will help the hygienist determine an appropriate schedule for each patient.[14]

Evaluation

Evaluation of care is an ongoing process for each maintenance appointment. Using specific, measurable goals will help the dental hygienist and the patient to determine whether the goals of implementation were met. Documentation of clinical signs of disease such as inflammation, bleeding on probing, and plaque assessment will guide future treatment needs. It must be documented if outcomes were met. The outcomes of the treatment will help the dentist, dental hygienist, and patient determine whether further treatment or referral to a specialist is needed, and the specific maintenance interval for the patient. The outcomes must be conveyed to the patient and documented in the chart.[23]

Documentation

The dental hygienist has the ethical and legal responsibility to document all procedures during the maintenance appointment. Documentation needs to cover the individualized dental hygiene care plan. Objective notation of all conversations with the patient should be documented, along with conversations with other care providers that pertain to the patient. This documentation is a legal document and needs to be neat and legible. Documenting what treatment is recommended next will help guide the next clinician in treatment choices.[23]

Case Study

Irene McCaw has recently moved in with her daughter and changed dentists. Irene indicates that she has to see the dental hygienist every 4 months. Her medical history indicates that she is under the care of a physician for diabetes, high blood pressure, and osteoporosis. Her daily medications are glucophage, nifedipine, and alendronate. Her last A1C was 12%, and her blood sugar today was 180 mg/dL. She made an appointment for today because the dark line on tooth 10 is bothering her and she wants it fixed. Due to the stress of moving, it has been 1 year since her last dental hygiene appointment. She reports that she had a "deep cleaning" 3 years ago. The dentist has completed an examination and has noted decay on tooth 21. Deposits are moderate plaque, light-moderate calculus. Vital signs are as follows: blood pressure—138/93, respiration—20 breath/min, pulse—75/min.

Case Study Exercises

1. Appropriate dental hygiene therapy for Irene would be which of the following?
   A. Prophylaxis
   B. Nonsurgical periodontal therapy
   C. Periodontal maintenance
   D. No dental hygiene therapy would be appropriate at this time.

2. The *most likely* cause of the generalized recession for this patient is
   A. use of calcium channel blocker.
   B. frenal attachment at gingival margin.
   C. aggressive brushing.
   D. age.

3. The dental hygiene diagnosis will include all of the following EXCEPT which one?
   A. Localized, moderate deposits—periodontal maintenance
   B. Active caries—restoration completed by dentist; fluoride treatment after dental hygiene therapy
   C. Generalized hyperplasia—referral to physician for possible medication change
   D. Generalized recession—fluoride treatment for prevention of root caries

4. This patient is at risk for progressive periodontal disease due to gender. Compliance for this patient has been ideal.
   A. Both statements are true.
   B. Both statements are false.
   C. The first statement is true, but the second statement is false.
   D. The first statement is false, but the second statement is true.

Case Study—cont'd

5. Irene has been prescribed a locally delivered antimicrobial that contains chlorhexidine due to contraindications with doxycycline derivative products.
   A. Both the statement and reason are correct and related.
   B. Both the statement and reason are correct but not related.
   C. The statement is correct, but the reason is not.
   D. The statement is not correct, but the reason is correct.
   E. Neither the statement nor the reason is correct.

6. Indications of possible uncontrolled diabetes include which of the following?
   A. A1C level
   B. Lack of bleeding on probing
   C. Increased inflammation
   D. Both A1C level and increased inflammation

Review Questions

1. Which three conditions are included in the definition of oral health?
   A. Absence of third molars
   B. No signs or symptoms of oral or pharyngeal cancer
   C. No active herpetic lesions
   D. No pain in the oral cavity
   E. Lack of restorations

2. Which of the following best describes a maintenance plan?
   A. Dental hygiene diagnosis
   B. Individualized care interval based on assessments
   C. Monitoring of the progression of periodontal disease
   D. Localized scaling and root planing

3. Order the following from the highest risk of oral and pharyngeal cancer to the lowest risk of oral and pharyngeal cancer.
   A. Alcohol use and tobacco use
   B. HPV
   C. Tobacco use alone
   D. Herpetic lesions

4. Caries and periodontal disease are _____ diseases.
   A. autoimmune
   B. acute
   C. chronic
   D. curable

5. Self-efficacy can be tied to homecare. It is best to give the patient many homecare aids to control plaque.
   A. Both statements are true.
   B. Both statements are false.
   C. The first statement is true, but the second statement is false.
   D. The first statement is false, but the second statement is true.

Active Learning

1. Have students gather appropriate tobacco cessation material for different patient types. Have them role play counseling a patient about tobacco cessation.
2. Have students journal/blog about their re-care patients. Have them identify relevant information relating to maintenance interval.
3. Have students diagram the role of the dentist, dental hygienist, and patient in the maintenance plan. ■

REFERENCES

1. U.S. Department of Health and Human Services. Oral health in America: A report of the Surgeon General. Available from: http://www.nidcr.nih.gov/nidcr2. nih.gov/Templates/CommonPage.aspx?NRMODE= Published&NRNODEGUID=%7b2B5A6D25-1226-4177- 96EA-4E2B3D9859AF%7d&NRORIGINALURL=% 2fDataStatistics%2fSurgeonGeneral%2fsgr%2fchap1% 2ehtm&NRCACHEHINT=Guest#base
2. Schätzle M, Faddy MJ, Cullinan MP, Seymour GJ, Lang NP, Bürgin W, Ånerud Å, Boysen H, Löe H. The clinical course of chronic periodontitis: V. Predictive factors in periodontal disease. *J Clin Periodontol*. 2009;36:365-371.

3. American Academy of Periodontology. Comprehensive periodontal therapy: a statement by the American Academy of Periodontology: *J Periodontol.* 2011;82: 943-949.

4. Little J, Falace D, Miller C, Rhodus N. *Dental management of the medically compromised patient.* 8th ed. Philadelphia, PA: Mosby Elsevier; 2012. Chapter 1, p. 11-15.

5. Elliot-Smith, S. The dental-medical connection: bridging the interdisciplinary communication gap to broaden patient care. *Access.* 2008:20-26.

6. Darby M, Walsh M. Application of human needs conceptual model to dental hygiene practice. *JDH.* 2000; 74(3):230-237.

7. American Cancer Society. Oral cancer and oropharyngeal cancer: early detection, diagnosis and staging topics. Available from: http://www.cancer.org/Cancer/OralCavityandOropharyngealCancer/DetailedGuide/oral-cavity-and-oropharyngeal-cancer-detection.

8. American Dental Association, Council on Dental Benefits. Council on Scientific Affairs. U.S. Department of Health and Human Services. Public Health Service Food and Drug Administration *The selection of patients for dental radiographic examination.* 2004.

9. Erdogan O, Incki KK, Benliday ME, Seydaoglu G, and Kelekci S. Dental and radiographic findings as predictors of osteoporosis in postmenopausal women. *Geriatr Gerontol Int.* 2009;9:155-164.

10. Chambrone LA, Chambrone L. Tooth loss in well maintained patients with chronic periodontitis during long-term supportive therapy in Brazil. *J Clin Periodontol.* 2006;33:759-764.

11. Ojima M, Kanagawa H, Nishida N, Nagata H, Hanioka T, Shizukuishi S. Relationship between attitudes toward oral health at initial office visit and compliance with supportive periodontal treatment. *J Clin Periodontol.* 2005;32:364-368.

12. Kakudate N, Morita M, Yamazaki S, Fukuhara S, Sugai M, Nagayama M, Kawanami M, Chiba I. Association between self-efficacy and loss to follow-up in long-term periodontal treatment. *J Clin Periodontol.* 2010; 37:276-282.

13. Stafford W, Edenfield S, Coulton K, Beiter T. Insurance as a predictor of dental treatment: a pilot study in the Savannah, Chattham County area. *JDH.* 2010;84(1): 16-21.

14. Sweeting L, Davis K, Cobb C. Periodontal treatment protocol (PTP) for the general dental practice. *JDH.* 2008;83(suppl 6):16-25.

15. Johnson G, Slach N. Impact of tobacco use on periodontal status. *JDE.* 2001;65(4):313-321.

16. Tobacco cessation protocols for the dental practice: ask. Advise. Refer. Available from: http://www.askadviserefer.org/downloads/Tobacco_Cessation_Protocols.pdf.

17. Guerenlian J, Ball WL, La Fontaine J. Diabetes mellitus: promoting collaboration among health care professionals. *JDH.* 2008;83(suppl):1-10.

18. American Academy of Periodontology. AAP parameters of care "periodontal maintenance." *J Periodontol.* 2000; 71:849-850.

19. Axelsson P, Nyström B, Lindhe J. The long-term effect of a plaque control program on tooth mortality, caries and periodontal disease in adults. Results after 30 years of maintenance. *J Clin Periodontol.* 2004;31:749-757.

20. Daniel S, Harfst S, Wilder R. *Mosby's dental hygiene concept, cases and competencies.* 2nd ed. St. Louis, MO: Mosby Elsevier 2008. Chapter 16, p. 327.

21. Lang N, Schatzle M, Loe H. Gingivitis as a risk factor in periodontal disease. *J Clin Periodontol.* 2009;(suppl 10):3-8.

22. Needleman I, Suvan J, Moles D, Pimlott J. Systematic Review of professional mechanical plaque removal for prevention of periodontal diseases. *J Clin Periodontol.* 2005;32(suppl 6):229-282.

23. American Dental Hygienists' Association. Standards for clinical dental hygiene practice. 2008. Available from: http://www.adha.org/downloads/adha_standards08.pdf.

24. American Dental Hygienists' Association. Dental hygiene diagnosis: an American Dental Hygienists' Association position paper. 2010. Available from: http://www.adha.org/governmental_affairs/downloads/DHDx_position_paper.pdf.

25. Vaugh L, Harvey L. Informed consent and the practice of dental hygiene. *Access.* 2008:10-15.

26. American Academy of Periodontology. Parameters of care, "periodontal maintenance." 2000. Available from: http://www.perio.org/resources-products/pdf/849.pdf.

27. American Dental Hygienists' Association. American Dental Hygienists' Association position on polishing procedures. Available from: http://www.adha.org/profissues/polishingpaper.htm.

28. U.S. Department of Human and Health Services, Agency for Healthcare Research and Quality. Health-Partners Dental Group and Clinic guidelines for the diagnosis and treatment of periodontal diseases. 2006. Available from: http://www.guideline.gov/content.aspx?id=10803&search=oral+health+and+periodontal.

29. Sison S. Implant maintenance and the hygienist. *Access.* 2003;(suppl). Available from: http://www.adha.org/downloads/sup_implant.pdf.

30. American Dental Association Council on Scientific Affairs. Professionally applied topical fluoride: evidence-based clinical recommendations. *JADA.* 2006;137(8):1151-1159.

31. Winston AE, Charig A, Patel V, McHale WA. Effect of prophy pastes on surface of tooth enamel. *J Dent Res.* 2005;84(Special Issue A), IADR Abstracts.

32. Burwell AK, Litkowski LJ, Greenspan DC. Calcium sodium phosphosilicate (NovaMin®): remineralization potential. *ADR Online First.* 2009 July 31.

33. Teles R, Patel M, Socransky S, Haffajee A. Disease progression in periodontally healthy and maintenance subjects. *J Periodontol.* 2008;79(5):784-794.

Part IX

Caring for Patients With Special Needs

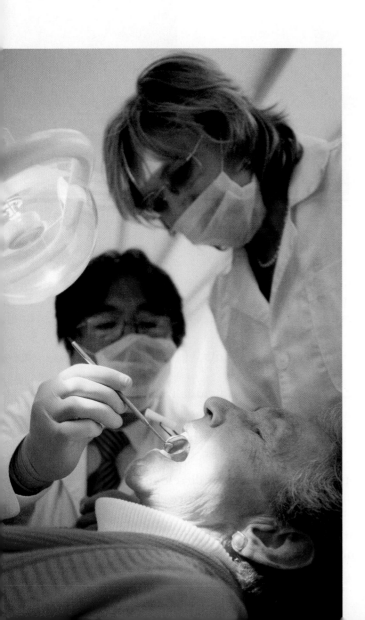

Chapter 36 | Introduction to Special Needs

Bernadette Alvear Fa, DDS • Allen Wong, DDS, EdD • Paul Subar, DDS, EdD • Douglas A. Young, DDS, MBA, MS, EdD

KEY TERMS

comorbidities

developmental disability

intellectual disability

people-first language

physical disability

psychosocial disability

self-care disability

sensory disability

special needs

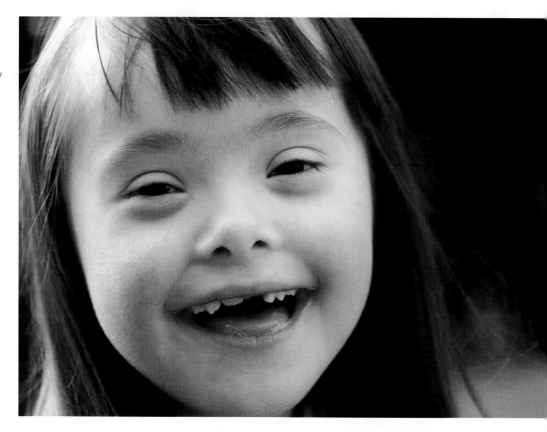

Learning Objectives

After reading this chapter, the student should be able to:

36.1 Identify terms appropriate for patients with special needs.

36.2 Manage patients with developmental disabilities or complex medical issues.

36.3 Describe best practices to interact with patients with special health-care needs.

36.4 Implement a strategy for determining an individualized treatment approach for patients with special needs.

Key Concepts

- Categorizing patients appropriately based on their developmental disabilities will help the clinician recognize best practices in formulating treatment plans.

- Having a clear understanding of behavioral and medical management allows the clinician to acknowledge that traditional methods of practice may not appropriate for the needs of patients with developmental disabilities.

- Understanding dental interventions that are suitable for patients with developmental disabilities aids in easier transition for the dental team.

RELEVANCE TO CLINICAL PRACTICE

It has been established that people with complex medical and developmental conditions experience more oral health problems than those who do not have these conditions.[1] Advances in medicine have increased the life expectancy of patients with complex medical and developmental disabilities. Thirty years ago, a person with Down syndrome had a life expectancy of about 12 years, compared with 60 years today.[1] For those with special health needs, dental care has been shown to be the number one unmet health-care priority. The many challenges of service delivery to this patient population include patient dexterity, patient cooperation, dependency on other care providers, and lack of available dental care facilities and access to care. Many offices and dental team members have not had adequate experiences in their dental education and elect not to treat this underserved population. As a result, increasing numbers of patients with complex medical and developmental conditions are seeking oral health-care providers with the appropriate knowledge, skills, and abilities to manage their treatment.[2]

DEFINING SPECIAL NEEDS

No single, universally agreed upon definition of the term **special needs** exists, because the terminology is ever changing. The following definition encompasses basic guiding principles common to dental patients with special needs: those patients with medical, physical, psychological, or social situations that make it necessary to modify normal dental routines to provide dental treatment for that individual.

Patients with special health-care needs can have congenital or acquired disabilities that are temporary or permanent in nature. The most obvious disabilities may be those accompanied by physical impairment; a person with loss of limb, sight, hearing, or mobility, for example, has outward signs. The less obvious may be emotional or psychosocial disabilities, which also may not be diagnosed or well managed. Mental illness, dementia, Alzheimer, attention deficit-hyperactivity disorder (ADHD), and organic brain disease are among the conditions that also are prone to comorbidities that influence oral health. Disabilities have no age limitations, but some syndromes are associated with or more common in a particular gender. For those patients with genetic or organic syndromes, there are accommodations to be considered. These individuals include, but are not limited to, people with developmental disabilities, complex medical problems, and significant physical limitations.[3,4] The U.S. Census Bureau graph in

Figure 36-1 categorizes civilian noninstitutionalized populations by age and type of disability; the types of disabilities listed are self-care, mental, sensory, difficulty with going outside, and physical.[5]

Changing Terminology

Various terms have been used to categorize patients with special health-care needs. Examples are *people with special needs, children with special health-care needs,* and *people with disabilities.* Terms to describe patients with special health-care needs are becoming more specific, and terminology has evolved to be more sympathetic and appropriate and to help break down social prejudices and barriers. In the late 1980s, a focus on political correctness led many people to adopt **people-first language**—for example, "person with a hearing impairment" rather than "hearing-impaired person" (Table 36-1). The purpose was to focus on the person as a person first and the diagnosis as a condition rather than defining an individual by a diagnosis. However, some groups reject the notion of political correctness or people-first language because they believe it suggests that the disability can be removed from the person when in fact it is part of the person and inseparable. The current trend is to focus on the patient as a person not with a disability but with a different ability. When treating patients with special needs, it is best to ask how they prefer to be described.

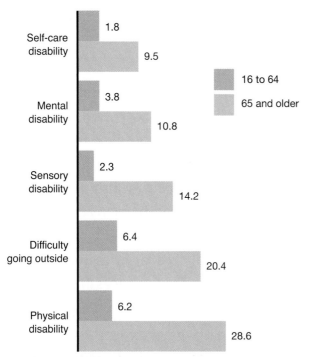

Percentage of the civilian noninstitutionalized population with a disability by age and type of disability: 2000

(For more information on confidentiality protection, sampling error, nonsampling error, and definitions, see: *www.census.gov/gov/cen2000/doc/sf3.pdf*)

Figure 36-1. U.S. Census Bureau categories of civilian noninstitutionalized population. (From U.S. Census Bureau. https://www.census.gov/people/disability/methodology/acs.html.)

HISTORY

In 1975, the Lanterman Act defined deinstitutionalization in California. Frank Lanterman, a state assemblyman, sponsored legislation that established regional centers charged with diagnosing individuals with disabilities and helping them access care. At the federal level, the rights movement for people with disabilities originated in the 1990s through the Americans with Disabilities Act, which was later amended in 1999 to mandate access for patients who require special accommodations. Before 2000, patients identified as having an acquired disability were institutionalized to concentrate services and care. The movement to deinstitutionalize patients and allow patients with a disability to receive services outside an institution was considered a human rights issue. According to Diversity Inc., "Segregating people with disabilities is a form of discrimination, as found in *Olmstead v. L.C.* This landmark disability-rights decision determined that isolating people with disabilities in institutional settings deprives them of the opportunity to participate in their communities, interact with individuals who don't have disabilities and make daily choices. The ruling also acknowledged that unnecessary institutionalization stigmatizes people with disabilities."[6]

Because of demographic changes, medical advancements, and deinstitutionalization, oral care for patients with special health-care needs is occurring more frequently in private-practice general dental offices.

Specific Categories

Medical science has defined thousands of syndromes and their variations. It would be impractical to provide an in-depth review of these conditions; therefore this section will discuss common categories. A dental hygienist who is familiar with a variety of conditions will be prepared to direct the patient interview. Further research can be conducted when patients present with specific diagnoses.

Proper care of patients with special needs begins with understanding how the medical or developmental condition may influence the delivery of dental services. Review current literature about the patients' conditions, and develop some familiarity with symptoms and drugs commonly prescribed for the conditions.

Table 36-1. *Categories of Disabilities: Definitions and Terms*			
Category of Disability	**Definition**	**Outdated Term**	**Preferred Term**
Self-care disability	Inability to care for self independently	Handicap, invalid	Person with challenge
Intellectual disability (ID)	Cognitive impairment, acquired or congenital	Mental retardation (MR)	Neurodevelopmental disability (ND) **Developmental disability** (DD)
Sensory disability	Any disability relating to a sensory organ, such as sight and sound	Blind, deaf, mute	Person with visual impairment Person with hearing impairment Person with speech impairment
Psychosocial disability	Behaviors inappropriate with social interrelations	Mad, crazy, senile	Person with X diagnosis (e.g., person with dementia)
Physical disability	Any impairment to physical activity	Handicapped, crippled, lame	Person who uses a cane

Consider the office environment and how it may affect the patient's experience. Is there room to maneuver a wheelchair or walker? Is the office noisy or are there noxious odors that might irritate the patient? What is the flow of patients through the office? If possible, make any accommodations before the patient arrives.

During the assessment process, determine the patient's current status of developmental delay and health stability for routine treatment (Table 36-2). Some patients with special needs will require routine oral hygiene care, whereas others may require general anesthesia for cooperation or for extensive work.

Management of Patients

Once the dental hygienist has identified the patient's needs and ability to be treated in an office, strategies can be implemented for greater productivity (Table 36-3).

Table 36-2. *Dental Hygiene Considerations*

Patient health stability	Medications	Patient Cognitive Ability
Patient cooperation level	Caregiver involvement	Legal guardian
Office setting	Support staff experience	Clinician experience
Number of times in routine setting	Last time hospital dentistry with general anesthesia (GA) performed	Local anesthesia
Patient reaction to oral sedation	Caries risk assessment	Periodontal risk assessment

Table 36-3. *Decisions for Office Treatment*

	Yes	Maybe	No
Patient health stability	Healthy, minor systemic, medication controlled	ASA 2 or mild ASA 3,	Medically unstable, requiring telemetry, ASA 3 and greater
Medications	Less than 3, nonanticoagulant except baby ASA	More than three meds needing monitoring	Anticoagulants and multiple medications
Patient cognitive ability	Able to verbalize and communicate	Nonverbal but follows commands; lacks ability to communicate	Nonverbal/not cognitively intact
Patient cooperation level	Willing to try anything/able to count teeth and some x-rays	Needs some coaxing	Aggressive and fearful
Caregiver involvement	Fully involved	New but willing/ able to count teeth	Disengaged
Legal guardian	Fully involved and responsible	Not responsive	Not responsive
Office setting	ADA compliant/ able to control noise, light, traffic in office	Some control of office environment	No control of office environment
Support staff experience	At least two trained or experienced individuals	At least one other experienced helper	No experienced helper
Clinician experience	Past experience didactic and clinical	Some experience, either didactic or clinical	No true experience with population
Number of times in routine setting (including local anesthesia)	1/3 years	1/5 years	Never
Last time hospital dentistry with general anesthesia (GA) performed	Within 5 years	5–8 years	Each time
Reaction to oral sedation	Valium makes patient cooperative	Meds cause patient anxiety	Paradoxical reaction
Caries risk assessment	Low/moderate	Moderate/high	High/extreme
Periodontal risk assessment	Low/moderate	Moderate	High/extreme

Patient Health Stability

A thorough and accurate health history is important to determine the fitness of the patient and whether dental procedures can or should be attempted in the office. All patients with a congenital or acquired disability should be under the care of a primary care physician, as their condition may influence treatment planning and care. Physician consults are valuable when the patient may not be able to fully provide pertinent information during the medical review process. As an oral health-care provider, it is important to share treatment objectives and possible dental procedures with the physician. Open communication with the patient's physician can result in more positive treatment outcomes. Because many patients with special needs have **comorbidities** (multiple chronic diseases), it is important to regularly update medical treatment regimens in the patient's chart. The patient's organ systems should be functional or have minimal effects on activities of daily living. Examples of conditions that may deter progress in a patient's treatment if not identified or discussed with physician include the following:

- Cardiovascular fitness: hypertension, hypotension, bleeding disorder
- Respiratory tolerance: breathing challenges (asthma, bronchitis, anatomical limitations)
- Neurological concerns: mood disorder, personality disorder, seizure history, behavioral control
- Hepatic (liver) function: bleeding concerns, hepatitis, medication clearance
- Renal (kidney) function: medication clearance

Medications

Many medications can be synergistic or have counter-effects to other medications. Some patients see multiple specialists for different medical conditions and are prescribed multiple medications. A consultation with the patient's primary care provider who coordinates the patient's overall care or a clinical pharmacist will help maximize the therapeutic goals of medication for the patient. Most important, dental hygienists and dentists should review drug interactions for analgesics, antibiotics, and anesthetics before administration or prescription to avoid potential side effects. One side effect that directly relates to dentistry is medication-induced xerostomia, or hyposalivary function (see Caries Risk Assessment later in this chapter).

Not all patients with special health-care needs require premedication with an anxiolytic (antianxiety drug such as Valium or Ativan). In some cases a reverse, or paradoxical, effect may result and the patient may become more agitated or alert. Ask about the patient's history with this type of medication before administering an anxiolytic.

Patient Cognitive Ability

Cognitive impairment can range from a mild to severe form of intellectual disability. A physician, psychiatrist, or court of law determines the patient's level of cognitive impairment. It is important for the dental hygienist to assess the level of understanding of the patient and caregiver/legal guardian to obtain accurate information and an informed consent. Even if patients can sign their names, they may not know why and what they are signing. Asking questions in multiple ways and having the patient paraphrase the risks, benefits, or procedures are methods of determining a patient's level of understanding. When in doubt, seek additional information.

Patient Cooperation Level

It takes time for patients to become familiar with the sights, smells, sounds, touch, and tastes of the dental office. Some patients will be cooperative, whereas others may be combative. Patients are most cooperative when trust is established. Take time to gather information about the patient's oral care history. Knowing about past experiences and actions that might make the patient anxious will help with establishing a trusting relationship.

Caregiver Involvement

The caregiver is essential to consistency and patient management. Often the caregiver is a family member and is very familiar with the patient's behavior. It is important to involve the caregiver with the dental hygiene goals for the patient and enlist the caregiver's cooperation. The most basic things should not be taken for granted. Many caregivers have never been given formal training on how to best provide oral care or modified oral care for the patient. The caregiver can provide information regarding the patient's likes and dislikes and help determine the best approach for a task. For example, the patient may not be willing to open his or her mouth for the dental hygienist but may readily open his or her mouth for the caregiver. The key is familiarity and trust.

Legal Guardian

The caregiver is not necessarily the legal guardian. Individuals of adult age are able to make their own decisions and sign their own consent forms unless they are deemed medically incompetent to give consent. In the event that patient cannot give consent for themselves, a legal guardian, conservator, or, in some states, an agency is assigned the responsibility of making the decisions for care. Determine whether there is a legal guardian before proceeding with dental treatment, and obtain proper consents.

Office Setting

The Americans with Disabilities Act (ADA) mandated that most public places and health-care offices must accommodate patients who use assistive devices, including wheelchairs, walkers, and, in some cases, gurneys. The dental operatory is usually not very spacious but can be modified to accommodate the patient. It would be prudent for the patient with special needs to visit the office before the day of a procedure to evaluate and identify any needed modifications and become familiar with the environment.

Support Staff Experience

The patient's experience is best when the dental team is working together. Some staff may have a great deal of experience with patients with special needs and can be a valuable resource. Some staff members may have never worked with patients with special needs. Familiarizing staff members with the patient's needs, behaviors, and concerns before the patient's appointment will help them understand and communicate with the patient. The goal is to be efficient and make the appointment a rewarding experience for the patient and staff.

Dental Hygienist Experience

The dental hygienist sets the tone and pace of the delivery of care. It is better to develop a trusting relationship with the patient than to try to achieve too much in one appointment. With experience, dental hygienists learn to tailor appointments to the patient's tolerance level rather than the procedure. This may require multiple shorter appointments initially to develop a relationship of trust.

Number of Times in Routine Setting /Last Visit

If the patient has had regular dental and re-care visits, the likelihood for routine care is favorable. Finding out what the patient likes and dislikes regarding dentistry is important to make the transition a smooth one. The proximity of the last dental visit can be a factor. The longer the time interval from the last visit, the more time it may take to reestablish a new routine in a new office setting.

Last Time Hospital Dentistry with General Anesthesia (GA) Was Performed

Dental work may be performed in a hospital setting with general anesthesia because the patient may need extensive work done at one time, may be uncooperative or combative, or both. For many patients, access to care is a challenge, and dental neglect is common. Patients with a history of hospital dentistry can be treated in the dental office, but it is important to learn when and why the patient last had hospital dentistry care. Much information can be gathered through a review of past episodes. The medications used, responsiveness of the patient, time since the last visit, and type of dentistry performed indicate what to expect with the patient.

Dental Local Anesthesia

The topic of anxiety and pain management is discussed in Chapter 31. Reviewing the patient's medical history and previous restorative dental visits provides information about the patient's past experience with local anesthesia. Before treatment, it is important to assess whether the patient's medical conditions or medications deter the use of a particular anesthetic agent or even the type of technique used to deliver the anesthesia. For example, patients taking tricyclic antidepressants are absolute contraindications for anesthetics containing levonordefrin or norepinephrine.[7]

Advances in dental local anesthesia, such as armamentarium that promotes painless, needleless, and/or reversible measures when treating individual patients, are available.[8] For example, phentolamine mesylate is a vasodilator used to reverse the feeling of numbness in soft tissue at the end of an appointment. This could benefit patients who have uncontrollable behaviors that potentially might cause trauma from biting the lip or cheek.[9] Research on the effectiveness of using these products with patients with special needs is ongoing.

Patient's Reaction to Oral Sedation

If oral sedation has been used before, has it been effective? Partnering with the patient's primary care provider to find an optimal medication could be beneficial. Oral sedation should be used as an aid, with the goal of curtailing its usage. Patients can become acclimated to medication, and it should not be a substitute for good patient management. The philosophy should be to minimize the amount of medication and segue to future appointments with a tapering of dosage over a period of time. This is accomplished through good patient care and patient–clinician familiarity.

Caries Risk Assessment

Patients with special health-care needs are among the most vulnerable and susceptible to dental caries disease.[10] Proper oral care is dependent on dexterity, management of risk, and consistency of care. The effects of medication-induced xerostomia cannot be underestimated, as saliva largely determines pH (to inhibit demineralization and promote remineralization) and provides necessary minerals needed to support remineralization. Comorbidities such as gastroesophageal reflux disease (GERD) can influence caries risk as well.

Testing for salivary flow, pH, and acidic bacteria provides helpful information for the caries risk assessment, for patient education, and to motivate behavioral change. Although any trained member of the dental team can perform these tests, the dental hygienist typically administers them.

Some medications and syndromes increase parafunctional habits such as grinding and clenching.

Visual cues such as acid-eroded teeth, advanced worn dentition, dry mouth appearance, ropey or stringy saliva, mouth breathing, and severe abfractions should be used in assessing caries risk.

Periodontal Risk Assessment

Addressing the oral biofilm in patients with special health-care needs is an essential step in determining the best approach to assess the periodontal condition of the patient. There has been much progression in periodontology to identify the host response to oral biofilm. It is understood that specific pathogens are the cause for the inflammatory process that is responsible for periodontal disease.[11]

Cooperative patients can undergo comprehensive periodontal examination to determine the need for prophylaxis, scaling and root planing, or extraction. Assess uncooperative patients to determine whether they can be treated in the routine care setting—and if so, the need for sedation—or whether dental care should be provided in a hospital setting.[12]

UNDERSTANDING BEST PRACTICES

Behavioral Management

There is no substitute for patience and understanding of the patient. Hygienists who listen to what is said—and often just as important, notice what is not said—will develop a useful relationship sooner than those who do not actively listen to their patients. Management of patients with special health-care needs requires careful observation of patient visual cues. Having the dental team ready and prepared for the patient's first experience is important to set a solid foundation. The tell-show-do method is a good starting point. Some patients prefer watching each step, whereas others just want to have the work done as quickly as possible. Look for and reward any effort toward the desired goals.

Desensitization

Many patients with developmental disabilities may experience hypersensitivity of their sensory organs or to a new environment. Allowing patients time to become familiar with equipment and materials will help them to accept the item or task. For example, at the beginning of most dental hygiene appointments, the patient is bibbed, the chair is positioned, and a bright light is turned on to inspect the teeth. For a person unfamiliar with the setting, it can be frightening to be placed in a reclined chair with a bright light shining into the eyes. A desensitization approach may be for the patient to touch and feel the bib, the chair, and the light, and even activate the chair and light.

Next, the patient would help place the bib, the dental hygienist would explain how the chair functions, and the patient would be allowed to tilt back slowly. The light would be turned on when facing away from the patient and slowly brought closer to the mouth. This technique may take a little more time initially but it will take less time at each subsequent appointment.

Visualization

Most individuals fear dentistry because they must give up control of their environment for a period of time.[13,14] The more a patient knows about the appointment and what to expect, the less stress the patient will have

regarding the next appointment. Explaining to the patient and caregiver what to expect at each appointment can lay the foundation for a future of positive dental experiences. Projecting an image of how the next appointment will proceed will help the patient mentally prepare for the visit through visualization and self-talk. Picture boards can be used to familiarize the patient with office procedures.

Time Management of Appointment

The timing of the dental hygiene appointment can affect its outcome. For many patients, early morning appointments are best to ensure that the patient is rested and ready for a new experience. Afternoon appointments may be less predictable, as fatigue lessens the patient's tolerance.

Keep initial appointments short and frequent and reward positive accomplishments to create a safe and positive environment. Future appointments may become longer through this desensitization technique.

Family and Caregiver Partnership

New situations or appointments in clinical settings can be stressful. To decrease the amount of stress, it is helpful to have a friend, family member, or caregiver accompany the patient to add support and help with improving the patient's health-care routine and aftercare instructions. Clinicians need to develop fluidity in their office space to address behavioral and medical management of patients with developmental disabilities.

Medical Management
Pharmacological Needs

Patients may be taking medications that alter mood and cause disorientation. Before adding to the patient's medication regimen, the clinician should obtain a complete list of prescription and nonprescription medications the patient is currently taking and consider how they will interact with the new medication. The dental hygienist should ask about any additions or changes to the patient's medication regimen that could affect clinical delivery. This includes over-the-counter medications and nutritional supplements.

Nitrous Oxide

Nitrous oxide is a good anxiolytic drug to lower anxiety but can cause the patient to feel claustrophobic or uncomfortable. One major drawback of nitrous oxide is the mask obstructing the view of the clinician. See Chapter 32, Nitrous Oxide/Oxygen Sedation, for more information.

Oral Sedation (by Mouth)

Oral sedation with medications such as diazepam (Valium) or lorazepam (Ativan) can be effective, but not all patients respond the same to medications. When using anxiolytics, consideration must be given to their synergistic effects with narcotics or mood stabilizers, particularly in the elderly population. For the new patient, a test dose is advised to see how the patient reacts.

Immobilization/Stabilization

In the past, the term *restraint* was used to describe equipment and techniques used to restrict a patient's movements. Due to its negative connotations, *restraint* was replaced with the term *restriction devices*. It is important to understand the patient's history with restriction devices. Some may find the experience traumatic, whereas others may enjoy the security it provides. Clinicians using any methods to restrict a patient's movement, even for the patient's protection, must be familiar with local state laws. Informed consent is needed from the patient's legal guardian for each application of stabilization; otherwise it can be considered battery. There is no generic blanket consent form that covers restraining a person as needed.

Mouth Props/Papoose Boards

Many patients are comforted by a stabilizing appliance such as a mouth prop to prevent the mouth from getting tired or the patient from biting down. Papoose boards or blankets can be used to help limit arm and leg movements by securing them to the patient's sides. Restrictive implementation should be used only as an adjunct to care, with permission, and should never replace good communication.

Dental Implications

Modifications to Oral Hygiene Products

Patients who are autonomous with their dental care should be educated regarding proper oral care. In cases where the patient lacks dexterity or strength, modifications may be necessary. It may be as simple as modifying the handle of a toothbrush for better grip using tape and wooden sticks or inserting a toothbrush through a ball. A mechanical toothbrush or Waterpick may also be useful after the patient is trained and desensitized.

Preventative and Disease Management Programs

Dental caries and periodontal disease are both treatable and preventable diseases. Contemporary care includes assessing the risk factors for disease and taking a proactive approach to manage underlying risk factors to halt the disease from progressing or to prevent disease onset. Risk factors for disease will change with time and thus require ongoing reassessment. Routine visits based on disease-specific risk can help minimize premature tooth loss from destruction of hard and soft tissue.

In the past, dental caries were treated with restoration only, which does not treat the underlying disease. The paradigm of treating the underlying disease based on the risk factors is sometimes called caries management by risk assessment (CAMBRA). Patients with special needs are often categorized as having high caries risk.[15] See Chapter 21, Cariology and Caries

Management, regarding the caries disease process and product recommendations.

Dental Management

Developing a Treatment Plan

Developing a treatment plan for a patient begins with the initial meeting with the patient and caregiver (Fig. 36-2). This experience, for the most part, may require gradual and steady movements from the oral health professional, and should also include the idea of "inform before you perform."[16] Oral health professionals may need to allocate more time to these appointments to emphasize and build upon a rapport between the oral health professional, the patient, and the caregiver.

Using the data collected from the initial patient interview and appointment, the dental hygienist develops an appropriate diagnosis or set of diagnoses. The dental hygienist then presents treatment recommendations to the patient and caregiver and explains the treatment plan and how it addresses the various diagnoses. As with all patients, the risks, benefits, and alternatives

Application to Clinical Practice

Overall teamwork helps to address individual patient needs. Dramatic changes have been made to accreditation standards within U.S. dental schools to educate dental professionals in treating populations with developmental disabilities and special needs.[17] These unique experiences that occur within dental education are helpful, but are only building blocks for the knowledge and understanding necessary for treating patients. There is still much that needs to be done to advance care and provide access, but the improvement has allowed for more practitioners to become involved. ■

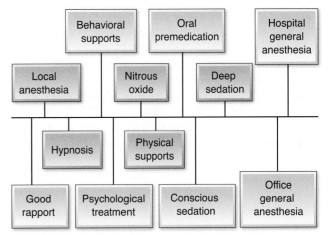

Treatment options continuum

Figure 36-2. Treatment options continuum.

should be included in the discussion. Emphasize that a maintenance program after the procedures and treatments are complete is beneficial to maintaining the patient's oral health. Informed consent must be obtained before treatment begins. See Application to Clinical Practice.

SUMMARY

There is a large population of patients with special health-care needs, and there is no single definition for each of the individual conditions. Patients are managed differently based on their individual oral health-care needs. Reviewing the patient's medical history and communicating with the patient's primary care physician are common examples of how to initiate best practices for the patient.

When patients seek care from the oral health-care provider, it is crucial for the provider to be prepared with the knowledge and information of the patient's condition, behavior, and previous treatments. Understanding this information allows the provider to prepare for the patient's appointment and formulate treatment plans that address the patient's oral health-care needs.

Case Study

A 34-year-old patient with autism presents at the clinic for root planing. The dental hygienist reviews the patient's health history and notices that the patient may have a history of subacute bacterial endocarditis. When asked about the finding, the patient's caregiver responds, "That heart thing was before I took care of him over 3 years ago. The other hygienist saw him last week for root planing of the other side and did not give antibiotics, so just go ahead and proceed."

Case Study Exercises

1. The dental hygienist should: (Choose two responses.)
   A. Consider recommendations provided by the primary care physician.
   B. Proceed with treatment before following up with patient's physician.
   C. Seek advice from the dental clinician as to the best course of action to obtain medical consult.
   D. Ask the legal guardian for more information.
   E. Ask only the patient regarding past appointments and need for antibiotics.

2. Which of the following would NOT affect the experience of an office environment for this patient?
   A. Noxious odors
   B. Parking availability
   C. Sound volume
   D. Brightness of room lighting

3. Desensitization is a process that helps introduce patients with special health-care needs to the environment of a dental office. This process involves all of the following EXCEPT which one?
   A. Positioning the dental light with quick and abrupt movements
   B. Slowly tilting back the chair
   C. Allowing the patient to feel the bib
   D. Allowing the patient to touch the operatory chair

Review Questions

1. All of the following statements regarding medical management are correct EXCEPT which one?
   A. Nitrous oxide is an anxiolytic drug that effectively lowers anxiety.
   B. Mouth props are an assisting aid to help keep patients from biting down.
   C. Oral sedation should be used for all patients.
   D. *Restraint* has negative connotations and is now termed *restriction devices*.

2. Time management of the appointment is an important aspect of treating patients with special health-care needs. Dental hygienists should consider which of the following?
   A. Morning appointments
   B. Short and frequent appointments initially
   C. Praising small positive accomplishments
   D. All of these choices

3. Before treating a patient with special health-care needs for the first time, the hygienist
   A. needs to thoroughly review the medical history.
   B. needs to familiarize the patient with the armamentarium that will be used.
   C. establishes rapport with both the patient and caregiver.
   D. All of these
   E. None of these

4. The _____ is essential for consistency and patient management.
   A. patient
   B. caregiver

C. dental hygienist
D. medical doctor

5. When considering treatment options, one aspect to consider as a starting point for interacting with patients with special health-care needs is which of the following?
   A. Ability to provide hospital dentistry
   B. Physical supports present in dental office
   C. Good rapport
   D. Behavioral supports

Active Learning

1. Working with a partner, chart out the various terms used to describe a patient with special health-care needs. Identify which terms are outdated and which are considered appropriate. Have a discussion about how the outdated terms may influence your rapport with your patient.

2. Working in groups of three, have each person play the role of patient, guardian, and dental hygienist. Assume the patient is a 70-year-old female in the early stages of dementia, and her caregiver is extremely knowledgeable of the patient's medical history and mildly combative behavior. The patient's treatment plan involves a prophy, extractions, and several glass ionomer restorations. Have a discussion to get the patient to consent to the prophy appointment. ■

REFERENCES

1. Glassman P, Subar P. Planning dental treatment for people with special needs. *Dent Clin N Am*. 2009;53(2):195-205.
2. Glassman P, Subar, P. Creating and maintaining oral health for dependent people in institutional settings. *J Pub Health Dent*. 2010;70:540-548.
3. Commission on Dental Accreditation. *Accreditation standards for dental education programs*. Chicago, IL: American Dental Association; June 30, 2004.
4. Waldman HB, Perlman SP. A special care dentistry specialty: sounds good, but. . . *J Dent Educ*. 2006;70(10): 1019-1022.
5. U.S. Department of Commerce, Economics and Statistics Administration, U.S. Census Bureau. *Census 2000. Disability Status 2000*. March 2003. Available from: https://www.census.gov/prod/2003pubs/c2kbr-17.pdf.
6. DiversityInc. Forced institutionalization of people with disabilities is illegal. 2010, June 6. Available from: http://diversityinc.com.
7. Jastak JT, Yagiela JA, Donaldson D, editors. *Local anesthesia of the oral cavity*. Philadelphia, PA: WB Saunders; 1995.
8. Malamed SF. Handbook of local anesthesia. St. Louis, MO: Mosby/Elsevier; 2013. p. 356-379
9. Saxena P, et al. Advances in dental local anesthesia techniques and devices: an update. *Natl J Maxillofac Surg*. 2013;4(1):19.
10. Jenson L, Budenz AW, Featherstone JD, et al. Clinical protocols for caries management by risk assessment. *J Calif Dent Assoc*. 2007;35(10):714-723.
11. Armitage GC, Robertson PB. The biology, prevention, diagnosis and treatment of periodontal diseases: scientific advances in the United States. *J Am Dent Assoc*. 2009;140(suppl 1):36S-43S.
12. Wong AW, Subar P. Management of the special needs patient. In *Hall's critical decisions in periodontology and dental implantology*. 5th ed. Harpenenau L, Kao R, Lundergan W, Sanz M, editors. Shelton, CT: People's Medical Publishing House; 2013. p. 163-164.
13. Wells, A. *Cognitive therapy of anxiety disorders: a practice manual and conceptual guide*. Chichester, England: Wiley; 2013.
14. Humphris G, Kristel K. The prevalence of dental anxiety across previous distressing experiences. *J Anxiety Disord*. 2011;25(2):232-236.
15. Young DA, Featherstone JDB, Roth JR. Curing the silent epidemic: caries management in the 21st century and beyond. *J Calif Dent Assoc*. 2007;35(10):681-702.
16. Wong, A. Treatment planning considerations for adult oral rehabilitation cases in the operating room. *Dent Clin N Am*. 2009;53(2):255-267.
17. Commission of Dental Accreditation. *Accreditation standards for dental education programs*. Chicago, IL: American Dental Association; 2007.

Chapter 37 | Cardiovascular Disease

Angelina E. Riccelli, BS, MS, RDH • R. Donald Hoffman, DMD, MEd, PhD

KEY TERMS

angina pectoris
anticoagulant therapy
arrhythmias
atheroma
atherosclerosis
atrial septal defect
bacteremia
bradycardia
cardiovascular surgery
congenital heart disease
coronary heart disease
cytokines
heart block
heart failure
hypertension
infective endocarditis
inflammation
ischemic heart disease
myocardial infarction
patent ductus arteriosus
periodontal disease
post–cardiovascular surgery
regurgitation
rheumatic heart disease
stenosis
tachycardia
thrombogenic
thrombus
ventricular fibrillation
ventricular septal defect
ventricular tachycardia

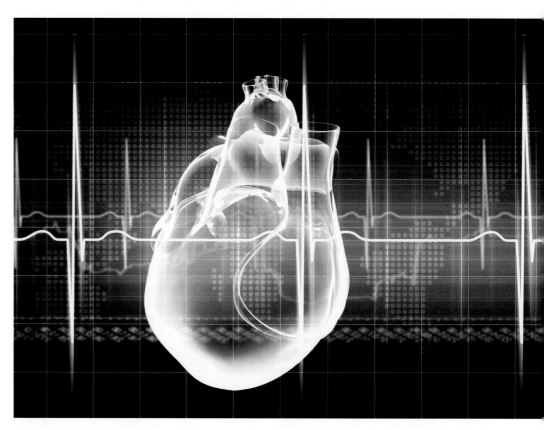

LEARNING OBJECTIVES

After reading this chapter, the student will be able to:

37.1 Identify cardiovascular diseases most commonly encountered in dental hygiene practice.
37.2 Explain the role of inflammation developed in response to the bacterial action in plaque and its link with cardiovascular disease.
37.3 Develop individualized dental hygiene care plans for patients with cardiovascular disease.
37.4 Implement the necessary dental hygiene treatment modifications for patients with various cardiovascular conditions.

KEY CONCEPTS

- Cardiovascular disease (CVD) is a leading cause of death in the United States.
- Dental hygienists must be aware of their patients' general health and recognize the signs and symptoms of CVD.
- Dental hygienists must be able to identify the cardiovascular conditions that prohibit or delay dental treatment, and assess, manage, and treat individuals with controlled cardiovascular disease.

- The assessment and treatment of the patient with CVD require an interdisciplinary approach by the dental hygienist, the dentist, and the patient's physician(s).
- Some of the risk factors associated with CVD are also identified as risk factors for periodontal disease.
- Chronic inflammation and tissue damage, which can result from periodontal disease, give bacteria an opportunity to disseminate to other organs and initiate infections in the host, including cardiovascular disease.
- Evidence-based studies are currently being conducted to determine whether the relationship between periodontal infections and CVD is a direct or an indirect relationship.
- Oral health can have profound consequences for cardiovascular health.
- An accurate medical history and knowledge of the patient's medications can assist the dental hygienist in recognizing and determining whether a patient has CVD.
- To help determine the type of CVD the patient suffers from, the dental hygienist should ask specific questions relative to the patient's medications.
- Dental hygiene treatment modifications should be made specifically to address the patient's type of CVD, medications, and symptoms experienced during treatment.
- Depending on the type of CVD and the patient's symptoms, dental hygiene treatment modifications for patients with CVD include measuring blood pressure before initiation of treatment and during treatment, minimizing the patient's stress and anxiety, careful consideration and use of local anesthesia, placing the patient in a reclined position rather than in a supine position, consulting the patient's physician before initiating treatment, and not treating the patient at this time.
- It is crucial for the dental hygienist to develop individualized oral health-care instructions and recommendations for patients with cardiovascular disease.
- Effective oral hygiene homecare is essential for patients with cardiovascular disease.

RELEVANCE TO CLINICAL PRACTICE

Due to increased life expectancy, dental hygienists are encountering and treating patients with a myriad of health disorders that not only affect their dental health, but also have profound effects on their dental treatment. Among the disorders that may be encountered is cardiovascular disease (CVD). According to the Centers for Disease Control and Prevention, cardiovascular disease is the leading cause of death in the United States for both men and women.[1] CVD encompasses many conditions, such as hypertension, heart failure, angina, infective bacterial endocarditis, valvular defects, and coronary heart disease. As a consequence of this, hygienists are more frequently encountering patients with implantable cardio-defibrillators and pacemakers, and patients with history of **cardiovascular surgery**. Moreover, multiple studies have shown a link between CVD and **periodontal disease**. Therefore, it is important that dental hygienists recognize the signs and symptoms of CVD, identify the cardiovascular conditions that prohibit dental treatment, and assess, manage, and treat individuals with controlled cardiovascular disease. Due to the risk factors associated with CVD, the assessment and treatment of individuals with CVD requires an interdisciplinary approach by the dental hygienist, the dentist, and the patient's physician(s).

This chapter addresses the association between oral and systemic health and the following cardiovascular diseases:

- Arrhythmias
- Atherosclerosis
- Congenital heart disease
- Heart failure
- Hypertension
- Infective endocarditis
- Ischemic heart disease
  - Angina pectoris
  - Myocardial infarction
  - Chronic ischemic heart disease
  - Sudden cardiac death
- Post–cardiovascular surgery
- Rheumatic heart disease

Suggestions for treatment modifications and dental hygiene considerations and precautions during treatment provided to these individuals are addressed, as is the link between CVD and periodontal disease.

CARDIOVASCULAR DISEASE

The term *cardiovascular disease* can be used to describe any disorder of the cardiovascular system (heart and blood vessels) that affects the ability of the heart and/or blood vessels to function normally. CVD is responsible for an estimated 17.1 million deaths each year.[2] Research supports the view that in most cases the risk of CVD can be decreased through lifestyle changes such as diet, exercise, stress reduction, smoking cessation, and cessation of harmful use of alcohol.[2] In addition, some of the risk factors associated with CVD also are identified as risk factors for periodontal disease (Fig. 37-1). Similarly, lifestyle strategies that are effective in the control of periodontitis can have a positive effect on cardiovascular disease, for example, reduction of bacterial load from the oral cavity via meticulous oral care, and modification of risk factors such as smoking cessation, improved nutrition, and stress reduction.

The prevalence of CVD is higher among men than women. According to the World Health Organization, in 2009, the prevalence for CVD was 81.1 cases per 1,000 for men, in contrast to only 49.6 cases per 1,000 per women.[3]

Physiology of the Heart

To comprehend CVD, it is crucial to first review the anatomy and physiology of the heart, the main organ involved in CVD. The heart is a muscular organ approximately the size of a fist, and is located just behind and slightly to the left of the breastbone. Simplistically stated, the heart is a pump that circulates blood through a network of arteries and veins called the cardiovascular system. The heart is a four-chambered

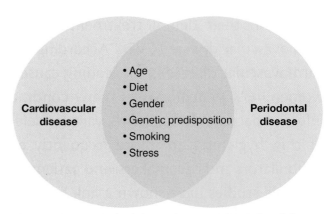

Figure 37-1. Associated risk factors for CVD and periodontal disease.

organ that contains two atriums and two ventricles. The right ventricle pumps deoxygenated blood received from the venous system of the body to the lungs for oxygenation, and the left ventricle pumps oxygenated blood returned from the lungs to the body through the aorta (Fig. 37-2). Thus, blood enters the heart through the superior and inferior vena cava, and travels into the right atrium, which then empties through a tricuspid valve into the right ventricle. From there the blood travels through the pulmonic valve to the pulmonary arteries, where it is oxygenated in the lungs. Blood returns from the lungs via the pulmonary veins into the left atrium. From there, it passes through the mitral valve to the left ventricle (the strongest chamber), which pumps oxygen-rich blood to the rest of the body. The left ventricle's vigorous contractions create the pressure essential to circulate blood throughout the cardiovascular system. The coronary arteries run along the surface of the heart and provide oxygen-rich blood to the heart muscle. A web of modified specialized cardiac muscle tissues, the Purkinje fibers (see Fig. 37-2), originates in the sinoatrial node and terminates in the Purkinje system. This system runs through the heart, conducting the complex signals that govern contraction and relaxation of the heart muscle (see Fig. 37-2). Any compromise to this system of veins and arteries can produce deleterious effects in the overall health of the cardiovascular system.

Association Between Oral and Systemic Health

The oral cavity harbors a large variety of microorganisms that not only include bacteria but also viruses, fungi, and protozoans. Bacteria mainly colonize as bacterial biofilm plaque on the surface of the teeth, the tongue, the gingival tissue around the teeth, and the buccal mucosa. (See Chapter 13, Biofilm, Calculus, and Stain, for a complete discussion of biofilm.) Among a large number of bacteria colonizing the oral cavity, only a few have been identified and only a small percentage of these are considered to be pathogenic. In the healthy oral cavity, the majority of the inhabiting bacteria are believed to be nonpathogenic; however, the localized or focal growth of pathogenic bacteria occurs during periodontal disease (PD), chronic periapical abscess (PA), dental pulp infections, and dental caries. Infections in the oral cavity can disseminate to other parts of the body via the circulatory system, as shown in Figure 37-3.

Oral infections are mostly treatable. However, when infectious microorganisms are allowed to colonize an oral site such as in the case of PD, bacterial products (proteolytic enzymes) secreted in the tissue initiate tissue damage around the infection. The tissue damage caused by bacterial products together with associated endotoxins that are secreted by the microbes initiates

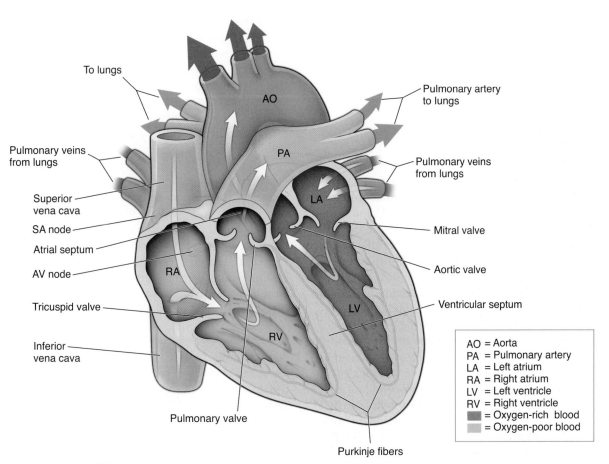

Figure 37-2. Normal heart.

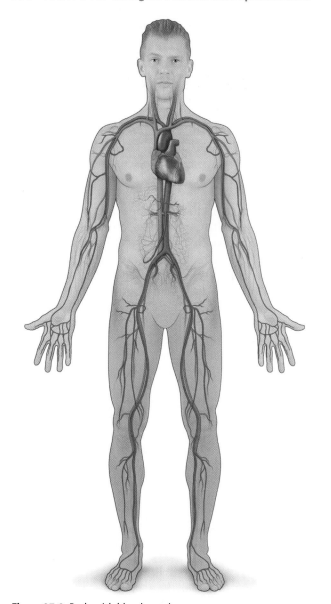

Figure 37-3. Body with blood vessels.

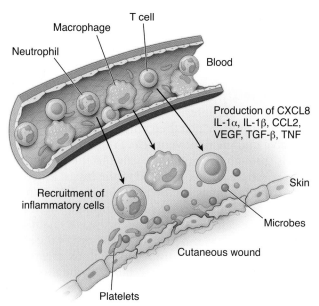

Figure 37-4. Pathogens eliciting immune response.

inflammatory responses in the host at the site of infection. Activation of the inflammatory response results in recruitment of immune cells—such as macrophages, neutrophils, and, later, lymphocytes—to eliminate the bacterial infection. If the infection is resolved, the soft tissue damage is repaired. However, if the infection is left unresolved, the infection and inflammatory response result in local inflammatory cell proliferation at the site of the infection. The body continues to deliver immune cells from the blood through capillaries. Activation of the immune cells results in the production of enzymes to kill bacteria and **cytokines** (signaling molecules that mediate the inflammatory response) to activate more immune cells (Fig. 37-4). Although this inflammatory response is very effective in killing bacteria, it also kills many bystander host cells, causing considerable soft tissue damage, and can initiate bone loss around the teeth, as is observed in PD. (For a complete discussion of inflammation, see Chapter 5, Immunology and the Oral–Systemic Link.)

The chronic **inflammation** and tissue damage in the oral cavity give bacteria an opportunity to disseminate to other organs and initiate secondary infections in the host, such as atherosclerotic plaques, and around the valves and endocardium of the heart, as in subacute bacterial endocarditis (BE) and CVD such as atherosclerosis (Fig. 37-5). Because a similar inflammatory process regulates PD and CVD, great emphasis has been placed on whether the circulating inflammatory mediators of PD are risk factors for or exacerbate insipient CVD[4] (see Fig. 37-4). Although considerable data support an association between PD and CVD,[5] evidence-based studies are currently being conducted to determine whether the relationship between periodontal infections and CVD is a direct or indirect relationship. Specifically, does the infectious and inflammatory PD process contribute causally to heart attacks and strokes, or are these two conditions coincidentally associated?[6–11]

The concept relating chronic oral infections with vascular disease is more than a century old.[12,13] This notion was based on frequent observations that relatively poor oral health (higher combined levels of caries, periodontitis, periapical lesions, and pericoronitis) was observed more often in patients with recent myocardial infarctions and strokes than in people who had not experienced a heart attack or stroke.[14] However, it was only recently that an association between PD and CVD has been revisited at the tissue, cellular, and molecular level.

It is believed that factors such as certain genetic indicators, family history, smoking, hormonal factors, and perhaps obesity that place individuals at high risk for oral infections can potentially place them at high risk for systemic diseases.[10] For example, the incidence of **bacteremia** (bacteria in the blood) following dental procedures such as tooth extraction, endodontic treatment, periodontal surgery, and root planing and scaling has been well documented.[15,16] The association between PD

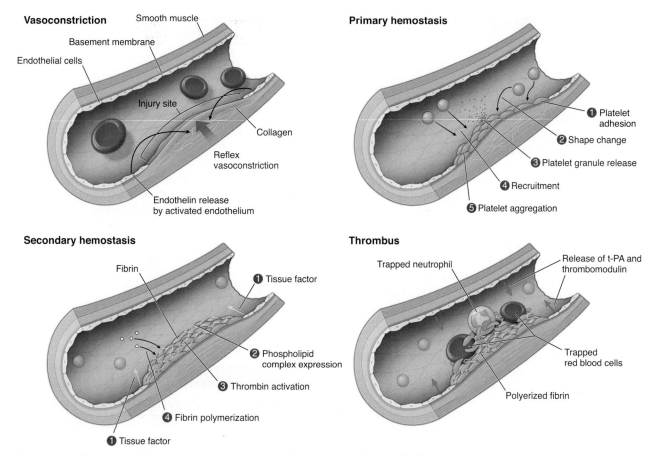

Figure 37-5. Microbes and inflammatory products in the pathogenesis of cardiovascular disease.

and CVD is also considered because both the presence of bacteria and the inflammation in response to microbes are believed to be critical components in both diseases. Specifically, subgingival biofilms are thought to act as reservoirs of gram-negative bacteria that serve as a source for bacterial dissemination and initiation of endocarditis. Additionally, the inflamed periodontium may act as a source of inflammatory mediators (cytokines and others) that can circulate and initiate cardiovascular tissue damage.[17]

Many molecular mechanisms have been proposed in which oral/periodontal pathogens serve as triggers for pathways leading to exacerbation of CVD through direct and indirect effects. Oral bacterial pathogens enter the bloodstream from diseased sites and enter systemic tissues such as carotid **atheroma** (lipid deposits in subendothelial tissue) (see Fig. 37-5). Periodontal microbes may also directly contribute to atherogenesis (atheroma formation or progression) and thromboembolic (clotting) events in the vessels via repeated challenges of inflammatory cytokines, microbes, and microbial products. In fact, oral bacteria such as *Streptococcus sanguis* and *Porphyromonas gingivalis* are shown to induce platelet aggregation, leading to **thrombus** formation in blood vessels.[18] Similarly, periodontal infections induce fibrinogen, a factor that initiates clot formation in vascular tissue.[19] In addition, periodontal infections stimulate the production of C-reactive protein (CRP) in the liver. This, in turn, may induce atheroma

formation in injured blood vessels and later initiate thromboembolic events. A study evaluating the relationship between CVD and CRP in adults showed that the mean level of CRP (8.7 g/mL) in patients with PD and CVD was significantly greater than that (1.14 g/mL) in controls exhibiting neither PD or CVD.[6] Further, treatment of PD caused a 65% reduction in the level of CRP at 3 months, linking CVD to periodontal inflammation. Thus, all of these factors and microbial product exposures may play significant roles in initiating or exacerbating chronic inflammatory responses in **coronary heart disease** and stroke. These observations have prompted extensive research to examine the existence of a definitive relationship between PD and CVD.[20]

Environmental factors are also suggested to be risk factors and indicators shared by periodontitis and systemic diseases, such as CVD. For example, tobacco smoking and stress affect the severity of periodontal infections and CVD.[21] Whether these risk factors are common to periodontal disease and CVD, or periodontal disease alone, the risk factors for the initiation of CVD remain unclear. Randomized intervention trials would be required before a relationship between periodontal disease and CVD could be established. Due to the correlation between oral health and cardiovascular health, the dental hygienist must be aware of the patient's health conditions to properly treat oral diseases.

DISEASE PROCESSES

Arrhythmias

Cardiac **arrhythmias** are the result of errors in impulse formation and/or impulse conduction that cause abnormal heart rhythms; the heart beats too fast (tachycardia) or too slow (bradycardia), or there can be asynchronous conduction. Arrhythmias can occur in both normal and diseased hearts. Common examples of arrhythmias include atrial fibrillation, premature ventricular contractions (PVCs), ventricular fibrillation, and heart block. Therefore, arrhythmias are caused by either a disturbance of the normal electrical conduction system of the heart or as a consequence of heart disease. The arrhythmias that affect a healthy heart may be associated with physical exercise and emotional stress, and usually diminish as the causative factor is removed. Arrhythmias can be associated directly with certain heart diseases, such as arteriosclerotic heart disease, rheumatic heart disease, and coronary artery disease. Consumption of certain foods, such as caffeine, or certain medications, especially medications for the common cold, can contribute to arrhythmias.[22]

Bradycardia

Bradycardia is defined as a sinus node dysfunction that results in a heart rate of less than 60 beats/minute. The reduced heart rate does not provide for adequate profusion of oxygenated blood to the body. Drugs, such as digitalis, sotalol, beta blockers, calcium channel blockers, and amiodarone, may also cause bradycardia.[22,23]

Because the brain and body do not receive enough blood to function well, the following symptoms may appear: fatigue and weakness, dizziness, lightheadedness, syncope, and shortness of breath. These symptoms may be confused with those of a myocardial infarction (MI) and other conditions. According to Advanced Cardiovascular Life Support (ACLS) algorithm guidelines, symptomatic bradycardia is treated with atropine sulfate and epinephrine.[23]

Dental Hygiene Considerations

Obtaining an accurate medical history and a list of the patient's medications will assist in identifying and determining whether a patient has arrhythmias. Ask specific questions relative to the medications taken, because some cardiovascular medications can be taken to treat different cardiovascular diseases. Take the patient's heart rate and blood pressure, and monitor both during treatment. If the patient experiences any symptoms of bradycardia during dental hygiene treatment, terminate treatment, alert emergency medical services (EMS), and monitor the patient's blood pressure and pulse. Slow heart rates are of greater concern than high heart rates. If a patient has a *new onset* of bradycardia symptoms and pulseless electrical activity occurs, the dental hygienist begins basic life support (BLS) while waiting for EMS to arrive. Be prepared for an incident of cardiac arrest.

Apply oxygen and an automated external defibrillator (AED), if indicated; activate EMS immediately if further deterioration occurs.

Tachycardia

Tachycardia is a condition that refers to a heart rate that is abnormally high, greater than 100 beats/minute and up to as many as 400 beats/minute. At these elevated rates, the heart is not able to pump oxygen-rich blood to the body. Symptoms of tachycardia include shortness of breath, dizziness, sudden weakness, fluttering in the chest, lightheadedness, and fainting. Tachycardia is classified as either atrial or ventricular depending on which chamber of the heart is affected.[22,23] Drugs used for the treatment of tachycardia are listed in Table 37-1.

Atrial Fibrillation

The rate for atrial tachycardia is 100 to 250 beats/min. Patients presenting with concomitant heart disease,

Table 37-1. *Antiarrhythmia Treatments*

Arrhythmia	Medication	Oral Side Effects
Atrial fibrillation	amiodarone (Cordarone) verapamil (Cronovera, Dilacoran) diltiazem (Cardizem) beta blockers esmolol (Brevibloc) metoprolol (Lopressor) propranolol (Inderal)	Abnormal salivation and taste Gingival hyperplasia Gingival hyperplasia Xerostomia
Supraventricular tachycardia	adenosine (Adenocard, Adenoscan)	
Ventricular fibrillation	amiodarone (Cordarone)	Abnormal salivation and taste
Unstable ventricular fibrillation	Use of automated external defibrillator (AED)	
Ventricular tachycardia	digoxin (Lanoxin)	Sensitive gag reflex

(From Mehta S, Mehta S, Meta S, Milder EA, Mirarchi AJ. *Step-up to USML, step 1.* 4th ed. Philadelphia, PA: Lippincott Williams and Wilkins; 2010; American Dental Association. How medications can affect your oral health. *JADA.* 2005;136. Available from http://www.ada.org/~/media/ADA/Publications/Files/patient_51.ashx; and PubMed Health, U.S. National Library of Medicine. Available from http://www.ncbi.nlm.nih.gov/pubmedhealth/.)

including coronary artery disease, valvular disease, cardiomyopathies, and congenital heart disease are more likely to experience atrial tachycardias.[22]

Premature Ventricular Contractions

Premature ventricular contractions (PVCs) may be perceived as a skipped heartbeat, a strong beat, or a feeling of suction in the chest. PVCs may also cause chest pain, a faint feeling, or fatigue. The frequency of PVCs may increase with age, and PVCs are also associated with fatigue, stress, and use of caffeine, tobacco, and alcohol. If more than five PVCs occur within a 60-second period, it may signal underlying coronary problems and could result in sudden cardiac death.[22]

Ventricular Tachycardia/Ventricular Fibrillation

Ventricular tachycardia (VT) is three or more consecutive depolarizations occurring at greater than 100 beats per minute. When there is a ventricular rhythm disturbance, it is important to determine whether it is ventricular tachycardia or supraventricular tachycardia (SVT) because the therapeutic and prognostic implications differ significantly. SVT is associated with a narrow complex electrocardiogram (ECG) rhythm because the impulse is generated above the ventricles. VT is associated with a wide complex rhythm that originates in the ventricles. VT that lasts more than 30 seconds in considered sustained. Sustained VT has the potential to result in hemodynamic instability, which could result in ventricular fibrillation.[22,23]

Uncoordinated contraction of the ventricle cardiac muscle is known as **ventricular fibrillation**. The ventricular cardiac muscle quivers rather than contracting properly. Ventricular tachycardia originates in one of the ventricles of the heart and is potentially life threatening because it may lead to ventricular fibrillation, asystole, and sudden death. If this condition continues for more than a few seconds, cardiogenic shock can occur, with death resulting in a matter of minutes.[22,23]

Dental Hygiene Considerations

Obtaining an accurate medical history with vital signs and a listing of medications taken by the patient will assist in identifying and determining whether a patient has history of arrhythmias. Ask specific questions relative to the medications taken, because some cardiovascular medications can be taken to treat different cardiovascular diseases. Local anesthesia considerations include evaluating the risk and benefits of using vasoconstrictors, modifying treatment, and assessing the use of low concentrations of epinephrine. If the patient experiences any symptoms of *new-onset* tachycardia during dental hygiene treatment, terminate treatment and monitor the patient's blood pressure and pulse and compare these values to the baseline values taken before the initiation of dental hygiene treatment. Be prepared to initiate BLS—activate EMS if further deterioration occurs; apply oxygen and AED, if applicable.

Heart Block

Heart block is a type of arrhythmia that is caused by the malfunction of the heart's electrical system. There are three degrees of heart block, with the third degree being the most severe and dangerous because the patient could potentially go into cardiac arrest. The three types of heart block are as follows:[22]

First-degree heart block—Patients with coronary artery disease and/or on beta blockers can demonstrate first-degree heart block. The patients may not be aware of their situation because symptoms may not be evident.

Second-degree heart block—Can result in the skipping a beat or beats. Patients may experience dizziness or fainting.

Third-degree (complete atrial ventricular [AV]) heart block—Patients with third-degree heart block have an absence of conduction between the sinoatrial node and the ventricles. A ventricular pacemaker maintains a ventricular rate between 25 and 40 (normal heart rate). This type of heart block is known as AV dissociation, is serious, and can result in sudden cardiac arrest/death.[22,23]

Dental Hygiene Considerations

Implantable pacemakers and automatic/artificial implantable defibrillators are used to maintain a regular heartbeat in patients who have experienced irregular heart rhythms. The dental hygienist may need to consult the physician/cardiologist before initiating treatment to determine whether any alterations to dental hygiene treatment are indicated. These may include antibiotic prophylaxis, choice of local anesthetic agents, and duration of treatment time. Another consideration for the dental hygienist is the use of ultrasonic scalers, as earlier models (ferromagnetic ultrasonic magnetostrictive scalers) are not properly shielded and may interfere with the operation of these devices. It has been determined that the piezoelectric dental scaler does not generate interference.[24] If in doubt, the dental hygienist should check with patient's physician regarding whether the pacemaker is shielded.

Power or battery-operated toothbrushes do not produce interference. However, a precaution was given by one of the leading cardiac implant manufacturers for the use of sonic toothbrushes with a battery charger. A patient needs to maintain a distance of at least 6 inches between the battery charger and the implanted device and needs to maintain a distance greater than 1 inch between the toothbrush and the implanted device.[25] Patients should check with the cardiologist to determine whether they can use power brushes.

ATHEROSCLEROSIS

Atherosclerosis is a buildup of fibro-fatty deposit or plaque consisting of several lipids on the internal walls

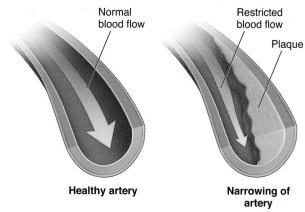

Figure 37-6. Blood vessels.

of medium and large arteries, which causes a narrowing of the lumen of the vessel (Fig. 37-6). Atherosclerosis is the main cause of angina pectoris, can lead to ischemic heart disease, and is the leading cause of death in the United States.[22]

Risk Factors

Risk factors for atherosclerosis include hypertension, smoking, diabetes, obesity, high cholesterol and levels of high-density lipoprotein (HDL) less than 45, high triglycerides, stress, family history of heart disease, and a sedentary lifestyle. Atherosclerosis is more evident in older individuals, males, and some racial groups. Discussing these risk factors with the patient is important, as atherosclerosis produces no symptoms until the damage to the arteries is extensive enough to restrict blood flood.

• Treatment—Lipid-lowering medications (Table 37-2), diet and lifestyle changes.
• Association with periodontal disease—Data suggest that the long-term, chronic inflammation associated with periodontal disease can exacerbate atherosclerosis.[13]

Dental Hygiene Considerations

There is a need for a thorough medical history and emphasis on the importance of excellent preventive care to treat and prevent periodontal disease. Therefore, the dental hygienist must provide individualized instructions on brushing, flossing, and use of any other oral physiotherapy aids that are needed.

HYPERTENSION

Hypertension is a commonly occurring disorder that affects about 60 million people in the United States and about 1 billion people worldwide, and is the leading cause of death.[26] Most hypertension is of unknown etiology, which is referred to as *essential hypertension*. For those with hypertension, 10% to 20% have an identifiable cause, such as renal diseases and endocrine causes, primary aldosteronism, pheochromocytoma,

Table 37-2. *Lipid-Lowering Medications*

Medication	Indications	Oral Side Effects
lovastatin (Altoprev, Mevacor) pravastatin (Pravachol) simvastatin (Zocor) atorvastatin (Lipitor)	High low-density lipoprotein (LDL) levels, preventive purposes after an MI or stroke	None
niacin (Niacor)	Increased LDL levels, slow progression of coronary artery disease, lower risk of MI	None
cholestyramine (Prevalite, Questran) colestipol (Colestid)	Increased LDL levels Management of primary hypercholesterolemia	None
ezetimibe (Zetia)	Increased LDL levels	
gemfibrozil (Lopid) clofibrate (Atromid-S) bezafibrate (Bezatrol, Bezalip) fenofibrate (Antara)	Increased triglyceride (TG) Increased LDL levels	Xerostomia and tooth disorder Xerostomia

(From Mehta S, Mehta S, Meta S, Milder EA, Mirarchi AJ. *Step-up to USML, step 1*. 4th ed. Philadelphia, PA: Lippincott Williams and Wilkins; 2010; American Dental Association. How medications can affect your oral health. *JADA*. 2005;136. Available from http://www.ada.org/~/media/ADA/Publications/Files/patient_51.ashx; and PubMed Health, U.S. National Library of Medicine. Available from http://www.ncbi.nlm.nih.gov/pubmedhealth/.)

hyperthyroidism, acromegaly, and Cushing syndrome.[22] Because of hypertension's asymptomatic nature, it is important that health-care professionals, including the dental hygienist, measure the patient's blood pressure at the initiation of each visit. This will assist with early detection of hypertension to minimize medical emergencies or the possibility of a serious health risk such as nonfatal or fatal cerebrovascular accident (stroke) and renal disease. The American Heart Association (AHA) defines hypertension as an elevated blood pressure of 140 mm Hg over 90 mm Hg. Healthy blood pressure levels are considered to be levels below 120 mm Hg over 80 mm Hg.

Values vary by individual, and it is important to establish a documented baseline.

Blood pressure is classified as normal, prehypertension, stage 1 hypertension, and stage 2 hypertension. Dental treatment with stage 2 hypertension should only be done after consultation with the patient's physician (Table 37-3).

Risk Factors

Risk factors for development of hypertension include genetic predisposition, family history, age, diet, weight, gender, race, stress, little or no exercise, and/or smoking. The incidence of hypertension increases with age, and hypertension has a greater prevalence in African Americans than Caucasians, in less educated populations of both races, and in women who have reached menopause.[27]

Treatment of Hypertension

Treatment of hypertension includes regular medical visits, use of prescription medications to maintain a systolic blood pressure below 120 mm Hg (Table 37-4), and lifestyle modifications. Educating the patient on the importance of reducing sodium intake, consuming a diet that is rich in fresh fruits and vegetables, and initiating lifestyle changes that include regular aerobic exercise, smoking cessation, moderation in alcohol consumption, and stress reduction is essential. Equally important is educating the patient on the adverse reactions that can affect oral and gingival health, and providing individualized oral health-care instructions to ensure optimal oral health.

Dental Hygiene Considerations

Dental hygiene treatment modifications include the following:

- Measure blood pressure (BP) at the initiation of treatment. If BP is within normal limits, the dental hygienist

Table 37-3. Classification of Blood Pressure

Blood Pressure Classification	Systolic Blood Pressure (mm Hg)	Diastolic Blood Pressure (mm Hg)
Normal	<120	<80
Prehypertension	120–139	80–89
Stage 1 hypertension	140–159	90–99
Stage 2 hypertension	≥160	≥100

(From National Heart, Lung, and Blood Institute. *The Seventh Report of the Joint National Committee on Prevention, Detection, Evaluation, and Treatment of High Blood Pressure. National High Blood Pressure Education Program.* Bethesda, MD: National Heart, Lung, and Blood Institute; 2004.)

Table 37-4. Antihypertensive Medications

Medication	Indications	Oral Side Effects
Diuretics		
hydrochlorothiazide (Esidrix, Microzide) furosemide (Lasix)	Hypertension, HF Hypertension, HF, pulmonary edema	None
Renin-Angiotensin-Aldosterone System		
captopril (Capoten) enalapril (Vasotec) fosinopril (Monopril) losartan (Cozaar)	Hypertension, HF, agents used after an MI, and as a vasodilator Hypertension	Loss of diminished perception of taste Abnormal taste
Sympatholytics		
metoprolol (Lopressor) atenolol (Tenormin) acebutolol (Sectral) esmolol (Brevibloc) propranolol (Inderal) carvedilol (Coreg) timolol (Cronovera, Dilacoran) prazosin (Minipress) clonidine (Catapres, Duraclon, Kapvay) methyldopa (Aldomet)	Hypertension, angina, MI, antiarrhythmic Hypertension, angina, MI, antiarrhythmic Pheochromocytoma, hypertension Hypertension, smoking, heroin, and cocaine withdrawal Hypertension	Xerostomia Xerostomia Xerostomia Xerostomia

(From Mehta S, Mehta S, Meta S, Milder EA, Mirarchi AJ. *Step-up to USML, step 1.* 4th ed. Philadelphia, PA: Lippincott Williams and Wilkins; 2010; American Dental Association. How medications can affect your oral health. *JADA.* 2005;136. Available from http://www.ada.org/~/media/ADA/Publications/Files/patient_51.ashx; and PubMed Health, U.S. National Library of Medicine. Available from http://www.ncbi.nlm.nih.gov/pubmedhealth/.)

can proceed with treatment. Careful attention should be directed toward minimizing stress and anxiety. In addition, there should be careful consideration of the use of local anesthesia.

- If the patient presents with severe stage 2 hypertension (BP greater than 180/110), do not initiate treatment; refer the patient directly to the physician/emergency room.
- Local anesthesia considerations include evaluating the risks and benefits of using vasoconstrictors, modifying treatment, and assessing the use of low concentrations of epinephrine.
- BP measurement varies throughout a 24-hour period. When measuring blood pressure, the dental hygienist needs to assure that the blood pressure is measured at least twice. The patient should be seated in an upright position, and the top of the blood pressure cuff is positioned at heart level.
- The use of antihypertensive drugs may cause orthostatic hypotension; therefore the dental hygienist should raise the chair slowly and allow the patient to wait a few minutes before rising from the chair.
- Xerostomia and gingival enlargement are associated with some antihypertensive drugs. The dental hygienist should be knowledgeable of the adverse reactions for each drug (see Table 37-4) and explain to the patient strategies to minimize the side effects. For xerostomia, instruct the patient to reduce the intake of caffeinated beverages, drink plenty of water, and suck on sugarless candy or gum. Instructions for gingival enlargement (associated with some of the calcium channel blockers) include decreasing the bacterial load, maintaining optimal oral hygiene, and scheduling regular maintenance appointments. See Application to Clinical Practice 37-1.

INFECTIVE ENDOCARDITIS

Infective endocarditis (IE) is a microbial infection, usually caused by gram-positive cocci, or fungi (*Aspergillus* and *Candida*), of the endocardial surface of the heart that typically affects one or more heart valves. The mitral and aortic valves are the valves that are frequently involved.[22]

Application to Clinical Practice 37-1

A 45-year-old African American male presents for his 6-month maintenance appointment. Review of his medical history reveals a history of hypertension, and the patient is taking the following medications: enalapril—10 mg/day, simvastatin—10 mg/day, low-dose aspirin—81 mg/day. What are the dental hygiene treatment considerations before the initiation of patient care? ■

Types of Endocarditis

Due to the serious nature of infective endocarditis, it is associated with significant morbidity and mortality. There are five types of endocarditis: acute, subacute, nonbacterial, Libman-Sacks, and carcinoid syndrome. The two that are of concern for the dental professional are acute and subacute endocarditis.

- Acute infective endocarditis
  - Caused most often by *S. aureus* and manifests a rapid onset, with clinical features such as fever, anemia, embolic events, and heart murmur.
  - Treatment for acute endocarditis is with IV antibiotics.
- Subacute infective endocarditis
  - Caused most often by *Viridians streptococci* and is the result of poor oral health or oral surgery in patients with preexisting heart disease or damage to the heart valves. The onset occurs over a period of 6 months.
  - Treatment for subacute endocarditis is with IV antibiotics.[22]

Dental Hygiene Considerations

Patients with inflammation of the periodontium are at risk for bacteremia, whether the dental hygienist or the patient performs procedures resulting in bleeding. Thus, premedication before dental treatment is a serious consideration for individuals who present with certain cardiac conditions (Table 37-5). Treatment considerations include taking a thorough medical history, consulting the physician/cardiologist before initiating treatment to determine whether any alterations to treatment are indicated, and having thorough knowledge of the cardiac conditions that require antibiotic prophylaxis for oral procedures. The dental hygienist must provide individualized oral hygiene instructions, and stress the importance of meticulous oral hygiene and the need for frequent recall appointments.

RHEUMATIC HEART DISEASE

Rheumatic heart disease (RHD) is a systemic inflammatory condition that demonstrates cardiac manifestations, and is caused by group A β-hemolytic streptococci. Rheumatic fever may, if left untreated, cause permanent damage to heart valves. RHD usually occurs after a streptococcal pharyngitis infection (strep throat) or scarlet fever. Rheumatic fever typically develops 2 to 3 weeks after the streptococcal infection, and often results in valvular damage, which can interfere with blood flow through the heart valves. The valvular damage may lead to the development of a heart murmur.

Dental Hygiene Considerations

The AHA no longer recommends routine antibiotic prophylaxis for patients with RHD.[28] Treatment considerations include taking a thorough medical history,

Table 37-5. *Premedication for Prevention of Infective Endocarditis Before Dental Treatment*

Situation Oral	Agent Amoxicillin	Adults 2 g	Children 50 mg/kg
Unable to take oral medication	Ampicillin	2 g IM or IV	50 mg/kg IM or IV
	or	1 g IM or IV	50 mg/kg IM or IV
	Cefazolin or ceftriaxone		
Allergic to penicillins or ampicillin-oral	Cephalexin	2 g	50 mg/kg IM or IV
	or	600 mg	20 mg/kg
	Clindamycin	500 mg	15 mg/kg
	or		
	Azithromycin or clarithromycin		
Allergic to penicillins or ampicillin and unable to take oral medication	Cefazolin or ceftriaxone	1 g IM or IV	50 mg/kg IM or IV
	clindamycin	600 mg IM or IV	20 mg/kg IM or IV

Regimen: Single dose 30 to 60 minutes before procedure.

(From American Heart Association, Inc. http://circ.ahajournals.org/content/116/15/1736.full.pdf.)

consulting the physician/cardiologist before initiating treatment to determine whether any alterations to treatment are indicated, and having thorough knowledge of the cardiac conditions that require antibiotic prophylaxis for oral procedures. The dental hygienist must provide individualized oral hygiene instructions, and stress the importance of meticulous oral hygiene and the need for frequent recall appointments.

ISCHEMIC HEART DISEASE

Ischemic heart disease (IHD) can be described as insufficient blood flow to the heart. The major cause of IHD is atherosclerosis. Ischemic heart disease can be categorized as angina pectoris, myocardial infarction, chronic ischemic heart disease (CIHD), and sudden cardiac death.[22]

Angina Pectoris

Angina pectoris is caused by a lack of oxygen supply to the myocardium, generally due to constriction of the coronary arteries as a result of coronary artery disease (CAD), specifically atherosclerosis. In males, it is typically characterized by severe chest pain. Symptoms vary in females.

Angina may be classified as either stable or unstable. Stable angina is precipitated by some physical activity, and symptoms typically lessen when the activity is discontinued. The anginal pain can be alleviated within 2 minutes with a use of a vasodilator such as nitroglycerin and does not return. Dental treatment can resume after determining the cause of the acute episode. If the patient reports that there is no change from previous episodes, the dental hygienist and dentist need to determine whether the incident was due to inadequate pain control or severe anxiety to ascertain if modification of

future treatment is warranted.[22] Unstable angina can exhibit any of the following three features:

- Can occur unpredictably at rest with minimal exertion and lasts longer than 10 minutes
- Is of new onset, and no prior history of chest pain
- Occurs with a crescendo pattern and can culminate in myocardial infarction

If the patient reports no prior history of chest pain and this is *new-onset* pain, the dental hygienist should terminate treatment and summon EMS, and an aspirin should be given to the patient. If the patient routinely experiences pain, the pain is alleviated within 2 minutes with use of a vasodilator, and the patient feels comfortable and consents to treatment, treatment can continue. Nitrates, nitrites, beta blockers, and calcium channel blockers are used in the treatment of angina (Table 37-6).

Dental Hygiene Considerations

Treatment considerations need to include a telephone call to the angina patient a day before treatment requesting the patient to bring his or her nitroglycerin and to check the medication expiration date because nitroglycerin loses its potency after it expires. In addition, provide a stress-free environment, schedule morning appointments, and have the patient's nitroglycerin readily available. Patients who are taking beta blockers or calcium channel blockers must be informed of the drug's oral adverse reactions, the importance of meticulous oral hygiene, and the need for frequent recall appointments. If chest pain occurs and is not alleviated by administration of sublingual nitroglycerin, and the pain continues, assume that the patient is experiencing a myocardial infarction and activate EMS immediately. The patient should be placed in a supine position if the blood pressure decreases or consciousness is lost.

Table 37-6. Medications Used to Treat Angina

Drug	Dose Form	Oral Side Effects
Nitrates		
Amyl nitrate	Ampule for inhalation	None
Short-Acting Nitrates		
nitroglycerin (NTC, Nitrostat) isosorbide dinitrate (Isordil)	Sublingual Sublingual	None
Long-Acting Nitrates		
isosorbide dinitrate (Isordil) isosorbide mononitrate (Ismo) nitroglycerin (Nitro-Bid) nitroglycerin (Nitro-Bid, Nitrol) nitroglycerin (Nitro-Dur, Transderm) pentaerythritol (Peritrate)	Oral Oral Sustained release, oral tablets Ointment Transdermal patches Oral	None

(From Haveles EB. *Pharmacology for dental hygiene practice.* Albany, NY: Delmar Cengage Learning; 1996; Nitrates. Available from: http://www.medicinenet.com/nitrates-oral/article.htm; and Mayo Foundation for Medical Education and Research. Available from: www.mayoclinic.org.)

Continuously monitor the patient's blood pressure and pulse. Oxygen and an AED should be administered if needed, and wait for EMS to arrive.

Myocardial Infarction or Acute Myocardial Infarction

Myocardial infarction (MI) is caused by lack of adequate blood flow to the cardiac tissue, leading to cell and tissue death of the affected areas of the heart muscle. MI is commonly referred to as a heart attack, and the symptoms include sudden severe to intolerable chest pain that typically radiates to the left side of the neck or left arm, shortness of breath, nausea and vomiting, palpitations, cold perspiration, dizziness, and sense of impending doom. In addition to the typical symptoms, women may present with atypical symptoms such as abdominal, back, arm, and shoulder pain.

A myocardial infarction is most often caused by atherosclerosis. An MI occurs when a vulnerable atherosclerotic plaque breaks off, causing the restriction of blood supply and oxygen shortage to the heart muscle

tissue. The patient may exhibit restlessness and acute distress, and the skin may appear cool, pale, and moist. The patient may exhibit bradycardia to tachycardia.[22]

Dental Hygiene Considerations

Should any of these symptoms occur, terminate treatment and monitor the patient's blood pressure and pulse. Reassure the patient, seat the patient in a comfortable upright position, and have the patient chew an aspirin. Oxygen and an AED should be made available and administered if needed, and EMS should be activated. See Application to Clinical Practice 37-2.

Cardiopulmonary resuscitation (CPR) should be initiated if the patient has no pulse or respiration; otherwise, rescue breathing should be initiated if the patient ceases breathing. Patients who have experienced an MI should not receive elective dental treatment for 6 months.

Chronic Ischemic Heart Disease

Chronic ischemic heart disease (CIHD) occurs commonly in the elderly as a result of atherosclerosis. As a consequence of atherosclerosis, the lumen of blood vessels narrows (see Fig. 37-6); thus the heart has to pump harder to move the same volume of blood as it did when the heart was healthy. Over time, this additional exertion causes the heart muscle to become ischemic. The risk of chronic ischemic heart disease increases not only with age, but also smoking, hypercholesterolaemia (high cholesterol levels), diabetes, and hypertension. This condition is more common in men and those with a history of heart disease.[22]

Dental Hygiene Considerations

The dental hygienist should take a thorough medical history and consult the physician/cardiologist before initiating treatment to determine whether any alterations to treatment are indicated. Provide as much of a stress-free environment as possible, reduce the amount of vasoconstrictors used, schedule short appointments, and monitor the patient's pulse rate.

Sudden Cardiac Death

Individuals who have CVA are at higher risk for sudden cardiac death (both in the diagnosed and nondiagnosed population). Sudden cardiac death can occur during or 2 hours post-MI. In addition atherosclerosis is usually present, and death is almost always caused by arrhythmia.[23]

Application to Clinical Practice 37-2

During treatment, the patient described in Application to Clinical Practice 37-1 reports that he is experiencing chest pain. List sequentially the procedures you should perform. ■

HEART FAILURE

Heart failure (HF), known previously as congestive heart failure (CHF), is a condition where the heart cannot pump enough blood to meet the body's needs under normal physiological conditions. Heart failure can be caused by lifestyle behaviors and/or genetics. The former includes things such as diet, activity level, smoking, and high levels of alcohol consumption.

Conditions such as narrowed arteries in the heart (CAD) or high hypertension gradually leave the heart too weak for the heart to fill and pump efficiently. HF can be categorized as left-sided or right-sided HF:

- *Left-sided HF:* Patients have difficulty receiving oxygenated blood from the lungs, resulting in dyspnea or orthopnea.
- *Right-sided HF:* Patients present with peripheral edema (foot and ankle swelling). For these patients, positioning is not critical.

The heart is a closed system, and thus both the left and right side need to function as a unit; otherwise, the efficiency of the heart's actions is diminished.[22]

Dental Hygiene Considerations

Patients who are monitored closely by a physician do not require any treatment modifications. Patients with left-sided HF should be placed in a reclined position rather than in a supine position to avoid fluid pooling in the lungs and breathing difficulties. Therapeutic agents in HF treatment include angiotensin-converting enzyme (ACE) inhibitors, angiotensin II receptor blockers, digitalis, diuretics, and dobutamine (Table 37-7).[22]

CONGENITAL HEART DISEASE

Congenital heart disease (CHD) is an abnormality of the heart structure and/or function caused by abnormal heart development before birth.

Congenital cardiac abnormalities occur in 0.8% of all live births and are a predominant cause of infant morbidity and mortality.[29] As a result of advances in pediatric cardiology and cardiothoracic surgery, a greater number of infants (85%) born with congenital heart disease can expect to survive into adulthood.[29] Therefore more adults with congenital heart disease present for dental treatment, and the dental hygienist must be knowledgeable in identifying procedures that may precipitate bacteremia and require antibiotic prophylaxis in these patients.

Common Forms of Congenital Heart Disease

Congenital heart disease may present in many forms. The forms observed most commonly include ventricular septal defect, atrial septal defect, and patent ductus arteriosus.

Table 37-7. Medications Used to Treat Heart Failure

Medication	Function	Oral Side Effects
Cardiac Glycosides		
digoxin (Lanoxin)	Increases the heart's contractibility	Sensitive gag reflex
Diuretics	Lower BP by eliminating excess sodium	Dry mouth
Beta Blockers propranolol (Inderal) atenolol (Tenormin) metoprolol (Lopressor) carvedilol (Coreg)	Lower BP by reducing heart rate	Dry mouth
ACE Inhibitors/ Angiotensin Receptor Blockers enalapril (Vasotec) fosinopril (Monopril) losartan (Cozaar)	Inhibit angiotensin converting enzyme Relax blood vessels	

(From American Heart Association, New York Heart Association.)

Ventricular septal defect presents as an opening in the septum between the ventricles, which allows oxygenated blood to flow from the left ventricle into the right ventricle (Fig. 37-7). The defect may be of varying size, with large ventricular septal defects causing hypertrophy of the ventricles, resulting in HF.[29]

Atrial septal defect presents as an opening between the left and right atria (Fig. 37-8). Blood volume overload eventually causes the right atrium to enlarge and the right ventricle to dilate. The patient is usually symptomatic. In adults, the patient experiences fatigue and shortness of breath after mild exertion.[29]

Patent ductus arteriosus is the most common congenital heart defect found in adults and is caused by the ductus arteriosus blood vessel, which connects the pulmonary artery to the descending aorta, not closing after birth (Fig. 37-9). This results in the recirculation of oxygenated blood through the lungs. Consequently, the left atrium and ventricle have increased workload from the increased pulmonary blood return, which can result in HF. The clinical manifestations include respiratory distress and susceptibility to respiratory tract infections.[29]

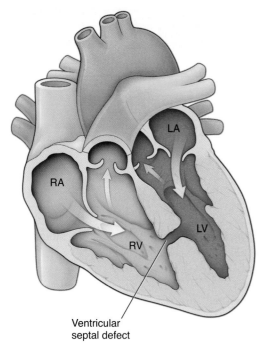

Figure 37-7. Ventricular septal defect.

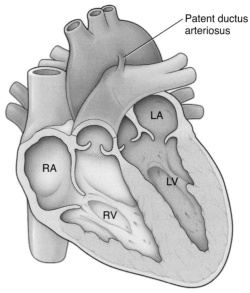

Figure 37-9. Patent ductus arteriosus.

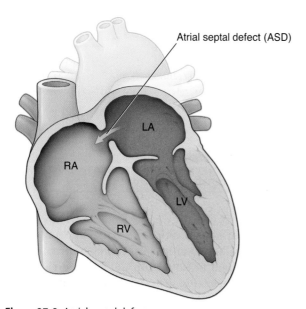

Figure 37-8. Atrial septal defect.

Dental Hygiene Considerations

Dental hygiene treatment modifications include the need for a thorough medical history, a physician consultation to confirm medical status, prophylactic antibiotic premedication to prevent infective endocarditis, and an assessment of any symptoms that are secondary to the disease, such as hypertension, heart failure, and arrhythmias, that may necessitate dental hygiene treatment modifications. When taking the patient's medical history, it is important to ask the patient the following questions: (1) type of repair, (2) timing of the repair, and (3) whether there are any residual effects of the congenital anomaly. The dental hygienist must provide individualized oral hygiene instructions, and stress the

importance of meticulous oral hygiene and the need for frequent recall appointments.

VALVULAR HEART DISEASE

Valvular heart disease includes aortic stenosis, aortic regurgitation, mitral stenosis, mitral regurgitation, and mitral prolapse. **Stenosis** is the incomplete opening of the valve, and **regurgitation** is the incomplete closure of the valve, leading to backflow of blood through the valve. Mitral valve prolapse occurs when the left ventricle pumps blood to the aorta and the mitral valve falls backward into the left atrium. Medical treatment for valvular defects consists of repair or replacement of the damaged valve(s). Over 4 million people worldwide have received prosthetic heart valves, and approximately 300,000 valves are implanted yearly worldwide for patients with severe valvular heart disease.[30] There are two major types of prosthetic heart valves: mechanical and bioprosthetic. The advantages and disadvantages of each are as follows:[29]

- Mechanical—Are more durable, but are more **thrombogenic** (causing or resulting in coagulation of the blood), and the patient may need long-term **anticoagulation therapy**.
- Bioprosthetic—Do not require long-term anticoagulation, are less thrombogenic, but are not as durable as the mechanical heart valves.[30]

Dental Hygiene Considerations

Dental hygiene treatment modifications include obtaining a thorough medical history and consulting with the patient's physician to confirm medical status and the need for premedication. If the patient is on anticoagulant therapy, it is important to know the patient's International Normalized Ratio (INR) value and prothrombin time (PT). PT is a blood test that measures how long it takes blood to clot, and may be used to monitor patients with prosthetic heart valves or who are prone to clotting. INR is the ratio between coagulation time of a sample of blood and the normal coagulation time. INR is a way of standardizing the results of prothrombin time tests, no matter the testing method. PT and INR measure the extrinsic and common pathways of coagulation. They are used to determine and/or monitor the clotting tendency of blood, liver function, and vitamin K status, and to monitor patients on anticoagulant therapy.

Normal INR values range from 1 to 2; normal PT values range from 10 to 12 seconds, and can vary from laboratory to laboratory. When a person is taking an anticoagulant, the physician will order periodic PT/INR testing to ensure the patient is being properly managed. Frequency of testing is determined by the patient's physician, with the goal of achieving an INR of 2.0 to 3.0 for basic "blood-thinning" needs (Box 37-1). Those patients with a higher risk of clotting will need to be maintained at an INR of 2.5 to 3.5 or higher.[31] To assure accuracy in data reporting, the hygienist needs to rely on information from the patient's physician, rather than self-reported INR values. Test results can be influenced by the consumption certain foods, such as beef and pork; the consumption of alcohol; some antibiotics and medications, such as barbiturates; hormone replacement therapies; and oral contraceptives. Due to changes in natural body functions during the day, laboratory tests may need to be performed at a certain time of the day.[31]

In addition, there should be an emphasis on the importance of excellent preventive care to reduce oral biofilms and the potential for bacteremia. Therefore, the dental hygienist must educate the patient about oral biofilms and the possible relationship between oral biofilms and infectious endocarditis. Proper brushing, flossing, and use of other oral physiotherapy aids is crucial. The dental hygienist's primary role of prevention specialist can influence the patient's health. Patients presenting with prosthetic valve replacement need to be premedicated according to the AHA's recommendations (Box 37-2).

ANTICOAGULANT THERAPY

Patients who are taking anticoagulants beyond aspirin may require physician consultation before the initiation

Box 37-1. *Therapeutic Range INR Testing*[31]

- Prevention of venous thromboembolism (VTE): 2–3
- Treatment of VTE, valvular heart disease: 2–3
- Treatment of mechanical heart valves, recurrent systemic embolism: 3–4.5

Box 37-2. *Cardiac Conditions Requiring Antibiotic Prophylaxis for Dental Treatment*

- Prosthetic cardiac valve
- History of infective endocarditis
- Cardiac transplantation
- Cardiac valvulopathy
- Congenital heart disease (CHD)
  - Unrepaired cyanotic CHD
  - Repaired CHD with prosthetic material (within 6 months of procedure)
  - Repaired CHD with residual defects at the site or adjacent to the site of prosthetic patch/device

(From Nishimura RA, Carabello BA, Faxon DP, et al. ACC/AHA 2008 guideline update on valvular heart disease: focused update on infective endocarditis. *Circulation.* 2008;118: 887-896. Available from: circ. ahajournals.org/content/118/8/887.)

of dental treatment. The two most commonly used anticoagulant drugs are heparin and warfarin. Heparin must be administered by injection and is used in hospitals and skilled-care facilities. Warfarin (Coumadin®) is administered orally. Because warfarin interferes with a number of clotting factors, with hemorrhage being the most common adverse reaction, dental professionals initiating deep scaling procedures need to be aware of the patient's INR.[30,32]

Dental Hygiene Considerations

Treatment considerations need to include a telephone call to the patient taking warfarin the day before treatment requesting the patient to bring his or her latest partial thromboplastin time (PT), a blood test that determines how long it takes for blood to clot. No reduction or dose changes in warfarin should be suggested without consultation with the patient's physician. Aspirin and NSAIDs are contraindicated for patients on anticoagulant therapy because of risk of increased bleeding.

POST–CARDIOVASCULAR SURGERY

Patients are **post–cardiovascular surgery**, such as patients who have had angioplasty, stent placement, or coronary bypass surgery, have no contraindications to dental hygiene therapy. Patients who have had valvular defects repaired must be premedicated, as must patients who have had heart transplantation. The American Dental Association (ADA) recommends premedication for patients with the following conditions:

- Artificial heart valves
- A history of an infection of the lining of the heart or heart valves, known as infective endocarditis
- A heart transplant in which a problem develops with one of the valves inside the heart

- Heart conditions that are present from birth, such as:
  - Unrepaired cyanotic congenital heart disease, including people with palliative shunts and conduit
  - Defects repaired with a prosthetic material or device—whether placed by surgery or catheter intervention—during the first 6 months after repair
  - Cases in which a heart defect has been repaired, but a residual defect remains at the site or adjunct to the site of the prosthetic path or prosthetic device used for the repair.

In regard to heart transplant patients, the major concern is infection as a consequence of the patient being placed on immunosuppressant medications. As in all dental hygiene treatment situations, adherence to infection control guidelines by the dental hygienist is paramount. The patient must be instructed on the importance of and necessity for meticulous oral hygiene to prevent bacteremia from oral pathogens and to prevent periodontal disease.

Dental Hygiene Considerations

There is a need for a thorough medical history, strict adherence to universal precautions, consultation with the physician, and emphasis on the importance of excellent preventive care to prevent periodontal disease. Therefore, the dental hygienist must provide individualized instructions on brushing, flossing, and use of any other oral physiotherapy aids that are needed.

SUMMARY

More medically compromised patients, particularly patients with cardiovascular disease, are presenting for dental treatment. Optimal oral care via individualized dental hygiene instructions is the goal for each patient, especially those with cardiovascular disease. Dental hygienists must possess knowledge of the disease processes and the indicated medications to provide optimal dental hygiene care. Dental hygienists must educate patients on the potential adverse effects of medications, including the oral effects that negatively affect oral health and how the patient can avoid or minimize these effects.

Case Study

A 60-year-old male presents for a dental hygiene appointment. A review of the medical history reveals that although the patient has a physician of record, it has been 3 years since his last visit. Upon questioning, the patient relates that he experiences shortness of breath while climbing stairs and performing other minor physical activities.

Case Study Exercises

1. What disease states could the patient be experiencing?
   1. Hypotension
   2. Atrial septal defect
   3. Heart failure
   4. Infective endocarditis
   5. Tachycardia
      a. 1, 2, 3
      b. 2, 4, 5
      c. 1, 4, 5
      d. 2, 3, 4
2. What dental hygiene treatment modifications are indicated?
   1. Consult physician before treatment
   2. Eliminate the use of ultrasonic instrument
   3. Place the patient in a supine position for treatment
   4. Verify that patient has taken his medication
   5. Limit treatment time
      a. 1, 2, 3
      b. 2, 4, 5
      c. 1, 4, 5
      d. 2, 3, 4

Review Questions

1. How many people in the United States are affected by hypertension?
   A. 20 million
   B. 55 million
   C. 67 million
   D. 79 million

2. Tachycardia is a condition where the heart rate is high; the rate is between _____bpm.
   A. 75 and 99
   B. 100 and 400
   C. 400 and 425
   D. 400 and 450

3. When treating patients who have an implanted pacemaker, dental hygienists need to be aware of the type of ultrasonic instrument they are using and should avoid use of a(n) _____ instrument.
   A. piezoelectric
   B. aluminamagnetic
   C. ferromagnetic in
   D. diazoelectric

4. Angina pectoris is caused by lack of oxygen supply to the
   A. myocardium.
   B. pericardium.
   C. endocardium.
   D. ventricular septum.

5. A ventricular septum defect permits blood to flow from the
   A. left ventricle to the right ventricle.
   B. right ventricle to the left ventricle.
   C. right atrium to the left atrium.
   D. left atrium to the right atrium.

Active Learning

1. Working with a partner, role-play the following scenario: A 20-year-old female patient presents for her initial dental hygiene visit. She reports a history of a corrected septal defect. What follow-up questions should be asked of the patient, and what precautions, if any, should be taken before initiating treatment?

2. Prepare a brief presentation explaining hypertension, medical treatments for the condition, and how dental hygiene treatment is modified for patients with the condition.

3. Taking turns with classmates, measure each other's blood pressure. Classify the readings as detailed in Table 37-3. ■

REFERENCES

1. Murphy SL, Xu J, Kochanek, KD, Centers for Disease Control and Prevention. Deaths: preliminary data for 2010. *National Vital Statistics Reports.* 2010;60(4):1-69.
2. World Health Organization. Cardiovascular diseases. 2012. Available from: http://www.who.int/cardiovascular_diseases/en/.
3. World Health Organization. Cardiovascular diseases: priorities. 2010. Available from: http://www.who.int/cardiovascular_diseases/priortities/en/.
4. Dietrich T, Jimenez M, Kaye E, Vokonas P, Garcia R. Age-dependent associations between chronic periodontitis/edentulism and risk of coronary heart disease. *Circulation.* 2008;117:1668-1674.
5. Vaishnava P, Narayan R, Fuster V. Understanding systemic inflammation, oral hygiene, and cardiovascular disease. *Am J Med.* 2011;124:997-999.
6. Beck J, Eke P, Heiss G. Periodontal disease and coronary heart disease: A reappraisal of the exposure. *Circulation.* 2005;112:19-24.
7. Libby P, Ridker P, Maseri A. Inflammation and atherosclerosis. *Circulation.* 2002;105:1153-1143.
8. Humphrey L, Fu R, Buckley D, Freeman M, Helfand M. Periodontal disease and coronary heart disease incidence: A systematic review and meta-analysis. *J Gen Int Med.* 2008;23(12):2079-2086.
9. Friedeweld V, Kornman K, Beck J, American Journal of Cardiology, Journal of Periodontology. The American Journal of Cardiology and Journal of Periodontology editors' consensus: periodontitis and atherosclerotic cardiovascular disease. *J Peridont.* 2009;80(7):1021-1032.
10. Genco RJ, Glurich V, Haraszthy JZ, DeNardin E. Overview of risk factors for periodontal disease and implications for diabetes and cardiovascular disease. *Compendium.* 1998;19:40-45.
11. Genco R, Van Dyke T. Prevention: Reducing the risk of CVD in patients with periodontitis. *Natl Rev Cardiol.* 2010;7(9):479-480.
12. Fong IW. Infections and their role in atherosclerotic vascular disease. *J Am Dent Assoc.* 2002;(suppl):13S.
13. Arbes SJ, Slade GD, Beck JD. Association between extent of periodontal attachment loss and self-reported history of heart attack: an analysis of NHANES III date. *J Dent Res.* 1999;78(12):1777-1782.
14. Genco RJ, Wu TJ, Grossi S, et al. Periodontal microflora related to the risk for myocardial infarction: a case control study. *J Dent Res.* 1999;78:457.
15. Weitz H. Invasive dental treatment and risk for vascular events: Have we bitten off more than we can chew? *Ann Int Med.* 2010;153:542-543.
16. Minassaian CDF, Hingoraani A, Smeeth L. Invasive dental treatment and risk for vascular events: A self-controlled case series. *Ann Int Med.* 2010;153:499-506.
17. Page, RC. The pathobiology of periodontal diseases may affect systemic diseases; inversion of paradigm. *Ann Periodontol.* 1998;3:108-120.
18. Chung, HJ, Champagne, CME, Southerland, JH, et al. Effects of *P. gingivalis* infection on atheroma formation in ApoE(+/-) mice [abstract]. *J Dent Res.* 2000;7:313.
19. Tonetti M, D'Aiuto F, Nibali L., et al. Treatment of periodontitis and endothelial function. *New Engl J Med.* 2007;356:911-920, 1668-1674.
20. Slade G, Ghezzi E, Heiss G, Beck J, Riche E, Offenbacher S. Relationship between periodontal disease and C-reactive protein among adults in the atherosclerosis risk in communities study. *Arch Int Med.* 2003;163:1172-1179.
21. Dorn BR, Dunn WA, Progulske-Fox A. Invasion of human coronary artery cells by periodontal pathogens. *Infect Immun.* 1999;67(11):5792-5798.
22. Mehta S, Mehta S, Meta S, Milder EA, Mirarchi AJ. *Step-up to USML, step 1.* 4th ed. Philadelphia, PA: Lippincott Williams and Wilkins; 2010. p. 87-91.
23. Neumar RW, Otto CW, Link MS, et al. Part 8: Adult advanced cardiovascular life support: 2010 American Heart Association guidelines for cardiopulmonary resuscitation and emergency cardiovascular care. *Circulation.* 2010;122(suppl 3):S729-S767.
24. Boston Scientific. ACL dental equipment. 2009. Available from: http://www.bostonscientific.com/templatedata/imports/HTML/CRM/A_Closer_Look/pdfs/ACL_Dental_Equipment_020209.pdf .
25. Boston Scientific. FAQ: living with a device. 2012. Available from: https://docs.google.com/viewer?a=v&q=cache:y7KzC6rU8BAJ:www.bostonscientific.

com/templatedata/imports/HTML/CRM/sgr/down-loads/FAQ-Living_with_a_device-C9-1091108.ppt+boston+scientific+pacemakers+and+electric+tooth brushes&hl=en&gl=us&pid=bl&srcid=ADGEESht sHGFSy0wXE7JmIv6f52UGXxTPoDsAJTJvdZc6k1OX7 3EEUWQuJ6YgjQmXUND2rXb_cxPEdy_b1fTpKcB8hMf-EA9f5vAoTNrqr2ikjDWJZhTw3v9kNhYdME5tq4ObFn 8hFjK&sig=AHIEtbQpuFjKjak7DwtfIce4Ys2GNkBxdg.

26. Vongpatanasin W, Victor RG. Vascular diseases and hypertension. In *Goldman's Cecil essentials of medicine.* 7th ed. Carpenter CJ, Griggs RC, Benjamin II, editors. Philadelphia, PA: Saunders Elsevier; 2007. p. 176

27. Haveles EB. *Pharmacology for dental hygiene practice.* Cincinnati, OH: Delmar; 1996. p. 189.

28. American Heart Association. Prevention of infective endocarditis. *J American Heart Association.* University of Pittsburgh—HSLS, August 31, 2011. http://circ.ahajournals.org/content/116/15/1736.full.pdf.

29. Whitehead KJ, Li DY. Congenital heart disease. In *Goldman's Cecil essentials of medicine.* 7th ed. Carpenter CJ, Griggs RC, Benjamin II, editors. Philadelphia, PA: Saunders Elsevier; 2007. p. 77-81.

30. Sun JC, Davidson MJ, Lamy A, Eikelboom JW. Antithrombotic management of patients with prosthetic heart valves: current evidence and future trends. *Lancet.* 2009;347(9689):565-576.

31. Giglia TM, Massicotte MP, Tweddell JS, et al. Prevention and treatment of thrombosis in pediatric and congenital heart disease: as scientific statement from the American Heart Association. *Circulation.* 2013; 128(24):2622-2703.

32. Torres R, Rinder HM. Disorders of hemostasis: thrombosis. In *Goldman's Cecil essentials of medicine.* 7th ed. Carpenter CJ, Griggs RC, Benjamin II, editors. Philadelphia, PA: Saunders Elsevier; 2007. p. 550-563.

Chapter 38 | Respiratory

Brooke Agado, RDH, BS

KEY TERMS

acute respiratory infection

asthma

chronic obstructive pulmonary disease

cystic fibrosis

tuberculosis

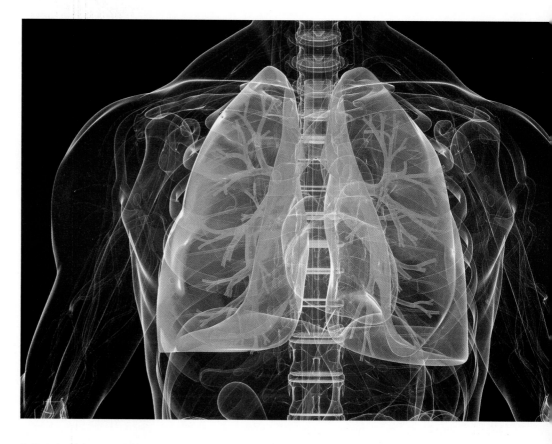

LEARNING OBJECTIVES

After reading this chapter, the student should be able to:

38.1 Describe the various respiratory diseases and conditions.

38.2 List signs and symptoms of respiratory complications of the various conditions.

38.3 Discuss proper stress reduction protocol measures for the respiratory patient.

38.4 Discuss proper management during a respiratory medical emergency.

38.5 Explain respiratory medications' mechanisms of action, potential side effects, and drug interactions.

38.6 Identify what patient interview questions regarding respiratory conditions are important for education, referral, and/or treatment alterations.

KEY CONCEPTS

• Respiratory pathogens responsible for acute respiratory infection reside in the oral cavity.

• Evaluation of health history, respiratory disease status, and medication usage, along with monitoring of vitals, are part of overall risk assessment for dental hygiene care.

- Precautions and treatment alterations for patients with respiratory disease need thorough consideration for prevention of respiratory complications and/or medical emergencies.

RELEVANCE TO CLINICAL PRACTICE

Respiratory diseases range from acute respiratory infections such as a cold, flu, or pneumonia to conditions such as asthma and cystic fibrosis. Dental hygiene procedures can release oral bacteria that can be swallowed or inhaled and cause infection. They can also be stressful, which can exacerbate respiratory problems. To prevent respiratory complications and manage care appropriately, the dental hygienist should be able to: (1) recognize the signs and symptoms of the various respiratory diseases and conditions; (2) understand the actions, side effects, and drug interactions of respiratory medications; and (3) implement stress reduction protocol measures.

OVERVIEW OF THE RESPIRATORY SYSTEM

The respiratory system consists of a series of organs that filters and prepares incoming air for gas exchange in the lungs. This system includes a complex defense mechanism that prevents harmful pathogens or particles from entering the body. It is one of the most complex organ systems in the body.[1] The respiratory system (Fig. 38-1) is divided into upper and lower tract systems. The upper system includes the oral cavity, nasal cavity, pharynx, and larynx and is primarily responsible for initial filtration of inhaled air or substances. The lower system includes the trachea, bronchial tree, and lungs.

The lungs have multiple roles, including supplying the blood with oxygen, removing toxins and waste, and defending against potential pathogens. The heart pumps blood into the lungs, where alveoli (small air sacs) exchange waste and toxins for nutrient-rich oxygen from pulmonary capillary blood (Fig. 38-2). This replenished blood with nutrient-rich oxygen is pumped from the heart back out to the body.

ORAL–RESPIRATORY DISEASE LINK

The oral cavity harbors many respiratory pathogens (e.g., *Staphylococcus aureus, Pseudomonas aeruginosa, Acinetobacter* species and enteric species) with the potential to initiate an infection.[2,3] All individuals inhale these pathogens on a regular basis during sleep and regular breathing.[2] The majority of individuals avoid respiratory infections by a combination of host defenses, including immune response and coughing. People with certain respiratory ailments or immunocompromising conditions might have a reduced ability to ward off these harmful pathogens, leading to respiratory complications.

Dental procedures such as scaling and root planing disrupt significant amounts of oral bacterial biofilm and their toxins, releasing them into the oral cavity, where they could enter the bloodstream and be swallowed or

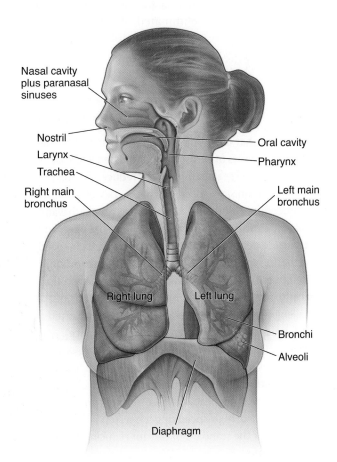

Figure 38-1. The respiratory system.

Nasal cavity plus paranasal sinuses

Nostril

Larynx

Trachea

Right main bronchus

Oral cavity

Pharynx

Left main bronchus

Right lung

Left lung

Bronchi

Alveoli

Diaphragm

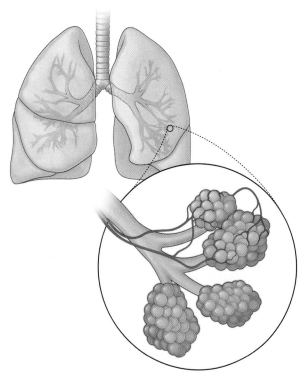

Figure 38-2. Alveoli.

inhaled. One concern is dental procedures that create *aerosols* (microscopic particles suspended in the air) contaminated with oral bacteria.[4] With proper precautions, the amount of bacteria and aerosol can be significantly reduced or eliminated during the dental appointment (see Advancing Technologies).[4]

Advancing Technologies

It is known that ultrasonic instrumentation creates significant amounts of aerosols contaminated with bacteria, and high-speed evacuation devices reduce aerosols more effectively than slow-speed evacuation devices.[4] For dental procedures producing aerosols (e.g., restorative and prosthetic procedures), a rubber dam can be used, and a chairside dental assistant often controls a high-speed evacuation tip. However, ultrasonic instrumentation is often restricted to use of a slow-speed evacuation tip, because use of a high-volume evacuation tip is too challenging for a single operator (i.e., hygienists often work independently without chairside assistance).

Hence, manufacturers have developed various adaptive devices for unassisted operators to utilize high-speed suction with ease. Although further research is needed to determine the efficacy of these devices compared with traditional high-speed tips, it is a step in the right direction for the standard of care for reducing aerosol contamination. ▪

In addition, stress can initiate or exacerbate respiratory problems, so appropriate stress reduction protocols must be considered.[5] The dental hygienist is responsible for interviewing patients about their respiratory disease, severity and control, and compliance with medications, and for consulting with the patient's physician when necessary. As with all patients, vital signs (including blood pressure, pulse, and respirations) should be assessed at baseline and routinely monitored to determine the patient's ability to tolerate the procedure(s) and/or identify an underlying issue.[5] A semisupine or upright chair position should be considered for those with difficulty breathing. Manufacturers recommend physician consultation for patients with severe respiratory disease to determine disease status before using air polishing devices.[6]

RESPIRATORY DISEASE

In individuals with respiratory disease (also called pulmonary disease or lung disease), the defense mechanism is compromised. Exchange of oxygen, removal of waste and toxins, or removal of pathogens is decreased, in turn affecting healthy functioning of the body and other organ systems. Respiratory disease can be acute (e.g., cough lasting less than 3 weeks) or chronic (e.g., cough lasting more than 3 weeks or recurrent) and has multiple etiologies and risk factors.[5]

The American Lung Association (ALA) recognizes more than 30 diseases or conditions related to the respiratory system that affect all ages.[1] When all respiratory diseases are combined in one entity, it is the third leading cause of death in the United States, following heart disease and cancer.[7] Approximately one in six people die of respiratory disease each year.[1] Common symptoms of respiratory diseases are listed in Box 38-1.

In addition to clinical signs and symptoms (e.g., cough, sputum, dyspnea), lung functioning capacity and blood gas levels are measured to determine the extent and severity of respiratory disease. Lung functioning capacity is measured by forced expiratory volume and represented by forced expiratory volume in 1 second (FEV_1). Arterial blood oxygen saturation levels are measured by

> ### Box 38-1. *Common Symptoms of Respiratory Disease*
>
> - Cough
> - Sputum (mucous production from the lungs)
> - Dyspnea (shortness of breath or difficulty breathing)
> - Wheeze (musical sounds heard on inspiration or expiration
> - Chest pain
> - Dizziness and fainting
> - Fever
> - Headache

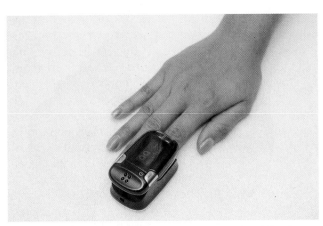

Figure 38-3. A pulse oximeter is used to measure arterial blood oxygen saturation levels.

Box 38-2. *Measurements of Lung Functioning Capacity and Blood Oxygen Levels*

- **Lung functioning capacity**
  - Forced expiratory volume in 1 second (FEV_1)
  - Disease categories:
    - Mild: greater than 80% FEV_1
    - Moderate: 60% to 80% FEV_1*
    - Severe: less than 60% FEV_1*
- **Blood oxygen level**
  - Pulse oximetry measures blood oxygen saturation level
  - Represented as partial pressure of oxygen (PO_2)
    - Greater than 95% PO_2: continue to monitor throughout appointment
    - 91–95% PO_2: requires supplemental oxygen
    - Less than 91%: PO_2 postpone treatment until better controlled

Note: Moderate and severe respiratory disease require a medical consult to assess level of control and need for dental treatment alterations.

---

pulse oximetry (Fig. 38-3) and represented as partial pressure of oxygen (PO_2). Monitoring and recording of PO_2 levels for patients with respiratory disease should accompany routine vitals.[5] Normal FEV_1 and PO_2 levels are shown in Box 38-2.

ACUTE RESPIRATORY INFECTIONS

Acute respiratory infections are communicable diseases (spread from one person to another) caused by bacteria, viruses, or fungi. Acute respiratory infections are one of the most prevalent microbial diseases in humans, leading to significant time missed from work and school.[8] Acute respiratory infections are classified as upper or lower respiratory tract infections (Box 38-3). See Spotlight on Public Health and Professionalism.

Box 38-3. *Acute Respiratory Infections*

A. Upper respiratory tract infections
  1. Influenza
  2. Common cold
  3. Strep throat
B. Lower respiratory tract infections
  1. Acute bronchitis
  2. Pneumonia

 Spotlight on Public Health

Respiratory pathogens can be found in oral bacteria; likewise, bacteria gathered and cultured from acute respiratory infections have also been found in the oral cavity.[15,16] These oral respiratory pathogens are responsible for causing nosocomial (i.e., hospital-acquired) infections leading to fatal pneumonia in high-risk individuals, such as those who are immunocompromised, hospitalized, ventilated, or residing in a nursing home or long-term care facility.[2] Interestingly, dentulous people (those with teeth) have a higher incidence of acute respiratory diseases compared with edentulous people (those without teeth). In addition, mortality from pneumonia appears to be associated with the presence of teeth and periodontal disease in the elderly.[15]

The incidence of nosocomial pneumonia can be significantly reduced with improved oral care (e.g., tooth brushing, flossing, and/or antimicrobial rinses) of these individuals.[2,17,18] Findings from recent studies and systematic reviews need to be considered when treating patients at high risk of developing pneumonia. It is crucial that dental hygienists working in public health settings collaborate with the other health providers responsible for the care of these individuals.

 Professionalism

Dental and dental hygiene students have a higher incidence of upper respiratory tract infections compared with their counterparts in medical and pharmacy schools.[8] As a health-care provider and clinician, it is crucial to *not* treat patients when you have signs and symptoms of an acute respiratory infection. Infected health-care workers should avoid (1) treating any patient while acute symptoms are present, (2) treating patients at higher risk of contracting infection, and (3) treating patients during community outbreaks of infection (e.g., respiratory viruses, influenza).[19]

ASTHMA

Asthma is a chronic lung disease characterized by inflammation and narrowing of the tracheobronchial tree (Fig. 38-4). Various stimuli, from allergens to exercise, exacerbate the inflammation, causing dyspnea (difficulty breathing). Nearly 25 million Americans, including 7 million children, have been diagnosed with asthma, making it one of the most common chronic childhood illnesses in the United States. Asthma is more prevalent in boys aged 5 to 17 and females over age 18.[9]

Etiology and Classification

Asthma is divided into five categories based on etiology: extrinsic (allergic), intrinsic, drug induced, exercise induced, and infectious.[5] *Extrinsic* (allergic) *asthma* is triggered by allergens such as seasonal pollens, pet dander, and environmental pollutants, and is the most common form of adult asthma, causing over 50% of asthma cases.[1] There is typically a family history of similar allergies and elevated serum immunoglobulin (IgE). *Intrinsic* asthma is associated with family history of allergy or other known cause. Intrinsic asthma differs from extrinsic because IgE levels are typically normal. Emotional stress, gastroesophageal acid reflux, and vagus nerve stimulation have been associated with onset of intrinsic asthma. *Drug-induced asthma* is caused by various substances. Common causes of drug-induced asthma include antibiotics, aspirin, NSAIDs, foods, and preservatives in food and drugs. *Exercise-induced asthma* occurs upon physical exertion or temperature changes. Exercise-induced asthma occurs more frequently in children and young adults.

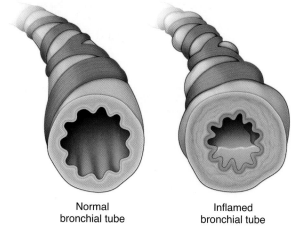

Normal bronchial tube

Inflamed bronchial tube

Figure 38-4. Asthma is characterized by inflammation and narrowing of the tracheobronchial tree.

Finally, *infectious asthma* occurs after an inflammatory response to infection caused by bacteria, viruses, or fungi.

Asthma can be further classified according to frequency and severity (i.e., mild, moderate, and severe).[5] People with *mild* asthma have wheezing less than 5 days per week, attacks occurring only a few times per month, and an FEV_1 greater than 80%. *Moderate* asthma consists of daily symptoms, attacks occurring at least once per week, some exercise intolerance, and an FEV_1 of 60% to 80%. People with *severe* asthma have frequent daily exacerbations, attacks more than four times per month, exercise intolerance, and an FEV_1 less of than 60%. Table 38-1 shows medications commonly used to treat asthma, their side effects, and their effects on dental hygiene practice.

Table 38-1. *Medications Commonly Used to Treat Asthma and Obstructive Lung Diseases*

Medication	Example Generic Drug Names	Purpose	Side effects Related to Dental Care	Drug Interactions Related to Dental Care
Bronchodilator—short acting (inhaled)	Albuterol, Bitolterol mesylate, Pirbuterol	Dilate the alveoli; prevention or quick relief of acute bronchospasm/asthma attack; daily control	Dry mouth, caries, gingivitis, headache, upper respiratory tract infection	None
Bronchodilator—long acting (inhaled)	Salmeterol, Formoterol, Theophylline	Long-term asthma control—not intended for asthma attack	Dry mouth, caries, gingivitis, anxiety, upper respiratory tract infection	Avoid macrolide antibiotics, erythromycin, and ciprofloxacin for patients taking theophylline
Corticosteroid (inhaled)	Beclomethasone dipropionate, Budesonide, Fluticasone propionate, Triamcinolone acetonide	Anti-inflammatory; daily control	Oral candidiasis, tachycardia	None

Table 38-1. Medications Commonly Used to Treat Asthma and Obstructive Lung Diseases—cont'd

Medication	Example Generic Drug Names	Purpose	Side effects Related to Dental Care	Drug Interactions Related to Dental Care
Corticosteroid (oral)	Prednisone Prednisolone Methylpred-nisolone	Anti-inflammatory; daily control	Impaired healing	Possible need for medical consult about additional corticosteroid for trauma or major invasive surgery
Antileukotriene (oral)	Zileuton Montelukast	Anti-inflammatory enzyme inhibitor; daily control	Headache, nausea	Increase in PT with warfarin Increased plasma levels of propanolol and theophylline

Signs and Symptoms

Each type of asthma is characterized by episodic obstruction of airflow caused by constriction of the airway by decreased diameter, increased resistance to airflow, and difficulty with expiration.[10] This is caused by smooth muscle spasms, inflamed mucosa, hypersecretion of mucus, and/or occlusion of the bronchi and bronchioles by thick, sticky mucus. Clinical symptoms include coughing (typically worse at night), wheezing, dyspnea, chest tightness, and flushed skin.

In addition, inhalers cause significant oral symptoms, including decreased salivary flow, decreased oral pH, increased caries, and gingival inflammation.[5] Oral candidiasis also can occur.[5] These symptoms can be reduced or eliminated by rinsing with water and/or brushing after each use of an inhaler.[5] The dental hygienist should inquire about the patient's usage of inhalers and educate the patient regarding recognition and prevention of potential oral side effects.

Dental Hygiene Considerations

Assessment

Before the appointment, request a medical consultation for patients with severe asthma to assess the patient's level of control and any treatment recommendations or alterations for dental care (including use of local anesthetics and alteration of corticosteroid medications needing supplementation).

Before beginning treatment, ask the patient about the treating physician, medications (usage and compliance), frequency and severity of attacks, date of last attack (and how it was managed), and triggers (if any). Assess current symptoms and reschedule elective dental treatment for patients with uncontrolled symptoms.

Planning

Ask the patient to bring his or her own inhaler to each appointment and keep it available in case of an emergency. Instruct patients with moderate to severe disease to use the inhaler before the appointment for prophylactic purposes.[5]

Implementation

Use pulse oximetry to monitor blood oxygen saturation. Administer supplemental oxygen during treatment to a patient with a PO_2 of 91% to 95%. A patient with a PO_2 of less than 91% should not receive treatment.

Nitrous oxide can be used for patients with asthma; however, PO_2 should be monitored closely.

Avoid using local anesthetics that contain sulfite preservatives, such as articaine and mepivacaine hydrochloride (Polocaine), in patients with moderate to severe asthma.[5] Instead, use local anesthetics without epinephrine or with levonordefrin, such as lidocaine 2% plain or mepivacaine 3%.

Aspirin, ibuprofen, and other NSAIDs are common allergens and may exacerbate an attack; advise patients with asthma to avoid them.[5] Dental management of the asthma patient is outlined in Box 38-4.

In the event of an asthma attack, have the patient use his or her inhaler. If one is not available, use the fast-acting bronchodilator (e.g., albuterol) from the emergency drug kit. Should the inhaler not alleviate the symptoms, administer subcutaneous epinephrine (0.3–0.5 mL 1:1000). See Application to Clinical Practice.

CHRONIC OBSTRUCTIVE PULMONARY DISEASE (COPD)

Chronic obstructive pulmonary disease (COPD) is the result of irreversible disease(s) that obstruct airflow from the lungs, and affects approximately 6% of the population.[11] COPD is preventable and treatable. Cigarette smoking is a major risk factor contributing to development and progression in 90% of COPD cases. As the number of cigarettes smoked per day and years of smoking increases, the risk of developing COPD significantly increases. Other causes of COPD include occupational exposure to industrial pollutants (e.g., metal workers, miners, and factory workers). COPD is the fourth leading cause of death in the United States, and incidence is increasing each year. It is more prevalent among male, non-Hispanic whites

Application to Clinical Practice

Asthma is a serious health problem affecting millions of people. Asthmatic attacks in the dental office are a common occurrence, and are frequently induced by stress. It is essential to know how to prevent and manage emergencies related to asthma. All patients with respiratory disease should bring their own inhaler(s) to their appointment. A short-acting bronchodilator (e.g., albuterol in the medical emergency kit) is not always effective for all asthmatic attacks. It is imperative to know the status of disease, triggers, and how frequently attacks occur. Should an asthma attack occur, all efforts to smoothly manage the situation should be taken, as follows:

- Recognize the symptoms early (i.e., sense of suffocation, tightness in chest, nonproductive cough and/or wheezing); severe asthma attack symptoms include cyanosis of the nailbeds, flushed skin, diaphoresis (profuse perspiration), confusion, and/or agitation.
- Discontinue treatment and position the patient comfortably for breathing.
- Administer short-acting inhaler.
- Administer supplemental oxygen (10 L/min).
- Monitor vital signs.
- If no improvement, activate EMS.
- Consider subcutaneous epinephrine 1:1000 (0.15–0.3 for children; 0.3–0.6 for adults). ■

Box 38-4. *Dental Management of the Asthma Patient*

1. Review and assess history
   a. Treating physician, medications (usage and compliance), frequency and severity of attacks, last attack (and how it was managed), and triggers (if any)
2. Avoid any triggers
3. Obtain medical consult for patients with severe asthma
4. Have patient bring his or her inhaler to each appointment and have readily available
5. Avoid aspirin and other NSAIDs
6. Consider local anesthetics without vasoconstrictors
7. Utilize adequate stress reduction protocol
8. Recognize signs and symptoms of an asthma attack and know how to manage
   a. Have patient use his or her own inhaler or fast-acting bronchodilator from the emergency kit
   b. If symptoms progress or are not alleviated by the bronchodilator, administer subcutaneous epinephrine (0.3–0.5 mL 1:1000)
   c. Activate EMS
   d. Repeat administration of bronchodilator every 5 minutes until EMS arrives ■

over the age of 65.[1] However, the number of females diagnosed with COPD is on the rise, and women are more likely to die of the disease. COPD includes two diseases, chronic bronchitis and emphysema. Some patients have one or the other, whereas others have both. Emphysema can only be officially diagnosed by autopsy.

Signs and Symptoms

COPD encompasses varying degrees of many of the signs and symptoms of respiratory disease, including cough, dyspnea, and sputum production.[10] Differences in signs and symptoms of chronic bronchitis and emphysema are outlined in Box 38-5. Lung functioning capacity (FEV_1) assists in the diagnosis and severity of COPD. People with mild COPD have an FEV_1 greater than 80%; with moderate COPD, an FEV_1 of 60% to 80%; and with severe (*end-stage*) COPD, an FEV_1 less than 60%. People with moderate to severe disease need a medical consult to determine level of control and any alterations necessary for dental treatment. In addition, radiographic changes are present with COPD.

People with COPD often have difficulty or tire easily when performing basic chores and walking short distances or up stairs. There is no cure for COPD. However, signs and symptoms can be managed to enhance quality of life and improve daily living. Treatment of COPD includes lifestyle modifications such as smoking cessation, diet and exercise modifications, and weight management. Medications, oxygen therapy, and inhalers or nebulizers can reduce the frequency and severity of symptoms.

Box 38-5. *Chronic Bronchitis and Emphysema*

- **Chronic Bronchitis**
  - Chronic inflammation of the bronchial tube lining, which leads to scarring and eventual obstruction of airflow; creates environment that is ideal for development of acute microbial infections
  - Mild dyspnea and frequent respiratory infections
  - Characterized by chronic productive cough with sputum production for 3 months in at least two consecutive years.
  - Patient tendency to be sedentary, overweight, cyanotic, edematous, and breathless ("blue boater")
- **Emphysema**
  - Destruction of the alveoli leading to decreased exchange of air flow and shortness of breath (dyspnea)
  - Severe dyspnea and few respiratory infections
  - Minimal nonproductive cough
  - Patient tendency to be barrel chested with weight loss; pursing of the lips on expiration ("pink puffers") ■

Dental Hygiene Considerations

Dental management of the COPD patient requires special consideration to prevent respiratory complications or emergency. Considerations include smoking cessation encouragement, assessing the severity and control of the disease, short appointments, semisupine or upright chair position, monitoring PO_2 (in addition to routine vital signs) at each appointment, and having the patient's inhaler(s) available during the appointment. The patient should prerinse with an antimicrobial (e.g., 15 mL of 0.12% chlorhexidine gluconate for 30 seconds) and may use an inhaler prophylactically before treatment begins. Supplemental oxygen (6 L/min) should be considered for a patient with a PO_2 of 91% to 95%. A patient with a PO_2 less than 91% is considered unstable and treatment should be postponed. Diligent homecare instructions and education about the oral–respiratory disease link should be discussed. See Evidence-Based Practice.

CYSTIC FIBROSIS

Cystic fibrosis is an inherited, lifelong disease that affects multiple organs, including the lungs, pancreas, and liver, resulting in a shortened life expectancy.[12] Production of thick, sticky mucus causes blockages in the airway, making it difficult to breath. Cystic fibrosis most commonly affects children and young adults. In the United States, approximately 30,000 people have cystic fibrosis. It is estimated that 10 million people are asymptomatic carriers of a defective cystic fibrosis gene. Cystic fibrosis occurs more frequently in whites and is distributed equally among males and females. There is no cure for cystic fibrosis, but various treatments can decrease symptoms and increase quality of life.[13]

Dental Hygiene Considerations

Cystic fibrosis and the medications used to treat it cause a decrease in saliva flow leading to a higher incidence of oral disease, including caries and periodontal disease. Recommendations to reduce caries risk may be necessary. Knowledge of cystic fibrosis and questioning the patient (or parent) about symptoms and current medications is essential for treatment planning and homecare modifications for the patient with cystic fibrosis. Scheduling issues might arise due to frequent lung infections and intermittent hospitalization. As with other respiratory diseases, a semisupine or upright chair position should be considered when the patient is experiencing difficulty breathing.

TUBERCULOSIS (TB)

Tuberculosis (TB) is an infectious and communicable pulmonary disease caused by *Mycobacterium tuberculosis* that is highly contagious. TB most frequently affects individuals in third-world countries (33% worldwide, versus 5–10% in the United States).[14] TB has two infectious forms: *TB infection* and *TB disease*. TB infection is present in individuals without symptoms; therefore individuals might not know they have been exposed. Individuals with TB disease have significant symptoms causing extreme illness.

TB is transmitted by aspiration of infected airborne droplets/aerosol. Individuals at higher risk include international travelers, anyone in close contact with an infected individual, and/or immunocompromised individuals.

Symptoms, Diagnosis, and Treatment

Initial symptoms of TB include appetite and weight loss, fever, fatigue, and night sweats. Symptoms may be vague and unnoticed or become dormant. Development of chronic symptoms of the disease includes chest pains and severe cough with bloody sputum. Additional organs also could become affected.

Screening for TB includes a skin test called purified protein derivative (PPD). Health-care providers should be tested regularly (i.e., at least yearly; more frequently if known exposure).[14] A positive PPD skin test requires being evaluated for active disease by physical examination and chest radiographs. With normal results and absence of active disease symptoms, the patient is considered to have latent TB and not be infectious. Prophylactic isoniazid may be prescribed for 6 to 9 months to prevent reactivation of disease. With abnormal physical or radiographic findings, additional testing (e.g., sputum sample, chest radiograph) is needed to confirm active TB. Once a patient is diagnosed with active TB based on bacterial culture or direct molecular tests, a physician will prescribe multiple antibiotics for a minimum of 6 months regardless of active symptoms. It is imperative to complete the entire course of prescribed medication or drug-resistant TB may develop.

Dental Hygiene Considerations

Patients with active TB disease should be deferred for treatment until a nonactive status is determined. For patients who report TB, further questioning is necessary to determine whether the proper treatment and follow-up testing for TB was completed. If a patient did not complete the full regimen of medications, a referral should be made for follow-up screening and treatment. Patients with a history of a positive PPD skin test and no active TB symptoms can be treated with normal standard precautions for infection control.

Case Study

Nancy is a 67-year-old patient diagnosed with COPD 2 months ago, when she also quit smoking after 40 years. She presents to her periodontal maintenance appointment reporting dry mouth and two new medications: (1) fluticasone propionate (inhaled corticosteroid) and (2) albuterol (short-acting bronchodilator). Vitals are blood pressure 138/86, pulse 90, respirations 17, and PO_2 97%. Her oral health includes loss of attachment 5 to 6 mm in the posterior sextants (probing depths of 4–5 mm in the posterior, recession 1–2 mm generalized) with light to moderate calculus and stain (coffee and tobacco). Gingival tissues are enlarged and fibrotic. She also has a recurrent carious lesion around a maxillary crown. She prefers and has always had the ultrasonic used during her past hygiene appointments.

CASE STUDY EXERCISES

1. Questions about all of the following should be asked during the health history interview of Nancy EXCEPT which one?
   A. Type of COPD diagnosed by physician
   B. Current treating physician and medical recommendations
   C. Current or past signs and symptoms
   D. Completion of 6- to 9-month multiple antibiotic regimen
2. Which of the following treatment considerations is warranted based on Nancy's vital signs?
   A. Physician consult before treatment
   B. Dietary and lifestyle recommendations
   C. Supplemental oxygen
   D. Referral to physician for assessment
3. Use of ultrasonic instrumentation for Nancy's care is contraindicated because contaminated aerosols are produced by ultrasonic instruments and potentially aspirated.
   A. Both the statement and the reason are correct and related.
   B. Both the statement and the reason are correct but not related.
   C. The statement is correct, but the reason is not.
   D. The statement is not correct, but the reason is correct.
   E. Neither the statement nor the reason is correct.
4. After 20 minutes of treatment, Nancy begins to cough and wheeze, and she is unable to catch her breath. All of the following actions should be taken EXCEPT which one?
   A. Call 911
   B. Administer oxygen
   C. Provide short-acting bronchodilator
   D. Upright chair position
5. All of the following conditions Nancy is experiencing could be attributed to her respiratory medications EXCEPT which one?
   A. Xerostomia
   B. Elevated pulse
   C. Recurrent decay
   D. Gingival enlargement

Review Questions

1. The oral cavity harbors pathogens with the potential to initiate a respiratory infection. The majority of healthy individuals avoid developing respiratory infection by host defense mechanisms.
   A. Both statements are true.
   B. Both statements are false.
   C. The first statement is true, the second statement is false.
   D. The first statement is false, the second statement is true.

2. All of the following are common symptoms of respiratory disease, EXCEPT which one?
   A. Dyspnea
   B. Chest pain
   C. Bloody sputum
   D. Fever
   E. Headache

3. Use of local anesthetics with sulfite preservatives (e.g., articaine or Polocaine) is preferred for patients with moderate to severe asthma because there is a greater possibility of allergic reaction to anesthetics without sulfites (e.g., mepivacaine).
   A. Both the statement and the reason are correct and related.
   B. Both the statement and the reason are correct but not related.
   C. The statement is correct but the reason is not.
   D. The statement is not correct, but the reason is correct.
   E. Neither the statement nor the reason is correct.

4. Dental management for the patient with COPD includes all of the following EXCEPT which one?
   A. Semisupine chair position
   B. Supplemental oxygen for PO_2 less than 91%
   C. Reappoint if acute symptoms are present
   D. Prerinse with antimicrobial (e.g., 15 mL chlorhexidine)
   E. Short appointments

5. Patients with a positive skin test for TB need follow-up tests to confirm the diagnosis and recommend the proper treatment regimen. Treatment of TB with multiple medications for a minimum of 6 months is only necessary if active symptoms are present.
   A. Both statements are true.
   B. Both statements are false.
   C. The first statement is true, but the second statement is false.
   D. The first statement is false, but the second statement is true.

Active Learning

1. Create a table comparing each respiratory disease and the dental hygiene considerations that should be made.
2. Investigate the rates of tuberculosis in countries outside of the United States. What are the global public health policies related to tuberculosis?
3. Create a video informing dental hygienists on respiratory conditions and what should be considered during a dental visit. ■

REFERENCES

1. American Lung Association. Lung disease data: 2008. 2008. Available from: http://www.lungusa.org.
2. Azarpazhooh A, Leake JL. Systematic review of the association between respiratory diseases and oral health. *J Periodontol.* 2006;77(9):1465-1482.
3. Scannapieco FA. Role of oral bacteria in respiratory infection. *J Periodontol.* 1999; 70:793-802.
4. Centers for Disease Control and Prevention. Guidelines for infection control in dental health-care settings. *MMWR Morb Mortal Wkly Rep.* 2003;52(RR-17):1-76.
5. Little J, Falace D, Miller C, Rhodus N. *Dental management of the medically compromised patient.* 8th ed. St. Louis, MO: Mosby Elsevier; 2012. p. 628
6. Dentsply Professional. *Cavitron® Plus(tm) ultrasonic scaler: directions for use.* York, PA: Dentsply Professional; 2008. Available from: http://www.dentsply.de/bausteine.net/file/showfile.aspx?downdaid=7929&sp=E&domid=1042&fd=2.
7. Medlineplus health topics. Lung diseases. 2015. Available from: http://www.nlm.nih.gov/medlineplus/lungdiseases.html.
8. Molinari J, Harte J. *Cottone's practical infection control in dentistry.* 3rd ed. Philadelphia, PA: Lippincott Williams & Wilkins; 2009. p. 400
9. National Center of Health Statistics. Asthma. 2014. Available from: http://www.cdc.gov/nchs/fastats/asthma.htm.
10. Heuer AJ, Scanlan CL. *Wilkin's clinical assessment in respiratory care.* 7th ed. St. Louis, MO: Mosby Elsevier; 2013. p. 476
11. National Center of Health Statistics. Chronic obstructive pulmonary disease. 2014. Available from: http://www.cdc.gov/nchs/fastats/copd.htm.
12. Medlineplus health topics. Cystic fibrosis. 2014. Available from: http://www.nlm.nih.gov/medlineplus/cysticfibrosis.html.
13. Kacmarek RM, Stoller JK, Heuer, AJ. *Egan's fundamentals of respiratory care.* 10th ed. Philadelphia, PA: Lippincott Williams & Wilkins; 2012. p. 1384
14. Centers for Disease Control and Prevention. Guidelines for preventing the transmission of *Mycobacterium* tuberculosis in health-care settings. *MMWR Morb Mortal Wkly Rep.* 2005;54(RR-17):1-147.
15. Awano S, Ansai T, Takata Y, et al. Oral health and mortality risk from pneumonia in the elderly. *J Dent Res.* 2008;87(4):334-339.
16. Gomes-Filho IS, Santos CM, Cruz SS, et al. Periodontitis and nosocomial lower respiratory tract infection: preliminary findings. *J Clin Periodontol.* 2009;36(5):380-387.
17. Paju S, Scannapieco FA. Oral biofilms, periodontitis, and pulmonary infections. *Oral Dis.* 2007;13(6):508-512.
18. Scannapieco FA, Bush RB, Paju S. Associations between periodontal disease and risk for nosocomial bacterial pneumonia and chronic obstructive pulmonary disease. A systematic review. *Ann Periodontol.* 2003;8(1):54-69.
19. Centers for Disease Control and Prevention. Guidelines for infection control in health care personnel. *Am J Infect Control.* 1998;26(3):289-354.

Chapter 39 | Sensory Disability: Vision and Hearing Impairment

Janet Jaccarino, CDA, RDH, MA

KEY TERMS

American Sign Language (ASL)

blind

cataract

cochlear implant

deaf

diabetic retinopathy

finger spelling (American Manual Alphabet)

glaucoma

guide dog

hearing aid

hearing dog

legal blindness

lipreading

macular degeneration

service animal

tactile finger spelling

tactile sign language (TSL)

telecommunications device for the deaf (TDD)

teletypewriter (TTY)

tinnitus

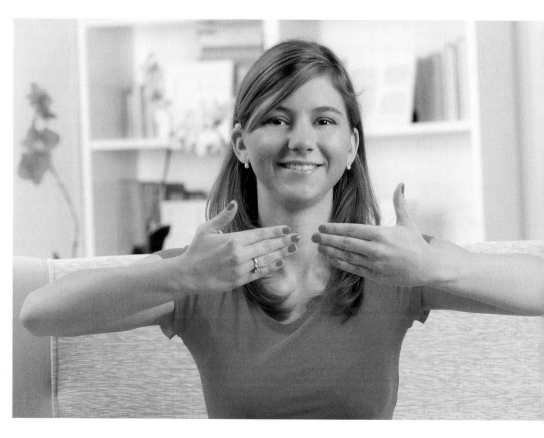

LEARNING OBJECTIVES

After reading this chapter, the student should be able to:

39.1 Describe blindness, low vision, and deafness.

39.2 Analyze the incidence of visual impairment in the United States.

39.3 Recognize the causes of blindness and hearing loss.

39.4 Identify the signs and types of hearing loss before and after birth and factors that contribute to lack of speech.

39.5 Distinguish the oral clinical findings commonly found in persons with sensory impairments.

39.6 Examine the personal and dental implications for care of patients with sensory impairments.

39.7 Explore strategies to communicate effectively with patients who have visual and hearing impairments.

39.8 Role-play seating and dismissal for the patient with visual impairment.

39.9 Develop management protocol that will enable you to provide safe and effective care for the patient with sensory impairments.

39.10 Plan an oral self-care program to improve the oral health of your patient with a sensory impairment.

KEY CONCEPTS

- Sensory disabilities alone do not require a change in treatment methods, just modifications in its provision.
- Sensory impairments alone have no direct effects on oral health; however, in patients with disabilities, there may be a greater incidence of dental disease because of lack of knowledge and communication about oral self-care or because of limited access.
- The Americans with Disabilities Act requires medical and dental offices to be made free of barriers to physical access and effective communication.
- Always ask patients with sensory disabilities what method of communication they prefer.
- Persons with sensory disabilities tend to rely more on their other senses.
- To prevent injury, ensure that the path to the dental operatory and the operatory itself are free of obstacles.
- Persons with a hearing disability may also have problems with speech.
- Appointments for patients with sensory impairments require extra time.
- Touch via hands is the primary method of communication for the person who is deaf and blind.

RELEVANCE TO CLINICAL PRACTICE

More than 20 million Americans report having loss of vision, including those who have trouble seeing even when wearing glasses or contact lenses, and those who are **blind,** or unable to see at all. Of those 20 million Americans, 6.2 million are seniors aged 65 years and older.[1] According to current U.S. Census Bureau Newsroom statistics, 1.8 million people aged 15 years and older report being unable to see printed words.[2] These figures translate to 1 of 20 dental patients having some degree of visual impairment.

Hearing impairment is often referred to as the invisible disability because there may be no visual clues that the person has an impairment. According to research studies, 35 million Americans are hearing impaired, corresponding to 11.3% of the U.S. population. Although hearing loss is considered a disability of the older adult, studies show that about 1 American school-aged child in 10 suffers from some form of hearing loss.[3] Those with hearing impairment are as individual as the cause and manifestation of their disability. Loss of function can be total or partial, affect one or both ears, and often impacts speech, language development, and even motor activity; communication is often a major challenge.[4] Many older persons have some degree of hearing impairment. As the baby boom generation (those born between 1946 and 1964) ages, the number of persons with vision and hearing loss will increase substantially.[5]

It is important for dental professionals to recognize the mental and physical aspects of having a sensory disability to use their resources and imagination to help furnish care. Sensory disabilities alone do not require a change in treatment methods, just modifications in its provision. Title III of the 1992 Americans with Disabilities Act requires medical and dental offices to be made free of barriers to physical access and effective communication.[6] Removing barriers for a blind person may involve adding raised letters or Braille to elevator control buttons, as well as providing written materials in Braille. For those with limited vision, the use of large-print materials is helpful. Effective communication for hearing-impaired persons may include auxiliary aids such as sign language interpreters, telecommunications devices such as a **teletypewriter (TTY)** for deaf persons, and the use of a reader.[6] Barriers to dental care for the patient with sensory impairments include physical access to the office, lack of transportation, lack of communication, and economic issues. Preparation, patience, flexibility, and consideration are essential and as valuable as technique in providing care.

VISION IMPAIRMENT

Legal blindness is defined as visual acuity of 20/200. A person who is legally blind even with optical correction can see at 20 feet what a person with normal vision can see at 200 feet. Approximately 800,000 persons are legally blind, but only 10%, or 80,000, are totally without sight. Not all visual impairments carry the same degree of blindness. Some individuals who are considered legally blind may be able to distinguish images, light, and colors, and may even be able to read large print. Low vision is different from legal blindness and covers a wide range of conditions. Low vision can interfere with a person's ability to perform everyday activities like reading, walking unassisted, and cooking.[1,7] These activities include oral self-care.

Causes

Children

Two percent of individuals with severe visual impairments are younger than 18 years. Any vision loss in children has the potential to affect their development as a whole. Vision impairment in children is caused by vitamin A deficiency, strabismus (eye turn), amblyopia (lazy eye), congenital cataracts, infantile glaucoma, and damage to the optic nerve and retina.[8] Children who are blind often have multiple developmental disabilities such as epilepsy, cerebral palsy, or deafness.[7]

Adults

The leading cause of vision impairments in adults is related to disorders such as **diabetic retinopathy** (from long-term diabetes), **macular degeneration** (affecting the center of visual field), **glaucoma** (no peripheral vision, from conditions that cause damage to the optic nerve), and **cataracts** (a cloud that develops over the lens of the eye). Other causes may be associated with

tumors, systemic diseases such as hypertension, arthrosclerosis, leukemia, Sjögren syndrome, a virus, hereditary factors, degenerative diseases of the optical system, or prolonged use of certain drugs to treat disease (Table 39-1).[7–10]

Oral Clinical Findings

Vision impairment does not have any direct effect on oral health; however, some may find it difficult to maintain a balanced diet or even visit the dentist. They may not detect dental disease symptoms that are typically recognized through vision at an early stage. Incidence of dental disease may be greater because of poor oral self-care because the patient is not able to see or from lack of effective oral self-care instruction.[11–14] Individuals may have impairment as a result of diseases such as diabetes and hypertension, which can affect dental treatment more than the impairment. Other oral symptoms that have been noted include lesions caused by lip and cheek biting, occlusal wear caused by bruxism, trauma due to accidents, and increased caries in the patient with Sjögren syndrome because of lack of saliva. Different types of visual impairments may contraindicate administration of certain dental drugs, for example, prescribing diazepam and atropine for patients with narrow-angle glaucoma.[11,12]

Patient Factors

Children

Visually impaired children, especially those who are totally blind, are deprived of the opportunity to learn by imitation. Because they do not have workable visual imagery in their memory, they must adjust to a world they have not seen or experienced. Blind children may learn to speak later and have an educational level behind that of a sighted child of the same age because they have started school later. They may take longer to cover the same amount of material as a sighted child.

Table 39-1. *Most Common Causes of Vision Loss*[9,10]

Condition	Effects
Diabetic Retinopathy 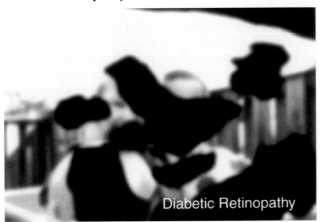 Diabetic retinopathy. (Courtesy National Eye Institute, National Institutes of Health.)	• Damage to the blood vessels in the retina • Risk factors include all people with diabetes, both type 1 and type 2, and pregnant women who have diabetes • 40%–45% of Americans diagnosed with diabetes have some stage of diabetic retinopathy • Early stages have no symptoms, so an eye examination is essential for all persons with diabetes • Better control of blood sugar levels slows the onset and progression • Treatment includes surgery or laser treatment
Macular Degeneration (age related) (AMD) 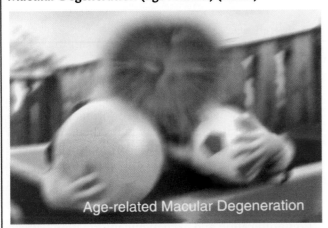 Macular degeneration (age related). (Courtesy National Eye Institute, National Institutes of Health.)	• Leading cause of vision impairment and legal blindness in individuals ≥50 years • Damage to the central visual area, the macula, which allows vision of fine detail; sharp central vision is blurred • Difficulty with straight-ahead activities like reading, sewing, and driving • Exact cause unknown • Treatment includes medications, laser treatments, and photodynamic therapy
Glaucoma 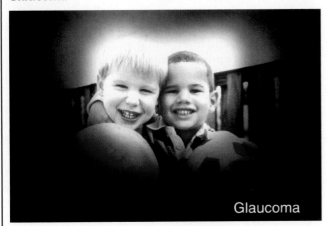 Glaucoma. (Courtesy National Eye Institute, National Institutes of Health.)	• Leading cause of blindness in the United States • Normal fluid pressure in the eye rises resulting in optic nerve damage • May result in vision loss and blindness • Risk factors include elevated eye pressure, age, African ethnicity, familial history, and nearsightedness • Symptoms: no peripheral vision, unusual trouble adjusting to dark rooms, challenges focusing on near or far objects, squinting or blinking due to unusual light, iris color change, encrusted or swollen lids, double vision, excessive tearing, dry eyes, and the appearance of ghost-like images • Can usually be controlled with medication

Continued

Table 39-1. *Most Common Causes of Vision Loss*[9,10]—cont'd

Condition	Effects
Cataract 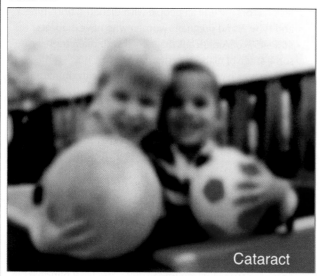 Cataract. (Courtesy National Eye Institute, National Institutes of Health.)	• Clouding of the lens preventing light from passing through • By age 80 years, more than half of Americans either have a cataract or have had surgery • Symptoms: blurred/cloudy vision, double vision, sensitivity to light, or a constant glare in the path of vision • Protection from ultraviolet B (UVB) light may prevent or slow the progression of cataracts • Treatment involves surgical removal of the lens and replacement with a human-made lens

Source: Photographs reprinted with permission from National Eye Institute, National Institutes of Health.

Some parents may be overindulgent and protective, which may foster emotional dependence. All children fear separation from their parents, but this is especially true for the blind child. Parents should be allowed to accompany the child into the operatory until the child feels comfortable with the dental team; this may take a little longer then for the child who is not blind. Equipment and sharp instruments present a safety concern because blind children may explore their environment by moving about, touching and feeling things, and putting their face close to an object to see or smell it; the child should never be left alone in the operatory. Mannerisms that interfere with treatment may include rubbing the eyes, rocking, and head bobbing. Those who are partially blind may stare at lights or try to pinpoint a light source by moving around with their arms held above the head or tilting their head upward. To gain a perspective on the child's behavior and personality, the dental team may need to consult with the child's pediatrician, school nurse, or teachers. Individuals who are blind from birth or a very early age eventually adapt to their condition; it becomes part of who they are.[7]

Adults

The person who experiences visual disability later in life often adjusts better to the world around them, but because they can remember what has been lost they may also have feelings of depression, helplessness, or frustration. Adjustment to blindness varies for each individual. All persons with visual disability tend to develop and use their other senses more. For example, they may rely on tone of voice to interpret what a sighted person may understand from a facial expression. Being well organized allows an individual to know exactly where things are located, and doing things deliberately and slowly helps them to gain perception and prevent accidents. Any new experience or concept will be understood easily if the person is told about it in detail.[7]

Communication

Communication and exchanging information between patient and hygienist is not only necessary for good clinical practice, it is essential for rapport and trust. Medical history, receiving instructions for oral self-care, and even making an appointment all depend on understanding without misinterpretation. The act of sending, receiving, and interpreting messages is complicated and often depends on seeing or hearing, or both. For the person with sensory disabilities, this process can become time-consuming and frustrating. Visually impaired persons may not pick up on nonverbal cues such as body posture, gestures, or facial expression, and they may be at a disadvantage. First, ask the person what is his or her preferred method of communication. Face the person and speak slowly and directly in a normal tone of voice. Give clear, concise instructions slowly. Speak directly to the patient, not the person who accompanies him or her, but include the caregiver if necessary. Avoid speaking to adults as if they are children; if necessary, repeat instructions. Keep it simple, stick to one topic, or ask one question at a time. The room should be well-lit; however, standing in front of strong backlighting from a window or light can interfere with any residual vision and make it difficult for the person with limited vision to see you. Let the person know when you move from one place to another or leave the room. Try not to startle the person, but first gain his or her attention by speaking or lightly touching his or her arm before speaking. The person with visual impairment needs to concentrate to understand directions or instructions, so limit distractions. Limit the number of people in the operatory and control noise by turning down the radio or closing a window.

Use of large-print material is helpful for the partially sighted person. Type size should be 16 to 18 point or larger, in a simple font, not thin, italic, or fancy typefaces, and double-spaced. Use yellow or off-white paper, which has less glare than plain white paper. Contrasting words on paper are easier to see; for example, blue letters against a yellow background. Using blue, green, and purple together makes it more difficult to distinguish words. Depending on the type of impairment, alternative ways of presenting information such as audio cassette or CD, Braille, or the use of a designated reader may also be used (see Application to Clinical Practice).[4,7,15,16]

Guiding and Seating the Patient

A dental visit starts at the front door to the office. Physical access for persons with disabilities is mandated by the Americans with Disabilities Act (Box 39-1).[6] Allow extra time for the appointment and have the room ready before the patient arrives. Make sure the dental chair is at the proper height for seating (chair at the level of the patient's knees). Greet the patient by introducing yourself. Ask the patient if he or she needs your help, and if so ask how. Before any physical contact with the patient, first explain what you are about to do. The best way to

Box 39-1. *Physical Access to the Dental Office*[7,11,15]

- Keep passages clear of clutter.
  - No loose rugs
  - No hanging plants
  - Ensure a clear passage to the chair in the operatory before the patient arrives: move operator and assistant chair, hoses for handpiece, suction and air, foot pedals, bracket tray, and any radiograph equipment
- All areas should be well-lit.
- Furniture should have no sharp edges.
- Door frames and handles and edges of steps should be well-defined in contrasting colors to prevent accidents. Contrast colors are also important to differentiate walls from floors.
- Staircases should have handrails and steps that are not too steep.
- Have tactile or Braille maps in the hall and elevator.
- The effects of glare may make it difficult to see.
  - High-intensity lighting
  - Sun shining directly through windows
  - Highly polished floors
- Use large-print signs.
  - Contrast colors for words against background

Application to Clinical Practice

Communication tips include:[4,7,15,16]
- Ask the person what is his or her preferred method of communication.
- Face the person and speak slowly.
- Keep conversation simple.
- Provide a well-lit room.
- Indicate when you move from one place to another or leave the room.
- Avoid startling the person by speaking or touching.
- Avoid distractions.
- Use large print material with:
  - 16-18 point type size or larger
  - Simple font, not thin, italic, or fancy typefaces
  - Double-space
  - Contrasting words on paper (yellow or off-white paper has less glare than plain white paper)
- Give clear, concise instructions slowly.
- Consider alternative ways of presenting information.

guide the patient is to have him or her take your arm just above the elbow. Children should hold your waist or your hand. As you guide the person to the operatory, be very specific when you point out obstacles in the path of travel. If there are steps, tell the patient how many, whether they go up or down, and describe which way the door opens before you let the person follow you through the doorway. Using clock directions in your description may be helpful, such as the door is at two o'clock. You may guide the person's hand to a stair railing or the back of a chair to help lead him or her to stairs or a seat. If the patient has a **service animal** or **guide dog,** walk on the side opposite of the dog. Do not touch, pet, or speak to the dog, or offer food; the dog is working and needs to concentrate. Never leave the dog unattended anywhere in the office; guide dogs may stay in the operatory with the person, but out of the way. While working, be aware of the tail and paws at all times.

To seat the patient, first place the patient's hand on the back of the chair and make sure he or she has physical contact with the chair for orientation. Position yourself near the chair as the person sits down, and be ready to help if necessary. Once the person is seated, give a verbal description of where the chair is located in relation to the rest of the room. Persons with disabilities consider any device they use to facilitate mobility and function an extension of themselves; therefore, it is important to keep items such as a cane or eyeglasses within the patient's view. Box 39-2 describes guiding and seating the patient[7,11,15] (see also Resources).

Box 39-2. *Guiding and Seating the Patient*

- Allow extra time.
- Have the operatory ready.
- Identify yourself and others who may be with you.
- Ask if the person needs help.
- Instruct the person to take your bent arm near your elbow.
  - Guide by walking as straight as possible a half step in front of the person.
  - Do not grab or pull the person by the arm; you may throw him or her off balance.
  - Do not hold on to or move a person's cane, it is part of the patient's personal space.
  - Let the person you are guiding set the pace.
  - Avoid sudden, unexpected movements.
  - Point out obstacles.
  - Be specific.
- Guide dog or service animal
  - When walking, walk on the side opposite of the dog.
  - Do not touch or pet the dog, or offer food.
  - The dog may stay in the operatory with the person but out of the way.
- Patient seating
  - When guiding the person to a chair put their hand on the back of the chair.
  - Position yourself near the chair as the person sits down; help if necessary.
  - Give a verbal description of where the chair is located in relation to the rest of the room.
  - If the person uses a cane, ask where he or she would like to keep it. ■

Dental Hygiene Considerations

It may be easy to recognize people with visual impairments because they have difficulty reading, wear glasses, use a white cane, or are accompanied by a guide dog. It is important to find out the degree of the patient's impairment, if the person needs assistance, and how he or she prefers to communicate. The environment should be relaxed. Let the person know before you change the position of the chair so the patient does not feel like he or she is falling. Some people may be sensitive to light, so be careful not to shine the dental light in the patient's eyes; dark safety glasses may be best. If you remove the patient's own glasses, ask where he or she would like you to put them. Explain every procedure in detail slowly and in terms that can be understood. Describe the texture, temperature, softness, or hardness of materials and instruments before you use them.

Because the patient's other senses may be more acute, warn him or her about smells and taste, including any medications and prophy paste. Tell the patient before using the air or water. Let the patient feel and hear the suction tip and let him or her know that the handpiece will vibrate. A moving rubber prophy cup can first be applied to a fingernail so the patient can get a sense of what it will feel like on the teeth. With assistance, the patient may feel some of the instruments. Tap the mirror and explorer together so the patient will recognize this sound because these instruments may touch each other in the mouth. Discuss rinsing options before it is necessary to rinse. There are several ways to do this. Place the cup in the patient's hand and have him or her rinse and spit the water into a second cup. Always take the cup away when the patient is finished. If using the saliva bowl, run the water as a sound cue and guide the patient's hand to the bowl or give the suction to the patient and let the patient clear his or her own mouth. Another option is to simply rinse the patient's mouth using the water spray and suction.

When administering local anesthetic, first describe the preinjection procedure, including the taste and feel of the topical anesthetic. Describe insertion of the needle as a sting or prick and caution the patient not to move during the procedure. Explain to the patient that any swelling he or she may feel is much less in his or her mouth. Tell the patient when you have finished. If you need to leave the operatory, let the patient know. When you re-enter the room, identify yourself because your voice may be confused with others who are working with you. When you are ready to dismiss the patient, let him or her know when changing chair position, reverse the guidelines for seating, and be ready to provide assistance out of the operatory if necessary.[4,7,11,15] Box 39-3 provides a summary of points to remember when caring for a patient with vision impairment.

Oral Self-Care Instruction

The strategy you use depends on the degree of impairment. In addition, the person's attitude and overall ability to cope with the impairment may cause a lack of motivation with home care. More plaque and calculus may be present because there may be little or no visual feedback when the teeth look dirty. Remember that the patient may not be able to learn by imitation, so be inventive with your instruction. As with any other patient, first have the patient demonstrate his or her current technique, then make any modifications to existing practice. For the partially sighted person who cannot see fine detail, position the chair for best visibility, have the patient wear his or her glasses, and use good lighting. A magnified mirror may provide better visibility. Use colored floss such as green, red, or black so that the patient may better identify plaque. Teach the patient to feel the plaque on the teeth with his or her tongue. Instruct the person to run his or her tongue over the teeth before brushing to recognize the "furry" feeling on dirty teeth. After brushing, have the patient feel the "glasslike" sensation of clean teeth. Another approach is to ask the patient to scrape a little plaque

Box 39-3. *Dental Management of the Patient With Vision Impairments*[4,7,11,15]

- Provide a relaxed environment.
- Warn the patient before any change in chair position.
- Do not expect the patient to see fine detail in radiographs or small models.
- If you remove the person's own glasses, find out where is the best place to keep them.
- Before using any visual aids, return the glasses to the patient.
- If the person is sensitive to light, use dark glasses.
- Avoid shining the light in the patient's eyes.
- Explain every procedure slowly using descriptive words.
- Describe any smell and taste.
- Avoid surprise applications of suction, air, water, moving rubber prophy cup, and the vibration of power-driven instruments.
- With assistance, the patient may feel some of the instruments.
- Discuss rinsing options before it becomes necessary.
- Reverse seating procedures for patient dismissal; guide the patient if necessary. ■

Table 39-2. *Types of Hearing Loss*[7,18]

Sensorineural	• Results from inner-ear or auditory nerve dysfunction • Reduces and/or distorts sound • Treatment with hearing aids
Conductive	• Involves the outer or middle ear • Blockage of the outer ear, damage to the eardrum • Diminished sounds • Surgery, drug treatment, possible hearing aid
Cochlear	• Involves the inner ear, cochlea, cochlear nerves, and eighth cranial nerve • Disease, injury, genetics, aging • Hearing aid
Mixed losses	• Contains both conductive and sensorineural components in the same ear

from the tooth, have the patient feel it and smell it, and then feel with his or her tongue how dirty the teeth are. Individuals with extremely limited vision, or no vision at all, can learn by using a tactile approach just as they would read using Braille. Explain toothbrush position and motion by placing the patient's hand over your hand as you move the brush in his or her mouth. Give a detailed verbal description while moving the brush. Make sure to watch patients perform procedures themselves, and have them feel with their tongue how clean the teeth are after brushing. Use similar methods for flossing instruction and point out that when the tooth surface is clean, the patient should hear a squeak as the floss moves on the tooth. Patients can record your oral hygiene instructions on audiotape; also, remember to reinforce the information in large-print or Braille instructions for them to take home.[7,11,14,17]

HEARING IMPAIRMENT

Causes and Types of Hearing Loss

The auditory system is delicate and complicated, and it can be affected by injury, disease or simply the aging process. Loss can be the result of damage to one or several parts of the outer, middle, or inner ear, as well as the sensory pathways from the ear to the brain. Different types of hearing loss are described in Table 39-2.[7,18] **Deaf** is a term used to refer to people with degrees of

hearing loss defined by the quietest sound a person can hear.[4,19,20] Hearing impairment is a broad term that covers the full range of hearing loss from mild to profound.[7] Congenital deafness, caused before birth, may be the result of genetic defects; prenatal infections in the mother such as rubella, influenza, and congenital syphilis; incompatible mother–child blood type; and certain drugs such as thalidomide, streptomycin, and neomycin. The more common causes of deafness after birth are infectious diseases including mumps, measles, chicken pox, influenza, and even the common cold. Other causes are trauma to the head or any part of the ear, and the toxic effects of drugs such as antibiotics and aspirin. Age of onset of deafness can affect the development of speech and language; however, there is evidence that normal language patterns are maintained when deafness occurs after age 5 years.[4,7] Notably, hearing loss can be the result of high noise levels. The length of exposure time and noise level determine the effects on hearing. Sounds greater than 80 dB, such as shop tools, a subway train, and loud rock music, are considered a danger to the hearing mechanism. Some sounds like a jet engine and firearms can even produce pain (Table 39-3).[19,21,22]

Millions of people listen to MP3 portable music players on a daily basis at noise levels that are near the danger zone. Especially vulnerable are young people who tend to use these devices more often. In one study, it was reported that 66% of those who use this type of device on a daily basis experienced ringing in the ears, a warning sign that the music is played too loud.[21] **Tinnitus** is the perception of sound or ringing in the ears or head when no external source is present. The sound may be continuous or intermittent, vary in pitch, and occur in one ear or both. If the noise is constant, it can be

Table 39-3. *What Is Too Loud?*	
85 dB	Prolonged exposure to this noise level can cause damage; e.g., heavy city traffic
100 dB	No more than 15 minutes of unprotected exposure is recommended; e.g., wood shop, snowmobile
110 dB	Regular exposure of more than 1 minute risks permanent hearing loss; e.g., rock concert
120 dB	Ambulance siren
150 dB	Firecracker

0 dB = threshold of normal hearing; 30 dB = whispered voice; 40 dB= refrigerator humming; 60 decibels = normal conversation.

Protect your ears. Wear earplugs when you are involved in a loud activity.

Source: National Institute on Deafness and Other Communication Disorders. Interactive Sound Ruler. www.nidcd.nih.gov/health/hearing/ruler.html.

distracting and cause trouble with hearing. The condition affects 50 million people in the United States. A deaf person can also have tinnitus. The cause is unknown. Noise exposure, head and neck trauma, tumors, jaw misalignment, wax buildup, cardiovascular disease, medications, and certain disorders such as hypothyroidism or hyperthyroidism and fibromyalgia are suspected causes. Treatments are aimed at the cause or may include the use of a hearing aid, drug therapy, and biofeedback. Alternative treatments such as diet and the use of herbs and vitamins may also be considered.[20,23]

Patient Factors

A problem with hearing, even a mild disability, has been shown to have an impact on a person's capacity to function socially. They may feel lonely, remote, or left out and have difficulty paying attention. Older people with hearing loss may be misunderstood as being cognitively impaired. Feelings of isolation and depression often result.[16,24] Some may actually try to hide their disability because they are self-conscious and may neglect to mention it during the health history interview. Lack of hearing is often accompanied by lack of speech. If the person cannot hear the sound of their own voice, they do not have the ability to learn to speak by imitating sounds; therefore, their voice may sound unpleasant and they may not be easily understood. A person may simply choose not to speak because he or she is shy about the sound of his or her voice. The patient with a hearing impairment may:

- Ignore or fail to respond to conversation.
- Exhibit strained facial expression during conversation.
- Turn the head to one side.
- Give unexpected answers unrelated to the question or do one thing when told to do another.
- Ask you to repeat what was said.

- Have an unusual speech tone or inaccurately pronounce words.
- Wear a hearing aid.
- Nod and agree with whatever you say.

Those who learned to speak at an early age before the disability occurred may have difficulty pronouncing medical or dental terms.[7] A **hearing aid** is a device that amplifies sounds, making the sound louder so that the person can hear better. Most new hearing aids are now digital technology.[25] A **cochlear implant** is an electronic device that consists of an external portion behind the ear surgically attached to a second part under the skin. It does not restore normal hearing but gives a representation of sound through a microphone and speech processor via signals sent directly to the auditory nerve of the brain. Cochlear implants offer help to those who are profoundly deaf or severely hard of hearing and cannot be helped by hearing aids.[18,25]

Communication

Hearing loss may range from mild to profound. Some deaf individuals are able to talk, whereas others cannot or choose not to. Note that people who wear a hearing aid may still have difficulty hearing. It is best to ask individuals with hearing disabilities how they prefer to communicate. Options include lipreading, **American Sign Language (ASL),** finger spelling, use of interpreters, or simply providing paper, pen, and a clipboard for writing. It is also helpful to ask the patient to repeat what you said to assure that he or she completely understood you.

Lipreading or Speech Reading

Lipreading or speech reading is a talent that requires practice and is developed over time. Spoken words are recognized by watching the lips, face, and gestures. Avoid standing in front of a light source or window, which makes it difficult for the person to see your face. If the patient is already seated in your operatory, place him or her in the upright position. It is difficult to lip-read when lying in the prone position. Face the person directly, maintain eye contact, and keep hands and other objects away from your mouth. If you are wearing a mask, be sure to remove it before speaking. Do not walk around the room or turn your back when speaking. If you look away the person might assume the conversation is over. Lipreading is often difficult to use because the majority of English speech sounds are not entirely visible or easily recognizable. This method should not be relied on for extended, complex discussions.

American Sign Language

ASL is a visual, gestural language that has its own vocabulary, grammar, and syntax; it is recognized as a language different from English. Hand movements, body postures, and facial expression serve as words of the language. Classes are widely available at community colleges, universities, and on the Internet. Figures 39-1 and 39-2 show examples of signing.[7,26]

Finger Spelling

Finger spelling (American Manual Alphabet) is the manual reproduction of English using the hands and fingers and is often combined with sign language.[28]

Interpreters

Interpreters translate from spoken language to ASL and vice versa and may be a better choice for communication involving a difficult and complicated consultation. The Americans with Disabilities Act mandates the use of interpreter services for patients who require them. Talk directly to the deaf person, not to the interpreter. For effective and full communication it is best to avoid using family or friends to interpret because the person may feel self-conscious discussing oral disease or habits. To find an interpreter and for information on fees, call the local speech and hearing clinic in your community, check the telephone directory, or search online. A directory of certified interpreters who are trained and passed a series of tests is available through the Registry of Interpreters for the Deaf, Inc.:

Registry of Interpreters for the Deaf, Inc.
333 Commerce Street
Alexandria, Virginia
http://www.rid.org/
(703) 838-0030 voice
(571) 384-5163 VP
(703) 838-0459 TTY
(703) 838-0454 Fax

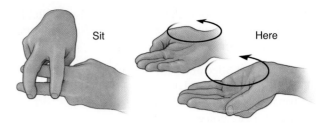

Sit — Here

Sit here - sit two fingers of the right hand over two fingers of the left hand. With palms facing up, move palms in small circles

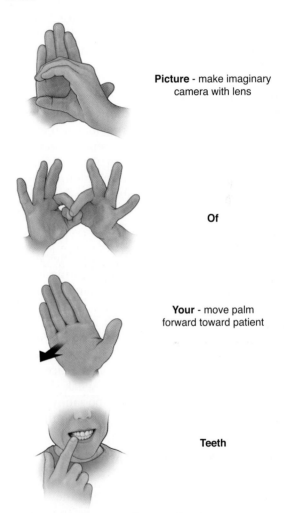

Picture - make imaginary camera with lens

Of

Your - move palm forward toward patient

Teeth

Figure 39-2. Sit here, picture of your teeth. (Reprinted with permission from the University of Washington. DECOD Program (Dental Education in Care of the Disabled). Module IX. Dental Management of patients with CNS and neurologic impairment (a series of 12 booklets). 2nd ed. Seattle, WA: DECOD, School of Dentistry, University of Washington; 1998.)

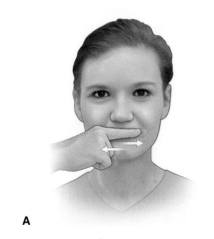

A

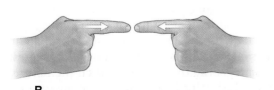

B

Figure 39-1. (A) Brush teeth. (B) Hurt/Pain. (©2006, www.Lifeprint.com. Adapted by permission.)

Electronic Aids

Telecommunications device for the deaf (TDD) provides relay services with a three-way call to an operator who serves as the communicator to the deaf person. When people use this device to place a call, be aware that there may be a delay or a series of electronic beeps, so wait a short amount of time before you hang up. A TTY sends text messages by telephone using a keyboard and visual display and/or printer. Telephone amplifiers can be installed on phones, and portable amplifiers for individual use are also available. For more information, contact the AT&T National Special Needs Center:

AT&T National Special Needs Center
2001 Route 46, Suite 310
Parsippany, NJ 07054-1315
(800) 233-1222 voice
(800) 833-3232 TDD

Hearing Dogs

Hearing dogs are used by the profoundly deaf and offer greater independence and confidence. The dog is trained to alert the person to sounds such as the doorbell, telephone, or smoke alarm, leading the person to the sound source.

Traditional Methods

If you are using a telephone to contact someone who is hard of hearing, let the phone ring longer than usual, speak clearly, and be prepared to repeat when necessary. For patients who have a personal computer, e-mail may be the best means of communication. Scheduling and confirming appointments should be done through e-mail or regular mail. If the patient is returning for an additional visit, provide a written card.

Resources are available through the U.S. Department of Justice Americans with Disabilities Act Fact Sheets.[6,26] Before you interact with hearing-impaired persons, make sure you have their attention. Wave your hand or use a light touch on the arm or other visual or tactile signals to gain their attention. Do not shout or use exaggerated facial expressions. Shouting distorts speech, and exaggerated expressions make it more difficult for the person to lip-read. Face the person whom you are addressing and speak slowly in a clear, normal tone of voice. Most importantly, if you do not understand something that is said, ask the person to repeat it or to write it down.[27]

Dental Hygiene Considerations

As mentioned earlier, be aware of patients' use of a TDD when they are using the phone. If they make an appointment in person, give them a written appointment card as a reminder. Be sure to follow up with a postcard or simply use e-mail to confirm an appointment. Plan before the appointment, and once the patient arrives, always ask what is his or her preferred method of communication. To summon the patient to the operatory, go out into the reception area rather than calling out the patient's name. When the patient is seated, avoid distractions by keeping interruptions and background noise, such as outside traffic or the radio, to a minimum. Remove your face mask or wear a clear face shield to facilitate lipreading. Ask the patient if a gentle tap on the hand or arm is an appropriate way to gain his or her attention. Explain each procedure to the patient and be prepared to repeat or rephrase sentences the person does not understand. Allow for extra time for the patient to respond. It may be helpful to demonstrate instruments and equipment. If the patient uses a hearing aid, make sure it is turned on for conversation. Because of noise amplification and possible discomfort during care, ask the patient to remove or turn off the hearing aid when using power-driven instruments. In addition, touching the hearing aid may create a whistle or buzz sound. Make an effort to avoid the unpleasant sound created by shuffling the instruments against one another. Some deaf patients, especially children, have trouble understanding the concept of local anesthesia. Make sure the procedure is thoroughly explained and understood and that anesthesia is complete before providing care. Watch the patient's facial expression to determine discomfort or other reactions. It may be useful to create several common dental phrases written on index cards to use during the appointment. Refer to Figures 39-1 and 39-2 for examples.[7,17,28]

Oral Factors, Self-Care, and Prevention

Impaired hearing has no direct effects on oral health; even so, patients with disabilities have a greater incidence of periodontal disease and missing or untreated carious teeth, possibly because of limited of access to dental care. In addition, homecare skills may be poor because of lack of communication between patient and caregiver.[7,26] Developmental defects, for example, enamel dysplasia, may be present in the person who is congenitally deaf and the patient may show signs of bruxism, especially those with other disabilities. Some children with disabilities have behavioral problems, and parents or caregivers may use candy or sweets as rewards; therefore, there may be increased potential for the development of caries. Nutritional assessment is part of any good prevention program and is critical when considering these facts. Teach by example and demonstrate brushing and flossing as you would with any other patient, in a step-by-step manner on the patient's own teeth while the patient is watching. Disclosing agents are useful to identify areas of plaque biofilm, and pictures and diagrams are helpful to explain the disease process. The patient should leave the visit with written instructions to reinforce the information you have provided.[7]

THE DEAF-BLIND PATIENT

Deaf-blind persons are those who have both vision loss and hearing loss. The degree of impairment varies from person to person. It has been estimated that 70,000 to 100,000 people in the United States are deaf-blind. In 50% of deaf-blind persons, the cause is the genetic disorder Usher syndrome.[7] Other causes include irradiation of the mother during the first trimester of pregnancy, drug use by the mother, premature birth, trauma during birth, eye disease, accidents, or illness. The majority of deaf-blind persons have multiple physical and mental disabilities. Patients with this condition present a special challenge to the dental professional. Communication with deaf-blind patients depends on the severity of the disability and their preference. Sign language and Braille may be used, but touch via the hands is the major method preferred. Deaf-blind individuals put their hands over the signers' hands to feel the movement of the signs. Examples are **tactile sign language (TSL)** or **tactile finger spelling** (TSL combined with ASL). Using a method called *print on palm,* the person communicating with the deaf-blind individual prints large block letters on his or her palm. Each letter is written in the same location on the palm. Speech vibration allows the patient to place his or her fingers on the speaker's lips while the speaker responds orally. Deaf-blind patients rely on touch and body movements to sense the world around them. Realize that the person may want to touch your face. With supervision, allow the patient to touch equipment and instruments. Your gentle touch may be reassuring to him or her. However, during treatment, avoid any unexpected stimuli to the person's head, face, or mouth.

This may be misinterpreted as a threat and may be met with resistance expressed as pursed lips, clenched teeth, and swinging of the hands. Many of the strategies used for dental management of persons with sensory impairments may be applied to the deaf-blind patient.[7,20,29]

SUMMARY

Persons with sensory impairments, especially those with combined disabilities, present challenges for the dental team. Most can receive care in the private office with a few modifications to treatment. It is vital that the dental hygienist be informed and confident in treating these patients. With knowledge, patience, and understanding, the dental hygienist can provide a stress-free, pleasant dental experience for everyone involved. Being prepared will save valuable treatment time and make the appointment safe, effective, and comfortable.

Case Study

Mr. Smith is a 90-year-old patient who has come to the office today for his 3-month re-care appointment. From a review of his medical history, the hygienist knows that Mr. Smith wears a hearing aid in his right ear, wears eyeglasses, and uses a cane. Mr. Smith tells the hygienist that his wife is with him today because he has been diagnosed with age-related macular degeneration.

Case Study Exercises

1. What are the oral effects of a sensory disability?
   A. Enamel defects
   B. Increased plaque biofilm distribution
   C. Increased dental disease
   D. A, B, and C
   E. None
2. Which of the following should the hygienist consider at the start of Mr. Smith's appointment?
   A. Make sure there are no physical barriers blocking the pathway to the dental operatory.
   B. Ask Mr. Smith if he needs assistance walking to the dental operatory.
   C. Ask Mr. Smith how he prefers to communicate.
   D. If removing Mr. Smith's glasses, ask where he would like to keep them.
   E. All of the above

3. Which of the following is NOT an appropriate strategy when communicating with Mr. Smith?
   A. Speak to Mr. Smith's wife because he has trouble seeing and hearing.
   B. Remove your face mask and in a normal tone speak slowly and clearly.
   C. When speaking to Mr. Smith, make sure he is wearing his hearing aid and that it is turned on.
   D. Provide a quiet, well-lit atmosphere.
4. When providing treatment for Mr. Smith, ask him to turn off or remove his hearing aid.
   A. True
   B. False
5. Which of the following is NOT a good strategy when providing oral self-care instruction for Mr. Smith?
   A. Stand in front of Mr. Smith and demonstrate flossing on a model.
   B. Include Mrs. Smith in oral self-care instruction.
   C. Use good lighting and instruct Mr. Smith to wear his glasses.
   D. Give Mr. and Mrs. Smith large-print materials to take home.

Review Questions

1. Sensory impairments alone have no direct effects on oral health. In patients with disabilities, there may be a greater incidence of dental disease because of lack of knowledge and communication about oral self-care or because of limited access.
   A. Both statements are true.
   B. Both statements are false.
   C. The first statement is true, but the second statement is false.
   D. The first statement is false, but the second statement is true.

2. Hearing impairments may affect:
   A. Older adults
   B. People of all ages
   C. Generally any child who has other disabilities
   D. Baby boomers

3. If necessary, an interpreter must be supplied by the dental office because the Americans with Disabilities Act requires medical and dental offices to be made free of barriers to physical access and effective communication.
   A. Both the statement and the reason are correct and related.
   B. Both the statement and the reason are correct but are not related.
   C. The statement is correct, but the reason is not.
   D. The statement is not correct, but the reason is correct.
   E. Neither the statement nor the reason is correct.

4. A cochlear implant:
   A. Amplifies sounds
   B. Restores normal hearing
   C. Gives a representation of sound
   D. Is digital

5. A cataract:
   A. Affects the optic nerve
   B. Affects the center of the visual field
   C. Is caused by diabetes
   D. Is a cloud that develops over the lens of the eye

Active Learning

1. Working in partners, use a blindfold or modified glasses to simulate vision impairment. (A pair of safety glasses can be modified to simulate vision impairment using nail polish or water-based lubricant. Allow both materials to thoroughly dry before use.) Use cotton balls to simulate hearing impairment. Practice patient seating, dismissal, and communication strategies.

2. Work in groups of four to five students. Brainstorm a list of common items used during a routine dental visit, for example, instruments, high- and slow-speed handpieces, oral evacuators, ultrasonic and piezoelectric scaling devices, prophy cups and brushes, and prophy paste. Discuss ways to describe the feeling, texture, temperature, and smell of each item. Do not forget to include rinsing options.

3. Create a cue card library that will allow a deaf patient to communicate how they are feeling during dental care. Combine pictures and drawings with words to create universally recognized symbols. For example, on an index card, draw a happy face and print the words "I'm OK." The symbols for American Sign Language (ASL) can be combined with words and pictures for the same purpose. Combining symbols, pictures, drawings, and words can also be used during discussion of treatment options. ■

REFERENCES

1. Facts and figures about blind & visually impaired individuals in the US. American Foundation for the Blind website. http://www.afb.org/Section.asp?SectionID=15&DocumentID=4398#numbers. Accessed December 2010.

2. Facts for features: 20th anniversary of Americans with Disabilities Act: July 26. U.S. Census Bureau website. http://www.census.gov/newsroom/releases/archives/facts_for_features_special_editions/cb10-ff13.html. Published May 26, 2010. Accessed December 2010.

3. 35 million Americans suffering from hearing loss. Hear-it.org website. http://www.hear-it.org/page.dsp?area=858. Accessed December 2010.

4. Dougal A, Fiske J. Access to special care dentistry, part 2. Communication. *Br Dent J.* 2008;205:11-21.

5. Macera L. Preparing for the baby boomer generation. *Geriatr Nurs.* November/December 2007:46-49. National Student Nurses website. http://www.nsa.org. http://www.nsna.org/Portals/0/Skins/NSNA/pdf/Imprint_NovDec07_Feat_Geriatric.pdf. Accessed Oct. 9, 2015.

6. Americans with Disabilities Act. U.S. Department of Justice website. http://www.ada.gov/t3hilght.htm. Accessed May 2009.

7. DECOD Program (Dental Education in Care of the Disabled). Module IX. *Dental Management of Patients with CNS and Neurologic Impairment. (A Series of 12 Booklets).* 2nd ed. Seattle, WA: DECOD, School of Dentistry, University of Washington; 1998.

8. Causes of childhood blindness. Lighthouse International website. Available from: http://www.lighthouse.org/about-low-vision-blindness/causes-of-blindness. Accessed November 2013.

9. Eye health information, A-Z diseases and disorders. National Eye Institute, National institutes of Health website. http://www.nei.nih.gov/health. Accessed December 2010.

10. Downs JZ, Lutins ND, Tybor DW. Common eye disorders encountered in the dental office. *Dimens Dent Hyg.* 2010;8(3):48-51.

11. Mahoney EK, Kumar N, Porter SR. Effect of visual impairment upon oral health care: a review. *Br Dent J.* 2008;204:63-67.

12. Shinh YH, Chang CH. Teaching oral hygiene skills to elementary students with visual impairments. American Federation for the Blind. *J Vis Impair Blind.* 2005;99. http://www.afb.org/jvib/jvibabstractNew.asp?articleid= JVIB990104 pdf. Accessed May 2009.

13. Simple steps to better dental health. Reviewed by the Faculty of Columbia University School of Dental Medicine. http://www.simplestepsdental.com/SS/ihtSSPrint/r.==/st.35394/t.35387/pr.3/c.365869.html#Visual_Impairments. Accessed December 2010.

14. Schembri A, Fiske J. The implications of visual impairment in an elderly population in recognizing oral disease and maintaining oral health. *Spec Care Dentist.* 2001;21(6):222-226.

15. DeAngelis S. Visual impairment in the older adult: breaking down the barriers to communication. *Access.* December 2002:36-39.

16. Chavez EM, Ship JA. Sensory and motor deficits in the elderly: impact on oral health. *J Public Health Dent.* 2000; 60:297-303.

17. Kumur DD, Ramasamy R, Stefanich GP. Science for students with visual impairments: teaching suggestions and policy implications for secondary educators. American Association for the Advancement of Science. *Electronic J Sci Educ.* 2001;5(3). http://wolfweb.unr.edu/homepage/crowther/ejse/kumar2etal.html. Accessed December 2010.

18. Aural Education and Counseling. Better Hearing Institute. Advocates for America's Ears(tm). http://www.betterhearing.org/aural_education_and_counseling/articles_tip_sheets_and_guides/communication_strategies.cfm. Accessed May 2009.

19. American Speech–Language–Hearing Association website. http://www.asha.org. Accessed December 2010.

20. Fiske J. Managing the patient with a sensory disability. In: *Special Care Dentistry.* London: Quintessence; 2007:27-41.

21. MP3 users risk hearing damage. Hear-It.org website. http://www.hear-it.org/page.dsp?page=3680. Accessed July 2009.

22. How loud is too loud? National Institute on Deafness and Other Communications Disorders, National Institute of Health website. http://www.nidcd.nih.gov/health/hearing/ruler.html. Accessed December 2010.

23. American Tinnitus Association website. http://www.ata.org. Accessed December 2010.

24. Wallhagen MI, Strawbridge WJ, Shema SJ, Kurata J, Kaplan GA. Comparative impact of hearing and vision impairment on subsequent functioning. *J Am Geriatr Soc.* 2001;49:1086-1092.

25. Hearing loss. Mayo Clinic Health Information. http://www.mayoclinic.com/health/hearing-aids/HQ00812. Accessed December 2010.

26. Americans with Disabilities Act. Fact sheet 2. Providing effective communication. U.S. Department of Justice website. http://adaptiveenvironments.org/neada/pubdocs/pub_352_t3fact2.pdf. Accessed May 2010.

27. American Sign Language Resource. Lifeprint website. http://www.lifeprint.com. Accessed December 2010.

28. Sarampalis A, Kalluri S, Edwards B, Hafter E. Objective measures of listening effort: effects of background noise and noise reduction. *J Speech Lang Hearing Res.* 2009;52(5):1230-1240.

29. American Association of the Deaf Blind website. http://www.aadb.org/FAQ/faq_aadb.html. Accessed December 2010.

*Note: Much of the original information for this chapter first appeared in the Journal of the American Dental Assistants Association, *The Dental Assistant,* in the following issues: Jaccarino J. Treating the special needs patient with a sensory disability—vision impairment. *Dent Assist.* 2009;78(4):8-10; Jaccarino J. Treating the special needs patient with a sensory disability—hearing impairment. *Dent Assist.* 2009;78(5):16-20.

RESOURCES

Providing effective communication. Fact sheet 2. American with Disabilities Act Fact Sheet Series. http://www.adata.org. Accessed December 2010.

Communicating with people with disabilities. Fact sheet 3. American with Disabilities Act Fact Sheet Series. http://www.adata.org. Accessed December 2010.

Communication with and about people with disabilities. U.S. Department of Labor. Office of Disability Employment Policy website. http://www.dol.gov/odep/pubs/fact/comucate.htm. Accessed December 2010.

Tact and courtesy. American Foundation for the Blind website. http://www.afb.org/Section.asp?sectionid=36&topicid=163&documentid=2263. Accessed December 2010.

Disability etiquette, tips on interacting with people with disabilities. United Spinal Association website. http://www.unitedspinal.org/pdf/DisabilityEtiquette.pdf. Accessed December 2010.

Treating adults with physical disabilities: access and communication. World institute on Disability website. http://www.wid.org. Accessed December 2010.

Mace RL. Removing barriers to health care. A guide for health professionals. The Center for Universal Design and The North Carolina Office on Disability and Health. http://www.fpg.unc.edu/~ncodh/rbar. Accessed December 2010.

Chapter 40 | Mental Health

Danielle Furgeson, RDH, EFDA

KEY TERMS

anorexia nervosa
autism spectrum disorder
binging
bipolar disorder
bipolar I disorder
bipolar II disorder
bulimia nervosa
cyclothymic disorder
dysthymic disorder
major depressive disorder (MDD)
mental disorder
mood disorder
schizophrenia

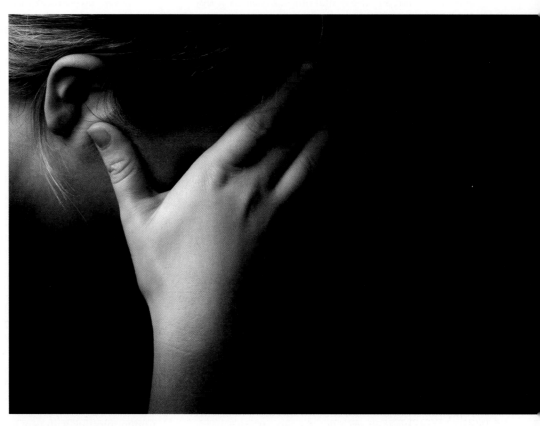

LEARNING OBJECTIVES

After reading this chapter, the student should be able to:

40.1 Describe the common mental disorders that may be encountered in dental hygiene care.

40.2 Discuss the implications of mental disorders on oral health.

40.3 Identify the common oral and dental manifestations of the mental disorders discussed.

40.4 Identify common oral manifestations associated with alcohol and illicit substance abuse.

40.5 Recognize the regularly prescribed medications for the mental disorders discussed and the oral/dental side effects.

40.6 Identify treatment preparation and planning modifications for patients with various mental disorders.

KEY CONCEPTS

• Evaluation of mental disabilities and psychiatric disorders as listed in patient medical histories is a part of risk assessment and treatment planning.

- There are treatment and homecare modifications that should be made for patients with various mental disorders
- It is essential for dental hygienists to identify common oral and dental issues that patients with mental disorders commonly have

RELEVANCE TO CLINICAL PRACTICE

Twenty-one percent of Americans suffer from some form of mental disorder in any given year.[1,2] Mental disorders affect all age groups from early childhood to geriatric populations. Usually a direct correlation exists between these disabilities and poor oral health. The majority of patients suffering from mental disorders are also likely to be prescribed medications with oral side effects and dental treatment implications. As a dental hygienist, it is imperative to have a basic understanding of the behaviors and needs of patients with mental disorders that are likely to be encountered. Appropriate treatment modification and planning, with a strong focus on preventive measures, is key to the oral health of patients with mental disorders.

WHAT ARE MENTAL DISORDERS?

Definition

The American Psychiatric Association defines **mental disorder** as "a clinically significant behavioral or psychological syndrome or pattern that occurs in an individual and that is associated with present distress (e.g., a painful symptom) or disability (i.e., impairment in one or more important areas of functioning) or with a significantly increased risk of suffering death, pain, disability, or an important loss of freedom."[1,3]

Categories

Mental disorders are not one-dimensional psychological disabilities. Biological factors such as genetics, systemic diseases, physiological disturbances, or injuries can trigger, contribute to, and exacerbate mental disorders.[1] Sociocultural experiences also impact mental disorders. The *Diagnostic and Statistical Manual of Mental Disorders*

(DSM) is a resource developed by the American Psychiatric Association. The current edition, DSM-5,[3] concisely classifies hundreds of mental disorders, provides descriptions, and gives examples of diagnoses. Patients who have been diagnosed with a mental disorder will also have been rated according to the Global Assessment of Functioning Scale (GAF). The GAF determines the severity of a patient's mental disorder by assessing his or her functionality.[3]

Pervasive Developmental Disorders

Autism spectrum disorders (ASDs) are classified as pervasive developmental disorders and include conditions such as Asperger syndrome and Rhett disorder. ASDs are not uncommon. The dental hygienist can expect to encounter a patient with an ASD, because statistics show 1 of every 150 eight-year-olds is diagnosed with autistic disorder.[1,4–6] ASDs begin in childhood and are characterized by severe impairment in social interaction and communication skills, repetitive behaviors, and strong aversion to change.[1,3,5–8] See Spotlight on Public Health.

Oral Manifestations

Characteristic ASD behaviors have several implications for overall oral health status (see Advancing Technologies). The inability to communicate, individualistic repetitive behaviors, and accompanying aversion to change frequently result in poor oral hygiene, increased caries rates, and active, advanced periodontal disease.[5] Many patients with ASD have a limited diet that favors soft, sugary foods. These conditions can be compounded by many of the psychotropic drugs prescribed to this population. Patients with ASD may also exhibit odd, repetitive body movements or sudden, unexpected movements, creating a potentially dangerous situation during dental hygiene treatment involving instrumentation. Some

Advancing Technologies

Advances in caries-prevention materials have progressed significantly in the last several years. Fluoride varnishes, chlorhexidine varnishes, xylitol, and casein phosphopeptide-amorphous calcium phosphate are all products to help minimize caries risk in patients. Patients with mental disorders are at greater risk for caries, and use of these products during clinical dental hygiene treatment and recommendations for home use should be carefully considered when tailoring treatment plans for these patients. ■

ATTITUDES REGARDING TREATMENT OF PATIENTS WITH AUTISM SPECTRUM DISORDERS

ASDs are lifelong conditions; therefore, patients in this population need dental care beyond childhood. Often these patients suffer from impaired communication and social interaction skills that may make treating this population a challenge. The literature indicates that although most pediatric dentistry practices routinely treat children with ASDs, a majority of general dentistry practices do not accept either adults or children with autism.[6] With the increased recognition and diagnosis of ASDs in the past two decades, there is a growing population of adults with these disorders who will need regular, preventive dental care.

Dental hygienists receive education on treating special needs populations as part of their undergraduate curriculum, including those patients who may have social or communication impairments, as well as physical impairments. This education focuses not only on the physical treatment needs, but the creation of tailored prevention strategies and homecare plans, as well as collaboration with primary caregivers. Dental hygienists should feel prepared and confident in treating this population of patients, whether adults or children. Actively seeking continuing education courses on the management and treatment of patients with ASD or other special needs can help bridge the gap in access to care for this population of patients. ■

You have an 8-year-old boy with ASD scheduled with you in clinic 3 weeks from now. Notes entered into the chart when the patient was scheduled indicate the patient has been resistant to dental visits and has not yet had a complete dental hygiene visit. In addition, the patient does not verbally communicate. You have concerns about being able to complete dental hygiene services on this patient. What are some things you can do to help increase the chances of having a successful appointment with this patient? ■

patients with ASD may also exhibit damaging oral habits such as bruxism, tongue thrusting, pouching of food, or self-harming habits.[2,5] Successful care of patients with ASD relies heavily on understanding the patient's functionality in these areas.

Dental Hygiene Considerations

Establishing the patient's communication ability is critical. Forty percent of all patients with ASD do not communicate verbally.[5,6] Lack of verbal communication can affect the patient's overall oral health by impairing not only dental hygiene treatment, but also home care (see Application to Clinical Practice). Some patients may not even communicate when they have dental pain. In fact, many reports show that more often than not, by the time a patient with ASD does have a dental visit, the extent of dental disease is so progressed that it frequently requires hospital dentistry.[5] Frequently, the caregiver's attention is monopolized by other behaviors and crises, leaving oral care low on the list of daily priorities. The dental hygienist must collaborate with the parent or caregiver to appropriately communicate with the patient.

Repetitive behaviors and resistance to change must be weighed heavily when treating the patient with ASD. The dental hygienist must understand that the sounds and smells encountered in the dental office may be overwhelming for the patient with ASD. Working closely with a parent or caregiver will alert the dental hygienist to necessary appropriate behavior management modifications. Creating visual aids such as flash cards with simple pictures for the caregiver to use at home can be helpful. Once these visuals have been introduced, the patient should be brought in for multiple tours of the dental office. These tours should include having the patient sit in the dental chair alone (although the patient may choose another place to sit to receive his or her treatment) to help desensitize him or her before actual treatment.[2,5] Other recommendations for treatment of the patient with ASD are included in Table 40-1. Also, the National Museum of Dentistry provides a guide to oral health care for children with ASD (available at: http://www.amchp.org/programsandtopics/CYSHCN/projects/spharc/Documents/autism_dental_from_national_museum_of_dentistry1.pdf).

The dental hygienist must realize that each patient with ASD will vary in his or her functionality. Treatment should focus heavily on prevention, as well as behavior modification and shaping. Treatment plans for the patient with ASD should be developed and altered in collaboration with the patient's caregiver and based on the patient's level of functionality and needs. Preappointment preparation is critical.

Mood Disorders and Bipolar Disorder

Mood disorders are disturbances in a person's mood or emotional state beyond what are considered normal, everyday variations.[1] These disorders are episodic, with episodes lasting anywhere from weeks to years. They may or may not recur. Because of the episodic nature of mood disorders, the dental hygienist must recognize that the patient's state of oral health may be indicative of a current or recent episode. A medical history update and careful assessments are necessary to plan appropriate treatment at each visit.

Table 40-1. Suggested Treatment Considerations for Patients With Autism Spectrum Disorders[5,6]
Collaboration with main caregiver • Establish patient's level of communication. • Establish behavior modifications that work well for the patient. • Create visual aids for the caregiver to use in preparation for the dental hygiene visit.
Preappointment visits to the office • Allow patient to become familiar with the sights, sounds, and smells of the office.
Consider limited appointments.
Allow for flexibility during appointments to accommodate the patient's comfort.
Provide oral hygiene instruction for the caregiver.

Major depressive disorder (MDD) is an acute occurrence of depression in which sufferers exhibit symptoms severe enough to limit everyday normal functioning. Those with **dysthymic disorder** suffer from chronic, less intense bouts of depression.[1] Symptoms may include lethargy, anxiety, withdrawal from social activities, indecisiveness or difficulty concentrating, anger, hopelessness, and psychosomatic aches and pains.[1,9] Mental health professionals define dysthymic disorders by specifiers that indicate things such as the severity of an episode or whether the event was triggered by an event such as a postpartum episode.[1]

Bipolar disorder is characterized by extreme mood swings between euphoria and depression.[1,10] Bipolar disorder is actually divided into two categories: bipolar I disorder and bipolar II disorder. **Bipolar I disorder** is diagnosed when a person experiences one or more manic episodes, without necessarily having experienced a subsequent depressive episode.[1] This form of bipolar disorder is referred to as manic-depression.[1,10] **Bipolar II disorder** differs in that the person suffers from at least one major depressive episode. Comparatively, persons suffering from **cyclothymic disorder** experience similar mood swings, just not as intensely as those seen in bipolar disorders. Although dental hygienists are likely to encounter a patient with bipolar I disorder, they are not likely to encounter a patient having a manic episode in practice, because they require in-patient treatment.

Oral Manifestations

Patients suffering from these mood disorders are likely to have poor oral hygiene because of lack of interest in personal care because of their disorder. In addition, they often have a greater incidence of smoking, decreased salivary flow, compromised immunity, and high carbohydrate and caffeine intake, increasing the risk for caries and periodontal disease.[10,11] These risk factors are frequently compounded by oral side effects of many psychotropic drugs typically prescribed for mood disorders. Side effects frequently include xerostomia, alterations in taste, bruxism, and stomatitis.

Dental Hygiene Considerations

Treatment planning for these patients should focus on preventive measures and homecare regimens such as prescription-strength fluoride toothpastes and saliva substitutes. Strategies to ensure patient compliance with appointments should also be put into place, as studies have shown that patients who report depression on their medical history are more likely to miss dental appointments.[12]

Schizophrenia

Schizophrenia is actually a group of disorders characterized by disturbed or distorted perceptions of reality, odd physical behaviors or speech, and random, illogical thinking. Frequently those suffering from schizophrenic disorders are delusional or have hallucinations. Schizophrenic episodes tend to follow a pattern of a prodromal stage leading to an active stage, followed by a residual phase.[1] During the prodromal phase, the person's behavior, actions, and thought patterns begin to deteriorate in an obvious manner. The active stage lasts a minimum of 6 months and is characterized by hallucinations and delusions, as well as disturbed social interaction and communication abilities, followed by the residual phase, in which a patient's symptoms may almost completely disappear.[1] Schizophrenia is also marked by either positive or negative symptoms. The positive symptoms are the symptoms noted in the prodromal stage that indicate a deterioration of the person's thought and behavior patterns.[1] Negative symptoms are inappropriate responses such as lack of facial expression, lack of verbal response, lack of motivation, and not enjoying activities that most people find appealing.[1] This may make dental hygiene treatment difficult, particularly when educating the patient on preventive home care. If the patient has a caregiver, it is important to go over homecare instructions with him or her.

People suffering from schizophrenic disorders may be hospitalized for long periods, but medication improvements have led to an increased number of patients being treated on an outpatient basis. This increases the probability of the dental hygienist providing dental hygiene treatment to a patient with a schizophrenic disorder. It is critical to obtain a consult with the patient's treating physician to confirm whether the patient has the mental capacity for consent and the ability to comply with proposed treatment and homecare procedures. In addition, the patient with schizophrenia who is taking clozapine should have a white blood cell (WBC) count evaluation of more than 3000/mm³ before dental treatment.[13] This WBC count is done weekly for the first 6 months the patient is taking the medication, which is reduced to every other week if the WBC count is stable after 6 months.[13] Clozapine has been known to cause bone marrow suppression, making the introduction of bacteria into the bloodstream potentially fatal. Therefore, it is critical to ensure the patient who is taking clozapine is having his or her regularly scheduled WBC counts and clearance verified by the patient's physician or psychiatrist. These steps will allow for safe and appropriate treatment.

Oral Manifestations

The nature of schizophrenia predisposes the patient to poor oral health, which is compounded by the side effects of the antipsychotic medications prescribed. Common negative side effects of the antipsychotic medications prescribed for treatment of schizophrenia include xerostomia; acute muscle spasms in areas such as the neck, face, and throat; symptoms that resemble Parkinson disease such as tremors that may make it difficult for patients to perform oral care well; and tardive dyskinesia, which causes repetitive tongue thrusting and lip smacking.[13]

Dental Hygiene Considerations

Preventive measures are key for this group of patients. A 3-month maintenance recall should be standard to help the patient with schizophrenia minimize the risk and incidence of oral disease. Treatment considerations should include fluoride treatments, saliva substitutes, and antimicrobial rinses. Periodontal therapy, restorative work, and extractions are common courses of dental treatment for patients with schizophrenia.[13]

Eating Disorders

Eating disorders are dangerous abnormalities in eating habits that tend to manifest more frequently in women. However, incidence in male individuals has been steadily increasing. The dental hygienist may be the first person to recognize an eating disorder and should not overlook the symptoms in male patients. **Anorexia nervosa** is an eating disorder in which the person sees herself as overweight no matter how dangerously underweight she becomes. This skewed body image is exacerbated by a fear of being overweight, causing the person to starve himself or herself. **Bulimia nervosa** is an eating disorder characterized by overeating, or binging, on large quantities of food. It differs from anorexia in that people with bulimia see their body weight realistically, but fear of gaining weight triggers them to compensate for the binge eating. **Binging** usually consists of consuming large quantities of simple carbohydrates, which the body craves because it is being deprived of nutrients; simple carbohydrates are easy for the body to break down. Many individuals with bulimia will purge by inducing vomiting to relieve the discomfort caused by binge eating. Not all individuals with bulimia purge; they may exercise excessively, fast, or overuse laxatives after binging.

Oral Manifestations

Both anorexia and bulimia affect the oral cavity in several ways (Table 40-2). The dental hygienist should be aware of the physical symptoms that can be observed during patient assessments. Because eating disorders directly impact nutrition, intraoral and extraoral manifestations of vitamin deficiencies such as cracked, yellow skin may be present. Some of the most prominent physical symptoms of anorexia and bulimia nervosa that can be observed in the oral cavity are enlarged parotid glands, severe enamel erosion, rampant caries, and bone and muscle deterioration caused by malnutrition and malabsorption of nutrients.[14] Patients with bulimia may also experience tooth sensitivity caused by dentin exposure from severe erosion. Studies have shown a decrease in bone density for patients with anorexia nervosa, which may directly impact the patient's periodontal health. In addition, the patient with anorexia may have excessive bleeding and swelling in the area of the maxillary incisors; bleeding may be induced by simple touch (see Professionalism).[15,16]

Dental Hygiene Considerations

Treatment for patients with eating disorders may be limited by their state. The priority is to relieve the patient of any dental pain. In general, aggressive preventive treatment planning, including anticaries strategies such as prescription-strength fluoride for home use, must be

Table 40-2. *Anorexia and Bulimia Comparison*

Anorexia	Bulimia
Irrational body image	Realistic body image
Fear of gaining weight	Fear of gaining weight
Person starves self	Binging/consumption of large quantities of food
May exercise excessively	Purging via vomiting, laxative abuse, fasting or excessive exercising
Oral and Physical Manifestations	
Enlarged parotid glands	Enlarged parotid glands
Severe enamel erosion	Severe enamel erosion
Rampant caries	Rampant caries
Bone and muscle deterioration	Bone and muscle deterioration
Bleeding upon touching the gingiva	Enamel erosion
Swelling/bleeding in the maxillary incisor area	Dentin sensitivity

Professionalism

Jennifer, your last patient before lunch, was your high school classmate. She is significantly thinner than she was in high school. After reviewing her medical and dental history and performing an oral inspection, you confirm that Jennifer has bulimia. Although you may know Jennifer outside of your clinical practice and may be tempted to share this with others who might be interested in hearing about Jennifer, Health Insurance Portability and Accountability Act (HIPAA) regulations, ethics, and professionalism require that you keep her disorder confidential. ■

pursued with these patients and their caregivers. The goal is to minimize current and future deterioration of oral health.[17] However, any preventive interventions may be neutralized by the continued nutritional deficiencies and other damaging behaviors associated with active eating disorders. Education and encouragement may be great motivators for the patient with an eating disorder.

Substance Dependence and Abuse

Substance abuse is a major contributor to dental and oral disease. In 2010, the Substance Abuse and Mental Health Services Administration (SAMHSA) released the National Survey on Drug Use & Health. This survey reported current use of illicit drugs (e.g., marijuana, cocaine, heroin, and inhalants), alcohol, and tobacco products in individuals older than 12 years. More than 22 million people reported using illicit drugs, whereas more than half of all Americans older than 12 years reported drinking alcohol. In addition, almost 70 million people reported themselves as being current tobacco product users.[18] This does not imply that all are addicts, but the high percentage of use means the dental hygienist is likely to encounter patients who are dependent on or abuse alcohol, tobacco, or another illicit drug.

Oral Manifestations: Alcohol Abuse

About 50% of patients with alcohol problems also have a mental disorder such as MDD and bipolar disorder. There is also a high incidence of simultaneous tobacco use in this population. This combination of alcohol and tobacco not only increases the occurrence and severity of periodontal disease, but may also predispose users to squamous cell carcinomas in the oral cavity (Table 40-3).[19] These patients therefore tend to present with poor oral health, particularly periodontal disease, because of a combination of lack of home care, poor nutrition, and tobacco use. These patients may also frequently present with dental trauma or history of mandible fractures from falls.[19,20]

Long-term alcohol use causes swelling of the parotid gland, significantly reducing salivary flow. This combination leaves the mouth in a constant state of vulnerability to acid attack. Alcohol also affects patients' oral health by affecting nutrition in two main ways: the bulk of their daily sustenance comes from the empty calories of alcohol and other drinks high in sugar; and their diets are lacking in vital nutrients such as protein, vitamins, minerals, and trace elements.[19,21] In addition, alcohol frequently interferes with, or alters the absorption of, vitamins and other nutrients while increasing the excretion of other key nutrients.[19,21]

Dental Hygiene Considerations: Alcohol Abuse

Like several other mental disorders, addictions such as alcoholism carry a stigma that keeps patients from revealing their condition on medical histories. It is therefore imperative that the dental hygienist recognize the oral and physical signs of alcohol addiction during assessments. Physical signs of current alcohol use include the odor of alcohol on the breath, an unsteady gait, slurred speech, involuntary eye movement, and inattention.[3] However, many patients suffering from addiction to alcohol will seek only emergency dental treatment. For those patients who do seek regular dental treatment, the literature suggests they be placed on 3-month recall. Products that contain alcohol, including mouthrinses, should be avoided. Dental hygienists should be aware that many over-the-counter fluoride rinses also contain alcohol and they should be able to suggest alternatives. The dental hygiene education and treatment plan should

Table 40-3. *Oral and Dental Manifestations of Commonly Abused Substances*[19,21–28]

Alcohol	Cannabis	Cocaine	Methamphetamines
Angular cheilosis	Xerostomia	Angular cheilosis	Poor oral hygiene
Glossitis	Leukoedema	Bruxism and/or wear facets	Rampant caries
Gingivitis/periodontitis	Leukoplakia	Occlusal wear	Xerostomia
Xerostomia	Candidiasis	Gold restoration corrosion	Bruxism
Erosion	Gingival hyperplasia	Candidiasis	Occlusal wear
Swollen parotid glands	Uvulitis	Oral ulcers	
Dental trauma	Gingivitis/periodontitis	Xerostomia	

focus on effective home care including a regimen that includes fluoride and other caries prevention such as xylitol and the recommendation of products that will help alleviate xerostomia.

Oral Manifestations: Cannabis Abuse

In addition to alcohol, the dental hygienist must be able to recognize oral manifestations of other illicit substance abuse. Those most likely to be encountered are cannabis (marijuana) and cocaine in various forms. Cannabis causes xerostomia and immunosuppression, which predisposes the chronic user to leukoedema, a grayish white lesion overlying edema in the tissues, usually found on the buccal and labial mucosa. Cannabis use also causes an increased risk for caries, periodontal disease, and oral infections such as *Candida albicans*.[22,23] Cannabis is also a known carcinogen. Patients who abuse cannabis may also present with red, swollen eyes, tachycardia, angular cheilosis, and respiratory infections.[3,24]

Dental Hygiene Considerations: Cannabis Abuse

Oral health recommendations should include avoiding products and drinks with alcohol, citrus, high sugar content, or sodium laurel sulfate, a synthetic ingredient commonly used in toothpastes to make it foam.[23] Such products can possibly cause aphthous ulcers and exacerbate the patient's dry mouth, which can increase the patient's already high risk for caries.[24]

Dental Hygiene Considerations: Cocaine Abuse

Patients who abuse cocaine present a more complicated risk to treatment because of its systemic effects, particularly on the cardiovascular system. Treatment should be avoided from 6 to 24 hours after cocaine use, although patients are not likely to disclose use. Use of local anesthetics that contain vasoconstrictors is particularly dangerous, because their effects are enhanced by cocaine use.[25] The dental hygienist should be familiar with the effects of cocaine in and around the oral cavity, as well as the physical manifestation of recent use. Physical signs and symptoms of cocaine use include dilated pupils, sweating, chills, nausea, vomiting, confusion, agitation, and possibly seizures.[3] Notation during assessment should alert the hygienist that treatment may be contraindicated or may need to be significantly modified.

Dental Hygiene Considerations: Methamphetamine Abuse

In 2010, the number of people aged 12 years and older who abused methamphetamines was almost 1.5 million, with an increase of use in those in their twenties and thirties.[18,26] Methamphetamine abuse has particular significance to the dental hygienist because it has a tendency to induce severe oral health issues. One of the most common signs of methamphetamine abuse is

"meth mouth," in which the person has rampant, severe caries (Figs. 40-1 and 40-2). This is because methamphetamine abuse not only causes xerostomia, it also induces severe cravings for sugary food and drinks and causes bruxism.[26] Methamphetamine abusers also tend to abuse other illicit drugs and pay little attention to oral hygiene. Notably, those who inject methamphetamines tend to have increased incidence of dental disease.[26]

The physical symptoms of recent or current methamphetamine use are the same as someone who abuses cocaine. These include dilated pupils, sweating, vomiting, confusion, among others. It is important to consider that the methamphetamine abuser may be abusing other illicit drugs as well and may display other physical symptoms. Therefore, the dental hygienist must be familiar with the common physical manifestations of various illicit substances (Table 40-4).

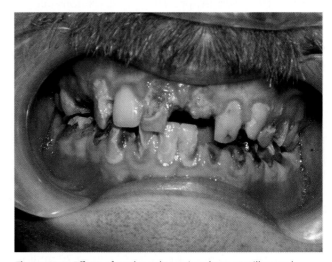

Figure 40-1. Effects of methamphetamine abuse; maxillary and mandibular arch. (Photo courtesy of Glenn J. Reside, DMD.)

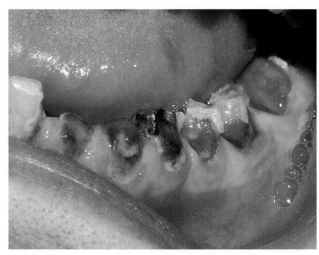

Figure 40-2. Effects of methamphetamine abuse; quadrant 3. (Photo courtesy of Glenn J. Reside, DMD.)

Table 40-4. Behavioral and Physical Manifestations of Commonly Abused Substances[3]

Alcohol	Cannabis	Cocaine	Methamphetamines
Slurred speech	Swollen, red eyes	Dilated pupils	Tachycardia/bradycardia
Uncoordinated	Increased appetite	Perspiration	Dilated pupils
psychomotor function	Dry mouth	Chills	Perspiration
Unsteady gait	Tachycardia	Nausea	Chills
Lack of attention or memory		Vomiting	Nausea
Stupor		Obvious weight loss	Vomiting
Involuntary eye movement		Psychomotor agitation	Obvious weight loss
		Weakness	Obvious psychomotor dysfunction
		Seizures	Weakness
		Confusion	Confusion
			Seizures

SUMMARY

Patients with mental disorders are at an increased risk for dental disease and poor oral health. The dental hygienist must have knowledge of these disorders, as well as an understanding of how the behaviors associated with them and the medications that may be prescribed for treatment can impact the patient's oral health (Table 40-5). The dental hygienist must use this knowledge and critical-thinking skills to tailor individual treatment, education, and recall plans. Major focus should be placed on prevention and education strategies. Both the patient and the caregiver must be included in all planning and education to ensure the success of the dental hygiene process of care for this population of patients.

Table 40-5 Common Medications Prescribed for Mental Disorders[9,10,13,29–32]

Drug	Disorder	Oral Side Effects/ Dental Concerns	Drug Class
Methylphenidate hydrochloride (Ritalin)	Autism	Caution using vasoconstrictors Xerostomia	CNS stimulant
Adderall XR	Autism		Amphetamine
Methylphenidate hydrochloride (Concerta)	Autism	Caution using vasoconstrictors Xerostomia	CNS stimulant
Methylphenidate hydrochloride (Metadate CD)	Autism	Caution using vasoconstrictors Xerostomia	CNS stimulant
Clomipramine (Anafranil)	Autism	Avoid use of epinephrine Avoid products that contain alcohol	Tricyclic antidepressant
Desipramine (Norpramin)	Autism Major depressive disorder	Avoid use of epinephrine	Tricyclic antidepressant
Haloperidol (Haldol)	Autism Antipsychotic Major depressive disorder	Avoid use of epinephrine Xerostomia	Antipsychotic
Fluoxetine (Prozac)	Autism Major depressive disorder	Xerostomia	Antidepressant

Continued

Table 40-5 *Common Medications Prescribed for Mental Disorders*[9,10,13,29–32]—cont'd

Drug	Disorder	Oral Side Effects/ Dental Concerns	Drug Class
Carbamazepine (Tegretol)	Autism Major depressive disorder	Xerostomia	Anticonvulsant
Fluvoxamine (Luvox)	Autism	Xerostomia	Selective serotonin reuptake inhibitor antidepressant
Paroxetine (Paxil)	Autism Major depressive disorder	Xerostomia	Antidepressant
Citalopram (Celexa)	Autism Mood disorder	Xerostomia	Antidepressant
Venlafaxine (Effexor)	Autism Major depressive disorder	Avoid use of epinephrine Xerostomia 3–4 month recall to monitor periodontal tissues	Bicyclic antidepressant
Thioridazine (Mellaril)	Autism Bipolar disorder Schizophrenic disorder	Use vasoconstrictors with caution	Antipsychotic
Chlorpromazine (Thorazine)	Autism Bipolar disorder Schizophrenic disorder	Xerostomia	Antipsychotic
Clozapine (Clozaril)	Autism Schizophrenic disorder	Xerostomia 3–4 month recall	Antipsychotic
Risperidone (Risperdal)	Autism Bipolar disorder Schizophrenic disorder	Xerostomia Use vasoconstrictors with caution	Antipsychotic
Olanzapine (Zyprexa)	Autism Bipolar disorder Schizophrenic disorder	Use vasoconstrictors with caution Xerostomia	Antipsychotic
Ziprasidone (Geodon)	Autism Bipolar disorder Schizophrenic disorder	Xerostomia	Antipsychotic
Quetiapine (Seroquel)	Autism Bipolar disorder Schizophrenic disorder	Avoid use of epinephrine Xerostomia 3–4 month recall	Antipsychotic
Aripiprazole (Abilify)	Autism Bipolar disorder Schizophrenic disorder	May cause side effects such as tardive dyskinesia and akathisia, which may interfere with home care and/or dental hygiene care	Antipsychotic
Lithium	Autism Bipolar disorder	Xerostomia	Antimanic
Valproic acid (Depakene)	Autism Bipolar disorder	Clotting may be affected	Anticonvulsant
Valproic acid (Depakote)	Autism Bipolar disorder	Clotting may be affected	Anticonvulsant
Carbamazepine	Bipolar disorder Autism	Xerostomia	Anticonvulsant

Table 40-5 *Common Medications Prescribed for Mental Disorders*[9,10,13,29–32]—cont'd

Drug	Disorder	Oral Side Effects/ Dental Concerns	Drug Class
Topiramate (Topamax)	Autism Bipolar disorder	Xerostomia	Anticonvulsant
Oxcarbazepine (Trileptal)	Autism Bipolar disorder	Xerostomia	Anticonvulsant
Lamotrigine (Lamictal)	Autism Bipolar disorder	Xerostomia	Antiepileptic
Levetiracetam (Keppra)	Autism	3–4 month recall	Antiepileptic

Case Study

Seth is a 19-year-old college student home for the summer. His mother has scheduled him for a recall dental hygiene appointment. During the medical and dental history review, Seth states that his "mouth and throat are sore." He also mentions that this last semester was very stressful. As the intraoral inspection is performed, the dental hygienist notes Seth's buccal mucosa has areas of bluish white appearance with some white folds, whereas the soft palate and tongue are erythematous, with white areas that can be wiped off with gauze. The dental hygienist also notes a significant decline in Seth's oral health, such as several areas of cervical demineralization and acute gingivitis.

Case Study Exercises

1. What is the likely cause of the white coating observed in Seth's mouth?
   A. Squamous cell carcinoma
   B. Benign migratory glossitis
   C. Aphthous stomatitis
   D. Candidiasis
2. What is the condition noted on Seth's buccal mucosa?
   A. Candidiasis
   B. Leukoedema
   C. Leukoplakia
   D. Reticular lichen planus
3. Based on the background information and assessments, what is the probable cause of Seth's oral conditions?
   A. Alcohol
   B. Cocaine
   C. Cannabis
   D. Methamphetamines

Review Questions

1. All individuals with bulimia purge by inducing vomiting after an eating binge. The dental hygienist can note erosion on the maxillary lingual of all individuals with bulimia.
   A. Both statements are true.
   B. Both statements are false.
   C. The first statement is true, but the second statement is false.
   D. The first statement is false, but the second statement is true.

2. The dental hygienist should include the caregiver in homecare and education plans for which of the following patients?
   A. Patients with autism spectrum disorders
   B. Patients with eating disorders
   C. Patients with bipolar disorder
   D. A and B
   E. B and C

3. Patients suffering from which disorder may need a blood test before dental hygiene treatment?
   A. Schizophrenic disorder
   B. Substance addiction
   C. Mood disorders
   D. Eating disorders

4. Which of the following mood disorders is chronic in nature, with less debilitating episodes?
   A. Major depressive disorder
   B. Bipolar I disorder

C. Bulimia
D. Dysthymic disorder

5. The dental hygienist is most likely to encounter a patient using which of the following substances?
   A. Cannabis
   B. Alcohol
   C. Cocaine
   D. Methamphetamines

Active Learning

1. Go into your clinic and to an empty operatory. Sit in the patient chair. Listen to the sounds in the clinic. What do you notice? What noises might be alarming to the patient with autism spectrum disorder (ASD)? Look around. Determine what equipment and armamentarium might be unsettling for the patient with ASD. What materials and armamentarium, such as gauze, might be a sensory issue for the patient with ASD?

2. Go through the Autism Speaks Family Services Dental Guide available at: http://www.autismspeaks.org/sites/default/files/documents/dentalguide.pdf. Write out a plan for a patient with ASD based on the materials in this toolkit that you could use in your clinic with your patients. Consider how this could be modified for teen and adult patients with ASD.

3. Using the previous two learning styles exercises, participate in a role-playing activity with some classmates. Have one classmate be the patient with ASD and one be the caregiver. Go through the plan you developed with your classmates. ■

REFERENCES

1. Halgin RP, Witbourne SK. *Abnormal Psychology: Clinical Perspectives on Psychological Disorders with DSM-5 Update.* 7th ed. New York: McGraw-Hill; 2013.
2. U.S. Department of Health and Human Services. *Mental Health: A Report of the Surgeon General—Executive Summary.* Rockville, MD: U.S. Department of Health and Human Services, Substance Abuse and Mental Health Services Administration, Center for Mental Health Services, National Institutes of Health, National Institute of Mental Health; 1999.
3. American Psychiatric Association. *Diagnostic and Statistical Manual of Mental Disorders (DSM-5).* 5th ed. Washington, DC: American Psychiatric Publishing; 2013.
4. Jepson B, Johnson J. *Changing the Course of Autism: A Scientific Approach for Parents and Physicians.* Boulder, CO: Sentient Publications; 2007.
5. Waldman HB, Perlman SP, Wong A. Providing dental care for the patient with autism. *J Can Dent Assoc.* 2011;36(9):663-670.
6. Weil TN, Inglehart MR, Habil P. Dental education and dentists' attitudes and behavior concerning patients with autism. *J Dent Educ.* 2010;74(12):1294-1307.
7. Jaber MA. Dental caries experience, oral health status and treatment needs of dental patients with autism. *J Appl Oral Sci.* 2011;19(3):212-217.
8. National Institute of Dental and Craniofacial Research National Oral Health Information Clearing House. *Practical Oral Care for People With Autism.* NIH Publication No. 09-5190. Bethesda, MD: National Institutes of Health; July 2009.
9. Friedlander AH, Mahler ME. Major depressive disorder: psychopathology, medical management and dental implications. *J Am Dent Assoc.* 2001;132(5):629-638.
10. Friedlander AH, Friedlander IK, Marder SR. Bipolar I disorder: psychopathology, medical management and dental implications. *J Am Dent Assoc.* 2002;133:1209-1217.
11. Clark DB. Dental care for the patient with bipolar disorder. *J Can Dent Assoc.* 2003;69(1):20-24.
12. Lin KC. Behavior-associated self-report items in patient charts as predictors of dental appointment avoidance. *J Dent Educ.* 2008;73(2):218-224.
13. Friedlander AH, Marder SR. The psychopathology, medical management and dental implications of schizophrenia. *J Am Dent Assoc.* 2002;133:603-610.
14. Mandel L, Abai S. Diagnosing bulimia nervosa with parotid gland swelling. *J Am Dent Assoc.* 2004;135:613-616.
15. Aranha AC, Eduardo CP, Cordás TA. Eating disorders part II: clinical strategies for dental treatment. *J Contemp Dent Pract.* 2008;9(7):89-96.
16. Lo Russo L, Campisi G, Di Fede O, Di Liberto C, Panzarella V, Lo Muzio L. Oral manifestations of eating disorders: a critical review. *Oral Dis.* 2008;14(6):479-484.
17. Christiansen GJ. Oral care for patients with bulimia. *J Am Dent Assoc.* 2002;133:1689-1691.
18. Substance Abuse and Mental Health Services Administration. Results from the 2010 National Survey on Drug Use and Health: summary of national findings. NSDUH Series H-41, HHS Publication No. (SMA) 11-4658. Rockville, MD: Substance Abuse and Mental Health Services Administration; 2011.
19. Friedlander AH, Marder SR, Pisegna JR, Yagiela JA. Alcohol abuse and dependence: psychopathology, medical management and dental implications. *J Am Dent Assoc.* 2003;134:731-740.

20. Bullock K. Dental care of patients with substance abuse. *Dent Clin North Am.* 1999;43(3):513-526.

21. Rifkind JB. What should I look for when treating an alcoholic patient (current or recovered) in my office? *J Can Dent Assoc.* 2011;77:b114.

22. Cho CM, Hirsch R, Johnstone S. General and oral health implications of cannabis use. *Austral Dent J.* 2005;50(2):70-74.

23. Versteeg PA, Slot DE, van der Velden U, van der Weijden GA. Effect of cannabis usage on the oral environment: a review. *Int J Dent Hyg.* 2008;6(4):315-320.

24. Veitz-Keenan A, Ferraiolo D. Cannabis use and xerostomia. *Dimens Dent Hyg.* 2011;9(11):65-67.

25. Maloney WJ. Significance of cocaine use to dental practice. *NY State Dent J.* 2010;76(6):36-39.

26. Ravenel MC, Salinas CF, Marlow NM, Slate EH, Evans ZP, Miller PM. Methamphetamine abuse and oral health: a pilot study of "meth mouth." *Quintessence Int.* 2012;43(3):229-237.

27. Harris CK, Warnakulasuriya KA, Johnson NW, Gelbier S, Peters TJ. Oral health in alcohol misusers. *Community Dent Health.* 1996;13(4):199-203.

28. Maloney WJ. Significance of cannabis use to dental practice. *NY State Dent J.* 2011;77(3):36-39.

29. Becker DE. Psychotropic drugs: implications for dental practice. *Anesth Prog.* 2011;58(4):166-172.

30. Thase ME, Kupfer DJ. Recent developments in the pharmacotherapy of mood disorders. *J Consult Clin Psychol.* 1996;64(4):646-659.

31. Handen BL, Lubetsky M. Pharmacotherapy in autism and related disorders. *Sch Psychol Q.* 2005;20(2):155-171.

32. Jeske AH, Ulbricht C, Seamon E. *Mosby's Dental Drug Reference.* 11th ed. St. Louis, MO: Mosby Elsevier: 2013.

Chapter 41 | Neurological Impairments

Anne H. Missig, RDH, MA, BA

KEY TERMS

akinesia

amyotrophic lateral
  sclerosis (ALS)

aphasia

asthenia

Bell palsy (BP)

biological marker

bradykinesia

bulbar muscles

cerebral palsy (CP)

chorea

diplopia

dysarthria

dysphagia

dysphonia

dystonia

familial

festination

hemianopsia

Huntington disease (HD)

hyperacusis

hypertonic

intention tremors

myasthenia gravis (MG)

neurological impairments

Parkinson disease (PD)

photophobia

ptosis

scoliosis

somnolence

stroke

tachycardia

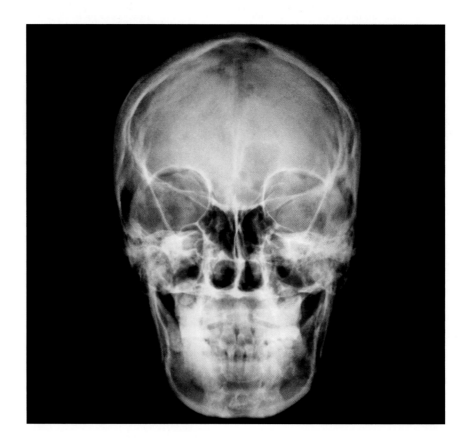

LEARNING OBJECTIVES

After reading this chapter, the student should be able to:

41.1 Identify the categories of neurological impairments.

41.2 Describe the common neurological impairments and their symptoms.

41.3 Identify common medications prescribed for neurological impairments including predominant contraindications or precautions, adverse reactions, and side effects.

41.4 Identify the effects of neurological impairments on the oral condition.

41.5 Assess patient/client needs based on data collection.

41.6 Develop an individualized treatment (care) plan including implementation strategies for modifications based on assessment of patient/client needs.

41.7 Develop individualized health-promoting goals and strategies for home care and maintenance.

41.8 Present and explain the home-care plan to the patient and caregiver.

KEY CONCEPTS

- Using critical thinking and sensitivity during the dental hygiene assessment is vital to developing adaptive methods of treatment delivery.
- Confidence in the dental hygienist's education and skill development enhances the comfort level of interacting and communicating with and treating the patient with neurological impairment.
- Modified treatment modalities maximize patient safety, comfort, and response.
- Interdisciplinary assessment and treatment planning results in comprehensive, total health outcomes.

RELEVANCE TO CLINICAL PRACTICE

Neurological disorders affect up to 1 billion people worldwide.[1] It is estimated that just more than 50 million Americans are affected by a neurological disorder, which equates to 1 in 6 people (World Health Organization [WHO], as reported by the American Academy of Neurology, A. Babb, Associate Director, Media and Public Relations, and D. Hoch, Department of Neurology, Massachusetts General Hospital, e-mail communication, September 2, 2010).[1] Some of the most common causes of neurological impairments are projected to increase substantially worldwide by the years 2017 and 2030.[1] Consequently, the number of patients with neurological impairments whom the dental hygienist will treat will also increase proportionately. The most recent survey results (2008) revealed that only 42% of dental hygiene programs require students to gain clinical experiences with patients with special needs.[2] It has and will become increasingly necessary for dental hygiene students to gain the experience and confidence in recognizing and treating patients with neurological impairments throughout the entire educational process. This chapter provides a comprehensive overview of the patient with neurological impairment and assists dental hygienists in developing a perspective of flexibility in modifying and adapting treatment modalities based on their patient assessments (see Chapter 8) and needs. It also focuses on enhancing effective communication skills among the patient, provider, and caregiver.

WHAT ARE NEUROLOGICAL IMPAIRMENTS?

Definition

Neurological impairments are disorders of the central nervous system[1] composed of the brain and spinal cord. They may include any loss or abnormality of psychological, physiological, or anatomical structure or function.[1]

Categories

Neurological impairments may be rated based on the level of impact that the condition has on the performance of activities of daily living.[3] When specific to the brain, they may be categorized as sensory and motor disturbances (Fig. 41-1), emotional disturbances, consciousness disorders, episodic neurological disorders, and sleep and arousal disorders. When specific to the spinal cord, they include station and gait, use of upper extremities, respiration, urinary bladder function, anal rectal function, and sexual function.[4] Symptoms are usually categorized more broadly in terms of physical or motor, cognitive or memory, affect or psychological, sensory, visual or perceptual, and communication.

COMMON NEUROLOGICAL IMPAIRMENTS

This chapter provides a broad overview of some of the most common neurological impairments and their

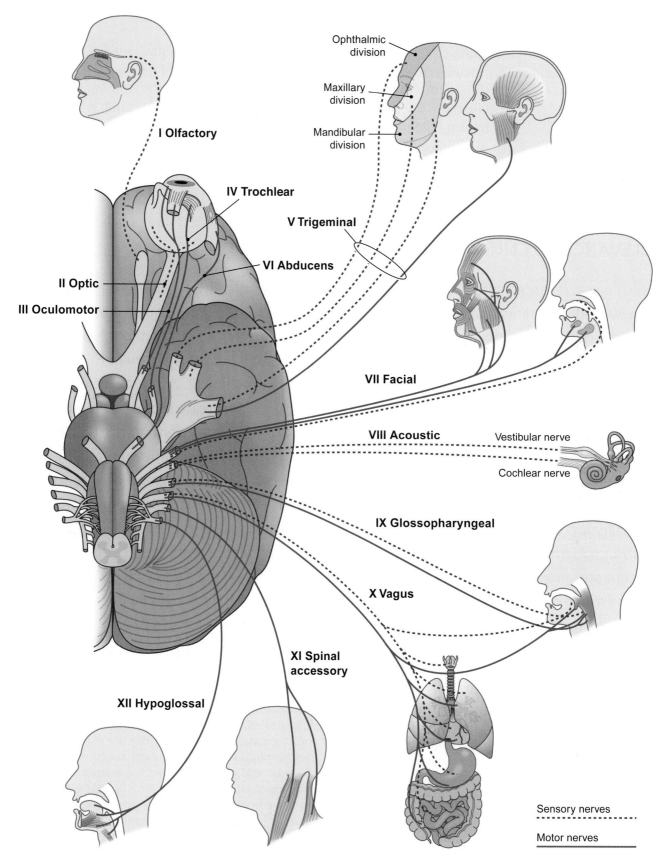

Figure 41-1. Sensory and motor nerves.

symptoms. Neurological impairments can occur from an anomaly or manifest suddenly such as from a stroke or brain injury. Some impairments may be temporary, resulting in partial paralysis of the face or limbs, whereas others may affect or limit speech or vision. The hygienist will need to be comfortable categorizing neurological impairments by symptom. Recognizing the symptoms of some of the most common neurological impairments will assist the dental hygienist in assessing patient needs. The dental hygienist will then be able to develop a treatment plan based on specific patient needs and modify the treatment delivery to optimize patient safety, comfort, and response.

Amyotrophic Lateral Sclerosis

Amyotrophic lateral sclerosis (ALS), often called Lou Gehrig disease,[5] is a serious neuromuscular disease resulting in muscle weakness, disability, and eventually death. No specific therapy exists for ALS, and the median survival time from onset is 25 months. Scientists have not yet identified a reliable **biological marker** (a biochemical abnormality shared by all patients with the disease) for ALS. As many as 20,000 Americans have ALS, and an estimated 5,000 people in the United States are diagnosed each year.[6]

Characteristically, some of the early signs and symptoms of ALS include weakness in legs, feet, or ankles; hand weakness or clumsiness; slurring of speech or trouble swallowing; muscle cramps and twitching in arms, shoulders, and tongue. It usually begins in the limbs and spreads to other parts of the body.[5] Eventually, all muscles under voluntary control are affected. When muscles in the diaphragm and chest wall fail, patients lose the ability to breathe without ventilator support.[7]

Dental Hygiene Considerations

Patient safety and comfort should be the hygienist's primary concern when considering any modifications to the delivery of dental hygiene services for patients with ALS. Given the rapid progression of the disease, the hygienist may notice an accelerated onset of symptoms from one visit to the next.

As the disease progresses, it is probable that all communication will be through a family member or caregiver. The patient may be transported to the office in a wheelchair and accompanied by a family member or caregiver. However, it is more likely that the patient will need to be treated at home or an alternate practice setting. To provide care in the patient's home, the hygienist will need to be equipped with portable devices, including a cordless slow-speed handpiece, a portable evacuation system, magnification loops with an illumination attachment, and an ultrasonic scaler with a reservoir. A hospital setting may provide easier access and have some of the equipment necessary. The hygienist with a direct access permit to patients in alternate practice settings will need to visit the patient's surroundings to do a complete assessment of supply and equipment needs (see Professionalism).

Professionalism

As a licensed oral health-care provider, you have a legal and ethical obligation to provide the highest standard of care while protecting the safety of your patients. As a licensed professional, you take these obligations very seriously. How are these obligations derived? Your professional association was created to ensure the long-term sustainability of the practice of dental hygiene and provide guidelines for the governance of your professional association. The right and scope of practice is predicated by each state's laws, as is the governance of your professional association. When you become a member, you take an active role in securing the future of your chosen profession. Although you may not choose to serve in leadership roles, your membership is an act of support. When you become a member of your professional association, you become a part of the collective that work to secure your future and your livelihood. As a member of your professional association, you have a voice. Your membership enables you to elect leaders who will represent you and the best interest of your profession. Your leaders take directives from you to the legislative body that creates the laws under which you practice. Because legislators are elected officials, they have an obligation to represent you. You are considered a "grassroots" member of your state or "constituent." Because the leaders of your professional association represent you, they can take not only your concerns but those of the entire membership to the legislators.

In 2009, California passed legislation to create the Dental Hygiene Committee of California. It became the first self-regulating committee for the profession of dental hygiene of its kind in the United States. This could not have been possible without the diligence and support of the members of the California Dental Hygienists' Association. In 2010, Ohio became the 38th state to pass direct access legislation, permitting the dental hygienist to be the first responder in an alternate practice setting. These two types of legislation are the result of dental hygienists working behind the scenes to secure and advance *your* profession.

Will *you* take an active role in securing your profession? All you have to do is become a member of your professional association. *You* have a voice. One person can make a difference. ■

It is important for the hygienist to review the prescribed medications the patient is currently taking and to evaluate the impact of side effects on treatment delivery. Patients with ALS may experience side effects such as dizziness, **somnolence** (severe drowsiness), and asthenia (weakness). Side effects such as dizziness or vertigo[5,6] will prevent the patient from being reclined too quickly or treated in a supine position.

The hygienist will need to use four-handed hygiene (the use of a dental auxiliary to assist the hygienist during treatment delivery) to prevent choking and aspiration, especially if the patient is bedridden or already on ventilator support.

Home Care

Considering the rapid progression of ALS, the primary focus of home care will be quality of life. Instructions will need to be directed to the caregiver while demonstrating on the patient. This is most important for proper technique to prevent any complications for the patient. Maintaining optimum oral hygiene will help to minimize or prevent any contributions to disease progression.

Bell Palsy

Bell palsy (BP) is caused by unilateral inflammation of the seventh cranial nerve, which results in weakness or paralysis of the facial muscles on the affected side.[6] It is associated with the herpes simplex or varicella virus infections, and more than 60,000 cases are diagnosed each year in the United States.[8] The paralysis is almost always confined to one side of the face and is subject to recurrence. Symptoms progress very quickly, with the individual waking up to dry eye or tingling around the lips that progresses to classic BP in the same day. Symptoms typically peak within a few days, but can take as long as 2 weeks.

General symptoms associated with facial paralysis include disappearance of forehead wrinkles, overall droopy appearance, nose runs or constant stuffiness, **dysarthria** (difficulty speaking), difficulty eating and drinking, **hyperacusis** (sensitivity to sound), facial swelling or soreness, and pain in or near the ear. Symptoms specific to the mouth include excessive or reduced salivation, diminished or distorted taste, and dry mouth or drooling. After paralysis, facial muscles have a tendency to become **hypertonic,** which means they become overactive, contracting when they should be at rest. Examples may be a squinty eye, difficult or impossible closure of the eyelid, lack of or excessive tears, or drooping eyebrow or lid. In addition, the patient will experience the mouth pulling up and **photophobia** (sensitivity to light).[9]

Dental Hygiene Considerations

When considering modifications to the treatment plan, the dental hygienist should exhibit a heightened sensitivity to the psychological impact of facial paralysis on patients with BP (see Application to Clinical Practice 41-1). Although the symptoms, their severity, and their duration may vary, the patient may exhibit residual effects if recovery is prolonged. It is important for the hygienist to communicate openly with the patient and inquire about both the symptoms the patient

---

Application to Clinical Practice 41-1

Mrs. Saunders arrived early for her 8:00 a.m. appointment. She is always joyful and ready to share her latest adventure. This morning, however, you notice a slightly agitated demeanor. You inquire if everything is all right. Mrs. Saunders indicates that "something just isn't right." She tells you that she woke up with tingling around her lips, but only on the left side, and she noticed that her left eye was a bit dry. She almost canceled her appointment because she thought she was getting a head cold. You document her symptoms and concerns in her chart, but initially you were not alarmed. Three quarters of the way through Mrs. Saunders's appointment, you notice she is becoming fidgety and asks if she can sit up. At this point you are fairly certain that Mrs. Saunders is exhibiting the symptoms of BP. As you sit her up, you observe that her face is noticeably droopy. Because all of your patients wear dark protective eyewear, you were not aware that Mrs. Saunders was having difficulty closing her left eye. This is what was causing her anxiety and desire to take a break. How will you effectively communicate your assessment of the symptoms she is exhibiting and help her to remain calm? What is your next course of action? ▪

---

is experiencing and the possible side effects from medications that have been prescribed.

If the patient is experiencing sensitivity to sound, or pain in or near the ears, consider treatment in a closed operatory to avoid excessive noise levels from surrounding activity. If salivation is excessive, the hygienist will either need to keep a saliva ejector in the patient's mouth throughout treatment or consider four-handed hygiene to prevent aspiration or choking. If salivation is reduced, then the hygienist will need to factor in frequent breaks to moisten the soft tissues and throat.

Protective eye wear or sunglasses should be available for patients who are unable to close their eyes or who experience sensitivity to light. Many patients will bring their own protective eyewear. The patient should be slowly reclined with brief pauses to accommodate side effects of medication such as dizziness.[9–11]

It is likely that Caries Management by Risk Assessment (CAMBRA) may reveal high risk for caries due to any combination of symptoms including swollen cheeks, reduced saliva, difficulty eating or drinking, and diminished taste. The hygienist may want to add nutritional counseling as part of the treatment plan to address types of food and drink that will be easier to digest and healthier for the patient experiencing difficulty eating or drinking.

Home Care

As part of the home-care plan, the hygienist should consider recommending or including products to increase salivation and daily fluoride rinses to help prevent or reduce caries. The use of an oral irrigation system will assist the patient in disrupting the biofilm and eliminating any undetected food debris.

Cerebral Palsy

Cerebral palsy (CP) is a nonprogressive neuromuscular disorder caused by brain abnormalities or damage. Resulting impairments may be characterized as sensory, motor, and emotional disturbances, and they include seizure disorders and cognitive disorders.[12-14] The four different types of CP are broadly classified according to associated motor impairments. They include spastic palsy, dyskinetic or athetoid palsy, ataxic palsy, and combined palsy.

- Spastic palsy is characterized by stiff or rigid muscles. It is identified by location or number of limbs affected. It may affect the arm and hand on one side of the body (hemi) and can also include the leg. The weakness may involve both legs (di) with less impact on the arms. The most severe form of spastic palsy involves all four limbs (quad) and is often associated with moderate-to-severe mental retardation.

  Physical symptoms may be confined to one side where the arm and leg of the affected side are shorter and thinner. Speech may be delayed. Children affected usually walk later and on tiptoe, and they may develop **scoliosis** (abnormal curvature of the spine) or experience seizures. When both legs are affected, tendon reflexes are hyperactive, toes point up, leg muscles tighten, and movement mimics the actions of scissors. Leg braces or a walker may be required. When spastic palsy becomes severe, the symptoms include stiffness of all limbs but with a floppy neck, frequent and uncontrollable seizures, and dysarthria, and patients are rarely able to walk.

- Dyskinetic or athetoid palsy is characterized by writhing movements. The physical symptoms of this palsy are characterized by slow and uncontrollable writhing movements of the hands, feet, arms, or legs. These patients may exhibit difficulty in coordinating speech, and drooling or grimacing may result from hyperactivity of facial muscles and tongue.

- Ataxic palsy is a rare form of CP that is characterized by poor balance, coordination, and depth perception. Physical symptoms are exhibited in a wide-based gait that may be unsteady and uncoordinated. Patients have difficulty with quick or precise movements and may also experience **intention tremors** (i.e., trembling during voluntary movement).

- Mixed palsy may exhibit a combination of any of the earlier described symptoms.[13,14]

Dental Hygiene Considerations

When considering modifications to the dental hygiene treatment plan, the hygienist should first consider which type of CP the patient has.

- Although the patient with spastic palsy may use a walker, it is likely that a wheelchair will be used for portability when experiencing weakness or spasticity in either or both of the legs. These patients may require assistance in transferring from the wheelchair to the treatment chair. The hygienist may assist the patient or use a transfer board to slide the patient into position (Fig. 41-2).

- Patients with severe spastic palsy will be confined to a wheelchair. It is possible that the hygienist will be treating the patient with severe spastic palsy in an alternate practice setting (see Teamwork). If the patient

Teamwork

The office where you are primarily employed has decided, as a team, to give back to the community by volunteering their services on a bimonthly basis. Various members of the team will be visiting a number of local group homes overseen by Community Alternative Programs/Department of Developmental Disabilities (formerly CAP/MRDD). One particular group home is dedicated to accommodating eight adult residents with CP. Both you and the dentist will be applying for an Access Supervision Permit and will be contracted with the Department of Developmental Disabilities. As the hygienist, you and the hygiene assistant will be the first responders to the home. Release forms will be forwarded to the office before scheduled hygiene appointments, together with the medical history of each patient, which you will update the day before. You will be responsible for creating all electronic patient files, completing assessments, updating medical and dental histories, and providing all preventive services. The hygiene assistant will be responsible for all electronic documentation and charting, assisting you with any four-handed hygiene services, and sterilization support. You will both share responsibilities of transporting portable equipment, supplies, and setup. The dentist will review all supporting and diagnostic documentation and formulate a preliminary treatment plan for each patient. In addition to the dentist, the team will be composed of an expanded functions dental auxiliary and a certified dental assistant. The team will spend 2 days completing patient examinations and all simple restorative treatment, and will begin those treatments that require multiple visits. Communication is crucial to the success of this type of community service project. What would you suggest as the best method for these two teams to communicate their plans and maintain cohesion? ■

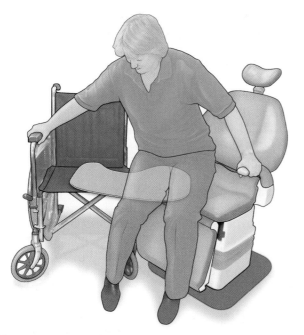

Figure 41-2. Transfer board.

is experiencing floppy head or uncontrollable seizures, an attachable headrest is advisable. Many headrests have attached head restraints that would also help to protect the patient during instrumentation. The patient may already have a motorized chair, many of which come with an attached headrest as standard equipment.

The hygienist will want to take advantage of any portable equipment to prevent strain and maintain an ergonomically correct posture during instrumentation. Portable equipment would include the use of loops with attachable illumination and a cordless handpiece. The hygienist will want to provide a calm, soothing environment to assist in minimizing seizures. The patient and hygienist may want to have the caregiver present for the patient experiencing dysarthria or have procedural/instructional picture boards available.

- The patient with dyskinetic or athetoid palsy experiences uncontrollable writhing and rigid muscles during the day and may benefit from a calm environment to help reduce the frequency. It may be necessary to cradle the patient's head during instrumentation. The hygienist will need to verbally communicate any change in procedure or patient position to minimize stress.[13]

If the patient has excessive drooling or a hyperactive tongue, the use of four-handed hygiene will prevent the patient from choking and keep the tongue retracted. These patients are also subject to malocclusion as a result of weakened facial muscles. It is likely that the patient is at risk for caries and should receive fluoride varnish treatments at every appointment; the patient may also benefit from sealants.

- The patient with ataxic palsy may have an unsteady gait and require the assistance of the hygienist in walking back to the operatory. If altered depth perception or dizziness from medications is an issue, the hygienist can assist the patient into the operatory chair and position the chair in slow increments. The hygienist may also advise the patient to keep his or her eyes closed during instrumentation and use four-handed hygiene to aspirate to help prevent the patient from being startled by any sudden movement. This will also eliminate any hand-to-mouth requirements of the patient.

Home Care

The goal of home care is to optimize total health through the prevention of caries and periodontal disease and by reducing the risk of damage to teeth. A family member or caregiver should be included during home-care instructions. The patient with severe CP who is subject to seizures will be at risk for chipped or broken teeth. Although caregivers may not be able to prevent a seizure, they can ensure that nothing is in the patient's mouth that will contribute to damage or choking.

Patients with malocclusion, or open bite, which contributes to mouth breathing, are at risk for caries and periodontal disease. In addition, xerostomia, which may be a negative side effect of medication, also increases the risk for caries. Daily fluoride rinses are advisable and over-the-counter products can be recommended to restore moisture to the mouth. The use of an electric toothbrush and oral irrigation system will disrupt the biofilm and ensure that no food debris is trapped in the vestibules. An antimicrobial rinse, such as chlorhexidine, can be diluted and used in the oral irrigation device to reduce the risk for periodontal disease. Demonstrate technique to the caregiver if the patient is not physically able to perform these activities. It would be advisable to educate both the patient and the caregiver about the potential for gingival hyperplasia as a negative side effect of antiseizure medications. This will need to be monitored and the patient may require more frequent cleanings.[10,14]

Huntington Disease

Huntington disease (HD) is a progressively degenerative, inherited brain disorder. It is **familial** (passed from parent to child). Each person who inherits the HD gene mutation will eventually develop the disease.[15] Approximately 30,000 Americans have HD, and it is currently estimated that 1 in every 10,000 people in the United States has this disease. As of 1993, genetic testing has made it possible for "at-risk" individuals to determine whether they are carriers of the disease.

Symptoms usually develop in individuals between the ages of 30 and 50 years and will progress over a 10- to 25-year period. They are characterized by progressive physical, cognitive, and psychological deterioration. Physical symptoms manifest as **chorea** (quick, dancelike, uncontrollable movements of the limbs). Movements tend to be grossly exaggerated. As the disease progresses, **dystonia** (constant writhing, twisting, uncontrollable movement) may involve the entire body. Eventually muscle stiffness or rigidity may occur, as well as **dysphagia** (difficulty in swallowing).

Cognitive changes result in hampered organizational skills. Patients may exhibit difficulty in processing information or remembering words. Speech becomes increasingly challenged. It may be slurred, hesitant, explosive, and eventually unintelligible.[6,16] Patients with HD may experience short-term memory loss and poor judgment. Psychologically, the patient may exhibit uncontrolled impulses or emotions, irritability, or anxiety. It is not uncommon for those individuals in a chronic condition to experience mild to severe depression.

Dental Hygiene Considerations

Modifications to the dental hygiene care plan will be determined based on the severity of the physical, cognitive, and psychological progression of the disease.[6] Because of ambulatory limitations and the degenerative nature of this disease, the patient with HD may be cared for at home with the assistance of respite care or in a long-term care facility or a hospital setting where multidisciplinary assistance is available (see Technology). The latter may be predicated on access to and the availability of dental hygiene services in alternate practice settings, and would be beneficial when considering side effects from medications such as seizures or **tachycardia** (abnormally rapid heartbeat).[10]

Patients with HD are not able to open their mouths very wide or for very long. Mouth props can be used to relieve tension and strain to the jaw and facial muscles. Patients should not be tilted or supine because of dysphasia and the possibility of choking.

Patients with HD experience uncontrollable movement in the face, tongue, and limbs. It is unlikely that they will be able to sit for long periods. Every precaution should be taken to prevent the patient from being harmed.

Preventive dental hygiene care should be provided more frequently based on risk assessments for caries and periodontal disease. This includes frequent applications of fluoride varnish. If frequent, short visits are not an option, it may be necessary for the patient to be sedated to afford the patient the most thorough treatment in one visit.[17]

Home Care

The goal for the home-care plan is to provide the caregiver with an overview of the devices available to accomplish the disruption of biofilm and plaque removal in the shortest period, or incorporating brief intervals. Demonstrating the use of a power toothbrush and a cordless irrigation device and handheld catch basin or bowl will assist the caregiver in achieving this primary goal.

Myasthenia Gravis

Myasthenia gravis (MG) is considered to be relatively rare, and there is still no certainty about the cause of this disease. Yet, it is the most common primary autoimmune disorder of neuromuscular transmission. MG is characterized by **asthenia** (varying degrees of weakness of voluntary muscles) that is usually progressive. Typically, muscles contract when receptor sites at the neuromuscular junction have been activated by

---

Technology

Technological advances in the dental field have increasingly served to remove barriers that, in the past, have hindered or prevented the hygienist from providing services to the disenfranchised populations across the country. Today, it is possible for the hygienist to overcome just about every barrier in meeting the needs of patients where they are located, including in the comfort of their own homes.

Virtual dentistry is one way in which the dental hygienist can provide optimum preventive services in the least invasive manner. In California, the concept of the virtual dental home has begun to emerge using teledentistry as a means of fostering collaboration between community-based oral health professionals and dental offices and clinics.[35]

Consider how the neurologically impaired patient can and will benefit from virtual dentistry. What are some of the current advances being introduced that can be incorporated into the treatment plan? For example, review the following list and think about how the dental hygienist would incorporate these tools into the treatment plan of a homebound patient with an advanced neurological disorder such as HD or PD. Develop a modified treatment plan incorporating the following items.

  Digital radiographs
  Intraoral camera
  Web cam
  Cordless prophy handpiece
  Voice-activated perioprobe
  Salivary DNA testing
  Magnification loops with an illumination attachment
  Portable evacuation system
  Dental software
  Caries detection devices
     What other equipment or devices might be added?. ■

acetylcholine. In patients with MG, as much as 80% of the acetylcholine receptor sites are destroyed or blocked by antibodies produced by the host. It is approximated that there are between 36,000 and 60,000 cases in the United States, and women are affected more frequently than men.[6,18–20]

Initially, the impairments manifest as ocular motor disturbances in approximately two thirds of patients. Symptoms include **diplopia** (double vision) and **ptosis** (drooping eyelids). However, a large majority of patients also experience impairments to **bulbar muscles** (mouth and throat muscles responsible for eating and talking), manifesting in facial or oropharyngeal muscles weakness. Symptoms include difficulty chewing or swallowing, **dysphonia** (speaking or voice impairments), and altered or bland facial expressions. A myasthenic crisis may occur when the disease process has been exacerbated. It is characterized by severe weakness of bulbar and respiratory muscles. These crises require immediate medical attention and ventilation assistance. They are most often caused by a respiratory infection. Additional precipitating triggers include change in medications, surgery, fever, or pregnancy.

Dental Hygiene Considerations

Modifications to the dental hygiene treatment plan will focus on the symptoms and side effects that directly impact the oral cavity. The first consideration is to assess the patient's ability to effectively communicate. If the patient experiences symptoms of dysphonia, the hygienist will want to provide an alternative, such as a writing pad or electronic keyboard.

Patients tend to have more strength in the morning and can endure activities with less stress. Muscles become progressively weaker throughout the day and may coincide with the durational effects of some medications.[21,22] The hygienist should schedule appointments in the morning, but for a shorter duration and more frequent intervals. If the patient is not able to accommodate more frequent appointments, then frequent breaks should be factored into the scheduled time. It may be advisable to schedule the patient's appointment 1.5 hours after he or she has taken an oral cholinesterase inhibitor, which will allow for optimized effects during the appointment time.[21]

Weakened facial muscles may prevent the patient from keeping his or her mouth open for long periods. The hygienist will want to use a bite block or mouth prop to prevent tension to the muscles and to relieve stress, which can aggravate MG.

Patients who have been prescribed pyridostigmine bromide may experience excessive salivation.[10] The patient may want to be in control of the saliva ejector to ensure that he or she is getting adequate aspiration during instrumentation.

The patient may experience any combination of symptoms such as difficulty swallowing and weakened respiratory muscles. When this is the case, the hygienist should consider reclining the patient to only a 45° angle or allowing the patient to remain in an upright position during treatment.

Vomiting is a common side effect of most of the medications the patient may be taking.[10] The hygienist will want to be aware of signs of teeth erosion and perform regular CAMBRA. If the patient has been prescribed cyclosporine, the hygienist will want to monitor the gingival tissue for indications of hyperplasia.

Home Care

The primary goal of home-care instructions for the patient with MG is optimized prevention. The hygienist will want to demonstrate the use of an oral irrigation device to ensure daily disruption of the biofilm and removal of trapped food debris as a result of weakened facial muscles.

Parkinson Disease

Parkinson disease (PD) is a neurological impairment that is part of a larger group of motor system disorders (see Application to Clinical Practice 41-2). The most common form of PD is identified as degenerative or idiopathic. It is a slowly progressing disease associated with decreased levels of dopamine produced in cells located in the basal ganglia region of the brain. The decreased levels of dopamine result from the destruction of pigmented neuronal cells, and clinical symptoms

Application to Clinical Practice 41-2

Workforce projections indicate that dental hygiene is one of the fastest growing professions. By the year 2018, the number of dental hygienists employed will increase by 36% over 2008 actual numbers.[34] Based on these projections, discuss nontraditional opportunities for the dental hygienist, such as research. Is it possible that you could be responsible for the next breakthrough that might have a direct impact on the neurologically impaired patient? For example, despite controversy regarding stem cell research, harvesting of stem cells from deciduous teeth has been proposed. Research the viability of this option. What would be the implications for the use of stem cells with a neurological impairment such as PD?

Feasibility studies were held during the American Dental Hygienists' Association's Annual Session held in Orlando, Florida, in June 2006 that pertained to educational requirements and credentialing for the profession of dental hygiene. Should the profession of dental hygiene expand the educational process to include specialty areas of study, such as treating the neurologically impaired patient? Should there be specific credentials for these specialty areas of study? ■

do not appear until 60% of these pigmented neurons are lost. The first symptoms of PD usually appear in individuals in their fifties; however, there have been cases as early as 30 years of age.[6,23,24]

The symptoms of PD appear over a prolonged period. Complex body movements are impaired, resulting in four major categories of primary motor symptoms: tremors, bradykinesia, akinesia, and postural instability.[6,24,25]

- Tremors are the earliest and most noticeable symptoms present in 75% of patients. They may manifest as localized, slow, rhythmic motion such as in the thumb and fingers of one hand. Over time, they may spread to the entire limb or may occur in the lips, feet, or tongue. Tremors often occur when the patient is at rest and increase while walking, concentrating, or feeling anxious.
- **Bradykinesia** (slowness of motion) is one of the most common symptoms of PD. Patients have difficulty initiating movement and take longer to complete activities. Movements may become increasingly slower and may randomly "freeze." This can be experienced with both bradykinesia and akinesia.
- **Akinesia,** or muscle rigidity, is resistance to passive limb movement. Akinesia causes the limbs to move in jerky increments, referred to as *cogwheeling.* Stiffness in posture or in the extremities is common. It may also affect the face, resulting in a masklike stare. Rigidity may cause pain and cramping.
- Patients may experience instability when standing or impaired balance and coordination, and may have difficulty in pivoting. Patients may walk with short, shuffling steps **(festination),** also known as propulsive gait (Fig. 41-3).

Various secondary symptoms are related to PD. Autonomic symptoms may include excessive or uncontrolled sweating (hot flashes), gastric dysfunction (inability to process food), constipation and urinary retention, or

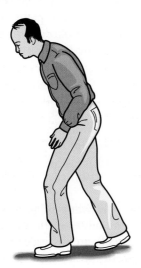

Figure 41-3. Patients with Parkinson disease may walk with propulsive gait, or short, shuffling steps.

sexual dysfunction. Symptoms of a psychological nature may include depression, dementia, sleep disturbances, and hallucinations. Symptoms specific to the oral cavity involve weakness in the coordination of muscles responsible for speech resulting in dysphonia or dysphagia, or both. Patients may exhibit a constant drool, increasing their risk for choking or aspiration.

Dental Hygiene Considerations

Modifications to the dental hygiene treatment plan for the patient with PD will depend on the progression of the disease. Because PD occurs most often in older individuals, there may be an increased probability that additional medical conditions exist, along with multiple medications. This may also be the case if the patient is exhibiting secondary symptoms from the disease, such as those that are autonomic or psychological. The hygienist will want to develop an interdisciplinary treatment plan based on consultation(s) with the treating physician(s). Because of the prevalence of tremors, the hygienist will need to exercise caution during instrumentation because these tremors can occur in the lip and tongue as well as the extremities. The hygienist can use a mouth prop to assist the patient in keeping his or her mouth open while relieving stress to the muscles and temporomandibular joint. It is important for the patient to be treated in a calm, quiet environment, such as a closed operatory.

Depending on the severity of the tremors, the hygienist may want to consider offering sedation as an option before treatment. The benefits to the patient are reduced stress, tremors, and need for multiple appointments.

The patient should be treated in an upright position, and the hygienist may want to consider four-handed hygiene for those patients who have difficulty swallowing, are at risk for choking, or who experience excessive drooling. Regular CAMBRA is recommended because of the high incidence of xerostomia and nausea as negative side effects from medications. This would also be an indication for increased fluoride applications. Other negative side effects from medications, such as dizziness or hypotension, may warrant caution when raising a patient from a supine position.[10,25]

Home Care

The goal for home care is to promote quality of life through the prevention of dental disease and periodontal infections. Daily disruption of biofilm with the use of an electric toothbrush and oral irrigation system will promote healthy gingival tissue. The benefits of an oral irrigation system are stimulation of the gingival tissues, disruption of the biofilm, and removal of any food debris that has been lodged or trapped in the vestibules. The addition of antimicrobials to the oral irrigation system will help with periodontal maintenance and assist in preventing infections, as well as destroying sulfides on the surface of the tongue. Many electronic devices are now equipped with attachments for flossing and tongue scraping. Products that restore moisture to the mouth or replace saliva can be recommended for patients who experience xerostomia. Products that contain xylitol can stimulate saliva and reduce the risk for caries. If the patient requires the assistance of a caregiver, it will be important to explain and demonstrate home-care instructions with the caregiver present.

Stroke

Stroke (ischemic or hemorrhagic) falls under the blanket term of cerebrovascular disorders resulting from a disruption of the blood supply to the brain, leading to neurological impairments of the central nervous system. It is considered the primary cerebrovascular disorder in the United States, with an estimated 795,000 cases occurring each year. Of those cases, one quarter will be recurrent. Stroke is also the third leading cause of death in the United States, which equates to approximately 137,000 deaths a year.[6,26–28] Cerebrovascular disorders comprise 55% of all neurological disorders globally. Based on projections by the WHO, it is expected that the incidents of cerebrovascular disease will increase to nearly 61 million cases by 2030.[1]

The two primary categories of stroke are ischemic stroke and hemorrhagic stroke. Ischemic strokes, also known as a cerebrovascular accident or a brain attack, result from a sudden interruption of blood flow to the brain.[29] Ischemic strokes account for approximately 87% of all cases. They are typically caused by an obstruction within the blood vessel, such as from a blood clot. Hemorrhagic strokes are caused by bleeding into the brain tissue. They occur when a weakened blood vessel ruptures, such as in an aneurysm or arteriovenous malformations.

Stroke victims may experience any number of neurological impairments, the effects of which depend primarily on the location and extent of brain tissue affected, broadly defined as right or left hemispheric. Right hemispheric effects produce paralysis on the left side of the body, left vision deficits, impulsive behavior or poor judgment, memory loss, and heightened distractibility. Left hemispheric effects produce paralysis on the right side of the body, right vision deficits, **aphasia** (speech or language deficits), altered intellectual ability, slow, cautious behavior, and memory loss. Should a stroke occur localized to the brainstem, both sides of the body can be affected. The best way to identify the most common symptoms is by category, as previously described in this chapter. Symptoms of motor impairment include hemiparesis, hemiplegia, ataxia, dysarthria, or dysphagia. Cognitive impairments may include short- or long-term memory loss, decreased attention span, an inability to concentrate, altered judgment, and diminished reasoning skills. Sensory impairments include paresthesia manifesting on the opposite side to where damage occurred in the brain. Visual impairments include diplopia, loss of peripheral vision, and **hemianopsia** (loss of half of visual field). Communication impairments include all manifestations of aphasia. Psychological impairments include depression; withdrawal; stress intolerance; emotional outbursts or expressions of fear, hostility, and anger; and loss of self-control.[6,26]

Dental Hygiene Considerations

A proactive approach to treatment planning is the key to preventing stroke or the recurrence of stroke. As the prevention specialist, the licensed dental hygienist is uniquely positioned to identify and educate his or her patients about modifiable and nonmodifiable risk factors for stroke. Nonmodifiable risk factors would include age, heredity, race, sex, and history of prior stroke or transient ischemic attacks. Modifiable risk factors include hypertension (high blood pressure), cigarette smoking, diabetes mellitus, carotid artery stenosis, arterial fibrillation, coronary heart disease, high blood cholesterol, poor diet, obesity, excessive alcohol consumption, drug abuse, and physical inactivity.[6,29]

Modifications to the dental hygiene treatment plan will focus on prevention. The hygienist will begin with assessment findings that identify risk factors that predispose the patient to stroke. The emphasis should be on patient education that correlates the risk factors for stroke with the risk factors for periodontal disease, as well as the systemic link to overall health and wellness. Periodontal disease not only predisposes the patient to stroke, but is also systemically linked to the risk factors for stroke including smoking, coronary heart disease, and diabetes. If the patient exhibits any of the risk factors for stroke, the hygienist should review the warning signs previously mentioned in this chapter. Because no risk factors can be modified, developing an interdisciplinary treatment plan will assist the patient in taking an active role in the treatment process, as well as helping the patient to comprehend the expected outcomes. Discuss patient risk factors and any recommendations with the patient's treating physician, and ask about any recommendations or programs he or she may have already suggested to the patient.

When the patient has high blood pressure, the hygienist will want to monitor and document findings at every appointment. Encourage patients who smoke to quit. Refer them to the smoking cessation hotline and provide fact sheets on the benefits and products available to assist them.

Patients with diabetes may need to be put on more frequent recare intervals because they are more susceptible to periodontal disease and impaired healing. Nutritional counseling and a low-impact exercise plan should be included in the dental hygiene treatment plan and monitored or reviewed at each visit for those patients with poor diet, who are physically inactive, or are obese.

The hygienist will want to be aware of dietary changes that have an adverse affect on anticoagulants. For example, dark leafy greens and some vegetables are high in vitamin K. Because warfarin blocks vitamin K to slow the clotting process, introducing it back in to the diet will counteract the effects of the medication and put the patient at risk. It is more advisable for the patient to maintain consistency in his or her diet.[30] The reverse effects can occur with patients taking antibiotics, such as tetracyclines, in combination with warfarin, causing the risk for increased bleeding. Because of the aggressive nature of anticoagulants, the patient's prescribing physician will be monitoring his or her clotting factor on a regular basis using the standardized system of International Normalized Ratio (INR). The hygienist will want to pay particular attention to these indicators when treating the patient for either acute or chronic periodontal disease where the patient experiences spontaneous bleeding. If the patient does not know his or her last reported INR, the hygienist will want to contact the patient's prescribing physician to confirm it is within an acceptable range. An acceptable range for patients considered to be high risk is 2.5 to 3.5.[6,10,26,30–32] This information should be updated in the patient medical history at every visit. Patients undergoing periodontal therapy or maintenance may require shorter appointments and more frequent visits.

Discuss alcohol consumption and drug interactions not only as predisposing factors, but also as they pertain to medications the patient may have been prescribed. For example, if aspirin has been prescribed as a preventive measure for secondary stroke, alcohol will have an adverse effect, increasing bleeding. The hygienist will want to discuss the risks of herbal supplements and self-medication with the patient who has been prescribed either anticoagulants or antiplatelets (see Evidence-Based Practice). Self-prescribing aspirin, taken as a preventive supplement, will increase the anticoagulation effects of warfarin and could increase the severity of a hemorrhagic stroke. The patient's prescribing physician should determine the dose, which could be anywhere from 30 to 325 mg/day. The hygienist will want to contact the prescribing physician to verify that the patient is taking an acceptable dose before proceeding with treatment.[10,31,32] Herbal supplements can also interfere with effects of prescribed medications. For example, the herbal supplement ginkgo can increase the risk for bleeding when taken in conjunction with aspirin.

Need-specific modifications are determined based on resulting impairments. For patients experiencing numbness of the face and/or dysphagia, the hygienist will want to include four-handed dental hygiene to ensure proper retraction of the tongue and cheek area, and aspiration for all procedures. Avoid positioning the patient completely supine to avoid any chance of choking. Dysphagia may increase the risk for caries requiring regular fluoride varnish applications. When ambulatory but using a cane or walker, patients will need more time and a clear path to the operatory. If experiencing residual weakness or numbness in one leg, the patient will likely be using a wheelchair and will need to be transferred to the treatment chair either

---

Evidence-Based Practice

HERBAL SUPPLEMENTS

The use of herbal supplements and remedies are not new to the dental hygiene community. It is estimated that more than 15 million Americans supplement their prescriptive medications with herbs, vitamins, or both. This has become a concern for both physicians and caregivers because approximately two thirds of individuals older than 65 years use at least 25% of all over-the-counter drugs. According to the U.S. Census Bureau, nearly one in five residents will be age 65 or older by the year 2030. This is largely due to the baby boomers' transition into this age group beginning in 2011. Projections indicate that by the year 2034, all of the baby boomers will be older than 70 years.[36] Considering the age of onset for many of the neurological impairments presented in this chapter, it is very likely that this same population may be under the care of multiple physicians or specialists because of advancing age and the complications that accompany it. As a result, multiple physicians could be prescribing multiple medications. Oftentimes, physicians are not aware that the patient is under additional care. To complicate matters, the patient may also be self-medicating with aspirin, vitamins, or herbal supplements. The term *polypharmacy* is used where multiple medications are prescribed. This can be in many forms and can lead to the increased risk for adverse drug reactions. This is seen most often with elderly patients.[32,37]

Any number of factors may precipitate the use of herbal supplements, but the two most evident are fear and cost concerns. Whether reviewing the medical history directly with the patient or with the caregiver, the hygienist will need to ask specific questions about all conditions for which the patient is currently being treated and all medications the patient is taking, including supplements. The hygienist needs to be aware of the interaction of medications and the effects of herbal supplements on medications the patient may have been prescribed. For example, the fear of ensuing memory loss may lead the patient or caregiver to add memory-enhancing supplements, such as the herb ginkgo, to the daily regimen of medications. Prescribed medications could include warfarin, corticosteroids, or tetracyclines. Research the interactions, contraindications, and side effects of the herbal supplement ginkgo with the earlier mentioned prescribed medications, as well as nonprescriptive medications such as aspirin, vitamin E, or fish oil.[32,37,38] ■

by physical assistance or by the use of a transfer board, transfer belt, or gait belt. When the patient's communication skills have been affected, the hygienist will need to speak slowly and clearly, and allow ample time for the patient to respond. It is advised to keep pen and paper handy in case the patient's verbal communication is permanently impaired. If the patient experiences dizziness, recline or raise the patient intermittently. Provide a stress-free environment by reducing noise factors and interruptions for the patient who experiences a heightened sense of distractibility. If the patient is experiencing cognitive impairments, such as memory loss or decreased reasoning skills, or has symptoms of psychological impairments, it is advisable to have a caregiver present during treatment.

Home Care

The overall goal for home-care instructions is to improve quality of life and reduce the risk for secondary stroke. Home-care instructions will be based on the specific needs of each patient. The hygienist will need to consider the severity of symptoms, as well as side effects from medications. Patients taking anticoagulants or antiplatelets should be instructed to watch for spontaneous or excessive gingival bleeding while eating or brushing. This should be reported to the treating physician immediately. A power toothbrush will provide optimum results with little effort on the patient's part. This is particularly important for the patient who is experiencing hemiplegia, such as on one side of the face or in the arm on one side of the body. The use of a power toothbrush in conjunction with an oral irrigation device will disrupt the biofilm, remove any trapped food debris the patient may not be aware of, and keep the tissue stimulated. The unaffected hand can easily manage either of these devices. In addition, many oral irrigation devices are equipped with interdental floss attachments and can also tolerate a diluted antimicrobial rinse solution such as chlorhexidine. Patients who are taking additional medications, such as antihypertensives, may experience xerostomia.[33] For those patients, the hygienist may need to recommend a saliva replacement. For the patient who relies on the assistance of a caregiver, home-care instructions should be demonstrated on both the caregiver and the patient. A home-care template should be saved on the computer to allow for modifications to instructions and recommendations specific to optimizing oral health outcomes for each patient. The hygienist should also be able to add comments for the caregiver that will emphasize why specific preferences or recommendations are made and provide the caregiver with a checklist to assist in compliance.

CRITICAL-THINKING PROCESS

The outcome of using a critical-thinking process is the primary goal of this chapter. Although many of the modifications to the dental hygiene treatment plan for

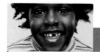

Spotlight on Public Health

In February 2009, both national and international leaders gathered in Washington, DC, in an attempt to formalize solutions to a decade of unmet concerns. This 3-day conference was held to discuss the U.S. Attorney General's findings, published in 2000, for this country's unmet oral health-care needs and access to care. The focus was on restructuring the health-care delivery system to meet the needs of underserved populations and on what the workforce would look like in the coming decade. During this forum, it was noted that the strengths of public health practitioners are in planning, implementation, and evaluation. This is especially true when it comes to integrating medicine and dentistry. One of the most innovative concepts being considered is that of a whole-health home. A whole-health home would be modeled after a community health center. A comprehensive delivery system could be formulated to incorporate collaborative assessment, diagnosis, and treatment planning between physician and dentist, nurse practitioner and advanced dental hygiene practitioner, and behavioral health and social work services. This approach would provide the most comprehensive treatment to underserved communities. Health Commons is one such model. It emphasizes the importance of an interdisciplinary team. Health Commons merges medical health, oral health, and behavioral health services to provide whole-health outcomes. These outcomes are specific to the needs of rural communities in New Mexico, where virtually all of the counties are designated as health professional shortage areas.[35] ■

the neurologically impaired patient are similar or repeated, the process of arriving at those modifications is what is important. As you become comfortable with the assessment process, you will also become more comfortable with the exchange of communication between all interested parties. Asking questions or probing further is an intricate part of discovery. Effective communication is the first step to accomplishing the desired outcomes for each patient based on facts and their needs. The next step is to ensure that each discovery is well documented. It is not reasonable to expect to remember every detail of every patient, but documentation is one of the most valuable sources of information. Based on documentation, the hygienist can develop the best dental hygiene treatment plan for the patient. Home-care instructions can incorporate devices and products that are specific to the patient's needs. Individual outcomes can be established and evaluated at each follow-up appointment.

Case Study

Mrs. Sharp is 53 years old and has been a patient of the office for 7 years. Her medical history reveals that she has type 2 diabetes and has smoked a pack of cigarettes a day for 30 years. The hygienist has discussed smoking cessation at numerous visits. Mrs. Sharp informed the hygienist that she has made several attempts to quit, but during every attempt she would gain so much weight that she gave up. Mrs. Sharp finally quit smoking last year with the help of hypnosis. Mrs. Sharp's dental history indicates that she has struggled with chronic periodontal disease for as long as she has been a patient in this office. She has generalized pocket depths of 4 to 5 mm and generalized bleeding on probing/bleeding on scaling. She visits the hygienist on a 4-month basis for periodontal maintenance. Soon after her last visit, she suffered a stroke and was hospitalized for a week. She scheduled her 4-month appointment at the time of her last visit. It is office policy for the receptionist to call and confirm patient appointments with the hygienist 48 hours in advance. The receptionist asked Mrs. Sharp if there were any changes in her medical history that the hygienist should be aware of. Mrs. Sharp disclosed her recent hospitalization and informed the receptionist that she had been prescribed warfarin (Coumadin) by her prescribing physician and was still being monitored by her cardiologist. The receptionist asked Mrs. Sharp for the name of her cardiologist and prescribing physician and the phone numbers where they can be reached. She then attached the information to the patient's chart in a note for the hygienist to follow up. After consulting with Mrs. Sharp's prescribing physician, the hygienist documents Mrs. Sharp's last INR, the physician's verbal release to treat his patient, and his concerns about some lasting symptoms: prolonged hemiplegia confined to her right hand and two middle fingers, and some incidents of troubled speech. Overall, he finds her to be stable and ready to resume her schedule of periodontal maintenance. He will have his staff fax this information in writing to be kept with the patient's documented medical history.

Case Study Exercises

1. Based on Mrs. Sharp's medical and dental history, identify the modifiable risk factors for stroke that were documented in her patient record.
   A. Age, weight, sex, periodontal disease
   B. Smoking, weight, sex, periodontal disease
   C. Smoking, weight, diabetes, periodontal disease
   D. Age, smoking, diabetes, weight

2. After escorting Mrs. Sharp to the operatory, the hygienist reviews the patient's medical history before beginning treatment. Mrs. Sharp reveals that she has seen a commercial about aspirin and how it can prevent stroke. She's been taking 350 mg aspirin a day for the last 2 weeks. Based on priority, what should be the hygienist's first course of action?
   A. Take Mrs. Sharp's blood pressure before beginning treatment.
   B. Document this information in Mrs. Sharp's chart.
   C. Ask Mrs. Sharp if her cardiologist knows she has added aspirin to her daily medications.
   D. Contact Mrs. Sharp's prescribing physician with this update before beginning treatment.

3. Based on the case information and the information revealed in question 2, what would be the effects of adding aspirin to Mrs. Sharp's prescribed medication(s), namely warfarin (Coumadin)?
   A. Increase the effects of warfarin
   B. Decrease the effects of warfarin
   C. Cause an adverse reaction
   D. Both A and C
   E. No effect

4. Based on Mrs. Sharp's medical and dental histories, what would be considered an acceptable target range for her INR readings to provide periodontal maintenance?
   A. 1.0–2.5
   B. 4.0–5.0
   C. 2.5–3.5
   D. 3.5–4.5

5. Based on Mrs. Sharp's noted symptoms, it is likely that she suffered a left hemispheric stroke. Identify some of the other symptoms associated with this type of stroke that the hygienist would need to consider in modifying the treatment plan.
   A. Altered intellectual ability
   B. Right visual field deficit
   C. Slow, cautious behavior
   D. All of the above
   E. None of the above

Review Questions

1. Which of the following neurological conditions would not impair mobility?
   A. Huntington disease
   B. Amyotrophic lateral sclerosis
   C. Bell palsy
   D. Cerebral palsy
   E. Both B and C

2. What modifications to the dental hygiene treatment plan might be considered for the neurologically impaired patient who is experiencing dysphagia?
   A. Make sure the patient is comfortable and completely supine.
   B. Use four-handed dental hygiene.
   C. Avoid ultrasonic instrumentation.
   D. Recline the patient to a 45° angle.
   E. Both B and C

3. When a neurologically impaired patient is complaining of "dry mouth" (xerostomia), what is the most likely cause?
   A. Side effects from prescribed medications
   B. Poor nutritional habits

   C. An excess of carbonated beverages in the patient's diet
   D. Both B and C
   E. None of the above

4. Which of the following neurological impairments would result in symptoms that require protective eyewear for the patient during dental hygiene procedures?
   A. Bell palsy
   B. Cerebral palsy
   C. Myasthenia gravis
   D. Huntington disease

5. Neurological impairments can occur from an anomaly, deficit, stroke, or brain injury.
   A. True
   B. False

Active Learning

1. Select two neurological impairments discussed in this chapter that are distinctly different in their characteristics and the way in which their symptoms manifest. Make a list of the characteristics and symptoms for each of the impairments. Search the internet for videos about patients who have the impairments you have selected and check off each of the characteristics and symptoms you have listed as you identify them in the videos.

2. Make a list of the products and equipment you think would be more adaptable in an alternate practice setting such as a home or long-term care facility when treating a patient with Huntington disease. Attend a trade show or exhibit hall featuring vendors who manufacture the products and equipment you have identified and test each item on your list. Make notations about your preferences. For example, is there more than one cordless prophy angle? Is one more comfortable than the other?

3. Look at various pictures of the mobile devices available to patients who are neurologically impaired. Compare and contrast the features available on a standard wheelchair, a motorized wheelchair, or a customized electric scooter. ■

REFERENCES

1. World Health Organization (WHO)/Brussels/Geneva, News release. Neurological disorders affect millions globally: WHO report. Geneva, Switzerland: WHO; February 27, 2007.
2. Dehaitem M, Ridley K, Kerschbaum W, Inglehart M. Dental hygiene education about patients with special needs: a survey of U.S. programs. *J Dent Educ.* 2008;72 (9):1010-1019.
3. Holmes EB. Impairment rating and disability determination. www.emedicine.medscape.com/article. Published May 14, 2008. Accessed September 25, 2010.
4. Neurological Impairment Section. http://www.cowork force.com/dwc/PhysAccred/Level%20II%20Accredita-tion/Level%20II/Neurological.pdf
5. Amyotrophic lateral sclerosis. Mayo Foundation for Medical Education and Research website. http://www.mayoclinic.org/diseases-conditions/amyotrophic-lateral-sclerosis/basics/definition/CON-20024397. Accessed September 30, 2015.
6. Williams LS, Hopper PD. *Understanding Medical-Surgical Nursing.* 4th ed. Philadelphia, PA: F.A. Davis; 2011.
7. Amyotrophic lateral sclerosis fact sheet. National Institute of Neurological Disorders and Stroke website. http://www.ninds.nih.gov/disorders/amyotrophiclateralsclerosis/detail_ALS.htm. Accessed September 30, 2015.
8. Steiner J. Treatment of Bell palsy: translating uncertainty into practice. *JAMA.* 2009;302(9):1003-1004.
9. Bell's palsy information site. www.bellspalsy.ws. Accessed August 14, 2010.
10. Vallerand AH and Sanoski CA. Davis's Drug Guide for Nurses®, 14th Edition (June 5, 2014), 1488 pages.

http://www.amazon.com/Daviss-Guide-Nurses-Hazard-Vallerand/dp/0803639767. Accessed September 30, 2015.

11. de Almeida J, Khabori M, Guyatt G, et al. Combined corticosteroid and antiviral treatment for Bell Palsy: a systematic review and meta-analysis. *JAMA* 2009; 302(9):985-993.

12. Simmer-Beck M. Providing care to individuals with special needs: the oral healthcare provider's guide to successfully treating special needs patients. *Dimens Dent Hyg.* 2010;8(5):64-67.

13. National Institute of Dental and Craniofacial Research. Practical oral care for people with cerebral palsy. www.nidcr.nih.gov. Accessed July 18, 2010.

14. National Institute of Neurological Disorders and Stroke. Cerebral palsy: hope through research. http://www.ninds.nih.gov/disorders/cerebral_palsy/detail_cerebral_palsy.htm. Accessed September 30, 2015.

15. Huntington's disease: hope through research. www.ninds.nih.gov/disorders/huntington. Accessed September 30, 2015.

16. Family Caregiver Alliance. Fact sheet: Huntington's disease. www.caregiver.org. Accessed October 6, 2010.

17. Columbia University College of Dental Medicine. Simple steps to better dental health. www.simplestepsdental.com. Accessed September 30, 2015.

18. Howard JF. Myasthenia Gravis Foundation of America, Inc. website. http://myasthenia.org/HealthProfessionals/ClinicalOverviewofMG.aspx. Published 2006. Accessed September 30, 2015.

19. Schulhof S, Kaminski H, Holtan T. Myasthenia Gravis Foundation of America (MGFA) correspondence to J.D. Porter, Executive Secretary, National Institutes of Neurological Disorders and Stroke (NINDS). 2009.

20. National Institute of Neurological Disorders and Stroke website. http://www.ninds.nih.gov/disorders/myasthenia_gravis/myasthenia_gravis.htm. Accessed September 30, 2015.

21. Rai B. Myasthenia gravis: challenge to dental profession. *Internet J Acad Physician Assistants.* 2007;6(1):18-20.

22. Myasthenia gravis. http://www.nhs.uk/Conditions/Myasthenia-gravis/Pages/Introduction.aspx. Accessed September 30, 2015.

23. NINDS Parkinson's Disease Information Page. National Institute of Neurological Disorders and Stroke website. www.ninds.nih.gov/disorders/parkinsons_disease. Accessed September 30, 2015.

24. Parkinson's Disease Information website. www.parkinsons.org. Accessed September 30, 2015.

25. Parkinson's Disease Foundation website. www.pdf.org. Accessed September 30, 2015.

26. American Stroke Association. http://www.strokeassociation.org/STROKEORG/. Accessed September 30, 2015.

27. National Stroke Association website. www.stroke.org. Accessed September 30, 2015.

28. Furie KL, Kasner SE, Adams RJ, et al; on behalf of the American Heart Association Stroke Council, Council on Cardiovascular Nursing, Council on Clinical Cardiology, and Interdisciplinary Council on Quality of Care and Outcomes Research. Guidelines for the prevention of stroke in patients with stroke or transient ischemic attack: a guideline for healthcare professionals from the American Heart Association/American Stroke Association. *Stroke.* 2011;42:227-276.

29. American Heart Association website. http://www.heart.org/HEARTORG/. Accessed September 30, 2015.

30. Understanding Coumadin. Cleveland Clinic. http://my.clevelandclinic.org/health/drugs_devices_supplements/hic_Understanding_Coumadin. Accessed September 30, 2015.

31. The Internet Stroke Center. www.strokecenter.org. Accessed September 30, 2015.

32. Spolarich AE, Andrews L. An examination of the bleeding complications associated with herbal supplements, antiplatelet, and anticoagulant medications. *J Dent Hyg.* 2007;81(3):67. http://jdh.adha.org/content/81/3/67.refs. Accessed September 30, 2015.

33. Friedman PK, Isfeld D. Uncover the cause. A review of the most common systemic health issues that contribute to the development of xerostomia. *Dimens Dent Hyg.* 2010;8(11):50-53.

34. U.S. Bureau of Labor Statistics. Occupational Outlook Handbook, 2010-2011 Edition.

35. IOM (Institute of Medicine). The U.S. oral health workforce in the coming decade: workshop summary. Washington, DC: The National Academies Press; 2009.

36. Vincent GK, Velkoff VA. Current population reports, U.S. Census Bureau. Taken from 2000 Census data. Projections completed 2008. Published May 2010.

37. American Council on Science and Health website. www.acsh.org. Accessed September 30, 2015.

38. Medline Plus website. www.nlm.nih.gov/medlineplus. Accessed September 30, 2015.

Chapter 42 | Endocrine System

Sandra Roggow, RDH, BA

KEY TERMS

A$_{1C}$

circadian rhythms

diabetes mellitus

endocrine system

glucagon

insulin

metabolic syndrome

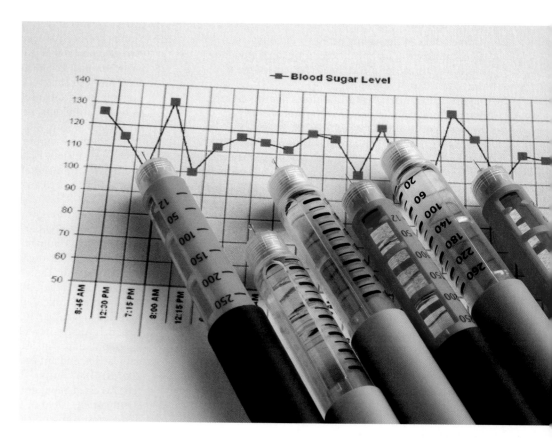

LEARNING OBJECTIVES

After reading this chapter, the student should be able to:

42.1 Identify endocrine system disorders most commonly encountered in dental hygiene practice.

42.2 Discuss the implications of endocrine disorders on oral health.

42.3 Develop individualized dental hygiene care plans for patients with endocrine disorders.

42.4 Implement the necessary dental hygiene treatment modifications for patients with various endocrine conditions.

KEY CONCEPTS

• The endocrine system is an important body health system with many complications.

• The diseases of the endocrine system have dental considerations.

• The dental hygienist must be aware of patients' medical health in relation to their oral health needs including periodontal disease and the oral–systemic connection.

RELEVANCE TO CLINICAL PRACTICE

The Centers for Disease Control and Prevention estimates that 29.1 million Americans, or 9.3% of the population, have diabetes. Of those people, 21.0 million have been diagnosed with diabetes and 8.1 million are undiagnosed. New cases of diabetes continue to be diagnosed, particularly among adults aged 45 years and older.[1] Patients with diabetes may also have other conditions, including periodontitis and hypertension. Links have been shown between diabetes and periodontitis. Diabetes is a risk factor for periodontitis, and periodontal inflammation negatively affects control of diabetes.[2] The National Diabetes Education Program recommends that dental professionals collaborate with primary care providers, nurses, diabetes educators, pharmacists, and other health-care professionals to provide patient-centered care to patients with diabetes.[3] For effective collaboration and positive patient outcomes, dental hygienists need to understand the diabetes disease process, its effect on the patient's oral health, and dental hygiene care modifications for the patient with diabetes.

Thyroid disorders are other common disorders of the endocrine system. It is estimated that 20 million Americans have a thyroid disorder, and more than 12% of Americans will experience development of a thyroid disorder.[4] Dental hygienists need to know how these diseases impact their patients' oral health and how to modify treatment for patients with these conditions.

ENDOCRINE SYSTEM

The **endocrine system** regulates the body's growth, metabolism, and sexual development and function. Glands of the endocrine system produce hormones that are released directly into the bloodstream and carried to tissues and organs throughout the body. The hormones stimulate the organs to function. Receptor sites in the single organ, gland, or tissue receive these precise signals via hormones. These are feedback loops. The endocrine system controls growth, sexual development, sleep, hunger, the way the body uses food, and metabolism. The system is scattered throughout the body, yet it is still one system with like functions (Fig. 42-1).[5,6]

Some of the endocrine system glands also have nonendocrine regions that have functions other than hormone secretion. These are referred to as exocrine glands. The exocrine glands use ducts to secrete their products directly. The salivary glands, sweat glands, and glands within the gastrointestinal tract are examples of exocrine glands.[5,6]

Pituitary Gland, Pineal Gland, and Hypothalamus

The pituitary gland, or hypophysis, is a small gland about 1 cm in diameter, or the size of a pea. The pituitary gland is connected to the hypothalamus, which is a group of neurons in the midbrain that secretes a variety of hormones that cause the pituitary gland to function. A

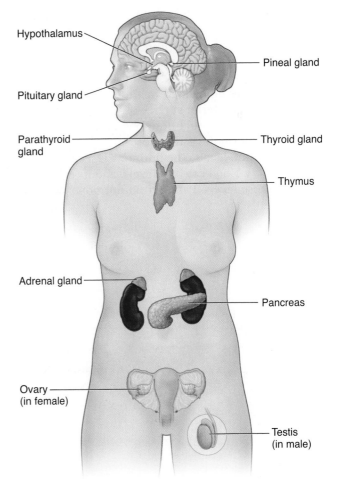

Figure 42-1. Major endocrine glands.

connection between the nervous system and the endocrine system is created. The hypothalamus releases its hormones into a tiny blood channel directly connected to the pituitary gland. These cause the pituitary gland to make its own hormones. The pituitary gland via the hypothalamus is considered the "master control gland" of hormone production because it regulates the activity of most other glands in the body (Fig. 42-2).[5,6]

The pineal gland is located near the center of the brain. This gland secretes melatonin, a hormone that affects the body's sleep-regulation apparatus. **Circadian rhythms** are regular changes in mental and physical characteristics that occur in the course of a day (*circadian* is Latin for "around a day"). Most circadian rhythms are controlled by the body's biological clock. The pineal gland responds to light-induced signals by switching off production of the hormone melatonin.[6]

Thyroid Gland and Parathyroid Glands

The thyroid gland is a very vascular organ that is located in the neck. It consists of two lobes, one on each side of the trachea, just below the larynx, or voice box. The two lobes are connected by a narrow band of tissue called the *isthmus*. Internally, the gland consists of follicles, which produce thyroxine and triiodothyronine hormones. These hormones contain iodine.

Calcitonin is secreted by the parafollicular cells of the thyroid gland. This hormone opposes the action of the parathyroid glands by reducing the calcium level in the blood. If blood calcium becomes too high, calcitonin is secreted until calcium ion levels decrease to normal.

The parathyroid gland is four small masses of epithelial tissue embedded in the connective tissue capsule on the posterior surface of the thyroid glands. They secrete parathyroid hormone or parathormone. Parathyroid hormone is the most important regulator of blood calcium levels. The hormone is secreted in response to low blood calcium levels, and its effect is to increase those levels. Parathyroid hormone works in

partnership with calcitonin from the thyroid gland. The two hormones have the opposite effect. Through negative feedback they keep calcium levels in the blood stable (Box 42-1).[5,6]

Adrenal Gland

The adrenal gland, also called the *suparenal gland*, is paired with one gland located near the upper portion of each kidney. Each gland is divided into an outer adrenal cortex and an inner medulla. The cortex and medulla of the adrenal gland, like the anterior and posterior lobes of the pituitary, develop from different embryonic tissues and secrete different hormones. The adrenal cortex is essential to life, but the medulla may be removed with no life-threatening effects. The hypothalamus of the brain

---

Box 42-1. *Control of Hormone Action*

Hormones are very potent substances, which means that very small amounts of a hormone may have profound effects on metabolic processes. Because of their potency, hormone secretion must be regulated within very narrow limits to maintain homeostasis in the body.[6]

Negative Feedback Mechanism
Many hormones are controlled by some form of a negative feedback mechanism. In this type of system, a gland is sensitive to the concentration of a substance that it regulates. A negative feedback system causes a reversal of increases and decreases in body conditions to maintain a state of stability or homeostasis.

Tropic Hormones
Some endocrine glands secrete hormones in response to other hormones. These are called *tropic hormones*. A hormone from gland A causes gland B to secrete its hormone.

Direct Nervous Stimulation
A third method of regulating hormone secretion is by direct nervous stimulation. A nerve stimulus causes gland A to secrete its hormone.[6]

Positive Feedback System
The production of some hormones is controlled by positive feedback. In such a system, hormones cause a condition to intensify, rather than decrease. As the condition intensifies, hormone production increases. Such positive feedback is uncommon but does occur during childbirth, where hormone levels build with increasingly intense labor contractions.[6] Oxytocin is the pituitary hormone that stimulates muscle contractions in the uterus during childbirth. These contractions cause the release of more oxytocin, creating a positive feedback system.[6] ■

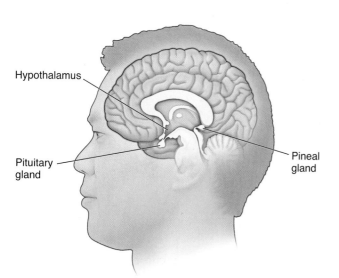

Figure 42-2. The pituitary gland, pineal gland, and hypothalamus.

influences both portions of the adrenal gland but by different mechanisms. The adrenal cortex is regulated by negative feedback involving the hypothalamus and adrenocorticotropic hormone (ACTH), the hormone released by the pituitary gland; the medulla is regulated by nerve impulses from the hypothalamus.

Hormones of the Adrenal Cortex

The adrenal cortex consists of three different regions, with each region producing a different group or type of hormones. Chemically, all the cortical hormones are steroid. Mineralocorticoids are secreted by the outermost region of the adrenal cortex. The principal mineralocorticoid is aldosterone, which acts to conserve sodium ions and water in the body.[5,6] Aldosterone inhibits the amount of sodium excreted in the urine, maintaining blood pressure and blood volume. Glucocorticoids are secreted by the middle region of the adrenal cortex. The principal glucocorticoid is hydrocortisone, also called *cortisol*, which increases blood glucose levels. Small amounts of corticosterone and androgen hormones are also secreted by the adrenal cortex. The third group of steroids secreted by the adrenal cortex is the gonadocorticoids, or sex hormones. These are secreted by the innermost region. Male hormones, androgens, and female hormones, estrogens, are secreted in minimal amounts in both sexes by the adrenal cortex, but their effect is usually masked by the hormones from the testes and ovaries. In females, the masculinization effect of androgen secretion may become evident after menopause, when estrogen levels from the ovaries decrease.[5,6]

Hormones of the Adrenal Medulla

The adrenal medulla develops from neural tissue and secretes two hormones, epinephrine and norepinephrine. These two hormones are secreted in response to stimulation by sympathetic nerve, particularly during stressful situations. A lack of hormones from the adrenal medulla produces no significant effects. Hypersecretion, usually from a tumor, causes prolonged or continual sympathetic responses.[5]

Pancreas—Islets of Langerhans

The pancreas is a long, soft organ that lies transversely along the posterior abdominal wall, posterior to the stomach, and extends from the region of the duodenum to the spleen. This gland has an exocrine system portion that secretes digestive enzymes that are carried through a duct to the duodenum. The endocrine portion consists of the pancreatic islets (islets of Langerhans), which secrete **glucagon,** a hormone secreted in response to low concentrations of glucose in the blood, and **insulin,** a hormone secreted in response to high concentrations of glucose in the blood.

Alpha cells in the pancreatic islets secrete glucagon.[5] Glucagon plays a vital part in maintaining the correct blood sugar level. When the blood sugar level starts to decline, glucogon makes cells release glucose and helps convert glycogen, the form of glucose stored in the liver, back to glucose and the blood sugar level increases. Blood has enough glucose to keep a person alive for just 15 minutes. However, as glucose is used up, more is released to take its place.[6] Beta cells in the pancreatic islets secrete insulin. Insulin reduces the level of sugar in the blood in two ways. The insulin takes up the glucose and makes the liver store glucose by turning it into glycogen. Insulin and glucogan have the opposite effects. Together they form a negative feedback system that keeps sugar levels within set limits.[5]

Cortisol is one of the glucocorticoids secreted by the middle cortex of the adrenal cortex that increases blood glucose levels.[5,6]

Gonads

The gonads, the primary reproductive organs, are the testes in the male and the ovaries in the female. These organs are responsible for producing the sperm and ova and for secreting hormones.

Testes

Male sex hormones, as a group, are called *androgens.* The principal androgen is testosterone, which is secreted by the testes. A small amount is also produced by the adrenal cortex. Production of testosterone begins during fetal development, continues for a short time after birth, nearly ceases during childhood, and then resumes at puberty. This steroid hormone is responsible for the growth and development of the male reproductive structures; increased skeletal and muscular growth; enlargement of the larynx (located just above the thyroid gland) accompanied by voice changes, growth, and distribution of body hair; and increased male sexual drive. Testosterone secretion is regulated by a negative feedback system that involves releasing hormones from the hypothalamus and gonadotropins from the anterior pituitary.[5,6]

Ovaries

Two groups of female sex hormones are produced in the ovaries, the estrogens and progesterone. These steroid hormones contribute to the development and function of the female reproductive organs and sex characteristics. At the onset of puberty, estrogen promotes the development of the breasts; distribution of fat evidenced in the hips, legs, and breast; and maturation of reproductive organs such as the uterus and vagina.

Progesterone causes the uterine lining to thicken in preparation for pregnancy. Together, progesterone and estrogens are responsible for the changes that occur in the uterus during the female menstrual cycle.[5,6]

DIABETES MELLITUS

Diabetes mellitus is a chronic metabolic disease caused either by the body's insufficient production of insulin or by the body's inability to respond to the insulin produced. Diabetes can lead to systemic complications such as hypertension, blindness and eye problems, kidney disease, and nervous system disease. Studies have also reported oral complications from diabetes. Recent research has shown an association with poor blood sugar control and the incidence and progression of periodontal disease in patients with diabetes, as well as inversely an association with uncontrolled periodontal disease affecting the control of blood sugar/diabetes.[7]

There are two types of diabetes mellitus, type 1 and type 2. Type 1 diabetes causes the immune system to destroy insulin-producing beta cells in the pancreas. This autoimmune disorder often develops in adolescence and may be triggered by a viral infection in combination with genetic susceptibility.

In type 2 diabetes, the pancreas produces adequate insulin but the body cells cannot respond normally to it and do not take up enough sugar from the blood. Often associated with obesity and an elevated risk for heart disease, type 2 diabetes has become a global health crisis. Worldwide, tens of millions of people exhibit a range of symptoms called **metabolic syndrome,** a cluster of conditions that includes high blood pressure and blood sugar levels, abnormal cholesterol levels, and excess body fat around the waist; metabolic syndrome is an early indicator of increased diabetes risk.[8]

Patients diagnosed with diabetes self-test their blood glucose levels. The goal is to maintain a blood glucose reading between 70 and 130 before meals. About 2 hours after a meal starts, the blood glucose level should be less than 180 (see Application to Clinical Practice). A person whose blood glucose is too low will feel shaky, sweaty, or hungry. People who take insulin need to check their blood glucose more often than people who do not.[9]

The most common oral problems from diabetes are gingivitis, periodontitis, thrush, burning mouth syndrome, and xerostomia, which result in increased caries risk. When diabetes is not controlled, high glucose levels in saliva help plaque grow. High glucose levels can also result in increased caries formation.[9]

Symptoms associated with diabetes include polydipsia (increased thirst), polyuria (increased quantity of urine passed and, often, the need to urinate frequently), and polyphagia (increased appetite).[9]

People with diabetes are at increased risk for high blood pressure. Diabetes can damage the blood vessels, making it more difficult for the blood to flow through the blood vessels and causing the blood pressure to increase. Controlling blood pressure is as important as controlling blood glucose in protecting against complications from diabetes. Blood pressure monitoring is critical for the patient with diabetes (Box 42-2).

Sleep apnea and diabetes are so closely linked that the International Diabetes Federation urges doctors who diagnose type 2 diabetes to also test for sleep apnea and vice versa. Sleep apnea causes a person to stop breathing briefly during sleep—sometimes hundreds of times—and it can cause blood sugar levels to rise. Snoring followed by gasping or choking sounds is the most common symptom; extreme daytime sleepiness is another symptom.[10]

Dental Hygiene Considerations

Patients with diabetes need to plan their dental visits carefully. Maintaining their blood sugar levels before, during, and after dental procedures will help avoid a medical emergency in the dental office (see Application to Clinical Practice). To avoid hypoglycemia during treatment, it is essential that patients with diabetes eat and take their medications before any dental procedures.[11] At each appointment the dental professional should ask patients with diabetes the following questions: When did you last eat? At what time did you take your medications? At what time did you last take your blood glucose reading? What was the result of that reading?

For patients with uncontrolled diabetes, a medical clearance may be necessary before any dental procedures (other than emergency care) are performed. Patients with diabetes, particularly uncontrolled diabetes, take longer to heal after invasive dental treatment; therefore, antibiotic premedication may be necessary before treating the soft tissues and bone, such as root planing, grafts, extractions, and implants. Patients with uncontrolled diabetes should be referred to their physician to evaluate and determine whether antibiotic premedication is required.[12]

Insulin shock, hypoglycemia, and low blood sugar are common risks during dental treatment of the patient with diabetes mellitus. Signs and symptoms

Application to Clinical Practice

A_{1C} is a laboratory test that measures average blood glucose level over the last 2 to 3 months. It shows whether blood glucose stayed close to the target range most of the time or was too high or too low. For people with diabetes, the A_{1C} test should be less than 7. An increased A_{1C} level increases the chances of having eye, kidney, nerve, and heart disease. ■

Box 42-2. *Blood Pressure Reading*

The systolic blood reading measures the pressure in the arteries when the heart is contracting. The diastolic reading measures the pressure in the arteries when the heart is relaxed. A reading of either systolic pressure greater than 130 mm Hg or diastolic pressure greater than 80 mm Hg, or both, is considered high blood pressure. A consistent reading three times or more at the high range must be shared with the patient's physician. ■

include confusion, sweating, shaking, and dizziness. An antihypoglycemic (a source of sugar) such as a tube of glucose gel should be included in the dental office emergency drug kit and be readily available when treating patients with diabetes.

Stress can cause a release of cortisol (glucocorticoid), resulting in a high concentration of glucose in the blood and a lack of sufficient insulin. Hyperglycemia can result, although it is slower to develop than hypoglycemia. Ketoacidosis (diabetic coma) could occur. Ketoacidosis is life-threatening and needs immediate treatment. Symptoms include shortness of breath, breath that smells fruity, nausea and vomiting, and/or a very dry mouth.[12] Dental hygienists must know the signs of hyperglycemia so it can be treated early.

Dental treatment by both the dental hygienist and the dentist on all patients with diabetes requires a protocol for prevention of hypoglycemia and hyperglycemia. A protocol for treatment of hypoglycemia and hyperglycemia also needs to be established and reviewed regularly by the entire dental team.

Blood pressure should be taken before the patient is prepared for dental treatment. Record the patient's last A_{1C} and glucose monitor reading and his or her last insulin injection if the patient is insulin dependent. Also document the patient's last meal before the dental appointment. The patient needs to have adequate carbohydrate intake before the appointment. Patients with diabetes should have dental treatment before or after peak insulin activity, not during peak insulin activity. Peak insulin activity varies according to the type of insulin used by the patient. The type of insulin and its peak activity need to be recorded and updated at each dental appointment. Shorter appointments or longer appointments with breaks are easier to tolerate for the patients with diabetes.[13]

DISEASE PROCESSES OF THE PITUITARY GLAND

A pituitary tumor is an abnormal growth of cells within the pituitary gland. Most pituitary tumors are benign, which means they are noncancerous, grow slowly, and do not spread to other parts of the body; however, they can make the pituitary gland produce either too many or too few hormones, which can cause problems in the body. Tumors that make hormones are called *functioning tumors,* and they can cause a wide array of symptoms depending on the hormone affected. Tumors that do not make hormones are called *nonfunctioning tumors.* Their symptoms are directly related to their growth in size and include headaches, vision problems, nausea, and vomiting.

Cushing Syndrome

ACTH-secreting tumors produce the hormone adrencoroticotropin. Diseases related to ACTH hormone abnormalites include Cushing disease, a disorder that occurs when the body is exposed to high levels of the hormone cortisol, a hormone made in the adrenal gland. The tumor on the pituitary gland causes too much of the hormone ACTH to be produced, signaling the adrenal glands to produce cortisol. Physical features include fat building up in the face, back, and chest, and the arms and legs becoming very thin.[14]

Dental Hygiene Considerations

Cushing syndrome causes a characteristic round or moon-shaped face. This may be observed when the dental hygienist is doing an oral cancer examination. The patient may not be aware that a change has occurred. The medical history needs to be documented and the patient should be referred to his or her primary physician for further evaluation (see Professionalism).

Patients who are receiving corticosteroids and those with adrenocortical insufficiency may require supplemental cortocosteroids during major dental prodecures. Patients with Cushing syndrome or those who are taking corticosteroids may have alveolar bone loss, delayed wound healing, and increased capillary fragility.

Acromegaly

A benign tumor of the pituitary gland, called an *adenoma,* produces excess growth hormone (GH). Pituitary tumors are labeled either microadenomas or macroadenomas, depending on their size. Acromegaly is a condition in which the hands, feet, and face are larger than normal.[8] In more than 95% of people with acromegaly, the benign tumor of the pituitary produces excess GH. The name *acromegaly* comes from the Greek words for

Professionalism

When contacting a medical office, be prepared with the correct spelling of the patient's first and last names and the patient's birthdate. The front desk administrator needs this information before transferring your call to a medical assistant, RN, nurse practitioner, physician's assistant, or physician. Identify yourself and explain that you have a mutual patient about whom you need to share or gather information. Record the name of the medical professional you speak with in the patient's dental record. Always ask if an e-mail address is also available to be able to communicate with the medical office in the future. A written, generic referral slip from the dental practice addressed to the patient's medical team with the medical concern you are asking to have evaluated will develop an opportunity for communication between the dental and medical teams and create a link between the patient's oral and systemic health care. ■

"extremities" and "enlargement," reflecting one of its most common symptoms: the abnormal growth of the hands and feet. Swelling of the hands and feet is often an early feature, with patients noticing a change in ring or shoe size, particulary shoe width.

Dental Hygiene Considerations

Gradually, bone changes alter the patient's facial features: The brow and lower jaw protrude, the nasal bone enlarges, and the teeth space out. This may cause a change in size of the jaw, causing night guards, retainers, teeth-whitening trays, and partial or full dentures to no longer fit properly. The tongue may also enlarge, affecting the way oral devices fit. Overgrowth of bone and cartilage often leads to arthritis. When tissue thickens, it may trap nerves, causing carpal tunnel syndrome, which results in numbness and weakness of the hands. If the hands swell, the patient may find he or she is having difficulty properly and comfortably holding dental floss or flossing adjuncts. The patient should be referred to his or her primary physician for further evaluation. The dental hygienist may also need to help the patient find other successful ways to maintain effective oral hygiene self-care. Body organs, including the heart, may enlarge, causing heart disease including hypertension.[15] (See Chapter 37 for a complete discussion on heart disease and hypertension.)

Thyroid Disorder

Approximately 95% of the active thyroid hormone is thyroxine, and most of the remaining 5% is triiodothyronine.[6] Both of these require iodine for their synthesis. Thyroid hormone secretion is regulated by a negative feedback mechanism. In this type of system, a gland is sensitive to the concentration of a substance that it regulates. Thyroid hormone secretion involves the amount of circulating hormone, the hypothalamus, and adenohypophysis. If there is an iodine deficiency, the thyroid cannot make sufficient hormone. This stimulates the anterior pituitary to secrete thyroid-stimulating hormone, which causes the thyroid gland to increase in size in a vain attempt to produce more hormones. But it cannot produce more hormones because it does not have the necessary raw material, iodine. This type of thyroid enlargement is called *simple goiter* or *iodine-deficiency goiter*.[6]

Thyroid dysfunction is the second most common glandular disorder of the endocrine system and its incidence is increasing, predominantly among women. Up to 5% of the female population has alterations in thyroid function, and up to 6% may have clinically detectable thyroid nodules on palpation. An estimated 15% of the general population has abnormalities of thyroid anatomy on physical examination, and an unknown percentage of these individuals do not receive a complete diagnostic evaluation. It has been suggested that the number of people affected may be twice as many as the undetected cases. This means that patients with undiagnosed hypothyroidism or hyperthyroidism are seen in the dental chair, where routine treatment has the potential to result in adverse outcomes. The dentist or dental hygienist may be the first person to suspect a serious thyroid disorder and aid in early diagnosis.

Dental Hygiene Considerations

If an undiagnosied thyroid disorder is suspected, modifications of dental care must be considered. The main complications of patients with hyperthyroidism and hypothyroidism are associated with cardiac comorbidity. Underactivity or overactivity of the thyroid gland can cause life-threatening cardiac events. Consultation with the patient's primary care physician or an endocrinologist is warranted if any sign or symptom of previously undetected thyroid disease is noted on examination. Patients who have hyperthyroidism have increased levels of anxiety, and stress or surgery can trigger a thyrotoxic crisis. Epinephrine is contraindicated, and elective dental care should be deferred for patients who have hyperthyroidism and exhibit signs or syptoms of thyrotoxicosis. A medically well-controlled patient will have no contraindications to dental treatment.

Subgingival irrigation with 10% povidone-iodine upon completion of a session of scaling and root planing for 5 minutes may be contraindicated in patients with iodine hypersensitivity, thyroid pathosis, as well as pregnant and nursing women to protect the infant. Povidone-iodine has the potential to induce hyperthyroidism because of excessive incorporation of iodine in the thyroid gland and, therefore, should be used only for short periods.

Cancer of the Thyroid

There are four main types of thyroid cancer: papillary, follicular, medullary, and anaplastic thyroid cancer. The four types are differentiated based on how the cancer cells look under a microscope. Cancer of the thyroid gland usually presents as a swelling in the thyroid gland. It is a relatively rare malignancy, and the majority of thyroid nodules will prove to be benign. More female than male individuals are diagnosed with thyroid cancer.

Hypoparathyroidism, or insufficient secretion of parathyroid hormone, leads to increased nerve excitability. The low blood calcium levels trigger spontaneous and continuous nerve impulses, which then stimulate muscle contraction.[5,6]

Dental Hygiene Considerations

To perform an extraoral cancer examination, observe the thyroid and then palpate it for any nodules, or irregular masses. The best way to become familiar with how the thyroid feels is to become familiar with the proper location of the thyroid in the neck. It is located below the larynx on the front of the neck. Gently palpitating the thyroid with the gloved fingertips will allow the dental hygienist to feel the butterfly shape of this gland.

Diseases of the Adrenal Gland

Cushing syndrome (see the earlier description of Cushing syndrome discussed with pituitary gland) is an example of a pituitary tumor producing hormones that cause the overproduction of hormones. The functioning tumor affects the adrenal gland. ACTH tumors produce the hormone adrenocorticotropin. The endocrine system needs to be a very balanced system. When something is not healthy with one of the glands, another one is affected negatively. The action between the pituitary tumor and the adrenal gland is a direct example of one gland in the endocrine system negatively affecting another gland.[5,6]

Dental Hygiene Considerations and Precautions

Obtaining an accurate medical history update from the dental patient at each dental visit is critical for the management of the patient's oral and systemic health during the dental hygiene appointment. (See Chapter 8 for a complete description of a comprehensive medical and dental history.)

Case Study

A female patient presents for her appointment at 10:00 a.m. She has a history of type 2 diabetes, which has always been controlled. She complains about sweating, shaking, and dizziness, but says it is not so bad. Her blood glucose level was normal when she checked it earlier in the morning, 110 mg/dL. She has her blood glucose testing kit with her. She also shares that she is preparing for her daughter's wedding in 1 month.

Case Study Exercises

1. What is the first order of business between the patient and the dental hygienist?
2. The symptoms the patient describes could be signs of what condition? What course of action should the dental hygienist take?
3. What else, if anything, can be affecting the patient's blood glucose levels?

Review Questions

1. Some of the endocrine system glands also have nonendocrine regions that have functions other than hormone secretion. The salivary glands, sweat glands, and pituitary glands are examples of exocrine glands.
   A. Both statements are true.
   B. Both statements are false.
   C. The first statement is true, but the second statement is false.
   D. The first statement is false, but the second statement is true.

2. Parathyroid hormone works in partnership with calcitonin from the thyroid gland. The two hormones have the same effect.
   A. Both statements are true.
   B. Both statements are false.
   C. The first statement is true, but the second statement is false.
   D. The first statement is false, but the second statement is true.

3. The adrenal cortex is essential to life. As well, removal of the medulla can have life-threatening effects.
   A. Both the statement and the reason are correct and related.
   B. Both the statement and the reason are correct but not related.
   C. The statement is correct, but the reason is not.
   D. The statement is not correct, but the reason is correct.

4. The adrenal cortex consists of three different regions, with each region producing a different group or type of hormones. For each symptom listed below, select the correct disorder from the list provided.
   1. Glucocorticoids
   2. Gonadocorticoids, or sex hormones
   3. Mineralocorticoids

   A. Secreted by the outermost region of the adrenal cortex
   B. Secreted by the innermost region of the adrenal cortex
   C. Secreted by the middle region of the adrenal cortex

5. The pancreas is a gland of the exocrine system. It has a portion that secretes digestive enzymes that are carried through a duct to the duodenum.
   A. Both the statement and the reason are correct and related.
   B. Both the statement and the reason are correct but are not related.
   C. The statement is correct, but the reason is not.
   D. The statement is not correct, but the reason is correct.
   E. Neither the statement nor the reason is correct.

Active Learning

1. Diabetes toolkit for principles and management of diabetes in the dental office: Create a 1-hour self-study PowerPoint presentation with a case involving a dental patient with diabetes. The presentation can be posted on Blackboard or other appropriate Internet-based education software program 1 month before the face-to-face meeting. It should include all aspects of diabetes management at a dental hygiene appointment. Dental hygienists can anonymously submit assessment and management strategies for the simulated patient with symptomatic descriptions and personal and family histories. Feedback is provided to other dental hygienists, and suggestions for improvement are expected. The case study and input provided can be discussed at a face-to-face meeting.

2. Endocrine system case presentation with errors: Have a group of five dental hygiene students create a 1-hour face-to-face presentation with numerous mistakes and inaccuracies. Have a face-to-face meeting where dental hygiene students will work in small groups, facilitated by a faculty member. Students should identify all inaccuracies in the case and indicate how to correct them and prevent future errors. Small groups can present to the larger group. Have the read/write students turn reactions, actions, charts, and so on into words.

3. Endocrine system medley: A faculty member or student appointed by a faculty member can collect students' questions about the management of patients (with endocrine disorders) who might visit the office for a dental hygiene appointment, 1 week before a face-to-face session. The face-to-face session could be conducted online. The faculty member or appointed student randomly chooses questions and facilitates a 1-hour discussion. Students are asked for their responses before answers are revealed, encouraging engagement in the learning process. Discussion points generally include variations in patient presentation, unique management by dental hygiene and dental caregivers, effects of medications on treatment, and a dental hygiene care plan. ■

REFERENCES

1. National Diabetes Statistics Report, 2014. Atlanta, GA: Centers for Disease Control and Prevention. http://www.cdc.gov/diabetes/pubs/statsreport14/national-diabetes-report-web.pdf. Accessed October 31, 2015.

2. Preshaw PM, Alba AL, Herrara D, et al. Periodontitis and diabetes: a two-way relationship. *Diabetologia.* 2012;55(1):21-31. http://www.ncbi.nlm.nih.gov/pmc/articles/PMC3228943. Accessed October 3, 2015.

3. What makes a team? Bethesda, MD: National Institute of Diabetes and Digestive and Kidney Diseases. http://ndep.nih.gov/hcp-businesses-and-schools/practice-transformation/team-based-care/what-makes-a-team.aspx. Accessed October 3, 2015.

4. General information/press room. Falls Church, VA: American Thyroid Association. http://www.thyroid.org/media-main/about-hypothyroidism. Updated 2014. Accessed October 3, 2015

5. Biology of the endocrine system. Whitehouse Station, NJ: Merck & Co. http://www.merckmanuals.com/home/hormonal_and_metabolic_disorders/biology_of_the_endocrine_system/endocrine_glands.html. Updated August 2013. Accessed October 3, 2015.

6. Endocrine system. Bethesda, MD: National Cancer Institute. http://training.seer.cancer.gov/anatomy/endocrine. Accessed October 3, 2015.

7. Complications due to diabetes. Atlanta, GA: Centers for Disease Control and Prevention. http://www.cdc.gov/diabetes/living/problems.html. Updated February 10, 2015. Accessed October 3, 2015.

8. Metabolic syndrome. Bethesda, MD: U.S. National Library of Medicine. http://www.ncbi.nlm.nih.gov/pubmedhealth/PMHT0024493. Accessed October 3, 2015.

9. National Diabetes Education Program. Bethesda, MD: The National Institute of Diabetes and Digestive and Kidney Diseases. http://ndep.nih.gov/index.aspx. Accessed October 3, 2015.

10. Guiding principles for the care of people with or at risk for diabetes. Bethesda, MD: National Institute of Diabetes and Digestive and Kidney Diseases. http://ndep.nih.gov/hcp-businesses-and-schools/guiding-principles/principle-01-identify-undiagnosed-diabetes-and-prediabetes.aspx. Accessed October 3, 2015.

11. Prevent diabetes problems: keep your diabetes under control. NIH Publication No. 14-4349. Bethesda, MD: National Diabetes Information Clearinghouse. http://diabetes.niddk.nih.gov/dm/pubs/complications_teeth/#sec5. Published February 2014. Updated April 23, 2014. Accessed October 3, 2015.

12. Gurenlian JR, Ball WL, La Fontaine J. Diabetes mellitus: promoting collaboration among health care professionals. *J Dent Hyg.* 2009;83(suppl 1):3-12. http://jdh.adha.org/content/83/suppl_1/3.full.pdf+html. Accessed October 3, 2015.

13. Malamed SF. *Medical Emergencies in the Dental Office.* 6th ed. St. Louis, MO: Mosby; 2007.

14. Cushing disease. Bethesda, MD: U.S. National Library of Medicine. http://www.nlm.nih.gov/medlineplus/ency/article/000348.htm. Updated November 7, 2013. Accessed October 3, 2015.

15. Acromegaly. NIH Publication No. 08-3924. Bethesda, MD: National Institute of Diabetes and Digestive and Kidney Diseases. http://endocrine.niddk.nih.gov/pubs/acro/acro.aspx. Published May 2008. Updated April 6, 2012. Accessed October 3, 2015.

Chapter 43 | Immune System

Kathryn Bell, RDH, MS

KEY TERMS

acute adrenal insufficiency

adaptive immune system

Addisonian crisis

Addison disease

adrenal insufficiency (AI)

antibody

antigen

apoptosis

autoantibody

autoimmune disease

bulbar weakness

cell-mediated immunity

chemokine

cholinergic crisis

complement

cytokines

demyelination

dysgeusia

erythema multiforme (EM)

fibromyalgia (FM)

fibrosis

HIV

humoral immunity

immune complex

immunodeficiency

immunoglobulin

immunological memory

innate immune system

lichen planus (LP)

major histocompatibility complex (MHC)

malar

microstomia

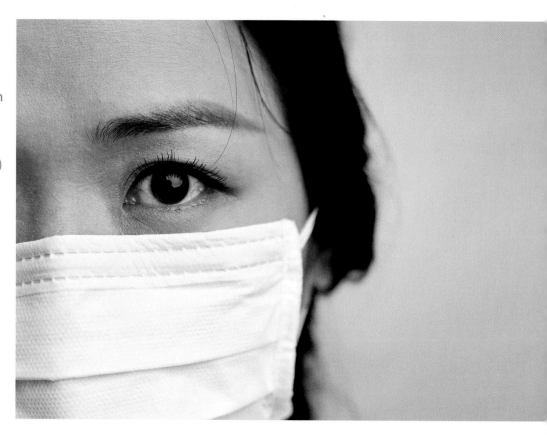

LEARNING OBJECTIVES

After reading this chapter, the student should be able to:

43.1 Discuss the general concepts of human immunity.

43.2 Describe the effects of each presented disease on general and oral health.

43.3 Identify precautions and modifications to dental hygiene care for each presented disease.

43.4 Critically evaluate a patient's medical history and list of medications in preparation for treating a patient with immune system dysfunction.

43.5 Provide safe and effective care for patients with immune system dysfunction.

KEY CONCEPTS

• Immune system dysfunction affects the patient's overall health, as well as their oral health.

• It is necessary for the dental hygienist to understand the progression and characteristics of a disease to safely treat a patient with immune dysfunction.

multiple sclerosis (MS)

myasthenia gravis (MG)

myasthenic crisis

palliative

paroxysmal pain
  syndromes

plasmapheresis

pleurisy

Raynaud phenomenon

rheumatoid arthritis (RA)

scleroderma (SC)

Sjögren syndrome (SS)

spasticity

systemic lupus
  erythematosus (SLE)

thymectomy

Wickham striae

xerophthalmia

- Evaluation of the medical history and medications is part of the assessment phase of dental hygiene treatment.
- Appropriate treatment modification for patients with immune dysfunction is a critical part of both the planning and the implementation phases of dental hygiene treatment.

RELEVANCE TO CLINICAL PRACTICE

Dental hygienists in clinical practice will see a wide variety of patients, typically ranging from the very young to the very old. Many of those patients will have some form of immune system disorder. Autoimmune diseases, immune complex diseases, and immunodeficiency diseases all negatively affect the performance of the immune system. Because these diseases are relatively common among the population at large, it is very important for the clinician to have a thorough understanding of how they affect the body, what types of treatments are available, and what modifications may be necessary for treatment planning and patient recommendations.

BASIC CONCEPTS OF IMMUNITY

To have a thorough understanding of the disease process, one must first understand the healthy state. The following information provides an overview of the immune system and its functions.

Self Versus Nonself and Immunological Memory

The human immune system serves as a defense system, protecting the host from invasion of foreign substances and potential pathogens such as bacteria, viruses, toxins, parasites, and transplanted tissues. The major concept around which the immune system functions is self versus nonself. The immunological concept of "self" is much what it sounds like and is relatively simple. In essence, this is the body's ability to recognize whether molecules, proteins, cells, or tissues belong to the body (self) or are of a foreign origin (nonself). The body's nucleated cells all have markers that express the cells as "self." These markers are called the **major histocompatibility complex (MHC)**. Histocompatibility issues arise when matching transplant donors and recipients. MHC proteins are matched for transplant donors and recipients before transplant surgery to help ensure that tissue rejection will not take place. Substances that the immune system identifies as nonself are known as **antigens.** If the immune system identifies an antigen, it will mount a defense to protect the body from potential pathogenesis. The human immune system has the ability to remember previous encounters with antigens, which enables the immune system to respond very quickly to a subsequent infection. This ability is called **immunological memory**. Sometimes, the immune system will identify parts of an individual's own body (self) as antigens and mount an immune response, resulting in **autoimmune disease.**[1–3]

Innate and Adaptive Immune Systems

The human body uses two main systems to combat infection: the **innate immune system** (nonspecific immune system) and the **adaptive immune system** (specific immune system). All individuals are born with defense mechanisms that comprise the innate immune system Examples of these include:

- Mechanical barriers (skin and mucous membranes)
- Physicochemical barriers (acidity of stomach fluid)
- Antibacterial substances present in external secretions (lysozyme)
- Normal movement of intestinal contents
- Bronchial secretions and urine
- **Complement** (a set of soluble molecules that can bind to certain molecules that are common among microbial cells)
- Some leukocytes (white blood cells [WBCs]) including phagocytic cells and granulocytic cells

The innate immune system is called nonspecific because these defense mechanisms are generally applicable to many different types of antigens. In contrast, the adaptive immune system targets specific organisms and generates what is typically thought of as the "immune response." The adaptive immune system will recognize a specific antigen and produce the cells and processes required to eliminate the antigen.[1,2]

Cells of the Immune Response

Many cells are involved in the immune response. The primary WBCs involved are lymphocytes. Two main types of lymphocytes mediate the immune response: B lymphocytes (B cells) and T lymphocytes (T cells).

B cells develop from bone marrow stem cells and mature in the bone marrow. When an antigen stimulates B cells, two main types of B cells will develop: the plasma cell and the B memory cell. The plasma cell will produce **antibodies,** also known as **immunoglobulins** (Igs). There are five types of Igs or antibodies: IgA, IgD, IgE, IgG, and IgM. Plasma cells are produced for a specific antigen; therefore, the plasma cell produces antibodies for the same specific antigen. Antibodies will bind to their specific antigen, forming an **immune complex,** which essentially identifies the antigen for destruction. The B memory cell will "remember" the antigen and circulate in the blood so that the body is prepared for future immune responses. B cells are a key component in **humoral immunity,** which is immune response that is mediated by soluble molecules such as complement and antibodies.[1,2] In autoimmune disease, B cells produce antibodies that attack the host tissues, which are called **autoantibodies.**

T cells also develop from the stem cells located in bone marrow, but they mature in the thymus. T cells have various roles in **cell-mediated immunity,** which refers to immune responses mediated by cells as opposed

to soluble molecules like antibodies. There two kinds of T cells: helper T cells (which have CD4 receptors and are sometimes referred to simply as CD4+ cells) that assist B cells in carrying out their function (producing antibodies) and cytotoxic T cells (which have CD8 receptors and are sometimes referred to as CD8+ cells) that are capable of directly attacking nonself or infected cells.[3] Because T cells essentially coordinate and control the immune response, MHC is a key factor in cell-mediated immunity.

In addition to B cells and T cells, several other leukocytes are involved in the immune response. These include antigen-presenting cells, phagocytic cells, and natural killer (NK) cells. Antigen-presenting cells trap antigens and present them for recognition by the lymphocytes. Examples of antigen-presenting cells include monocytes, macrophages, and dendritic cells. (Note: Mononuclear phagocytes are known as monocytes when they are circulating in the blood; once they migrate into the tissues, they are referred to as macrophages.) Phagocytic cells (phagocytes) eliminate antigens that have been identified by engulfing and degrading them with enzymes. Monocytes, macrophages, and granulocytes are all examples of phagocytes. Granulocytes include polymorphonuclear leukocytes (also known as neutrophils or PMNs—the most numerous WBC), basophils, eosinophils, and mast cells. NK cells function in surveillance, playing an important role in innate immunity, by directly identifying and eliminating infected and malignant cells. NK cells can recognize reduced MHC surface molecules (this signifies the molecule/protein/cell/tissue as an antigen), thus allowing them to identify antigens. NK cells and cytotoxic T cells perform similar functions, but NK cells function in the innate immune system and cytotoxic T cells function in the adaptive immune system.[1–3]

Chemokines and Cytokines

Chemokines are a large group of small proteins that guide WBCs to sites where they are needed. **Cytokines** are proteins made by cells that affect the behavior of other cells; in essence, they are controlling cells that help mediate the immune response.[3]

Autoimmune Diseases

Autoimmune diseases result from the misdirection of the adaptive immune response toward normal components of the human body. When this happens, the adaptive immune system will produce a response (autoimmune response) that attacks the cells or tissue, resulting in a disease state. An example of this is insulin-dependent diabetes mellitus (type 1 diabetes mellitus). The β cells of the islets of Langerhans are destroyed via an autoimmune response, rendering the patient unable to produce insulin.[3] For information regarding type 1 diabetes mellitus, see Chapter 42.

Immunodeficiency Diseases

Sometimes components of the immune system are missing or dysfunctional. This usually leads to increased susceptibility to infection. This state of immune dysfunction is termed **immunodeficiency.** Immunodeficiency can be caused by genetic mutation or by pathogens. An example of immunodeficiency caused by a pathogen is AIDS, which is caused by infection with HIV.[3]

DISEASES THAT AFFECT OVERALL AND ORAL HEALTH

This chapter introduces the student to several diseases of the immune system that affect both overall and oral health. Most of the diseases are autoimmune in nature, but some stem from immunodeficiency and others are of unknown origin.

Sjögren Syndrome

Sjögren syndrome (SS) is an autoimmune disease that affects the salivary and lacrimal glands. Immune cells (primarily T cells) attack the glands, causing tissue destruction, which impairs the patient's ability to produce saliva and tears.[4] SS is categorized as primary SS when it appears independently and as secondary SS when it accompanies another autoimmune disease (e.g., **rheumatoid arthritis [RA], systemic lupus erythematosus [SLE],** or **scleroderma [SC]**). SS occurs primarily in patients 40 years or older, and women are nine times more likely to have SS than men. The hallmark symptoms of SS are dry mouth (xerostomia) and dry eyes **(xerophthalmia),** which are sometimes referred to as "sicca symptoms" or "sicca syndrome" (Fig. 43-1). Dryness of the skin, nose, mucous membranes, and vagina may also be present. SS typically causes fatigue and may also affect the lungs, central and peripheral nervous systems, and kidneys.[5]

Pathogenesis

The inability to produce saliva and tears stems from the destruction of epithelial cells that line the salivary and lacrimal glands. The epithelial cells are excretory cells that actually produce the liquid that comprises saliva and tears. The destruction of epithelial cells within the glands happens as follows: The epithelial cells produce chemokines that attract T cells, which, in turn, produce cytokines that induce **apoptosis** (also known as programmed cell death) in the epithelial cells. B cells also invade the glandular tissue and will produce autoantibodies that attack the gland.[6,7]

Treatment

There is no known cure for SS, and treatment is primarily **palliative** (provides relief without curing).[6] Artificial tears are commonly used to alleviate dry eye symptoms. Saliva replacement products and sugar-free chewing gums may provide effective relief for mild-to-moderate dry mouth. Use of xylitol-containing products will also stimulate salivary flow. For patients with some remaining salivary gland function, sialogogues such as oral pilocarpine (Salagen) and cevimeline (Evoxac) are effective medications.[8]

Dental Hygiene Considerations

Oral dryness is the main dental finding of SS. Oral dryness may also lead to dry and cracked lips, oral mucosal sores, and tongue depapillation. Salivary gland swelling can be an extraoral sign of salivary dysfunction and is common among patients with SS (Fig. 43-2). Because there is a marked lack of saliva, patients with SS will have increased rates of decay and an increased incidence of oral infections, particularly oral candidiasis.[6] It is vital that patients with SS maintain meticulous oral hygiene to help prevent dental decay.

During the dental hygiene appointment, special attention should be paid to the provision of oral hygiene instructions (OHI). Clinicians should record a plaque index and use the information to individualize OHI, focusing on plaque-retention areas. The clinician may

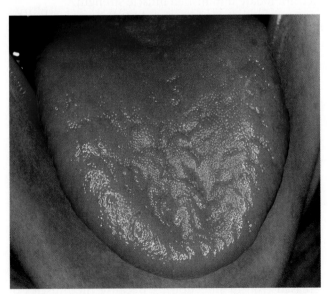

Figure 43-1. Sjögren syndrome. This patient had severe xerostomia. The filiform papillae are lacking. (From Ibsen OAC, Phelan JA. *Oral Pathology for the Dental Hygienist.* 6th ed. St. Louis, MO: Saunders; 2014.)

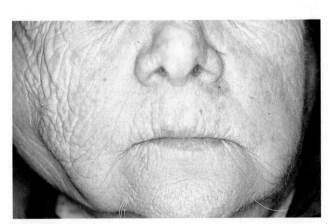

Figure 43-2. Bilateral parotid gland swelling seen in Sjögren syndrome. (From Ibsen OAC, Phelan JA. *Oral Pathology for the Dental Hygienist.* 6th ed. St. Louis, MO: Saunders; 2014. Courtesy Dr. Louis Mandel.)

recommend xylitol gum and candy to help stimulate salivary flow. Additional sources of xylitol, such as XyloSweet (a sugar substitute), may also prove beneficial. Fluorides should be prescribed to help with remineralization of enamel. Over-the-counter fluoride rinses are an inexpensive way to boost remineralization, but a more effective therapy is a custom fluoride tray to be used with prescription fluorides. Prescription-strength fluorides (1.1% solutions, e.g., PreviDent 5000) will be very beneficial to the patient when used regularly as a part of oral home care. These gels can either be worn in a custom tray or brushed onto the teeth for 2 minutes. If brushing the gel on, patients should be instructed not to rinse after application. In addition, professional fluoride treatments (in-office) should be recommended. Neutral sodium fluoride varnish is an effective option for professional fluoride delivery. For more information on fluorides and preventive agents, see Chapter 21.

Myasthenia Gravis

Myasthenia gravis (MG) is an autoimmune disorder that negatively affects the transmission of synapses at the neuromuscular junction (NMJ), resulting in muscle weakness and fatigue. MG occurs in all ethnic groups and in both men and women. MG more commonly affects women younger than 40 years and men older than 50 years.[9]

MG can be classified as ocular MG (patients have problems with extraocular muscles only) or generalized MG (patients experience problems in other areas of the body in addition to the eyes). In ocular MG, patients will experience characteristic droopiness of the upper eyelid (ptosis) and diplopia (double vision).[10] Patients with generalized MG will report muscle fatigue and weakness of the eyes, limbs, and possibly respiratory weakness. They will also demonstrate **bulbar weakness,** which refers to weakness of the facial muscles, difficulty chewing and swallowing, difficulty speaking, and weakness of the neck muscles. This group of symptoms is called *bulbar weakness* or *bulbar symptoms* because the affected nerves originate on the bulblike portion of the brainstem.[11]

Pathogenesis

In 85% of cases with MG, B cells will produce autoantibodies to the nicotinic acetylcholine (ACh) receptors (AChRs) at the motor end-plate, rendering them dysfunctional either by direct destruction of the receptors, by blockade of the receptors, or by complement-mediated destruction.[5,10] As the synapse at the NMJ is essentially blocked, patients with MG experience the characteristic fatigue and muscle weakness in voluntary muscles. The fatigue will worsen with use and will improve with rest; therefore, patients typically feel stronger in the morning and weaker as the day progresses.[11] Eighty-five percent of patients with MG also have some type of thymus abnormality. This can present as a non-neoplastic condition (hyperplasia) or neoplastic condition (thymoma).[10]

Treatment

There are five approaches of treatment for MG: cholinesterase inhibitors, corticosteroids, immunosuppressive drugs, plasmapheresis, and thymectomy. The use of cholinesterase inhibitors is the most common treatment modality, with pyridostigmine (Mestinon) as the most widely prescribed medication.[10] Cholinesterase inhibitors prevent the breakdown of available ACh. Oral corticosteroids and immunosuppressive agents are used to diminish or prevent the destruction of the AChRs. Plasmapheresis is used to treat patients with severe bulbar symptoms or myasthenic crisis. **Plasmapheresis** is a method of treating the blood plasma to try and remove the AChR antibodies from the plasma to decrease the autoimmune response. **Thymectomy** is the surgical removal of the thymus gland, which is performed to improve weakness in patients with MG who are unresponsive to other therapies and to remove thymomas.[5,10,12]

Dental Hygiene Considerations

Patients with MG who remain stable and who have limited or mild neuromuscular involvement may be safely treated in a private dental practice. Patients with uncontrolled MG (who have frequent exacerbations or significant weakness) may receive the safest care in a hospital setting where there is emergency intubation and respiratory support. It is recommended that the dental hygienist consult with the patient's physician before treatment to ensure that the individual can be safely treated in the dental office.[11] Special management considerations should be well-understood by all members of the dental team when treating patients with MG. The dental professional should be able to identify myasthenic weakness or crisis, avoid harmful drug interactions, recognize oral side effects of drugs prescribed for MG, and modify treatment to help accommodate diminished muscle strength.[13]

Dental appointments should be scheduled for the morning, when muscle strength is typically the best, and should be relatively short. Also, appointments should be scheduled when the patient's cholinesterase inhibitors are providing maximum effectiveness, typically 1 to 2 hours after they are taken. If dental treatment is lengthy (e.g., scaling and root planing), multiple short appointments are best.[11,13]

Special care should be taken when reviewing the patient's medical history. Several of the drugs used in dentistry pose possible negative interactions with medications used to treat MG. Refer to Table 43-1 for a list of safe and contraindicated medications.

The clinician should consult with the patient's physician to determine whether there is a need for antibiotic prophylaxis before dental treatment (patients taking corticosteroids or immunosuppressants may be at increased risk for infection).[11] Because the muscles of the oropharynx may be weakened, patients with MG may be at high risk for aspiration. Therefore, the use of powered scalers and air polishers is contraindicated.

Table 43-1. Potential Complications of Dental Medications in Patients With Myasthenia Gravis

Type of Medication	Relatively Contraindicated	Use With Caution	Safe
Local anesthetics	Procaine (Novocaine)*	Lidocaine* Mepivacaine* Bupivacaine* Prilocaine*	
Analgesics and sedatives		Morphine and derivatives[†] Narcotics[†] Benzodiazepines[†] Hypnotics[†] Barbiturates[†]	Acetaminophen NSAIDS[‡] Aspirin N_2O/O_2 sedation
Antibiotics	Erythromycin* Gentamycin* Neomycin* Polymyxin B* Bacitracin* Clindamycin*	Metronidazole Tetracycline Vancomycin	Penicillin and derivatives
Other		Corticosteroids[§]	

*Drugs that may acutely potentiate myasthenic weakness.

[†]Use with caution in patients with respiratory difficulty or depression.

[‡]Significant drug interaction with cyclosporine.

[§]May induce exacerbation of myasthenia gravis.

Source: Adapted from the Myasthenia Gravis Foundation of America. Dental treatment considerations; 2010.[13]

High-speed suction should be used to help prevent aspiration during the appointment. Mouth props may be used to help prevent excess muscle fatigue. For patients with ocular MG, it is important to minimize exposure to the dental light. Dark glasses will help minimize eye strain for the patient.[11]

Two types of crises can occur in patients with MG: myasthenic crisis and cholinergic crisis. It is vital that the dental hygienist be familiar with the signs and symptoms of myasthenic and cholinergic crises so that immediate action can be taken should one occur. **Myasthenic crisis** is defined as the need for respiratory assistance and is due to muscle weakness. Signs to look for include the inability to swallow, speak, or maintain an open airway, double vision, tachycardia, and profound muscle weakness. It is imperative that the patient's first complaint of dyspnea (difficulty breathing) be taken seriously.[11] A **cholinergic crisis** typically results from overmedication. Signs and symptoms of cholinergic crisis include excess salivation, abdominal pain, vomiting, diarrhea, and respiratory distress.[10,11]

Oral hygiene instruction should be very supportive and respective of the patient's muscle weakness. An electric toothbrush or manual toothbrush with a modified, easy-to-grasp handle should be recommended to help reduce muscle fatigue. Toothbrush handle modification may include elongation or widening. Oral rinsing may be difficult if the patient has diminished muscular control. For these patients, toothettes dipped in the rinse or oral irrigators may be recommended. For patients with ocular MG, written education materials should be enlarged.[11]

Scleroderma

SC is a debilitating disease of the connective tissue with no known cause, although it is suspected to be autoimmune in nature. In patients with SC, excessive amounts of collagen are produced and deposited into the connective tissue, producing a hard appearance of the skin.[14] SC can be broken down into two major categories: localized and systemic. Localized SC is generally limited to the skin and underlying tissues, whereas systemic SC also affects the vasculature and internal organs. Although SC affects both sexes and patients of all ages, it is more prevalent in women than men (2:1 to 3:1), and the disease most commonly develops between 40 and 60 years of age. Approximately 50,000 Americans are affected with SC.[14]

Hallmark characteristics of SC include **fibrosis** (thickening and hardening) of the skin of the hands and face and Raynaud phenomenon. **Raynaud phenomenon** describes an intensified reaction to cold or anxiety that elicits discoloration and numbness in the fingers, toes, ears, and nose. Fingers will characteristically become white, then blue, due to spasm of the vasculature and the resulting diminished blood supply.[15] Fibrosis of the skin typically begins in the fingers and the skin surrounding the mouth. Eventually, the skin fuses with the underlying structures, and patients will develop ulcerations at the joints. Patients will develop **microstomia** (abnormal smallness of the mouth) as the skin around the oral cavity hardens and tightens. Patients will experience itchiness because of dryness. Fibrosis may also affect the major salivary glands, resulting in xerostomia. Systemic involvement issues include renal problems, cardiac problems, interstitial lung disease, gastrointestinal problems such as gastroesophageal reflux disease (GERD), and pulmonary hypertension.[16]

Pathogenesis

There are three main facets to the pathogenesis of SC: (a) vascular dysfunction that leads to damaged endothelial cells; (b) activation of T cells, cytokines, and inflammation; and (c) fibrosis.[5,16]

Treatment

Treatment of SC typically consists of pharmacological interventions, which are aimed at immunosuppression, vasodilation, increasing blood flow, and treating organ problems. Methotrexate (Rheumatrex, Trexall) and cyclosporine (Gengraf, Sandimmune) are immunosuppressants that are commonly prescribed for patients with SC. Patients who are taking these medications may need to take prophylactic antibiotics before dental treatment.[16] Nifedipine (Procardia, Adalat CC, Afeditab CR, Nifediac CC) and amlodipine (Norvasc) are often prescribed for treating Raynaud phenomenon and may cause gingival overgrowth. Patients may also be taking a regimen of corticosteroids, which again may cause immunosuppression. Consultation with the patient's physician is recommended before treatment.

Dental Hygiene Considerations

Oral manifestations of SC include microstomia, xerostomia, fibrosis of the hard and soft palate, widening of the periodontal ligament (PDL) space affecting all teeth, enamel erosion, mandibular resorption, and trigeminal neuropathy (disease of the trigeminal nerve).[16] Trigeminal neuropathy commonly precedes systemic involvement of systemic SC. It is characterized by gradual facial muscle inactivity, pain, and paresthesia (abnormal sensations like prickling or pins and needles). These symptoms may appear years before diagnosis of SC. Dental professionals should suspect SC if there is no dental cause for this type of pain. Referral to the patient's physician is an appropriate step should the dental hygienist note this finding. Widening of the PDL space involving all teeth is another red flag for dental professionals. If there is no evidence of occlusal trauma, the dental professional should suspect SC. Resorption of the mandible results from facial skin tightening and compression of the vasculature and musculature that applies constant force to the mandible. Areas of resorption are often asymptomatic and increase the risk for mandibular fractures, trigeminal neuropathy, and osteomyelitis.

The dental hygienist should plan to perform routine panoramic radiographs to monitor the mandible.[16] Patients with SC will often demonstrate decreased function of the temporomandibular joint, which limits the movement of the mandible.[17,18]

Fibrosis of the facial skin and skin of the fingers will highly affect the patient's ability to perform oral self-care. Deficient manual dexterity and limited opening ability negatively affect the efficiency of oral hygiene practices, leading to an increased risk for periodontal disease and dental decay (see Professionalism).

Stretching exercises have been demonstrated to be effective in helping patients with SC maintain elasticity.[19] Some simple stretching exercises are outlined in Table 43-2.

Oral hygiene instructions should be very individualized and should focus on meeting the patient's needs in light of his or her state of disease progression. Because of limitations of manual dexterity, enlargement or extension, or both, of a toothbrush handle may improve the patient's ability to remove plaque biofilm. In addition, powered toothbrushes and floss holding devices may facilitate improved oral hygiene. For patients with Raynaud phenomenon, wrapping floss around the ends of the fingers may prove to be painful. Patients will likely need a compact toothbrush head, pediatric toothbrush, or an end-tuft brush to access the oral cavity when the opening is limited.[16] In patients with xerostomia and GERD, the enamel may be demineralized, leading to decay and hypersensitivity. Fluorides should be recommended to combat these problems.

Before dental treatment, a thorough review of the patient's medications is necessary. If there are any concerns regarding immunosuppression, consultation with the patient's physician is recommended. The dental hygienist should provide nutritional counseling to decrease the risk for decay. Fibrosis in the oropharyngeal region may lead to dysphagia (difficulty swallowing); therefore, the use of powered scalers and air polishers is contraindicated and the use of high-speed suction is recommended. Because of limited mandibular function, a mouth prop may prove to be helpful in facilitating

Professionalism

Treating patients with scleroderma provides the dental hygienist a good opportunity to act professionally. The patients will have some form of debilitation, as well as changes to their physical appearance. When working with these patients to provide OHI and direct care, it is extremely important for the dental hygienist to demonstrate empathy and provide support. Demonstrating an understanding of the patient's debilitation, as well as being supportive, will facilitate the development of a trusting and respectful relationship. ■

Table 43-2. *Stretching Exercises for Increasing Range of Motion for the Patient With Scleroderma*

Oral Exercises

Exercise 1: Do three sets of five stretches, holding each for 3–5 seconds.
1. Purse your lips.
2. Open your mouth as wide as you can.
3. Puff out your cheeks.
4. Make an exaggerated smile.
5. Move lower jaw down and forward, right and left.

Exercise 2: Repeat at least two times a day.
1. Stack four tongue blades together and secure with a clean rubber band.
2. Open mouth and place stack between the teeth.
3. Determine the number of blades that can comfortably fit in the stack.
4. Add one additional tongue blade to the middle of the stack and let it gently stretch the mouth.
5. Gradually increase the number of blades in the stack to stretch the mandibular opening.

Hand Exercises

Exercise 1: Perform in three sets of five stretches, holding each for 3–5 seconds.
1. Make a fist.
2. Press the fingers flat against each other.
3. Touch the thumb to the base of the little finger.

Exercise 2: Repeat 10 times a day.
1. Place arms at sides with fingers pointed toward the toes, palms facing the body.
2. Curl fingers and attempt to touch your finger tips to your palm.
3. Slowly uncurl and straighten fingers as much as possible.

Source: Adapted from Poole J, Conte C, Brewer C, et al. Oral hygiene in scleroderma: the effectiveness of a multi-disciplinary intervention program. *Disabil Rehabil.* 2010;32(5):379-384; and Tolle SL. Scleroderma: considerations for dental hygienists. *Int J Dent Hyg.* 2008;6(2):77-83.

Teamwork

Advanced SC presents the dental hygienist with an opportunity for interprofessional collaboration with an occupation therapist (OT). OTs work with patients who have disabilities that affect activities of daily living. Referring a patient to an OT, as well as working collaboratively with the OT to make adaptations to oral self-care aids or find adaptive devices necessary to meet the patient's needs, will maximize the success of oral self-care regimens. ■

dental hygiene treatment. The patient may experience some discomfort during and after the appointment because of the need to keep the mouth open for an extended period. Analgesics may be recommended as needed, provided that there is no drug interaction with the patient's prescribed medications. Raynaud phenomenon is typically triggered by cold temperatures and stress; therefore, it is imperative that the appointment remain as stress-free as possible. Adequate pain control is paramount. Also, it is prudent to have a blanket on hand to facilitate patient comfort (see Teamwork).[5,16,17]

Multiple Sclerosis

Multiple sclerosis (MS) is a chronic, inflammatory autoimmune disease that results in **demyelination** (destruction of the myelin sheath) in the central nervous system (CNS). MS is two times more common in women than men, and it affects approximately 400,000 people in the United States.[20,21] Symptoms of MS include fatigue; numbness; balance, coordination, and walking problems; bladder dysfunction; bowel dysfunction; vision problems; dizziness and vertigo; sexual dysfunction; pain; cognitive dysfunction; emotional changes; depression; and **spasticity** (muscular spasms).[21] Symptoms of MS may lead to an inability to manage activities of daily living, ambulation, and/or mobility.

There are four clinical types of MS: (a) relapsing/remitting, in which the disease is episodic in nature with acute attacks of worsening condition; (b) primary progressive, in which there is gradual progressive deterioration of neurological function; (c) secondary progressive, in which the disease begins with relapsing/remitting course followed by changes in the clinical course of the disease to progressive deterioration; and (d) progressive relapsing, in with there is steady deterioration of neurological function exacerbated by periodic acute attacks. Relapsing/remitting is the most common presentation of MS.[21,22]

Pathogenesis

MS is inflammatory and degenerative. Pathogenesis involves the stimulation of T cells and macrophages that attack oligodendrocytes, which are glial cells that comprise the myelin sheath. B cells are also stimulated to produce an autoantibody response that contributes to demyelination.[2,22]

Treatment

Treatment for MS can be divided into three categories: treatment of acute attacks, disease-modifying treatment, and symptomatic treatment. For treatment of acute attacks, corticosteroids are commonly prescribed to shorten the duration of an attack and accelerate recovery. Examples of commonly used corticosteroids include prednisone (PredniSONE Intensol) and methylprednisolone (Depo-Medrol, Medrol).[22] Several types of medications are used in disease-modifying treatment. They include beta interferons (Betaseron, Rebif, Avonex,

Extavia), copolymer 1, which is also known as glatiramer acetate (Copaxone), the immunosuppressant mitoxantrone (Novantrone), and natalizumab (Tysabri), which is a relatively new antibody-based treatment.[20] Symptomatic treatment is used as needed, and common examples of medications used in this way are anticonvulsants, tricyclic antidepressants, and benzodiazepines for spasticity and analgesics for pain.[22]

Dental Hygiene Considerations

There are several orofacial manifestations of MS. The most common of these are intermittent unilateral facial numbness or pain, facial palsy or spasm, visual disturbances, and impaired articulation. **Paroxysmal pain syndromes** may develop in the orofacial region as well. These are characterized by short-duration, intense, electric or shocklike pains that occur at a high frequency.[22] Patients with these signs and symptoms with no obvious dental cause and with no previous diagnosis of MS should be referred to their physician for evaluation.

Exacerbations of MS may negatively impact the patient's ability to maintain a good oral self-care regimen as well as their ability to visit a dentist. For patients with reduced mobility visiting a dentist can be particularly challenging. Patients who are wheelchair bound may need assistance transferring to the dental chair (see transfer procedure in Chapter 49). Appointment times and appointment lengths should be adjusted to suit the patient's individual needs.

Before treating the patient, it is imperative to perform a thorough review of the medical history and evaluate the medication list. There may be potential drug interactions with medications commonly used in dentistry, as well as oral side effects of medications prescribed for MS. Oral side effects of MS medications include xerostomia, gingival hyperplasia, mucositis/ulcerative stomatitis, **dysgeusia** (impaired sense of taste), and overgrowth of opportunistic infections such as candidiasis.[22]

A mouth prop should be used during treatment to help prevent muscle fatigue and spasm. Some patients experience difficulty swallowing. If so, avoid placing the patient in a supine position. OHI should be tailored to the patient's specific needs. Some patients experience a loss of manual dexterity, and for these patients a modified toothbrush handle or electric toothbrush can be recommended. Xerostomia is a common side effect of medications prescribed for MS, so nutritional counseling and prescription of fluoride use is appropriate. Oral moisturizers and xylitol gum can be recommended to help with dry mouth. Sialogogues such as pilocarpine and cevimeline may also prove to be effective.[22]

Rheumatoid Arthritis

RA is an autoimmune disease that results in pain, swelling, and loss of function in the joints. RA affects approximately 1.3 million people, and affects women two to three times more often than men. The initial presentation of the disease typically occurs in middle age, but it is possible for the disease to develop in younger people.[23]

Characteristic features of RA include tender, warm, and swollen joints occurring in a symmetrical pattern (both right and left sides are affected, like mirror images). RA most often affects finger and wrist joints, and sometimes affects the neck, shoulders, elbows, hips, knees, ankles, and feet. Patients with RA typically experience fatigue, occasional fevers, and general malaise. Pain and stiffness will generally last longer than 30 minutes after a long rest or upon first waking. Patients typically experience symptoms for many years.[23]

Systemic effects of RA also exist, the most common of which is anemia (decreased number of red blood cells). Less commonly experienced systemic effects are neck pain and dry eyes and mouth. Rarely, patients with RA will experience vasculitis, **pleurisy** (inflammation of the pleura, characterized by a dry cough and pain on the affected side), and pericarditis. The mental health of patients with RA is commonly affected, and patients may experience depression, anxiety, low self-esteem, and feelings of helplessness. RA may progress to the degree that the patient's activities of daily living are affected.[23]

Pathogenesis

WBCs travel to the synovial membranes, causing inflammation, and the inflamed synovium destroys bone and cartilage in the joint. Supporting muscles, tendons, and ligaments then become weak and dysfunctional. The exact pathogenesis of RA is unknown, but several factors are believed to impact the development of the disease. It is accepted that genetics plays a role in the development of RA, as certain genes that are known to play a role in the immune system are associated with the tendency to develop RA. Scientists believe that there is some sort of trigger, either viral or bacterial, that initiates the development of disease in RA-prone individuals, but the exact trigger is unknown. Also, hormones may contribute to the development of the disease.[23]

Treatment

Treatment for RA consists of lifestyle management and medications and, in certain cases, surgical therapy. Patients with RA need a good balance of exercise and rest, resting more during exacerbations. Exercise is important for overall health, as well as maintaining strong muscles and joint mobility. Self-help devices are recommended (e.g., zipper pullers and shoe horns), as well as stress reduction and a healthy diet.

Medications for RA fall into several categories: medications for symptoms (analgesics for pain, corticosteroids and NSAIDs for inflammation), disease-modifying antirheumatic drugs (DMARDs) to slow the course of the disease, and biologics to interrupt the cascade of events that drive inflammation.[23]

In some instances, patients will undergo surgical treatment for RA. Joint replacement surgery, arthrodesis (joint fusion), tendon reconstruction, and synovectomy (removal of synovial membranes—usually only used as part of reconstructive surgery) are possible surgical options for some patients.[23]

Dental Hygiene Considerations

Decreased manual dexterity is the main factor that affects the oral health of patients with RA. RA will often cause joint deformity that results in the inability to use the hands efficiently. Because the decreased manual dexterity negatively affects oral hygiene practices, patients with RA are at increased risk for periodontal disease and caries. Patients with RA may also experience changes to the gingiva, xerostomia, and acid reflux as negative side effects of medications prescribed for RA. OHI should be individualized for the patient, paying particular attention to the patient's manual dexterity. Modified toothbrush handles, electric toothbrushes, and floss holders may be appropriate recommendations for oral self-care aids. Fluorides should be recommended as well. For the dental hygiene appointment, the clinician must complete a thorough review of the medications the patient is taking. Oral side effects are prevalent, and there is the potential for drug interaction with medications often used in dentistry.[23,24]

Systemic Lupus Erythematosus

SLE is the most common form of lupus, and the form of lupus to which most people are referring when they simply say "lupus." SLE is an autoimmune disease in which there is inflammation and damage to various tissues in the body. Common symptoms of SLE include arthritis and muscle pain, extreme fatigue, unexplained fever, red skin rashes most commonly on the face (called **malar** or butterfly rash), chest pain upon deep breathing, unusual hair loss, Raynaud phenomenon, mouth ulcers, swollen glands, and kidney problems. The lungs, CNS, blood vessels, blood, and heart can also be affected.[25] SLE is more common in women than men, and more prevalent among African American, Asian, and Hispanic women than those of Caucasian descent. This disease typically manifests between the ages of 10 and 50 years.[25]

Pathogenesis

The specific pathogenesis of SLE is unknown, but the immune system produces autoantibodies and immune complexes that mediate destruction of host tissue cells via the inflammatory process.[25,26]

Treatment

There is no cure for SLE, and the goal of treatment is to control symptoms. Because the disease typically involves multiple body systems, treatment usually requires collaboration between the patient's physician and specialists to develop a comprehensive care plan. Corticosteroids are a mainstay of SLE therapy. Corticosteroids will rapidly suppress the inflammatory response. NSAIDs will also be recommended to treat joint pain, chest pain, and fever. Antimalarials (e.g., hydroxychloroquine) are used to treat fatigue, joint pain, skin rashes, and inflammation in the lungs. For patients whose SLE affects their kidneys or CNS, immunosuppressants are often prescribed. B-lymphocyte stimulator–specific inhibitors are sometimes prescribed to reduce the abnormal number of B cells. DMARDs are also used to treat SLE.[25]

Dental Hygiene Considerations

Oral involvement in SLE is common. Patients with SLE may experience the following complications: dry mouth, cracked lips, bleeding gums, sore jaws, cracked tongue, oral lesions and ulcers, and candidiasis. Patients may also have a second autoimmune disease (e.g., SS or SC) and experience the oral effects of the additional disease as well.[27] Because of dry mouth, oral hygiene should be meticulous, and fluoride supplements should be recommended. Baking soda rinses may be appropriate as well. For patients experiencing dry mouth, oral moisturizers, xylitol gum or candy, and sialogogues may prove to be effective. To ease pain from oral sores, patients can use topical benzocaine ointments such as Orabase or Orajel. Alcohol-containing mouthrinses should not be recommended for patients with oral sores.[27]

For the dental hygiene appointment, the clinician should take special care when reviewing the patient's medication list and planning treatment. Certain antibiotics (e.g., tetracycline) or analgesics (e.g., aspirin and NSAIDs) used in dentistry can adversely affect kidney function, and therefore should not be prescribed for patients with SLE who experience kidney involvement.[27] Many patients with SLE also have Libman–Sacks endocarditis (noninfective endocarditis). Consultation with the patient's physician regarding the use of antibiotic prophylaxis is recommended before dental treatment.[27] For patients with lung involvement, the use of nitrous oxide may be contraindicated. As always, the clinician needs to have a good understanding of the side effects of medications prescribed for SLE, as well as potential drug interactions with medications prescribed by or used in the dental office.[27]

Adrenal Insufficiency

Adrenal insufficiency (AI) is a hormonal disorder that occurs when the adrenal glands are not functioning properly to produce needed hormones. AI can be classified as primary AI (**Addison disease**) or secondary AI. In Addison disease, the adrenal glands are damaged and cannot produce enough cortisol and, in many cases, not enough aldosterone either. In secondary AI, the pituitary gland fails to produce enough adrenocorticotropin. Adrenocorticotropin stimulates the adrenal gland to produce cortisol and, without sufficient stimulation, the adrenal glands will eventually atrophy. Addison disease affects approximately 1 to 4 individuals in every 100,000 people of all ages and all races. Secondary AI is much more common than Addison disease.[28]

Cortisol is responsible for maintaining blood pressure (BP) and vascular function, slowing the inflammatory response, maintaining blood glucose levels, and regulating metabolism of carbohydrates, proteins, and fats. Aldosterone helps to maintain BP as well as regulate the salt/water balance by influencing the kidneys to retain sodium and excrete potassium. The main symptoms of AI include chronic, worsening fatigue, muscle weakness, loss of appetite, and weight loss. Other less common symptoms include nausea, vomiting, diarrhea, low BP that drops upon standing (orthostatic hypotension), irritability, depression, craving for salty foods, hypoglycemia, headache, sweating, and irregular or absent menstrual cycles.[28] Patients with AI may experience what is known as an **Addisonian crisis** or **acute adrenal insufficiency.** This crisis situation is characterized by severe worsening of symptoms, including sudden penetrating pain in the lower back, abdomen, or legs; severe vomiting or diarrhea; sudden drop in BP; and/or loss of consciousness.

Pathogenesis

Eighty percent of cases with Addison disease result from autoimmune disease in which lymphocytes and plasma cells invade the adrenal cortex (outer layer of the adrenal gland) and produce autoantibodies that attack and destroy it.[5,28] In less than 20% of Addison disease cases, infection with tuberculosis (TB) can destroy the adrenal gland. Less common causes of Addison disease include chronic infections (typically fungal in nature), cancer, AIDS-associated infections, bleeding into the adrenal gland, surgical removal, and genetic defects. Secondary AI is generally caused by a lack of adrenocorticotropin. Less common causes of secondary AI are tumors or infections, loss of blood to the pituitary gland, radiation therapy for pituitary tumors, surgical removal of the hypothalamus, or surgical removal of the pituitary gland.[28]

Treatment

Treatment of AI consists of replacing or substituting the deficient hormones. For patients who are producing insufficient amounts of cortisol, a synthetic glucocorticoid (e.g., hydrocortisone [A-Hydrocort, Cortef], prednisone [PredniSONE Intensol], or dexamethasone [Baycadron, Dexamethasone Intensol, DexPak]) is prescribed. For those who are deficient in aldosterone, a mineralocorticoid (e.g., fludrocortisone acetate [Florinef]) is prescribed. Addisonian crisis can be life-threatening, and in this instance, intravenous glucocorticoids and saline are administered.[28]

Dental Hygiene Considerations

Patients with AI should be scheduled at the time of day that they feel the best. Thorough evaluation of the patient's medication list is imperative to evaluate for side effects of medications and possible drug interactions. Evaluating the patient's BP before treatment is an essential procedure for the dental hygienist. Dropping BP is a sign of Addisonian crisis, and a baseline level should be established before treatment. The dental hygienist needs to be aware of the signs and symptoms of Addisonian crisis, and the entire dental team needs to be ready to respond to a medical emergency should one arise. Patients may require extra dosing or additional medications (e.g., hydrocortisone) before major dental work (such as root canal treatment or extractions). Consultation with the patient's physician before major dental work is recommended.[29]

Fibromyalgia

Fibromyalgia (FM) is a disorder that causes muscle pain and fatigue. Patients with FM typically have "tender points" that experience pain when pressure is applied to these areas. Typical tender points are the neck, shoulders, back, hips, arms, and legs.[30] Other symptoms of FM include difficulty sleeping, stiffness upon waking, headaches, painful menstrual periods, tingling or numbness in the hands and feet, and trouble with thought processes and memory (commonly called "fibro fog"). FM may occur as a lone disease, but it is commonly found alongside another condition, such as RA or SLE. An estimated 5 million Americans suffer from FM. Approximately 80% to 90% of cases are women, and most are diagnosed in middle age.[30]

Pathogenesis

The exact cause of FM is unknown, although it has been linked to traumatic events, repetitive injuries, and illnesses.[30]

Treatment

Treating FM may require a team approach, with the team composed of the patient's physicians and specialists. Lifestyle adaptation is a large part of treatment. Lifestyle changes include eating a healthy diet, getting exercise, and following a good sleep regimen (e.g., going to bed and getting up at the same time daily).[30,31] Several medications have been approved by the U.S. Food and Drug Administration for the treatment of FM, including pregabalin (Lyrica), duloxetine (Cymbalta), and milnacipran (Savella). Symptoms may also be treated with nonnarcotic pain relievers and low doses of antidepressants or benzodiazepines. Complementary and alternative medicine (CAM) therapies have also proved to be effective in treating FM. Examples of CAM therapy include physical therapy, massage, acupressure, acupuncture, yoga, and relaxation techniques.[31]

Dental Hygiene Considerations

The dental hygienist should be very thorough in the medical history review and have a good understanding of the side effects of any medications prescribed for FM. Patients should be scheduled at a time when they feel less fatigued. The patient may need pillows or other positioning aids to remain comfortable throughout the appointment. If patients experience tender points in the arms, a wrist BP cuff may prove to be more comfortable.

HIV/AIDS

HIV is a virus that attacks CD4+ helper T cells, resulting in impaired immune function. Because CD4+ helper T cells are responsible for assisting plasma cells in producing antibodies, patients with this disease will demonstrate a decreased capacity for fighting infection.[32] Infection with HIV eventually leads to the development of AIDS. AIDS is the most advanced stage of HIV infection and is diagnosed when the patient presents with a CD4+ count of less than 200 cells/mm³ or has an AIDS-defining disease. Examples of AIDS-defining diseases are *Pneumocystis jiroveci* pneumonia, TB, and toxoplasmosis.[33] HIV is most commonly spread via unprotected sexual contact and sharing intravenous drug needles with a person infected with HIV. Blood, semen, genital fluids, and breast milk are body fluids that contain HIV.[33] At the end of 2008, an estimated 1,178,350 people in the United States aged 13 years or older were living with HIV infection, including 236,400 (20.1%) whose infection had not been diagnosed.[34]

Pathogenesis

HIV binds to and fuses with CD4+ T cells. After fusion, the virus releases RNA into the cell. Then reverse transcriptase (HIV enzyme) converts the RNA to a double-stranded HIV DNA. The HIV DNA enters the cell's nucleus where another enzyme, called *integrase,* incorporates the foreign DNA into the host cell's DNA. When the host cell receives a signal to become active, a process called *transcription* takes place in which copies of the HIV genetic material are made and long chains of HIV proteins are produced. Then the long chains are cut into smaller, individual pieces by an enzyme called *protease.* These smaller pieces combine with HIV genetic material to form viral particles. These viral particles will then exit the host cell using a process called *budding* in which they steal a portion of the cell's membrane that serves as a covering. The virus is then ready to spread and infect other cells.[35]

Treatment

To date, there is no cure for HIV/AIDS. Patients are managed through a regimen of multiple drugs that is called highly active antiretroviral therapy (HAART). HAART protocols can consist of several different classes of drugs. These include protease inhibitors, nucleoside reverse transcriptase inhibitors, non-nucleoside reverse transcriptase inhibitors, integrase inhibitors, and fusion inhibitors.[36]

Dental Hygiene Considerations

There are several common oral problems among patients with AIDS. Patients with AIDS can present with oral warts, herpetic lesions, hairy leukoplakia, oral candidiasis, aphthous ulcers, dry mouth, linear gingival erythema, necrotizing ulcerative gingivitis, necrotizing ulcerative periodontitis, Kaposi sarcoma (Fig. 43-3), and intraoral and head and neck lymphomas. Patients with AIDS are prone to infection

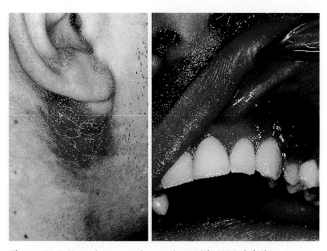

Figure 43-3. Kaposi sarcoma in a patient with AIDS. (A) Skin. (B) Gingiva. (From Ibsen OAC, Phelan JA. *Oral Pathology for the Dental Hygienist.* 6th ed. St. Louis, MO: Saunders; 2014. Courtesy Dr. Fariba Younai.)

with herpes simplex virus (HSV), cytomegalovirus, Epstein-Barr virus, varicella zoster virus, and human papillomavirus.[36] Children with AIDS may demonstrate delayed dental development.[37]

Before treating a patient with HIV/AIDS, the clinician should consult with the patient's physician to establish that it is safe for the patient to undergo treatment. Patients with immunosuppression may need to take antibiotic premedication before treatment.[36] Some patients may experience increased bleeding times, so consultation regarding this issue is important as well. As always, thorough review of the patient's medications for side effects and possible drug interactions is imperative. HAART can significantly alter the metabolism and elimination of drugs by the liver. Consultation with the patient's physician or pharmacist is recommended before prescribing medications for patients receiving HAART treatment. In general, the most commonly prescribed antibiotics for dental infections (e.g., amoxicillin and clindamycin) are not affected by HAART.[36] For patients with advanced AIDS, dental care may be more focused on urgent needs such as pain control and control of infection. Some patients may be seen most safely in a hospital or other specialized setting.

For patients with xerostomia, saliva substitutes and fluorides should be recommended. Some medications for HIV/AIDS contain sugar and can therefore increase the risk for decay even more when paired with dry mouth. Prescription-strength fluorides (1.1% solutions, e.g., PreviDent 5000) are very beneficial to the patient. Xylitol candies and gums can also be recommended. Individualized OHI and nutritional counseling are important aspects of preventive dental treatment for patients with dry mouth.[36] Patients with oral sores may experience relief through the use of Orajel or Orabase, or other topical lidocaine applications. For oral candidiasis, topical or oral antifungals may be prescribed. Consultation with the patient's physician is recommended before prescribing any medications (see Spotlight on Public Health).

Spotlight on Public Health

The Oregon Health and Science University (OHSU) Russell Street Dental Clinic is located in downtown Portland, Oregon, and is part of the Coalition of Community Health Clinics. The dental clinic opened on August 1, 1975, and provides a wide range of dental services at reduced cost to low-income patients. The Russell Street Clinic is unique in that the dental team sees many patients who are HIV-positive (about 40% of their patients) and specializes in providing care to this special needs population. The Russell Street Clinic has received grant funding through the Ryan White HIV/AIDS program to support its mission of serving patients with HIV/AIDS. During the early years of the clinic, the dental team saw most of the HIV-positive population in the state of Oregon. In more recent years, the clinic continues to see more than 1,000 HIV-positive patients annually, providing an important resource to HIV-positive patients in the Portland area. The dental team at Russell Street is composed of dentists, dental hygienists, patient care coordinators, and a dental laboratory technician. ■

Lichen Planus

Lichen planus (LP) presents as a rash on the skin or painful oral lesions (Fig. 43-4). Typically LP affects middle-aged adults. Cases usually resolve within 2 years, although one in five will have a second outbreak, and some patients may experience outbreaks off and on for years.[38] Oral lesions can be tender or painful and can appear on the sides of the tongue and insides of the cheeks. Occasionally, lesions may appear on the gingiva. Lesions characterized by a network of lines are called **Wickham striae,** which are lacy in appearance (Fig. 43-5). The lesions will sometimes progress into painful ulcers.[39] The skin rash is usually located on the inner wrist, legs, torso, or genitals. It has a symmetrical appearance and may appear as a single lesion or a cluster of lesions. LP lesions typically have distinct borders, are shiny or scaly in appearance, and may develop blisters (Fig. 43-6). Lesions may occur at the site of an injury. Other symptoms of LP may include dry mouth, hair loss, ridges in the nails, and a metallic taste in the mouth.[39]

Pathogenesis

The exact pathogenesis of LP is unknown, but it is thought to be allergic or immune in nature. Exposure to certain chemicals can place an individual at risk for development of LP. Examples of these include gold, arsenic, iodides, chloroquine (Aralen), phenothiazines, and diuretics. Infection with hepatitis C may also place an individual at risk for development of LP.[39]

Treatment

Treatment for LP attempts to reduce symptoms and to speed healing and resolution of lesions. Antihistamines,

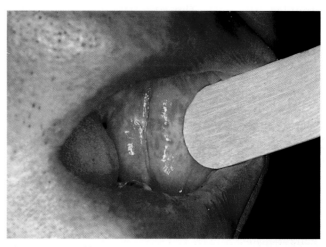

Figure 43-5. Wickham striae. (Courtesy of Ricardo Padilla, DDS, University of North Carolina Oral and Maxillofacial Pathology.)

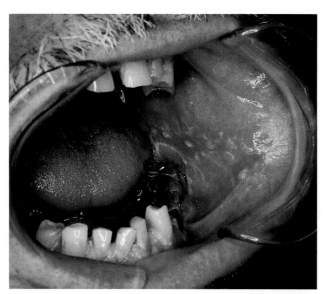

Figure 43-4. Wickham striae in lichen planus. Erosion of the mucosa appears as erythema adjacent to white striae. (From Ibsen OAC, Phelan JA. *Oral Pathology for the Dental Hygienist.* 6th ed. St. Louis, MO: Saunders; 2014.)

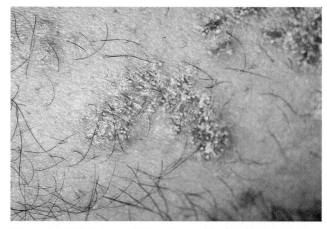

Figure 43-6. Skin lesions of lichen planus. (From Ibsen OAC, Phelan JA. *Oral Pathology for the Dental Hygienist.* 6th ed. St. Louis, MO: Saunders; 2014.)

immunosuppressants (in severe cases), lidocaine-based mouthrinse, topical or oral corticosteroids, topical retinoic acid cream, topical immunosuppressives, oral retinoids, and ultraviolet treatments may be used to treat LP.[39]

Dental Hygiene Considerations

If patients experience dry mouth, a fluoride regimen should be recommended. Patients may also need oral moisturizers. For patients with extensive oral lesions, a lidocaine-based mouthrinse may be used to help facilitate eating. This may be prescribed by the patient's physician or dentist. Mouth ulcers that remain for prolonged periods may eventually turn into cancerous lesions, so a thorough intraoral examination is imperative every 6 months.[39] Nutritional counseling is important for patients with LP, because certain foods can aggravate the condition. Patients should be advised to avoid spicy and acidic foods and beverages, caffeine, and crispy or salty foods. Tobacco cessation counseling is extremely important for patients with LP. Patients are already at a higher risk for development of oral cancer because of prolonged tissue changes; therefore, tobacco and alcohol cessation should be encouraged (see Advancing Technologies).[38]

Erythema Multiforme

Erythema multiforme (EM) is a skin disorder that occurs primarily in children and young adults and presents as multiple types of skin lesions. EM occurs as an allergic reaction or as a reaction to infection. Several medications can induce EM, including barbiturates, penicillins, phenytoin (Dilantin), and sulfonamides. Infection with HSV or mycoplasma can also cause EM.[40]

There are two forms of EM: EM minor and EM major. EM minor is not a serious condition and is most often caused by infection with HSV or mycoplasma (Fig. 43-7). EM major, which is also known as Stevens-Johnson syndrome, is more severe and is usually caused by a reaction to medications rather than infection (Fig. 43-8). Symptoms of EM include fever, general malaise, itching, joint pain, and multiple skin lesions. The skin lesions may appear as a macule, nodule,

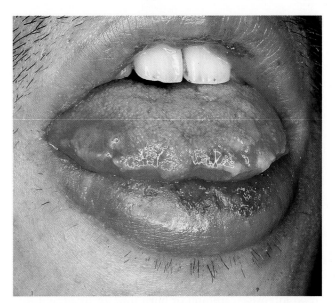

Figure 43-7. Oral lesions of erythema multiforme. Crusted lip lesions with edema, ulceration, and erythema. (From Ibsen OAC, Phelan JA. *Oral Pathology for the Dental Hygienist.* 6th ed. St. Louis, MO: Saunders; 2014.)

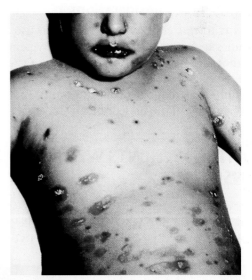

Figure 43-8. Stevens-Johnson syndrome. (From Ibsen OAC, Phelan JA. *Oral Pathology for the Dental Hygienist.* 6th ed. St. Louis, MO: Saunders; 2014. Courtesy Dr. Sidney Eisig.)

Advancing Technologies

Oral cancer screening is an important part of the assessment phase of the dental hygiene appointment. In the past several years, advances in technology have led to the development of devices to aid the clinician in detecting oral cancer. The VELscope Vx is an example of this emerging technology. It is a handheld tool that emits a blue-spectrum light that causes the oral tissues to appear fluorescent. Changes in the tissue indicative of oral cancer will fluoresce differently from healthy tissue. This provides the clinician with an enhanced visual examination. ■

papule, or may look like hives. There is often a central sore surrounded by pale red rings, giving the lesion a target-like appearance. This type of appearance is often referred to as "target," "bull's-eye," or "iris." There may be vesicles or bullae of various sizes, and typically the lesions have a symmetrical appearance. EM may affect the face and lips. Other symptoms include oral sores, bloodshot eyes, dry eyes, eye pain, burning and itching in the eyes accompanied by discharge, and vision problems.[40]

Pathogenesis

The exact pathogenesis of EM is unknown. The disorder is believed to be caused by damage to the blood vessels in the skin, which subsequently leads to damage in the skin tissues themselves.[40]

Treatment

The goals of treatment for EM include controlling the illness that causes EM, preventing infection, and treating symptoms.[40] Treatment options are different for EM minor and EM major. For mild cases of EM, treatment options include discontinuing suspect medications; taking antihistamines for itching; using moist compresses for the skin; taking oral antivirals if a viral infection is suspected; taking over-the-counter medications to help control fever and relieve discomfort (e.g., NSAIDs or acetaminophen); and using topical anesthetics for oral lesions (lidocaine-based mouthrinse for diffuse lesions, Orajel or Orabase for isolated lesions; Fig. 43-9).[40]

For severe cases of EM, antibiotics may be prescribed to control skin infections. Corticosteroids may be used to control inflammation, and patients with severe cases and Stevens-Johnson syndrome may be hospitalized or placed in an intensive care unit or burn unit for treatment. Intravenous immunoglobulin may be used as a treatment modality to stop the disease process. Patients may also need skin grafting in cases where large areas are affected.

Dental Hygiene Considerations

Patients with this condition may need to use topical anesthetics to facilitate eating and oral hygiene practices. Lidocaine-based mouthwash, Orajel, or Orabase may be used, and the clinician needs to inquire about usage (amount, frequency, and duration) and record this information in the patient medical history.

TREATING PATIENTS WITH TRANSPLANTS

Patients who have undergone organ transplantation have special needs that should be addressed when planning and providing dental treatment. Organ transplantation is often a procedure that is life-saving for a patient. If a patient undergoes organ transplantation, the dysfunctional organ will be removed and a healthy organ from a donor will be put in its place. Organs that can be transplanted include the heart, intestine, kidney, lung, liver, and pancreas.[41]

Dental Hygiene Considerations

The dental hygienist should take into account several factors before treating a patient who has received an organ transplant. Patients with transplants are placed on antirejection medications that suppress the immune response. Although effective, this course of treatment places the patient at increased risk for infection. Because patients with transplants face an increased risk for infection, they may need to have antibiotic premedication before dental treatment (see Evidence-Based Practice).[42]

Consultation with the patient's physician or specialist is strongly recommended before providing treatment. If the patient has any additional special needs, his or her medical provider can help the dental hygienist plan to accommodate those needs. An example of an additional need would be a change in regimen of the patient's ongoing medications before treatment.[42]

Antirejection medications can cause negative oral side effects that can lead to oral health problems. Accordingly, the patient needs to be as healthy as possible before transplant surgery. Any decay should be restored and periodontal disease arrested before the transplant operation. The dental evaluation is an important part of the preoperative transplant surgery workup.[42]

Side effects of antirejection medications include dry mouth, mouth ulcers, opportunistic infections (e.g., candidiasis), and gingival overgrowth. Transplant patients, particularly patients with a history of smoking, may be at increased risk for oral cancer.[42] Because of dry mouth and decreased immune response, it is imperative that the patient maintain excellent oral hygiene. OHI should be individualized to help the patient access any problem areas. Conducting a plaque index is helpful in assessing missed areas that may need special attention (see Application to Clinical Practice).

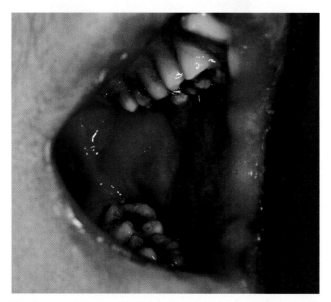

Figure 43-9. Oral lesions of erythema multiforme. Erythematous and ulcerated lesions of the lips and buccal mucosa. (From Ibsen OAC, Phelan JA. *Oral Pathology for the Dental Hygienist.* 6th ed. St. Louis, MO: Saunders; 2014.)

Evidence-Based Practice

It is important that the dental hygienist remain current regarding his or her knowledge of antibiotic prophylactic regimens. As evidence emerges, the American Heart Association and the American Academy of Orthopaedic Surgeons will update their respective guidelines for the use of antibiotic premedication for dental treatment. Keeping current with the guidelines will facilitate a safe and caring practice for all patients. ■

Application to Clinical Practice

Mr. Jordan arrives at your office for his new patient visit. As with any appointment, you begin with a review of the patient's medical history. You come across a few medications with which you are unfamiliar, and your review in a drug guide reveals several potential concerns regarding dental treatment. You decide that it is important to contact the patient's physician to make sure it is safe to proceed with treatment. What are some specific areas of concern that you would like to address? ■

Case Study

Ms. Johansson, a 38-year-old white female, is a new patient who is seeking dental hygiene services and a basic dental examination. During the dental hygienist's review of Ms. Johansson's medical history, Ms. Johansson reports that she has had some changes in her health over the last several months. She complains of weakness in her hands and occasional droopiness of her eyelids. She has more strength in the morning, and her weakness gets worse as the day progresses. She also says that her hands seem to be a little better after she takes her lunch break at work. Ms. Johansson is an accountant and spends most of her day at a computer. The hygienist asks Ms. Johansson if she has seen a physician about this problem, and she responds that she has not. The hygienist recommends that Ms. Johansson see her physician, because these symptoms seem indicative of a systemic health issue.

The hygienist proceeds with the appointment and records a plaque index to tailor OHIs specifically for Ms. Johansson. The plaque index score is 45%. Plaque retention is located mostly at the gingival margin, with specifically heavy areas on #2, #3, #14, #15, #18, #19, #30, and #31. Ms. Johansson reports that she brushes twice daily and flosses once daily.

Case Study Exercises

1. Based on the described symptoms, from what disease is the patient most likely suffering?
   A. Rheumatoid arthritis
   B. Scleroderma
   C. Multiple sclerosis
   D. Myasthenia gravis
2. Which of the following drug categories is/are most likely to be effective in treating this disease?
   A. Cholinesterase inhibitors
   B. NSAIDs
   C. Corticosteroids
   D. A and B
   E. A and C
3. Which of the following would be the best oral self-care aid for Ms. Johansson?
   A. Floss holder
   B. Electric toothbrush
   C. Interproximal brush
   D. Floss threader
4. All of the following are appropriate to use when treating Ms. Johansson EXCEPT:
   A. Air polisher
   B. Hand scalers
   C. Fluoride varnish
   D. Polishing paste
5. If Ms. Johansson needs antibiotics, which of the following options would be the safest to prescribe based on her condition?
   A. Clindamycin
   B. Erythromycin
   C. Amoxicillin
   D. Tetracycline

Review Questions

1. Your patient has an upper respiratory virus. Which of the following will NOT be active in mounting an immune response to the virus?
   A. Helper T cells
   B. Autoantibodies
   C. Plasma cells
   D. Immunoglobulins

2. Which of the following best describes the pathogenesis of Sjögren syndrome?
   A. Autoantibodies destroy acetylcholine receptors at the neuromuscular junction.
   B. Chemokines attract T cells that induce apoptosis of epithelial cells in the salivary glands.
   C. T cells and macrophages attack oligodendro-cytes, contributing to demyelination of nerves.
   D. Pathogenesis is unknown.

3. Widening of the periodontal ligament space involving all teeth is an oral manifestation of which of the following diseases?
   A. Multiple sclerosis
   B. Myasthenia gravis
   C. Scleroderma
   D. Adrenal insufficiency

4. Patients with which of the following diseases experience paroxysmal pain syndromes?
   A. Multiple sclerosis
   B. Myasthenia gravis
   C. Lichen planus
   D. HIV/AIDS

5. What type of treatment modifications may need to be made for a patient with systemic lupus erythematosus?
   A. Appointment scheduled for morning
   B. Use of powered scaler is contraindicated
   C. Local anesthetics are contraindicated
   D. Antibiotic prophylaxis

Active Learning

1. Create a table listing hallmark symptoms, commonly used medications, and dental hygiene considerations for each condition discussed in this chapter.

2. Consult a drug guide and prepare a presentation on six medications listed in this chapter. Include the drug category, specific medication, and oral side effects. ■

REFERENCES

1. Doan T, Melvold R, Waltenbaugh C. *Concise Medical Immunology.* Baltimore, MD: Lippincott Williams & Wilkins; 2005.
2. Virella G. *Medical Immunology.* 6th ed. New York: Informa Healthcare USA; 2007.
3. Parham P. *The Immune System.* 3rd ed. New York: Garland Science, Taylor and Francis Group; 2009.
4. National Institute of Neurological Disorders and Stroke, National Institutes of Health. Sjögren's syndrome information page. http://www.ninds.nih.gov/disorders/sjogrens/sjogrens.htm. Accessed October 3, 2015.
5. Lahita RG, Chiorazzi N, Reeves WH. *Textbook of the Autoimmune Diseases.* Lahita RG, Chiorazzi N, Reeves WH, eds. Philadelphia, PA: Lippincott Williams & Wilkins; 2000.
6. Mathews SA, Kurien BT, Scofield RH. Oral manifestations of Sjögren's syndrome. *J Dent Res.* 2008;87(4):308-318.
7. Scully C, Langdon J, Evans J. Marathon of eponyms: 19 Sjögren syndrome. *Oral Dis.* 2011;17(5):538-540.
8. Ramos-Casals M, Tzioufas AG, Stone JH, Siso A, Bosch X. Treatment of primary Sjogren syndrome: a systematic review. *JAMA.* 2010;304(4):452-460.
9. National Institute of Neurological Disorders and Stroke, National Institutes of Health. Myasthenia gravis fact sheet. http://www.ninds.nih.gov/disorders/myasthenia_gravis/detail_myasthenia_gravis.htm. Published October 17, 2011. Accessed October 3, 2015.
10. Jamal BT, Herb K. Perioperative management of patients with myasthenia gravis: prevention, recognition, and treatment. *Oral Surg Oral Med Oral Pathol Oral Radiol Endod.* 2009;107(5):612-615.
11. Tolle L. Myasthenia gravis: a review for dental hygienists. *J Dent Hyg.* 2007;81(1):12.
12. Myasthenia Gravis Foundation of America. Thymectomy. pp. 1-5. 2010. http://www.myasthenia.org/LinkClick.aspx?fileticket=BIVoreOXJGo%3d. Accessed October 3, 2015.
13. Myasthenia Gravis Foundation of America. Dental treatment considerations. pp. 1-6. 2010. http://myasthenia.org/LinkClick.aspx?fileticket=-T58YmALjmc%3d&tabid=84. Accessed October 3, 2015.
14. National Institutes of Health. Scleroderma fact sheet. http://report.nih.gov/nihfactsheets/ViewFactSheet.aspx?csid=68&key=S. Published February 14, 2011. Accessed October 3, 2015.
15. National Institutes of Health. Raynaud's phenomenon. National Library of Medicine website. http://www.nlm.nih.gov/medlineplus/ency/article/000412.htm. Published March 21, 2012. Accessed October 3, 2015.
16. Tolle SL. Scleroderma: considerations for dental hygienists. *Int J Dent Hyg.* 2008;6(2):77-83.
17. Scleroderma Foundation. *Dental Care in Scleroderma.* Danvers, MD: Scleroderma Foundation; PP 1-10, 2009.

http://www.scleroderma.org/site/DocServer/Dental.pdf ?docID=313. Accessed October 3, 2015.

18. Ferreira EL, Christmann RB, Borba EF, Borges CT, Siqueira JT, Bonfa E. Mandibular function is severely impaired in systemic sclerosis patients. *J Orofac Pain.* 2010;24(2):197-202.

19. Poole J, Conte C, Brewer C, et al. Oral hygiene in scleroderma: the effectiveness of a multi-disciplinary intervention program. *Disabil Rehabil.* 2010;32(5):379-384.

20. National Institutes of Health. NIH fact sheet—multiple sclerosis. http://report.nih.gov/nihfactsheets/ViewFact Sheet.aspx?csid=103&key=M. Published February 14, 2011. Accessed October 3, 2015.

21. National Multiple Sclerosis Society. What we know about MS. http://www.nationalmssociety.org/about-multiple-sclerosis/what-we-know-about-ms/index. aspx. Accessed October 3, 2015.

22. Fischer DJ, Epstein JB, Klasser G. Multiple sclerosis: an update for oral health care providers. *Oral Surg Oral Med Oral Pathol Oral Radiol Endod.* 2009;108(3):318-327.

23. National Institutes of Health. Handout on health: rheumatoid arthritis. http://www.niams.nih.gov/ Health_Info/Rheumatic_Disease/default.asp. Published April 2009. Accessed October 3, 2015.

24. Kelsey JL, Lamster IB. Influence of musculoskeletal conditions on oral health among older adults. *Am J Public Health.* 2008;98(7):1177-1183.

25. National Institutes of Health. Handout on health: systemic lupus erythematosus. Published August 2011. http://www.niams.nih.gov/Health_Info/Lupus/default. asp. Accessed October 3, 2015.

26. Powers DB. Systemic lupus erythematosus and discoid lupus erythematosus. *Oral Maxillofac Surg Clin North Am.* 2008;20(4):651-662.

27. Galusha-Phillips H, Lupus Foundation of America. *Lupus Guide to Dental Care.* http://pdfsr.com/pdf/lupus-guide-to-dental-care. Accessed October 3, 2015.

28. National Endocrine and Metabolic Diseases Information Service. Adrenal insufficiency and Addison's disease. Published April 6, 2012. http://www.niddk.nih.gov/ health-information/health-topics/endocrine/adrenal-insufficiency-addisons-disease/Pages/fact-sheet.aspx. Accessed October 3, 2015.

29. Addison's Clinical Advisory Panel. Surgical guidelines. http://www.addisons.org.uk/comms/publications/ surgicalguidelines-bw.pdf. Accessed October 3, 2015.

30. National Institutes of Health. Fast facts about fibromyalgia. Published July 2011. http://www.niams.nih.gov/ Health_Info/Fibromyalgia/fibromyalgia_ff.asp. Accessed October 3, 2015.

31. National Fibromyalgia Association. About fibromyalgia: treatment. http://www.fmaware.org/about-fibromyalgia/. Accessed October 3, 2015.

32. Centers for Disease Control. Basic information about HIV and AIDS. http://www.cdc.gov/std/hiv/stdfact-std-hiv.htm. Accessed October 3, 2015.

33. National Institutes of Health. HIV/AIDS: the basics. http://aidsinfo.nih.gov/contentfiles/HIVAIDS_the Basics.pdf. Published November 2011. Accessed October 3, 2015.

34. Centers for Disease Control. MMWR: HIV surveillance—United States, 1981-2008. http://www.cdc.gov/mmwr/ preview/mmwrhtml/mm6021a2.htm. Published June 3, 2011. Accessed October 3, 2015.

35. National Institutes of Health. HIV life cycle. http:// aidsinfo.nih.gov/contentfiles/HIVLifeCycle_FS_en.pdf. Published May 2005. Accessed October 3, 2015.

36. University of Washington DECOD Program. Special needs fact sheets: oral health fact sheet for dental professionals: adults with human immunodeficiency virus (HIV). http://dental.washington.edu/wp-content/media/sp_need_pdfs/HIV-Adult.pdf Accessed October 3, 2015.

37. University of Washington DECOD Program. Special needs fact sheets: oral health fact sheet for dental professionals: children with human immunodeficiency virus (HIV). http://www.thecenterforpediatricdentistry. com/intranet/special_needs_fact_sheets/dental_provide rs/HIV-Dental.pdf. Accessed October 3, 2015.

38. American Academy of Dermatology. Lichen planus. http://www.aad.org/skin-conditions/dermatology-a-to-z/lichen-planus. Accessed October 3, 2015.

39. National Institutes of Health. Lichen planus. http://www.nlm.nih.gov/medlineplus/ency/article/ 000867.htm. Published October 10, 2010. Accessed October 3, 2015.

40. National Institutes of Health. Erythema multiforme. http://www.nlm.nih.gov/medlineplus/ency/article/ 000851.htm. Published October 10, 2010. Accessed October 3, 2015.

41. National Institutes of Health. Organ transplantation. http://www.nlm.nih.gov/medlineplus/organtrans plantation.html. Published March 28, 2012. Accessed October 3, 2015.

42. National Institutes of Health. Organ transplantation and your mouth. http://www.nidcr.nih.gov/OralHealth/ Topics/OrganTransplantationOralHealth/Organ TransplantPatient.htm. Published April 2011. Accessed October 3, 2015.

Chapter 44 | Hematological Considerations

Janet Weber, RDH, MEd

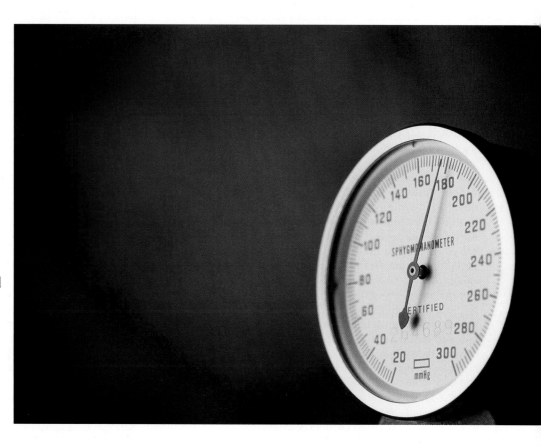

KEY TERMS

anemia

bleeding time

celiac sprue

complete blood cell count (CBC)

fibrin

hemophilia

hemostasis

hepatitis

Hodgkin disease

International Normalized Ratio (INR)

leukemia

partial thromboplastin time (PTT)

prothrombin time (PT)

sickle cell anemia

thrombocytopenia

von Willebrand disease

warfarin

LEARNING OBJECTIVES

After reading this chapter, the student should be able to:

44.1 Identify medical conditions associated with increased bleeding.

44.2 Define types of bleeding disorders.

44.3 Determine whether treatment modifications are necessary for conditions with increased bleeding.

44.4 Identify medications that affect clotting.

44.5 Describe the management of a hematological emergency in the dental hygiene services.

44.6 Differentiate between red blood cell disorders and white blood cell disorders.

KEY CONCEPTS

• All individuals have the right to seek treatment for their dental needs. It is the responsibility of the dental team to determine how best to manage any individual who presents with health considerations.

- The dental team collaborates with other health-care practitioners to offer the best possible treatment. Understanding how the body's clotting mechanism works, what various laboratory values might indicate, their potential complications, and how to manage complications will ensure proper care and reduce the risk of an emergency.
- When treating patients with hematological conditions, the dental hygienist considers what the patient needs to do before the appointment, what the hygienist needs to do (treatment considerations) before the appointment, whether the hygienist can identify warning signs that would affect management of the dental hygiene appointment, and what the protocols are for handling an emergency with a patient who has a hematological condition.

RELEVANCE TO CLINICAL PRACTICE

The body is a complex system of organs and other tissues maintained by the hematological system. The human body would not be able to sustain itself if it were not for the complex "highways" of veins and arteries that provide needed nutrients to all of the organs in the body. Although it is very complex, the purpose of the hematological system is very simple: to transport nutrients to the organs in the body (through the arteries) and transport waste out (via the veins). Should injury occur anywhere along its many pathways, the body's defense mechanism is the formation of blood clots that help to slow down and stop the flow of blood out of the injured blood vessel. Blood clotting is a critical factor in ensuring the survival of the individual. Blood clotting is influenced by conditions such as blood disorders, bone marrow disorders, and blood diseases, as well as medications. Dental hygienists need to understand clotting principles and how various conditions and medications may affect clotting to plan and implement appropriate dental hygiene services for patients.[1]

CLOT FORMATION

Bone marrow is responsible for the formation of blood platelets, which are small cell fragments that contain no DNA. Blood platelets are essential for **hemostasis,** or clotting of the blood, within the vessels of the body should an injury occur. Blood platelets are also a natural source of growth factors, which are responsible for stimulating cell growth, proliferation, and differentiation.[2]

When bone marrow releases platelets into the bloodstream, the platelets travel throughout the body, transporting oxygen to the body's organs and transporting carbon dioxide out. Should an injury occur, a chemical reaction is activated, which changes the surface of the platelet, making it sticky. This sticky substance is known as **fibrin** (Fig. 44-1). When a platelet becomes "activated," the fibrin coating helps the platelet adhere to the walls of the injured blood vessel. The activated platelets also begin to adhere to each other. Within a few minutes, the platelets form clumps,

continuously attaching to each other. This formation of clumps appears white to the naked eye and is known as "white clots." The white clots continue to band together until the injured area is sealed and blood can no longer exit out of the blood vessel. This defensive action of closing an open area so the body does not drain itself of all of its blood enables the human body to survive. Unfortunately, some injuries are too extensive for the body to seal itself in a timely manner, resulting ultimately in death.

The body is extremely dependent on its clotting function. Otherwise, uncontrolled blood loss could occur at the slightest bump during physical activity. When blood takes too long to clot, blood loss can be overwhelming (Fig. 44-2). In contrast, blood that clots too quickly can cut off the flow of oxygen and nutrients to organs, resulting in organ shutdown. A stroke is an example of an organ shutting down because of a blockage. A clot that is too large will actually seal off the artery, blocking the flow of blood to the organ.[3] The organ can only maintain itself so long before it will shut

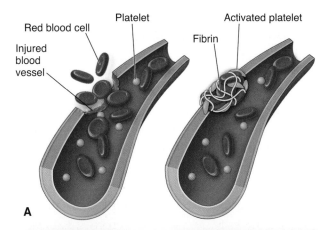

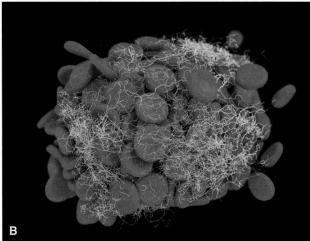

Figure 44-1. (A) When the body sustains an injury, a chemical reaction causes the platelets to become sticky and adhere to each other and the injured blood vessel, producing a fibrin coating, which forms a mesh that stabilizes the clot and seals off the injured area. (B) Blood clot with white fibrin.

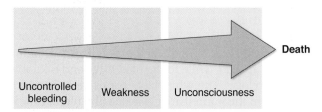

Figure 44-2. Uncontrolled bleeding is the first stage of a hematological emergency. If bleeding continues too long, the patient will become weak and eventually unconscious, resulting ultimately in death.

down. Therefore, normal clot formation in a timely manner is essential for survival.

CLOTTING DETERMINATION

A **complete blood cell count (CBC)** test is requested by the patient's physician to determine the number of red blood cells, white blood cells, and platelets in the body, to determine whether blood is clotting normally. Normal platelet formation is 150,000 to 400,000 cells/mm.[1] A count less than 150,000 is

considered **thrombocytopenia.** Spontaneous bleeding problems will occur when platelet count is less than 50,000 to 60,000 cells/mm (Table 44-1). The **International Normalized Ratio (INR)/prothrombin time (PT)** and **partial thromboplastin time (PTT)** tests determine bleeding time. These tests can be affected by abnormalities with the blood platelets themselves or with the body's ability to clot.

Bleeding Time

Bleeding time determines how well the blood platelets function. It measures how long it takes a standardized skin incision to stop bleeding. Normal readings are between 1 and 6 minutes.

International Normalized Ratio

The INR measures the body's ability to clot and compares it with an average. The higher the INR, the longer it takes blood to clot. It takes the average person 1 to 6 minutes to clot. Normal clotting has an INR count of 1.0. People who are taking medications that thin the blood (anticoagulants) should typically have an INR count of 2.0 to 3.0, and those with atrial fibrillation or mechanical heart valves will have readings normally between 3.0 and 4.0. Values greater than 4.0 indicate that the blood is not clotting enough to prevent bruising

Test	Range	Clinical Implication
Bleeding time	Normal: 1–6 minutes	Not a reliable screening test
International Normalized Ratio (INR)	<2	May proceed with routine care
	2–3	May proceed with routine care but should monitor patient regarding bleeding status
	3–4	Medical consult should be obtained before care
Platelet count	>150,000/mm	Normal
	<50,000/mm	Spontaneous bleeding—do not perform elective procedures
Hemoglobin	Males: 13.6– 17.2 g/100 mL	
	Females: 12– 15 g/100 mL	
Hematocrit	Male: 39%–49%	
	Female: 33%–43%	

Table 44-1. *Laboratory Values and Clinical Implications*

or uncontrolled bleeding should the person be injured. Depending on the person's medical status, there is a fine line between keeping the blood thin enough (low number of platelets) so that the blood flows freely through the body, but thick enough (high number of platelets) that it has the ability to clot if and when needed because of injury.

Prothrombin Time

PT also evaluates the body's ability to clot. However, PT uses different reagents (additives) than the INR test. Normal range for clotting to occur using this test is between 11 and 16 seconds.[4]

The INR and PT tests are very similar to each other in that they determine how long it takes the body's blood to clot. Both tests compare results with a controlled sample in the laboratory. The INR also compares it with other laboratory results for standardization. For this reason, most physicians prefer the INR test over the PT test.

Partial Thromboplastin Time

The PTT also measures clotting time. However, the reagent is added to the patient's skin at the time of testing. Normal readings are between 25 and 40 seconds. Severe bleeding problems are indicated when the readings are longer than 50 seconds.

Thrombocytopenia[5]

Thrombocytopenia is any condition in which the blood platelet counts is abnormally low (≤150,000/mm). Thrombocytopenia can be caused by:

- Decrease in platelet production due to:
  - Cytotoxic drugs
  - Bone marrow irradiation or replacement
  - Vitamin deficiencies (vitamin B_{12}, iron, and folic acid)
- An increase in platelet destruction or consumption
  - Autoimmune (decreased survival time of the blood platelets)
    - Autoimmune thrombocytopenic purpura[6]
- Increase in spleen sequestration (the trapping of sickled red blood cells in the spleen)
  - Capturing of circulating platelets in the spleen
    - Hypersplenic thrombocytopenia
    - Pregnancy
    - Drug use[5]

BLOOD-THINNING DRUGS

Almost all medical conditions require the use of medications to help correct dysfunction or maintain adequate function. Some medications are prescribed for preventative purposes. Some examples of common medications that affect clotting are:

- Aspirin
- Plavix
- Warfarin (Coumadin)

- Antibiotics
- Birth control pills/progesterone–estrogen combination pills
- Statins

Acetylsalicyclic Acid (Aspirin)[7]

The dental hygienist should be acutely aware if the patient is taking any medication(s) that affect clotting (see Application to Clinical Practice). The patient's medical history or the medications the patient is taking, or both, may signal the presence of a hematological condition. With careful inquiry, the hygienist can determine whether a blood-thinning drug such as aspirin is taken specifically for its blood-thinning properties, such as to prevent stroke, or for its analgesic properties to alleviate pain. If aspirin is taken for its blood-thinning properties, the dental hygienist will notice an increase in bleeding during scaling and periodontal debridement procedures.[7] Aspirin is classified as a NSAID with antiplatelet properties. Aspirin (acetylsalicyclic acid) is an over-the-counter (OTC) drug often taken in small doses for the long-term prevention of blood clot formation to reduce risk for strokes or heart attacks. Aspirin can also be given at the time of a suspected stroke or heart attack because of its immediate antiplatelet action, thus restoring blood flow. Antiplatelet means that the drug (in this case, aspirin) reduces platelet aggregation. Platelet aggregation is the clotting process that takes place at a site of injury. When a stimulus is activated, after an injury occurs, the production of thromboxane, a substance that is needed to formulate fibrin, is affected. Fibrin is the sticky substance needed to "stick" or adhere the platelets to each other to form a clot—basically, no fibrin, no clot. This action permanently affects the platelet. The decrease in platelet aggregation will be seen clinically as an increase in bleeding during invasive dental procedures. Patients who are taking low-dose aspirin for the prevention of heart attack should not be taken off of it

Application to Clinical Practice

The dental hygienist should update and confirm the patient's medical status at each and every dental hygiene appointment. Verbal interviewing during the updating of the medical history is extremely important because it could suggest conditions that may influence the dental hygiene appointment. For example, the medical history may not indicate that a blood condition is present. Open-ended questioning is a good way to ascertain additional information. Patients often do not draw a correlation that OTC or herbal medications, or both, may influence their health status. It is recommended to specifically ask the patient if he or she may or may not be taking OTC medications. Citing specific medications often helps the patient with recall. ■

before dental procedures, because this may increase the original risk that the aspirin is being used to prevent. Because of its antiplatelet properties, aspirin effects can remain in the body until 7 days after its discontinued use.

Dental Hygiene Considerations

Complete and thorough medical history interviews must be taken at a minimum once a year along with updates at each dental visit in between. Be sure to inquire whether the patient is taking both prescription and OTC medications by asking open-ended questions to gather complete information; for example: "What medications do you take?" "Do you ever take any 'over-the-counter' medications such as aspirin?" Patients often forget to mention OTC medications in the medical history interview. Patients often think that because OTC medications do not require a prescription, they are not as important as their "other" medications. Stating a specific time frame will help determine whether the patient is taking aspirin daily for its blood-thinning properties or if it is taken sporadically as a pain reliever; for example, "Have you taken any aspirin in the past 7 days?" This information helps with management of the dental hygiene appointment. The blood-thinning properties of aspirin can be apparent in the body up to 7 days after its ingestion, so increased bleeding may be observed.[4]

Gingival health coupled with aspirin intake will determine the severity of noted bleeding. Under normal conditions, healthy gingiva does not bleed when a mildly invasive procedure, such as probing, is performed. However, the patient who is taking aspirin over a period of time may exhibit an exaggerated response to instrumentation in areas of gingival disease. This may cause concern with both the patient and the dental hygienist if the cause of the bleeding is not understood. Therefore, education is an extremely important service. If the patient has moderate-to-severe gingivitis, the dental hygienist and the patient may be acutely aware of spontaneous bleeding during the procedure. At home, the patient may become alarmed while performing oral care such as tooth brushing, flossing, or both. The patient may notice bleeding takes longer than expected to stop. In either scenario, the patient should be advised of the increased bleeding and its causes (i.e., gingivitis coupled with the blood-thinning medication is causing an exaggerated response). To control spontaneous bleeding during instrumentation, the dental hygienist may apply firm pressure to the area using gauze and then firmly apply lateral pressure with a finger.[3] Pressure should continue to be applied for up to 5 minutes or until bleeding has stopped. The patient should be advised that the area may be tender for the next 24 hours and that he or she should observe it for bleeding. The patient should be taught how to control bleeding should it begin again at home. If unable to control the bleeding, the patient should be directed to call a dental professional.

Clopidogrel (Plavix)

Plavix (clopidogrel) is also an antiplatelet drug that affects platelet aggregation and platelet function. However, Plavix can only be given in prescription strength. Plavix, like aspirin, affects the production of thrombin, which then negatively affects the production of fibrin, the sticky substance needed to cause the platelets to adhere to each other. The patient who presents for dental hygiene services is not normally taken off of this medication before the procedures because taking him or her off the medication may increase the risk for aggravating the condition for which the patient is being treated. In some cases, the patient with an atrial stent or a new joint replacement (less than 1 month) may need to take premedication before initiating invasive dental hygiene services such as probing, scaling, and periodontal debridement. Antibiotic prophylaxis will not adversely affect Plavix because of its mechanism of action regarding platelet aggregation. However, close consultation with the patient's physician is necessary to determine the best course of action for this patient. Requesting INR values for the patient taking Plavix will not indicate whether there is a potential bleeding problem. Remember, INR tests indicate how well the body clots by determining the number of platelets. It answers the question: Are there enough platelets to cause a clot if needed. Plavix affects the body's ability to clot (production of fibrin), not the actual number of platelets. Instead, a bleeding time test, which is measured in minutes, will help determine how well the blood platelets function and the potential for severe bleeding. However, this test is often not requested because it is known that the patient taking Plavix will experience clotting; however, it will take longer. Observing blood flow during invasive procedures is a better indicator as to when the procedure(s) should be discontinued.

Dental Hygiene Considerations

The dental hygienist should be aware of the potential for prolonged bleeding in the patient taking Plavix. Appropriate measures should be available should the need arise to control bleeding during the dental hygiene procedures. Applying pressure to the site with a moistened gauze square for several minutes (up to 5 minutes) is very effective. In cases where bleeding continues, the dental hygienist can inject in the area a small amount of anesthetic containing a vasoconstrictor such as lidocaine with epinephrine (1:100,000) until blanching occurs (Box 44-1). Other anticoagulating agents such as fibers or pads designed to aid in the clotting mechanism can be inserted into the sulcus to produce the desired effect. Treatment should be terminated if bleeding is too heavy, generalized, and too spontaneous. Every effort should be made to help the patient achieve effective home-care strategies for biofilm removal. The healthier the gingiva, the less likely bleeding will be severe and spontaneous. Follow-up consultation with the patient's physician is recommended (see Teamwork).

Box 44-1. *Treating a Hematological Emergency*

To control a hematological emergency:

- Apply very firm pressure with gauze and your finger to the area of bleeding for a minimum of 1 to 2 minutes.
- Continue applying pressure as long as the site continues to bleed. Usually 1 to 2 minutes is enough for satisfactory clotting to occur.
- If bleeding extends beyond 15 minutes, infiltrate the area with an anesthetic containing epinephrine such as lidocaine with epinephrine (1:100,000) until blanching occurs.
- After bleeding has stopped, observe the patient to ensure the clot formation will not become dislodged. ■

Teamwork

Based on medical history responses, preliminary consultation with the patient's physician may be necessary before initiating invasive procedures. The dental hygienist should be clear as to the intent of the inquiry by specifically citing patient's current medical status and any medications (along with OTC medications if applicable) the patient is taking. ■

Coumadin (Warfarin)

Warfarin (coumadin) is another example of a prescription-strength, blood-thinning drug. Warfarin is often prescribed for patients who have experienced:

- A heart attack or stroke
- Irregular heartbeat
- Prosthetic (replacement or mechanical) heart valves
- Short-term treatment for prosthetic joint replacement such as total knee or hip replacement
- Treatment or prevention of venous thrombosis (swelling and blood clot in a vein)
- Pulmonary embolism (a blood clot in the lung)

Warfarin is classified as a vitamin K antagonist, which means that its blood-thinning properties come from its ability to break down vitamin K. Vitamin K is a necessary component in the product of fibrin, the sticky substance that is activated when injury occurs. Fibrin causes the platelets to stick to each other, forming a clot. All dental patients on warfarin should initially have a medical consultation with their physician to determine their health status and specifically their INR count. The physician may or may not recommend that the patient refrain from taking the drug 72 hours before the invasive procedure. Recent literature suggests that taking the patient off the blood-thinning medication may not be advisable

because it increases the risk for blood clotting, which may aggravate the condition being treated or prevented. It should be made clear during the medical consultation that the potential for severe bleeding may occur because of the nature of the deep scaling and periodontal debridement procedures. Dental hygiene procedures may proceed if the patient's INR values are less than 3, or if taken for atrial fibrillation/mechanical heart valves, the count should be no higher than 4 (see Table 44-1). If the INR count is higher than the recommendations for that condition, then elective procedures, such as probing, scaling, among others, should be delayed until the INR count is within the reference range for that condition.

If a patient is taking a blood thinner because of a very recent joint replacement (within 35 days), the physician will most likely advise antibiotic premedication before the dental hygiene instrumentation. However, consultation with the patient's physician is necessary to confirm the need for premedication and, if appropriate, the regimen. Antibiotics affect the bacteria in the gut that produce vitamin K.[8] This will negatively affect the body's ability to produce fibrin. Coupling the antibiotic with warfarin will greatly influence the negative production of fibrin. In essence, it will increase the blood-thinning properties beyond the desired level for the patient. The need to continue with antibiotic premedication before dental hygiene services at subsequent recare visits should be confirmed with the patient's physician. In 2012, the American Dental Association and the American Association of Orthopedic Surgeons updated the antibiotic prophylaxis (premedication) guidelines for patients with orthopedic implants undergoing dental procedures. These new guidelines no longer recommend antibiotics for everyone with artificial joints. The need for continued antibiotic premedication should be evaluated, on a case-by-case basis, with the patient's physician especially in cases where the patient is taking warfarin.

All patients should be educated about their condition and the effects of their medication on the blood and how this may affect the dental hygiene appointment. Patients should also be warned of the serious effects of taking warfarin with other anticoagulation medications. The dental hygienist can increase the patient's dental literacy by making this an integral part of all home-care education. The following anticoagulation medications should not be taken with warfarin unless specifically prescribed by the patient's physician:

- Aspirin
- Antidepressants
- Natural health products such as coenzyme Q_{10}, ginseng, vitamin K
- Certain foods such as avocados, flax, and onions
- Statins: a class of drug used to reduce cholesterol levels

Dental Hygiene Considerations

If any of the conditions mentioned earlier are present in the patient's medical history, the dental hygienist should consult the dental record for a Medical Consult that would provide recommended treatment guidelines from the patient's physician. If a consult is not present, one should be sent before actual treatment. **Invasive procedures should NOT be initiated at this time until the consult is returned with the physician's recommendations.**

- It is important to inquire about the patient's condition and the INR count used for the management of these conditions. Current INR values are taken every 3 months by the patient's physician to monitor blood values and should be available at every dental/dental hygiene appointment. Patients who are compliant with this regimen will often know their value and can provide it at the time of the appointment. If not, the dental hygienist can make a call to the patient's physician's office to obtain the most current values. People who are taking anticoagulation medications should typically have an INR count of 2.0 to 3.0, and those with atrial fibrillation or mechanical heart valves should normally have readings of 3.0 to 4.0. **Do not treat the patient if values are greater than 4.0 because this indicates that clotting will not occur quickly enough to prevent an emergency.** However, emergencies to this extent are rare during dental hygiene procedures. Patients taking warfarin who have more severe gingival inflammation may experience bleeding for a very extended period. Bleeding longer than 15 minutes can be treated by infiltrating the affected area with an anesthetic containing a vasoconstrictor such as lidocaine with epinephrine (1:100,000) until blanching occurs. Other anticoagulating agents such as fibers or pads designed to aid in the clotting mechanism can be inserted into the sulcus to produce the desired effect. All patients taking warfarin should be continuously monitored during procedures for exaggerated bleeding. It is recommended that treatment be terminated if bleeding is too heavy and excessive because INR values at that time might not be consistent with the previous values.

During routine dental hygiene care, if the patient states he or she is taking an antibiotic, this should alert the dental hygienist that an acute, underlying condition is present. The patient should be questioned as to the nature of the condition and whether he or she has been advised to discontinue the warfarin treatment. Invasive dental hygiene services should be terminated at this point and consultation with the patient's physician is highly recommended. If the patient is taking any medication that affects the production of vitamin K in the body, further consultation with the physician is necessary.

Other "Blood-Thinning" Medications

Additional blood-thinning medications are continuously being developed and marketed. However, their general properties remain the same. As with all medications, it is important to have a good understanding of the drug, its interactions, and how it might or might not affect treatment. The hygienist must consult with the patient's physician before scaling and periodontal debridement procedures to determine blood count values and clotting count (INR). The physician will often recommend that the patient continue with the blood-thinning medication because stopping the drug may cause the condition the drug is preventing.

Antibiotics

Antibiotics can also interact with warfarin or other blood-thinning medications by influencing the bacteria in the gut that produce vitamin K.[8] Vitamin K influences the production of prothrombin. Therefore, a decrease in vitamin K decreases prothrombin production. Decreased prothrombin production negatively affects the body's ability to form thrombi, the enzyme that converts to fibrin, the "glue" that binds the platelets together to form a blood clot. With less fibrin coupled with the blood-thinning properties of warfarin or other blood-thinning medications, platelets have little ability to attach to each other to form clots, leading to uncontrolled bleeding.[8]

Antibiotics with the ability to affect vitamin K production, in descending effect, are:

- Cotrimoxazole
- Ciprofloxacin
- Amoxicillin
- Ampicillin
- Nitrofurantoin
- Norfloxacin

Dental Hygiene Considerations

Hygienists should be aware that not all antibiotics are created equal, and they should evaluate each antibiotic for the risk it poses when combined with blood thinners. Consultation with the patient's physician is recommended to determine whether elective procedures, such as scaling and periodontal debridement, should be postponed until the patient has completed antibiotic therapy. INR values should be obtained as close to the dental hygiene appointment as possible, and the hygienist should monitor the patient closely to determine whether and when treatment should be terminated to prevent an emergency.[8]

As discussed previously, the hygienist should discuss all medications and their interactions with the patient. The more educated patients are, the more willing they are to accommodate requests and provide needed information.

Statins

Statins, or cholesterol-lowering drugs, have been shown to reduce the ability of thrombin to produce fibrin. Statins are normally prescribed to people with high cholesterol, specifically when low-density lipoprotein (or "bad" cholesterol) levels are less than 130. Cholesterol is the plaquelike substance that adheres to the walls of the veins. As this sticky plaque becomes thicker, it reduces the blood's ability to flow freely through the veins, increasing the patient's risk for heart attack or stroke. Statins have also been shown to effectively reduce the blood's ability to clot.

Dental Hygiene Considerations

The dental hygienist should always verify with the patient that cholesterol-reducing and blood-thinning medications are being taken together. Consult with the patient's physician to confirm this therapy and inquire about the INR count. Advise the patient's physician that the patient may be undergoing invasive procedures such as scaling and periodontal debridement, as well as the potential effects of the statins and the blood-thinning medications.[9]

Table 44-2 provides examples of additional drugs that require a thorough review and consultation with the patient's physician before invasive procedures.

Herbal Medications

It is important for the dental hygienist to consider that the patient may be taking OTC medications together with other prescription medications or that the patient may be taking herbal medications as an alternative to his or her physician's recommendations. When herbal medications are taken together with prescription blood thinners, the patient may be at risk for increased bleeding, bleeding that is difficult to stop, hemorrhaging, headaches, dizziness, and weakness.[10] The exact mechanism of action on its blood-thinning properties is not yet understood. It is highly recommended that patients be specifically asked whether they are taking any herbal medications. As in the case of those patients who are taking aspirin, the patients may not be aware of the blood-thinning properties of some herbal medications. They may assume the herbal medication has no adverse effects because it is an OTC drug. However, the interaction between the herbal drug and other medications may produce undesirable affects. The following OTC herbal medications have blood-thinning properties and should not be taken with other blood-thinning medications:[10]

- Devil's claw
- Dong quai
- Feverfew
- Ginger
- Ginseng
- Garlic
- Gingko
- Cinnamon

BLEEDING DISORDERS[11]

Von Willebrand Disease

Von Willebrand disease is the most common inherited bleeding disorder. Because of a lack of glycoprotein Ib (von Willebrand factor), platelets are not able to stick to tissue surfaces, thereby reducing the body's ability to clot. Under normal circumstances, spontaneous bleeding occurs after a surgery or trauma and then clotting begins to form within minutes. Unfortunately, the individual with von Willebrand disease will experience prolonged bleeding because of the blood's inability to adhere to the surrounding tissue surfaces. This will prolong the bleeding until the clot is able to form eventually. Signs of von Willebrand disease are as follows:

- Petechiae of the skin: Petechiae are small hemorrhages the size of a pinhead. They are often red, but larger petechiae often appear more purplish. Petechiae are normally found clustered together as a result of trauma. However, in von Willebrand disease, the petechiae are often disbursed about the oral cavity.
- Gastrointestinal bleeding
- Epistaxis (nosebleeds)

Table 44-2. *Other Blood-Thinning Medications*

Drug Name	Use	Mechanism of Action
Dipyridamole	Reduces risk for blood clots after heart valve replacement	Inhibits thrombus formation long term and causes vasodilation short term
Aggrenox (aspirin and dipyridamole)	Prevents transient ischemic attacks ("mini-strokes")	When combined with low-dose aspirin and extended-release dipyridamole, platelets become less sticky, affecting their ability to clump together and form clots
Pradaxa (dabigatran etexilate mesylate)	Prevents strokes and blood clots in patients with atrial fibrillation	Inhibits thrombin formation
Plavix (clopidogrel)	Prevents blood clot formation that causes heart attacks or strokes	Inhibits platelet aggregation and thrombus formation

Dental Hygiene Considerations

When managing the patient with von Willebrand disease, the dental hygienist should consult with the patient's physician for the following reasons:

- Blood platelet levels: It is important to know the INR count before instrument implementation to determine whether the patient is within a manageable range to prevent excessive bleeding. INR count should be determined before every instrumentation session with this patient.
- Need for additional medical treatments before oral health care is provided

Hemophilia[12]

Hemophilia refers to a group of inherited bleeding disorders in which the person suffers from the inability to form clotting factors.[13] As a result, spontaneous bleeding occurs and the body cannot produce clots quickly enough to stop bleeding.

Hemophilia A

Hemophilia A is also known as factor VIII deficiency or classic hemophilia. It is largely an inherited disorder in which one of the proteins needed to form blood clots is missing or reduced. Approximately 1 in 5,000 male individuals born in the United States has hemophilia. All races and economic groups are affected equally. When a person with hemophilia is injured, he does not bleed harder or faster than a person without hemophilia, but instead, he will bleed longer. Hemophilia is inherited from the mother. A woman who gives birth to a child with hemophilia often has other male relatives who also have hemophilia. Sometimes, a baby will be born with hemophilia when there is no known family history. This means either that the gene has been "hidden" (i.e., passed down through several generations of female carriers without affecting any male members of the family) or the change in the X chromosome is new (i.e., a "spontaneous mutation").[8]

Dental Hygiene Considerations

Dental hygiene considerations for patients with hemophilia are as follows:

- The patient's physician should be consulted before invasive procedures to determine INR value and special risk factors.
- Replacement factor should be given according to the patient's physician's recommendations just before instrumentation.
- Full-mouth scaling is not recommended because of the high risk for heavy and prolonged bleeding. The mouth should be scaled in small sections over several appointments.
- Treat small wounds with regular first aid: Clean the cut, then apply pressure until bleeding stops, and place a bandage over the area if needed.
  - Individuals with mild hemophilia can use desmopressin acetate (DDAVP), a nonblood product, to treat minor bleeds.

- Deep cuts or internal bleeding, such as bleeding into the joints or muscles, require more complex treatment. The missing clotting factor (VIII or IX) must be replaced so the child can form a clot to stop the bleeding. Patients may have to be seen only in the hospital.
- In cases of severe hemophilia, physicians sometimes recommend giving a regimen of regular factor replacement treatments (a therapy called *prophylaxis*) to prevent bleeding episodes before they happen. The Medical and Scientific Advisory Council of the National Hemophilia Foundation recommends prophylaxis as optimal therapy for children with severe hemophilia A and B.

As with all bleeding disorders, consultation with the physician is necessary before any invasive procedure (see Professionalism). Some patients with severe hemophilia may be required to have these procedures performed in a controlled environment such as a hospital.

Hemophilia B

Hemophilia B can also be known as factor IX deficiency, or Christmas disease. It was named "Christmas disease" for Stephen Christmas, the first person diagnosed with the disorder in 1952.

Dental Hygiene Considerations

Patients with hemophilia B should be managed in the same manner as described for hemophilia A.

RED BLOOD CELL DISORDERS

Red blood cells are responsible for carrying oxygen to the various organs within the body and carrying waste material out. Red blood cells also contain an iron-containing biomolecule, which gives them their red color.

Anemia

Anemia is a condition that occurs when the body does not produce enough healthy red blood cells, resulting in the possible lack of oxygen to the organs. Red blood cells carry oxygen to the various organs in the body via

Professionalism

Patients with bleeding disorders will require laboratory values the same day as treatment, so the patient should be advised of this before the appointment. Depending on the patient's status, premedication or factor replacement therapy, or both, before the dental hygiene appointment may be required as well. The dental hygienist should be cognizant of the acceptable laboratory blood values and how it will affect the management of the dental hygiene appointment. ■

a protein called *hemoglobin*. If the red blood cells are deficient in hemoglobin, then the organs within the body are not getting enough oxygen. Anemia can be caused from certain deficiencies in:

- Iron
- Vitamin B$_{12}$ (pernicious anemia)
- Folic acid
- Vitamin K

Iron Deficiency

Iron deficiency causes red blood cell production to decline. Individuals with iron-deficiency anemia will often display a bluish tint in the whites of their eyes and experience a loss of appetite or unusual cravings for particular foods such as celery, carrots, peanuts, seeds, crackers, pretzels, and tomatoes. Fatigue, headaches, and irritability often are present. Individuals may also have brittle nails and a pale look to their skin. They may complain of a sore tongue. Overall malaise may be present. The dental hygienist may notice that the filiform papillae on the dorsum of the tongue have disappeared. The tongue looks smooth and glossy. Patients may also exhibit angular cheilitis or chapping of the commissures.

Encourage patients with anemia to supplement their diet with iron or eat foods rich in iron such as fish, legumes, red meats, poultry, raisins, and whole-grain bread.

Dental Hygiene Considerations

Dental hygiene considerations for patients with anemia include:

- Encourage patients to seek medical advice if symptoms of anemia are present. Poor iron absorption may be caused by:
  - Celiac disease
  - Crohn disease
  - Gastric bypass surgery
  - Taking antacids
  - Women's health issues such as endometriosis or recent pregnancy
- Dietary analysis and education is of utmost importance. Patients should be referred to their physician for nutritional counseling and education. The dental hygienist can enhance this education by offering additional information on how nutrition affects the oral environment.
- The dental hygienist should work closely with the patient on home-care strategies that will improve the overall health of the periodontium. Follow-up strategies need to be continually re-evaluated and modified where necessary. Reinforce those strategies that are effective.
- Elective procedures may have to be rescheduled for those patients who are experiencing symptoms of anemia.

B$_{12}$ Deficiency

Red blood cell count may also decrease because of a lack of sufficient vitamin B$_{12}$. The body needs B$_{12}$ for normal nervous system function and blood cell production.

Patients may exhibit confusion, diarrhea, malaise, loss of appetite, numbing and tingling of the hands and feet, shortness of breath, and mouth/tongue soreness. The dental hygienist will notice that the patient may have angular cheilitis (cracking at the commissures of the mouth). This patient will exhibit a loss of filiform papillae as well. The mucosa may be ulcerated, painful, inflamed, and atrophic.[14]

Vitamin B$_{12}$ deficiency can be caused by:

- Abdominal or intestinal surgery that affects intrinsic factor production or absorption
- Strict vegetarian diets that exclude all meat, fish, dairy products, and eggs
- Celiac disease
- Chronic alcoholism
- Crohn disease

Dental Hygiene Considerations

Dental hygiene considerations for patients with vitamin B$_{12}$ deficiency are as follows:

- Dietary analysis and education is of utmost importance. Dietary supplements may be recommended.
- Encourage patient to seek medical advice if symptoms of anemia present. Elective procedures may have to be rescheduled for those patients who are experiencing symptoms of anemia.
- Treatment with vitamin B$_{12}$ injections may be necessary.

Pernicious Anemia

Pernicious anemia is the inability of the red blood cell to absorb vitamin B$_{12}$. This deficiency in B$_{12}$ is caused by a lack of, or deficiency of, the intrinsic factor. Intrinsic factor is needed so that the body can absorb vitamin B$_{12}$. Vitamin B$_{12}$ is needed to make red blood cells, which carry oxygen to the tissues in the body. Without enough oxygen being supplied to the tissues, an individual will experience fatigue and shortness of breath. Patients with pernicious anemia require vitamin B$_{12}$ injections.

Early symptoms of pernicious anemia are:

- Weakness
- Fatigue
- Palpitations
- Syncope
- Tingling of the fingers and toes
- Numbness
- Lack of coordination

Oral manifestations of pernicious anemia include:

- Burning tongue
- Glossitis
- Painful swallowing
- Pale gingiva

Many patients may exhibit no symptoms.

Dental Hygiene Considerations

Management of pernicious anemia is the same as that for vitamin B$_{12}$ deficiency.

Celiac Sprue

Celiac sprue is a red blood cell disorder that is associated with the body's inability to properly metabolize gluten. Gluten is a protein found in wheat and wheat products such as breads and pastas. This inability to metabolize gluten properly causes intestinal mucosa injury, resulting in malabsorption of nutrients such as vitamin B_{12}. The patient with celiac sprue will experience nervousness, diarrhea, and extremity paresthesia. The dental hygienist may notice loss of papillae on the tongue, sore and ulcerated oral mucosa, and the patient may complain of painful burning of the tongue.[14]

Dental Hygiene Considerations

Dental hygiene considerations for patients with celiac sprue are as follows:

- Dietary counseling is most important, and patients should be referred to their physician for possible referral to a nutritionist. Patients must be made aware of the limitations in their diet that are needed to enable vitamin absorption.
- Do not use prophy pastes unless specifically noted as "gluten-free."
- Do not use rinses with alcohol in them (if patient is experiencing burning mouth syndrome).

Sickle Cell Anemia

Anemia can present because of abnormalities with the red blood cell itself. This is noted particularly in the following conditions:

- Sickle cell anemia
- Celiac sprue
- Aplastic anemia
- Polycythemia

Sickle cell anemia presents as a crescent-shaped red blood cell that is quite different from the disc shape of a normal red blood cell. It becomes sickled shaped because of an abnormal form of hemoglobin, a substance within the blood cell that carries oxygen. Unlike the disc-shaped red blood cell, the sickled red blood cell is stiff and fragile. These cells break down much quicker and do not last as long in the bloodstream as disc-shaped cells. This creates an anemic state within the body. Sickle cell anemia is an inherited disorder that develops mostly in individuals with African or Mediterranean ancestry.

Symptoms of sickle cell anemia are:

- Overall malaise
- Joint pain
- Shortness of breath
- Nausea
- Delayed eruption, malocclusion, and dentin hypomineralization
- Facial and dental pain

The dental hygienist will notice a loss of trabeculation and large, irregular-shaped spaces of marrow loss on the patient's radiographs. Lamina dura often appears to be dense.

Dental Hygiene Considerations

Dental hygiene considerations for patients with sickle cell anemia include:

- Recommend close monitoring with the patient's physician. Medical consult must indicate whether the patient's condition is stable enough for treatment. Routine dental care is usually provided for those patients in noncrisis state. The medical consult should also indicate whether the patient needs to be premedicated. Prophylactic antibiotics may be necessary for major surgical procedures, as well as some scaling/periodontal debridement procedures, if the oral environment is not healthy.
- Supportive services will most likely be recommended by the patient's physician. The dental hygienist should encourage this with the patient.
- Elective procedures may have to be rescheduled based on how the patient is feeling (during noncrisis periods).
- Home-care strategies should be discussed with the patient. These strategies should include oral hygiene instruction for plaque removal, diet control, and fluoride application.
- Appointments should be short.
- Monitor oxygen intake; the patient's saturation levels should be greater than 95%.
- If local anesthetic is needed, use without epinephrine. Diazepam (Valium) may be used if sedation is preferred.
- Generally, patients with sickle cell anemia can be treated in the dental office at low risk if the patient is in a noncrisis state. The patient who presents with a severe infection, severe dehydration, or severe hypoxia should not have elective procedures done. They should be referred to their physician for possible blood transfusion.

Aplastic Anemia

Aplastic anemia occurs when bone marrow does not produce enough red blood cells, white blood cells, or blood platelets. This form of anemia is rare and is due to bone marrow damage. It can develop suddenly or slowly. The disorder tends to get worse over time, unless its cause is found and treated. Treatments for aplastic anemia include blood transfusions, blood and marrow stem cell transplants, and medications. Individuals with aplastic anemia are at high risk for infections because their immune system is unstable. Therefore, patients with aplastic anemia should not undergo elective treatments. The dental hygienist should postpone any dental hygiene services that are considered invasive and consult with the patient's physician. Routine dental procedures should not occur until the patient's condition is resolved. The dental hygienist should give the patient oral hygiene care instructions to help the patient maintain her oral health status until treatment can be given.

Polycythemia

Polycythemia indicates that too many red blood cells are being produced. This can be caused by an increase in the mass of red blood cells or a decrease in the volume of plasma from some abnormality of the bone marrow. The individual with polycythemia will experience quicker clotting of the blood because of the slow rate it travels throughout the body.

Orally, the dental hygienist might notice purplish or red areas on the tongue, cheeks, lips, and gingiva. Polycythemia may be noted in people who are heavy smokers, have emphysema, or live in areas very high in altitude. When treating the patient with polycythemia, INR values should be obtained from the patient's physician before treatment to determine clotting values.[15]

WHITE BLOOD CELL DISORDERS

White blood cells provide the primary defense against infections through its activation of the immune system. White blood cells are produced primarily in bone marrow and are then released to circulate throughout the body, ready to activate the immune system when needed. When the white blood cells are weakened or altered structurally, theses mutated white blood cells, or cancers, will affect the body's ability to fight off infection. The condition itself along with its treatment can have devastating effects on the oral cavity. Leukemia and Hodgkin disease are two examples of white blood cell cancers.

Leukemia

Leukemia is a cancer of the white blood cells in bone marrow and the circulating blood. Leukemia is the most common type of cancer in children. Patients who have leukemia will often have recurrent infections, enlarged spleen, enlarged lymph nodes, and fever. They often exhibit signs of fatigue, weakness, and weight loss.

Oral manifestations of leukemia include the following:

- Enlarged tonsils
- Enlarged lymph nodes
- Gingival hyperplasia or enlarged gingiva
  - Progressive generalized gingival enlargement when oral hygiene is poor
  - Loss of stippling
  - Gingiva appears pale red to deep purple
  - Bleeds easily
  - Gingival ulcerations may occur as a result of infections

Hodgkin Disease

Hodgkin disease is a white blood cell disorder in which there is uncontrolled growth (neoplasm) of B lymphocytes that do not actually mature into plasma cells. B lymphocytes are involved in the production of plasma cells and immunoglobulin in the production of antibodies (humeral immunity). The condition is named after the pathologist Thomas Hodgkin. Hodgkin disease presents as firm, enlarged lymph nodes that are not tender and may be accompanied with fever, weight loss, fatigue, and night sweats.

As with all forms of cancer, patients experience various complications, especially in the oral cavity. Chemotherapy often impairs the function of bone marrow, suppressing the formation of white blood cells, red blood cells, and platelets (myelosuppression) and frequently resulting in toxic effects to the oral tissues.

Some common oral complications of both chemotherapy and radiation are:

- *Oral mucositis:* inflammation and ulceration of the mucous membranes; can increase the risk for pain, oral and systemic infection, and nutritional compromise
- *Infection:* viral, bacterial, and fungal; results from myelosuppression, xerostomia, and/or damage to the mucosa from chemotherapy or radiotherapy
- *Xerostomia/salivary gland dysfunction:* dryness of the mouth because of thickened, reduced, or absent salivary flow; increases the risk for infection and compromises speaking, chewing, and swallowing; medications other than chemotherapy can also cause salivary gland dysfunction; persistent dry mouth increases the risk for dental caries
- *Functional disabilities:* impaired ability to eat, taste, swallow, and speak because of mucositis, dry mouth, trismus (involuntary contraction of the muscles used in mastication), and infection
- *Taste alterations:* changes in taste perception of foods, ranging from unpleasant to tasteless
- *Nutritional compromise:* poor nutrition from eating difficulties caused by mucositis, dry mouth, dysphagia, and loss of taste
- *Abnormal dental development:* altered tooth development, craniofacial growth, or skeletal development in children secondary to radiotherapy and/or high doses of chemotherapy before age 9 years

Complications specific to chemotherapy include:

- *Neurotoxicity:* persistent, deep aching and burning pain that mimics a toothache, but for which no dental or mucosal source can be found; this complication is an adverse effect of certain classes of drugs, such as the vinca alkaloids
- *Bleeding:* oral bleeding from the decreased platelets and clotting factors associated with the effects of therapy on bone marrow

If the patient is receiving chemotherapy, consultation with the oncology team must take place 24 hours before the dental treatment. Blood work 24 hours before treatment is needed to determine the patient's current platelet count, clotting factors, and absolute neutrophil count. There must be sufficient numbers to recommend oral treatment. Postpone oral surgery or other oral invasive procedures in the following situations:

- Platelet count is less than 75,000/mm³ or abnormal clotting factors are present

- Absolute neutrophil count is less than 1,000/mm³ (or consider prophylactic antibiotics)

Dental Hygiene Considerations

Dental hygiene considerations for patients with Hodgkin disease include:

- Consult with the patient's oncologists to determine blood platelet levels. Patient should only use soft gauze to gently cleanse until these levels increase. As INR values stabilize, encourage the patient to gently cleanse teeth and gums after every meal with a soft toothbrush. Soaking the toothbrush in warm water to soften bristles is highly recommended. Brush teeth at bedtime as well. The patient should be encouraged to always evaluate the severity of blood flow and its spontaneity to determine the appropriate oral cleansing device.
- Recommend fluoride gel for use after meals and before bedtime.
- Recommend flossing at least once a day.
- Recommend rinsing with water throughout the day. Recommend a saliva substitute in cases where xerostomia is more severe.
- Do not recommend rinses that contain alcohol. They may irritate already sensitive mucosa and increase the burning sensation.
- The patient's diet may need to be more bland. Avoid spicy foods, hard foods like bread crusts or pretzels, and acidic foods like oranges. Very hot and very cold foods should be avoided as well.
- Highly recommend smokers and tobacco chewers to quit.
- Recommend salt water rinses of 1/8 tsp. salt and ¼ tsp. baking soda in 1 cup of warm water.
- Reinforce continued professional dental care before, during, and after dental treatment.[16]

OCCUPATIONAL EXPOSURE RECOMMENDATIONS

Hepatitis

Hepatitis is an inflammation of the liver caused by a virus. When the virus attacks the liver, it impairs the liver's ability to clot by reducing its ability to produce fibrin, the sticky substance that bonds blood platelets together at the site where injury occurs. This results in increased bleeding. Thrombocytopenia often results as well, because of the spleen's inability to remove platelets from the body's blood system. Individuals who suffer from liver impairment usually will show signs of jaundice, or yellowing of the skin. Complete liver shutdown will result in death.

There are at least eight known types of hepatitis; however, only the bloodborne strands are discussed in this chapter because of their high risk for transmission. These strands include hepatitis B, C, D, non-ABCDE, and TT.[12]

Hepatitis B and C

Hepatitis B and C have the ability to develop into a carrier state, which means that the individual will not only experience the infection itself but will then develop the ability to "carry" the virus within his or her hematological system. Because of the body's ability to carry this virus, there is a definite possibility that another individual will contract hepatitis during a specific type of contact with the infected individual. Chronic infection will eventually destroy the liver and its ability to cleanse or detoxify the body, synthesize proteins, and produce the biochemicals necessary for digestion.

Hepatitis B is transmitted through injection drug use or from transmission of body fluids from another person. Hepatitis B is the most transmissible form of hepatitis. Hepatitis poses an extremely high risk for those in the health field, especially dentistry. Transmission in this environment occurs from instrument lacerations, needlestick injuries, and blood droplet contamination onto open mucous membranes. As in all treatment conditions, complete personal protective equipment should be worn if treatment for this individual is necessary. Because of the high risk of infection to the health-care provider, it is also highly recommended by the Occupational Safety and Health Administration that vaccination against the virus be administered. Vaccine against hepatitis B requires three injections, the second injection occurring 1 month after the first, and the third one occurring 6 months after the second. A booster may be recommended if titer levels are too low.

Hepatitis C also will develop into a carrier state once contracted. Unfortunately, no vaccine is available to prevent contracting the disease. Also, no treatment is available once an individual has contracted the virus.

Hepatitis D

Contraction of hepatitis D often occurs with drug users and individuals with hemophilia. Hepatitis D also has the ability to develop into a carrier state, which will eventually cause cirrhosis of the liver. Immunity through the hepatitis B vaccine confers immunity to hepatitis D.

Non-ABCDE and Hepatitis TT

Non-ABCDE and hepatitis TT are grouped together in this section because of the specific conditions that are necessary for contraction of the virus to occur. This type of infection occurs during transfusions.

Dental Hygiene Considerations

If the patient indicates he or she has or has had hepatitis, the dental hygienist should ask what type and whether it was successfully treated. Medical consult with the patient's physician to determine the presence of serum marker HBsAg and HBeAg will indicate whether patient is infectious with hepatitis B.

Universal precautions should be followed on all patients, regardless of medical status, to minimize the risk for transmission of infectious disease. When using ultrasonic instrumentation on a patient with hepatitis, it is recommended to use high-speed suction because it will greatly reduce the amount of aerosol that is created during the procedure. Should an incident occur during which the dental hygienist is exposed to the patient's blood, basic first aid should be the first line of defense for the dental hygienist. Thorough cleansing of the wound and the surrounding area with a mild soap and tepid water should be done immediately after the injury occurs. If bodily fluids come in contact with the eyes or other mucous membranes, the area should be flushed with water. It is not necessary to force the wound to bleed more than it is doing already. "Bleeding" a wound does not cleanse it nor does it prevent bacteria/viruses from entering the host. More caustic detergents such as bleach are not recommended because they may actually cause further damage. Once the wound is cleansed, allow it to "help" itself. The body will initiate its immune system by sending white blood cells to the area to encourage clotting. The clotting mechanism can be encouraged by depressing the wound so that the bleeding is not so spontaneous. Applying pressure to the site will actually slow down the bleeding and allow the blood cells to stick to each other and form clots. It is this accumulation of clots that will slow down and eventually stop the site from losing any more blood.

When the exposure is contained, the dental hygienist should see a health-care provider qualified to evaluate the exposure and who recognizes the unique nature of and implications of this type of exposure to the dental provider. The following information should be recorded at this time:

- Date and time of the incident
- Detailed description of the incident, along with the procedures being performed at the time
- Any and all instruments used in the incident should be clearly listed along with type of fluids involved

- A detailed description of the other individual involved in the incident should be provided
- Both parties involved in the incident should be encouraged to obtain further blood testing along with possible counseling and postexposure follow-up and management

HIV/AIDS

This chapter does not discuss the patient with HIV/AIDs because it is primarily an immunologic disorder caused by a virus that attacks the individual's immune system. Please note that exposure to the patient with HIV/AIDS during treatment should be handled in the same way as discussed earlier in the Occupational Exposure Recommendations section. Any incident that occurs where the dental hygienist is exposed to a patient's body fluids should *always* be treated with basic first aid. This would include stabilizing the injury first, basic cleansing of the site, and then follow-up visits to a health-care provider who is qualified to evaluate the unique nature of this incident and take appropriate actions for possible treatment. Refer to Chapter 43 for further discussion of HIV/AIDS.

SUMMARY

The dental hygienist can influence the oral health status of patients by encouraging them to achieve as healthy an oral health status as possible. Educating the patient on specific personal oral health strategies will help the patient achieve and maintain this goal. A healthy oral environment reduces the risk for unforeseen complications or emergencies, or both, that may occur while treating the patient with blood conditions.

Case Study

Mrs. X is a 65-year-old, white female patient who presents for her scaling and root planing appointment. She is currently under the care of a physician for hemophilia A. She must take 2,500 units of clotting factor VIII three times per week. When she has a dental appointment, Mrs. X takes her clotting factor VIII just before the procedure(s). In 2006, Mrs. X had bilateral knee replacements and has had no resulting complications. Mrs. X has a history of hepatitis C. In addition to her clotting medication, Mrs. X takes vitamin D and a multivitamin daily. Her vitals today are: BP: 118/62, Respiration: 65 bpm, and Pulse: 16 pm.

Case Study Exercises
1. Why does Mrs. X need to take clotting factor VIII right before her dental appointments?
   A. Clotting factor VIII positively influences clotting in the patient with hemophilia A.
   B. Clotting factor VIII will increase the amount of white blood cells that are needed to fight possible infection that may occur during the dental appointment.
   C. Clotting factor VIII is a mild pain reliever and will be more effective if taken right before invasive procedures.

Case Study

D. There is no reason Mrs. X needs to take clotting factor VIII right before her dental appointment.

2. The dental hygienist should ensure all of the following have been attended to before Mrs. X's scaling and root planing EXCEPT:
   A. The patient's physician has been consulted to determine special precautions and risk factors.
   B. The patient has been treated with replacement factor before the appointment.
   C. Universal precautions for disease transmission are adhered to.
   D. The patient has taken prophylaxis premedication.

3. Mrs. X should be treated in a hospital setting best equipped for handling bleeding emergencies.
   A. True
   B. False

4. Consulting with Mrs. X's physician regarding her hepatitis status is necessary to:
   A. Determine whether the hepatitis has negatively influenced the ability of her liver to help with clotting.
   B. Determine whether Mrs. X is a carrier of hepatitis C.
   C. Determine Mrs. X's INR values.
   D. All of the above are appropriate reasons to consult with Mrs. X's physician.

5. Due to Mrs. X's hemophilia and other contributing factors, it would be best to schedule her dental appointments:
   A. In shorter durations but more frequently
   B. In longer durations and less frequently
   C. In one very long appointment to do all needed work, then not at all for 1 year
   D. Not at all, she should be treated in the hospital only

Review Questions

1. Which of the following blood disorders has a distinct, characteristic blood cell shape that reflects a defect in its anatomy?
   A. Hemophilia
   B. von Willebrand disease
   C. Sickle cell anemia
   D. Thrombocytopenia

2. An International Normalized Ratio (INR) count of 1 is indicative of:
   A. Normal blood clotting
   B. Very low blood clotting ability
   C. Unusually shaped blood cells
   D. The size of individual blood cells

3. Thrombocytopenia is any condition in which blood platelet count is less than:
   A. 250,000/mm
   B. 200,000/mm

C. 150,000/mm
D. All of the choices are correct

4. Use of antibiotics should be evaluated when combined with which of the following drugs because of its effect on vitamin K production?
   A. Warfarin
   B. Plavix
   C. Acetaminophen
   D. Statins

5. Anticoagulants differ from antiplatelet agents in that they
   A. Should be discontinued before invasive procedures such as scaling and root planing
   B. Can be safely used along with antibiotics
   C. Increase fibrin production
   D. Do not inhibit platelet aggregation

ACTIVE LEARNING

1. Working with a partner, take turns role-playing gathering a medical history for a patient who takes warfarin. In particular, ask the patient about other medications, including over-the-counter (OTC) and herbal supplements she takes. Explain how you would manage the appointment based on the patient's

responses. For example, what would you do if the patient states that she is taking an antibiotic?

2. Create a table listing the dental hygiene considerations for each of the conditions listed in this chapter; for example, which conditions require prophylactic treatment or laboratory tests before the dental hygiene appointment.

REFERENCES

1. Ibsen OAC, Phelan JA, Oral manifestations of systemic disease. In: Ibsen OAC, Phelan JA, eds. *Oral Pathology for the Dental Hygienist.* 6th ed. St. Louis, MO: Saunders Elsevier; 2014:282-296.

2. Stefanou LB, Wilkins EM. The patient with a blood disorder. In: Wilkins EM, ed. *Clinical Practice of the Dental Hygienist.* 11th ed. Baltimore, MD: Lippincott Williams & Wilkins; 2013:1025-1041.

3. Pickett FA, Gurenlian JR. Blood-related abnormalities and diseases. In: Pickett FA, Gurenlian JR, eds. *The Medical History: Clinical Implications and Emergency Prevention in Dental Settings.* 2nd ed. Lippincott Williams & Wilkins Baltimore, MD: 2010:114-135.

4. Brennan MT, Wynn RL. Aspirin and bleeding in dentistry: an update and recommendations. *Oral Surg Oral Med Oral Pathol Oral Radiol Endod.* 2007;104(3): 316-323.

5. Lesser D. Thrombocytopenia: what the dental hygienist should know. *CDHA J.* 2000; 15(3):9-15.

6. Mann M, Grimes E. Treating patients with immune thrombocytopenia purpura. *Dimens Dent Hyg.* 2011:20-25.

7. Royzman D, Recio L, Badovinac RL, et al. The effect of aspirin intake on bleeding on probing in patients with gingivitis. *J Periodontal.* 2004;75:679-684.

8. Baillargeon J, Holmes HM, Kuo Y. Concurrent use of warfarin and antibiotics and the risk of bleeding in older adults. *Am J Med.* 2012;125(2):183-189.

9. Gupta A, Epstein JB, Cabay RJ. Bleeding disorders of importance in dental care and related patient management. *J Can Dent Assoc.* 2007;73(1):77-83a.

10. Kaweckyj N. Eastern medicine meets dentistry: the use of herbal supplements in dentistry today. Crest Oral B Continuing Ed., December 2010:1-25.

11. Israels S, Schwetz N, Boyer R, McNicol A. Bleeding disorders: characterization, dental considerations and management. *J Can Dent Assoc.* 2006;72(9):827A-827L.

12. Riley L, Womack M. Hepatitis and hemophilia. In: Nursing Working Group, ed. *Nurses' Guide to Bleeding Disorders.* National Hemophilia Foundation; 2012:1-20.

13. Brewer A, Correa ME. Guidelines for Dental Treatment of Patients with Inherited Bleeding Disorders, Treatment of Hemophilia. World Federation of Hemophilia, Montréal, Québec; 2006:40:1-13.

14. National Hemophilia Foundation website. http://www.hemophilia.org. November 9, 2015.

15. Warfarin Dosing Calculator. http://www.globalrph.com/warfarin_calc.htm.

16. Little JW, Falace DA, Miller CS, Rhodus NL. *Dental Management of the Medically Compromised Patient.* 7th ed. St. Louis, MO: Elsevier Mosby; 2008.

Chapter 45 | Cancer

Tara Johnson, RDH, PhD

KEY TERMS

adjunctive screening techniques

cancer

chemotherapy

field cancerization

metastasis

mucositis

multidisciplinary team (MDT)

nadir

oral squamous cell carcinoma (OSCC)

osteoradionecrosis (ORN)

radiation caries

risk factor

salivary diagnostics

tumor

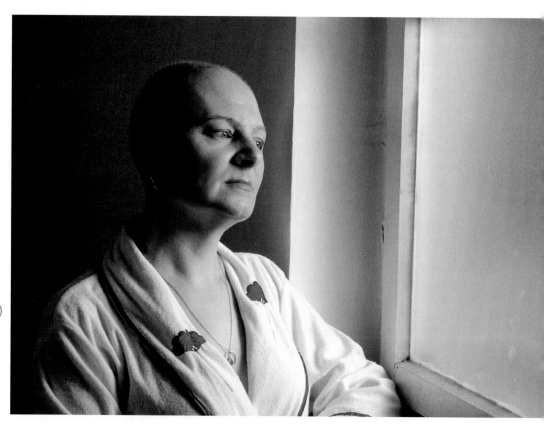

LEARNING OBJECTIVES

After reading this chapter, the student should be able to:

45.1 Define the terms *cancer* and *staging,* and explain how cancer is staged.

45.2 Discuss the incidence, risk factors, therapies, and potential oral complications related to treatment for all cancers.

45.3 Discuss the incidence, risk factors, therapies, and oral complications unique to head and neck cancers.

45.4 Identify behavioral interventions recommended for reducing the incidence of oral cancer.

45.5 Identify the common signs and symptoms of oral cancer.

45.6 Discuss dental hygiene care plan treatment alterations or precautions to be taken with patients with cancer.

KEY CONCEPTS

• Risk assessment for cancer is a critical part of comprehensive health care for all patients.

• Dental hygiene care of patients with cancer requires individualized consideration of systemic and oral complications.

• Types of treatment for cancer and oral cancer include chemotherapy, radiation therapy, surgery, and/or bone marrow and stem cell transplantation, all of which require consideration of precautions in dental hygiene care.

RELEVANCE TO CLINICAL PRACTICE

Because of improvements in health care and asepsis, expected life span is increasing worldwide. Along with this longer life expectancy, the incidence of cancer has increased over the past 50 years. **Cancer** is a general term that applies to a group of more than 100 diseases in which cells in a part of the body begin to grow out of control. Although there are many kinds of cancer, they all start because these abnormal cells proliferate uncontrollably. Untreated cancers can cause serious illness and even death.[1] Early detection and treatment should reduce mortality rate and morbidity from cancers and their treatment. Cancer care can be complex, and more recently, it is being directed by a **multidisciplinary team (MDT)** of health-care professionals. People cared for by a MDT are more likely to: (a) receive accurate diagnosis and staging, (b) be offered a choice of treatments, (c) receive appropriate and consistent information, and (d) have their psychological and social needs considered.[2] The dental hygienist can play an important role on that team. Treatment improvements are largely directed at targeted therapy designed to treat the cancer cells with minimal effects on healthy cells; however, reducing complications from treatment remains a major issue in both general cancers of the body and those specific to oral cancer.

WHAT IS CANCER?

All cancers involve the malfunction of genes that control cell growth and division. It is helpful to compare normal cells with cancer cells when trying to understand cancer. The genetic material (DNA) of a cell is the regulatory mechanism that controls all functioning of that cell. Normal cells grow and divide in a controlled way to produce more cells. Over time, cells degenerate or are damaged, die, and are replaced with new cells. A series of mutations of the DNA can affect normal cell growth and division, resulting in loss of regulatory control, moving a normal cell toward a cancerous one. When this happens, cells do not die when they should and these abnormal cells proliferate, forming a mass of tissue called a **tumor.** Tumors may be benign or malignant. Malignant tumors overcome normal tissue boundaries by losing cell adhesion (binding to other cells or tissues) and metastasizing, or spreading to other tissues. **Metastasis** is a distinct form of cancerous spread that occurs when malignant cells enter blood or lymphatic vessels and travel to distant sites. Metastatic tumors are difficult to remove surgically and can recur when removed or treated. Benign cells or tumors do not have the capacity to invade tissues or travel to distant sites, although they can grow. Benign cells and tumors are typically able to be removed surgically and do not usually recur. When cancer metastasizes, the new tumor has the same type of cancer cells as the primary (original) tumor. For example, if breast cancer spreads to the lung tissues, the cancer cells there are actually breast cancer cells. The disease is metastatic breast cancer rather than lung cancer, and it is treated as breast cancer, not lung cancer.[1,3]

Staging

Staging describes the extent or spread of the disease at the time of diagnosis. Proper staging is essential in determining the choice of therapy and assessing prognosis. When malignant cancers are diagnosed, they are assigned a stage (I, II, III, or IV) by the medical team on the basis of the size of the tumor and how far it has spread. Tests such as radiographs, computed tomography scans, magnetic resonance imaging, endoscopy, and positron emission tomography scans may be used for diagnosis and staging. Generally speaking, stage I is localized and defined to the site of origin. Stage II is regional in nearby structures. Stage III is extensive beyond the regional site crossing several tissue layers. Stage IV is widely disseminated. These general stages can be further delineated to include specific information about each type of cancer. The Tumor, Node, Metastasis (TNM) System comprises the most widely used internationally agreed-on standards to describe and categorize cancer stages and progression. The TNM staging system assesses tumors in three ways: (a) extent of the primary tumor (T), (b) absence or presence of regional lymph node involvement (N), and (c) absence or presence of distant metastasis (M).[4–6] Table 45-1 presents an overview of the TNM Clinical Classification of Carcinomas for the lips and oral cavity.

Grading

Tumor grade is a measure of the changes in cells that are affected by cancer compared with similar healthy

Table 45-1. *Tumor, Node, Metastasis (TNM) Clinical Classification and Staging of Oral Carcinomas*

Stage	Primary Tumor (T)	Regional Lymph Nodes (N)	Distant Metastasis (M)
Stage 0	T (carcinoma in situ)	N0 (no regional lymph node involvement)	M0 (no distant metastasis)
Stage I	T1 (tumor ≤ 2 cm)	N0 (no regional lymph node involvement)	M0 (no distant metastasis)
Stage II	T2 (tumor 2 to ≤ 4 cm)	N0 (no regional lymph node involvement)	M0 (no distant metastasis)
Stage III	T3 (tumor > 4 cm)	N0, N1, N2 (no regional lymph node involvement, single lymph node ≤ 3 cm, or lymph node(s) > 3 cm)	M0 (no distant metastasis)
Stage IV	Any T	Any N	M1 (distant metastasis)

Source: National Cancer Institute. Cancer staging. http://www.cancer.gov/cancertopics/factsheet/detection/staging. Accessed November 9, 2015.

cells. Tumor grade is an indicator of how quickly the tumor is likely to grow and spread. Tumor grading systems differ depending on the type of cancer and may be one of the factors considered when planning treatment for a patient. If the cells of the tumor and the organization of its tissue are similar to those of normal cells and tissue, the tumor is called "well-differentiated." These tumors have a tendency to grow and spread at a slower rate than tumors that are "undifferentiated" or "poorly differentiated," which have abnormal-looking cells and may lack normal tissue structures.[6,7]

CANCER INCIDENCE, RISK FACTORS, AND MOST COMMON TYPES

Millions of people worldwide are living with a cancer diagnosis. Incidence rates in the United States are higher in male than in females individuals across all racial and ethnic populations. Among male individuals, African Americans have the highest incidence followed by white individuals, and the current risk for developing cancer over their lifetime for all men in the United States is one in two. Racial differences in cancer incidence among women are less notable, although white women have the highest incidence rates. Approximately one in three women in the United States will develop cancer in her lifetime. The overall 5-year survival rate for cancer among whites is 59% and among African Americans is 50%. The most common types of cancer in the United States, as of 2012 statistics, are prostrate, breast, lung, and colorectal.[8]

Researchers are learning more about cancer's causes, prevention, and treatment. It is often difficult to elucidate why one person will develop cancer and another will not. Research findings show that certain **risk factors,** or variables, increase the chance of development of cancer, and many of the risk factors can be avoided through lifestyle changes. Tobacco and alcohol use are considered primary risk factors in both men and women across all cancer types.

It was estimated worldwide that more than 1,600,000 men and women were diagnosed with and 572,000 men and women died of cancer of all sites in the year 2012. From 2004 through 2008, the median age for cancer of all sites was 66 years and the median age at death from cancer was 73 years. African American men followed by white men had the highest age-adjusted incidence rate.[1,3] Box 45-1 provides a summary and brief explanation of varying risk factors associated with cancer. Tobacco-cessation initiatives are discussed in Professionalism.

Professionalism

The American Dental Hygienists' Association's (ADHA) Public Health and Advocacy Forums facilitate an exchange of ideas and support State Liaisons, dental hygienists, and any interested party in promoting smoking cessation and tobacco quitlines. Ask, Advise, and Refer, ADHA's national smoking-cessation initiative, is designed to promote cessation interventions by dental hygienists. The Ask, Advise, Refer approach integrates the 5 A's (Ask, Advise, Assess, Assist, Arrange) into a prescribed reasonable time-frame intervention that remains consistent with recommended guidelines. Quitlines are telephone-based tobacco-cessation services that have existed since the late 1980s. Most are accessed through a toll-free number and provide callers with a myriad of services including educational materials, referral to formal cessation programs, and individualized telephone counseling. They are a significant resource that is universally available to dental hygienists and can be easily accessed online during a dental hygiene appointment. Evidence has revealed that quitlines are convenient, effective, and preferred by smokers.[22,23] ■

Box 45-1. *Risk Factors Associated With Cancer*

- *Growing older:* most cancers occur in people older than 65 years
- *Tobacco:* cigarette, smokeless, environmental, or secondhand
- *Alcohol:* heavy consumption serves as a solvent for tobacco carcinogens, as well as numerous other risks for alcohol as a carcinogen
- *Betel leaves/Areca nut:* chewing of these is a particular risk factor for oral cancer
- *Some viruses and bacteria:* strongest evidence to date is the association of *Helicobacter pylori* and stomach cancer; several viruses have been identified as risk factors; the Epstein-Barr virus has been linked to Burkitt's lymphoma; hepatitis B and C have been linked to liver cancer; human papillomaviruses (HPVs) are linked to cervical cancer and more recently to oral cancer
- *Sunlight exposure:* ultraviolet radiation from sunlight, sun lamps, or tanning booths
- *Ionizing radiation:* radioactive fallout, radon gas, x-rays, and other sources
- *Certain chemicals and other substances:* benzene, chlorinated hydrocarbons, asbestos, and hexavalent chromium have all been shown to be carcinogenic
- *Certain hormones:* estrogens and progestins are related to breast cancer
- *Family history:* history of certain cancers, especially breast, ovarian, colorectal, and prostate malignancies, within families puts persons with these family histories at increased risk
- *Poor diet, lack of physical activity, and obesity:* these three factors are interrelated and all are involved in the body's proinflammatory state, which is also shown to play a part in the development of cancer

CHEMOTHERAPY-ASSOCIATED COMPLICATIONS

Cancer **chemotherapy** is a systemic drug regimen designed to specifically kill rapidly dividing cells. The number of patients who experience oral complications from anticancer treatment varies. Estimates according to therapy include 10% receiving adjuvant chemotherapy, or treatment that is given in addition to primary or initial therapy; 40% receiving primary chemotherapy; 80% receiving stem cell transplantation; and 100% receiving head and neck radiation therapy directly to areas in the oral cavity. Oral side effects can interfere with the ability of some patients to receive all of their cancer treatment. Sometimes treatment has to be delayed because of the severity of the oral side effects. This

disruption can directly affect a patient's chances for survival. Preventing and controlling oral complications is vital to enhancing a patient's quality of life and to ensuring they get the most benefit from cancer therapy.[9]

Assessing a patient's oral status and stabilizing any existing oral disease before any cancer therapy are critical to overall patient care. Preventing and treating oral complications after cancer therapy has started include identifying and educating patients who may be at risk, taking preventive action before anticancer treatments are started, and treating any complications promptly.

CANCER THERAPY AND ACUTE ORAL COMPLICATIONS

Poor oral health has been associated with increased incidence and severity of oral complications in patients with cancer; therefore, an aggressive approach to stabilizing oral care before cancer treatment begins is considered a primary first step. Primary preventive measures such as appropriate nutritional intake, effective oral hygiene practices, and early detection/treatment of oral disease are important pretreatment interventions. In addition, patients should be educated relative to the range and management of oral complications that may occur during subsequent phases of therapy. Baseline oral hygiene instructions should be provided. To maximize outcomes, the oncology team and the dental team should communicate treatment plans before, during, and after therapy. The overall objective of interdisciplinary care from a dental hygiene perspective is to complete a comprehensive evaluation and oral care plan to help prevent or alleviate oral disease that could otherwise produce complications during or after chemotherapy.[6] Systemic chemotherapy and head and neck radiation therapy often result in acute oral complications. The oral cavity is highly susceptible to anticancer treatment for a variety of reasons, including:

- Radiation therapy and chemotherapy target cells that rapidly divide, whether they are cancerous or healthy. The cells of the mucosal lining of the mouth reproduce quickly, to heal the trauma that occurs to normal tissues from oral activity. Anticancer treatment interferes with these rapidly reproducing cells, because it cannot determine the difference between healthy cells and abnormally proliferating cells. Radiation therapy does not affect the oral cavity unless administered in the head and neck region, whereas systemic chemotherapy affects the oral cavity more than 40% of the time.
- The mouth contains hundreds of different bacteria, some beneficial, some not. Normally these bacteria remain in balance. However, chemotherapy and radiation therapy can upset this balance and can also affect saliva production. These factors can lead to mouth sores, infection, and tooth decay.

Oral lesions are principally related to chronic cancer regimen–associated (chemotherapy with or without radiation therapy) toxicity. Cytoreductive therapy (decrease in tumor size through chemotherapy, radiotherapy, or initial surgery) generally leads to low white blood cell count and, in particular, low neutrophil counts (neutropenia), which increases susceptibility to infection, particularly bacterial infections. Because most oral infections such as deep caries, periodontal disease, and pericoronitis around third molars are usually of bacterial origin, elimination of potential sources of infection in the oral cavity is essential.[9,10]

Mucositis

Mucositis is the most common acute complication following chemotherapy or head and neck radiation therapy, or both. **Mucositis** is inflammation of the mucous membrane lining the digestive tract from the mouth to the anus. When such inflammation occurs in the mucous membranes of the oral and oropharyngeal region, it is termed oral mucositis (OM). OM is a common side effect usually beginning 7 to 10 days after initiation of cytotoxic therapy and it remains present for approximately 2 weeks after cessation of that therapy. Removal of sharp edges of teeth or restorations may help to reduce trauma to the mucosa and reduce the severity of mucositis and corresponding pain and discomfort. Patients receiving systemic chemotherapy or radiation therapy to the chest/head/neck area should examine their mouths at least once a day for redness, sores, or signs of infection. The oral health-care provider should be notified if worsening sores, white patches, pus, a "hairy" or thick feeling tongue, and/or bleeding in the mouth is noticed. Undetected or inadequately treated OM can lead to pain, discomfort, and inability to tolerate foods or fluids with increased propensity for opportunistic infections in the mouth, resulting in a reduction of the patient's quality of life. Poorly managed OM is one of the leading causes for unplanned treatment interruptions and, therefore, increases in overall cancer treatment time. Prolongation of cancer treatment time adversely affects the treatment's ability to control the tumor; it also increases the overall cost of the treatment.[9,10] Early diagnosis and effective treatments are needed to prevent or reduce the incidence and severity of OM. Table 45-2 presents a brief index for assessing the severity of OM. Signs and symptoms of mucositis include:

- Red, shiny, or swollen mouth and gingiva
- Blood in the mouth
- Sores in the mouth or on the gums or tongue
- Soreness or pain in the mouth or throat
- Difficulty swallowing or talking
- Feeling of dryness, mild burning, or pain when eating food
- Soft, whitish patches or pus in the mouth or on the tongue
- Increased mucus or thicker saliva in the mouth (Fig. 45-1)

Treatment

Treatment of mucositis is mainly supportive. Oral hygiene is the mainstay of treatment. Clinical management using current therapies is aimed at reducing the severity of mucositis. General oral care protocols include:

- Rinse mouth (swish and spit) before and after meals and at bedtime with either:
  - Normal saline (1 tsp. table salt to 1 quart [32 oz.] water)
  - Salt and soda (1/2 tsp. salt and 2 tbsp. sodium bicarbonate in 1 quart of warm water)
- Use an ultrasoft-bristle toothbrush after meals and at bedtime. Replace brush frequently. Use of powered toothbrush ONLY if technique does not contribute to trauma of oral tissues (if the brush causes pain, toothettes may be used).
- Use a nonabrasive toothpaste (or mix 1 tsp. baking soda in 2 cups water). Avoid toothpastes with whiteners.
- Keep lips moist with moisturizers. Avoid using Vaseline (the oil base can promote infection).
- Avoid products that irritate the oral tissues:
  - Avoid commercial mouthwashes and those with alcohol.
  - Limit use of dental floss, DO NOT use with platelets less than 40,000.
  - Do not use lemon or glycerin swabs or toothbrushes without soft bristles.
- Increase fluid intake to at least 3 L/day.
- Include high-protein foods in diet.
- Avoid hot, spicy, or acidic foods, alcohol, and hard or coarse foods (crusty bread, chips, crackers).
- Partial or full dentures:
  - Remove whenever possible to expose oral tissues to air.
  - Loose-fitting dentures can irritate the oral tissues and should not be worn.
  - Do not wear dentures if mouth sores are severe.

Table 45-2. *Oral Mucositis Assessment Scale*

Grade	0	1	2	3	4
World Health Organization criteria of symptoms	None	Soreness and/or erythema	Erythema or ulcers but patient can swallow solid food	Ulcers with extensive erythema and patient cannot swallow solid food	Mucositis to the extent that intake of any nutrition is not possible

Source: The World Health Organization (WHO) oral toxicity scale. http://www.gelclair.net/Institutional.aspx?Pagina=239&SM=230&Lingua=EN

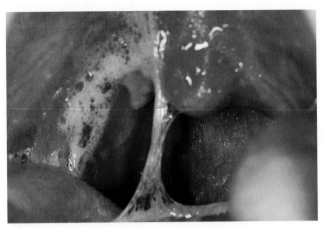

Figure 45-1. Saliva changes. (Source: Rosenthal DI, Mendoza TR, Chambers MS, Burkett VS, Garden AS, Hessell AC, Lewen JS, Ang KK, Kies MS, Gning I, et al. The M.D. Anderson symptom inventory-head and neck module, a patient-reported outcome instrument, accurately predicts the severity of radiation-induced mucositis. *Int J Radiat Biol Phys.* 2008;72(5):1355-1361. Reprinted with permission.)

Although many interventions used for the treatment or prevention of OM have some evidence supporting their use, no intervention has been conclusively validated by research. Consequently, the following discussion of targeted therapies is not intended to be all-inclusive, but rather highlights agents and strategies that are at the forefront of clinical practice.[10,11] These interventions have been categorized in Table 45-3 to aid the discussion and/or implementation of procedures.

Early Infections

Viral, fungal, and bacterial infections may arise; however, frequency of infection declines upon resolution of OM and regeneration of neutrophils. Candidiasis is the most common clinical infection of the oropharynx in irradiated patients and presents as an opportunistic infection. *Candida* species are frequently part of the

Evidence-Based Practice

It is difficult for the clinician to choose from a bewildering array of treatment options for OM. It appears many interventions show conflicting evidence supporting their effectiveness, whereas others have a moderate amount. No intervention has been conclusively shown to be effective. For instance, alcohol-free chlorhexidine rinse is commonly used and recommended, although its effectiveness remains uncertain in the research. Controversy exists about the effectiveness of chlorhexidine in preventing radiochemotherapy-induced OM in patients with cancer. Chlorhexidine mouthrinse may have a role in the prevention of OM in adult patients with solid tumors treated with chemotherapy in conventional doses. Evidence suggests that amifostine (chemoprotectant), benzydamine oral rinse (locally acting NSAID with local anesthetic and analgesic properties), calcium phosphate, Chinese medicine, honey, hydrolytic enzymes, ice chips, iseganan hydrochloride (broad-spectrum antimicrobial solution), and oral care provide some benefit in preventing or reducing the severity of mucositis associated with cancer treatment; however, caution is advised as benefits may apply to specific cancer types and treatment. The ease of use of low-level laser therapy, high patient acceptance, and the positive results achieved suggest this therapy as an alternative for the prevention and treatment of OM in young patients. Natural honey is a safe, simple, and inexpensive alternative for preventing OM resulting from radiochemotherapy in patients with head and neck cancer. Povidine-iodine and cryotherapy can be effective in the prevention of radiochemotherapy-induced OM in patients with cancer.[24] ■

Table 45-3. *Therapeutics for Oral Mucositis*

Reduce Toxicity to Mucosa	Mixed Action Topicals	Pain Control
Cryotherapy: involves sucking on ice chips during chemotherapy administration, has shown some effect in preventing mucositis	**Sodium hyaluronate (Gelclair):** lubricant, restores moisture and prevents abrasion **OTC Zilactin:** bioadhesive protectant and aspirin	**Topical pain relievers** (lidocaine, benzocaine, dyclonine hydrochloride [HCl], and Ulcerease [0.6% phenol]): unable to effectively coat all areas and the pain relief is brief
Sodium hyaluronate (Gelclair) and OTC Zilactin: mucosal protectants that work by coating the mucosa, forming a protective barrier for exposed nerve endings	**Benzydamine hydrochloride:** drug with anti-inflammatory, pain-relieving, antipyretic, and antimicrobial activities and has been used as a gargle or mouthwash to prevent and treat oral mucositis	**Low-level laser therapy (light amplification by stimulated emission of radiation):** produces pure light in a single wavelength; noninvasive treatment modality uses a low-intensity laser to produce photochemical reactions in the cells
Amifostine (Ethyol): protects against the damage to the mucosa caused by radiation, is approved by the FDA for patients receiving radiation therapy for cancers of the head and neck	**Calcium phosphate rinse (NeutraSal):** prevents and reduces the severity of oral mucositis caused by radiation and high-dose chemotherapy	**Narcotic pain relievers:** opioids can help the patient with moderate-to-severe mucositis become relatively comfortable

Continued

Table 45-3. *Therapeutics for Oral Mucositis—cont'd*

Reduce Toxicity to Mucosa	Mixed Action Topicals	Pain Control
MuGard: FDA-approved mucoadhesive oral protectant that forms a protective hydrogel coating over the oral mucosa while a patient is undergoing chemotherapy and/or radiotherapy to the head and neck		

FDA, U.S. Food and Drug Administration; OTC, over the counter.

human body's normal oral and intestinal flora, yet a weakened immune system can predispose a patient to overgrowth of this common yeastlike fungus. Patients receiving head and neck radiation are frequently colonized with *Candida,* as demonstrated by an increase in rates of clinical infection. Candidiasis may exacerbate the symptoms of oropharyngeal mucositis as well. Treatment of oral candidiasis has primarily used topical antifungals such as nystatin (Bio-statin) and clotrimazole (Lotrimin). Compliance can be compromised secondary to OM, nausea, pain, and difficulty in dissolving nystatin pastilles (tablet to be chewed) or clotrimazole troches (lozenges). Use of systemic antifungals including ketoconazole and fluconazole to treat oral candidiasis has proved effective and may have advantages over topical agents for patients experiencing OM and candidiasis. Bacterial infections may also occur early in the course of head/neck radiation and, following culture and sensitivity tests, should be treated with appropriate antibiotics. Herpes virus infections may also occur after head and neck radiation in patients who are prone to breakouts.[9,12]

Taste Dysfunction (Dysgeusia)

Taste receptors become damaged from oral exposure to radiation and taste discrimination becomes increasingly compromised. After several weeks of radiation, it is common for patients to complain of no sense of taste. It will generally take upward of 6 to 8 weeks after the end of radiation therapy for taste receptors to recover and become functional. Zinc sulfate supplements (220 mg two or three times a day) have been reported to help with recovery of the sense of taste.

Frequency and severity of acute oral complications typically begin to decrease approximately 3 to 4 weeks after cessation of chemotherapy. Long-term survivors of cancer treated with high-dose chemotherapy alone or chemoradiotherapy (if radiotherapy is not directed at oral cavity) will generally have few significant permanent oral complications.[9] Once all complications of chemotherapy have been resolved, patients may be able to resume their normal dental care schedule.

Dental Hygiene Considerations

Goals of dental management before the inception of cancer therapy are to eliminate or stabilize oral disease and to minimize local and systemic infection during and after cancer therapy (Box 45-2).[12]

Specific interventions are directed toward:

- Mucosal lesions
- Dental caries and endodontic disease
- Periodontal disease
- Ill-fitting dentures
- Temporomandibular dysfunction
- Short-term considerations (decreased immune response and infection)

ORAL CANCER AS A SUBSET OF HEAD AND NECK CANCERS

Oral cancer is part of a group of cancers commonly referred to as head and neck cancers. Of all head and neck cancers, the group known as oral cancer comprises about 85% of that category. True oral cancers

Box 45-2. *Pretreatment Oral Evaluation*

Review recent medical history:
　Social history
　Family history
　Medications
　Drug Allergies
Review current cancer diagnosis:
　Previous treatment (if any)
　Planned treatment
Dental history:
　Frequency of past visits, including dental hygiene
　History of extractions, endodontics, infections
Current chief complaint:
　Recommended management of complaint
Oral examination:
　Extraoral (including nodes, salivary glands, swelling, temporomandibular joint)
　Intraoral (including fit and function of any appliances, soft tissue abnormalities, caries, extent of plaque and calculus, complete periodontal charting, complete dental charting including periapical/periodontal infections, faulty restorations and fractures)
Radiographs:
　Panoramic and full-mouth radiographic series

include the lips, tongue, gingiva, buccal mucosa, floor of the mouth, retromolar areas, hard and soft palates, and nasopharynx and oropharynx. Brain, eye, and thyroid cancer, as well as those of the scalp, skin, muscles, and bones of the head and neck, are not included in the group of head and neck cancers. More than 90% of head and neck cancers are **oral squamous cell carcinoma (OSCC).** Squamous cell carcinoma is a histologically distinct form of cancer deriving from epithelium. It arises from mutated ectodermal or endodermal cells that line body cavities. OSCC occurs in the squamous cell epithelium that covers the oral cavity, lips, and throat. It originates from the oral keratinocytes where DNA mutations can be spontaneous, and carcinogens from tobacco and alcohol increase the mutation rate. The remainder of head and neck cancers includes salivary gland tumors, lymphoma, and sarcoma. Head and neck squamous cell carcinomas can be found in the nasopharynx, larynx, thyroid and parathyroid, throat, oral cavity, and lips; however, the most common site in both American men and women is the tongue, particularly the posterior lateral surfaces (Fig. 45-2). Estimated new cases and deaths from oral cancer in the United States in 2014 were 42,000 and 8,300, respectively. If the definition is expanded to include cancer of the larynx, for which the risk factors are the same, the numbers of diagnosed cases grow to approximately 55,000 individuals and 11,900 deaths.

Worldwide, OSCC is the sixth most common cancer. The 5-year survival rate for oral cancer has remained between 50% and 60%, not because oral cancer is difficult to discover or difficult to diagnose, but because the cancer is usually seen in late stages of development.[13,14] Often, oral cancer is discovered only when it has metastasized to another location, most likely the lymph nodes of the neck. Prognosis at this stage is significantly worse than when it is caught in a localized intraoral area. Oral cancer, in its early stages, does not make itself readily apparent to the patient, although, as it progresses, signs and symptoms can become evident (Box 45-3; also see Advancing Technologies).[13] Dental hygienists should

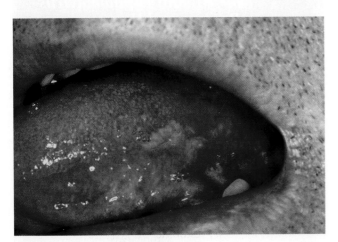

Figure 45-2. Tobacco-related tongue cancer. (Source: Mirbod SM, Ahing SI. Tobacco-associated lesion of the oral cavity: part II. Malignant lesions. *J Can Dent Assoc.* 2000;66:308-311. Reprinted with permission.)

Advancing Technologies

Even the most thorough visual examination cannot classify oral lesions as benign or cancerous; therefore, other modes of identification and diagnoses are necessary. Identification of precancer/cancer will dramatically improve treatment outcomes. Today technologies are available to assist in the early screening or identification of precancerous or cancerous lesions within the oral cavity. These technologies enable practitioners to alert the patient to the need for a more definitive diagnosis and are considered screening tools only. When appropriately integrated into clinical assessment, these screening options may provide a means for early identification and intervention. There are currently no hard data to support the contention that these technologies can help the clinician to identify premalignant lesions before they are detectable by visual screening alone; studies are under way to determine their utility in the dental setting.[25]

Adjunctive screening techniques include:
Toluidine blue staining: preferential staining of oral premalignant lesions and oral malignancies (selective dye uptake by abnormal cells)
VELscope Vx: handheld device to identify abnormal oral tissue through fluorescence by direct visual examination using blue light source
ViziLite Plus: rinse with a 1% acetic acid solution followed by direct visual examination of the oral cavity using a blue-white light source
Oral CDx: cell sample specimen collected with specially designed brush to collect cells; cells are fixed to a slide and sent to specialty laboratory for analysis

CHARACTERISTICS OF A GOOD SCREENING TEST
A screening test should have the following characteristics:
1. Be simple, safe, and acceptable to the public.
2. Detect disease early in its natural history.
3. Preferentially detect those lesions that are most likely to progress.
4. Detect lesions that are treatable or where an intervention will prevent progression.
5. Have a high positive predictive value and low false negatives (high sensitivity).

Adjunctive oral cancer screening options should not be confused with salivary diagnostics. **Salivary diagnostics** involve the use of saliva to look for indicators of health conditions or diseases. Currently available salivary diagnostic tests include various hormonal, HIV, and alcohol tests; however, studies are in progress to identify salivary biomarkers for early oral cancer detection.[26] ■

Box 45-3. Signs and Symptoms of Oral Cancer

- White and/or red patches in the mouth, lips, or on the sides of or under the tongue
- A sore or blister lasting longer than 2 weeks or does not heal
- Difficulty swallowing
- Swelling/thickening, lumps or bumps, or eroded areas on the lips, gingiva, or other areas inside the mouth
- Difficulty chewing, swallowing, speaking, or moving the jaw or tongue
- Hoarseness, chronic sore throat, or changes in the voice
- Ear pain
- A change in the way teeth or dentures fit together
- Unexplained bleeding in the mouth
- Unexplained numbness or loss of feeling, or pain/tenderness in any area of the face, mouth, or neck

teach all patients, especially those at high risk for oral cancer, to perform self-examinations for identification of early signs of oral cancer to enhance detection at an early stage. Much like breast or skin self-examinations, an oral self-examination is easy to do and does not require any special equipment. In addition, it will help familiarize individuals with their mouths (Box 45-4).[15]

Demographics

The demographics of those who develop oral cancer have been stable for quite some time. Historically, age at time of onset or diagnosis has been noted in people aged 40 years or older who exhibit the primary risk factor behaviors of tobacco and alcohol use or exposure

Box 45-4. Oral Cancer Self-Examination

1. Press along the sides and front of your neck and feel for any tenderness or lumps.
2. Pull your upper lip up and look for any sores and/or color changes on your lips or gums. Repeat this on your lower lip.
3. Use your fingers to pull out your cheek on each side and look for any color changes such as red, white, or dark patches.
4. Tilt your head back and open your mouth wide to see if there are any lumps or color changes. Look at the top, back, and each side of your tongue for sores or color changes.
5. Touch the roof of your mouth with your tongue; look at the underside of your tongue and the floor of your mouth for sores or color changes. Using one finger, feel inside your mouth for unusual bumps, swelling, or tenderness.

to other traditional risk factors such as occupation, sun exposure, or a family history of oral cancer.

Recently, oral cancers are being diagnosed in a much younger population (people between 20 and 40 years of age) without a history of traditional risk factors. Research directed at exact causes of those affected at an earlier age has revealed a viral cause, specifically the human papillomavirus (HPV). HPV, particularly strain 16, has been shown to be sexually transmitted between partners and is conclusively implicated in the increasing incidence of oral cancer in young, nonsmoking individuals. This is the same virus as the causative agent in more than 90% of all cases of cervical cancer. Even though the majority of head and neck cancer cases are still generally related to tobacco and alcohol use (75%), high-risk HPV-related oral cancers account for many of the remaining 25%. Not only do the two types of oral cancer differ in risk factors, they differ in common locations in the oral cavity as well (Table 45-4).[16] In addition, persons with HPV-related oral cancer have a higher survival rate than those with HPV-negative oral cancer. The concept, first noted by Slaughter et al in 1953, proposed to explain the development of multiple primary tumors and locally recurrent cancer associated with high-risk behaviors of tobacco and alcohol use. These lesions appear in the context of the existence of mutated cells at multiple sites.[17] These tumor-associated genetic alterations have been attributed to exposure of the entire oral cavity, oropharynx, and larynx to carcinogens from tobacco and alcohol, resulting in mutation in multiple areas and the predisposition to second primary tumors. This complicated process has been termed **field cancerization.** Better known today as *cancer fields,* the concept encompasses four general ideas: (a) abnormal tissue surrounds the tumor that may not be apparent clinically, (b) potentially cancerous cells can arise at multiple locations simultaneously, (c) oral cancer can consist of several independent lesions

Table 45-4. Common Oral Cancer Sites for Human Papillomavirus–Positive and Human Papillomavirus–Negative Oral Cancer

Cancer Type	Common Sites
HPV-negative oral cancers	Lateral borders of the tongue Floor of the mouth Buccal mucosa Soft and hard palates Gingiva
HPV-positive oral cancers	Tonsils Posterior lateral borders (base) of the tongue Oropharynx

HPV, human papillomavirus.

Application to Clinical Practice

Oral cancer is associated with severe morbidity and high mortality. On average, only half of those with the disease will survive more than 5 years. With early detection and timely treatment, deaths from oral cancer could be dramatically reduced and early detection is often possible. Tissue changes in the mouth that might signal the beginnings of cancer often can be seen and felt easily. *What you can do:* A cancer risk assessment and complete head and neck examination should be a routine part of each patient's dental hygiene visit. First, *take a thorough history* of their alcohol and tobacco use. Clinicians should be particularly vigilant in checking those patients who show evidence of high-risk behaviors. If your patient smokes, calculate a *pack-year** for them. Quantification of pack-years smoked is important in clinical care where degree of tobacco exposure is closely correlated to risk for disease.[27] *Examine* your patients

using the standardized visual head and neck examination recommended during your clinical training. *Inform* your patients of the association among tobacco use, alcohol use, and oral cancer. *Follow up* to make sure a definitive diagnosis is obtained on any possible signs/symptoms of oral cancer. This important examination should take no longer than 5 minutes. ■

*A pack-year is a quantification of cigarette smoking. It is a way to measure the amount a person has smoked over a long period. It is calculated by multiplying the number of packs of cigarettes smoked per day by the number of years the person has smoked. For example, if a person smokes a pack of cigarettes a day (20 cigarettes) for 1 year, 1 pack-year equals 365 packs of cigarettes (or 7,300 individual cigarettes). The formula for a pack-year is:

Number of pack years = (packs smoked per day) × (years as a smoker)

OR

Number of pack years = (number of cigarettes smoked per day × number of years smoked)

Spotlight on Public Health

Oral cancer includes major morbidity and mortality attributable to the disease and to the various forms of treatment. All areas of health status are affected. The focus of a public health program related to oral and pharyngeal cancer is to improve early detection and provide prevention strategies in target populations. East Side Health District in East St. Louis, Illinois, has been intricately involved in an Oral Cancer Prevention Program since 2006. This program has been instrumental in solidifying community partnerships and planning interventions for early detection and prevention of oral and pharyngeal cancers. East Side Health District's goal is to develop and implement interventions that reduce the incidence of late-stage diagnosis of oral cancers in the community to less than 50% and to increase the number of adults in the community who report that

they have had an oral cancer examination in the past year to 20%. Strategies used to accomplish this goal include: (a) building sustainable partnerships with ownership in the intervention strategies devised and implemented; (b) improving awareness of oral cancer among the target population to ensure a decline in the incidence of late-stage diagnosis and oral cancer, and to encourage steps to reduce risk and foster early detection; (c) making the community more aware of the associated high-risk factors such as smoking, drinking, and chewing tobacco products; (d) enhancing the capacity of local health-care providers to detect oral cancer and to counsel patients about risk; and (e) making oral cancer screening examinations a priority of the provider community, and conducting special promotional and screening events at appropriate venues throughout each fiscal year.[28] ■

that can coalesce into one tumor, and (d) the incomplete removal of abnormal tissue borders after surgery may explain recurrences. These second primary tumors are a significant problem in treating oral and oropharyngeal squamous cell carcinoma and have a negative impact on survival. However, research has shown HPV-positive oral cancer to have a higher survival rate and better response to therapy. It has been hypothesized that the higher survival rate and better response to therapy of HPV-related tumors may be related to reduced multiple mutations of the oral cavity that are

created from exposure to the primary risk factors of tobacco and alcohol.[18] See Application to Clinical Practice and Spotlight on Public Health.

ORAL CANCER THERAPIES AND ORAL COMPLICATIONS

After a definitive diagnosis has been made and the oral cancer has been staged, treatment may begin. Treatment of oral cancers is ideally a multidisciplinary approach that involves the efforts of surgeons, oncologists, dental and dental hygiene practitioners, nutritionists, and rehabilitative and restorative specialists.[2] The actual curative treatment modalities are usually surgery and radiation with chemotherapy added to decrease the possibility of metastasis, to sensitize the malignant cells to radiation, or for those patients who have confirmed distant metastasis of the disease. Before the commencement of curative treatment, it is likely that other oral health needs will be addressed to decrease the likelihood of development of post-therapeutic complications.

Whether a patient has surgery, surgery and radiation, or surgery, radiation, and chemotherapy is dependent on the stage of development of the cancer. Each case is individual. Those with cancer treated in the early stages may have little in the way of disfigurement; nevertheless, oral tissues can be profoundly affected. Injury to normal oral tissues can be either reversible or irreversible. Because oral epithelium is highly active tissue with replication times estimated at 9 to 16 days, chemotherapy and radiation may be directly toxic to the oral mucosa, resulting in acute symptoms of dysgeusia (taste dysfunction), OM, pain, abnormal bleeding, and compromised normal function. The dental/periapical, periodontal, or salivary gland tissues may also suffer acute injury. Radiotherapy can cause both serious destruction to bone and permanent salivary gland disturbances.[19] Dental hygienists play an important role in addressing these issues both in oral health and in quality of life.

Head and neck radiation therapy may cause some of the same acute oral side effects that were discussed earlier. These can lead to serious indirect complications, including tooth decay, periodontitis, bone or tissue loss, systemic infections, delayed healing, dehydration, and malnutrition. Acute complications occur while treatment is ongoing. Patients undergoing chemotherapy usually experience acute complications that heal after treatment ends, whereas patients receiving direct radiation therapy to the head and neck region may have extended or lifelong (chronic) complications.[9] Surgical management of oral cancer typically includes both the primary lesion and the cervical lymph nodes. The risks of surgery develop directly from the extent of the tumor and its relationship to surrounding oral structures. Problems may include disfigurement and compromise of vascularity and nerve tissue, as well as disruption of taste sensation, mastication, speech, and swallowing functions. Once the patient has completed head and neck cancer therapy and acute oral complications have abated, the patient should be evaluated regularly (every 4–8 weeks) by a dental hygienist for the first 6 months. Most importantly, this provides an opportunity to educate the patient about the role of dental health in systemic disease. Thereafter, a schedule based on the patient's needs should be determined. However, oral complications can continue or emerge long after radiation therapy of the head and neck region

has ended. Patients should be informed about why a dental evaluation is important before cancer therapy, what to expect during cancer therapy (such mucositis and xerostomia), and measures that can be taken to minimize side effects of therapy.[20,21] The importance of long-term follow-up should be stressed, and dental hygienists should provide information resources for cancer survivors (Box 45-5).

Long-Term Oral Complications

Radiation to the head and neck has the potential for increased caries risk and reduced healing capacity (particularly of the bone) in the long term. Identification and elimination of dental disease (especially removal of teeth with poor prognosis) by thorough dental and dental hygiene care are important preventive strategies to avoid future dental extractions, a significant risk factor for postradiation **osteoradionecrosis (ORN).** Postradiation ORN represents nonhealing, dead bone and is the result of functional and structural bony changes that may not be expressed for months or even years. Because radiation therapy works by destroying cancer cells through the deprivation of oxygen and vital nutrients to both normal and cancer cells, it causes damage to the small arteries, reducing blood circulation to the alveolar ridges. Insufficient blood supply, and thus inadequate oxygen to irradiated bone, diminishes the bone's ability to heal, especially in the mandible where the blood supply is more concentrated. Although ORN may develop spontaneously, it most frequently occurs in response to trauma to irradiated areas subsequent to surgery, tooth extractions, or denture irritations. ORN may be reduced through early intraoral evaluation, treatment, and adequate healing time for surgical procedures before beginning radiation therapy to the head and neck. Hyperbaric oxygen (HBO) therapy has been beneficial in the prevention and treatment of ORN. It is of paramount importance for the medical and dental community to recognize the factors that may reduce ORN incidence, endorse oral care protocols, and acknowledge the value of HBO therapy in the prevention and treatment of this disease. In addition, patients treated with intravenous bisphosphonates or long-term oral bisphosphonates are at risk for developing bisphosphonate-related osteonecrosis of the

---

Box 45-5. *Information Resources for Cancer Survivors*

- Cancer Survivors Network | CancerHopeNetwork.org
- Cancer Survivors | MDAnderson.org
- LIVESTRONG.org
- Centers for Disease Control and Prevention: Cancer Survivorship—Basic Information (www.cdc.gov/cancer/survivorship/basic_info)
- Oral Cancer Foundation: Information, Support, Advocacy (oralcancerfoundation.org) ■

jaws (BRONJ). Bisphosphonates are a class of drugs used to prevent bone loss demineralization (weakening or destruction) caused by osteoporosis and to decrease bone pain from the spread of cancer to bone tissue. Some of these drugs can be taken by mouth, whereas others must be given intravenously at a hospital or clinic. Examples include drugs such as risedronate (Actonel), zoledronic acid (Zometa and Reclast), alendronate (Fosamax), and ibandronate sodium (Boniva). Bisphosphonate-related osteonecrosis of the jaw is caused by trauma to alveolar structures that have a limited capacity for bone healing because of the effects of intravenous bisphosphonate therapy. Because invasive dental procedures such as extractions are a risk factor for both ORN and BRONJ, an important aspect of patient management is elimination of dental disease to reduce the necessity of surgical dental procedures in the long term.[9]

The following chronic complications are also common after radiation therapy to the head or neck has ended and should be addressed with appropriate protocols: dry mouth, radiation caries, infections, impaired sense of taste, and difficulty with use of the muscles of the mouth and temporomandibular joint because of permanent damage to the tissues.[9,10]

Caries

Because of the damage to the salivary glands during radiation and the ensuing xerostomia that follows, these patients are at higher risk than the average person for the development of dental caries. Caries risk increases from a number of factors associated with xerostomia, including an increase in cariogenic bacteria, reduced concentrations of salivary antimicrobial proteins, and loss of mineralizing components. **Radiation caries** is defined as tooth decay of the cervical regions, incisal edges, and cusp tips secondary to xerostomia induced by radiation therapy to the head and neck. Optimal oral hygiene must be maintained using a soft-bristled toothbrush after softening it further under hot water. Treatment strategies must be directed to each component of the caries process. Xerostomia should be managed via salivary substitutes, sugar-free mints, and frequent sips of water. Caries susceptibility can be enhanced with application of in-office fluoride varnish every 3 to 4 months. Efficacy of topical agents for use at home is improved by increased contact time on the teeth (4 minutes for 2% neutral NaF gel in custom trays) and mineralizing agents such as casein phosphopeptides with amorphous calcium phosphate (CPP-ACP). Those patients not able to comply with use of fluoride trays should be instructed to use brush-on gels and rinses.[19,20] CPP-ACP has shown to reduce demineralization and enhance remineralization of the enamel subsurface of carious lesions. It is also believed to have an antibacterial and buffering effect on plaque and interfere in the growth and adherence of *Streptococcus mutans*. Combined with fluoride, CPP-ACP may have an additive effect on caries activity. Xylitol is a commonly used sugar substitute, especially in chewing gum and mints. This nonfermentable sugar alcohol acts as a carrier for calcium phosphates and may inhibit the cariogenicity, adhesivity, and acidogenic potential of plaque. Optimal oral hygiene and consistent use of the anticaries agents listed earlier must be maximized for caries reduction following head and neck radiation therapy. Exposure to fluoride from over-the-counter dentifrices and rinses is generally considered inadequate to meet the needs of this high-risk population, although fluoride use should be determined for each patient based on age, physical abilities, health awareness, and attitude.[9,10,12]

Tissue Necrosis

Necrosis and secondary infection of previously oral irradiated tissue is a serious complication. Chronic changes involving bone and mucosa are a result of the process of vascular inflammation, and scarring may ultimately cause a hypovascular, hypocellular, and hypoxic state. The process is confounded by infection and tissue injury with resulting ORN, or death of bone tissue. Trauma and injury are often associated with nonhealing lesions. This situation most often involves the mandible, and presenting features involve pain, foul odor, exposure of bone, infection, and fistula. Ideally, oral disease where teeth have a poor prognosis should be addressed by extracting indicated teeth at least 7 to 14 days before initiation of radiation. The patient should take extreme care not to traumatize areas of the oral cavity for prevention of this serious situation as well. Topical antibiotics (tetracycline) and antibacterial rinses (chlorhexidine) may contribute to wound resolution. Analgesics for pain control and local resection of affected bone may be possible. HBO therapy is recommended for management of the hypoxic condition associated with ORN, although it has not been universally accepted. The mandible can be reconstructed to provide for aesthetics and function. A multidisciplinary cancer team including oncologists, prosthodontists, general dentists, dental hygienists, and physical therapists are all needed for management of the patient with ORN (see Teamwork).[9,10,12]

Dysfunction of the Temporomandibular Joint

Musculoskeletal syndromes rarely may develop secondary to head and neck radiation and surgery. The risk for developing jaw stiffness (trismus) from radiation therapy increases with higher doses of radiation and with repeated radiation treatments. The stiffness usually begins near the end of radiation treatments and may get worse over time, remain the same, or get somewhat better on its own. Treatment should begin as soon as possible to keep the condition from getting worse or becoming permanent. Patients can be instructed in physical therapy interventions including mandibular stretching exercises, as well as the use of prosthetic aids designed to reduce severity of fibrosis. It is important that these approaches be instituted before

Teamwork

Patient-centered methods for managing oral cancer emphasize an MDT approach to coordinate surgery, radiation therapy, chemotherapy, and associated complications from oncology treatment. Considering the extensive morbidity related to this type of cancer, expertise from many disciplines is needed for provision of comprehensive care. The team may include medical oncologists, radiation oncologists, surgeons, otolaryngologists (ear, nose, and throat doctors), maxillofacial prosthodontists (specialists who perform restorative surgery to the head and neck area), general dentists and dental hygienists, physical therapists, speech pathologists, mental health professionals, nurses, dietitians, and social workers. It is crucial that a comprehensive treatment plan is established before treatment begins, and patients may need to be seen by several specialists before such a plan can be created. Dental and dental hygiene practitioners need to understand current treatment modalities for oral and pharyngeal cancers to determine to whom they should refer patients for the most appropriate treatment, to evaluate oral conditions before, during, and after cancer treatment, to provide safe and effective oral care, and to make recommendations regarding complications associated with these cancers. ■

trismus development. If clinically significant changes develop, several approaches including stabilization of occlusion, trigger-point injections and other pain-management strategies, muscle relaxants, and/or tricyclic medications (an alternative pharmacological intervention for chronic pain) can be considered.[9]

TREATMENT-PLANNING STRATEGIES

Treatment planning for patients with cancer or oral cancer is initially guided by several principles: (a) risk for infection during neutropenia, (b) risk for ORN, and (c) risk for infection/bleeding after dental procedures. The following treatment plan suggestions are ideal before, during, and after cancer therapy.[10]

Before Cancer Therapy or After Diagnosis of Oral Cancer

- A thorough oral examination should be completed including procedures listed in Box 45-2.
- All carious teeth should be restored.

- All teeth with a poor prognosis should be extracted as soon as possible for maximum healing time.
- Nonsurgical periodontal therapy should be completed.
- Oral hygiene education should be given regarding possible oral complications associated with treatment and need for continued dental care.

During Cancer Therapy

- Ask the patient about his or her blood levels (red, white, and platelet). When cells divide and mature, and live out their life span, the circulating supply is depleted by chemotherapy and the blood counts decline to a low point, the **nadir.**
- Evaluate the need for antibiotic prophylaxis.
- Manage OM by frequent checks.
- Manage acute infection from the cytopenic (reduction in the number of blood cells) stages of cancer chemotherapy.
- Treat severe dental infections with appropriate antibiotics and pain medications until blood counts allow for appropriate dental interventions.

After Cancer Therapy or With a History of Oral Cancer

Here are some protocols to follow after a patient undergoes cancer therapy or has a history of oral cancer.

- Continue follow-up and routine dental care.
- Schedule frequent recall appointments with head and neck radiation.
- Encourage maintenance of ideal oral health by home-care measures and consistent recare intervals.
- Manage long-term side effects.
- Screen carefully for local recurrence and second primary tumors of oral cavity cancer (approximately 30% recurrence).

SUMMARY

The oral cavity has the potential to be a major source of short-term and long-term complications from cancer therapy. Appropriate evaluation and elimination of potential sources of oral infection before cancer therapy is vital because oral bacteria are a known source of bacteremia and septicemia during cancer therapy. Cancer diagnosis with previous and planned treatment, current medications, drug allergies, social history, family history, laboratory values, extraoral findings, intraoral findings, and radiographic findings must be evaluated in planning dental and dental hygiene treatment for these complex cases. Patients with cancer, especially oral cancer, are thus faced with a range of troublesome symptoms, from pain and anxiety to dry mouth to disturbed taste, eating, swallowing, and speech. The importance of minimizing adverse effects from treatments and of good support for patients with oral cancer from dental health professionals is a major focus of this chapter.

Case Study

Mr. Simpson, 62 years old, is a new patient at your dental office. His chief complaints are a broken, jagged tooth on the mandibular right side and severe staining of his teeth. Mr. Simpson has smoked a pack of cigarettes a day for 40 years. He has tried to quit on several occasions but has not been successful. His health history indicates hypertension, a history of prostate cancer (5 years ago), and type 2 diabetes. He is currently receiving pharmacological therapy for hypertension and diabetes and was treated with chemotherapy for a year after his prostate cancer was diagnosed. He has chronic advanced periodontitis with very few areas of bleeding.

Case Study Exercises

1. All of the following are considered risk factors for head and neck cancer with Mr. Simpson EXCEPT:
   A. Cigarette smoking
   B. Age
   C. Hypertension
   D. Sex
2. Which is the most widely accepted method of screening for head and neck cancer for this patient?
   A. Visual examination and palpation
   B. Brush biopsy using Oral CDx

C. Toluidine blue staining
   D. ViziLite
3. All of the cancers listed below are considered to be cancers of the head and neck EXCEPT:
   A. Salivary gland tumor
   B. Oropharynx tumor
   C. Lymph node cancer
   D. Thyroid cancer
4. Mr. Simpson's type 2 diabetes puts him at a greater risk for oral cancer. Because of his higher risk for head and neck cancer, he should perform an oral self-screening for the signs of oral cancer.
   A. The first statement is true, but the second statement is false.
   B. The first statement is false, but the second statement is true.
   C. Both statements are true.
   D. Both statements are false.
5. If Mr. Simpson were to develop a premalignant or malignant oral lesion, a *common* intraoral site for the lesion would be the:
   A. Lateral borders of the tongue
   B. Oropharynx
   C. Tonsils
   D. Posterior borders of the tongue

Review Questions

1. A patient with oral squamous cell carcinoma of the floor of the mouth exhibits metastatic disease in the lungs. What is the clinical stage of oral carcinoma for this patient?
   A. Stage I
   B. Stage II
   C. Stage III
   D. Stage IV

2. Which of the following is NOT associated with malignant transformation of cells?
   A. Sunlight
   B. Family history
   C. Fungal infections
   D. Viral infections

3. Which of the following is the most common oral complication of cancer chemotherapy and oral cancer therapies?
   A. Osteonecrosis
   B. Mucositis
   C. Xerostomia
   D. Infection

4. A patient presents for her dental hygiene appointment and states she has been referred by her oncologist because of painful lesions on her oral mucosa and tongue. Her last chemotherapy infusion was 1 week ago and her next one is scheduled in 3 weeks. Following the complete assessment, what is the most important educational component you should **initially** address at this appointment?
   A. Complications related to early infection
   B. Caries theory and prompt treatment of all carious lesions
   C. Use of an antimicrobial rinse for reduction of bacterial infection
   D. Gentle but thorough oral hygiene techniques

5. A patient has been diagnosed with stage III oral cancer. What does stage III indicate about tumor size (T), nodal involvement (N), and metastasis (M)?
   A. T2, N0, M0
   B. T3, N0 or N1, M0
   C. T3, N1, M1
   D. Any T, any N, M0

Active Learning

1. Organize a panel discussion and invite an oncology nurse, oncology physician, radiation oncologist, and oral and maxillofacial surgeon to sit on the panel. Individual or student groups would formulate one or two questions/points of discussion for a panel of experts to address, including each professional's view on how to best incorporate the dental hygienist's expertise in the provision of oral care for patients with cancer.

2. Role-play scenarios for using the 5 A's to address tobacco cessation with a patient. Take turns playing the tobacco user and the dental hygienist addressing tobacco cessation during a dental hygiene appointment.

3. Formulate a table comparing and contrasting the demographics of HPV-related oral and pharyngeal cancers, oral cancers, and head and neck cancers.

4. Create a dental hygiene treatment plan for a patient with recently diagnosed cancer and a patient undergoing therapy for oral cancer.

5. Rank various treatments of oral mucositis based on the amount of evidence in the literature for efficacy of those treatments. ■

REFERENCES

1. Cancer facts & figures. Atlanta. GA: American Cancer Society. http://www.cancer.org/research/cancerfactsfigures/cancerfactsfigures/cancer-facts-figures-2012. Updated 2012. Accessed October 3, 2015.

2. Taylor C, Munro AJ, Glynne-Jones R, et al. Multidisciplinary team working in cancer: what is the evidence? *BMJ*. 2010;340:c951.

3. Cancer overview. Palo Alto, CA: Stanford Cancer Institute. http://cancer.stanford.edu/information/canceroverview.html. Updated January 2012. Accessed October 3, 2015.

4. Cancer staging. Bethesda, MD: National Cancer Institutes. http://www.cancer.gov/about-cancer/diagnosis-staging/staging/staging-fact-sheet. Updated January 6, 2015. Accessed October 3, 2015.

5. American Joint Committee on Cancer. Lip and oral cavity. *AJCC Cancer Staging Manual.* 7th ed. New York: Springer; 2010:29-35.

6. American Joint Committee on Cancer. Pharynx. *AJCC Cancer Staging Manual.* 7th ed. New York: Springer; 2010:41-49.

7. Tumor grading. Bethesda, MD: National Cancer Institutes. http://www.cancer.gov/cancertopics/factsheet/detection/tumor-grade. Updated May 3, 2013. Accessed October 3, 2015.

8. Siegel R, Naishadham D, Ahmedin J. Cancer Statistics, 2012. *CA Cancer J Clin.* 2012;62:10-29.

9. Oral complications of chemotherapy and head and neck radiation. Bethesda, MD: National Cancer Institutes. http://www.cancer.gov/cancertopics/pdq/supportivecare/oralcomplications/HealthProfessional. Updated February 28, 2013. Accessed October 3, 2015.

10. Little J, Falace D, Miller C, Rhodus N. Cancer and oral care of the patient. In: *Dental Management of the Medically Compromised Patient.* 7th ed. St. Louis, MO: Mosby Elsevier; 2008:433-461.

11. Treister NS, Sook-Bin W. Chemotherapy-induced oral mucositis treatment and management. *Medscape Medical News.* http://emedicine.medscape.com/article/1079570-treatment. Published April 23, 2013. Accessed October 3, 2015.

12. Ibsen OA, Phelan JA. *Oral Pathology for the Dental Hygienist.* 5th ed. St. Louis, MO: Elsevier; 2008:261-264.

13. National Cancer Institute fact sheet: head and neck cancers. Bethesda, MD: National Cancer Institute. http://www.cancer.gov/types/head-and-neck/head-neck-fact-sheet. Reviewed: February 1, 2013. Accessed October 3, 2015.

14. Oral cancer facts. Newport Beach, CA: The Oral Cancer Foundation. http://oralcancerfoundation.org. Updated February 2012. Accessed October 3, 2015.

15. Oral cancer. Rosemont, IL: American Association of Oral and Maxillofacial Surgeons. http://aaoms.org/images/uploads/pdfs/oralcancerfacts.pdf. Accessed October 3, 2015.

16. Ang KK, Harris J, Wheeler R, et al. Human papillomavirus and survival of patients with oropharyngeal cancer. *N Engl J Med.* 2010;363(1):24-35.

17. Braakhuis BJ, Tabor MP, Kummer JA, et al. A genetic explanation of Slaughter's concept of field cancerization: evidence and clinical implications. *Cancer Res.* 2003;63(8):1727-1730.

18. Tsui IF, Garnis C, Poh, CF. A dynamic oral cancer field: unraveling the underlying biology and its clinical implication. *Am J Surg Pathol.* 2009;33(11):1732-1738.

19. Bsoui SA, Huber MA, Terezhalmy GT. Squamous cell carcinoma of the oral tissues: a comprehensive review for oral healthcare providers. *J Contemp Dent Pract.* 2005;4:1-16.

20. Messadi DV, Wilder-Smith P, Wolinsky L. Improving oral cancer survival: the role of the dental professional. *J Calif Dent Assoc.* 2009;37:789-798.

21. Rhodus NL. Oral cancer and precancer: improving outcomes. *Compendium.* 2009;30:486-504.

22. Stead LF, Lancaster T, Perera R. Telephone counseling for smoking cessation (Cochrane Review). In: The Cochrane Library. Chichester, UK: John Wiley & Sons, Ltd; 2004, Issue 1.

23. Fiore MC, Croyle RT, Curry SJ, et al. Preventing 3 million premature deaths and helping 5 million smokers quit: a national action plan for tobacco cessation. *Am J Public Health.* 2004;94(2):205-210.

24. Harris DJ, Ellers J, Harriman A, Cashavelly BJ, Maxwell C. Putting evidence into practice: evidence-based interventions for the management of oral mucositis. *Clin J Oncol Nurs.* 2008;12(1):141-152.

25. Rethman MP, Carpenter W, Cohen EE, et al. Evidence-based clinical recommendations regarding screening for oral squamous cell carcinomas. *Tex Dent J.* 2012; 129(5):491-507.

26. NIH Research Portfolio Online Reporting Tools (RePORT): salivary diagnostics. Bethesda, MD: National Institutes of Health. http://report.nih.gov/nihfact sheets/ViewFactSheet.aspx?csid=65. Accessed October 3, 2015.

27. Pack year. San Francisco, CA: Wikimedia Foundation, Inc. https://en.wikipedia.org/wiki/Pack-year. Accessed October 3, 2015.

28. East Side Health District Preventive Health and Education Services. Oral cancer prevention program. East St. Louis, IL: East Side Health District. http://www.ihrp.uic.edu/study/east-side-health-district-oral-cancer-prevention-program-evaluation-phase-ii. Accessed October 3, 2015.

Chapter 46 | Pediatric Patient

Lisa Handa, MS, RDH, RDHAP • Amy Molnar, RDH, MS

KEY TERMS

anticipatory guidance

desensitization

early childhood
    caries (ECC)

malocclusion

medical model

non-nutritive habits

partial participation

protective stabilization

surgical model

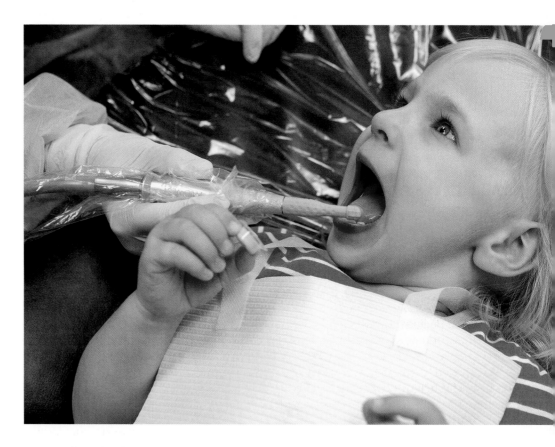

LEARNING OBJECTIVES

After reading this chapter, the student should be able to:

46.1 Discuss the importance of positive dental experiences for the pediatric patient as they relate to achieving a lifetime of good oral health.

46.2 Outline the differences between the surgical model and the medical model approach to oral health.

46.3 Provide appropriate anticipatory guidance to a child's parent or caregiver.

46.4 List several methods to positively engage or develop rapport with the pediatric patient.

46.5 Define the term *dental home* and its significance to oral health.

KEY CONCEPTS

• There has been a paradigm shift in pediatric dentistry from a surgical model to a medical/preventive approach.

• A lifetime of oral health begins before birth.

• Oral-care plans are tailored to each patient's needs and abilities.

• Anticipatory guidance is a part of every child's dental visit.

• Communication with the child's parent or caregiver is essential at every visit.

RELEVANCE TO CLINICAL PRACTICE

The goal of dentistry is the health and preservation of the human dentition—a lifetime of oral health. The child's potential to achieve a lifetime of oral health is largely dependent on the environment he or she lives in and the guidance and manner in which dental care is provided. Understanding and utilizing the knowledge gained in this chapter will allow the dental hygienist to deliver preventive services that are appropriate and cultivate successful oral health behaviors over the child's lifetime.

EVOLUTION AND GOALS OF PEDIATRIC DENTISTRY

Pediatric dentistry was introduced in the 1900s as a means of addressing the oral pain or dental trauma that occurred in children's dentition. Children are treated according to the following categories: early childhood, ages 0 to 6 years; later childhood, ages 7 to 12 years; and adolescent and young adult, ages 13 to 18 years.

The American Dental Association (ADA) defines the specialty of pediatric dentistry as follows: "An age specialty that provides both primary and comprehensive preventive and therapeutic oral health care to infants and children through adolescence, including those with special health care needs."[1] This chapter focuses on the different age groups and their developmental stages. This knowledge will enable the dental hygienist to choose the best treatment approach for children and adolescents.

A Paradigm Shift: Surgical Model Versus Medical Model

In the past, dental care focused on treating dental disease by eliminating carious or diseased tissue and restoring the tooth. In other words, the surgical model solely involves treating the problem. In recent years, dental health providers have embraced that treatment does not end with restoring the teeth (**surgical model**). A **medical model** approach supports the idea of prevention of dental diseases and, if present, early and minimally invasive treatment. In the medical model, a risk assessment is needed to determine the individual's risk for dental disease, and preventative treatment and recommendations follow. Table 46-1 demonstrates the common characteristics of each model for comparison.[2]

PUBLIC HEALTH RATIONALE ON PEDIATRIC ORAL HEALTH

Many publications have cited the impact poor oral health has had on children's development. From self-esteem issues and speech delay to more missed days of school, which affect academic performance, oral health plays a significant role in the lives of children. See Spotlight on Public Health.

UNIQUE ASPECTS OF PEDIATRIC DENTISTRY

The clinical approach to providing oral care to the pediatric patient does not vary greatly from that of the adult patient, which is the prevention and elimination

Spotlight on Public Health

HELPING CHILDREN THROUGH GIVE KIDS A SMILE
The ADA launched the Give Kids A Smile (GKAS) program nationally in 2003 as a way for dentists across the country to join with others in their community to provide dental services to underserved children. The program began as a 1-day event and grew to include local and national events year-round. At each event, dental health professionals, teachers, parents, school nurses, and other community health professionals volunteer to provide screenings, treatments, and education to children. In 10 years nearly 4.5 million children have been cared for in GKAS events by almost half a million volunteers. Volunteers participate to serve their community and to help children avoid needless suffering from dental pain by teaching them good oral health habits. ■

Table 46-1. *New Approach to Dental Care*	
Surgical Model	**Medical Model**
Drilling and filling	Risk assessment
Extraction	Preventive care
	Minimally invasive
	treatment

of periodontal disease and tooth decay. However, the ramifications of an unpleasant dental experience or lack of professional foresight in treating the pediatric patient, or both, can create a lifetime of dental anxieties for the impressionable youth.

The Dental Home

In a December 2008 policy statement,[3] the American Academy of Pediatric Dentistry (AAPD) describes the concept of the dental home as follows:

> A medical home to improve families' care utilization, seeking appropriate and preventive services with optimal compliance to recommendations. The concept of the dental home is based on this model and is intended to improve access to oral care. A dental home provides the ongoing relationship between the dentist and the patient, inclusive of all aspects of oral health care delivered in a comprehensive, continuously accessible, coordinated, and family-centered way.

AAPD recommends a dental home be established at the eruption of the first tooth or by the age of 1 year. ADA and American Public Health Dentistry (APHD) recommend that children be scheduled for initial dental evaluation within 6 months of the first eruption and no later than 12 months of age.[3]

Anticipatory Guidance

The AAPD defines **anticipatory guidance** as "the means of providing practical, developmentally appropriate information about children's health to prepare parents and patients for the significant physical, emotional, and psychological milestones."[4] Appropriate discussion and counseling should be an important part of each pediatric patient's dental visit. Initially, caregivers are responsible for the child's daily oral hygiene, and they are the primary source of a child's dental knowledge.[4] As a result, failure to appropriately educate caregivers at an early stage can lead to dental disease for the child. Topics to be discussed include proper oral hygiene, limiting high-carbohydrate foods, limiting the frequency of snacking, use of mouth guards for trauma prevention, non-nutritive habits, substance abuse, intraoral/perioral piercing, and the importance of dental development to speech and language development.[5]

Role of the Dental Hygienist

The role of the dental hygienist in creating the foundations for a child's oral health is paramount. Unlike the adult patient, the changes in the pediatric patient are dynamic. As the patient grows and matures, the dental hygienist must be aware of the changing interests and developmental norms of each age group and adapt the manner in which care and education are delivered to meet the child's needs (Table 46-2). Examples

Table 46-2. Childhood Characteristics

Age	Anatomical Characteristics	Pathological Characteristics	Physiological Characteristics
Prenatal	Primary teeth begin forming in the 14th week of pregnancy	Illness and medications taken during pregnancy can affect tooth formation	Enamel formation begins in utero
Birth to 6 months	Eruption of the first primary tooth may occur by the age of 6 months	Decreased birth weight increases prevalence of enamel defects	Permanent teeth begin forming 3–4 months after an infant's birth
6–12 months	By the age of 1 year, a baby may have 4–8 primary teeth	Medications taken for chronic or periodic use may affect oral health; dental visits should begin at the eruption of the first tooth or at age 1 year	Caregiver should begin infant oral hygiene with the eruption of the first tooth. Anticipatory guidance to the child and family should begin at the first dental appointment
12–18 months	By the age of 18 months a child may have 12 primary teeth	Infants sleeping with a bottle are at increased risk for tooth decay	Weaning to a cup by age of 1 year is desirable; walking begins as does the possibility of trauma
2–3 years	All 20 primary teeth should be present	Dental visits should occur every 6 months	Fluoride adequacy should be evaluated
3–6 years	All 20 primary teeth should be present	Dental visits should occur every 6 months	Non-nutritive oral habits should be counseled[7]

Table 46-2. *Childhood Characteristics—cont'd*

Age	Anatomical Characteristics	Pathological Characteristics	Physiological Characteristics
7 years (See American Association of Orthodontics website: www.braces.org)	Problems to monitor are anterior and posterior cross-bite, crowding, open bite, protrusion, ectopic eruption, complete class III, diastema, and oral habit	Consider sealants on first molars to aid in decay prevention	Use of mouth guards during sports is needed to help prevent trauma

Source: Adapted from U.S. Department of Health and Human Services. *Oral Health in America: A Report of the Surgeon General— Executive Summary.* Rockville, MD: U.S. Department of Health and Human Services, National Institute of Dental and Craniofacial Research, National Institutes of Health; 2000.

of developmental changes include diet; physical, emotional, and intellectual growth; and peer influence. Dental hygienists have an opportunity to create and develop the oral health patterns, tools, and education that will influence their patients' health behavior choices. The dental hygienist educates the caregiver and the child and makes age-appropriate recommendations, such as fluoride use, supplements, or both, limiting thumb sucking and pacifiers, and limiting juice and simple carbohydrate intake.

Physical, Emotional, and Mental Development

Before providing care to children, dental hygienists need to understand emotional, physical, and mental development. As a child matures, the hygienist's approach to patient care will change to accommodate the child's maturity level. Developmental psychologist Erik Erikson identified psychosocial milestones that can aid the hygienist in gauging the potential abilities of pediatric patients. Table 46-3 provides a summary of Erikson's psychosocial stages and the management techniques that dental hygienists can use during each stage.[4,5]

THE DEVELOPING DENTITION

Primary Dentition

The primary dentition begins to form during the seventh week of development in utero. During this time, a mother's health or use of medications, or both, can have an effect on the condition of the developing

Table 46-3. *Erikson's Psychosocial Stages and Relevance to the Dental Hygienist*

Stage	Basic Conflict	Important Events	Outcome	Relevance to the Dental Hygienist
Infancy (birth to 18 mo)	Trust vs. Mistrust	Feeding	Children develop a secure attachment to their caregivers and a sense of trust when their needs are met consistently. A lack of trust will lead to mistrust.	This age is crucial to establishing the dental home as a safe and caring environment.
Early childhood (2–3 yr)	Autonomy vs. Shame and Doubt	Toilet training	Children begin to assert themselves and explore their abilities as they develop control over physical skills and a sense of independence. Success leads to feelings of autonomy; failure results in feelings of shame and doubt.	Children during this stage may benefit from communication management techniques such as tell-show-do, distraction, and positive reinforcement.
Preschool (3–5 yr)	Initiative vs. Guilt	Exploration	Children begin to assert control and power over the environment. Success in this stage leads to a sense of purpose. Children who try to exert too much power experience	Children during this stage may benefit from communication management techniques such as tell-show-do, distraction, and positive reinforcement. Partial participation may help

Continued

Table 46-3. *Erikson's Psychosocial Stages and Relevance to the Dental Hygienist—cont'd*

Stage	Basic Conflict	Important Events	Outcome	Relevance to the Dental Hygienist
			disapproval, resulting in a sense of guilt.	these children gain a positive attitude toward oral health. Use voice control, but be careful when expressing disapproval.
School age (6–11 yr)	Industry (Competence) vs. Inferiority	School	Children begin to develop skills and a sense of pride in accomplishments. Success leads to a sense of competence, whereas failure results in feelings of inferiority.	Positive reinforcement and partial participation can help these children feel comfortable. Distraction techniques, such as talk of school and/or friends, can help establish rapport.
Adolescence (12–18 yr)	Identity vs. Role Confusion	Social relationships	Teens need to develop a sense of self and personal identity. Success leads to a sense of fidelity, whereas failure leads to role confusion and a weak sense of self.	Positive reinforcement and age-appropriate discussion can lead to a successful dental appointment. Avoid using "baby" talk or terms such as "honey," "sweetie," or "cutie."

child's primary dentition. For example, the mother's use of the antibiotic tetracycline during pregnancy may cause tooth discoloration in the developing child's teeth. Also, the incident of high fever(s) with the mother may cause enamel hypoplasia of the developing child's teeth. Eruption of the primary teeth usually begins at 7½ months and is completed by 24 to 36 months; enamel formation is complete by 1 year, and root development is complete by 3 years (Table 46-4).[6]

Mixed Dentition

Exfoliation of the mandibular central incisors denotes the transitional phase, which begins at 6 to 7 years of age and continues through the eruption of the mandibular second molar at age 11 to 13 years (see Table 46-4).[6]

Permanent Dentition

The permanent dentition begins to form as early as birth, and the enamel formation is completed by the seventh to eighth birthday. Eruption of the first permanent tooth (mandibular first molar) occurs around 6 to 7 years of age, and root development is complete at approximately 14 to 15 years.[6] Third molars, also known as wisdom teeth, erupt as early as 17 years and into adulthood. Table 46-5 shows the average eruption and exfoliation patterns.

ORAL HEALTH CONSIDERATIONS FOR PEDIATRIC PATIENTS

Dental Caries

Dental caries is defined as a "common chronic infectious transmissible disease resulting from tooth-adherent specific bacteria, primarily mutans streptococci, that metabolize sugars to produce acid, which, over time, demineralizes tooth structure."[6] In children younger than 6 years, the presence of one or more decayed, missing, or restored primary teeth is termed **early childhood caries (ECC),** and is also referred to as baby

Table 46-4. *Eruption Patterns Primary Dentition*

Maxillary (primary)	Erupt	Shed	Mandibular (primary)	Erupt	Shed
Central incisor	8–12 mo	6–7 yr	Central incisor	6–19 mo	6–7 yr
Lateral incisor	9–13 mo	7–8 yr	Lateral incisor	10–16 mo	7–8 yr
Canine	16–22 mo	10–12 yr	Canine	17–23 mo	9–12 yr
First molar	13–19 mo	9–11 yr	First molar	14–18 mo	9–11 yr
Second molar	25–33 mo	10–12 yr	Second molar	23–31 mo	10–12 yr

Table 46-5. Eruption Patterns Permanent Dentition

Maxillary (primary)	Erupt	Mandibular (primary)	Erupt
Central incisor	8–12 mo	Central incisor	6–7 yr
Lateral incisor	9–13 mo	Lateral incisor	7–8 yr
Canine	16–22 mo	Canine	9–10 yr
First premolar	13–19 mo	First premolar	10–12 yr
Second premolar	25–33 mo	Second premolar	11–12 yr
First molar		First molar	6–7 yr
Second molar		Second molar	11–13 yr
Third molar		Third molar	17–yr

bottle decay. As the term implies, this type of decay is often the result of the prolonged feeding an infant or child a high-carbohydrate liquid, such as juice, soda, or formula, or breast milk in a bottle or training cup.

However, ECC is not solely associated with poor feeding practices. As previously mentioned, dental caries is a transmissible disease, and bacteria such as mutans streptococci can be vertically transmitted from caregiver to child through saliva. If the caregivers have high levels of mutans streptococci as a result of untreated decay, the infant is at a greater risk for development of dental caries.[7] Dietary examination and the role of dietary choices on oral health should be addressed through nutritional and preventive oral health discussion at periodic dental visits.

Caries Risk Assessment

Dental caries is one of the most common preventable diseases among children.[8] A caries risk assessment is a key concept of contemporary (medical model) preventive care for infants, children, adolescents, and persons with special health-care needs. The goal of a risk assessment is to prevent disease by determining and decreasing causative factors (dietary habits, plaque biofilm) and increasing protective/preventative factors (fluoride, proper oral hygiene, sealants). A caries risk assessment form can simplify the process and guide the dental hygienist to create individualized oral health interventions that will provide the greatest benefit to that patient. A new risk assessment should be completed anytime there is a new carious lesion, change in medication, or change in health status. Sample AAPD caries risk assessment forms can be found at: http://www.mchoralhealth.org/flvarnish/documents/AAPD_CAT.pdf.

Non-nutritive Habits

A child's habits in the early years of life can affect the development of the oral architecture (i.e., positioning of the primary and permanent dentition). These behaviors, defined as **non-nutritive habits,** include thumb/digit sucking, use of pacifiers, tongue thrusting, bruxism, fingernail biting, and intraoral/perioral piercings. The use of pacifiers and digit sucking are considered normal early in life, but continual frequency, force, and time pose a risk for changes in occlusion and facial development. Dental hygienists have the opportunity at early dental visits to encourage parents to wean their children from sucking habits by age 3 years or younger, as recommended by the AAPD.[9]

Pain, infection, and tooth fracture are all complications that can occur from intraoral/perioral piercings. Although piercings are more common in the older pediatric patient, the dental hygienist can educate preteen child/parent on the potential pathologies before a piercing is present.

Malocclusion

Malocclusion is defined as a misalignment or an incorrect relation between the two dental arches. Anterior and posterior crossbite, crowding, open bite, protrusion, and diastema are common problems that may be observed in the developing mixed dentition of children (Figs. 46-1 to 46-4). If identified early in growth, these malocclusions may be corrected with minimal intervention depending on their cause.

Dental Trauma

Injury to a child's mouth can have long-lasting effects. Teeth can become discolored or malpositioned, or

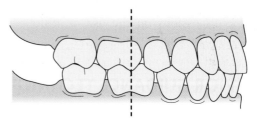

Figure 46-1. Normal occlusion.

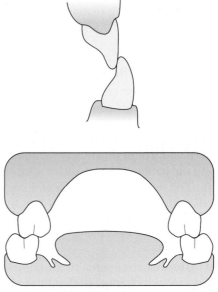

Figure 46-2. Crossbite.

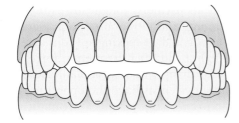

Figure 46-3. Open bite.

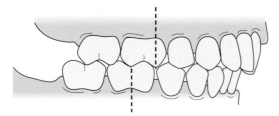

Figure 46-4. Protrusion.

potentially permanent tooth loss may occur. The most commonly injured teeth in the child are the maxillary incisors. By the time a child reaches 5 years of age, approximately 30% of boys and 25% of girls have experienced some type of trauma to their teeth. The toddler years are a common period of increased trauma due to their developing ability to walk. Other causes of dental trauma are car accidents, sports, and abuse.[8] Dental hygienists should counsel children and their caregivers on injury prevention, including the use of safe play objects. As the child grows older and begins sporting activities, discussions on the use of athletic mouth guards would be appropriate.

BEHAVIOR GUIDANCE TECHNIQUES

Providing oral health care to infants, children, adolescents, and patients with developmental disabilities may require the use of behavior guidance techniques. Various techniques are used to manage patient behaviors in pediatric dentistry and must be individualized to each patient.

Communicative Management

Proper communication is essential to establishing a relationship with a pediatric patient and allowing for the successful completion of necessary dental procedures.[10] Specific techniques, including tell-show-do, voice control, positive reinforcement, and distraction, can all be used to help the patient gain a positive attitude toward oral health. The dental hygienist should consider the cognitive development of the patient when choosing appropriate communication techniques.

Desensitization

Desensitization means gradually introducing objects or procedures to an individual so that he or she will become accustomed to them and begin to accept them.[11]

When helping children overcome fears, remember to go slowly. Never force someone to do something that he or she fears (Fig. 46-5). A specific desensitization technique is referred to as *tell-show-do*. This technique involves verbal explanation of the procedure in age-appropriate terminology (tell), followed by visual, auditory, and tactile demonstrations for the patient (show), and finally completing the procedure on the patient (do). Desensitization can help establish trust and eliminate fear in the following ways:

- Familiarizing the child with the object or procedure
- Avoiding overwhelming the child with too many new things at once
- Focusing on achieving success at each visit

Voice Control

A dental hygienist can influence a patient's behavior by altering the volume, tone, and pace of their voice. A deep, controlled voice helps the child understand that the health professional is in control and increases patient compliance. Another technique is using a soft, quiet voice with a loud child in an effort to get the child to calm down so he or she can hear what the practitioner is saying.[10]

Positive Reinforcement

Giving feedback is necessary to build appropriate patient behavior. Positive reinforcement is a technique that rewards desired behaviors by using social and nonsocial reinforcers. Social reinforcers include positive voice alteration, pleased facial expression, praise, and physical demonstrations of approval (e.g., high-five, fist pound). Nonsocial reinforcers include physical rewards such as stickers, tokens, and toys.[10]

Distraction

The behavior guidance technique of distraction is used to divert a patient's attention from the current situation, which may be perceived as unpleasant. Giving the child a break during a stressful procedure can help the child perceive the appointment less negatively.[10] The distraction technique can also be used at the

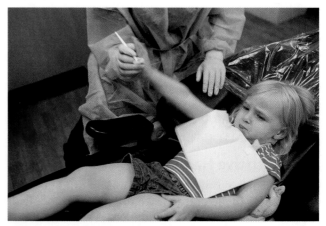

Figure 46-5. Child refusing care.

beginning of an appointment with an apprehensive child. For example, after the apprehensive or fearful child is seated, the dental hygienist can delay treatment and distract the child by discussing the patient's favorite coloring, complimenting his or her outfit, or talking about his or her favorite sport or singer.

Other Communication Recommendations

Other communicative management techniques include:

- Establish eye contact. When starting the dental appointment, begin by establishing eye contact. Try to place yourself at eye level with the patient, if possible.
- Speak in a calm, friendly, but firm voice, using the individual's name frequently: "Liz, be sure to swish the mouthrinse."
- Use simple declarative sentences: "Liz, please open wide." "Turn your head toward me."
- Offer choices whenever possible, but make sure that the choices all lead to completing the task: "Liz, I am going to polish your teeth now. Would you like mint-flavored paste or bubble gum flavor?"
- Use words and phrases that are perceived as helping, not giving orders: "Remember how good it feels to have a clean mouth. After brushing we will use some of that good-tasting rinse." Avoid giving orders such as: "Liz, go and brush your teeth now."
- Give one instruction at a time. Avoid giving multiple instructions in one phrase; for example, "Liz, please show me how you brush your teeth and be sure to brush all three surfaces—front, back, and top."[11]

Physical Techniques

Partial participation and protective stabilization are physical techniques for managing patient behavior. According to Erikson's psychosocial stages, early childhood (ages 2–3 years) and preschool (ages 3–5 years) children are beginning to gain independence and want to assert control over a situation.[4] **Partial participation** is a technique that nurtures these stages and can help the dental hygienist reduce fears and anxiety toward the unfamiliar tools used during the dental visit.[11] Partial participation allows the child to have a role in the dental appointment and act as the hygienist's helper. The child can assist the hygienist by holding the low-volume suction or the prophy paste (Figs. 46-6 and 46-7). Partial participation can also be a tool for redirecting a child to focus on the task at hand rather than his or her anxiety.

Protective stabilization (also known as behavioral support) is the restriction of a patient's movements to decrease the risk for injury to the patient and dental hygienist and allow for safe completion of treatment.[10] Restrictive devices can include the use of another person such as a health-care professional or caregiver, or a patient stabilization device such as a papoose board or mouth prop to protect the patient, practitioner, staff, or caregiver from harm while providing necessary dental treatment. The dental hygienist must evaluate the need for complete or partial protective stabilization and

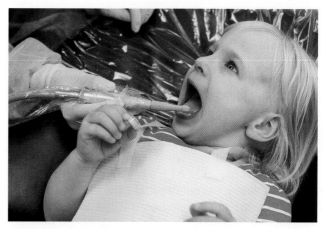

Figure 46-6. Child holding prophy paste.

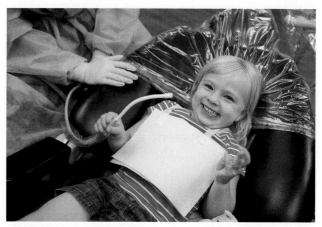

Figure 46-7. Child holding suction.

always use the least restrictive method that provides safe and effective stabilization. Most importantly, the dental hygienist must have written, informed consent in the patient's record from the caregiver to perform protective stabilization, with or without the use of a restrictive device.[10]

THE DENTAL APPOINTMENT

Before Dental Hygiene Care

Before the child's appointment, the hygienist reviews the patient chart for the medical and dental histories, as well as for information regarding previous dental encounters and the outcomes of the visits. If this is the patient's first time to the office, the hygienist should ask the parent and/or child, depending on the child's age, if there are existing phobias or anxieties associated with dental appointments. The hygienist may also want to ask the following questions: What is the level of parental or caregiver involvement in the child's dental health? Do the parents or caregivers have negative beliefs about dental care that they may have conveyed to the child? What is the caregiver's oral health status? Another issue to consider is whether the parent or caregiver should accompany the child to the operatory. Children younger than 3 years often behave better if the parent or caregiver is present in the operatory.[10] After this age, most children do not require the parent's or caregiver's presence, and the independence allows the hygienist an opportunity to develop better patient rapport. The decision to have parents or caregivers in the treatment room is ultimately based on office policy, the dentist, and the parents' level of comfort and safety for their child.

Greet each patient with warmth and friendliness (Fig. 46-8). A hygienist with a negative attitude toward treating a young patient can make the visit uncomfortable and more challenging than it needs to be. Body language can relay significant information via nonverbal signals. Confidence, compassion, and respect can all be conveyed to the child (see Application to Clinical Practice). Three essential messages are conveyed to the pediatric patient primarily through nonverbal means:[12]

1. "I see you as an individual and will respond to your needs as such."
2. "I am thoroughly knowledgeable and highly skilled."
3. "I am able to help you and will do nothing to hurt you needlessly."

During Dental Hygiene Care

The AAPD has developed guidelines for the provision of preventive dental services.[9] Table 46-6 highlights anticipatory guidance guidelines that should be discussed at the age-appropriate visits.

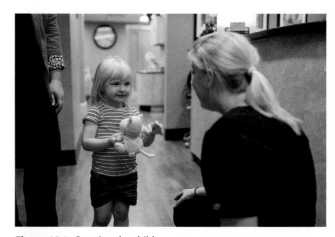

Figure 46-8. Greeting the child.

Application to Clinical Practice

You have decided to participate in oral health screenings at a local Head Start program. The children you will see this morning range in age from 3 to 5 years. Many of these children have never been to the dentist before. What can you do to make their time with you a positive experience? How will you get them to cooperate? ■

Table 46-6. **Anticipatory Guidance by Age**				
	6–12 mo	**12–24 mo**	**2–6 yr**	**6–12 yr**
Oral development	Eruption of primary dentition	All primary teeth erupted	Loss of first primary tooth and eruption of permanent molars	Primary tooth loss and permanent eruption continues
Fluoride/ Caries Risk	Assess exposure frequency and source Discuss use of child paste	Assess exposure, frequency and source Discuss toxicity/ingestion Appropriate paste amount	Assess exposure, frequency and source; discuss toxicity/ingestion Appropriate paste amount/smear	Assess exposure, frequency, and source; if able to spit, child may now use pea-sized amount of paste when brushing
Oral hygiene/ caries risk	Swab mouth with soft cloth or use soft toothbrush after eating and drinking Demonstrate proper brushing Discuss infectious nature of dental decay and transmission routes	Discuss parent's role in daily oral care Encourage use of songs and play to engage child's cooperation in brushing Introduce flossing Reinforce importance of good oral habits	Child may now brush with supervision and assistance from adult Child may be ready for dental sealants	Child still brushes with supervision and assistance until 8–9 years of age; continue with sealants as needed
Habits	Discuss non-nutritive habits such as thumb-sucking, pacifiers, etc.	Discuss/review non-nutritive habits, including sippy cups	Discuss/review non-nutritive habits; encourage and assist with cessation of habit	Discuss tobacco, drug use, intraoral and perioral piercings, and their oral effects

Table 46-6. *Anticipatory Guidance by Age—cont'd*

	6–12 mo	12–24 mo	2–6 yr	6–12 yr
Nutrition	Discuss sugars and their role in the decay process; identify areas of hidden sugars in diet Discuss baby bottle tooth decay and sleep-time bottle use	Discuss sugars and their role in the decay process; identify areas of hidden sugars in diet Discuss continued bottle use and sippy cups	Discuss sugars and their role in the decay process; identify areas of hidden sugars in diet; assess frequency of snacking	Monitor snacking, food selection, sport/soft drink consumption
Injury prevention	Look for and discuss oral trauma; provide information on what to do if oral trauma occurs	Look for and discuss oral trauma; provide information on what to do if oral trauma occurs	Encourage helmet and mouth guard use to prevent orofacial trauma	Encourage helmet and mouth guard use to prevent orofacial trauma

Sources: American Academy of Pediatric Dentistry. *Guideline on Periodicity of Examination, Preventive Dental Services, Anticipatory Guidance/Counseling, and Oral Treatment for Infants, Children and Adolescents.* Reference manual, 2009/10, 31, 6, 118-125; O.M. Sanchez, DMD, MS, and N.K. Childers, DDS, MS, PhD, University of Alabama School of Dentistry. Anticipatory guidance in infant oral health: rationale and recommendation. *Am Fam Physician.* 2000 Jan 1;61(1):115-120.

6 to 12 Months

This early visit is most important for the parent/caregiver. It is an opportunity to provide early education and intervention that has the potential to change high-risk to low-risk oral behaviors early in the dental development process. At this age, the infant can be assessed while in a knee-to-knee position. This position allows the child to rest simultaneously in the laps of the parent and the dental provider. It also allows for good visualization of the oral cavity by the parent and dental hygienist while providing stabilization of the child.

12 to 24 Months

This is another opportunity to assess the child's risk status and discuss preventive measures with the parent/caregiver. Assess feeding practices, such as whether and how a bottle is used, and counsel as necessary. Counsel the parent/caregiver regarding the use of supplemental fluoride. Provide topical fluoride treatment every 6 months or more frequently depending on the patient's needs (Procedure 46-1).

Procedure 46-1 Application of Fluoride Varnish

MATERIALS AND PREPARATION

Familiarity with the necessary materials and proper preparation for applying fluoride varnish is essential in utilizing time and resources. Being prepared for the procedure will eliminate stress and difficulty during the treatment. Gather and organize the necessary materials before the patient's arrival.

Materials

Fluoride varnish
Applicator

Preprocedure

PATIENT EDUCATION

The patient, parent, or both must be educated on what varnish is, how it will be applied, and the reason for varnish application.

INFORMED CONSENT

Informed consent is required before applying varnish on all patients. When treating pediatric patients, it is essential to obtain consent from the parent or guardian before proceeding with treatment.

Procedure

1. Open fluoride varnish.

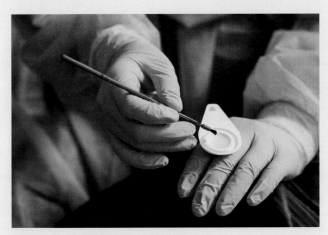

Mix varnish with applicator.

2. Mix varnish with applicator.

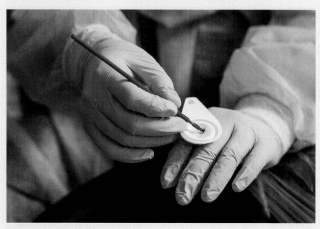

Open fluoride varnish.

3. Dry teeth if indicated by manufacturer.
   a. Drying of the teeth before varnish placement is not required of all varnishes.

4. Apply a thin coat of varnish to the teeth.

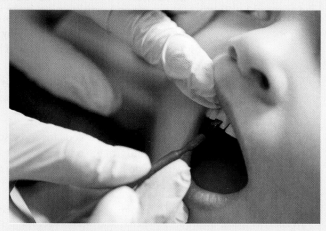

Apply a thin coat of varnish to the teeth.

5. Give patient instructions.
   a. The patient may feel the varnish on his or her teeth until it is removed by brushing.
   b. Avoid eating for 30 minutes and avoid brushing the teeth for at least 4 hours.

Postprocedure

After any dental procedure, the patient and, if the patient is a minor, the parent or guardian should be informed about the results of the procedure and given postprocedure instructions.

2 to 6 Years

Scale and clean the teeth every 6 months or more frequently depending on the patient's needs. Children of this age may be most cooperative in the knee-to-knee position (Fig. 46-9). Assess the child's eating habits and provide nutritional counseling. Apply sealants to primary and permanent molars, premolars, and anterior teeth, which are susceptible to caries. Recommend the use of protective devices such as a mouth guard or helmet when biking. Assess speech and language development and refer to a specialist if needed.

6 to 12 Years

Continue to provide care and age-appropriate counseling. In addition, educate the patient and parent/caregiver about substance abuse, including smoking and smokeless tobacco, and intraoral and perioral piercings.

12 Years and Older

Continue to provide care and age-appropriate counseling. Assess the presence, position, and development of third molars, and counsel regarding their removal.

After Dental Hygiene Care

Before dismissing the patient from the chair, it is beneficial to review the findings of the appointment. If the child is old enough to understand the importance of the dental visit, the hygienist can review the appointment and prepare the child for the expectations of future visits. Emphasize the child's strengths, encourage his or her efforts, and express belief in his capabilities. For example, "Kevin, I'd like to thank you for being a wonderful patient today. Do you remember the things we talked about today that you can do to keep your mouth healthy? Do you remember how pink your teeth were when we looked for sugar bugs? Kevin, today you

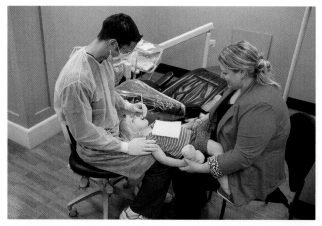

Figure 46-9. Knee-to-knee position.

showed me what a great tooth brusher you can be and I know we won't find as many bugs next time, right?" This is also a time to review the visit, oral findings, and recommendations with the parent. Care should be taken to avoid the appearance of being a "tattletale" in front of the child. It is best to report to the parent while the child is selecting a prize from the toy box and away from the conversation. If a situation occurs where the parents or caregivers are not available, a phone call or note informing them of the visit can be effective and appreciated. Remember to end the session on a positive note. This will reduce the potential for future dental anxieties.

Case Study

Sally is 6 years old and in the first grade. She and her 4-year-old brother, Sean, are seeing you for their first dental visit. Their mother tells you that Sean is very excited to see all the "cool things" in the office, whereas Sally is a bit uncertain about the visit. Their mother comments that she, herself, has never liked going to the dentist and does not understand why there are people who actually enjoy it.

Case Study Exercises

1. Which primary teeth are likely to be missing from Sally's mouth?
   A. D, E
   B. S, T
   C. O, P
   D. A, B

2. What is the main concern you have after hearing from the mother that this is their first dental visit?
   A. The children do not drink enough water.
   B. The children do not know how to brush their teeth.
   C. The children may be lacking in fluoride exposure.
   D. The children will not like you.

3. What techniques will you use to engage Sally and develop rapport?
   A. Approach her with confidence and a firm handshake.
   B. Ask her if she would like to have her teeth cleaned today.
   C. Give her a tour of the office.
   D. Greet her at eye level and be friendly.

4. How many teeth would you expect to see in Sean's mouth?
   A. 20
   B. 18
   C. 16
   D. 14

5. What would be the most appropriate anticipatory guidance topic(s) to discuss with the mother?
   A. Breastfeeding and pacifier use
   B. Prenatal oral health
   C. Use of sealants
   D. Use of sealants and infectious nature of tooth decay

Review Questions

1. What is the term used to describe the current approach to dental care?
   A. Surgical model
   B. Treatment model
   C. Desensitizing model
   D. Medical model

2. What is the purpose of a dental home?
   A. Improves access to oral care
   B. Provides continuity of care
   C. Provides preventive care
   D. All of the above

3. At what age is it advised a child have a dental home?
   A. 2 years
   B. 3 years
   C. 1 month
   D. At the eruption of the first tooth

4. Anticipatory guidance addresses all areas of patient education EXCEPT:
   A. Habits
   B. Fluoride
   C. Exercise frequency
   D. Diet

5. When should the dental hygienist begin to educate mothers about oral health?
   A. When the child is born
   B. Prenatally
   C. The child's first visit
   D. Before the child starts school

Active Learning

1. Working with a partner, take turns role-playing giving anticipatory guidance to the parent of an 18-month-old child, a 5-year-old child, and an 11-year-old child.

2. Create a brief PowerPoint presentation reviewing Erikson's psychosocial stages and how they influence dental hygiene treatment of children at each stage. ■

REFERENCES

1. Pediatric dentistry definition. Chicago, IL: American Dental Association. Adopted 1995. http://www.ada.org/en/education-careers/careers-in-dentistry/dental-specialties/specialty-definitions. Accessed October 22, 2015.

2. Malcmacher L. *Minimal Intervention Dentistry and Caries Prevention: A Peer-Reviewed Publication.* Academy of Dental Therapeutics and Stomatology, a division of PennWell; 2008. http://ineedce.com/courses/1553/PDF/MinimalIntervention.pdf.

3. American Academy of Pediatric Dentistry. Preventive Oral Health Intervention for Pediatricians, Policy Statement. *Pediatrics.* 2008;122(6):1387-1394.

4. Erikson EH. Erikson's theory of psychosocial development: psychosocial development in infancy and early childhood. *Childhood and Society* (2nd ed.). New York: Norton; 1963. http://psychology.about.com/od/theoriesofpersonality/a/psychosocial_2.htm.

5. Erikson EH. Erikson's Stages of Development Summary: an eight stage theory of identity and psychosocial development. *Identity: Youth and Crisis.* New York: Norton; 1968. http://www.learning-theories.com/eriksons-stages-of-development.html.

6. Vick VC, Goldie MP, Shay K. *Life Stages.* In: Daniel SJ, Harfst SA, Wilder RS. *Mosby's Dental Hygiene Concepts, Cases, and Competencies.* 2nd ed. Philadelphia, PA: Mosby; 2008:205.

7. National Institutes of Health (NIH). *A National Call to Action to Promote Oral Health* [Publication no. 03-5303]. May 2003. http://www.nidcr.nih.gov/datastatistics/surgeongeneral/nationalcalltoaction/nationalcalltoaction.htm.

8. Glassman P, Miller CE, Baker K, Helgeson M. *Overcoming Obstacles to Oral Health: A Training Program for Caregivers of People & Adults with Disabilities and Frail Elders.* 5th ed. 2010. University of the Pacific, San Francisco, CA. http://dental.pacific.edu/Community_Involvement/Pacific_Center_for_Special_Care_%28PCSC%29/Education_/Overcoming_Obstacles.html

9. American Academy of Pediatric Dentistry. *Guideline on Periodicity of Examination, Preventive Dental Services, Anticipatory Guidance/Counseling, and Oral Treatment for Infants, Children and Adolescents.* Reference Manual. 2013; 36(6):118-125. http://www.aapd.org/media/Policies_Guidelines/G_Periodicity.pdf.

10. American Academy of Pediatric Dentistry. *Guideline on Behavior Guidance for the Pediatric Dental Patient.* Reference Manual. 2009;30(7):118.

11. Pinkham JR, et al. *Pediatric Dentistry: Infancy through Adolescence.* 4th ed. Philadelphia: Elsevier; 2005:405.

12. Sanchez OM, Childers NK. Anticipatory guidance in infant oral health: rationale and recommendation. *Am Fam Physician.* 2000;61(1):115-120.

Chapter 47 | Men's and Women's Health Issues

Maria Perno Goldie, RDH, BA, MS

KEY TERMS

adolescence

bisphosphonates

bisphosphonate-related osteonecrosis of the jaw (BRONJ)

epulis gravidarum

gender

interconceptual

menopause

osteonecrosis

osteopenia

osteoporosis

osteoradionecrosis

preconceptual

puberty

sex

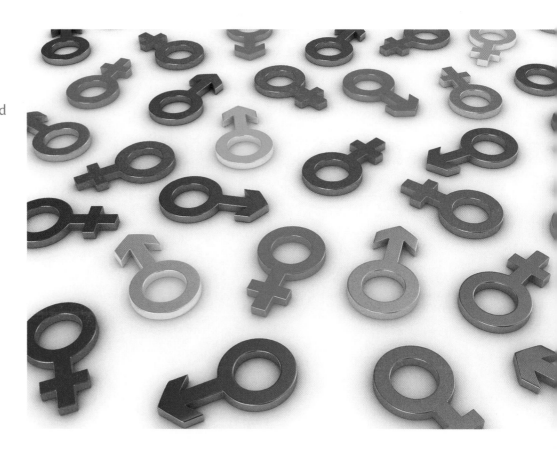

LEARNING OBJECTIVES

After reading this chapter, the student should be able to:

47.1 Define the terms *sex* and *gender,* and explain how they are different.

47.2 Discuss dental hygiene care plan treatment alterations or precautions to be taken during pregnancy.

47.3 Discuss the incidence, risk factors, therapies, and oral complications unique to bisphosphonate-related osteonecrosis of the jaw and osteoradionecrosis.

47.4 Discuss dental hygiene care plan treatment alterations or precautions to be taken with patients with prostate cancer.

47.5 Identify the common signs and symptoms of domestic abuse.

KEY CONCEPTS

• Insight into men's and women's health issues is vital for health-care professionals to understand which issues require consideration of precautions in dental hygiene care.

- Dental hygiene care of patients with prostate cancer requires individualized consideration of systemic and oral complications.
- Risk factors for bisphosphonate-related osteonecrosis of the jaw and osteoradionecrosis include use of IV bisphosphonates, oral bisphosphonates to a lesser degree than IV, patients with or at risk for osteoporosis, and previous radiation therapy, all of which require consideration of precautions in dental hygiene care.
- Although periodontal therapy has been shown to be safe and leads to improved periodontal conditions in pregnant women, case-related periodontal therapy, with or without systemic antibiotics, does not reduce overall rates of preterm birth and low birth weight.
- Regarding domestic violence, 75% of the physical injuries are to the head, neck, and/or mouth.

RELEVANCE TO CLINICAL PRACTICE

Good oral health involves prevention of disease, in both male and female individuals. It is vital to overall health and well-being at all stages of life. Poor oral health has been linked to heart disease, diabetes, oral cancer, and preterm delivery. Common oral diseases include tooth decay and periodontal diseases, which are caused by bacterial infections. These infections cause an immune response that destroys the gingival tissue and bone that surround the teeth in periodontal disease and, in combination with other factors, cause tooth decay. Dental hygienists should be prepared to understand men's and women's general patterns of growth and development to provide dental hygiene care. Many of the concepts discussed in this chapter will allow the dental hygienist to approach the patient's needs specific to his or her sex and gender, and apply dental hygiene therapies to maintain and improve oral health.

SEX VERSUS GENDER

In humans, biological sex is determined by five factors present at birth: the presence or absence of a Y chromosome, the type of gonads (testes or ovaries), the sex hormones, the internal reproductive anatomy (such as the uterus in females), and the external genitalia.[1] A distinction is sometimes made between sex and gender. Sex differences in physical sciences tend to refer solely to people according to their biological sex, regardless of the person's self-perceived gender. Sex differences in other fields, such as when studying social roles, may use the person's gender, regardless of whether the person is intersexed or biologically the other sex. *Intersex* is a group of conditions where there is a discrepancy between the external genitals and the internal genitals (the testes and ovaries).[2]

Sex differences in medicine include sex-specific diseases, which are diseases that occur only in people of one sex, and sex-related diseases, which are diseases that are more common to one sex or which manifest differently in each sex. For example, certain autoimmune diseases may occur predominantly in one sex, for unknown reasons. Ninety percent of primary biliary cirrhosis cases occur in women, whereas primary sclerosing cholangitis is more common in men. Gender-based medicine, also called "gender medicine," is the field of medicine that studies the biological and physiological differences between the human sexes and how that affects differences in disease. Traditionally, medical research has mostly been conducted using the male body as the basis for clinical studies. The findings of these studies have often been applied across the sexes, and health-care providers have assumed a uniform approach in treating both male and female patients. Recently, medical research has started to understand the importance of taking the sex of a person into account because the symptoms and responses to medical treatment may be very different between males and females.[3]

How do you know when to call something a sex difference rather than a gender difference? Using the definitions given for **sex** (biological differences between males and females) and **gender** (socially defined differences between men and women), sex differences refer only to those differences that can be attributed solely to biological difference. Medical literature most commonly addresses biological sex differences. Gradually we find that medical evidence is published with sex as a variable of analysis.

Gender differences define differences that exist between men and women in society. They allow for the fact that it is impossible to control for the interactions between people and their environment. Outcomes data demonstrate gender difference because it is impossible to tell whether health outcomes are 100% attributable to the biology of males and females or whether they are some mixture of the interaction between biology and the environment within which men and women experience them. It is more common to use *gender differences* as an all-encompassing term for sex and gender difference when speaking about people because individuals cannot be separated from their environment. The generic rule is: If a difference is 100% biological, it is a sex difference. Everything else is considered to be a gender difference.[4]

LIFE CYCLES

In addition to bacteria, a woman's periodontal health may be affected by a variety of factors. The biological changes that occur in tissues of the periodontium during puberty, pregnancy, menopause, and oral contraceptive use have heightened interest in the relationship between sex hormones and periodontal health. Gingival tissues contain receptors for androgens, estrogen, and progesterone, and it was documented that these hormones have effects on the oral mucosa and the periodontium.[5] Estrogen and progesterone changes seem to modify the gingival tissues, leading to a higher vascular permeability and decreased keratinization of the gingival epithelium. The changes in the circulating levels of female sex hormones also affect the host response, resulting in an exaggerated response against dental biofilm.[6] It was hypothesized that sex hormones have an impact on the periodontium by alteration of the immune system. Interleukin (IL)-6, a key mediator in periodontal inflammation, is decreased by progesterone in gingival fibroblasts.[7] Also, polymorphonuclear leukocytes and phagocytosis are decreased. The need for meticulous oral care, both professionally and at home, will provide for the best result when facing these factors.

Puberty

Puberty is the developmental stage when an individual is capable of reproduction, typically between ages 11 and 14 years in girls and 13 and 16 years in boys. During puberty in females, an increased level of sex hormones, such as progesterone and possibly estrogen, causes increased blood circulation to the gingival tissues. This may cause an increase in gingival sensitivity and lead to a greater reaction to any irritation, including food particles and plaque. During this time, the soft tissues may become swollen, turn red, and feel tender. Studies show that although women tend to take better care of their oral health than men do, women's oral health is not significantly better than men's oral health.[8,9] This can be caused by hormonal fluctuations throughout a woman's life cycle that affect many body tissues, including oral tissues. Microbial changes in the gingival sulcus can cause a shift from a healthy microbial flora to a more pathogenic microbial flora. This change has been attributed to those increased levels of hormones in the blood, namely, estrogen and progesterone, which certain pathogenic bacteria can use for nutrition, growth, and proliferation. The presence of plaque biofilm and calculus can increase this marked response.

In addition to general health consequences, poor nutrition, fad diets, and eating disorders in young women and men affect the oral environment in a negative manner. Diets high in sugars can contribute to dental decay, and nutritional deficiencies can cause changes in the lips, oral mucosa, and periodontal tissues. High levels of caffeine, protein, and sodium may increase bone loss.[10] Pubescent girls who diet may be more likely to begin smoking than those who are not dieting. Women, from teenagers to young adults, gain an average of 8 to 10 pounds after they quit smoking.[11]

Many epidemiological surveys have shown that gingivitis is more prevalent in males than in females.[8] One study showed that females had greater knowledge, a more positive attitude, a healthier lifestyle, and higher level of oral health behaviors than males.[8] There were significant differences in lifestyle, knowledge, and attitude about oral health behaviors and oral health status between boys and girls.[8] Sex-based differences in gingivitis in young people can be explained, in part, by oral health behaviors and hygiene status, which are influenced by lifestyle, knowledge, and attitude. To prevent gingivitis, different approaches to care in males and females may be useful.[12]

Both males and females in puberty demonstrate statistically significant proportional increases in the levels of *B. intermedius* relative to prepubertal children. Colonization by other species of Bacteroides, spirochetes, and other motile forms is well established in individuals with poor oral hygiene by late **adolescence** (the period from puberty to adulthood), without clinically detectable bone loss.[13]

Dental Hygiene Considerations

Dental hygienists should understand the changes that occur during adolescence to better direct patient education and home-care instructions. During puberty, adolescents should be instructed to brush more often, perform interdental cleaning daily, and rinse with antimicrobials as directed by the dental hygienist or dentist. The dental hygienist should focus on prevention and health promotion, including dietary counseling and tobacco cessation.

Because oral health behaviors and oral hygiene status are influenced by lifestyle, knowledge, and attitude, different approaches to males and females may be necessary to really connect with the patient. An example is that eating disorders are more common in females, and smoking is more common in adolescent males. With both sexes, reinforce the importance of good oral hygiene. Focus on healthy eating and screening for eating disorders in females. Discourage all forms of tobacco use in males and females, and discuss peer pressure in this age group. Discuss the risks of oral piercings. Adolescents, especially males, are at increased risk for trauma to the mouth and teeth because of their active lifestyle and increased risk-taking behaviors. Oral and facial trauma can occur secondary to falls, violence, athletics, or motor vehicle and other accidents. Encourage the use of protective face and mouth gear for athletes. Discussing the effects of soft drinks, especially energy drinks, would be especially helpful with males.

Childbearing Years

Menstruation

Fluctuations in sex hormones, which are noticeable throughout the menstrual cycle of women, may affect periodontal health. The aim of one study was to evaluate the effect of hormonal changes occurring in the menstrual cycle on gingival inflammation and the gingival crevicular fluid (GCF) levels of IL-6, prostaglandin E_2, tissue plasminogen activator, and plasminogen activator inhibitor-2. The results were that the percentages of sites with bleeding on probing were significantly higher during menstruation than in the premenstrual phase (days 22–24) in the gingivitis group. The results were similar for all phases in the healthy group. GCF levels of IL-6 were significantly elevated in patients with gingivitis compared with healthy subjects in all phases. GCF levels of IL-6, prostaglandin E_2, tissue plasminogen activator, and plasminogen activator inhibitor-2 were unchanged in different menstrual phases in both groups.[14]

Other disorders that affect mainly women vary with biological development and intake of exogenous sex hormones. For example, sex differences in experience of orofacial pain arise at puberty, peak during reproductive years, and decline at menopause.[15] The use of oral contraceptives and hormone replacement therapy has been associated with a higher prevalence of temporomandibular disorders (TMD).[16] TMDs are more common and severe in women, especially in those who are in their reproductive years.[17] However, no correlation exists between using oral contraceptives and development of TMDs in healthy menstruating women.[17] Even though the etiology and pathogenesis of TMD remain unclear, sex and age suggest a possible link between the mechanism of the disease and the female reproductive system.

Many recurrent pain disorders, especially those with a higher female prevalence, are of unknown origin, and sex-specific pains can be due to anatomical and hormonal differences. These include nonpathological pain, such as during menstruation, ovulation, pregnancy, and childbirth.[18] Distinct anatomic, physiological, and hormonal features in women and men provide important clues about how their pains might be controlled in a different manner by a number of biological factors. Sometimes, when a female is experiencing pain, she is told that it is common among women, especially in the presence of stress, and therefore "could be psychosomatic." Observations about differences in pain management between men and women should help minimize prejudicial attitudes toward female patients, which can lead to inadequate care.[19]

Few data have addressed the features of gastroesophageal reflux (GERD) in women compared with men. The clinical impression from the few existing studies is that the common presentations of GERD are similar regardless of sex.[20] Heartburn is present in about 20% of pregnancies during the first trimester, 40% during the second trimester, and 70% during the third trimester.[21] Anatomical changes, such as a decrease in lower esophageal sphincter pressure, slowed gastric emptying, and higher intra-abdominal pressure from the enlarging uterus likely play a role. Some of these changes might be caused by progesterone.[22] There is a distinct relationship between body mass index and GERD in women. Reflux symptoms are common in pregnancy but can be safely and successfully managed.[23]

Dental Hygiene Considerations

Try to make patients with GERD as comfortable as possible. A semisupine position in the dental chair may be necessary. Educate males in particular about GERD-related Barrett's esophagus. In one study, significantly more men (23%) than women (14%) with GERD had Barrett's esophagus.[24] If gingivitis is present, more frequent recare appointments should be suggested.

Preconception

Preconceptual (before pregnancy) and **interconceptual** (between pregnancies) counseling by health-care professionals should incorporate oral health as an essential intervention for a healthy pregnancy. These recommendations should include information on establishing good oral hygiene practices and seeking professional care. Although largely preventable through evidence-based interventions, both periodontal disease and caries in women of childbearing age are highly prevalent, particularly among low-income women and members of racial and ethnic minority groups.[25] Dental care during pregnancy may be too late to intervene as a means of reducing the systemic inflammation of periodontal disease that has been related to adverse birth outcomes.[26] Oral health interventions are optimal during the preconceptual period.[27] Preconception health care focuses on protecting the health of a future baby. However, preconception health is important for all women and men. The dental hygienist can provide anticipatory guidance. Expectant mothers should be made aware of the importance of their own oral health and learn how to improve it. Educate about the warning signs of oral disease, how to prevent disease, and provide information on early childhood caries (ECC).[28]

Pregnancy

Every body system is influenced by the physiological changes that occur during pregnancy, and the mouth is no different. Pregnancy outcomes for both the mother and the embryo are greatly influenced by the mother's overall state of health at the time of conception and continuing after delivery. Early interventions by health-care professionals can result in optimum periodontal health and hygiene (see Application to Clinical Practice).

Existing research in the areas of maternal and fetal physiology indicates that the benefits of providing dental care during pregnancy compensate for any likely risks. Prevention, diagnosis, and treatment of oral diseases, dental radiographs, and use of local anesthesia can be part of oral care during pregnancy with no additional fetal or maternal risk compared with the risk of not providing care. Control of oral diseases in pregnant women has the potential to reduce the transmission of oral bacteria from mothers to their children.[25]

Pregnancy may be associated with an increased risk for periodontal disease. Estrogen, progesterone, and chorionic gonadotropin, during pregnancy, affect the microvasculature by producing the following changes: swelling of endothelial cells and pericytes of the venules (contractile cells that wrap around the endothelial cells of capillaries and venules throughout the body), adherence of granulocytes and platelets to vessel walls, formation of microthrombi, disruption of the perivascular mast cells, increased vascular permeability, and vascular proliferation.[29,30]

This increase in gingivitis is thought to be partially connected to an alteration in the subgingival microflora. This includes the presence of *Prevotella intermedia,* which can substitute estrogen and progesterone for vitamin K, an essential bacterial growth factor.[29,30]

Application to Clinical Practice

Dental hygienists play an important role in patient education throughout the life span. Anticipatory guidance is important for both sexes. To be most effective, it is important that dental hygienists understand how a patient's sex affects his or her development and oral health. Consider what guidance you would give to a newly pregnant female patient about how the changes in her body may affect her oral health. ■

Pregnancy sometimes has adverse outcomes including low birth weight (less than 2,500 g), preterm birth (<37 weeks), growth restriction, pre-eclampsia, miscarriage, and/or stillbirth. Maternal periodontitis directly and/or indirectly has the potential to influence the health of the fetus and the pregnant woman. Low birth weight, preterm birth, and pre-eclampsia have been associated with maternal periodontitis. Two major pathways have been identified, one direct, in which oral microorganisms and/or their components reach the fetal–placental unit, and one indirect, in which inflammatory mediators circulate and impact the fetal–placental unit. Although periodontal therapy has been shown to be safe and leads to improved periodontal conditions in pregnant women, case-related periodontal therapy, with or without systemic antibiotics, does not reduce overall rates of preterm birth and low birth weight.[31] Various treatment strategies could be evaluated that consider specific target populations, as well as timing and intensity of treatment.[31] For instance, studies could investigate the use of local or systemic antimicrobials at various times during a pregnancy to determine whether adverse pregnancy outcomes are affected.

Periodontal pathogens and by-products may reach the placenta and spread to the fetal circulation and amniotic fluid. Their presence in the amniotic fluid and placenta can stimulate a fetal immune or inflammatory response characterized by the production of IgM antibodies against the pathogens and the secretion of elevated levels of inflammatory mediators. This can then cause miscarriage or premature birth.[32] Also, infection, inflammation, or both may cause structural changes in the placenta, which may lead to pre-eclampsia and impaired nutrient transport, causing low birth weight. Fetal exposure to infection may also result in tissue damage, increasing the risk for illness or death of the fetus. Finally, the stimulated systemic inflammatory response may exacerbate local inflammatory responses at the feto-placental unit and further increase the risk for adverse pregnancy outcomes.

In spite of all the research, debate still continues regarding potential relationships between maternal periodontitis during pregnancy and adverse pregnancy outcomes. The purpose of one systematic review was to synthesize the available epidemiological evidence on this association to date.[33] Pregnant women with or without periodontal disease and with or without adverse pregnancy outcomes were assessed either during pregnancy or postpartum. No intervention studies were included.

Maternal periodontitis was shown to modestly but significantly be associated with low birth weight and preterm birth, but the use of a definite or continuous exposure definition of periodontitis appears to impact the findings. Although significant associations emerge from case–control and cross-sectional studies using periodontitis case definitions, these were substantially weakened in studies assessing periodontitis as a continuous variable. Data from prospective studies followed a similar pattern, but associations were generally weaker. Maternal periodontitis was significantly associated with pre-eclampsia. There is a high degree of inconsistency in study populations, recruitment, and assessment, as well as differences in how data are recorded and handled. As a result, studies included in meta-analyses show a high degree of heterogeneity (differences within a group).

A critical question might be the effect of periodontal treatment on pregnancy outcomes, because that is a controllable factor. To date, all published trials included nonsurgical periodontal therapy; only two included systemic antimicrobials as part of test therapy. The trials varied considerably in sample size, obstetric histories of subjects, study preterm birth rates, and the periodontal treatment response. The largest trials, considered high quality and at low risk for bias, have shown dependable results and indicate that treatment does not alter rates of adverse pregnancy outcomes. The conclusion is that nonsurgical periodontal therapy, scaling and root planing, does not improve birth outcomes in pregnant women with periodontitis.[34] However, because periodontal care has been shown to be safe and effective in reducing periodontal disease and periodontal pathogens, it should be provided during pregnancy. No evidence has linked early miscarriage to dental treatment in the first trimester.[34]

Dental Hygiene Considerations

It is important to practice good oral hygiene during all the life cycles, including during pregnancy and breastfeeding. The American Dental Association (ADA) provides a patient handout regarding oral health during pregnancy.[35] Issues discussed in the document indicate that control of oral diseases in pregnant women has the potential to reduce the transmission of oral bacteria from mothers to their children; there is no evidence relating early spontaneous abortion to first-trimester oral health care or dental procedures; and pre-eclampsia is a challenging condition in the management of the pregnant patient, but pre-eclampsia is not a contraindication to dental care. While research is continuing, the bulk of the evidence shows that periodontal treatment has no effect on birth outcomes of preterm labor and low preterm birth weight, and it is safe for the mother and the fetus. Periodontal care has been shown to be safe and effective in reducing periodontal disease and periodontal pathogens and should be provided during pregnancy.[36]

Establishing a healthy oral environment is the most important objective in planning oral care for the pregnant patient. Adequate plaque control, brushing, flossing, interdental cleaning devices, rinsing, and professional prophylaxis including coronal scaling, root planing, and polishing are indicated.[36]

Use of radiographs or diagnostic radiographic imaging of oral tissues is not contraindicated in pregnancy and should be used as necessary to carry out a full examination to prepare a diagnosis and treatment plan.[37] The clinician should provide protection from radiation exposure for the pregnant woman's abdomen and neck using an abdominal and neck shield. Digital radiographs offer the advantage of a reduction in radiation. Regarding the use of nitrous oxide/oxygen analgesia, if other methods to control anxiety fail, nitrous oxide may be used as the sedation agent of choice.[38] However, it is recommended to avoid administration in the first trimester and to consult with the patient's obstetrician before administering any drug. See Chapter 32 for information on nitrous oxide. Use a standard informed consent form. A special form is not required due to pregnancy.

In the third trimester, when a pregnant woman lies flat on her back, the uterus can press on her inferior vena cava and impede venous return to the heart.[39] This can cause supine hypotensive syndrome, which occurs in 15% to 20% of pregnant women. This can be avoided during treatment by placing the patient in a semireclining position, encouraging frequent position changes, and placing a wedge underneath one of her hips to displace the uterus. A small pillow or folded blanket under the right hip, rolling the patient to the left side, changes the position of the uterus, taking pressure off the vena cava to prevent postural hypotensive syndrome. Keeping a semiseated position will also help to prevent possible aspiration caused by reduced gastroesophageal sphincter tone during pregnancy.

Epulis Gravidarum

Epulis gravidarum, or pregnancy granuloma, are single, tumor-like growths of gingival tissue that occur most frequently in an area of inflammatory gingivitis or other areas of recurrent irritation, or from trauma or any source of irritation.[40] They are usually painless, less than 2 mm, in areas of misalignment of teeth and malocclusion, can occur in healthy women, but are often a result of poor oral hygiene. They can vary in color from light red to purple. They can be pedunculated or broad based, highly vascularized, smooth, edematous, hemorrhagic, soft, red with glossy surface, and hardened when they have been in the mouth for a long time. (An elongated stalk of tissue is called a *peduncle*. A mass such as a cyst or polyp is said to be *pedunculated* if it is supported by a peduncle.) These tumors can be excised if the patient requests that option, but they normally resolve soon after delivery of the baby. They may recur after excision.

Medications

Oral health professionals should be familiar with the risks and benefits for pregnant or breastfeeding patients posed by five types of medications: analgesics and anti-inflammatories, antibiotics, local anesthetics, sedatives, and emergency medications. When medications are prescribed to pregnant women, the risk to the fetus is weighed against the benefit to the mother, and the decision to prescribe a medication reflects current evidence.

The U.S. Food and Drug Administration's Pregnancy and Lactation Final Rule helps explain what is known about using medicine during pregnancy and lactation.[41] This system replaces the letter categories formerly assigned to all prescription medicines. In some cases, medication should be avoided or altered. There may also be situations when it is unnecessary to stop the use of medications.[42] Breastfeeding also represents a clinical challenge, the risks and benefits of which need to be understood by both the patient and the practitioner before any medication is administered (Table 47-1).

Postpartum

The American Academy of Pediatric Dentistry (AAPD) recognizes the importance of perinatal oral health as the basis for the oral health of an infant. AAPD's 2011 guidelines on perinatal and infant oral health care provide a scientific basis for preventing and managing ECC and the more severe and rampant form of the disease.[43] In addition to professional guidelines, research supports simple solutions to avoid bacterial transmission from mother to infant. One example is having mothers chew xylitol-containing gum, or other xylitol-containing products, after eating, to reduce the transmission of caries from mother to child, a relatively simple, low-cost strategy to incorporate into a patient's oral health education. Six to 8 g xylitol daily is necessary to be effective.[44–46]

Oral health professionals are encouraged to provide necessary treatment for children assessed to be at increased risk for oral disease or in whom carious lesions or white spot lesions are identified. Offer anticipatory guidance to increase the possibility of changing oral health behaviors. Assess the risk for oral diseases in children starting by age 1 by identifying risk indicators. See Chapter 21 for information on Caries Management by Risk Assessment (CAMBRA) and Chapter 46 for detailed information about identifying risk indicators.

Table 47-1. Resources for Drug Safety in Pregnancy and Breastfeeding

Breastfeeding Online	www.breastfeedingonline.com/meds.shtml
National Library of Medicine Drugs and Lactation Database (LactMed)	http://toxnet.nlm.nih.gov/cgi-bin/sis/htmlgen?LACT
Organization of Teratology Information Specialists	www.otispregnancy.org
SafeFetus.com	www.safefetus.com
Texas Tech University Health Sciences Center Infant Risk Center	http://www.infantrisk.com
U.S. Food and Drug Administration	www.fda.gov

Menopause and After Menopause

Women in **menopause** (the stage when menstruation ceases, typically between ages 45 and 55) or postmenopause may experience changes in their mouths. They may notice discomfort in the mouth, including dry mouth, pain and burning sensations in the gum tissue, and altered taste, especially salty, peppery, or sour. Bone levels may decline as well.

Bone Loss

In menopause, estrogen levels decline rapidly, which can lead to systemic bone loss in the form of **osteopenia** (condition of decreased bone calcification or bone density, or reduced bone mass) or **osteoporosis** (condition in which bones become more porous and brittle, increasing the likelihood of fracture).[47] The same processes that lead to loss of bone in the spine and hips can also lead to loss of the alveolar bone of the jaws, resulting in increased risk for periodontal disease, loose teeth, and tooth loss. **Bisphosphonates,** the class of drugs most often prescribed for osteoporosis, have been linked by case reports to **osteonecrosis** (bone tissue death) of the jaw. This low-evidence-level information, its extensive interpretation, and misinformation in the lay media about hormonal changes associated with menopause have led to confusion among women. To acquire clarification and reliable information, patients often ask their physicians challenging questions related to oral health.[48]

The ADA considers osteoporosis to be a risk factor for periodontal disease.[49] Healthy postmenopausal women with high bone mineral density seemed to retain teeth better than those with low bone density or those with osteoporosis, even if they had deep periodontal pockets.[50] Hormone therapy preserves bone, but it may have adverse effects, such as an increased risk for breast cancer in some women. Postmenopausal women who were estrogen deficient had a higher frequency of sites with a net loss of alveolar bone density at recare.[51]

Women receiving hormonal therapy had significantly less gingival inflammation, lower plaque scores, and less loss of attachment than those not taking hormones.[52] Women who take hormonal therapy as directed may also comply with oral hygiene instructions. This compliance could explain the lower gingival inflammation scores, lower plaque scores, and reduced loss of attachment found in these women.[53] Hormone therapy significantly reduces the amount of clinical attachment loss and periodontal disease.[54] The apparent inconsistency of women having fewer teeth despite better periodontal health than men is related to an increased bone turnover rate and socioeconomic conditions such as low education and low social status. Periodontal health is even worse if these factors are combined.

Low estrogen production after menopause is associated with increased production of IL-1, IL-6, IL-8, IL-10, tumor necrosis factor α, granulocyte colony-stimulating factor, and granulocyte-macrophage colony-stimulating factor, which stimulate mature osteoclasts, modulate bone cell proliferation, and induce resorption of both skeletal and alveolar bone.[55] Progesterone levels decline after menopause, and luteinizing hormone levels increase.[56] Although the current osteoporosis model for women is focused on lower levels of estrogen, progesterone is considered an important hormone that collaborates with estrogen. In vitro studies of human osteoblasts in culture, prospective studies in adolescent, premenopausal, perimenopausal, and postmenopausal women show that progesterone has an active role in maintaining women's bone health and in osteoporosis prevention. Although progesterone does not prevent bone loss, progesterone as cotherapy with an antiresorptive agent (such as a bisphosphonate) may show promise.[57]

Dental Hygiene Considerations

Oral health-care providers should encourage patients to discuss the benefits and risks associated with hormone therapy with their physician. Health-care providers should keep the physical and mental changes of a patient in menopause in mind when evaluating for risk factors. No specific relationship to menopause needs to be emphasized. Patients should be encouraged to seek regular dental evaluation for prevention and early management of oral diseases.[48]

Bisphosphonate-Related Osteonecrosis of the Jaw

There are two categories of osteoporosis medications: antiresorptive medications that slow bone loss and anabolic drugs that increase the rate of bone formation.[58] Bisphosphonates are a class of drugs that prevent the loss of bone mass. High-potency IV bisphosphonates have been shown to modify the progression of malignant bone disease in several forms of cancer, especially breast and frequently prostate cancer. Oral bisphosphonates are used to treat osteoporosis, osteitis deformans (Paget disease of the bone), and other conditions that lead to bone fragility.[58]

After they are taken orally or IV, bisphosphonates bind tightly to the surface of the bone directly beneath the osteoclasts, which actively dissolve bone. The drugs then become incorporated into the osteoclasts, stopping them from dissolving bone. As a result, bone production continues, bone loss decreases, bone density is improved, and the risk for fracture is reduced. Bisphosphonates help in the fight against malignant bone disease. When used with chemotherapy agents, bisphosphonates have been shown to significantly reduce skeletal complications in patients with bone cancers.

The drugs have also proven effective when taken orally by patients with or at risk for osteoporosis. Treatment in these cases increases the density of the patient's bones and reduces the risk for fracture. The benefits of bisphosphonate therapy for osteoporosis sufferers are still evident several years after treatment. Monoclonal antibody drugs such as denosumab (Prolia) are also used to treat osteoporosis in postmenopausal women at high risk for fractures and to reduce bone weakening

or loss in patients with cancer.[59] Denosumab has been identified as just as high a risk factor for osteonecrosis as bisphosphonates.

Bisphosphonate-related osteonecrosis of the jaw (BRONJ) can be described as an area of bone in the jaw that has died and been exposed in the mouth for more than 8 weeks in a person taking any bisphosphonate. Patients treated with bisphosphonates subsequently develop osteonecrosis of the jaw or maxillary bone after minor local trauma including dental work. Although the exact cause is unknown, BRONJ is considered to be an adverse effect of bisphosphonate therapy.[60]

Symptoms of BRONJ include exposed bone, localized pain, swelling of the gum tissues and inflammation, and loosening of previously stable teeth. BRONJ is most often seen in patients who have received bisphosphonates through IV therapy, but cases have been reported in patients who are taking oral bisphosphonates. Prevention is always the best treatment. Recognize the risk factors. High cumulative doses of bisphosphonates, poor oral health, and dental extractions may be significant risk factors for BRONJ development.[61] The dosage and length of therapy are risk factors for BRONJ. IV bisphosphonates used in cancer treatment are much more potent than the oral bisphosphonates used to manage osteoporosis, thus increasing the risk for BRONJ in these patients. The risk for developing BRONJ appears to increase in relation to the number of treatments with an IV bisphosphonate. The third part of the equation is undergoing routine dental surgical procedures, including tooth extraction, periodontal surgery, or dental implant placement. These procedures in patients being treated with bisphosphonates comprise about 60% of BRONJ cases.[62]

Preventive strategies include removing all areas of dental infection before starting bisphosphonate therapy. Treatment is focused on control of pain and infection and local debridement of dead bone, but not wide excision of lesions. Good oral hygiene is critical. There is no published evidence to support or oppose discontinuation of bisphosphonate therapy once osteonecrosis develops or before required dental surgery. Because of the long half-life of bisphosphonates, recovery of normal osteoclast function and bone turnover after drug withdrawal may be too gradual for this measure to have clinical significance.[62]

Osteoradionecrosis

Osteoradionecrosis (ORN) is the most serious possible complication facing the patient with oral cancer. A condition of the nonvital bone in a site of radiotherapy, osteoradionecrosis is bone that has died as a complication of radiotherapy. Because radiation works to destroy cancerous cells through the deprivation of oxygen and vital nutrients, it unavoidably destroys normal cells as well, damaging small arteries and reducing circulation to the area of the mandible. Not an infection itself, it is the bone's reduced ability to heal, resulting in lesions, pain, and fragility. Insufficient blood supply to the irradiated areas decreases the ability to heal, and any subsequent infections to the jaw can pose a huge risk to the patient. Although it is possible that it will develop spontaneously, ORN most frequently occurs when an insult to the bone is sustained in the irradiated area, such as related subsequent surgery or biopsy, tooth extractions, or denture irritations.[63] Complete dental authorization before treatment is no longer necessary. Controversy exists regarding the management of osteoradionecrosis of the maxillofacial skeleton because of the variability of this condition. The treatment of osteoradionecrosis has included local wound care, antibiotic therapy, surgical procedures, and the administration of hyperbaric oxygenation.[64]

DOMESTIC VIOLENCE

Domestic or intimate partner violence occurs when a partner in a relationship uses behaviors such as physical and psychological abuse to establish control over the other person. Domestic abuse is not confined to a specific population; it occurs in people of all races, ethnicities, social classes, religions, sex, and genders. It affects people of all ages and can occur throughout the life span.[65]

Seventy-five percent of the physical injuries are to the head, neck, and/or mouth. Bruises, bites, burns, lacerations, abrasions, head injuries, and skeletal injuries are some of the common forms of domestic violence trauma that are detectable in the dental office.[66] See Spotlight on Public Health.

Dental Hygiene Considerations

Dental professionals are responsible for reporting suspected child abuse and neglect, elder abuse and neglect, and domestic violence involving physical assault. Screen patients for signs and symptoms of abuse or neglect, including bruises, fractures, tooth loss, bite marks, untreated caries, and untreated pain, infection, or trauma affecting the orofacial region. Ask direct questions in a kind, compassionate manner. Document your findings. If the patient seems to be in imminent danger or the situation is an emergency, call 911. Otherwise,

Spotlight on Public Health

Dental professionals must report suspected abuse, neglect, and domestic violence. Some resources for reporting include:
- Childhelp USA National Child Abuse Hotline: 1-800-422-4453 or 1-800-4-A-CHILD
- The National Domestic Violence Hotline: 1-800-799-7233 or 1-800-799-SAFE
  In a particular state: http://www.thehotline.org/get-help/help-in-your-area/ ■

follow local guidelines and report the situation to the appropriate authorities.[66]

MEN'S HEALTH

Early detection and treatment of diseases in men begins with awareness of preventable health problems, screenings, and regular oral care. Heart disease, diabetes, stroke, and cancer are chronic conditions that present serious obstacles to providing care for patients. Healthcare professionals should better understand the dental hygiene considerations of men facing various diseases of the prostate and cancer.

Diseases of the Prostate

Prostate disease is a general term that describes a number of medical conditions that can affect the prostate gland. The prostate gland is a small gland that is found only in men; it is located between the penis and bladder, and it surrounds the urethra. The prostate gland helps with the production of semen and produces a thick white fluid that is liquefied by a special protein called *prostate-specific antigen*. The fluid is mixed with sperm, produced by the testicles, to create semen. A number of conditions can affect the prostate gland including prostate enlargement, prostatitis (inflammation of the prostate gland), and prostate cancer.

Medications

Two classes of drugs are commonly used to treat prostate enlargement and benign prostatic hyperplasia (BPH): alpha-blockers and 5-alpha-reductase inhibitors. Alpha-blockers are generally used first because they act fast, relieving urination problems in a matter of days or weeks, whereas reductase inhibitors can take several months to provide relief. Sometimes the two types of drugs are used in combination. Indications for treating BPH include reversing signs and symptoms or preventing progression of the disease. Long-acting alpha blockers approved for the treatment of BPH in the United States are: terazosin, doxazosin, tamsulosin, and alfuzosin.[67] Adverse events may be dizziness or hypotension, so the medical history should always be updated.

Prostate cancer is predominantly a tumor of older men. Most treatments do not have oral side effects, with the exception of chemotherapy. The most common chemotherapy drug, docetaxel (Taxotere), is very well tolerated, and some men find that many disease-related symptoms, such as pain, fatigue, and loss of energy, improve as therapy continues. Docetaxel does have some negative side effects, such as fever, low white blood cell count, infection, fatigue, and numbness or weakness in the toes or fingers that interferes with function (neuropathy). Other negative side effects of docetaxel include low platelets that can result in bleeding (1%), anemia (5%), reduced heart function (10%), hair loss (65%), diarrhea (32%), nail changes (30%), loss of appetite (20%), shortness of breath (15%), and fluid retention (10%–20%). Many of these are mild, reversible, and treatable and should not be a reason to avoid chemotherapy if it is needed.[68]

Dental Hygiene Considerations

Poor oral health has been associated with increased incidence and severity of oral complications in patients with cancer, hence the adoption of an aggressive approach to stabilizing oral care before treatment. Primary preventive measures such as appropriate nutritional intake, effective oral hygiene practices, and early detection of oral lesions are important pretreatment interventions. When treating a patient who is undergoing chemotherapy or radiation, it is important to know his medical status. Necessary information is the white and red blood cell counts, platelet count, and whether the patient has a port or indwelling venous line, through which chemotherapy drugs are delivered. See Table 47-2 for National Cancer Institute Guidelines.[69] For more information, see Chapter 45.

DENTAL DECAY AND THE SEXES

Sex differences in oral health have been widely documented through time and across cultures. Women's oral health declines more rapidly than men's. The magnitude of this disparity in oral health by sex increases throughout the life span. Representative studies of sex differences in caries, tooth loss, and periodontal disease were critically reviewed.[70] Surveys conducted in Hungary, India, and in an isolated traditional Brazilian sample provide additional support for a significant sex bias in dental caries, especially in mature adults. Compounding hormonal and reproductive factors, the sex difference in oral health in India appears to involve social and religious causes such as preferring a male child to a female child, ritual fasting, and dietary restrictions during pregnancy.

Like the sex difference in caries and decay, tooth loss in women is greater than in men and has been linked to caries.[70] Results of genome-wide association studies have found caries-susceptible and caries-protective loci (specific location of a gene or DNA sequence on a chromosome) that impact disparities in taste, saliva, and

Table 47-2. *Management Guidelines Relative to Invasive Dental Procedures*[69]

Medical Status	Guideline	Comments
Patients with chronic indwelling venous access lines (e.g., Hickman)	AHA prophylactic antibiotic recommendations (low risk)	There is no clear scientific proof detailing infectious risk for these lines after dental procedures. This recommendation is empiric. Order CBC with differential.
Neutrophils >2,000/mm^3 1,000–2,000/mm^3	No prophylactic antibiotics AHA prophylactic antibiotic recommendations (low risk)	Clinical judgment is critical. If infection is present or unclear, more aggressive antibiotic therapy may be indicated.
<1,000/mm^3	Amikacin 150 mg/m^2 1 h presurgery; ticarcillin 75 mg/kg IV 30 min presurgery; repeat both 6 hr postoperatively	If organisms are known or suspected, appropriate adjustments should be based on sensitivities. Order platelet count and coagulation tests.
Platelets* >60,000/mm^3 30,000–60,000/mm^3	No additional support needed Platelet transfusions are optional for non-invasive treatment; consider administering preoperatively and 24 hr later for surgical treatment (e.g., dental extractions); additional transfusions are based on clinical course	Use techniques to promote establishing and maintaining control of bleeding (i.e., sutures, pressure packs, minimize trauma).
<30,000/mm^3	Platelets should be transfused 1 hr before procedure; obtain an immediate postinfusion platelet count; transfuse regularly to maintain counts >30,000–40,000/mm^3 until initial healing has occurred; in some instances, platelet counts >60,000/mm^3 may be required	In addition to above, consider using hemostatic agents (i.e., microfibrillar collagen, topical thrombin). Aminocaproic acid may help stabilize nondurable clots. Monitor sites carefully.

CBC, complete blood cell count; AHA, American Heart Association.

*Assumes that all other coagulation parameters are within normal limits and that platelet counts will be maintained at or above the specified level until initial stabilization/healing has occurred.

enamel proteins. These affect the oral environment and the microstructure of enamel. Genetic variation, some of which is linked to the X chromosome, may partly explain how sex differences in oral health begin to develop. An important, but often overlooked, factor in explaining the sex discrepancy in oral health is the multifaceted and synergistic changes associated with female sex hormones, pregnancy, and women's reproductive life history. Caries etiology is complex and impacts understanding of the sex difference in oral health. Both biological (genetics, hormones, and reproductive history) and anthropological (behavioral) factors such as culture-based division of labor and gender-based dietary preferences play a role. Recent studies suggest that a sex-linked gene may explain why rates of dental decay may be higher in women.[71]

Case Study

A female patient arrives at your general dental office for a preventive prophylaxis and examination. The medical history reveals the following: age, 63 years; blood pressure, 120/75; medications: alendronate sodium (Fosamax), levothyroxine, vitamin C, and oral atenolol. No significant medical issues were disclosed. Dental examination reveals periodontal pockets: 3 to 5 mm; 4 restorations; no active decay or restorative needs; alveolar bone loss noted on radiographs; partially impacted #32 that is infected.

Case Study Exercises

1. Based on the patient's medications, what medical conditions are present, whether controlled or uncontrolled?
   i. Osteoporosis
   ii. Low thyroid
   iii. Hypertension
   iv. Rheumatoid arthritis
      A. i and ii
      B. i and iii
      C. i, ii, and iv
      D. i, ii, and iii

2. The dentist diagnoses #32 as needing to be extracted. What steps should be taken?
   A. Schedule the patient for the extraction.
   B. Refer the patient to her physician before scheduling the extraction.
   C. Prepare the patient for the extraction at this appointment.

3. Preventive prophylaxis:
   A. Should be delayed until after a consultation with the patient's physician.
   B. Should be done by a periodontist.
   C. Should be offered in the treatment plan.
   D. Should not include root planing.

Review Questions

1. In humans, biological sex is determined by five factors present at birth. Which one is incorrect?
   A. The presence or absence of an X chromosome
   B. The type of gonads
   C. The sex hormones
   D. The internal reproductive anatomy
   E. The external genitalia

2. Gender-based medicine, also called "gender medicine," is the field of medicine that studies the biological and physiological differences between the human sexes and how that affects differences in disease. Traditionally, medical research has mostly been conducted using the male body as the basis for clinical studies.
   A. Both statements are true.
   B. Both statements are false.
   C. The first statement is true, but the second statement is false.
   D. The first statement is false, but the second statement is true.

3. A woman's periodontal health may be impacted by a variety of factors. Gingival tissues contain receptors for androgens, estrogen, and progesterone, and it was documented that these hormones have effects on the oral mucosa and the periodontium.
   A. Both the statement and the reason are correct and related.
   B. Both the statement and the reason are correct but *not* related.
   C. The statement is correct, but the reason is *not*.
   D. The statement is *not* correct, but the reason is correct.
   E. *Neither* the statement *nor* the reason is correct.

4. Estrogen and progesterone changes seem to modify the gingival tissues. This leads to decreased vascular permeability and decreased keratinization of the gingival epithelium.
   A. Both the statement and the reason are correct and related.
   B. Both the statement and the reason are correct but *not* related.
   C. The statement is correct, but the reason is *not.*
   D. The statement is *not* correct, but the reason is correct.
   E. *Neither* the statement *nor* the reason is correct.

5. The changes in the circulating levels of female sex hormones affect the host response, resulting in all of the following EXCEPT:
   A. An exaggerated response against dental biofilm
   B. Alteration of the immune system
   C. Interleukin-6, a key mediator in periodontal inflammation, was found to be increased by progesterone in gingival fibroblasts
   D. Higher vascular permeability
   E. Decreased keratinization of the gingival epithelium

Active Learning

1. Working with a partner, take turns role-playing treating a 5-year-old child, 87-year-old woman, and 25-year-old man with Down syndrome who you suspect are being abused. Ask questions to elicit information from the patient and/or caregiver. Discuss with the class how you feel handling the situation.
2. Create a brief presentation for adolescents on oral health promotion. ■

REFERENCES

1. Knox D, Schacht C. *Choices in Relationships: An Introduction to Marriage and the Family.* 12th ed. Boston, MA: Cengage Learning; 2015.
2. Intersex. Bethesda, MD: U.S. National Library of Medicine. http://www.nlm.nih.gov/medlineplus/ency/article/001669.htm. Updated August 22, 2013. Accessed September 27, 2015.
3. Cuozzo K, Bratman S (reviewer). Women, men, and medicine: we're not equal. EBSCO Publishing; September 2005.
4. Exploring the biological contributions to human health: does sex matter? Washington, DC: National Academy Press. http://www.iom.edu/~/media/Files/Report%20Files/2003/Exploring-the-Biological-Contributions-to-Human-Health-Does-Sex-Matter/DoesSexMatter8pager.pdf. Published 2001. Accessed September 27, 2015.
5. Mariotti A. Sex steroid hormones and cell dynamics in the periodontium. *Crit Rev Oral Biol Med.* 1994;5:27-53.
6. Influence of estrogen and osteopenia/osteoporosis on clinical periodontitis in postmenopausal women. *J Periodontol.* 1999;70:823-828.
7. Lapp CA, Thomas ME, Lewis JB. Modulation by progesterone of interleukin-6 production by gingival fibroblasts. *J Periodontol.* 1995;66:279-284.
8. Furuta M, Ekuni D, Irie K, et al. Sex differences in gingivitis relate to interaction of oral health behaviors in young people. *J Periodontol.* 2011;82(4):558-565. doi: 10.1902/jop.2010.100444.
9. *ADA Survey Results Reveal Oral Hygiene Habits of Men Lag behind Women.* Chicago, IL: American Dental Association; May 2004.
10. Ross AC, Taylor CL, Yaktine AL, et al., eds. Institute of Medicine (US) Committee to Review Dietary Reference Intakes for Vitamin D and Calcium; Dietary Reference Intakes for Calcium and Vitamin D. Washington, DC: National Academies Press; 2011.
11. National Academies Press. A lethal diet. *Dying to Quit.* Washington, DC: National Academies Press; 1998. http://www.nap.edu/html/dying-to-quit/chapter6.html.
12. Ericsson JS, Abrahamsson KH, Ostberg AL, Hellström MK, Jönsson K, Wennström JL. Periodontal health status in Swedish adolescents: an epidemiological, cross-sectional study. *Swed Dent J.* 2009;33:131-139.
13. Wojcicki CJ, Harpert DS, Robinson PJ. Differences in periodontal disease-associated microorganisms of subgingival plaque in prepubertal, pubertal and postpubertal children. *J Periodontol.* 1987;58(4):219-223. doi: 10.1902/jop.2010.090590.
14. Becerik S, Ozçaka O, Nalbantsoy A, et al. Effects of menstrual cycle on periodontal health and gingival crevicular fluid markers. *J Periodontol.* 2010;81(5):673-681. doi: 10.1902/jop.2010.090590.
15. LeResche L, Mancl LA, Drangsholt MT, Saunders K, Korff MV. Relationship of pain and symptoms to pubertal development in adolescents. *Pain.* 2005;118(1-2):201-209.
16. LeResche L, Saunders K, Von Korff MR, Barlow W, Dworkin SF. Use of exogenous hormones and risk of temporomandibular disorder pain. *Pain.* 1997;69(1-2):153-160.
17. Madani AS, Mirmortazavi A, Ghazi N, Ziaee S. The possible role of oral contraceptives in the development of temporomandibular disorders. *Indian J Stomatol.* 2010;2(3):149-152.
18. Berkley KJ. Sex differences in pain. *Behav Brain Sci.* 1997; 20(3):371-380.
19. Dao T. Sex differences in pain. *J Am Dent Assoc.* 2012; 143(7):764-765.
20. Nilsson M, Johnsen R, Ye W, Hveem K, Lagergren J. Prevalence of gastro-oesophageal reflux symptoms and the influence of age and sex. *Scand J Gastroenterol.* 2004;39:1040-1045.
21. Marrero JM, Goggin PM, de Caestecker JS, Pearce JM, Maxwell JD. Determinants of pregnancy heartburn. *Br J Obstet Gynaecol.* 1992;99:731-734.
22. Richter JE. The management of heartburn in pregnancy. *Aliment Pharmacol Ther.* 2005;22:749-757.
23. Katz PO, Lehrer JK. GERD in women. *NEJM Journal Watch.* November 16, 2006.

24. Lin M, Gerson LB, Lascar R, Davila M, Triadafilopoulos G. Features of gastroesophageal reflux disease in women. *Am J Gastroenterol.* 2004;99:1442-1447.

25. Boggess KA, Edelstein BL. Oral health in women during preconception and pregnancy: implications for birth outcomes and infant oral health. *Matern Child Health J.* 2006;10(1):169-174.

26. Goldenberg RL, Culhane JF. Preterm birth and periodontal disease. *N Engl J Med.* 2006;355:1925-1927.

27. Xiong X, Buekens P, Vastardis S, Yu SM. Periodontal disease and pregnancy outcomes: state-of-the-science. *Obstet Gynecol Surv.* 2007;62(9):605-615.

28. Integration of oral health and primary care practice. Rockville, MD: U.S. Department of Health and Human Services, Health Resources and Services Administration. http://www.hrsa.gov/publichealth/clinical/oralhealth/primarycare/integrationoforalhealth.pdf. Published February 2014. Accessed January 26, 2015.

29. Markou E, Eleana B, Lazaros T, Antonios K. The influence of sex steroid hormones on gingiva of women. *Open Dent J.* 2009;3:114-119.

30. Xie Y, Xiong X, Elkind-Hirsch KE, et al. Change of periodontal disease status during and after pregnancy. *J Periodontol.* 2013;84:725-731.

31. Sanz M, Kornman K. Periodontitis and adverse pregnancy outcomes: consensus report of the Joint EFP/AAP Workshop on Periodontitis and Systemic Diseases. *J Periodontol.* 2013;84(4 Suppl.):S164-S169.

32. Madianos P, Bobetsis YA, Offenbacher S. Adverse pregnancy outcomes and periodontal disease: pathogenic mechanisms. *J Periodontol.* 2013;84(4 Suppl.):S170-S180.

33. Ide M, Papapanou PN. Epidemiology of association between maternal periodontal disease and adverse pregnancy outcomes—systematic review. *J Periodontol.* 2013;84(4 Suppl.):S181-S194.

34. Michalowicz BS, Gustafsson A, Thumbigere-Math V, Buhlin K. The effects of periodontal treatment on pregnancy outcomes. *J Periodontol.* 2013;84(4 Suppl.):S195-S208.

35. Oral health during pregnancy: what to expect when expecting. Chicago, IL: American Dental Association. http://www.ada.org/~/media/ADA/Publications/Files/for_the_dental_patient_may_2011.ashx. Published May 2011. Accessed January 26, 2015.

36. *Oral Health during Pregnancy and Childhood: Evidence-Based Guidelines for Health Professionals.* Sacramento, CA: CDA Foundation. http://www.cdafoundation.org/portals/0/pdfs/poh_guidelines.pdf. Published February 2010. Accessed November 13, 2015.

37. American Dental Association, U.S. Food and Drug Administration. The selection of patients for dental radiograph examinations. http://www.ada.org/~/media/ADA/Member%20Center/FIles/Dental_Radiographic_Examinations_2012.ashx. Accessed September 27, 2015.

38. Becker DE, Rosenberg M. Nitrous oxide and the inhalation anesthetics. *Anesth Prog.* 2008;55:124-131.

39. Wasylko L, Matsui D, Dykxhoorn SM, Rieder MJ, Weinberg S. A review of common dental treatments during pregnancy; implications for patients and dental personnel. *J Can Dent Assoc.* 1998;64(6):434-439.

40. Demir Y, Demir S, Aktepe F. Cutaneous lobular capillary hemangioma induced by pregnancy. *J Cutan Path.* 2004;31:77-80.

41. Pregnancy and lactation labeling final rule. Silver Spring, MD: U.S. Food and Drug Administration. http://www.fda.gov/Drugs/DevelopmentApprovalProcess/DevelopmentResources/Labeling/ucm093307.htm. Updated December 4, 2014. Accessed January 27, 2015.

42. Donaldson M, Goodchild JH. Pregnancy, breast-feeding and drugs used in dentistry. *J Am Dent Assoc.* 2012;143(8):858-871.

43. American Academy of Pediatric Dentistry, Clinical Affairs Committee. Guideline on Infant Oral Health Care. Clinical Guidelines. http://www.aapd.org/media/Policies_Guidelines/G_InfantOralHealthCare.pdf. Adopted 1986. Revised 2014. Accessed November 13, 2015.

44. Isokangas P, Söderling E, Pienihäkkinen K, Alanen P. Occurrence of dental decay in children after maternal consumption of xylitol chewing gum: a follow-up from 0 to 5 years of age. *J Dent Res.* 2000;79(11):1885-1889.

45. Soderling E, Isokangas P, Pienihakkinen K, Tenovou J. Influence of maternal xylitol consumption on acquisition of mutans streptococci by infants. *J Dent Res.* 2000;79(3):882-887.

46. Thorild I, Lindau B, Twetman S. Caries in 4-year-old children after maternal chewing of gums containing combinations of xylitol, sorbitol, chlorhexidine, and fluoride. *Eur Arch Paediatr Dent.* 2006;7(4):241-245.

47. North American Menopause Society. *Menopause Practice: A Clinician's Guide.* 3rd ed. 2007.

48. Buencamino MCA, Palomo L, Thacker HL. How menopause affects oral health, and what we can do about it. *Cleve Clin J Med.* 2009;76(8):467-475.

49. American Dental Association Council on Access, Prevention and Interprofessional Relations. Women's Oral Health Issues. November 2006.

50. Klemetti E, Collin HL, Forss H, Markkanen H, Lassila V. Mineral status of skeletal and advanced periodontal disease. *J Clin Periodontol.* 1994;21:184-188.

51. Payne JB, Reinhardt RA, Nummikoski PV, Patil KD. Longitudinal alveolar bone loss in postmenopausal osteoporotic/osteopenic women. *Osteoporos Int.* 1999;10:34-40.

52. Civitelli R, Pilgram TK, Dotson M, et al. Alveolar and postcranial bone density in postmenopausal women receiving hormone/estrogen replacement: a randomized, double blind, placebo-controlled trial. *Arch Intern Med.* 2002;162:1409-1415.

53. Albandar JM, Kingman A. Gingival recession, gingival bleeding, and dental calculus in adults 30 years of age and older in the United States, 1988–1994. *J Periodontol.* 1999;70:30-43.

54. Meisel P, Reifenberger J, Haase R, Nauck M, Bandt C, Kocher T. Women are periodontally healthier than men, but why don't they have more teeth than men? *Menopause.* 2008;15:270-275.

55. Pacifici R. Estrogen, cytokines and pathogenesis of postmenopausal osteoporosis. *J Bone Miner Res.* 1996;11:1043-1051.

56. Menopause: time for change. Bethesda, MD: National Institute on Aging, National Institutes of Health, U.S. Department of Health and Human Services. http://www.nia.nih.gov/sites/default/files/menopause_time_for_a_change_0.pdf. Updated August 2010. Accessed January 27, 2015.

57. Seifert-Klauss V, Prior JC. Progesterone and bone: actions promoting bone health in women. *J Osteoporos.* 2010;2010:845180.

58. Types of osteoporosis medications. Washington, DC: National Osteoporosis Foundation. http://www.nof.org/articles/22. Accessed September 27, 2015.

59. FDA approval for denosumab. Bethesda, MD: National Cancer Institute. http://www.cancer.gov/cancertopics/druginfo/fda-denosumab. Updated July 2, 2013. Accessed September 27, 2015.

60. Sharma D, Ivanovski S, Slevin M, et al. Bisphosphonate-related osteonecrosis of jaw (BRONJ): diagnostic criteria and possible pathogenic mechanisms of an unexpected anti-angiogenic side effect. *Vascular Cell.* 2013;5:1. http://www.vascularcell.com/content/pdf/2045-824X-5-1.pdf. Accessed September 27, 2015.

61. Hoff AO, Toth BB, Altundag K, et al. Frequency and risk factors associated with osteonecrosis of the jaw in cancer patients treated with intravenous bisphosphonates. *J Bone Miner Res.* 2008;23(6).

62. Woo S, Hellstein JW, Kalmar JR. Systematic review: bisphosphonates and osteonecrosis of the jaws. *Ann Intern Med.* 2006;144:753-761. http://www.aaomp.org/papers/Bisphosphonates%20and%20Osteonecrosis%20of%20the%20Jaws.pdf. Accessed September 27, 2015.

63. Chrcanovic BR, Reher P, Sousa AA, Harris M. Osteoradionecrosis of the jaws—a current overview—part 1: physiopathology and risk and predisposing factors. *Oral Maxillofac Surg.* 2010;14(1):3-16. doi: 10.1007/s10006-009-0198-9.

64. Chrcanovic BR, Reher P, Sousa AA, Harris M. Osteoradionecrosis of the jaws—a current overview—Part 2: dental management and therapeutic options for treatment. *Oral Maxillofac Surg.* 2010;14(2):81-95. doi: 10.1007/s10006-010-0205-1.

65. Enhancing dental professionals' response to domestic violence. Sacramento, CA: National Health Resource, Center on Domestic Violence. A Project of the Family Violence Prevention Fund Enhancing Dental Professionals' Response to Domestic Violence. http://www.futureswithoutviolence.org/userfiles/file/HealthCare/dental.pdf. Accessed September 27, 2015.

66. Shanel-Hogan KA. Dental professionals against violence. California Dental Association Foundation, Inc.; 2004. http://www.vdh.virginia.gov/ofhs/prevention/dsvp/projectradarva/documents/older/pdf/dentalmanual.pdf. Accessed September 27, 2015.

67. Lepor H. Alpha blockers for the treatment of benign prostatic hyperplasia. *Rev Urol.* 2007;9(4):181-190.

68. Side effects of chemotherapy. Santa Monica, CA: Prostate Cancer Foundation. http://www.pcf.org/site/c.leJRIROrEpH/b.5836637/k.D89F/Side_Effects_of_Chemotherapy.htm. Accessed September 27, 2015.

69. National Cancer Institute. Oral complications of chemotherapy and head/neck radiation, table 3. Bethesda, MD: National Cancer Institute. http://www.cancer.gov/about-cancer/treatment/side-effects/mouth-throat/oral-complications-hp-pdq. Accessed September 27, 2015.

70. Lukacs JR. Sex differences in dental caries experience: clinical evidence, complex etiology. *Clin Oral Investig.* 2011;15(5):649-656. doi: 10.1007/s00784-010-0445-3.

71. Ferraro M, Vieira AR. Explaining gender differences in caries: a multifactorial approach to a multifactorial disease. *Int J Dent.* 2010;2010:649643. http://dx.doi.org/10.1155/2010/649643.

RESOURCES

MedLine Plus—Women's Health: http://www.nlm.nih.gov/medlineplus/womenshealth.html

Monash University: http://www.med.monash.edu.au/gendermed/difference.html

livescience: http://www.livescience.com/37053-depression-gender-differences.html

American Association of Oral and Maxillofacial Surgeons: http://www.aaoms.org/conditions-and-treatments/bronj http://www.aaoms.org/images/uploads/pdfs/mronj_position_paper.pdf All accessed September 27, 2015.

Chapter 48 | The Elderly

Kay Murphy, CDA, RDH, MS

KEY TERMS

achlorhydria

activities of daily living (ADL)

Alzheimer disease

angular cheilitis

arthritis

biological age

chronic obstructive pulmonary disease (COPD)

chronological age

dementia

diabetes mellitus

functional age

osteoporosis

Parkinson disease

pathophysiology

presbycusis

presbyopia

senescence

stroke

tinnitus

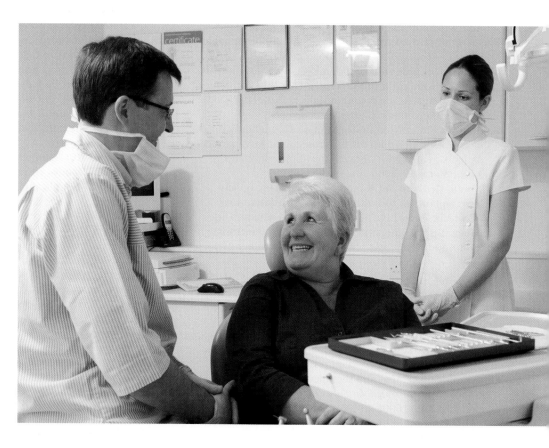

LEARNING OBJECTIVES

After reading this chapter, the student should be able to:

48.1 Identify demographic changes over the past century in American society and discuss how these changes impact current and future oral health-care needs of an aging society.

48.2 Explain the difference between chronological age and functional age.

48.3 Discuss pathophysiological changes associated with age, as well as age-related conditions and systemic diseases common to the elderly.

48.4 Differentiate between normal aging and pathophysiological oral conditions of the elderly.

48.5 Discuss the importance of assessment of the elderly dental patient for treatment planning, patient management, dental hygiene care, and maintenance of oral health.

48.6 Discuss educational and preventive oral health considerations for the elderly patient.

KEY CONCEPTS

- Demographic data project substantial increases in all age brackets of older populations aged 65 and older.
- In older adults, a disparity between a person's chronological age and functional age is common.

- Many older adults require multiple medications for a variety of diseases, challenging both overall health and oral health.
- The dental professional needs to understand both medical and dental complexities of older adults, as well as how complex conditions such as diabetes, multiple medications, and self-care limitations impact oral health and oral care.
- Older adult patients have an increased incidence and prevalence of root caries because of underlying risk factors such as xerostomia.
- When treating older adult patients, dental professionals should focus on prevention rather than restorative care.

RELEVANCE TO CLINICAL PRACTICE

During the past century, the United States has witnessed advancements in both medicine and dentistry, allowing people to live longer and keep their teeth for a lifetime. Vaccines, antibiotics, improved nutrition, and healthier lifestyle practices have helped to increase life expectancy. In addition, systemic and topical fluorides, advanced dental procedures, and better oral hygiene self-care have decreased tooth loss and lowered the edentulous rate. Although these improvements have made significant contributions to the overall health of the U.S. population, they have also introduced a new set of problems caused by a rapidly growing number of aging Americans that have placed increased demands on the medical and dental health-care system in the United States.[1]

DEMOGRAPHICS OF AGING

The changing demographics in the United States, particularly the rapidly growing number of adults aged 65 years and older, have become a key issue in determining how to meet their oral health needs. In 1900, 3.1 million people, or 4% of the U.S. population, were 65 years and older; in 2008, this same age group grew to 38.9 million, or 12.8% of the U.S. population.[2] By 2050, this number is expected to reach 71 million, with older adults comprising almost 20% of the U.S. population. The driving force behind the population increase of older adults is the aging baby boom generation, those born from 1948 to 1964. Considered the largest U.S. cohort, the "boomers" are expected to make a major impact on oral health delivery systems because of their growing numbers and need for care (see Application to Clinical Practice).[1–3]

Chronic Conditions

Today's older adults experience more chronic medical and dental problems than the generations who preceded them. Diseases once considered terminal such as heart disease, diabetes, and cancer are now managed with medications and have become chronic. In 2007, the Centers for Disease Control and Prevention (CDC) reported more than 50% of those aged 75 years and older as having, on average, three or more chronic diseases and taking five or more different medications.[4,5]

Medications for chronic diseases commonly have unintended oral side effects such as xerostomia, which sometimes result in oral complications such as coronal or root caries. As the number of older adults diagnosed with chronic diseases increases, the number of oral complications also rises.

Physical and Cognitive Disabilities

Further affecting the oral health of older adults is the increasing number of those who have physical and cognitive disabilities. According to the Institute of Medicine, the two most prevalent disabilities in older adults are arthritis and dementia, both of which limit the individual's ability to perform certain **activities of daily living (ADL).** ADL are tasks an individual performs that involve self-care such as eating, bathing, and dressing.[6] Patients who suffer from arthritis have limited dexterity, making brushing and flossing difficult, whereas patients afflicted with Alzheimer disease may not remember how to perform specific activities. In 2007, roughly 40%, or 14 million, of adults aged 65 years and older showed some type of limitation that impacted their daily living, and this number is expected to double to 28 million by 2030 (see Teamwork).[6]

Homebound and Institutionalized Adults

The number of homebound and institutionalized older adults is increasing. Patients with limited mobility and residents in long-term care facilities are not

Application to Clinical Practice

When treating the elderly, the dental hygienist must first be aware of the general stereotypes that exist to avoid them. For example, using language such as "having a senior moment" when an older patient is being forgetful or confused, or "being a demanding patient" when someone is making requests or asking questions can appear condescending or belittling to an elderly patient. Elderly patients need to be treated with the same care and respect as all patients and thought of as individuals. Every patient has his or her own unique circumstances, concerns, and needs, and the elderly patient is no exception.

To successfully treat elderly patients, the dental hygienist needs to understand and attend to each patient's individual needs such as using a neck support for an arthritic neck, allowing for frequent restroom breaks for those taking diuretics, or treating a patient in a semiupright position because of respiratory problems. In addition, dental hygienists may need to verbally repeat or write down information for patients suffering from hearing loss. They also need to be aware that elderly patients in general move at a slower pace and usually require longer appointments to complete all the necessary dental hygiene assessments and procedures.

Spending the extra time and providing individual care for elderly patients can be challenging but as rewarding for the dental hygienist. Elderly patients know they require extra attention and, at times, are frustrated that they can no longer do the things they used to do. By showing patience, kindness, and empathy to elderly patients during dental care visits, the dental hygienist shows the respect that they deserve. ■

Teamwork

Providing comprehensive dental care to elderly patients can be a challenge for many dental professionals; elderly patients struggle not only from an array of medical and dental problems, they also struggle with problems related to transportation, scheduling conflict, and multiple caregivers. To meet their varying needs and provide proper care, the entire dental office, which includes dentists, hygienists, assistants, and front office staff, needs to collaborate and work together.

Elderly patients increasing rely on others as they age. Some patients no longer drive and depend on caregivers or transportation services to get to and from their appointments. When scheduling appointments, it may be best to schedule one long appointment rather than several short appointments to decrease the number of dental visits. Although elderly patients may have difficulty tolerating longer appointments, if given frequent breaks, the longer appointment times can prove to be more beneficial to both the patient and the dental team. The dental team should also keep in mind that elderly patients may have several care providers, so when scheduling multiple appointments, it is important to contact all care providers. If applicable, a list of care providers should be part of patients' dental records.

In addition, well-organized dental offices maintain open and continuous communication among patients, care providers, and dental team members to provide successful patient care appointments. Many of the scheduling challenges that elderly dental patients face can be eased by a dental team who works together efficiently, for example, by calling and reminding patients to take their premedication before appointments or e-mailing patients and care providers appointment times and dates. These are just a few examples of an efficient dental office that makes teamwork a priority while providing comprehensive dental care to elderly patients. ■

receiving the necessary oral care services required to meet the residents' oral needs. According to U.S. Census Bureau projections, the population of the oldest old, those aged 85 years and older, is expected to grow by 377% by the year 2050.[2] To ensure that adequate oral health care for immobilized older adults occurs, the dental community needs to embrace new paradigms in dental education, prevention, and treatment. Some dental communities have begun this paradigm shift by creating new curriculum in geriatric dentistry for dental and dental hygiene schools, implementing oral hygiene education into long-term care facilities, and educating the existing dental community on best practices when treating elderly patients (see Spotlight on Public Health).[2,7,8]

Because demographics are projecting a rapid increase in the number of older adults, the dental profession needs to be prepared. Providing dental care to

Spotlight on Public Health

Traveling to and from a dental office can be challenging for many elderly patients, especially those living in assisted care facilities. Some may require a medical transport vehicle and special transfer assistance to travel to and from the office. Others with walkers, canes, or motorized scooters may have difficulty navigating the stairs, hallways, and examining rooms of the dental office.

Providing transportation to appointments strains the care facility's resources, and the high cost of medical transport may result in the patient delaying or forgoing treatment. The patient's ability to pay for transportation services or coverage by Medicare or other insurance may determine the patient's access to dental care.

To combat these problems, Apple Tree Dental, a nonprofit organization, brings the dental office to the patient's care facility and provides all necessary dental care. Started more than 20 years ago by cofounder Dr. Michael Helgeson in Minneapolis, Minnesota, Apple Tree Dental consists of dental professional teams who travel to the patient using a mobile dental office system. The dental team, consisting of general and specialty dentists and hygienists, performs comprehensive dental care on patients who may not readily tolerate treatment at a traditional dental office or have the resources to get there.

Using large trucks, the Apple Tree Dental team transports mobile dental offices including all necessary dental equipment and supplies to the care facilities where elderly patients undergo urgent, restorative, and preventive dental care. At the care site, the visiting dentists and hygienists work with the patient's care facility staff to screen patients and collaboratively develop an individualized, comprehensive treatment plan for each patient. This team approach not only places importance on the patient's medical and dental needs but allows the responsibility of treatment decisions to be shared.

Before the initial and subsequent treatment visits, all members of the team are assigned specific tasks. For example, the care facility physician evaluates and monitors the patient's medical history for drug interactions and contraindications before and during treatment. The hygienist completes the dental hygiene assessments, demonstrates oral hygiene education to the patient and caregivers, and performs preventive treatments such as an oral prophylaxis and fluoride varnish. The dentist then reviews the assessments and conducts the dental examination to diagnose and complete all necessary dental treatment.

On-site dentistry not only increases dental care access for elderly patients, it allows for a more collaborative treatment approach and a higher quality of care. Apple Tree Dental provides mobile dental delivery services to more than 100 communities across Minnesota. It is expanding to several other states including North Carolina and Florida. On-site dentistry provides the elderly patient with a more efficient, cost-effective, and comfortable treatment experience delivered by professionals well-versed in understanding medical and dental needs of the elderly. ■

Sources: Elliott-Smith S. Teledentistry: a new view on oral health care. *Access.* 2007;21(2):8-15; and Helgeson M. Oral health in healthcare reform. Institute for Oral Health. 2010. IOHWA.org. Accessed October 9, 2011.

older adults with complex medical and dental conditions can be challenging. The dental professional needs to understand and identify the involved medical and dental conditions of older adults to anticipate, respond, and care for their oral health needs.[7,8]

WHAT IS AGING?

The definition of the term *older person* has been inconsistent and problematic for many researchers when studying the oral effects of aging. The three most commonly used definitions of age are chronological age, biological age, and functional age. **Chronological age,** the number of years a person has lived, is usually categorized into the following age brackets: younger old (ages 65–75), older-old (ages 75–85), and oldest old (ages 85+).[3] Although a person's chronological age may define how many years a person has lived, this number fails to describe the biological and functional changes a person can experience over the years. Most researchers agree that definition of age should be based on a person's physiological changes, as well as his or her ability to perform certain tasks. Although the majority of older adults are healthy and perform at a high degree of independent function, many adults older than 65 years have compromised health and limited abilities.[3,7,8]

A person's **biological age** describes how a person's body ages physiologically.[8] Medical assessments such as vital signs, bone density, basal metabolic rate, hearing, vision, balance, and flexibility are examples of instruments used to measure a person's biological age. Most risk factors are lifestyle choices that can be altered, such as nutrition, exercise, and smoking, and can impact a person's biological age.[3,7] Therefore, how individuals manage their life choices can either increase or decrease their biological aging process in varying degrees.

Functional age describes how a person interacts mentally and physically with his or her surroundings and is measured by the ability to perform certain ADL.

The following three functional age groups show the different levels of ADL:[3,7,8]

- **Functionally independent older adult** can independently perform ADL.
- **Functionally dependent older adult** can no longer survive without direct and daily help from others.
- **Frail older adult** can no longer live independently and must rely on help from others for food, daily chores, and transportation.[2,7,8]

When managing and treating older adults, the dental hygienist needs to assess a patient's biological and functional age to provide the best preventive and restorative options based on the person's abilities, capabilities, and need. Although many older adults have good oral habits and are capable of maintaining oral health throughout their lives, many others have complex medical, physical, and social limitations that hinder oral care. Regardless of how a person's chronological, biological, and functional age are defined, the goal of dental hygienists is to maintain or improve the person's quality of life.

PHYSIOLOGICAL AGING

Senescence (the aging process) progresses at different rates within different body systems in different individuals. Therefore, age-related changes in one system are not predictive of changes in other systems or other people.[9] For example, an older adult experiencing hearing loss can have excellent cardiovascular function, whereas someone with short-term memory loss may still be able to play tennis on a daily basis. For some researchers, it is still unclear what is considered age-related versus disease-related aging. For example, for people who have short-term memory loss, when does forgetting where you parked the car progress from being normal to **dementia** (brain disorder that results in deterioration of memory, concentration, and judgment)? Because everyone ages differently, understanding the aging process is a challenge for many researchers.[9,10]

Although it is still unknown exactly how the aging process occurs, many theories exist. Several studies show the effects of aging on the body's cells, organs, and organ systems, but how these effects come about is still in debate. At the cellular level, one theory discusses the accumulation of waste products in cells causing toxicity, dysfunction, and early cell death. Brown spots on the skin are a common result of waste product accumulation in skin cells. Another theory reviews

cellular changes in the connective tissue of organs and organ systems, which results in the loss of elasticity. This can impact a person's physical and sensory functions, such as muscle movement, hearing, and sight.[9] Researchers will continue to study the effects of aging on the body and develop additional treatments to manage age-related diseases.

Although a number of physiological changes occur as a person ages, the rate at which changes occur depends on the person's health. Age-related physiological changes occur in healthy individuals as opposed to pathological, or disease-related, changes that occur in unhealthy individuals. As noted earlier, a person's chronological age is not necessarily their physiological age.[7] For example, a healthy and active 75-year-old can be more functionally capable than a 60-year-old person with diabetes who smokes. For the dental hygiene professional, it is important to be able to recognize the normal changes of aging versus the effects of disease. Untreated disease can result in "excess disability" and reduce the quality of life of individuals.

The following section gives a brief summary of the physiological aging process for each system of the body. The brief overview focuses on the components that may be affected by age-related changes.

Cardiovascular System

The normal age-related changes that occur in the cardiovascular system do not significantly decrease the heart's main function, which is to circulate the blood throughout the body. However, the changes that occur in older adults cause an increase in heart contractions, which forces the heart to pump the same volume of blood as someone younger.[9] As a person ages, the heart, arteries, and veins lose elasticity, becoming stiff and hard. This causes an extra workload on the heart, and over time the heart increases in size. These vascular changes cause an increase in blood pressure, retention of tissue fluids, and a decrease in blood volume to vital organs such as the liver and kidneys. Although the resting heart rate and the cardiac output may remain the same, the working heart rate and blood pressure of a 70-year-old adult take longer to return to resting level following stress than someone who is 30 years old.[9] In addition, hypotension, the sudden drop in heart rate and blood pressure, commonly occurs in older adults who stand too quickly after sitting or lying down for a lengthy period.[9,11,12] See Chapter 37 for more information.

Respiratory System

As a person ages, the lung tissue progressively loses its elasticity, and the respiratory muscles weaken, causing the individual to breathe less efficiently. Alveoli, the saclike bundles located within the lungs, become enlarged and flattened, which reduces the surface area available for the gas exchange of oxygen and carbon dioxide.[9] At the age of 70, the lung capacity in a healthy individual declines by 50% from its peak functional ability, which occurs at approximately age 30.

This decrease in the complete exchange of oxygen and carbon dioxide makes inspiration (breathing in) and expiration (breathing out) more difficult. In healthy older adults, reduced gas exchange is not a sign of disease and usually does not hamper a person's daily living activities.[9,11,12] Only when the adult is fighting a respiratory infection or performing a physical activity does the diminished breathing capability become apparent. See Chapter 38 for more information.

Gastrointestinal System

In general, aging affects only minor physiological changes in the gastrointestinal system. The most notable change is **achlorhydria,** the insufficient production of gastric acid in the stomach. Achlorhydria decreases the absorption of important nutrients, which puts a person at risk for nutritional deficiencies.[9,11] For example, a vitamin B_{12} deficiency is the most common result of achlorhydria. For vitamin B_{12} to be absorbed in the stomach, an adequate amount of gastric acid, along with a protein and an enzyme, must be produced. A deficiency of vitamin B_{12} can cause permanent neurological damage and symptoms including tingling of the arms and legs, fatigue, and dementia.[9] Although achlorhydria is considered a normal age-related condition, it is important to recognize the symptoms early for the correct diagnosis and treatment.

The large intestines are also affected by age. Peristalsis, wavelike muscular contractions, pushes ingested food and waste through the large intestines and colon. With age, the contractions are reduced and the movement of waste products is slowed, leading to constipation. Even though constipation is a common complaint in many healthy older adults, poor eating habits, lack of exercise, and medications are also factors that contribute to the problem.[9,11] A healthy diet and daily exercise can decrease gastrointestinal problems along with many other conditions of aging.

Urinary System

During the aging process, both the kidneys and the bladder undergo significant changes. Beginning at approximately age 40 years, the function of the kidneys begins to decline, reducing the body's ability to filter blood and dispose of wastes and excess fluids.[9] By the age of 80, blood flow to the kidneys is reduced by 50%, whereas kidney mass is reduced by 40%. Both reductions decrease the rate at which the blood is filtered by the kidneys.[10] With age, maintaining fluid homeostasis becomes problematic. With a decrease in function, the kidneys are less able to maintain fluid concentrations. Older adults will have either too much or not enough body fluids, causing either swelling or dehydration. Dehydration is commonly seen in older adults because their recognition for thirst diminishes and their body's signal to replenish fluids declines. Dehydration symptoms include sleepiness, irritability, and in severe cases, delirium. These symptoms can also mimic many disease conditions.[9,11]

Endocrine System

Normal aging alters the amount of hormones produced and secreted by the endocrine system's glandular tissues, including the pituitary, pineal, thyroid, and reproductive glands, as well as the hypothalamus, thymus, and pancreas.[9,11] The change in hormone levels produced by these glands decreases the body's ability to regulate various bodily functions.[9] Examples of altered functions include body temperature, nutrient resorption, stress response, target cell response to insulin, and heart function. Many older adults adapt to the changes and function well.[9,11] See Chapter 42 for more information.

Brain and Nervous System

Age-related physiological changes to the brain and nervous system show a slow decline in the size of the brain after the age of 35.[9] Research shows that after the mid-30s, individuals lose approximately 0.4% of brain matter annually until age 65 years and 1% annually after the age of 65.[10] In addition, older neuron cells may become demyelinated and have fewer dendrites as people age, which may slow message transmission at the synapse. Although most of these neurological changes do not appear to affect daily living activities in those aged 65 to 85 years, after the age of 85, the incidence of cognitive impairment increases substantially.[10,12]

Research studies have shown a degree of cognitive impairment in approximately one third of individuals 85 years and older. These impairments include the inability to stay focused, difficulty correctly combining words, short-term memory loss, and a slower reaction time.[10] Although long-term memory and verbal intelligence remain relatively stable in healthy older adults and extend well into their later years, short-term memory is often lost first. The ability of older adults to recall information from the past such as where they grew up or worked may remain intact, but their ability to recall what happened the day before is a struggle.[10,12] See Chapter 41 for more information about neurological impairments.

Immune System

With age, immune system function decreases as the body's production of effective antibodies diminishes, reducing a person's ability to fight infections. Antibodies are "memory cells" such as T cells and B cells that travel through the body looking for infectious agents such as the influenza virus or streptococcus bacteria that previously invaded the body.[10] A body with ineffective antibodies has difficulty fighting virulent pathogens. Therefore, older adults with diminished immune systems are more susceptible to pathogenic diseases such as pneumonia and influenza.[10,12]

In addition, adults are at an increased risk for developing autoimmune diseases because of the immune system's autoantibodies, which increase in prevalence as people age. Autoantibodies are antibodies that attack parts of the body instead of the invading pathogens when the body's immune system has difficulty recognizing itself.[10] Examples of autoimmune diseases include lupus, rheumatoid arthritis, and multiple sclerosis. Although autoimmune diseases may occur at any age, older adults have shown a higher incidence and prevalence of the diseases.[12]

The immune system is the body's defense system. It protects the body from viral, bacterial, and autoimmune diseases.[10] With advancing age, the immune system function decreases in older adults, increasing their risk for infections and diseases. When treating older adults, it is important to identify changes in their immune system for early intervention and modifications to treatment.[10,12] See Chapter 43 for more information.

Musculoskeletal System

Age-related changes that occur to the musculoskeletal system result in a decline in bone density and muscle mass. Beginning at approximately age 40 years, the bone's osteoblasts (cells that grow bone) and osteoclasts (cells that destroy bone) gradually begin to decline, causing the bones to become thinner, more spongelike, and less dense.[10] Reduced bone density weakens the bones and increases the risks for gait problems, falls, and fractures in older adults. Bone loss also occurs in the body's structural support system, the vertebra column, resulting in a curvature of the spine and loss of height.

Muscle mass also decreases as a person ages. By the age of 80 years, a person typically loses about 23% of muscle mass because of the decrease in both the number and the size of the muscle fiber.[10] Loss of muscle mass in older adults reduces muscle strength, resulting in weakness, fatigue, and a reduced ability to perform ADL. However, it should be noted that older adults who engage in daily physical activities or exercises are able to maintain or even strengthen their muscle mass and tone.[10,13]

Sensory System

Hearing

Several age-related physiological changes occur in the ear. Located within the middle ear, the eardrum and the three small bones called the *ossicles* become sclerotic, or hardened, which can lead to a decrease in hearing acuity. In addition, excessive cerumen (ear wax) results in the auditory canal becoming narrower, which can interfere with the conduction of sounds. If left untreated, both the hardening of the middle ear tissues and bones and the buildup of cerumen can eventually lead to hearing loss.[10,12]

Common auditory problems that affect aging older adults include presbycusis and tinnitus. **Presbycusis,** age-related hearing loss, progresses over many years and usually affects hearing high-frequency sounds. By the age of 70 years, more than 50% of adults have some presbycusis.[10] **Tinnitus,** a continuous ringing or buzzing in the ear, can be caused by presbycusis, anemia, or a thyroid hormone imbalance. Tinnitus can also be a negative side effect of many common medications such as NSAIDs, diuretics, and benzodiazepines.[10] Because tinnitus is a symptom rather than a disease, it can be difficult to treat, especially if the underlying cause is not apparent. Most patients suffering from tinnitus manage their symptoms using low-tone sounds to block out ringing or electrical devices made especially for tinnitus.[10,12]

Many older adults with hearing loss symptoms complain of difficulty discriminating the different sound pitches and understanding another person's speech, especially when there is background noise. Hearing loss can lead to isolation and, if it continues without treatment, depression and a decreased quality of life. Older adults may not recognize their hearing loss symptoms because their hearing declines slowly. By the time older adults realize they have a hearing problem, the symptoms have progressed well beyond the early stages.[10,12] See Chapter 39 for more information on auditory impairments.

Vision

As people age, their vision is affected by eye changes. One of the most common age-related changes of the eyes is **presbyopia**, a condition that makes it difficult to see things at close range. For most people, the condition starts around the age of 45 years and becomes noticeable when reading small print is a challenge.[10] Presbyopia occurs when the lens of the eye loses its elasticity and subsequently its ability to change shape. For the eyes to focus on small objects at close range, the lens of the eye needs to be able to change its shape. When this ability declines, focusing on nearby objects becomes more difficult. In addition, the ability of the pupils to contract and dilate declines, making adjustments to changes in light more difficult. For example, many older adults have difficulty driving at night and adjusting their eyes to glaring headlights and streetlights. Clarity in seeing certain colors, especially blues and greens, also decreases because of the yellowing of the eyes' lens. Even though these changes are considered a normal process of aging, they can affect older adults' daily living activities, such as reading, cooking, and driving, and increase the need for assistance.[10–12] See Chapter 39 for more information on visual impairments.

Integumentary System

The integumentary system consists of the skin, hair, nails, and glands, and it undergoes many physiological changes as a person ages. Although these changes are considered normal in older adults, these changes can also produce pathological effects. The integumentary system functions to protect the body from external damage as well as maintain homeostasis such as temperature regulation, hormone synthesis, and sensory perception, so any age-related changes to the system can increase the risk for injury, infection, and diseases.[9–11] For example, older adults are at a greater risk for skin cancer because they produce less melanin, have a slower cell turnover rate, and have a longer history of sun exposure than those who are younger.

The skin is the largest organ in the body and experiences significant changes during the aging process. The skin's outer epidermal cells change shape, become more irregular, and lose their function to retain water, causing the skin (epidermis) to gradually become thin and dry. The inner layer of the skin, called the *dermis*, consists of collagen and elastic fibers, sensory receptors, sweat, and sebaceous glands. With age, the collagen fibers harden while the elastic fibers lose their elasticity, resulting in wrinkles. The thinner, drier, and wrinkled skin is now more susceptible to trauma and infection. Common skin infections in the elderly include herpes zoster, pressure ulcers, bacterial cellulitis, and methicillin-resistant *Staphylococcus aureus*.[9,10]

In addition to skin infections, older adults also have an increased susceptible to heat strokes because the body's sweat gland function has decreased. Sweat glands regulate the body's temperature by transporting water to the skin's surface and cooling it down. When this function decreases, older adults can quickly become overheated. Older adults also struggle to stay warm. A diminishing number of blood vessels and a reduced amount of subcutaneous fat lead older adults to wear layers of clothing to compensate for their inability to regulate their body temperature. Their nerve endings have also diminished in number, altering their temperature sensation and increasing their risk for burns and skin lacerations.[9,10]

It is important for the dental hygiene professional to understand the changes that occur to the integumentary system during the aging process. In healthy older adults, the changes to the integumentary system are mostly superficial, a few more wrinkles and gray hairs. In unhealthy older adults, the changes to the integumentary system can be a sign of disease.

COMMON PATHOPHYSIOLOGICAL DISEASES OF THE ELDERLY

Pathophysiology is the study of the functional changes associated with diseases.

Alzheimer Disease

Definition and Etiology

Alzheimer disease is an irreversible, degenerative brain disease that affects 1 in 10 adults older than 65 years. A form of dementia, Alzheimer disease accounts for approximately 60% to 80% of all dementia cases, making it the most common.[13,14] The disease progresses gradually, and over time slowly diminishes a person's ability to think, remember, and eventually perform simple daily tasks such as dressing and bathing. Although the progression rate of the disease varies greatly from person to person, as some live with the disease for only 3 years and others survive for well

more than 20, the disease never improves. There is no known cure for Alzheimer disease, and it is always fatal.[13,14]

Alzheimer disease progresses gradually as protein amyloids called *plaques* and *tangles* accumulate in the brain and eventually kill the brain's cells.[14] The brain cell destruction begins at the synapse, the juncture where two neurons meet. Neurons are the pathway for the brain to communicate to the rest of the body. At the synapse, in healthy individuals, chemicals are exchanged signaling messages, such as to breathe, blink, cough, or raise a hand.[14] In patients with Alzheimer disease, a slow buildup of amyloid plaque proteins slowly forms on the brain's neuron synapses, and messages sent and received become muddled, delayed, or eventually cut off. Although a definitive diagnosis for Alzheimer disease occurs only after death with a brain autopsy, most physicians diagnose a patient using clinical observation.[14–16]

Epidemiology (Incidence and Prevalence)

Alzheimer disease rate is rapidly growing as the U.S. population continues to grow older. In 2010, it was reported that 5.4 million Americans suffered from Alzheimer disease; of those, 5.1 million, or 13%, were aged 65 and older. By 2020, this number is expected to double largely because of the aging baby boomers, who began to turn 65 in 2011. Unless new treatments are developed to decrease the likelihood of developing Alzheimer disease in the United States, the number of individuals with the disease is expected to be 14 million by the year 2050.[14]

Risk Factors

Although there are no definitive tests to determine who will or will not develop Alzheimer disease, having one or more risk factors can certainly increase the likelihood. The primary risk factors for Alzheimer disease include advancing age, family history, and genetics. The number one risk factor is advancing age. Ten percent of individuals older than 65 years and more than 50% of those older than 85 years have Alzheimer disease.[14,15] Although those younger than 65 years can be afflicted with Alzheimer disease, this type of early onset rarely occurs. Alzheimer disease is not a normal part of aging and is not something that inevitably happens in later life. Many people live to be more than 100 years of age and never develop the disease.[14,15] However, Alzheimer disease is a concern for our aging population, as well as those who care for them.

Research has shown that those who have a parent or siblings with Alzheimer disease are at an increased risk of 2- to 3-fold for developing the disease compared with those who do not have a relative with the disease. Moreover, if more than one family member has the disease, the risk continues to increase. It is important to also know that having a family history is not a guarantee that an individual will get the disease.[14,15]

Signs and Symptoms

Because there are no definitive tests for Alzheimer disease and the symptoms usually develop gradually over time, physicians find the disease difficult to diagnose.[14] Physicians routinely assess and evaluate a patient's past and present memory as well as cognitive and psychomotor functions to detect for abnormal memory loss and behaviors. Although most people older than 65 years display some form of forgetfulness, such as a person's name or where they placed their car keys, a person with Alzheimer disease progresses far beyond this occasional memory lapse (Table 48-1).[14,16]

After the initial diagnosis of Alzheimer disease, the patient's memory, cognitive, and psychomotor abilities generally progress through stages. Although the duration of each stage of the disease varies considerably from patient to patient, the symptoms always follow the same progression, from mild to severe.[14,16]

Early/Mild Stage (Duration: 2–4 Years)

In the earlier stages of Alzheimer disease, when the symptoms are mild, individuals with the disease can live independently, particularly when taking prescription medications that manage the symptoms and prolong the early stage of the disease. During this first stage, the patient with Alzheimer disease tends to show minor memory loss by forgetting names of familiar faces, placing everyday items in odd locations, and repeating answered questions, such as the date and time. Individuals at this stage may exhibit mild coordination problems, such as writing illegibly or stumbling when they walk. They may become confused, get easily lost, and have difficulty performing daily tasks. Mood swings are common as their temperament can change from anger to tears for no apparent reason. Hobbies that once brought them joy no longer interest them as they become withdrawn and depressed.[14,16,17]

Middle/Moderate Stage (Duration: 2–10 Years)

As the patient enters the second stage of Alzheimer disease, his or her need for assistance becomes more apparent as the ability to live independently becomes increasingly difficult. Symptoms revealed during the first stage become more noticeable at the middle stage as patients rapidly lose cognitive function. Memory loss progresses, and recognizing familiar faces becomes more difficult. Patients often forget personal information like their home address and telephone number while being unaware that they do not remember things. Also at this stage, most with Alzheimer disease lose the ability to communicate coherently and experience personality changes, becoming withdrawn, exhibiting paranoid behavior, and having hallucinations. Toward the end of this stage, they become increasingly dependent on others for help and need live-in care to monitor their daily living activities, which can include eating, dressing, and bathing.[14,16,17]

Late/Severe Stage (Duration: 1–3+ Years)

During the final stage of Alzheimer disease, patients gradually lose control of body functions and begin to sleep often. Their memory loss progresses to the point that they won't recognize others or know their own name. Language and the means to communicate have also diminished, decreasing the ability to convey their pain. At this time, the patient with Alzheimer requires round-the-clock care and assistance for all daily activities. As Alzheimer runs its course, the bedridden patient weakens and becomes more vulnerable

Table 48-1. *Signs of Normal Aging Changes Versus Early Alzheimer Symptoms*	
Normal	**Early Alzheimer Disease**
Misplaces keys	Routinely places important items in odd places, such as keys in the fridge or wallet in the dishwasher
Searches for casual names and words	Forgets names of family members and common objects, or substitutes words with inappropriate ones
Briefly forgets conversation details	Frequently forgets entire conversations
Feels the cold more	Disregards the weather when dressing; e.g., wears several layers of clothes on a warm day or shorts in a snowstorm
Cannot find a recipe	Cannot follow recipe directions
Forgets to record a check	Can no longer manage checkbook, balance figures, solve problems, or think abstractly
Cancels a date with friends	Withdraws from usual interests and activities, sits in front of the TV for hours, sleeps far more than usual
Makes an occasional wrong turn	Gets lost in familiar places, does not remember how he or she got there or how to get home
Occasionally feels sad	Experiences rapid mood swings, from tears to rage, for no discernible reason

to illnesses and infections. Pneumonia or respiratory failure is the leading cause of death in patients with Alzheimer.[14,16,17]

Dental Hygiene Considerations

Patients with Alzheimer disease often lose the ability to brush their teeth effectively, which can rapidly lead to caries, dental abscesses, and multiple tooth loss. Their appetite and diet also changes, further increasing their risk for caries and oral lesions. In addition, the multiple medications they take to manage their disease frequently have oral side effects, which include xerostomia, and again lead to oral complications, such as caries.[18]

In addition to a high caries risk, Alzheimer disease patients with poor oral hygiene also are at high risk for contracting aspiration pneumonia. Studies have shown that institutionalized patients with poor oral hygiene have an increased risk for contracting bacterial aspiration pneumonia, especially those patients on a ventilator.[19] Because pneumonia is one of the leading causes of death for an Alzheimer disease patient, caregivers and dental hygiene professionals need to be aware of this risk and attend to patient's health-care needs accordingly.

As Alzheimer disease progresses, the patient may not be able to communicate feelings of discomfort or pain, and dental infections may progress to a severe stage before the patent is brought in for a dental examination. Patients with Alzheimer disease should be scheduled for frequent dental appointments to detect potential problems before they become untreatable.[18] The following are dental management recommendations that coincide with the three stages of Alzheimer disease (Table 48-2).

Early/Mild Stage

Patients in the mild stage of Alzheimer disease should schedule routine dental appointments for preventive and restorative care while they are still able to perform basic oral hygiene procedures and cooperate in the dental chair.[18] During these appointments, it is essential for the dental health professional to educate and instruct both the patient and their personal care providers (PCPs) on how to use additional oral hygiene aids to maintain and preserve oral health. Many products such as the electric toothbrush, electric flosser, and water pic can help the patient and PCP when challenged with the patient's declining psychomotor and cognitive functions. Supplemental products such as chlorhexidine rinses and fluoride varnishes are also recommended as both preventive and treatment regimens.[18]

Middle/Moderate Stage

Patients in the moderate stage of Alzheimer disease are more anxious and less cooperative during dental procedures than those in the mild stage. The patient may need to be sedated using oral medications before the dental appointment to enable the dental professionals

Table 48-2. *Three Stages of Alzheimer Disease*		
Stage	**Characteristics**	**Dental Hygiene Care**
Early Duration: 2–4 years	Frequent recent memory loss, particularly of recent conversations and events; repeated questions, some problems expressing and understanding language; mild coordination problems with writing and using objects; depression and apathy can occur, accompanied by mood swings; need reminders for daily activities, and may have difficulty driving	Recommend electric toothbrush and flosser and a video on how to use these oral hygiene aids. Need verbal or written reminders (recommend patient to post notes on bathroom mirror to brush and floss).
Middle Duration: 2–10 years	Pervasive and persistent memory loss, unable to recognize friends and family; rambling speech, unusual reasoning, and confusion about current events, time, and place; more likely to become lost in familiar settings, experience sleep disturbances, and changes in mood and behavior; mobility and coordination is affected by slowness, rigidity, and tremors; need structure, reminders, and assistance with the activities of daily living	Instruct care providers on how to provide adequate oral hygiene for patients, such as using an electric toothbrush, and chlorhexidine or fluoride swabs. Schedule routine dental visits for examinations if patient is compliant or teledentistry and mobile visits if available.
Late Duration: 1–3+ years	Loss of ability to remember, communicate, or process information; generally incapacitated with severe-to-total loss of verbal skills; problems with swallowing, incontinence, and illness; extreme problems with mood and behavior; support and care needed 24 hr/day	Care providers should continue oral-care regimen, if able. Continue chlorhexidine or fluoride swabs. Emergency palliative dental treatments routinely require sedation.

to complete the necessary treatment. At this stage, dental treatment should be focused on extracting teeth that are causing or will eventually cause pain, such as large carious lesions and aggressive periodontal disease.[18] As patients' symptoms and disease progresses, their performance and dexterity decreases along with their ability to maintain adequate home care. Forgetting to brush and floss or how to accomplish either becomes common at this stage. Because the patient's PCPs may struggle with the patient to complete adequate oral hygiene care, it is recommended to use chlorhexidine or fluoride swabs daily to decrease bacterial count in oral flora.[18]

Late/Severe Stage

Dental treatment during the last stage of Alzheimer disease is predominantly palliative care.[18] Patients at this stage are generally incapacitated and exhibit extreme mood swings. Care providers will continue to struggle to complete daily personal home care including oral hygiene care. Daily use of chlorhexidine or fluoride swabs is recommended to decrease bacterial count in oral flora. If available, teledentistry or mobile dentistry should be scheduled for oral examinations.[18] See Chapter 50 for information on mobile dentistry.

OTHER COMMON SYSTEMIC DISEASES IN THE ELDERLY

The systemic diseases and conditions commonly experienced by the elderly population include arthritis, cancer, **chronic obstructive pulmonary disease (COPD),** diabetes, heart disease, osteoporosis, Parkinson disease, and stroke (Table 48-3).[6,19–22] A brief description of each disease or condition together with suggestions for dental management, treatment, and preventive considerations follows.

Table 48-3. *Common Age-Related Diseases and Conditions in the Elderly*

Disease or Condition	Patient Education	Dental Hygiene Treatment Considerations
Arthritis	Adapt toothbrush handles with larger grips Recommend electric toothbrushes and oral irrigators	Increased bleeding caused by medications Reduced dexterity for oral hygiene Joint discomfort in the dental chair—change chair position Possible need for corticosteroid supplementation and antibiotic Coverage for joint prostheses
Head and neck cancer	Smoking and tobacco chewing cessation Reduce alcohol intake, if heavy Limit sun exposure Recommend saliva substitutes, at-home fluoride dentifrices, gels, or rinses	In-office brush biopsy (OralCDx) and fluoroscope (VELscope) Need for oral health before cancer therapy Patient may experience reduced saliva—xerostomia, increased caries, and painful ulcerations In-office fluoride applications
Chronic obstructive pulmonary disease	Decrease in oral health can increase respiratory infection	Management depends on extent of dyspnea Medications include bronchodilators and/or corticosteroids Patient best treated in upright position Use of ultrasonic instruments is contraindicated Avoid nitrous oxide sedation
Diabetes	Eating and taking medications before appointments Maintaining blood sugar before and after appointments Association between periodontal disease and uncontrolled blood sugar levels	Risk for hypoglycemia is main concern during dental treatment Blood glucose level at the peak should be <180 mg/dL and Hb A_{1c} level <7% Patients with poorly controlled diabetes require medical clearance; may be immunocompromised; patient is more susceptible to infections and may require more aggressive infection management
Ischemic heart disease Angina Myocardial infarction	Taking NSAIDs can increase the effects of anticoagulants (drugs used to prevent blood clot formation) Patient to bring nitroglycerin medication	Defer elective care for 6 months after myocardial infarction Schedule short morning appointments Use stress-reduction protocols

Table 48-3. *Common Age-Related Diseases and Conditions in the Elderly—cont'd*

Disease or Condition	Patient Education	Dental Hygiene Treatment Considerations
		Limit use of epinephrine Ask patients about their prothrombin time—Internation Normalized Ratio should be 2.0–3.0
Hypertension	Prehypertension stage: 120–149/ 80–89 mm Hg Discuss risk factors (smoking, high-sodium diet, lack of exercise, and weight gain) with patient Discuss importance of medication compliance	Take patient's blood pressure before treatment. Control before treatment—medical consult Avoidance of anxiety and pain—local anesthetics Increased risk for orthostatic hypotension Allow for restroom breaks for long appointments because of diuretic medications
Dementia Alzheimer disease	Educate caregivers on oral care for patients Recommend 0.12% chlorhexidine and prescription fluoride gels and rinse	Behavioral problems Decrease in cognitive and motor skills increases oral disease In-office 5% fluoride varnish application—caries prevention Reduced cooperation as disease advances
Osteoporosis	Bisphosphonate-related osteonecrosis of the jaw (BRONJ)—90% of the cases occur due to IV bisphosphonate therapy	Increase risk for BRONJ—complete dental treatment before bisphosphonate therapy begins
Parkinson disease	Patients may exhibit difficulty with small motor skill function such as brushing and flossing Recommend electric toothbrush with large handle Educate caregivers on oral care for patients	Involuntary movements, restorative care increasingly difficult as the disease progresses
Stroke	Patients may exhibit a decrease in motor skill function Recommend electric toothbrush with large handle Caregiver assistance may be necessary Educate caregivers on oral care for patients Patients who wear dentures may need assistance with their placement and maintenance	Defer elective care for 6 months after stroke Patient can experience confusion, mobility and/or communication problems, deterioration of oral hygiene Short sessions and treat patient upright
Xerostomia	Home fluoride dentifrices, gels, and rinses Over-the-counter saliva substitutes Electric toothbrushes and flossers Oral irrigators Xylitol products	In-office 5% fluoride varnish application—caries prevention Ulcers and other sores caused by dentures and partials

Sources: Optimal oral health for frail older adults: best practices along the continuum of care. Ottawa (ON): Canadian Dental Association Committee on Clinical and Scientific Affairs. http://www.cda-adc.ca/_files/dental_profession/practising/best_practices_seniors/optimal_oral_health_older_adults_2009.pdf. Published July 2009. Accessed January 28, 2015; Szarejko M. Dental considerations for geriatric patients. http://www.netce.com/coursecontent.php?courseid=842. Released June 1, 2012. Accessed January 28, 2015.

Arthritis

Arthritis is a chronic condition that is characterized by pain, swelling, and stiffness in the joints. Primarily affecting the body's muscles, bones, and joints, arthritis can also systemically affect the whole body by compromising the immune system. Approximately 50% of, or 16 million, U.S. adults older than 65 years are afflicted with arthritis, and this number is expected to increase to 60 million by 2020.[6,22] The two most prevalent forms of arthritis are osteoarthritis and rheumatoid arthritis. Both arise from an inflammatory mechanism that causes pain and swelling in the joints, which can limit an individual's daily living activities. Arthritis commonly affects the hands, feet, knees, and hips, and can become severe enough to manifest into degenerative joint disease that requires joint replacement surgery.[6,23,24]

Dental Hygiene Considerations

When treating older adults with arthritis, the dental professional should consider several factors to adequately treat and manage their patients' oral-care needs. Dental appointments should be routinely scheduled to monitor patients' oral hygiene care. Appointment times are best scheduled for the late morning or early afternoon because joint stiffness tends to improve during the day. Supine positioning may be uncomfortable for patients with arthritis, and they may need neck and leg supports.[6,18]

Patients with arthritis who experience dexterity limitations in their hands may have difficulty maintaining adequate plaque control. These patients may benefit from using an electric toothbrush and flosser or a manual toothbrush with specially adapted handles, such as a ball added to a toothbrush handle to help the patient grip.[6,18,23] See Chapter 49 for more information on adapting dental hygiene tools for patients with physical challenges.

Many patients with arthritis take NSAIDs for pain control and to manage joint inflammation. Because NSAIDs can cause increased bleeding, the patient's bleeding tendency needs to be monitored during invasive treatment. Also, supplemental corticosteroids or antibiotic coverage may be necessary for patients with rheumatoid arthritis before performing any invasive procedures because of their compromised immune systems.

Chronic Obstructive Pulmonary Disease

COPD is a progressive lung disease that obstructs airflow and interferes with breathing. COPD includes asthma, chronic bronchitis, and emphysema.[6] In 2010, about 12 million people older than 65 years were reported to have COPD, with another 12 million estimated undiagnosed cases.[6,24]

Dental Hygiene Considerations

Before providing dental care to patients with COPD, it is important for the dental hygienist to understand the breathing difficulties patients can experience and the recommended modifications for treatment. There are three risks categories—low, moderate, and high—based on patients' breathing difficulties:[18]

1. Low-risk patients may experience breathing difficulties but have normal exchange of oxygen and carbon dioxide. All necessary dental or dental hygiene care services can be performed on these patients with minor modifications.
2. Moderate-risk patients experience breathing difficulties when climbing stairs and are treated with bronchodilators, corticosteroids, and/or partial pressure of oxygen. Before any dental or dental hygiene treatment begins, it is advised to seek a medical consultation with the patient's physician.
3. High-risk patients experience symptomatic COPD that is either undiagnosed, untreated, or both. A medical consultation is necessary before starting any dental or dental hygiene care.

Treatment modifications for patients with COPD include sitting patients in an upright position because of their increased breathing difficulties when in supine position, and scheduling appointments at midmorning or in the early afternoon after medications have taken effect and breathing has improved. Patients who are taking corticosteroids for COPD should be treated with appropriate consideration because they do not heal well or tolerate stress well.[6,18]

Diabetes

Diabetes mellitus is a chronic metabolic disease caused either by the body's insufficient production of insulin or the body's inability to respond to the insulin produced. In 2010, the CDC reported 10.9 million, or 26.9% of, adults aged 65 years and older had diabetes. Diabetes can lead to systemic complications such as hypertension, blindness and eye problems, kidney disease, and nervous system disease.[25] Studies have also reported oral complications from diabetes. Recent research has shown an association with poor blood sugar control and the incidence and progression of periodontal disease in patients with diabetes, as well as inversely an association with uncontrolled periodontal disease affecting the control of blood sugar/diabetes.[6]

Symptoms associated with diabetes include polydipsia (increased thirst), polyuria (increased quantity of urine passed and, often, the need to urinate frequently), and polyphagia (increased appetite).[20] In older adults, these symptoms can be exacerbated when the diabetes is poorly controlled. Older adults with well-controlled diabetes have fewer oral health problems than adults with poorly controlled diabetes. At each appointment the dental professional should ask patients with diabetes the following questions: When did you last eat? At what time did you take your medications? At what time did you last take your blood glucose reading? What was the result of that reading?

Dental Hygiene Considerations

Patients with diabetes need to plan their dental visits carefully. Maintaining their blood sugar levels before, during, and after dental procedures will help avoid a medical emergency in the dental office. To avoid hypoglycemia during treatment, it is essential that patients with diabetes eat and take their medications before any dental procedures. Older patients are especially prone to hypoglycemic episodes because dental appointments can disrupt their normal pattern of food and medication intake.[6,20]

For patients with uncontrolled diabetes, a medical clearance may be necessary before any dental procedures (other than emergency care) are performed. Patients with diabetes, particularly uncontrolled diabetes, take longer to heal after invasive dental treatment; therefore, antibiotic premedication maybe necessary before treating the soft tissues and bone, such as root planing, grafts, extractions, and implants. Patients with uncontrolled diabetes should be referred to their physician to evaluate and determine whether antibiotic premedication is required.[6,20] For more information on treating patients with diabetes, see Chapter 42.

Cardiovascular Disease

Cardiovascular disease is discussed in Chapter 37; therefore, refer to that chapter for detailed explanations of cardiovascular disease and its relation to oral health.

Dental Hygiene Considerations

Many older adults with heart conditions take multiple medications, which can affect dental treatment. It is important for the dental hygienist to review each medication for dental considerations and follow the appropriate management.[20] For example, patients who are taking warfarin (Coumadin), a blood thinner, may need to have their dosage adjusted before any invasive dental procedures such as extractions, implants, and root planing are performed. Serious complications can arise if invasive treatment is performed on patients taking warfarin (Coumadin) or other blood thinners if their International Normalized Ratio (INR) is greater than 3.5. A safe INR range to perform both invasive and noninvasive dental procedures is between 2.0 and 2.5.[4,6,21] INR measures the time it takes for a patient's blood to clot; an INR of 3.5 may indicate the blood is clotting too slowly. Medication reference books and online sources are available to research medications. Ideally, it is best to contact the patient's physician before treatment.

Osteoporosis

Osteoporosis is a disease characterized by a thinning and weakening of the bones resulting in bone fractures of the hip, wrist, and spine. In aging adults, bone mass decrease occurs when the activity of the bone's building cells (osteoblasts) decrease while the bone's destroying cells (osteoclasts) stay the same. This imbalance in bone growth can lead to osteoporosis. Menopausal women are at an increased risk for the disease and have an incidence rate that is four times greater than men. Older adults afflicted with osteoporosis have reduced mobility.[19]

Dental Hygiene Considerations

Older adults with osteoporosis are routinely prescribed medications called *bisphosphonates* for their condition. Bisphosphonates, pamidronate and zoledronate, which are primarily used intravenously, are concerns for the dental professional because they can lead to osteonecrosis of the jaws (ONJ). ONJ is a painful refractory bone exposure in the jaws that is observed after invasive dental procedures involving the alveolar bone, such as tooth extractions or implants (see Advancing Technologies).[6,20]

Therefore, whenever possible, dentists should avoid performing extractions and elective oral surgery in patients taking intravenous bisphosphonates. If surgery is essential, the dentist must counsel the patient and the patient's physician about the risks of intravenous bisphosphonate treatment.[6,20] For more information on treating patients who are taking intravenous bisphosphonates, see Chapter 48.

Parkinson Disease

Parkinson disease is a progressive neurological disorder that affects more than 1.5 million people in the United States. Because the disease is degenerative (i.e., gets worse over time), older adults, those 65 years and older, are impacted the most. Parkinson disease is caused by a reduction in the brain cells that produce the chemical dopamine, which plays a major role in muscle control. The disease is characterized by involuntary muscle movements and tremors of the head, arms, and legs, which cause fine motor skill, balance, and gait problems. For example, many people with Parkinson disease shuffle in a stooped position when they walk and have difficulty using their hands to complete tasks such as writing or brushing their teeth.

Dental Hygiene Considerations

Treating patients with Parkinson disease can be both challenging and problematic because the patient's involuntary head movements and excessive drooling may compromise the completion of dental services. Using sharp dental instruments on patients with involuntary head movements can make treatment hazardous to both patient and dental hygienist. Because the disease is degenerative, patients should schedule routine dental care appointments to closely monitor oral hygiene care and treatment needs. Recommended oral hygiene aids include the electric toothbrush and flosser along with a prescription fluoride for home use. For patients who need assistance at home, it is critical for the dental professional to give the PCP instructions on how to perform oral hygiene care on patients.[6,18,22]

Stroke

A **stroke** is a sudden disruption of blood supply to the brain after a blockage of an artery or a hemorrhage. In the United States, approximately 8% of adults 65 years and older has a history of stroke. A stroke occurs when the neurons in the stroke area are deprived of oxygen and glucose and within minutes start to die. Depending on the area of the brain that is affected, the patient may have cognitive, motor, or sensory deficits.[20,22] Many older adults who experience a stroke are initially confused and may experience emotional distress and depression. Physical therapy along with persistence and encouragement can help stroke patients improve their functions, although they rarely recover 100% of their prestroke functions.[6,18]

Dental Hygiene Considerations

Support with preventive care is critical for stroke patients; oral hygiene tends to deteriorate on the paralyzed side, and impaired manual dexterity may interfere with tooth brushing. Use of an electric toothbrush or adaptive holders may help.[6,18]

Dentists should defer elective and invasive dental care for patients who have had transient ischemic

Advancing Technologies

New technologies in tissue engineering continue to advance with the use of cultivated stems cells to grow new teeth. Infused with a growth factor and layered over a scaffold, the stem cells over a period of just 9 weeks can produce an anatomically correct tooth. Animal studies conducted by Dr. Jeremy Mao, a professor of Dental Medicine at Columbia University Medical Center, has pioneered this technique by using a biocompatible scaffold covered with stem cells and implanted in the mouth to grow a new tooth within the alveolar bone. This advanced technology—to grow and regenerate dental tissue from stem cells—could replace the need for dental implants in the future.

Although the use of stem cells in the medical and dental field is still years away, researchers continue to study for viable, cost-effective, and ethical justifications to replicate stem cells. One such way is for people to bank and save their own personal stem cells. Researchers at the National Institutes of Health discovered that potent stem cells found in the pulp of primary teeth and the dental follicle sack surrounding forming third molars are excellent sources for stem cell replication. If people could save or bank their own stem cells, this could potentially reduce cost and dissipate ethical concerns that surround these issues today.

Dental stem cells also have the potential to save many lives because teeth are not the only tissue that can be replicated. Studies have shown that stem cells from primary teeth multiply rapidly and differentiate into a wide array of tissues, and thus hold promise in many cell-based therapies such as spinal cord injury, cardiovascular disease, Parkinson disease, and even diabetes because of its early 6-week embryonic development stage.

Several companies in the United States and internationally provide services for patients to bank dental stem cells for future use in both medicine and dentistry. Before a planned office visit for the removal of a primary tooth or third molar, the patient or parent contacts the stem cell banking service to receive a Food and Drug Administration–approved and American Dental Association–accepted kit. After the tooth is removed, it is medically stored at chairside and shipped to facilities where the tissues undergo cryopreservation.

There are several advantages to retrieving and banking dental stem cells compared with other stem cells. Retrieving dental stems cells is a less invasive procedure than harvesting bone marrow stem cells, has fewer ethical considerations than embryonic cells, and is easier and less costly than umbilical cord blood collection and storage. The added benefit of banking dental stem cells for future use is the potential for research to progress to offer clear options for tissue repair and regeneration for both medical and dental patients. ■

Sources: Tissue engineering technique yields potential biological substitute for dental implants. http://www.sciencedaily.com/releases/2010/05/100524111724.htm. May 10, 2010; National Institutes of Health, U.S. Department of Health and Human Services. Stem cell information. http://stemcells.nih.gov. Accessed December 12, 2011; Peng L, Ye L, Zhou XD. Mesenchymal stem cells and tooth engineering. *Int J Oral Sci.* 2009;1(1):6-12; and Spolarch A. The regenerative process. *Dimens Dent Hygiene.* 2009;7(2):38-41.

attacks or strokes for 3 months after the event. It is important to communicate clearly with the stroke patient by facing the patient without a mask on, speaking slowly and clearly, and using language that is not complex.[6,18] It is recommended to schedule short treatment sessions for either the late morning or early afternoon. Patients who have difficulty swallowing should be treated in an upright position, if possible, to prevent foreign objects from entering the pharynx.[6,18]

For preventive care, support is critical. Most stroke patients have impaired manual dexterity and are unable to maintain adequate oral hygiene, especially on their paralyzed or partially paralyzed side, which shows the biggest decline. It is recommended to educate and instruct the patient's care provider in oral care techniques, such as the use of an electric toothbrush and flosser. Supplement prescription fluorides are also recommended.[6,18]

NORMAL AND PATHOLOGICAL ORAL CHANGES IN THE ELDERLY

Most healthy older adults do not experience significant destructive changes in their mouths as they age. Research shows that age alone is not a factor in development of diseases and conditions of the oral cavity.[6,20] Although some individuals may encounter oral changes such as chipped and yellowing teeth or aging dental restorations, these changes, for the most part, are considered normal wear and occur from regular use.[26] Older adults who develop and maintain a healthy lifestyle increase their likelihood of having a healthy body, including the oral cavity.

Conversely, unhealthy older adults are at risk for many oral diseases and conditions. The most common include caries, periodontal disease, and oral cancer. Many factors, including decreased saliva function, inadequate oral hygiene self-care, and irregular dental examinations, contribute to the severity and occurrence of these pathological conditions.[20,21,26] Older adults with pathological oral conditions are also more likely to have financial difficulties, be homebound or institutionalized, and suffer from physical disabilities.[20] When managing and treating older adult patients, it is important for the dental professional to differentiate between normal and pathological oral conditions, assess oral health risks, and identify barriers that may impede patients' oral health care.

Lips

Lips that appear cracked and dry are not necessarily related to disease and are primarily due to dehydration. Aging adults tend to lose their thirst sensation and drink less. Because many older adults are not drinking enough daily fluids, it is important to encourage them to rehydrate with water throughout the day even if they are not thirsty.[27,28]

Oral Mucosa

In healthy older adults, lips and oral mucosa generally appear no different than those in younger adults. Clinically, the dental hygienist should see no changes on the inner lining of the lips, cheek, and floor of mouth or any area composed of stratified squamous epithelial cells. Histologically, though, there are age-related changes as the mucosal lining loses both its resiliency and elasticity and becomes thinner. As the epithelium thins, the tissue becomes more prone to injury, predisposing the older adult patient to infections.[20,26,28]

Tongue

Clinically, in older adults, the most noticeable age-related changes to the tongue are the sublingual varicosities. Located on either side of the midline on the ventral surface of the tongue, the sublingual varicosities appear deep red or blue and, at times, enlarged. With age, the tongue shows a decline in both taste and function as the renewal rate of the taste buds decreases.[27]

Taste buds, which are associated with the foliate, fungiform, and circumvallate papillae, are located on the tongue and function to give the sensations of sweet, salty, bitter, and sour. Of the four taste perceptions, the only one that declines in older adults is salty. Yet, aging older adults still complain of a diminishing taste in foods and add flavoring agents or spices to enhance flavor. The decline in taste comes largely from the dramatic decrease in the sense of smell rather than taste. A decline in an older adult's olfactory acuity has a direct effect on the sense of taste.[9]

Salivary Glands

Salivary flow should remain unchanged as a healthy person ages. Noticeable changes in the amount and flow of saliva signal a pathological condition. These conditions can be induced by medications, tumor, radiation, and systemic diseases and cause a reduction in salivary flow as well as nutritional deficiencies.[26,27]

COMMON PATHOLOGICAL ORAL CONDITIONS

Xerostomia

Xerostomia, or dry mouth, is not a normal part of aging. It is often a side effect of certain medications but can also develop from other causes. Multiple factors contribute to dry mouth, with multiple treatment options available (see Evidence-Based Practice). Sjögren syndrome is a disorder of the immune system that is identified by dryness in the mouth. Medications that cause xerostomia include diuretics such as furosemide (Lasix), antihypertensives, antidepressants, and antihistamines.[29]

Oral Candidiasis

Many species of *Candida* are present in the normal oral flora of healthy older adults. When an overgrowth of *Candida* occurs, the result is a fungal infection called *candidiasis* or *candidosis*. The most common fungal organism in the oral cavity is *Candida albicans*.[26] Risk factors that increase the incidence of candidiasis in older adults include local factors (e.g., xerostomia, ill-fitting dentures, and steroid inhalers) and systemic factors (e.g., malnutrition, endocrine disorders, and compromised immune system).[4] Examples of diseases that can compromise the immune system are diabetes and HIV. The presence of oral candidiasis is a signal to look for underlying factors to find the cause.[26,30]

Oral candidiasis may be difficult to recognize and diagnose because the signs and symptoms of the disease vary in individuals. Some individuals experience no symptoms, whereas others experience a burning sensation or a salty or bitter taste sensation. Clinically, white curdlike plaques that can be removed by wiping firmly with gauze are the most recognizable sign. Treatment involves application of a topical antifungal agent, most often nystatin (Mycostatin) oral rinse. Oral candidiasis found in the commissures of the lips is known as angular cheilitis; in the palate of patients who wear dentures, it is known as denture stomatitis.[30]

Angular Cheilitis

Angular cheilitis is an oral mucosa condition that occurs bilaterally at the commissures of the lips. It appears as deep red cracks or inflamed ulcerated fissures with or without symptoms of discomfort.[26,30] Older adults with one or more of the following risk factors for angular cheilitis have a higher incidence: *Candida albicans*, vitamin B_2 (riboflavin) deficiency, or ill-fitting dentures. Accurate diagnosis of the underlying cause leads to proper treatment options such as new dentures, nutritional supplements, or antifungal regimen. If left untreated, angular cheilitis may persist with reoccurring remissions and exacerbations.[26,30]

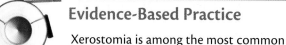

Evidence-Based Practice

Xerostomia is among the most common side effects associated with prescription and nonprescription drugs. More than 500 medications list xerostomia as a side effect, including antihistamines, antihypertensive medications, decongestants, pain medications, diuretics, and antidepressants. Although medications may be the most prevalent cause of xerostomia, other factors can also cause dry mouth including head and neck cancer radiation treatments, autoimmune diseases such as Sjögren, and systemic disease. Because 80% of adults 65 years or older take one or more mediations and suffer from at least one chronic disease, this age group is the most at risk for xerostomia.

When treating elderly patients who experience dry mouth, it is important for the dental hygienist to recognize the clinical signs of xerostomia, as well as question patients about dry mouth symptoms. During patient care the hygienist can check the patient's salivary flow and observe the oral tissues for clinical signs including cracked dry lips, red, fissured tongue, and dry mucosa lining. The hygienist should also ask the patient about dry mouth symptoms such as burning and tingling sensations, difficulty with chewing and swallowing, and dryness in the mouth, throat, and nasal passages.

Early assessment of prolonged xerostomia is especially important because dry mouth can have a profound effect on hard and soft tissues. Although patients' chief complaint about dry mouth is discomfort, most are unaware of the effects on the dentition and how it increases plaque buildup, leading to an increase in caries. This is especially true for the elderly who have a high incidence of root caries caused by gingival recession and poor oral hygiene. Hygienists using evidence-based research can educate elderly patients on plaque-control modifications, perform caries prevention treatments, and recommend products to relieve patient's dry mouth symptoms.

An ideal choice for plaque removal for elderly patients is the electric toothbrush. The large handle makes it easier to grip, and the mechanical action of the brush allows the patient to focus only on placement of the brush head. Flossing alternatives such as a water flosser or air flosser have been clinically proved to be easier and more effective than flossing. Because change is difficult for older patients, personal preferences as well as dexterity issues need to be taken into account when selecting a new plaque-control aid. Demonstrating the new product and giving a pamphlet or brochure with home-care instructions leads to better patient compliance.

The best caries prevention products for treatment in-office and at home list fluoride as an active ingredient. Research clearly demonstrates that fluoride not only prevents caries from occurring but can also remineralize and repair the tooth surface. Hygienists can help reduce dry mouth complications of caries by educating elderly patients on the benefits of fluoride, applying in-office fluoride varnishes, and recommending home rinse and dentifrice products that contain fluoride.

Patients have several options to relieve dry mouth symptoms, but most provide minimum or short-term relief. Saliva stimulants such as sugarless gum, lozenges, and mints are recommended to chew or suck on to encourage patient's own salivary production. Hygienist should especially encourage products that contain xylitol because xylitol has been shown to have anticaries properties. Patients should also be advised to take frequent sips of water throughout the day and suck on ice chips. Another source for dry mouth relief are artificial salivary substitutes, which can help mimic patient's natural saliva, although they provide only short-term relief. Prescription drugs approved by the U.S. Food and Drug Administration are also available for severe cases such as radiation therapy–induced xerostomia. These drugs induce salivary production in patients and have demonstrated xerostomia symptom relief, but they have considerable adverse effects and should be used with caution. ■

Sources: Beebe S. Zeroing in on xerostomia. *Dimens Dent Hygiene.* 2008;6(11):40-43; Fox PC. Xerostomia: recognition and management. *Access.* 2008;22(2). www.adha.org/CE_courses/. Accessed Oct. 1, 2011; and Spolarich AE. Xerostomia and oral disease. *Dimens Dent Hygiene.* 2011;9(11; special suppl):43-54.

Oral Cancer

Oral cancer can occur in any part of the oral cavity including the oral pharynx. It most frequently appears on the lateral borders of the tongue, lips, and floor of mouth, respectively, and the most prevalent type is the squamous cell carcinoma. Like most cancers, the likelihood of developing oral cancer increases with age. Research shows that those 60 years of age and older have the highest incidence rate of oral cancer.[31] The risk factors for the disease include tobacco, the primary risk, followed by alcohol intake. There is also growing evidence showing the sexually transmitted human papillomavirus, particularly genotype 16, as a risk factor.

In 2010, approximately 37,000 new cases of oral cancer were reported in the United States, with 8,000 of those cases resulting in death. Although these numbers have scarcely changed over the last 50 years because of the challenge in early detection, studies are now showing that early detection is saving lives. According to the Oral Cancer Foundation, the overall survival rate for patients diagnosed early with stage I oral cancer is between 80% and 90%, whereas those diagnosed late with stage IV is close to 50%.[31]

The challenge of detecting oral cancer during the early stages is that the patient usually does not experience any symptoms of pain. The signs that do appear are clinical and include ulcerated lesions that do not heal and white or reddish patches that ultimately grow into a tumor or mass.[31] The dental hygienist plays a central role in detecting oral cancer because the most frequent dental appointments are for dental hygiene care. At each dental care appointment, it is essential for the dental hygienist to perform a thorough intraoral examination to identify, document, and communicate findings with the patient. The dental hygienist should refer the patient for a definitive diagnosis if any lesion persists more than 2 weeks.[6,31] See Chapter 10 for more information.

Dentition

In the dentition of older adults, normal age-related changes can be attributed to both functional and environmental factors. Attrition, abfraction, and abrasion are forms of functional wear that occur from chewing, brushing, or grinding the dentition, causing enamel loss and, in more severe cases, exposing the underlying dentin. Erosion occurs when extrinsic sources such as acidic beverages and citrus fruits, and intrinsic sources such as gastroesophageal reflex and vomiting chemically dissolve the tooth's enamel surface.[28] Depending on the amount or severity of enamel loss or dentinal exposure, attrition, abfraction, abrasion, and erosion can be considered either normal or pathological conditions.

Teeth undergo a color change and appear yellow or darkened because of a thickening and composition change of underlying dentinal tissues. A reduction in tooth sensitivity occurs as dentin's thermal, osmotic, and electric properties decrease, which affects the patient's perception of pain. The blood vessels entering the pulp chamber decrease, resulting in a decrease in tooth sensitivity. In some elderly patients, by the time tooth pain is identified, severe damage has occurred.[27,28] Regularly scheduled preventive appointments are imperative to combat this problem.

Dental caries is still a major concern in older adults, especially those with root exposures who are at high risk for developing root caries. The three most common risk factors include inadequate oral hygiene, infrequent dental office visits, and decreased salivary function. Other influencing factors consist of insufficient fluoride use and removable partial dentures that trap plaque and food around teeth. The initial phase of caries can be asymptomatic and, if left untreated,

can quickly lead to pulpal involvement in an older adult patient because of a decrease in dentinal pain receptor sensitivity.[27,28]

Tooth loss due to extraction is a pathophysiological condition that is caused primarily by severe dental caries and periodontitis.[28] Older adult patients have a high susceptibility for both dental caries and periodontal disease, and therefore an increased risk for tooth loss. Losing teeth can affect the older adult's overall health and lifestyle. They may experience temporomandibular joint problems, shortened vertical dimension of the face, and have difficulty chewing and speaking.[28]

Periodontal Structures

Increasing evidence shows that oral health is associated with overall health. Few periodontal age-related changes occur in older adults who have few medical conditions and practice healthy lifestyles. The gingiva, periodontal ligament fibers, cementum, and alveolar bone can remain relatively unchanged during a healthy person's lifetime. The changes that do occur are minimal and have little effect on the functions of the periodontal structures.[27,28] The periodontal ligaments lose their elasticity and the spaces between the teeth and alveoli widen, which are considered normal age-related changes.[27]

Older adults with existing medical conditions and unhealthy lifestyles are at a higher risk for pathological changes to their periodontal structures than those who are healthy. Increasing evidence links oral health to general health and shows an association between medical conditions such as diabetes, cardiovascular diseases, and chronic respiratory diseases and oral conditions such as periodontal disease.[6,22] For example, in patients with diabetes, the alveolar bone may show an increase in porosity because of the body's metabolism inhibiting the bone from regenerating, and thus reducing the bone's density. Destructive pathology changes to cementum, periodontal fibers, gingiva, and alveolar bone are dependent on various factors and affect different structures in different people.[32]

Periodontal Diseases

Two common diseases of the periodontium are gingivitis and periodontitis. Gingivitis is an inflammatory response that occurs when bacterial biofilm and its endotoxins accumulate along the gingival margins. The untreated accumulation of bacterial endotoxins signals the body's immune response to fight the infection, resulting in inflammation. If the inflammation progresses into the underlying tissues and bone, periodontitis occurs. Although age alone is not a risk factor for either gingivitis or periodontitis, both are more common in older adults than those of younger cohorts. Factors that increase the risk for periodontal disease in older adults include medical conditions that require multiple medications, physical and sensory limitations, and residing in long-term care facilities.[32]

Case Study

Background and Personal History: Mrs. J.D. is a 79-year old white female who is 5'5" and weighs 160 lbs. She says, "My mouth is always dry and I'm having sensitivity on my right side when I eat sweets or drink cold water." Mrs. J.D. takes the following medications: metoprolol tartrate (Lopressor) 12.5 mg bid and furosemide (Lasix) 20 mg daily for high blood pressure; simvastatin (Zocor) 10 mg daily for high cholesterol; metformin (Glucophage) 25 mg bid for type 2 diabetes; levothyroxine (Synthroid) 0.1 mg bid for hypothyroidism; and celecoxib (Celebrex) for arthritis in her hands and knees. Mrs. J.D. also revealed that she sometimes skips a day when taking her blood pressure medications because they are so expensive.

Vital Signs: Blood pressure 148/89, Pulse 72, Respirations 16.

Dental History: Mrs. J.D. states that she brushes and flosses daily and uses a mouthrinse but does not know if it contains fluoride. She reports that her teeth and gums are important to her and she wants to keep them for a lifetime. However, because of her husband's illness and death, she has not seen a dentist for 5 years and is concerned that she is in need of a great deal of dental work.

Extraoral/Intraoral Examination: Right and left commissures on lips are cracked, dry, and bleeding. Patient states they have been this way for 6 months. Her physician told her she needs to drink more water.

Periodontal: Patient has healthy gingiva with generalized 1- to 2-mm recession. Probe readings generalized 3 to 4 mm except one 6 mm on mesial of tooth #3. No bleeding upon probing and class I mobility on #24 and #25. Radiographically, patient exhibits generalized 30% horizontal bone loss and her American Academy of Periodontology classification is moderate periodontitis.

Hard Tissue: Dental charting noted patient is missing #1, #3, #12, #16, and #19 and replacement bridges and crowns covering posterior teeth. Caries examination revealed several areas of root caries on exposed root surfaces and mesial caries tooth #2 crown abutment.

Case Study Exercises

1. Which of the patient's medications is MOST likely contributing to her xerostomia?
   A. Synthroid
   B. Lipitor
   C. Metformin
   D. Furosemide

2. Which of the following oral hygiene aids is recommended for a patient with arthritis?
   A. Electric toothbrush
   B. Flossing instructions
   C. Manual toothbrush

3. Which of the following is the LEAST likely treatment modification for dental hygiene care for this patient?
   A. Early-morning appointment
   B. Using a local anesthetic without epinephrine
   C. Medical clearance for high blood pressure (HBP)
   D. Slowly raise dental chair for patient to exit

Review Questions

1. During the past century, people in the United States are living longer and keeping their teeth for a lifetime because of advancements in both medicine and dentistry such as vaccines, antibiotics, and improved nutrition.
   A. Both the statement and reason are correct and related.
   B. Both the statement and reason are correct but are *not* related.
   C. The statement is correct, but the reason is *not*.
   D. The statement is *not* correct, but the reason is correct.
   E. *Neither* the statement *nor* the reason is correct.

2. Which of the following age definition categories describes how a person interacts mentally and physically with his or her surroundings?
   A. Biological age
   B. Functional age
   C. Chronological age
   D. Physiological age

3. Which of the following physiological changes of the dentition occurs normally as a person ages?
   A. An increase in volume of the cementum
   B. An increase in volume of the enamel
   C. An increase in volume of reparative dentin
   D. An increase in volume of the pulp chamber

4. Which of the following factors is associated with a higher incidence of root caries in older adults?
   A. Increased salivary flow
   B. Lack of medications
   C. Xerostomia
   D. Use of xylitol products

5. Physiological aging changes to the heart include which of the following?
   A. Decrease in heart size
   B. Increase in heart contractions
   C. Decrease in fluid retention
   D. Increase in blood volume to vital organs

Active Learning

1. Research drugs used to treat Alzheimer disease and create a table showing their side effects and impact on dental hygiene. Include their effects on oral self-care, as well as the dental hygiene appointment.
2. Prepare a presentation for caregivers at a long-term care facility, outlining oral care challenges older adults with conditions discussed in this chapter may experience and steps caregivers can take to assist patients in maintaining their oral health. ■

REFERENCES

1. U.S. Department of Health and Human Services. *Oral Health in America: A Report of the Surgeon General—Executive Summary.* Rockville, MD: U.S. Department of Health and Human Services, National Institute of Dental and Craniofacial Research, National Institutes of Health; 2000.
2. Ettinger RL. Oral health and the aging population. *J Am Dent Assoc.* 2007;138(suppl): 5S-6S.
3. Vincent GK, Velkoff VA. The next four decades, the older population in the United States: 2010 to 2050. U.S. Government Census. http://www.census.gov/prod/2010pubs/p25-1138.pdf. Published May 2010. Accessed May 2010.
4. Mulligan R. *Geriatrics: Contemporary and Future Concerns. Dental Clinics of North America.* Philadelphia, PA: Saunders; 2005.
5. Centers for Disease Control and Prevention. The state of aging and health in America, 2007. Whitehouse Station, NJ: The Merck Company Foundation; 2007. http://www.cdc.gov/Aging/pdf/saha_2007.pdf. Accessed September 27, 2015.
6. Scully C, Ettinger RL. The influence of systemic diseases on oral health care in older adults. *J Am Dent Assoc.* 2007; 138(suppl):7S-14S.
7. Ettinger RL. Meeting oral health needs to promote the well-being of the geriatric population: educational research issues. *J Dent Educ.* 2010;74:29-35.
8. Ettinger RL. Rational dental care: part 1. Has the concept changed in 20 years? *J Can Dent Assoc.* 2006; 71(5):441-445.
9. AgeWorks, a division of the Ethel Percy Andrus Gerontology Center, University of Southern California. http://gero.usc.edu/.
10. Loue S, Sajatovic M. Biology of aging. *Encyclopedia of Aging and Public Health.* New York, NY: Springer Science; 2008:1-10.
11. Stassi ME. Certified In-Home Aide Student Manual. Missouri Center for Career Education, Central Missouri State University, Warrensburg, Missouri. 2006. http://mcce.org/. Accessed October 22, 2015.
12. Aldwin CM, Gilmer DF. Aging and the regulatory systems. *Health, Illness, and Optimal Aging: Biological and Psychosocial Perspectives.* Thousand Oaks, CA: SAGE Publications; 2004:163-253.

13. Alzheimer's Association. Alzheimer's facts and figures. http://www.alz.org/alzheimers_disease_facts_figures.asp. Accessed September 27, 2015.
14. National Institutes of Health, National Institute of Aging. 2010 Alzheimer's disease progress report: a deeper understanding. Bethesda, MD: U.S. Department of Health and Human Services. https://www.nia.nih.gov/alzheimers/publication/2010-alzheimers-disease-progress-report-deeper-understanding. Accessed September 27, 2015.
15. Alzheimer's Association. Alzheimer's disease: risk factors. http://www.alz.org/alzheimers_disease_causes_risk_factors.asp. Accessed September 27, 2015.
16. Alzheimer's symptoms and stages. Alzheimer's Health Assistance Foundation. http://www.ahaf.org/alzheimers/about/symptomsandstages.html. Accessed September 27, 2015.
17. Guideline for Alzheimer's disease management: final report. California Workgroup on Guidelines for Alzheimer's Disease Management. California Council of the Alzheimer's Association. http://www.cdph.ca.gov/programs/Alzheimers/Documents/professional_GuidelineFullReport.pdf. Published 2008. Accessed September 27, 2015.
18. Szarejko MJ. Dental considerations for geriatric patients. 2009 CME Resource. http://www.netce.com/courseoverview.php?courseid=1193. Accessed September 27, 2015.
19. Scannapieco FA. Pneumonia in nonambulatory patients. The role of oral bacteria and oral hygiene. *J Am Dent Assoc.* 2006;137(suppl):21S-25S.
20. Lamster IB, Crawford ND. The oral disease burden faced by older adults. In: Lamster IB, Northridge M, eds. *Improving Oral Health for the Elderly: An Interdisciplinary Approach.* New York, NY: Springer; 2008.
21. Ship JA. Oral medicine and geriatrics. *Clinician's Guide: Oral Health in Geriatric Patients.* 2nd ed. Hamilton, ON: BC Decker Inc.; 2006:1-5.
22. Szarejko MJ. Dental care for special needs patients. 2010 CME Resource. http://www.netce.com/coursecontent.php?courseid=924. Accessed September 27, 2015.
22. Montandon AA, Pinelli LA, FaisLM. Quality of life and oral hygiene in older people with manual function limitations. *J Dent Educ.* 2006;70(12):1261-1262.
24. Centers for Disease Control and Prevention. National Center for Chronic Disease Prevention and Health Promotion. The power of prevention 2009. Available from: www.cdc.gov/chronicdisease/pdf/2009-power-of-prevention.pdf. Accessed September 27, 2015.
25. Centers for Disease Control and Prevention. Diabetes Public Health Resource. 2011 National Diabetes Fact Sheet. http://www.cdc.gov/diabetes/pubs/pdf/ndfs_2011.pdf. Updated May 23, 2011. Accessed September 27, 2015.
26. Gonsalves WC, Wrightson AS, Henry RG. Common oral conditions in older persons. *Am Fam Physician.* 2008;78(7):845-852.
27. Greenberg MS, Glick M, Ship JA. Geriatrics. *Burket's Oral Medicine.* 11th ed. Lewiston, NY: BC Decker Inc.; 2008:605-619.
28. Guiglia R, Musciotto A, Compilato D, et al. Aging and oral health: effects in hard and soft tissues. *Curr Pharm Des.* 2010;16(6):619-630.

29. Turner MD, Ship JA. Dry mouth and its effects on the oral health of elderly people. *J Am Dent Assoc.* 2007;138(suppl 1):15S-46S.

30. Silverman S. Mucosal lesion in older adults. *J Am Dent Assoc.* 2007;138(suppl 1):41S-46S.

31. The Oral Cancer Foundation. Oral cancer facts. 2011. http://www.oralcancerfoundation.org/facts. Published 2015. Accessed September 27, 2015.

32. Tobias KB, Frank AS. The epidemiology, consequences and management of periodontal disease in older adults. *J Am Dent Assoc.* 2007;138(suppl 1):15S-46S.

Chapter 49 | Physical Impairment

Kristin Wolf, BA, RDH, MSHS

KEY TERMS

attitudinal barrier

autosomal recessive

barrier-free design

cystic fibrosis (CF)

hydrocephalous

hypertonic

hypotonic

lower motor neurons

meninges

motor neurons

muscular dystrophies (MD)

myelomeningocele

paralysis

paraplegia

paresis

quadriplegia

spina bifida (SB)

spinal cord injury (SCI)

spinal muscular atrophy (SMA)

traumatic brain injury (TBI)

upper motor neurons

ventriculoatrial shunt

ventriculoperitoneal shunt

vertebra

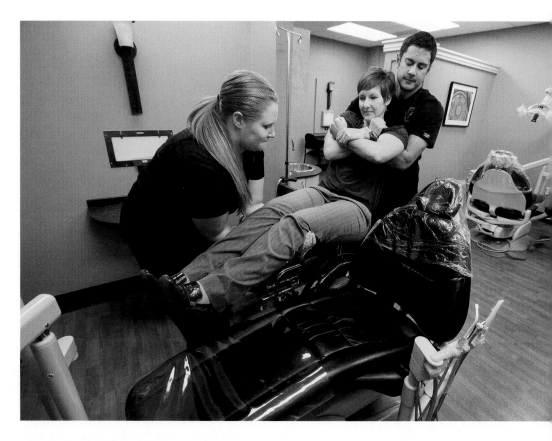

LEARNING OBJECTIVES

After reading this chapter, the student should be able to:

49.1 Identify barriers for people with physical impairments.

49.2 Describe the causes and age of onset of common physical impairments.

49.3 List various physical conditions of people with physical impairments.

49.4 Describe the clinical considerations for treatment for people with physical impairments.

49.5 Describe treatment modalities and adaptations for people with physical impairments.

49.6 Describe modifications that the dental hygienist may make when providing care to people with physical impairments.

49.7 Describe the conditions, causes, and incidence of various impairments.

49.8 Perform a two-person wheelchair transfer.

KEY CONCEPTS

- Lack of access to dental care is a critical problem for people with physical impairments.
- Maintaining good oral health is particularly important for the overall health of people with physical impairments.

- Successful provision of oral hygiene care for people with physical impairments requires a basic general knowledge of conditions resulting in degrees of impairment.

RELEVANCE TO CLINICAL PRACTICE

With an increasingly older population and medical advances, the prevalence of people with physical impairments is increasing. Chronic disabling diseases affect millions of Americans and compromise oral health and functioning. Those who seek care may be faced with health practitioners who lack the training and cultural competence to communicate effectively to provide needed services.[1] The dental hygienist must have the knowledge and ability to effectively serve people with physical impairments.

PHYSICAL IMPAIRMENT

Definition

A physical impairment is defined as:

Any physiological disorder or condition, cosmetic disfigurement, or anatomical loss affecting one or more of the following body systems: neurological, musculoskeletal, special sense organs, respiratory (including speech organs), cardiovascular, reproductive, digestive, genitourinary, hemic and lymphatic, skin, and endocrine.[2]

Physical impairment includes the following conditions:

- Medical impairments resulting from disease (e.g., polio)
- Musculoskeletal conditions involving the joints, limbs, and associated muscles
- Neurological conditions involving the central nervous system (the brain, spinal cord, or peripheral nerves) that affect the ability to move or to coordinate the control of movement
- Sensory impairments involving hearing, vision, or speech[3]

A person with a physical impairment has a disabling condition that requires an adaptation to the person's environment to perform activities of daily living. Persons with physical disabilities often rely upon assistive devices such as wheelchairs, crutches, canes, artificial limbs, helping dogs, hearing aids, and alternative language to function in their environment.[3]

Prevalence

The world population of persons with physical impairments is estimated at 6.5 billion. In the United States, 54 million adults reported difficulty with basic movement actions such as walking, bending, reaching overhead, or using their fingers to grasp something. About 13% of the adult population reported vision or hearing difficulties (hearing is measured without the use of hearing aids). These estimates continue to rise as the population ages.[4]

Historical Perspective

Before the 1960s most people with physical impairments lived in institutions such as sanitariums or nursing homes, where they were totally dependent on their caregivers. The social reform ideology of the 1960s and early 1970s changed the focus from a person's impairments to the person's abilities. This shift in thinking led to the idea that people with impairments could live independently or with assistance in the community and play a functional role in society. Deinstitutionalization began in the 1970s. Spurred by dilapidated facilities, overcrowded institutions, and the rising costs associated with providing total care, the former homes for the majority of persons with impairments closed their doors. The practices of normalization (training individuals with impairments to lead more independent lives) and mainstreaming (including persons with impairments in societal activities such as schools and work) became the norm.

People with impairments faced many barriers as they were assimilated into society.[3] Legislation has been successful in removing some barriers (Table 49-1), but more obstacles remain (see Spotlight on Public Health).

BARRIERS TO HEALTH-CARE ACCESS

Access to health care, dentistry in particular, is difficult for many individuals with physical impairments due to financial, architectural, transportation, and attitudinal barriers.

Financial Barriers

Cost is the primary obstacle that people with impairments face in regard to health care. Financial resources

Table 49-1. *Disability Timeline*

Year	Law	Barrier Addressed
1973	The Rehabilitation Act of 1973	Provided equal opportunity for employment in the federal government and federally funded programs; also established the Architectural and Transportation Barriers Compliance Board, mandating equal access to public services
1975	The Education of All Handicapped Children Act (later renamed the Individuals With Disabilities Education Act [IDEA])	Required free, appropriate public education in the least restrictive setting; mandated the inclusion of children with disabilities in mainstream classrooms unless the child's disability prevented a satisfactory level of education
1988	The Fair Housing Amendments Act	Prohibited housing discrimination based on race, color, religion, sex, disability, familial status, and national origin, and established minimum standards of adaptability for newly constructed multiple-dwelling housing
1990	The American with Disabilities Act (ADA)	Mandated that local, state, and federal governments and programs must be accessible and make "reasonable accommodations" for disabled workers, and that public accommodations such as restaurants and stores must ensure access for those with disabilities; also mandated access in public transportation, communication, and other areas of public life
1993	The National Voter Registration Act of 1993	Made it easier for all Americans to exercise their right to vote; aimed to increase the low registration rates of minorities and persons with disabilities due to discrimination; requires all offices of state-funded programs that are primarily engaged in providing services to persons with disabilities to provide all program applicants with voter registration forms, to assist them in completing the forms, and to transmit completed forms to the appropriate state official
1996	The Telecommunications Act	Required manufacturers of telecommunications equipment and providers of telecommunications services to ensure that such equipment and services are accessible to and usable by persons with disabilities, if readily achievable
1999	The *Olmstead* Decision	U.S. Supreme Court ruling on June 22, 1999, in *Olmstead v. L.C. and E.W.* that the "integration mandate" of the Americans with Disabilities Act requires public agencies to provide services "in the most integrated setting appropriate to the needs of qualified individuals with disabilities"
2000	Developmental Disabilities Assistance and Bill of Rights Act Amendments of 2000	Recognizes the basic precept of disability policy that disability is a natural and normal part of the human experience that does not diminish the rights of individuals with disabilities to exert control and choice over their own lives and to fully participate in and contribute to their communities through full integration and inclusion in the mainstream
2001	New Freedom Initiative	Goals are to increase access to assistive and universally designed technologies, expand educational opportunities, promote homeownership, and integrate Americans with disabilities into the workforce
2008	ADA Amendments Act of 2008	Clarifications of the law as it related to Supreme Court hearings challenging areas of the original law
2010	ADA Standards for Accessible Design	Revised standards for new construction and alterations
2014	Achieving a Better Life Experience (ABLE) Act	Allows people with disabilities and their families to create a tax-exempt savings account that can be used for maintaining health, independence, and quality of life

(From U.S. Department of Justice. *A guide to disability rights*. Washington, DC: U.S. Department of Justice; 2009, July. Available from: http://www.ada.gov/cguide.htm#anchor66477; U.S. Department of Justice. *2010 ADA standards for accessible design*. Washington, DC: US Department of Justice; 2010 Sept 15. Available from: http://www.ada.gov/regs2010/2010ADAStandards/2010ADAstandards.htm; and Library of Congress. *ABLE Act of 2014*. Washington, DC: Library of Congress. Available from: https://www.congress.gov/bill/113th-congress/house-bill/647.)

Spotlight on Public Health

Access to care is a more prevalent problem for people with physical impairments than the general population. Many states have passed legislation to attempt to rectify this problem. Although slightly different for each state, new laws expand the supervision requirements for dental hygienists to enable them to provide dental hygiene care in alternative settings such as nursing homes and geriatric centers. This removes a barrier to dental care for those who might have difficulty securing transportation to a dental office. ■

Professionalism

The ultimate goal of the dental hygiene profession is to improve oral health. Where a problem such as access to care exists, we search for creative ways for improvement. Where barriers to care are vast, we seek to remove them. The most effective way to approach these issues is to be well informed of the situation in your particular area and what steps, if any, are in place to correct problems. Involvement in your professional association is the most effective place to begin to gain this knowledge on the local, state, and national levels. Legislative initiatives begin within the association, with knowledge of what other states have done to alleviate these problems, and with knowledge of the issues facing the profession on the national level. ■

are needed for all basic needs, including food, shelter, clothing, rehabilitation, education, job training, and transportation. Most people with impairments live on subsidized incomes from the Social Security Disability program. Those able to find employment usually earn the minimum wage. Health care is limited to Medicare and Medicaid. Beyond basic coverage, the cost for health care is the responsibility of the patient.[6] The Patient Protection and Affordable Care Act (ACA) requires dental coverage for children up to age 19. Dental benefits are included in health insurance exchanges run by the federal government; however, they must be purchased in the individual and small-group markets. Some states will expand Medicaid dental benefits for adults, but many will not expand coverage.[7]

Architectural Barriers

The Americans with Disabilities Act of 1990 mandated that all local, state, and federal facilities are required by law to conform to **barrier-free design**, meaning a universal design that allows accessibility for people with or without physical impairments. New facilities must follow a strict building code allowing access to those relying on assistive devices (mobility and sensory). Existing facilities were mandated to remove barriers when such removal was readily achievable. Building owners argue that such renovations are financially impossible. Consequently, many older buildings housing dental and medical offices lack elevators, accessible restrooms, doorways wide enough for a wheelchair to pass through, ramps, or an electronic-operated door to gain entrance to the structure itself.[6]

Transportation Barriers

Many clinicians choose not to participate with the Medicare and Medicaid programs because of their inadequate reimbursement for fees for services. As a result, individuals with physical impairments often are forced to travel a considerable distance to find a facility where their insurance is accepted. Public transportation is commonly used, but schedules, inclement weather, expense, and inaccessible stations may make travel difficult. Some people with physical impairments must rely on family members and caregivers for transportation, adding another burden to those accompanying the individuals to appointments.[6]

Attitudinal Barriers

Attitudinal barrier is a term used to describe the difficulties or challenges experienced by a person with physical impairments as a the result of another individual's misunderstanding or ignorance of the disability, dismissal of the individual as a "person" due to the disability, or unjust decisions about the individual's capabilities. Attitudinal barriers include discrimination, pity, stereotypes, and fear of the impairment. Another barrier is the fear that extra time must be allotted for accommodating the individual in the dental chair and any physical sequelae that might lengthen treatment. These include spasms, poor salivary control, and **hypotonic** (decreased muscle tone) or **hypertonic** (increased muscle tone) oral musculature. Fear of interacting with people who have impairments may cause the practitioner to avoid accepting them into the health-care facility. Inadequate knowledge of the different conditions that can cause physical impairments and the extent of physical involvement may also cause avoidance.[6]

Other Barriers to Care

The person with a physical impairment may be coping with other challenges, such as depression, which may create a barrier to accessing dental care. Lack of knowledge of available resources can also be a barrier. Some individuals may not realize the importance of a healthy mouth to overall health and social acceptance and not consider it a priority.[6]

Table 49-2. *Conditions Resulting in Physical Impairment*

Inherited/Generic	Congenital	Developmental	Acquired	Age Related
Muscular dystrophy	Spina bifida	Any physical impairment manifested before age 22	Any physical impairment manifested after age 22	Any physical impairment manifested after age 50
Cystic fibrosis	Traumatic birth (cerebral palsy, hydrocephalus)	Medical—polio Trauma—accident Autoimmune—rheumatoid arthritis Degenerative—sensory	Medical Trauma Autoimmune Degenerative (e.g., macular degeneration)	Medical Trauma Autoimmune Degenerative (e.g., Alzheimer disease)
Spinal muscular atrophy	Abnormal or missing structures (e.g., cleft palate)			

ETIOLOGY

The etiology (cause) of physical impairments may be genetic, congenital (present from birth), developmental, acquired, age associated, or of multiple origins (Table 49-2). Some of the most common etiologies resulting in physical and health impairments are genetic and chromosomal defects, teratogenic causes (from an agent such as alcohol that affects an embryo), prematurity, and complications of pregnancy. Acquired causes include infectious disease, congenital conditions, and developmental problems or chronic health problems that are poorly understood. Impairments associated with traumatic brain injury can be the result of vehicular accidents, gunshot wounds, burns, falls, and poisoning. Substance abuse and physical abuse by caretakers, infectious diseases, and substance abuse by the mother during pregnancy result in impairment. Advances in medicine and related treatments are reducing or eliminating physical impairments resulting from some diseases, injuries, and chronic conditions. However, advances in medicine also increase the number of individuals surviving congenital anomalies, accidents, and diseases with severe impairments.[3]

Certain physical and health impairments have multiple etiologies. For example, prenatal abnormalities, biochemical abnormalities, genetic causes, congenital infections, environmental toxins, prematurity-associated complications, or postnatal events can cause cerebral palsy. The exact cause of other physical and health impairments is unknown.[3]

Physical and health impairments can also be progressive or nonprogressive. This refers to whether or not the condition increases in extent or severity.[3]

CLASSIFICATION OF IMPAIRMENTS

Impairments are classified in several different ways depending on the purpose for classification. The government has developed classifications to determine the need for federal assistance. Physical impairments are also classified by etiology or grouped by similar manifestations. In addition, individuals can be classified by functional status and to what level they can perform basic activities.[8]

For health-care providers, the most useful means of classifying a physical impairment is by functional status using activities of daily living as a measure. Several tools that ask questions about the patient's level of function are available. Basic activities of daily living (BADLs) include activities required for personal care, such as feeding, dressing, grooming, and toileting. Instrumental activities of daily living (IADLs) encompass more complex tasks for independent living, such as using the telephone, preparing a meal, cleaning the house, driving a car, and using public transportation. Impairments can affect five areas of function: communication, movement, mental ability, medical health, and sensory perception.[9] It is imperative that a dental hygienist be aware of the functional status of a patient with a physical impairment to determine the patient's ability to perform BADLs and IADLs, especially in the area of personal oral hygiene care.

DISABILITY ETIQUETTE

The primary goal of the Americans with Disabilities Act was to integrate individuals with disabilities into every aspect of life. As a result, sensitivity toward people with impairments is necessary. Familiarity with the following guidelines will help dental hygienists treat patients with disabilities.

Communication

Disability advocacy groups have created guidelines referred to as *people-first language* to establish appropriate communication strategies. When speaking to a person with a physical impairment, it is important to focus on the person rather than the disability. See Table 49-3 for examples of people-first language.[7]

Table 49-3. *People-First Language*

Labels Not to Use	People-First Language
Afflicted with, suffers from, victim of	Person who has...
The handicapped or disabled	People with disabilities
Handicapped parking	Accessible parking
The mentally retarded or he's retarded	People with intellectual disabilities
She is developmentally delayed	She has a developmental delay
Is learning disabled or LD	Has an intellectual disability
She's in Special Ed	She receives Special Ed services
My son is autistic	My son has autism
She's a Down's; she's mongoloid	She has Down syndrome
Birth defect	Has a congenital disability
Epileptic	A person with epilepsy
Wheelchair bound or confined to a wheelchair	Uses a wheelchair or a mobility chair or is a wheelchair user
Quadriplegic, paraplegic, etc.	He has quadriplegia, paraplegia, etc.
He's cripple, lame	He has an orthopedic disability
She's a dwarf (or midget)	She has short stature
Mute	Is nonverbal
She's emotionally disturbed; she's crazy	She has an emotional disability
Normal and/or healthy	A person without a disability

(From National Center on Birth Defects and Developmental Disabilities, Centers for Disease Control and Prevention. *Communicating with and about people with disabilities.* Atlanta, GA: National Center on Birth Defects and Developmental Disabilities, Centers for Disease Control and Prevention. Available from: http://www.cdc.gov/ncbddd/disability andhealth/pdf/DisabilityPoster_Photos.pdf)

Other communication guidelines include:

- Accept that a disability exists; not acknowledging this fact is the same as denying the person.[8] If you are uncertain about how to interact with a person who has a disability, ask the person. Do not assume that the person with a disability needs help.
  - If the setting is accessible, people with disabilities can usually get around without assistance.
- Offer assistance only if the person appears to need it.
  - Adults with disabilities want to be treated as independent people. If the patient does want help, ask how you can be of assistance before you act.[9]

- Always speak directly to the person with the disability.
  - Avoid speaking directly to the companion, caregiver, or interpreter instead of the patient.
- Focus on the individual, not the disability.
  - Tailor recommendations to what the patient can do, rather than activities the patient cannot perform.
- Make small talk before easing into more personal questions.

Wheelchair Etiquette

If a patient uses a wheelchair, never assume he or she needs help and automatically push the wheelchair. Stand in front of the person and ask if he or she would like assistance maneuvering into the operatory. If a person uses a wheelchair, conversations at different eye levels are difficult. If a conversation continues for more than a few minutes and if it is possible to do so, sit down, kneel, or squat and share eye level. A wheelchair is part of a person's body space. Do not hang on it; doing so would be similar to leaning on the person. People who use wheelchairs may not always be confined to them; they may easily transfer to the car or use a walker, cane, or braces. Depending on the situation, the wheelchair may make it more comfortable.[9]

Physical Contact

When treating patients with a physical impairment, be sensitive about physical contact. Many individuals who require assistance with mobility depend on their arms for balance. Grabbing a person's arm, even when the intention is to help, may cause him or her to lose balance and fall. Although some people may not have a visible disability, they might have limited range of motion with their hands or wrists.[9]

Other Considerations

People with physical impairments represent the largest range of specific disability types (Table 49-4). Individuals with a physical impairment may have difficulty with musculoskeletal control, weakness, and fatigue, in addition to neurosensory or musculoskeletal dysfunction (e.g., walking, talking, sensing, grasping, reaching). Physical impairments make activities that require multiple simultaneous actions, such as turning and pushing (e.g., opening a door using a door knob) difficult.[10]

THE DENTAL HYGIENE APPOINTMENT

When treating a person with physical impairments in the clinical setting, there are some common oral and clinical treatment concerns to be addressed (Table 49-5). See Teamwork for some general guidelines to be observed by clinicians for a successful outcome. More in-depth issues particular to specific conditions are listed with the descriptions of conditions that follow.[11]

Table 49-4. Oral Characteristics More Common to Persons with Physical Impairments Than the General Population

Periodontal disease	**Poor oral hygiene, lack of dental care, lengthy hospital stays, oral habits, malocclusion, musculoskeletal deformities, poor neuromuscular control, the ability to hold the toothbrush, the inability to reach all areas of the mouth, and medications all contribute to the periodontal condition.**
Dental caries	Poor oral hygiene, lack of dental care, malocclusion medication, enamel hypoplasia, mouth breathing, and food pouching can lead to caries.
Malocclusion	Musculoskeletal conditions, mouth breathing, oral habits, trauma, the inability to close the lips, excessive drooling, an anterior open bite, and enamel dysplasia are often the cause of malocclusion.
Bruxism	Uncontrollable movements of the mouth are common.
Hyperactive gag reflex	Introduced instruments, radiographs, and drooling can cause gagging.
Trauma	Persons with physical impairments fall and have accidents frequently. Instruct the patient or caregiver what to do in case of broken or avulsed teeth, and the importance of immediate attention. Often physical abuse may present as trauma. Persons with physical disabilities have a higher rate of abuse. Know the numbers of the appropriate agencies to call if you suspect abuse.

Table 49-5. Common Clinical Concerns for the Practitioner

Before the Appointment	
Physician Consult **If the patient has seizures:**	• Record information in the chart about the frequency of seizures and the medications used to control them. • Determine before the appointment whether medications have been taken as directed. • Know and avoid any factors that trigger your patient's seizures. • Be prepared to manage a seizure. If one occurs during oral care, remove any instruments from the mouth and clear the area around the dental chair. • Attaching dental floss to rubber dam clamps and mouth props when treatment begins can help you remove them quickly. • Do not attempt to insert any objects between the teeth during a seizure. • Stay with your patient, turn him or her to one side, and monitor the airway to reduce the risk of aspiration.
Understand the patient's abilities. **Will the patient be bringing a caregiver?** **Does the patient have sensory issues?** **Is the patient hearing impaired?**	• People with physical impairments have varying degrees of involvement with movement and posture. • Allow enough space in the operatory to accommodate others. • The patient may want to turn off hearing aids so that the sounds of the instruments are not too loud or frightening. • If the patient is completely deaf but reads lips, speak in a normal tone and cadence. Make sure when you are speaking that the patient can see your lips (take off mask) and the light is not making a glare over the face. • If the patient signs, ask the patient to bring an interpreter to the appointment.
Is the patient visually impaired?	• People with facial neuromuscular impairments who have involvement of the facial muscles may have strabismus, which looks like the eyes are misaligned due to abnormal muscle tension. • Determine the level of assistance the patient will require to move safely through the office and operatory. • Rely on the patient's other senses to establish trust. Tactile feedback such as a warm handshake can help the patient feel comfortable. • Face the patient when you speak and keep him or her aware of all procedures in advance, particularly those involving air and water.

Table 49-5. *Common Clinical Concerns for the Practitioner—cont'd*

Before the Appointment

Is the patient able to communicate?	• Ascertain whether an interpreter will be needed. • The patient may use an adaptive device for communication, such as an electronic board that can be used with fingers or a mouth stick. A mouth stick is molded to fit in the patient's mouth (like a mouth guard) and has a stick protruding from it that the patient can use like a finger.
Does the patient have visual limitations?	• Allow space for a caregiver or assisting dog in the operatory.
Is the patient mentally impaired?	• Speak to the patient as you would any other patient. Determine whether the person understands and can follow directions. • Discuss communication with the caregiver. Unless the patient does not respond, do not speak to the caregiver, speak to the patient. • Use clear and concise directions. • Try to be consistent at all appointments—the same staff, the same room, etc. • Listen actively; communication may be slow, and the person may use an adaptive device for communication such as an electronic board or a bite stick.
Schedule short appointments.	• It takes a lot of energy for a person with a physical impairment to prepare for, transport to, and adjust to the dental chair. Short appointments are easier on the patient and the clinician.

During the Appointment

	• Maintain clear paths for movement throughout the treatment setting. • Keep instruments and equipment out of the patient's way.
If you need to transfer your patient from a wheelchair to the dental chair:	• Ask about special preferences such as padding, pillows, or other things you can provide to ease the transition. • The patient or caregiver can often explain how to make a smooth transfer.
If the patient has dysarthria:	• Depending on the extent of the impairment, there may be problems involving the muscles that control speech and mastication. • Be patient. Allow time for your patient to express him- or herself. • Remember that many people with dysarthria have normal intelligence. • Consult with the caregiver if you have difficulty understanding your patient's speech.
If the patient has primitive reflexes:	• These are common in many people with neuromuscular disorders and may complicate oral care. • These reflexes often occur when the head is moved or the patient is startled, and efforts to control them may make them more intense. • Three types of reflexes are most commonly observed during oral care: **Asymmetric tonic neck reflex:** When a patient's head is turned, the arm and leg on that side stiffen and extend. The arm and leg on the opposite side flex. **Tonic labyrinthine reflex:** If the neck is extended while a patient is lying on his or her back, the legs and arms also extend, and the back and neck arch. **Startle reflex:** Any surprising stimuli, such as noises, lights, or a sudden movement on your part, can trigger uncontrolled, often forceful movements involving the whole body. • Be empathic about your patient's concerns and frustrations. • Minimize the number of distractions in the treatment setting. • Movements, lights, sounds, or other stimuli can make it difficult for your patient to cooperate. • Tell him or her about any such stimulus before it appears. For example, tell the patient before you move the dental chair. • Some impairments affect the oral-facial muscles; the patient may have difficulty opening the mouth and/or keeping it open.
If the patient has tremors:	• Uncontrollable tremors require a steady hand and often an extra oral fulcrum. • Special attention must be paid to absolute control over the instrument.

Continued

Table 49-5. *Common Clinical Concerns for the Practitioner—cont'd*

During the Appointment	
If the patient has drooling:	• Hypotonia contributes to drooling, as does an open bite and the inability to close the lips. • Manage oral secretions with careful evacuation techniques, avoiding the loose oral tissues that can get caught and cause loud sounds.
Use care when positioning patients in the dental chair.	• People with musculoskeletal disorders cannot be forced into some positions that would be advantageous for the clinician.
Do not put the patient in a totally supine position.	• To maintain an open airway, keep the patient reclined at a 45° angle or more.
Use padding to help the patient be comfortable.	• Ulcers of the skin are common in people who cannot control their own movements. • Have the patient shift positions frequently.
If the patient is ambulatory, provide frequent breaks.	• Those with musculoskeletal and neuromuscular disorders find it difficult to remain still for an extended period.
Persons who have no bowel or bladder control must utilize a catheter attached to a bag.	• Always check to ensure that the bag remains below the level of the chair to prevent backflow.
Utilize a mouth prop.	• Those with musculoskeletal and neuromuscular disorders find it difficult to keep the mouth open for an extended period.
Whenever possible, utilize an assistant.	• When patients have uncontrollable reflexes, tremors, seizure disorders, or have a bladder bag, an assistant can minimize injury to the patient and/or the clinician.
At the End of the Appointment	
Watch the patient closely.	• Be alert for postural hypotension • Is the bag in place? • Is the patient secure?
Establish short re-care intervals.	
Use critical thinking to determine adaptive aids for homecare.	• Include the caregiver in all homecare instructions
Consider the use of prescription dentifrice and rinses.	

Oral Hygiene Instructions

Oral hygiene care for people with physical impairments that involve the upper extremities or the oral-facial structures can be challenging. All instructions given either to the patient or caregiver must be geared to the particular patient's abilities, but do not assume that the patient with a physical impairment also has a cognitive impairment. Instructions will vary depending on the particular impairment.[11]

Teamwork

Teamwork and interdisciplinary collaboration are an integral part of providing care for all patients, especially those with special needs. It is essential to involve the physician in all cases. Individual needs for the inclusion of other allied health personnel may vary. It may be necessary to consult with occupational therapists, physical therapists, psychologists, or social workers. Often a case worker or family member will be able to provide guidance about such consults. ▪

Teaching the Patient

Employ the "tell-show-do" approach to simplify instructions.

1. Tell the patient what you want him or her to do.
2. Show the patient; use a model to demonstrate the action.
3. Do the action for the patient in his or her mouth.
4. Have the patient perform the action.
5. Give positive feedback.

Set up a routine with the patient, so the person follows the same steps at the same times every day.

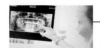

Advancing Technologies

New technology as applied to the individual with physical impairments involves making the appointment quick and noninvasive with the least chance of defect. Any new technology in dentistry will improve the dental experience for both the patient and clinician. Lasers and air abrasion techniques show great promise for treating patients with physical impairments. Advancements in sedation, anesthesia, and dental materials will ease treatment for all individuals. New wheelchair design and aids to assist transfer, such as vests and belts, are helpful for patients with specific conditions. Environmental technology such as audiosensation and noise-cancelling headphones can improve the desensitization process. Products for adaptation of toothbrushes, floss, and other oral hygiene aids continue to evolve. Newer and better power brushes, and newer moldable silicones for adaptation, are continually being released. ■

Modifying Recommendations

Patients with a physical impairment may have dexterity complications. For example, a person with rheumatoid arthritis may have difficulty gripping the small handle of a toothbrush or wrapping floss around the fingers. An electric toothbrush may be a solution for these patients. The handle of an electric toothbrush is much larger than that of a manual brush, and the vibrating action can simplify the motions needed to brush. Floss holders and interdental brushes are also helpful for people who have dexterity issues.[11] See Chapter 19, Devices, for more information on toothbrushes, floss holders, and other tools.

If the person is able to brush on his or her own but needs some help, there are some creative ways to modify the brush and floss to make it easier. There are also some commercial products available online.[11]

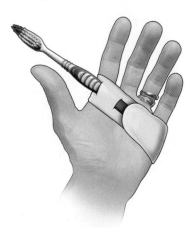

Figure 49-1. A Velcro strap can be attached to a toothbrush and wrapped around the hand to make it easier for a person with a physical impairment to brush the teeth.

To make the toothbrush easier to hold:[11]

- A Velcro strap can be attached to the handle of the toothbrush and around the hand (Fig. 49-1).
- The handle can be held in place with a rubber band (Fig. 49-2).

To make the handle larger:[11]

- A bicycle handlebar grip can be slid onto the handle (Fig. 49-3).
- A washcloth can be wrapped around the handle of the toothbrush and secured into place with a rubber band.

Teaching the Caregiver

1. Wash hands and put on disposable gloves. Sit or stand where all of the patient's teeth can be seen.
   - The bathroom is not the only place for brushing and flossing. The kitchen or dining room may have more room. Instead of leaning over the bathroom sink, it is often easier to have the patient at a table. Place the toothbrush, toothpaste, floss, a bowl, and a glass of water on the table within easy reach. Ensure that there is adequate light; it is impossible and unsafe to help someone when you cannot see.
   - If the patient is in a wheelchair, ensure that the wheels are locked. Stand or sit behind the patient, and have the patient lift his or her chin to provide an adequate visual field and clear access to the mouth (Fig. 49-4). It may be necessary to lean against a wall for support. Use an arm to hold the

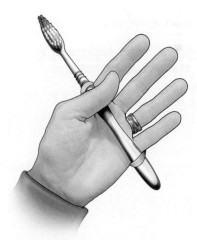

Figure 49-2. A rubber band can be used to hold the toothbrush in the patient's hand. The rubber band should not be too tight.

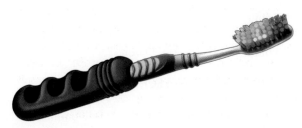

Figure 49-3. A bicycle grip can be slipped onto the toothbrush handle to make it easier to grip the toothbrush.

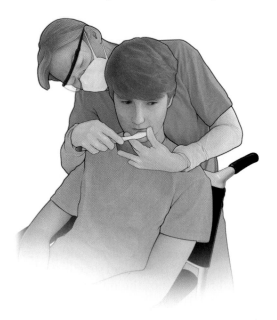

Figure 49-4. Sit behind the patient when treating a patient in a wheelchair.

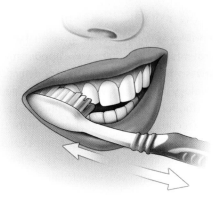

Figure 49-5. Angle the brush at the gumline and brush gently with a circular motion or short strokes.

patient's head against the caregiver's body for support. If the patient is unable to lift the chin, tip the wheelchair back against the caregiver.[11]
- Always use a soft toothbrush or electric toothbrush.
2. Apply a pea-size amount of toothpaste with fluoride. If the patient is likely to choke or swallow, use water only.

3. Brush all surfaces of the teeth. Angle the brush at the gumline and brush gently with a circular motion or with short strokes (Fig. 49-5).
4. Gently brush the tongue after the teeth are brushed.
5. Help the patient rinse with plain water. If the patient is unable to rinse and there is not too much saliva, a sweep of the mouth with gauze may work to remove the debris, or the patient can drink the water.

Procedure 49-1 lists the steps for transferring a patient from a wheelchair to the dental chair.

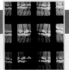

Procedure 49-1 Wheelchair Transfer[11]

1. DETERMINE THE PATIENT'S NEEDS
- Ask the patient or caregiver about the preferred transfer method; the patient's ability to help; the use of special padding or a device for collecting urine; any straps, belts, or vests; and the probability of spasms.
- Reduce the patient's anxiety by announcing each step of the transfer before it begins.

2. PREPARE THE DENTAL OPERATORY
- Remove the dental chair armrest or move it out of the transfer area.
- Relocate the hoses, foot controls, operatory light, and bracket table from the transfer path.
- Position the dental chair at the same height as the wheelchair or slightly lower.

3. PREPARE THE WHEELCHAIR
- Remove the footrests.
- Position the wheelchair close to and parallel to the dental chair.

- Lock the wheels in place and turn the front casters forward.
- Remove the wheelchair armrest next to the dental chair.
- Check for any special padding or equipment.

4. PERFORM THE TWO-PERSON TRANSFER
- Never perform a single-person transfer, even if it is the patient's preferred method. Always have another clinician available to provide assistance.
- Support the patient while detaching the safety belt.
- Transfer any special padding or equipment from the wheelchair to the dental chair.
- *First clinician*: Stand behind the patient. Help the patient cross his or her arms across the chest. Place your arms under the patient's upper arms and grasp the patient's wrists.

- *Second clinician*: Place both hands under the patient's lower thighs. Initiate and lead the lift at a prearranged count (1-2-3-lift).

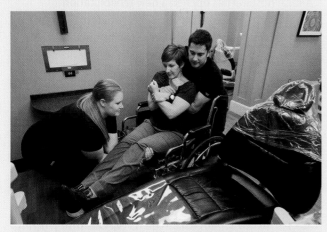

First clinician: Stand behind the patient. Help the patient cross his or her arms across the chest. Place your arms under the patient's upper arms and grasp the patient's wrists. Second clinician: Place both hands under the patient's lower thighs.

- *Both clinicians*: Using your leg and arm muscles while bending your back as little as possible, gently lift the patient's torso and legs at the same time.

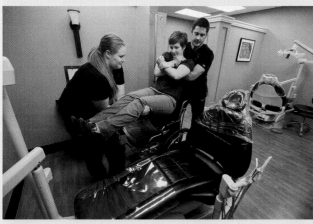

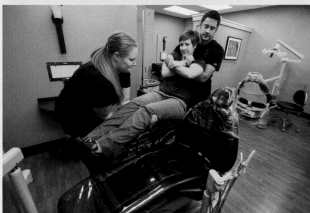

Both clinicians: Using your leg and arm muscles while bending your back as little as possible, gently lift the patient's torso and legs at the same time.

- Securely position the patient in the dental chair and replace the armrest.

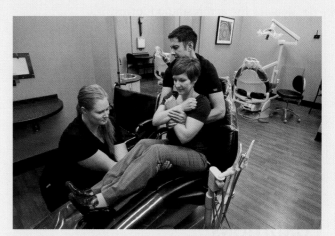

Securely position the patient in the dental chair and replace the armrest.

Use of a sliding board for a person with paraplegia (paralysis of the lower limbs)
- The board is made of hardwood with smooth, tapered ends.
- Use the board with a patient who can transfer him- or herself.
- Be prepared to assist.

5. POSITION THE PATIENT AFTER THE TRANSFER
- Center the patient in the dental chair by lifting, not sliding, the patient.
- Reposition the special padding and safety belt as needed for the patient's comfort.
- If a urine-collecting device is used, straighten the tubing and place the bag below the level of the bladder.

6. TRANSFER FROM THE DENTAL CHAIR TO THE WHEELCHAIR
- Position the wheelchair close to and parallel to the dental chair.
- Lock the wheels in place, turn the casters forward, and remove the armrest.
- Raise the dental chair until it is slightly higher than the wheelchair and remove the armrest.
- Transfer any special padding.
- Transfer the patient using the two-person transfer.
- Reposition the patient in the wheelchair.

- Attach the safety belt (if there is one), check the tubing of the urine-collecting device (if there is one), and reposition the bag.
- Replace the armrest and footrests.

A skilled and sensitive dental staff can instill confidence during the wheelchair transfer and encourage the patient to maintain a regular appointment schedule[11] (see Application to Clinical Practice).

If the wheelchair transfer is too difficult, the patient can be treated in the chair.[11]

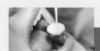

Application to Clinical Practice

A local hospital has opened a new rehabilitation facility with a state-of-the-art dental operatory for patients with physical impairments. The hospital has contracted with your office to provide dental services for the hospital's patients. You will not have the opportunity to view each patient's medical history until the day of treatment. What can you do in advance to enhance your patient management skills? ■

CONDITIONS

Inherited and Genetic Conditions

Muscular Dystrophy

The term **muscular dystrophy (MD)** refers to a group of more than 30 genetic diseases characterized by progressive weakness and degeneration of the skeletal muscles that control movement. Some forms of MD are seen in infancy or childhood, whereas others may not appear until middle age or later. The disorders differ in terms of the distribution and extent of muscle weakness (some forms of MD also affect cardiac muscle), age of onset, rate of progression, and pattern of inheritance. The incidence is approximately 1 in every 3,500 births. Descriptions of the most common types follow:

- Duchenne is the most common form and primarily affects boys. Onset is between 3 and 5 years, and the disorder progresses rapidly.[12]
- Facioscapulohumeral usually begins in the teenage years. It causes progressive weakness in muscles of the face, arms, and legs, and around the shoulders and chest. It progresses slowly and can vary in symptoms from mild to disabling.[12]
- Myotonic MD is the disorder's most common adult form and is typified by prolonged muscle spasms, cataracts, cardiac abnormalities, and endocrine disturbances. Individuals with myotonic MD have long and thin faces, drooping eyelids, and a swan-like neck. People with myotonic dystrophy may have trouble chewing, moving their lips, and turning their heads.[12]

Certain orofacial characteristics are unique to facioscapulohumeral muscular dystrophy (Table 49-6).[12]

Cystic Fibrosis

Cystic fibrosis (CF) is an inherited chronic disease that affects the lungs and digestive systems of about 30,000 children and adults in the United States (70,000 worldwide). A defective gene and its protein product cause the body to produce unusually thick, sticky mucus that clogs

the lungs and leads to life-threatening lung infections, and obstructs the pancreas, which stops natural enzymes from helping the body break down and absorb food.

People with cystic fibrosis are extremely susceptible to lung infections. About 60% of people with cystic fibrosis have a chronic respiratory infection caused by bacteria called *Pseudomonas aeruginosa* that settles into the thick

Table 49-6. Oral-Facial Characteristics of Muscular Dystrophy

Condyles inclined backward	Mandibular arch deviated to left
Delayed tooth eruption	Posterior cross-bite
Depressed nasal bridge	Anterior open bite
Enlarged tongue	Altered chewing and swallowing patterns
Facial asymmetry	Loss of head control and stabilization
High narrow palate	Muscle flaccidity
Palatal plane inclined upward	Muscle rigidity
Hypocalcification	Muscle weakness
Supernumerary teeth	Poor facial expression
Underdevelopment of ramus	Poor muscle control
Wide mandible	Poor salivary control
Malar hypoplasia	Speech may be unintelligible
Mandible rotated backward	Speech patterns altered due to poor muscle tone

(From National Institute of Dental and Cranial Research, National Institutes of Health. Strategies for providing oral care to people with developmental disabilities. Available from: http://www.nidcr.nih.gov/EducationalResources/HealthCareProviders/EdMaterials.htm.)

mucus trapped in the airways. Once it invades the respiratory tract, *P. aeruginosa* is difficult to eliminate. Respiratory failure caused by the infection is often the ultimate cause of death in many people with CF. Another common infection in persons with CF is methicillin-resistant *Staphylococcus aureus* (MRSA). Immaculate infection control procedures must be followed to avoid cross-contamination to protect the CF patient from acquiring an infection from the aerosols in the dental office.[11,13]

Spinal Muscular Atrophy

Spinal muscular atrophy (SMA) is an **autosomal recessive** hereditary disease, which means an identical gene is received from each parent. It is characterized by progressive hypotonia (decreased muscle tone) and muscular weakness. The characteristic muscle weakness occurs because of a progressive degeneration of the alpha motor neuron from anterior horn cells in the spinal cord. The weakness is more severe in the proximal musculature than in the distal segments. In certain patients, the **motor neurons,** the nerve cells that control the muscles of cranial nerves (especially the CNV–CNXII), can also be involved. Sensation, which originates from the posterior horn cells of the spinal cord, is spared, as is intelligence. Several muscles are spared, including the diaphragm, the involuntary muscles of the gastrointestinal system, the heart, and the sphincters. The three different types of SMA are genetically similar but differ in patient age at presentation, severity of muscle weakness, and disease progression.[11] The three types of SMA are as follows:

- Type I (Werdnig–Hoffmann disease): This acute infantile SMA is usually identified in patients from birth to age 6 months.
- Type II: This chronic infantile SMA is diagnosed in infants aged 6 to 12 months.
- Type III (Kugelberg–Welander disease): This type of SMA is diagnosed in children aged 2 to 15 years.[11]

Children with mild to moderate forms of SMA (SMA types II and III) generally live into adulthood and can have normal life expectancy. Good multidisciplinary care, including physical therapy, occupational therapy, respiratory therapy, and nutritional support, can improve quality and length of life.[11]

The incidence of SMA is about 1 in 15,000–20,000 (5–7 per 100,000) live births. The prevalence of persons with the carrier state is 1 in 80. SMA is the most common degenerative disease of the nervous system in children. It is the second most common disease inherited in an autosomal recessive pattern, after cystic fibrosis, to affect children. It is the leading heritable cause of infant mortality.[5,11]

Congenital Conditions

Spina Bifida

Spina bifida (SB), also known as **myelomeningocele**, is a birth defect in which the backbone and spinal canal do not close before birth. It is a neural tube defect in which the bones of the spine do not completely form, resulting in an incomplete spinal canal. This causes the spinal cord and **meninges,** the tissues covering the spinal cord, to stick out of the child's back. It may affect as many as 1 out of every 800 infants. **Hydrocephalus,** an abnormal accumulation of cerebrospinal fluid in the ventricles of the brain that may cause enlargement of the skull, may affect as many as 90% of children with myelomeningocele.[5]

The cause of myelomeningocele is unknown. However, low levels of folic acid in a woman's body before and during early pregnancy are thought to contribute this type of birth defect. The vitamin folic acid (or folate) is important for brain and spinal cord development.[9,10]

Individuals with SB have neuromuscular involvement below the level of the lesion, causing **paresis** (partial or slight paralysis), paralysis, muscle tone changes, and sensory problems. Musculoskeletal issues may include scoliosis and bone deformities causing the inability to sit or walk. Sometimes there are respiratory problems, bowel and bladder incontinence, and skin lesions due to pressure points causing epidermal breakdown.[10]

Clinical considerations include scheduling short appointments to prevent stress. To avoid pressure sores and pain, add some padding in the dental chair. Change the patient's position during the appointment to help minimize sores. Depending on the procedure, a wheelchair transfer (see Procedure 49-1) may be necessary, although it is advisable to treat in the wheelchair whenever possible. It may be difficult for the patient to keep his or her mouth open for a long period of time, and he or she will have difficulty controlling the tongue. A rubber bite block or a mouth prop may be of benefit to keep the mouth open for the duration of the treatment. This appliance also reduces the stress on the muscles. A tongue retractor can be used so that the tongue is kept in place. Latex allergy is prevalent among those with SB due to multiple hospitalizations and surgeries, which increases their exposure to latex products. There is controversy over whether antibiotic premedication is necessary for those with surgically placed tubes or shunts. Generally, patients with a **ventriculoatrial shunt** (a port placed in patients with hydrocephalus to allow cerebrospinal fluid to flow from the cerebral ventricular system to the cardiac atrium) require antibiotic premedication, whereas those with a **ventriculoperitoneal shunt** (a port placed in patients with hydrocephalus to remove excess cerebrospinal fluid from the brain's ventricles and transfer it into the peritoneal cavity of the abdomen), do not. A medical consult is always recommended before treatment.[10]

Oral hygiene procedures may be difficult or impossible depending on the level of the lesion. Several adaptive dental aids are available to maintain oral health. A caregiver should be included in the oral hygiene instructions when necessary. Additionally, medications may cause xerostomia or gingival hyperplasia.[10]

Developmental and Acquired Conditions

Many medical conditions can result in physical impairments. In some cases the pharmacological treatment is the cause of any oral sequelae, such as xerostomia or candidiasis (Table 49-7). Two physically compromising conditions caused by traumatic injuries are described here.

Traumatic Brain Injury

Traumatic brain injury (TBI), a form of acquired brain injury, occurs when a sudden trauma causes damage to the brain. TBI can result when the head suddenly and violently hits an object, or when an object pierces the skull and enters brain tissue. Symptoms of a TBI can be mild, moderate, or severe, depending on the extent of the damage to the brain. A person with a mild TBI may remain conscious or may experience a loss of consciousness for a few seconds or minutes. Other symptoms of mild TBI include headache, confusion, lightheadedness, dizziness, blurred vision or tired eyes, ringing in the ears, bad taste in the mouth, fatigue or lethargy, a change in sleep patterns, behavioral or mood changes, and trouble with memory, concentration, attention, or thinking. A person with a moderate or severe TBI may also have a headache that gets worse

Table 49-7. *Medications Commonly Taken by Persons With Physical Impairments*

Some Common Drugs Used	Adverse Effects	Oral Sequelae
Corticosteroids (prednisone)	Nervousness Increased appetite Glucose intolerance Indigestion Increases toxic gastrointestinal effects of NSAIDs Increases possibility of adrenal suppression Immunosuppressant Hyperlipidemia Cataracts Glaucoma Osteoporosis	Xerostomia Increased fungal infections Aphthous ulcers
Antiseizure **Dilantin** **Tegretol** **Depakote** **Klonopin** **Phenobarbital**	Dizziness, nausea, vomiting Tremor Hair loss Weight gain Depression Reduced attention span Osteoporosis Swelling of the ankles Irregular menstrual period Hearing loss Liver damage Decreased platelets Hyperactivity	Gingival hyperplasia Drooling Xerostomia
Anticholinergic **Levodopa** **Atropine** **Dicycloverine**	Nausea Vomiting Dizziness Headache Chest pain Seizures Glaucoma	Xerostomia Facial swelling Swelling of mouth and tongue Bruxism
Chemotherapeutics **Imuran** **Endoxana** **Novantrone**	Alopecia Thrombocytopenia Leukopenia Nausea Vomiting	Xerostomia Gingivitis Periodontitis Osteonecrosis Dysphagia Osteomyelitis
Antidepressants	—	Xerostomia

or does not go away, repeated vomiting or nausea, convulsions or seizures, an inability to awaken from sleep, dilation of one or both pupils of the eyes, slurred speech, weakness or numbness in the extremities, loss of coordination, and increased confusion, restlessness, or agitation.

Disabilities resulting from a TBI depend on the severity of the injury, the location of the injury, and the age and general health of the individual. Some common disabilities include problems with cognition (thinking, memory, and reasoning), sensory processing (sight, hearing, touch, taste, and smell), communication (expression and understanding), and behavior or mental health (depression, anxiety, personality changes, aggression, acting out, and social inappropriateness). More serious head injuries may result in stupor (the individual is unresponsive but can be aroused briefly by a strong stimulus such as sharp pain); coma (the individual is totally unconscious, unresponsive, unaware, and unarousable); vegetative state (the individual is unconscious and unaware of his or her surroundings but continues to have a sleep-wake cycle and periods of alertness); and a persistent vegetative state (PVS), in which an individual stays in a vegetative state for more than a month.[14,15]

Spinal Cord Injury (SCI)

A **spinal cord injury (SCI)** usually begins with a sudden, traumatic blow to the spine that fractures or dislocates vertebrae. The damage begins at the moment of injury when displaced bone fragments, disc material, or ligaments bruise or tear into spinal cord tissue. Most injuries to the spinal cord don't completely sever it. Instead, an injury is more likely to cause fractures and compression of the vertebrae, which then crush and destroy the axons, extensions of nerve cells that carry signals up and down the spinal cord between the brain and the rest of the body. An injury to the spinal cord can damage a few, many, or almost all of these axons. Some injuries will allow almost complete recovery. Others will result in complete paralysis.[14]

The spinal cord is about 18 inches long and extends from the base of the brain, down the middle of the back, to about the waist. The nerves that lie within the spinal cord are **upper motor neurons** (UMNs), and their function is to carry messages back and forth from the brain to the spinal nerves along the spinal tract. The spinal nerves that branch out from the spinal cord to the other parts of the body are called **lower motor neurons** (LMNs). These spinal nerves exit and enter at each vertebral level and communicate with specific areas of the body. The sensory portions of the LMN carry messages about sensation from the skin and other body parts and organs to the brain. The motor portions of the LMN send messages from the brain to the various body parts to initiate actions such as muscle movement.[14,16]

The spinal cord is surrounded by rings of bone called **vertebra**. These bones constitute the spinal column (backbone). In general, the higher in the spinal column the injury occurs, the more dysfunction a person will experience. The vertebrae are named according to their location. The eight vertebrae in the neck are called the cervical vertebrae. The top vertebra is called C-1, the next is C-2, and so on. Cervical SCIs usually cause loss of function in the arms and legs, resulting in quadriplegia. The 12 vertebrae in the chest are called the thoracic vertebrae, and injury to these vertebrate could cause inability to control abdominal muscles and trunk instability. The first thoracic vertebra, T-1, is the vertebra where the top rib attaches.[14]

A person can "break" the back or neck yet not sustain a spinal cord injury if only the bones around the spinal cord (the vertebrae) are damaged, but the spinal cord is not affected. In these situations, the individual may not experience paralysis after the bones are stabilized.[14]

The effects of SCI depend on the type of injury and the level of the injury. SCI can be divided into two types of injury: complete and incomplete. A complete injury means that there is no function below the level of the injury, no sensation, and no voluntary movement (**paralysis**). Both sides of the body are equally affected. An incomplete injury means that there is some functioning below the primary level of the injury. A person with an incomplete injury may be able to move one limb more than another, may be able to feel parts of the body that cannot be moved, or may have more functioning on one side of the body than the other. With the advances in acute treatment of SCI, incomplete injuries are becoming more common.[16]

The level of injury is very helpful in predicting what parts of the body might be affected by paralysis and loss of function. Remember that in incomplete injuries there will be some variation in these prognoses.

Approximately 450,000 people in the United States live with SCI. There are about 10,000 new SCIs every year; the majority of them (82%) involve males between the ages of 16 and 30. These injuries often result from motor vehicle accidents (36%), violence (28.9%), or falls (21.2%). **Quadriplegia** (paralysis of all four limbs) is slightly more common than **paraplegia**.[15,16]

For information on degenerative diseases such as amyotrophic lateral sclerosis and Parkinson's disease, refer to Chapter 40. For information on autoimmune disorders such as multiple sclerosis, myasthenia gravis, and rheumatoid arthritis, refer to Chapter 42. For information on Alzheimer disease and other dementias, refer to Chapter 47.

Case Study

A 36-year-old male calls your office complaining of pain in the lower left teeth. He is added to your schedule for that afternoon. When reading the medical history you see that he was born with spina bifida. You go to the reception area and see that he is in a wheelchair equipped with several attachments. You bring the patient into your operatory for data gathering. The medical history reveals that the location of the injury is at T8. The patient states that he has some arm and hand weakness, and bowel and bladder involvement. He is excited about his new wheelchair that can adjust his sitting position, which helps prevent skin lesions. He also has hydrocephalus and has a ventriculoperitoneal shunt. The visual examination reveals a parulis on the attached gingiva buccal to tooth 19. Radiographic imaging reveals an interradicular radiolucency. The dentist prescribes a 14-day regimen of antibiotics followed by periodontal debridement.

Case Study Exercises

1. Spina bifida can also be termed myelomeningocele. Individuals with myelomeningocele also have hydrocephalus.
   A. Both statements are true.
   B. Both statements are false.
   C. The first statement is true, but the second statement is false.
   D. The first statement is false, but the second statement is true.

2. Before implementation of dental hygiene procedures, consultation with all of the following EXCEPT which one is advised?
   A. Family or caregiver
   B. Occupational therapy
   C. Physical therapy
   D. Social services
   E. The hospital operating room staff

3. Information gleaned from the medical history indicates that the level of involvement is at T8 and that the patient has a ventriculoperitoneal shunt and incontinence. Treatment planning will include which of the following?
   A. Antibiotic premedication
   B. A two-person wheelchair transfer
   C. Short appointments
   D. A communication aid, such as a mouth stick

4. The treatment plan should include all of the following EXCEPT which one?
   A. The patient's daily schedule
   B. The use of a mouth prop
   C. The patient's manual dexterity
   D. Introduction of adaptations to self-care aids
   E. A long appointment to minimize the number of appointments required

5. Adaptations to oral self-care devices may be necessary for successful biofilm removal at home. Several considerations should be made when designing or recommending adaptations. Assessments should NOT include which of the following?
   A. Range of motion
   B. Grip strength
   C. Skill level and manual dexterity
   D. Current oral health status
   E. Adaptations proven useful for others with the same disability

Review Questions

1. Cost is the primary obstacle that people with impairments face in regard to health care. The Patient Protection and Affordable Care Act (ACA) requires dental coverage for adults and children.
   A. Both statements are true.
   B. Both statements are false.
   C. The first statement is true, but the second is false.
   D. The first statement is false, but the second is true.

2. From the following list, select three basic activities of daily living.
   A. Dressing
   B. Preparing dinner
   C. Making a phone call
   D. Feeding
   E. Grooming

3. The dental hygienist who is uncertain about how to act with a patient who has a disability should do which of the following?
   A. Avoid treating the patient.
   B. Treat the patient like any patient without a disability.
   C. Ask the patient's caregiver what to do.
   D. Ask the patient about how to proceed.

4. Avoiding grabbing the arms of a person with a physical impairment because it may cause the person to fall.
   A. Both the statement and reason are correct and related.
   B. Both the statement and reason are correct, but they are not related.
   C. The statement is correct, but the reason is not.
   D. The statement is not correct, but the reason is correct.
   E. Neither the statement nor the reason is correct.

5. Order the steps in the tell-show-do approach to patient teaching. Match each letter with its proper sequence number.
   __1. A. Use a model to demonstrate the action.
   __2. B. Have the patient perform the action.
   __3. C. Explain what you want the patient to do.
   __4. D. Give positive feedback.
   __5. E. Perform the action in the patient's mouth.

Active Learning

1. Create a collection of customized oral self-care devices. Try attaching plastic rulers and rods to toothbrushes and floss holders to make handles longer. Heat the handle of a brush or floss holder and bend it to create an angle, making it easier to reach lingual surfaces. Washcloths, Styrofoam balls, bicycle grips, and putty-like compounds can be added to make handles thicker for added grip strength. Use your imagination to experiment with other types of modifications.

2. Choose a type of physical impairment and create a dental hygiene care plan based on the needs associated with the impairment. Include information about the condition, its cause, related medical conditions, medications, oral health, assistive devices necessary, and adaptations for dental hygiene care.

3. Spend a day using a wheelchair or walker to experience the challenges associated with being impaired. Write a reflection about your experiences.

4. Form groups of three and practice wheelchair transfers. Students should alternate roles so that each student has the experience of being the transferee and the transferor. ■

REFERENCES

1. Altman B, Bernstein A. *Disability and health in the United States, 2001–2005.* Hyattsville, MD: National Center for Health Statistics; 2008.
2. Islets of Hope. Diabetes and civil rights law: An overview of your legal right to equal access to programs, benefits, opportunity, accommodations, education, and employment. Publication PA-04-2006. 2006. Available from http://www.isletsofhope.com/pdf/diabetes-and-the-law.pdf.
3. Jaeger PT, Bowman CA. *Understanding disability: inclusion, access, diversity, and civil rights.* Westport CT: Praeger; 2005.
4. U.S. Department of Health and Human Services. *Oral health in America: A Report of the Surgeon General.* Rockville, MD: U.S. Department of Health and Human Services, National Institute of Dental and Craniofacial Research, National Institutes of Health; 2000. p. 2-3.
5. Muzzin K. Persons with disabilities. In *Dental hygiene theory and practice.* 3rd ed. Darby ML, Walsh MM, editors. St. Louis: Saunders; 2010. p. 813-832.
6. Albrecht GL, Steelman KD, Bury M. *Handbook of disability studies,* London: Sage; 2001.
7. American Dental Association. Affordable Care Act: dental benefits examined. Aug 19, 2013. Available from: http://www.ada.org/en/publications/ada-news/2013-archive/august/affordable-care-act-dental-benefits-examined.
8. United Spinal Association. Disability etiquette. Available from: http://www.unitedspinal.org/pdf/Disability Etiquette.pdf.
9. Smith BJ, Henry RC. Neurological and sensory impairment. In *Dental hygiene: concepts, cases, and competencies.* 2nd ed. Daniel SJ, Harfst SA, Wilder R, editors. St. Louis, MO: Mosby; 2008. p. 815-833.
10. National Institute of Dental and Cranial Research, National Institutes of Health. Strategies for providing oral care to people with developmental disabilities. Available from: http://www.nidcr.nih.gov/Educational-Resources/HealthCareProviders/EdMaterials.htm.
11. U.S. National Library of Medicine, U.S. Department of Human Services, National Institutes of Health. Neuromuscular disorders. Available from: http://ghr.nlm.nih.gov/condition/spinal-muscular-atrophy.
12. Thayer HH, Crenshaw J. Oral manifestations of myotonic muscular dystrophy: report of case. *J Am Dent Assoc.* 1986; 72(6):1405-1411.
13. Aaron SD, Vandemheen KL, et al. Infection with transmissible strains of pseudomonas aeruginosa and clinical outcomes in adults with cystic fibrosis. *J Am Med Assoc.* 2010;304(19):2145-2153.
14. National Institute of Neurologic Disorders and Stroke, National Institutes of Health. Available from: http://www.ninds.nih.gov/.
15. Elliot-Smith S. Treating patients with special needs. *Access.* 2011;Jan.
16. Stiefel, D. Dental care considerations for disabled adults. *Spec Care Dent.* 2002;22(3):26S-39S.

Chapter 50 | Alternative Practice Settings

Noel Kelsch, RDHAP

KEY TERMS

Advanced Dental Hygiene Practitioner (ADHP)

alternative practice setting

direct access

direct supervision

general supervision

mobile dental clinic

portable unit

Registered Dental Hygienist in Alternative Practice (RDHAP)

simplified portable unit

wellness model

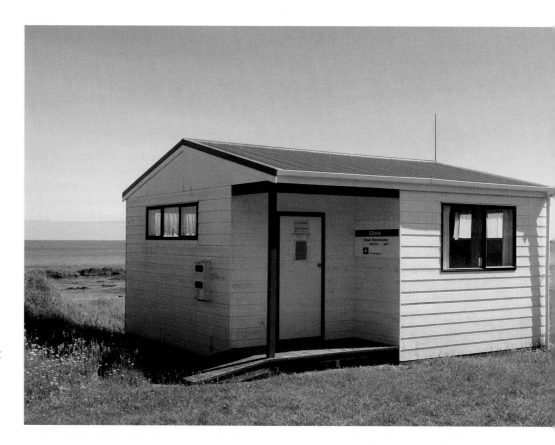

LEARNING OBJECTIVES

After reading this chapter, the student should be able to:

50.1 Define the issues in access to oral health prevention measures and care.

50.2 Identify venues beyond the traditional office setting where dental hygienists provide access to care.

50.3 Describe alternative setting methods and identify resources for delineating state laws related to those settings.

50.4 List the equipment necessary to facilitate delivery of care in alternative practice settings.

50.5 Identify the roles dental hygienists play in alternative settings.

50.6 Discuss the protocols and techniques for delivering care in alternative settings.

KEY CONCEPTS

• Access to a Registered Dental Hygienist is vital to clients' overall health, and there are many settings for delivery of care.

- Preventive and operative dental hygiene services can be delivered in a variety of settings by adapting practices to the location and using proper equipment.
- Availability of dental care in alternative settings allows all patients to receive preventive strategies and operative care.

RELEVANCE TO CLINICAL PRACTICE

Many Americans lack access to adequate dental care, resulting in extensive dental disease.[1] Traditional models for increasing access to care expand delivery systems such as private dental offices and community clinics. Newer models that utilize nonoffice settings and expand the role of dental hygienists are proving effective in eliminating many of the obstacles to access to care. In states that allow **direct access,** dental hygienists can "initiate dental treatment based on their assessment of the patient's needs without authorization from a dentist, treat the patient without the presence of a dentist, and maintain a provider-patient relationship."[1] Since 1995, the number of states that allow direct access has increased from 5 to 36 states.[2]

As the dental profession embraces the **wellness model** of guiding patients toward risk reduction and disease prevention, dental hygienists play a major role in the prevention of disease, from dental caries to aspiration pneumonia. Dental hygienists continue to expand the venues in which they serve and develop methods of service to meet their clients' needs.

ACCESS TO CARE

Community water fluoridation and health promotion and disease prevention efforts such as encouraging individuals to brush and floss daily have led to improved oral health for many Americans. However, poor oral health continues to affect the lives of some Americans. Individuals who face barriers to oral health care include those who:

- Lack dental insurance and funds to pay for dental care
- Lack transportation to dental care providers
- Hold a job that does not allow time off for appointments
- Reside in an area where there are no dental practices
- Reside in a long-term care facility or nursing home where dental care is not provided
- Are disabled or have complex health problems

Public and policymaker awareness of the importance of oral health can also create barriers to oral health. When oral health is deemed less important than other health needs, individuals may neglect dental care, and policymakers may not create and fund programs that would improve access to care.[3]

ALTERNATIVE PRACTICE

Among the responses to the access-to-care issues are the initiatives to create a midlevel oral health provider and expand the dental hygienist's scope of practice. The American Dental Hygienists' Association (ADHA) proposed creation of new dental care provider, the **Advanced Dental Hygiene Practitioner (ADHP)**, and later adopted competencies for the ADHP.[4,5] In California, the state legislature created the license category of **Registered Dental Hygienist in Alternative Practice (RDHAP)** to deliver dental hygiene care in settings outside a dental office, such as residential facilities, schools, and areas where there is a shortage of dental care providers. Requirements and scope of practice vary in states that allow direct access.[2] Consult state regulations for details. See Chapter 54, Lifelong Learning, for more information about alternative practice models.

ALTERNATIVE PRACTICE SETTINGS

Alternative practice settings include mobile dental clinics, nursing homes, assisted living facilities, hospitals, schools, community health centers, and retail clinics. The methods of delivery of services are as varied as the services themselves. Adapting to the different settings involves understanding the services that are needed, the patients' needs, and the equipment necessary to meet those needs.

Mobile Dental Clinics

Description: **Mobile dental clinics** are self-contained dental operatories with all equipment necessary for delivery of treatment. Equipment ranges from a generator for power to a radiography unit. These units are dental offices on wheels.

Equipment and instruments: Any dental equipment the hygienist uses in a clinical setting can be utilized here.

Serving: Underserved populations from schools; community centers; federal Women, Infants, and Children (WIC) sites; senior centers; work sites; and a variety of other settings. WIC is a federal program for low-income pregnant and postpartum women and children under age 5 who are at nutritional risk.

Limitations: Mobile dental clinics require a large amount of space to set up and a solid area of ground to level on. They cannot be set up on unstable ground due to weight. The state may require the operator to have a special permit for driving and relocating the unit. Establishing a mobile dental clinic can be as expensive as setting up a complete dental office. Moving the unit can be very costly.

Benefits: Mobile dental clinics can bring dental services into communities with residents who cannot travel to the traditional dental setting. School-age children whose parents have limited time off from work are able to receive treatment on the premises. All dental treatment can be delivered in one setting.

Portable Units

Description: **Portable units** are lightweight, self-contained units, and have a compressor for suction. They usually require a separate power source. They require very little space and can be configured to fit almost anywhere.

Equipment and Instruments: The units may require use of specific handpieces and equipment. It is important to make sure equipment is compatible.

Serving: A great variety of populations can benefit from the use of these self-contained units, which can be set up adjacent to a bedside or reclining chair, or in a school or community center. Portable units enable delivery of care in situations where space and weight are potential obstacles.

Limitations: Portable units can be quite loud. Check the noise level before purchasing. Difficulty in setting up the unit can vary greatly. Some do not have the power to deliver complete care. Sterilization of instruments must be outsourced or a sterilization unit must be set up at the care delivery site.

Benefits: Portable units are lightweight, easy to transport, and affordable. Most can be plugged directly into a 110-volt outlet.

Simplified Portable Units

Description: The **simplified portable unit** utilizes available resources (such as the Devilbiss pump for suction that is bedside in most hospitals) and a self-contained ultrasonic scaler along with a cordless handpiece and basic dental hygiene instrument setup to meet the needs of those who cannot come to the dental office. The simplified portable unit

allows hygienists to provide care at the bedside in cramped spaces to patients who cannot sit in a regular dental chair.

Equipment and Instruments: Simple dental hygiene setup for examination and prophylaxis, and portable handpiece.

Serving: This is especially advantageous to those who have difficulty leaving the bed or changing positions.

Limitations: The hygienist is required to maintain a position that can be uncomfortable while delivering care. Procedures that require larger pieces of equipment cannot be performed.

Benefits: Provides access to care for those who cannot go into the dental setting and those who are in a confined setting such as those in a halo cast or ventilator. Costs are limited and setup is simple.

Independent Practice Hygienist Karine Strickland, RDHAP

Karine Strickland delivers care in a variety of venues reaching far beyond the traditional setting. Seeing patients in skilled nursing facilities, residential care facilities, and intermediate care facilities allows her to reach the elderly, disabled, and infirm, among others.

What are the challenges of working in this venue?

Karine: If you have forgotten the distilled water for your unit, your camera, your extra battery for your LED [light-emitting diode], extra polish, the new box of fluoride varnish, or the handpiece, or dropped the package of extra saliva ejectors on the floor, you work without them. This creates increased stress in an already stressful workday and work environment.

What obstacles have you faced that would not be encountered in the traditional setting?

Karine: Creating and maintaining relationships with executive directors, social services, directors of nursing, and the nursing and support staff is essential to gaining access to provide care. It requires time, energy, and negotiation skills. A positive demeanor and approach are required. Connecting with other organizations can also help with the development of relationships. I find that related industries such as Visiting Nurses, Senior Help, and the Alzheimer's Association are extremely supportive and appreciative.

Mobile equipment: The RDHAP has to make a decision on equipment and supplies based on the type of care that she intends to provide. My personal opinion is that a dental chair, a dental unit, an operator chair, and cabinets full of disposable supplies are mandatory for the provision of comprehensive care. Some RDHAP practices require hygiene instruments, paper cups, and toothbrushes for polishing. [Karine's start-up costs were approximately $15,000.] Equipment requires maintenance, and repairs can be time intensive and costly. Learning to repair equipment can save time and money.

Additional responsibilities: The independent practice hygienist is responsible for administrative tasks such as billing, employees, infection control, and paperwork. Not all insurance companies recognize dental hygienists as providers, and therefore they do not pay for the hygienist's services. Insurance billing is another aspect of this type of work that is time intensive.

What are the rewards of being an independent practice hygienist?

Karine: As an RDHAP we can spend as much time as we feel is appropriate with our patients. We are not bound by a 50- to 60-minute schedule, which reduces stress. Improvement in the oral health of your patients is extremely rewarding. Pain is alleviated. Oral inflammation is reduced. My skills as a hygienist are fully utilized. Many of the patients are very appreciative. There are great personal and professional rewards.

Freestanding Building

Description: Dental hygienists in some states can establish their private practice in a **freestanding building**.[2] They are able to deliver services directly to the public, giving the community direct access to a dental hygienist.

Equipment and Instruments: Full dental hygiene services and equipment.

Serving: Depending on the state's dental practice act, dental hygiene private practices may be limited to areas that are qualified as underserved. It is essential to check the state laws before developing the model for creating a practice.

Limitations: The cost is high, and frequently the hygienist is only able to offer services in the office.

Benefits: This allows communities direct access to a dental hygienist in areas where they are not able to get dental services.

Shelby Kahl, Owner and Operator of a Freestanding Clinic

What type of setting do you work in to deliver treatment?

Shelby: I own and operate a freestanding dental hygiene practice that includes a school-based mobile component and an implemented collocated oral medicine model. The collocation model situates the dental hygienist alongside a pediatrician and physician office.

How does this venue differ from working in a traditional dental office setting?

Shelby: This professional venue differs from a traditional dental office setting by virtue of conceptual design and implementation strategies for optimal patient outcomes. This dental hygiene model incorporates integrating patient resources, services, and providers into a comprehensive experience.

What challenges does this setting present?

Shelby: The challenge with integration of health services is in communication and relationships both with the patient and the patient's health-care providers. Definitive diagnostics and thorough treatment planning is the crux of integrative services. There must be ease of communication access among the providers, prompt provider response, and meticulous attention to diagnostic details.

What are the advantages of working in this setting?

Shelby: The advantage to owning a dental hygiene practice is the tremendous creativity one is allowed—creativity in direct access to patients, that is, bringing the services to specific populations; creativity in the equipment and protocols a dental hygienist chooses to follow; the freedom to purchase specialty equipment to provide more comprehensive diagnostics and provide specific treatment modalities.

How are you received by the community and other health-care professionals working in this setting?

Shelby: We are well received by both the community and consumers. Economics can be a positive factor in why consumers seek preventive care. When funds are restricted the consumer returns to basic health prevention to avoid costly restoration or adjunctive dental procedures. Currently more opportunities exist for creative dental hygiene practices than there are willing and available dental hygienists. The practice receives referrals from a variety of health providers; this large network includes but is not limited to acupuncturists, clinical nutritionists, chiropractors, registered nurses, physicians, and dentists.

What are the requirements to perform in this setting as far as equipment and supplies? Was this a major investment?

Shelby: Any business venture requires a commitment of financial resources. This includes equipping the business, funding to run the business and maintain operations, and savings for future endeavors. Equipping this comprehensive model ranges from a complete dental hygiene operatory to portable dental hygiene equipment. A significant feature of the integrative dental hygiene practice is a commitment to the environment. This office is committed to reducing the carbon footprint and materials used by purchasing used dental operatory equipment, used appliances, and recycled cabinetry and furnishings. The new purchases made include dental hygiene instruments and the steam sterilizer. This particular model utilizes existing plumbing combined with self-filtering fresh water to remove minerals for steam sterilizing. This omits storage of distilled water containers, maximizing space. It also significantly reduces overhead costs because it isn't necessary to have distilled water delivered to the office location.

Are you working under the supervision of a dentist?

Shelby: No. There are three procedures that require a dentist to have knowledge that I may perform them with a patient. The procedures require supervision; the dental hygienist is not supervised.

What duties are you allowed to perform?

Shelby: Every procedure is allowed to be performed in this model—from radiographs to local anesthesia to dental hygiene diagnosis and treatment planning. The dental hygienist makes the decision regarding which services to provide that will require supervision.

What tips would you like to share with someone who wants to work in this setting?

Shelby: Hurry up. Consider this model if you are healthy and happy now. This is a choice for those who want to utilize their professional skills as a dental hygienist to their fullest potential. It is also a chance to gain a new perspective on contributing to the health of individual patients—a chance to view how influencing a patient's health affects the patient's family, and how that affects your community, the state, the nation, the world as a whole.

How is this model financed?

Shelby: This model accepts third-party reimbursement from private insurance companies, Medicaid, and CHP+. The office has a large population of uninsured clients who pay cash or through credit card. A small portion of the school-based and collocation model is supported with grant funding.

Do you work with any assistants? If so, what duties do they perform?

Shelby: This office utilizes dental assistants with the school-based model. They provide administrative and instrument-processing support. The office utilizes an office administrator who manages all aspects of daily business.

What are the special needs of clients who are receiving access to care as a result of your being in this setting?

Shelby: The practice is inclusive of all patients, young and elders, whether systemically or physically challenged. We do specialize in services for patients who have a nonresponsive history to periodontal therapy. Through the use of specialized equipment, such as the Perioscope® [a periodontal endoscope], this dental hygiene practice has an emphasis on clinical nutrition, adrenal health, and salivary diagnostics.

What challenges do you have in meeting the needs of these patients?

Shelby: Many of these patients are fearful because of previous dental experiences. To make them feel comfortable, the office dental chair has bolsters and warm blankets for patients, and we encourage patients to take their shoes off. The school-based model has improvised by using a reclining lawn chair made of mesh fabric to keep children in the best position.

Shelby concluded by sharing a vital thought: "The challenge those in the dental hygiene profession have in front of them is to fulfill the obligation we created with policymaking. Along with changes in regulation comes the profession's commitment to provide the services dental hygienists are available to do."

Backpack

Description: With the use of a model that nurses have implemented for years, dental hygienists can provide preventive care to populations that have typically not received treatment. Many populations do not have a means of transportation or the resources to gain access to a registered dental hygienist. Loading up a backpack with needed supplies and visiting those who have no access allows dental hygienists to meet the needs of those who cannot come to them.

Equipment and Instruments: Limited to lightweight supplies for evaluation and distribution. Kits typically contain 2 x 2 gauze pads, tongue depressors, disposable mirrors, single-use supplies such as fluoride varnish, and supplies to be distributed.

Serving: Low income, homeless, those with limited transportation

Limitations: Everything has to fit into a single bag and be lightweight enough for a single person to carry. Services offered are limited to simple procedures and preventive measures such as fluoride varnish.

Benefits: Prevention can be taken to those who in the past did not have access. This is an inexpensive, simple model that is very easy to develop.

Flying Hygienists

Description: This model brings dental hygiene to rural areas that are not accessible by other means of transportation. Dental hygienists fly in with all of their supplies and equipment on prop planes. This system successfully delivers care in rural settings such as outlying villages in Alaska.

Equipment and Instruments: Flights are limited to lightweight supplies and equipment. Facilities range from full clinics with some equipment to school gyms with no dental equipment.

Serving: Rural areas that have no access to care.

Limitations: Flights may be very costly, and supplies are limited due to weight constrictions.

Benefits: Populations that had no access to care because of transportation are supplied direct access to a dental hygienist.

Kelly Nance, Flying Hygienist

Kelly Nance left her job in a traditional dental office to practice in rural Alaska. Practice settings range from full clinics with two to three dental chairs; to health clinics with one chair, a dental unit, and basic equipment; to school gyms. The dental team brings portable equipment and jugs of distilled water with them when they travel to locations without a clinic.

Kelly: Our clients' special needs here are the incredibly high caries rate and their geographical location. There are no roads in or out of the villages. All travel is by plane or boat. Lots of villages are an hour or more away by plane. With the high caries rate, the importance of getting out to these people is huge.

Here in Bethel we have a large 14-chair clinic. Patients can only be seen by the hygienist if they have had a full comprehensive examination. To get a full comprehensive examination you have to call the clinic Monday mornings between 7:45 a.m. and 8:00 a.m. to schedule that examination. The full examination is good for a year. Depending on the village you go to, each setup is different. Cassie, the other hygienist here, went to a village where they set up their portable equipment in the gym at the school. She and a dentist stayed in that village for 5 days and would sleep in the library of the school. Some villages have health clinics that have a dental chair in them. In those villages we don't have to bring the portable equipment; they keep a chair, dental unit, ultrasonic, Cavitron, and autoclave in the clinic. There are also sub-regional clinics (SRCs) that are full clinics with 2 to 3 chairs. We have five of the SRCs in the area we cover. The whole Yukon-Kuskokwim Delta is the size of the state of Oregon.

Working in public health is much different than private practice. For one, your focus seems to be more on the community rather than individuals. It is really interesting to see true problems with access to care. Most of the people have to take a plane into Bethel (which can be expensive) to see a dentist or get their teeth cleaned. I believe if someone is in enough pain Medicaid will pay for a trip in. There is not much concern for "cosmetic dentistry," to say the least, or whitening of the teeth. I think because there is such a lack of care, people don't understand the importance of getting their teeth cleaned two times a year. The women of the villages who are pregnant need to come to Bethel 4 weeks before their babies are due, so we spend 1 day a week at the Prematernal Home providing education and services to these soon-to-be moms. With all the portable equipment, it isn't as comfortable for the clinician or the patient, really.

Cassie Williams: We often have to do our own scheduling in the villages. Sometimes we don't have access to computers, radiographs, or medical history charts. You also have to bring *all* the equipment you may need with you. If you forget anything (gloves, instruments, adapters), it can cost upwards of $40 to get it to you and you lose time while waiting. One of the biggest challenges I am seeing is the cultural changes that would really need to happen to make changes complete. Tobacco use is very common. Babies are often given chew for teething. A hygienist whom I had lunch with yesterday said she saw a "tobacco pouch" on an 8-year-old boy. You see 2- to 3-year-old kids walking around with a Mountain Dew. I think access to care is really another huge problem. People in some villages may only see a dental health provider, at most, once a year. Then the dentist or hygienist really need to triage who needs to be seen first... so you still don't get seen if you have "small" cavities; it is usually only when you are in pain. That is why I love the program I am working with, getting native people from the villages to help educate and get fluoride on teeth.

You learn to plan ahead and also ways to improvise when you don't have the equipment that you need. You learn to be a "mechanic" for your own gear.

I think a lot of the advantage of working in this setting is personal. I have learned to live in a small town where things are much slower... I am learning so much about an amazing group of people with a wonderful culture that they are really proud of and trying to keep true. I am learning there are so many more important things in this world—really—like helping people keep their teeth through high school. I see so many kids getting first molars extracted at age 7 and 8.... It breaks my heart as well as that of the dentist who has to do it. We had a meeting this morning, and two-thirds of the kids in this area are being seen in the OR [operating room] under general anesthesia for dental treatment. There is an average of 600 births a year, with 400 kids at age 2 being seen in the OR. The advantage is that it is rewarding. Each community differs. Some are really glad to see you, whereas some school staff see you as a hassle because you get kids out of class. I have had good feedback from the people I see...I think it will be important to try to really get native people involved and educate them so they can work and live in the villages and provide services. Working here, it seems like all the health-care professionals want to work together! It has been really encouraging! We even had the pediatric nurses asking us for fluoride and how to use it.

When we don't have a clinic we bring out chairs, portable units, compressors as well as instruments, masks, gloves, and other items. We also have to bring the water and sterilizing equipment. We work under the supervision of a dentist but it doesn't have to be direct. Most village trips are just a hygienist and an assistant. We can and sometimes will travel with a dentist depending on how much room is available.

I love working out here! There is a huge need! I have talked about and heard about problems with access to care since school.... However this is really a problem with access to care. Most plane trips from a village are about $450 round trip. Most people are not going to come in for preventative care, only when they are in pain...

BEYOND THE DENTAL OFFICE: VENUES AND SERVICES

The clinical functions of a dental hygienist have been typically defined as the functions that occur in an office setting. Practicing in venues beyond the dental office expands the dental hygienist's role in obtaining full-body health for the patient.

Skilled Nursing Facilities and Intermediate Care Facilities

Access to proper oral health care has proven to be one of the most profound issues for health care in seniors residing in a long-term care facility. According to the Surgeon General's report, "nursing homes and other long-term care institutions have limited capacity to deliver needed oral health services to their residents, most of whom are at increased risk for oral diseases."[3]

In long-term care facilities, the absence of a comprehensive oral assessment upon intake and at regular intervals prevents the proper identification of dental disease, therefore creating a barrier to appropriate care. Currently, oral health assessments of the elderly and disabled residing in skilled nursing facilities are generally completed by nursing staff who lack the necessary dental training to do so.[6]

The federal government requires skilled nursing facilities (SNFs) and intermediate care facilities (ICFs) to provide each resident with "access to dental services," specifically mandating "an oral examination annually." Further, regulations state that if dental care "is not included in the facility's per diem fees and the resident is unable to pay for care then the facility must attempt to find alternative sources to fund services."[7]

The lack of daily preventive care from direct-care staff is paramount. One study found that only 16% of the residents in an SNF received oral care, and the average toothbrushing time was 16.2 seconds.[8]

The roles of the dental hygienist working in an SNF include the following:

1. **Delivery of direct patient care**: Many SNFs have a dental operatory on site or a beauty salon that can be used to provide privacy and limit the risk of cross-contamination. Dental equipment must be transported to facilities that use a beauty salon to deliver care. It is important to comply with the Health Insurance Portability and Accountability Act (HIPAA) and infection control regulations and standards in any setting. Privacy and infection control are sometimes difficult to accomplish in facilities where patients share rooms. Having a designated area that is private and free from the risk of cross-contamination assures that hygienists are complying with state regulations and keeping the patient safe in this setting. In this setting the hygienist can deliver any care within the state dental practice act and the regulations governing venues. Hygienists are able to deliver the same care they deliver in the office in an SNF.

2. **Education**: Many SNFs and ICFs have no system for oral care of patients or training for staff in oral care. Teaching administrators, nursing staff, direct-care staff, patients, and family members or conservators about the importance of oral care, the chain of infection, contagion of dental diseases, and daily care

is the first step to combating the discrepancy in care. Dental hygienists can deliver care every 3 months, but if the patient is unable to perform daily care and the staff does not value it, the patient will never achieve a state of health.

3. **Advocacy**: The oral health of patients residing in SNFs and ICFs may be neglected because of the number of health issues these patients face. One study in the United Kingdom discovered that only 5% of residential home dwellers who requested assistance with oral care received it.[8] However, oral health may be the cause of other health issues. For example, aspiration pneumonia has been associated with lack of oral care and is one of the leading causes of death in SNFs.[9]

A dental hygiene advocate can affect the care of those residing in facilities. Advocates ensure that patients have direct access to a dental hygienist and dental care. They work with facilities to develop a protocol for oral health care that includes stocking needed supplies for optimum oral care, training staff, and holding staff accountable for patient oral care. They also make evidence-based recommendations for staff training and development in oral health (see Spotlight on Public Health 50-1).

Hospitals

With increased understanding of the synergy between oral and general health, the role of the dental hygienist in the hospital has expanded to include the following responsibilities:

1. Providing comfort care for cancer patients and end-of-life patients

Spotlight on Public Health 50-1

Lettecia Reyes, RDH, worked with clients with special needs in a traditional setting and took a course on serving clients with special needs. She soon discovered that this culture was one of the most underserved populations that did not have a voice in their care, and she went to work for the Lanterman Center in Los Angeles, California. She oversees the evaluation and delivery of care of over 10,000 developmentally delayed adults living in SNFs, ICFs, residential care facilities, and private homes. She delivers and secures staff training and development in oral health care. Her duties include reviewing treatment plans, evaluating patient needs, and securing providers for services. Lettecia stated, "There is not a day that goes by that I am not blessed for doing this job! I see the smiles of those who were once destined to be edentulous and think how wonderful it is that I could be a small part of the solution to access to care." ■

2. Treating ventilation, aspiration pneumonia, and pulmonary patients to lower the bioburden
3. Treating hospitalized patients before surgery to ensure a good outcome and lower the chance of infection
4. Treating long-term patients who are not able to leave the hospital
5. Delivering preventive supplies to patients
6. Training staff to deliver daily care and develop a protocol.

See Spotlight on Public Health 50-2.

Schools

Dental hygienists in the school setting perform preventive services such as fluoride and sealant programs. They also educate students, parents, teachers, and staff. See Spotlight on Public Health 50-3.

Private Homes

Providing care to patients in their homes has advantages for both the dental hygienist and the patients. The dental hygienist can evaluate the dynamics of the care the patient is receiving and educate and train caregivers and family members. Becoming familiar with the environment the patient lives in helps the dental hygienist make clinical decisions, including those regarding product choice and preventive measures. The patient does not have to leave home and be exposed to outside risks such as cross-contamination, exposure to the elements, and diseases. See Spotlight on Public Health 50-4.

Street Outreach

Just as nurses have brought preventive care to patients living on the streets with programs such as needle

Spotlight on Public Health 50-2

Susan McLearn visited a hospital facility during a manpower project she was working on. As she developed a relationship with a subacute hospital, she soon discovered that members of the nursing staff were overwhelmed with duties and had a very limited understanding of the necessary preventive measures to aid patients. Utilizing her expanded license and scope of practice, Susan developed a protocol, trained the direct care staff, and brought in her portable unit to give direct care to clients who were unable to leave the facility due to health issues. Susan's comprehensive program, which addressed access to care and included an educational component for the direct-care staff, created a long-term solution. The program has met the need of patients who may not have received care otherwise. "It is very rewarding to work with other health professionals and to be considered an important part of the health-care team," Susan notes. ■

Spotlight on Public Health 50-3

Susan McCracken, Robin Shaffer, and Dr. Stacey Eastman lived in a rural area where children did not receive preventive care. They created a grant program that maximizes the scope-of-practice laws that allow Registered Dental Hygienists in Alternative Practice (RDHAPs) and Registered Dental Hygienists (RDHs) in public health settings to deliver preventive services without the supervision of a dentist. Dental hygiene and dental assisting students from a nearby school help deliver care. They conduct oral assessments, provide fluoride varnish treatments, and deliver other preventive services in public and private preschools and elementary schools.

Some challenges of providing care in schools include having to have depend on the van driver to deliver all of the portable equipment ahead of time, scheduling time to set up a dental office on a stage or in a library, and finding an appropriate space to sterilize equipment. Also, services must be scheduled on days when there are no school holidays, assemblies, or other conflicts to interfere with the 3 days they are on campus.

School nurses are their greatest advocates. Developing relationships with teachers, administrators, and families also ensures a successful turnout. Teachers send home permission slips, and the front office collects them and makes sure the school will have the requisite 60% student participation the week before dental hygiene team arrives. Program staff members visit the school the week before the program to educate the students about what to expect and to review oral hygiene and nutrition with the help of puppets.

Susan and Robin: "First and foremost, you must have a love of small children and loads of patience to work in the schools. You must be flexible and resourceful because public health is not at all like delivering dentistry in a typical dental office. You really have to think for yourself and be able to problem solve the many obstacles that may come up during a day. It also helps to be comfortable meeting and training school nurses and working with administration who generally know nothing about the challenge of delivering dental services to schoolchildren. You must also familiarize yourself with the process of writing a grant or working with a trained grant-writer to obtain funds to purchase dental equipment and supplies."

Their program is very committed to making the whole experience educational and fun for the children.

Susan: "This is often their first experience receiving dental services, so some of them are nervous as they come into the clinic for the first time. Once they watch their classmates getting treatment and smiling, they

Continued

calm down right away and join in the fun! We can adjust our chairs to make both patient and clinician comfortable. The students wear sunglasses to keep the lights out of their eyes, and we are very careful to keep the saliva ejectors handy so the kids can spit out frequently. With patience, a sense of humor, and a caring staff, we are able to provide treatment to thousands of 4- and 5-year-old kids each year." ■

Spotlight on Public Health 50-4

Brenda Kibbler started her private dental hygiene practice to reach out to meet the needs of the homebound. Unable to find resources or materials to meet the needs of patients who were living with tracheostomies, ventilators, and other breathing equipment, Brenda researched and developed a program to meet the needs of those patients. She also began teaching continuing education courses on the subject.

Brenda shared the rewards of this work: "My trach patients' rooms are equipped with oxygen tanks, ventilator machines, suction units, hospital beds, nebulizers, wheelchairs. This setting is completely different from a dental office setting. Ergonomics is not ideal, but you do the best you can. Patient comfort is now the key element, and I do whatever is necessary to prevent a medical emergency. Having a hygienist available to these patients is literally a matter of life and death." ■

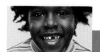

Spotlight on Public Health 50-5

Because he had worked in a free clinic for many years, Noel Kelsch knew that most people without secure housing did not show up to the clinic unless they were in pain. He notes, "Dental disease prevention is not a priority when you do not know where you are going to lay your head at night or where the next meal is coming from." Noel decided to take preventive services to the streets by initiating a toothbrush exchange program. "Utilizing small grants and donations, I can gather supplies for this program. I am able to provide a fluoride varnish program, nutrition counseling, xylitol distribution, education, referrals, and triage. I am no longer just sticking my finger in the dike! I am starting to see patients on the street who are maintaining their oral health in the high-risk environment they are living in." ■

exchange and condom distribution for disease prevention, dental hygienists can also provide preventive care to homeless patients. Programs for the homeless may provide fluoride varnish, xylitol distribution, and care kits that give patients the equipment to properly care for their oral health. These programs are frequently funded by grants and gifts in kind. See Spotlight on Public Health 50-5.

Institutions and Prisons

The dental hygienist's role in institutions and prisons is the same as that in the traditional service model. Preventive care is performed and existing conditions are treated. The hygienist's role is vital in this setting because most prisons have crowded living conditions, and dental disease can be spread through these close contacts.

Workplace

It is often difficult for companies to give their staff time off to go to dental appointments. To meet their employees' needs, some companies now have medical and dental operatories at their work sites. This model allows patients to receive treatment without leaving work. It limits time away from the job and helps to maintain staff health and productivity.

ADMINISTRATION OF CARE

Charting

All charting and record-keeping requirements that apply in the clinical dental setting are also required in other venues. Utilizing paperless systems is essential in the limited space supplied in these situations and allows for easy transfer of records. All laws governing the portability and sharing of patient records are governed by the 1996 HIPAA regulations. Privacy and security rules must be adhered to in all venues. See Chapter 2, Legal and Ethical Considerations, for detailed information on HIPAA.

Allowable Duties, Venues, and Supervision

There are many laws and regulations that govern the practice of dental hygiene. It is vital to become aware of the state's dental practice act or dental hygiene practice act and any other laws that govern the practice of dental hygiene. State business and professional codes, local laws, occupational safety and hazard laws, Environmental Protection Agency (EPA) regulations, and Centers for Disease Control and Prevention (CDC) recommendations must all be addressed. These laws and regulations determine the dental hygienist's scope of practice, location, and need for supervision, and understanding of them is essential.

Dental Hygiene Practice Act, Level of Supervision, and Scope of Duties

Each state has laws governing the practice of dental hygiene. These laws include the following:

1. The level of supervision required from a dentist, which often includes direct supervision, general supervision, and indirect supervision. With **direct supervision,** most states require the dentist to be present when the patient is receiving the direct-supervision-duty treatment. The duty must be performed pursuant to the order, control, and full professional responsibility of the supervising dentist. Such procedures must be checked and approved by the supervising dentist before dismissal of the patient from the office of said dentist. **General supervision** is defined as duties that are based on instructions given by a licensed dentist, but not requiring the physical presence of the supervising dentist during the performance of those procedures.

2. The scope of practice, which governs the allowable duties a dental hygienist may perform and the location where those duties may be performed.

It is important to note that some states now have a separate board for dental hygiene. An overview of each state dental practice/dental hygiene practice act, scope of practice, and level of supervision as it relates to dental hygiene can be found at https://www.adha.org/resources-docs/7513_Direct_Access_to_Care_from_DH.pdf.

Restorative

The scope of practice in many states now includes restorative care. Two-thirds of the states currently allow hygienists to deliver restorative care in their scope of practice. A factsheet reviewing restorative care services provided by dental hygienists is available at http://www.adha.org/resources-docs/7517_Restorative_Services_Factsheet.pdf.

Case Study

Sara has been working as a dental hygienist in a private dental practice for 5 years. She knows that many long-term care facilities are not equipped to deliver oral health care to their patients. She has started researching how she can provide services in those facilities and advocate for the residents.

Case Study Exercises

1. Obstacles to residents of long-term care facilities receiving oral health care include which of the following?
   A. Daily oral care is provided for residents who cannot perform their own care.
   B. The plan for oral health care created when patients enter the facility does not include time for regular dental hygiene appointments.
   C. Nursing staff lack the necessary training to perform oral health assessments on patients.

2. Sara could work with a long-term care facility to develop a protocol for oral health care and make evidence-based recommendations for staff training and development in oral health. Which role encompasses these responsibilities?
   A. Educator
   B. Advocate
   C. Independent practice hygienist
   D. Advanced Dental Hygiene Practitioner

3. Sara decided to create an oral health training presentation for staff members at long-term care facilities. All of the following topics should be included in the presentation EXCEPT which one?
   A. The importance of oral care
   B. The chain of infection
   C. The process for delivering preventive care
   D. The process for assessing the dental needs of patients

Review Questions

1. The wellness model is based on
   A. risk reduction and disease prevention.
   B. disease identification and treatment.
   C. direct access to a dental hygienist.

2. Where can dental professionals find their scope of practice?
   A. Health Insurance Portability and Accountability Act (HIPAA) Privacy Rule
   B. State dental practice act or dental hygiene practice act
   C. federal Dental Practice Act

3. Mobile dental clinics
   A. are self-contained.
   B. require a large amount of space and solid ground.
   C. are high-cost investments
   D. All of these choices

4. Direct access is a general term that the American Dental Hygienists' Association (ADHA) uses to describe policies that allow hygienists to initiate patient care in settings outside the private dental office. Nursing staff in skilled nursing facilities are qualified to assess patients' oral health and deliver oral health care.
   A. Both statements are true.
   B. Both statements are false.
   C. The first statement is true, but the second is false.
   D. The first statement is false, but the second is true.

5. Every state allows dental hygienists to own their own practice in a freestanding building. Public and policymaker awareness of the importance of oral health can also create barriers to oral health.
   A. Both statements are true.
   B. Both statements are false.
   C. The first statement is true, but the second is false.
   D. The first statement is false, but the second is true.

Active Learning

1. Arrange to visit a nursing home or long-term care facility to talk to the director about the residents' oral health-care needs and how they are met.
2. Research dental hygiene practice acts to determine which states allow dental hygienists to practice independently. Present your findings to the class. ■

REFERENCES

1. American Dental Hygienists' Association. Advocacy. 2012. Available from: http://www.adha.org/direct-access.
2. American Dental Hygienists' Association. Direct access states. 2013. Available from: http://www.adha.org/resources-docs/7513_Direct_Access_to_Care_from_DH.pdf.
3. Department of Health and Human Services, National Institute of Dental and Craniofacial Research. Oral health in America: a report of the Surgeon General. 2000. Available from: http://silk.nih.gov/public/hck1ocv.@www.surgeon.fullrpt.pdf.
4. American Dental Hygienists' Association. Facts about the Dental Hygiene Workforce in the United States. Revised 2015. Available from https://www.adha.org/sites/default/files/75118_Facts_About_the_Dental_Hygiene_Workforce.pdf.
5. American Dental Hygienists' Association. Competencies for the Advanced Dental Hygiene Practitioner (ADHP). 2012. Available from: https://www.adha.org/resources-docs/72612_ADHP_Competencies.pdf.
6. California Dental Association Foundation's Geriatric Oral Health Access Program (GOHAP) final report 8/2009.
7. Code of Federal Regulations, section 42:483.55.a.
8. Simons D, et al. Relationship between oral hygiene practices and oral status in dentate elderly people living in residential homes. *Comm Dent Oral Epidemiol.* 2001;29(6):464-470.
9. Terpenning MS, et al. Aspiration pneumonia: dental and oral risk factors in an older veteran population. *J Am Geriatr Soc.* 2001;49(5):557-563.

Part X

Emergency Management

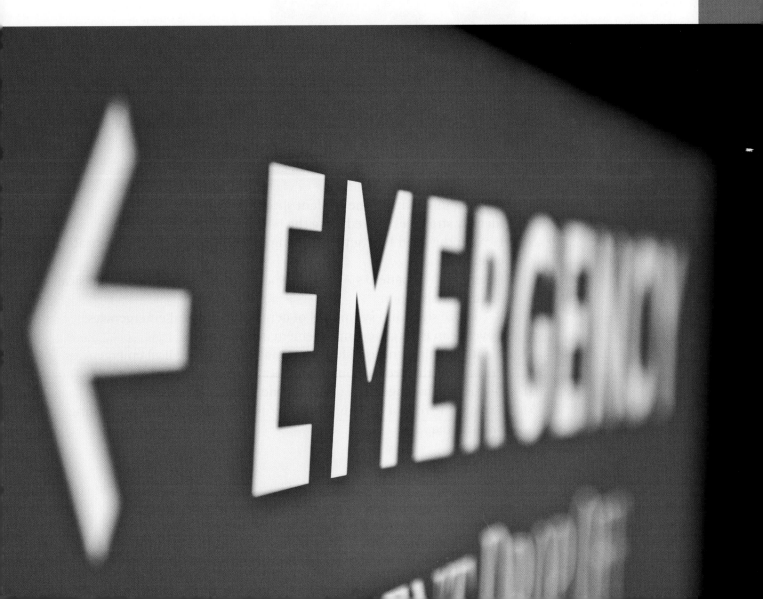

Chapter 51 | Dental and Medical Emergencies

Mark G. Kacerik, RDH, MS • Renee G. Prajer, RDH, MS

KEY TERMS

anaphylaxis

angioedema

aromatic ammonia

automated external
defibrillator (AED)

avulsed tooth

basic life support (BLS)

bronchodilator

cyanosis

diphenhydramine

hyperinsulinism

ipecac syrup

luxation

protective oral appliance

rescue breathing

urticaria

vasodilator

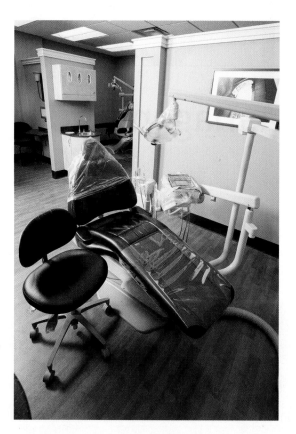

LEARNING OBJECTIVES

After reading this chapter, the student should be able to:

51.1 Identify strategies for reducing the risk of a potential emergency.

51.2 Explain the need for routine training in the management of medical emergencies.

51.3 Determine the patient's American Society of Anesthesiologists Physical Status Classification.

51.4 Recognize signs and symptoms of dental and medical emergencies.

51.5 Develop an emergency management action plan.

51.6 Identify equipment used for the management of medical emergencies.

51.7 Prepare for the prevention of a medical emergency.

51.8 Discuss the management of dental and medical emergencies.

51.9 Explain the role of oral appliances in overall safety and in preventing oral trauma.

KEY CONCEPTS

- Prevention is the first component in managing an emergency.
- Appropriate training and preparation are key aspects of emergency management for all office personnel.
- Recognition and management of emergencies is an element of comprehensive care.

RELEVANCE TO CLINICAL PRACTICE

As a health-care professional, the dental hygienist assumes the responsibility to take the necessary measures needed to prevent or minimize the risk of an emergency occurring during treatment. However, it must be anticipated that an emergency will occur at some point in one's career. It is therefore critical that the dental hygienist be prepared to recognize and manage medical emergencies (see Professionalism box).

The first component in managing medical emergencies is prevention. It is the hygienist's responsibility to identify potential emergencies. This is accomplished through patient observation and the completion of a comprehensive medical history at each appointment. These steps provide the hygienist with an opportunity to identify those patients who are medically compromised or present with risk factors that may increase the likelihood of an emergency. With this knowledge the hygienist can make appropriate modifications regarding treatment and patient management to reduce the risk of emergencies.

The second component of successful management of medical emergencies is preparedness. All members of the dental team should be aware of their role in the event of an emergency. Accomplishing this includes appropriate and routine training, a clear action plan for dealing with emergencies, and regular review of policies and procedures regarding emergency management (see Spotlight on Public Health).

Professionalism

As professionals, dental hygienists are obligated to maintain a standard of care that promotes the well-being of the individuals they serve. Maintaining currency through membership in the American Dental Hygienists' Association, participating in continuing education, making choices that demonstrate integrity and sound judgment, and collaborating with other health-care professionals are key elements in ensuring the safety and well-being of patients, colleagues, and community. ■

EMERGENCY PREVENTION

Medical History Assessment

The medical history assessment is generally viewed as an integral step in care planning and as a legal obligation, but it can also prove to be a pertinent step in preventing medical emergencies. When a thorough dialogue transpires between the dental hygienist and the patient/caregiver, the hygienist is able to interpret and evaluate the need for further clarification of positive responses indicated on the medical history questionnaire. In addition, when effective dialogue is created, the patient may ask the dental hygienist for clarification of medical terminology and be more forthcoming with significant medical information (see Application to Clinical Practice).[1]

Application to Clinical Practice

Your 9-year-old patient presents with a history of asthma. The patient's mother dropped her child off for the appointment and reviewed her medical history with the office receptionist. The patient's mother indicated that there have been no medical history changes since the child's last visit. You ask the child if she brought her inhaler with her to the appointment. The child responds "no" and continues to explain that her inhaler was empty because she had three asthma attacks over the weekend. How will you proceed? ■

Physical Observation

Observing the patient's physical status is another vital component in preventing medical emergencies. Overall physical characteristics and the patient's vital signs, gait, communication, and motor skills should also be evaluated to determine the need for further investigation and/or medical referral.

Psychological Assessment

Through the completion of the medical history, observation, and dialogue, an appropriate venue is established to assess the patient's outlook on dental treatment. Stressors associated with dental fear or anxiety increase the risk of acute medical emergencies. Dental hygienists must be attentive to the patient's anxiety level and determine an appropriate plan of action for safe treatment. There are a variety of approaches available for managing patients who experience dental anxiety, including education, pharmaceuticals, and natural alternatives, to assist them in anxiety reduction during dental treatment. Reducing a patient's stress level is an essential component in preventing an acute medical emergency.[1] See Chapter 31, Anxiety and Pain Control Management, for detailed information on strategies to reduce a patient's anxiety.

The American Society of Anesthesiologists (ASA) Physical Status (PS) Classification System is a valuable process in determining the patient's surgical and anesthetic risk before dental treatment (Table 51-1).[2]

Medical Consultation

Dental hygienists should consult with the patient's physician when concerns regarding the patient's physical or psychological health arise. Gathering specific information from the patient's physician allows for a decreased risk of a medical emergency, and in turn a safe dental experience. Dental hygienists are now working in a variety of nontraditional settings such as hospitals, nursing homes, mobile dental units, and school-based clinics, and must prepare differently for emergencies in these settings.

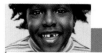

Spotlight on Public Health

As the dental hygiene community works to address the need for access to care, more dental hygienists are finding employment in nontraditional settings such as hospitals, nursing homes, mobile dental units, and school-based clinics. Many of the sites with access-to-care issues are located in remote areas; because of this the response time of emergency personnel is greater. Individuals providing care in such locations should anticipate the delay in response time and prepare for emergencies accordingly. ■

Table 51-1. *American Society of Anesthesiologists Physical Status Classification System*[1,2]

Classification	Conditions	Treatment Modifications
ASA PS 1	Normal, healthy patient; little or no dental anxiety	No modifications indicated
ASA PS 2	Patient with mild systemic disease or extreme dental anxiety	Medical consultation when indicated, possible sedative techniques, pain control
ASA PS 3	Patient with severe systemic disease	Exercise caution during treatment, allow patient to rest, monitor patient closely, sedative techniques, pain control
ASA PS 4	Patient with severe systemic disease that is a constant threat to life	Postpone elective dental care, treat emergency dental care in a hospital setting
ASA PS 5	A moribund patient who is not expected to survive without an operation	Palliative treatment for pain management only
ASA PS 6	A patient declared brain dead whose organs are being removed for donor purposes	Treatment not indicated

Oral Trauma Prevention

Dental hygienists are in the position to educate and advocate regarding the importance of **protective oral appliances** for the prevention of dental trauma. The use of mouthguards can prevent many sports-related dental emergencies. Although inexpensive over-the-counter mouthguards can be purchased, compliance is poor due to their ill-fitting nature, and protection is minimal. Custom-fabricated mouthguards offer optimum protection and the greatest comfort because of their proper fit. According to the American Academy of Pediatrics, 10% to 39% of dental injuries are sports related, and approximately 50% of children will experience a tooth injury by the time they are adolescents. Mouthguards not only protect the teeth from trauma but also decrease the chances of facial bone fractures, injury to the temporomandibular joint (TMJ), and head injuries. Other safety measures and equipment such as seatbelts, facemasks, and helmets serve as dental trauma prevention tools when used appropriately. Following recommended safety guidelines can prove to be instrumental in avoiding a dental emergency.[3,4]

EMERGENCY PREPARATION AND ORGANIZATION

Proper management of an emergency requires preparation and organization. All office personnel should be appropriately and adequately trained to manage an emergency in the dental setting. Preparation should include routine certification in **basic life support (BLS)**, continuing education related to the recognition and management of medical emergencies, team review of emergency policies, an action plan, and maintenance of emergency equipment.

Training

The training of office personnel should include one- and two-person cardiopulmonary resuscitation (CPR) for adults, children, and infants; the use of an **automated external defibrillator (AED)**; management of an obstructed airway; and **rescue breathing**. Knowledge of CPR is the most critical skill because the need to supply oxygen to the heart and brain is vital in the early management of almost all emergencies. The American Heart Association 2010 BLS guidelines stress the importance of compressions: pushing hard and fast at a rate of at least 100 compressions per minute for all victims, with minimal interruptions, and allowing full chest recoil between compressions. The BLS sequence follows the steps C-A-B for all victims: **c**hest compressions, **a**irway, **b**reathing (see Advancing Technologies; Table 51-2).[5,6]

Advancing Technologies

Technology innovations in dental hygiene practice have enhanced patient care in several areas. The World Wide Web assists practitioners in obtaining current information on medical conditions and pharmacological agents. Equipment such as the automated external defibrillator and other advancements assist the oral health-care professional in maintaining a safe treatment environment. In this age of emerging technology, it is important that dental professionals remain current. ■

Table 51-2. *Basic Life Support Emergency Care Reference Guide*[5,6]

	Adult	Child (1–8 years of age/puberty)	Infant (Less than 1 year of age)
Assess for responsiveness	Unresponsive, no breathing, no pulse Activate EMS/get AED.	Unresponsive no breathing, no pulse Observed collapse: Activate EMS/get AED. Unobserved collapse: Perform 2 minutes of CPR, then activate EMS/get AED.	Unresponsive no breathing, no pulse Observed collapse: Activate EMS/get AED. Unobserved collapse: Perform 2 minutes of CPR, then activate EMS/get AED.
Airway	Perform head-tilt, chin-lift technique. If head or neck injury is suspected, utilize the jaw-thrust technique.	Perform head-tilt, chin-lift technique. If head or neck injury is suspected, utilize the jaw-thrust technique.	Perform head-tilt, chin-lift technique. If head or neck injury is suspected, utilize the jaw-thrust technique.
Rescue breathing	1 breath: every 5–6 seconds	1 breath: every 3–5 seconds	1 breath: every 3–5 seconds
CPR	**Compression rate:** at least 100 per minute	**Compression rate:** at least 100 per minute	**Compression rate:** at least 100 per minute

Continued

Table 51-2. *Basic Life Support Emergency Care Reference Guide*[5,6] —cont'd

	Adult	Child (1–8 years of age/puberty)	Infant (Less than 1 year of age)
	Depth: at least 2 inches (5 cm) **Compression-to-breath ratio:** 30:2 (for 1 or 2 rescuers)	**Depth:** at least 1/3 anterior posterior diameter, about 2 inches (5 cm) **Compression-to-breath ratio:** 30:2 (1 rescuer) 15:2 (2 rescuers)	**Depth:** at least 1/3 anterior posterior diameter, about 1 1/2 inches (4 cm) **Compression-to-breath ratio:** 30:2 (1 rescuer) 15:2 (2 rescuers)
AED	Attach AED as soon as available, **use adult pads only**, minimize interruptions in chest compressions, resume CPR after each shock.	Attach AED as soon as available; **use child pads when available, otherwise use adult pads**; minimize interruptions in chest compressions; resume CPR after each shock.	**Manual defibrillator is preferred.** If unavailable use AED with pediatric dose attenuator. If neither is available, you may use an AED without a pediatric dose attenuator. Minimize interruptions in chest compressions; resume CPR after each shock.
Choking	**Mild obstruction:** Observe patient until obstruction is relieved. If obstruction persists, activate EMS. **Severe obstruction:** Utilize abdominal thrusts until obstruction is relieved or patient becomes unresponsive. If patient becomes unresponsive, begin steps of CPR starting with compressions. If a patient is pregnant or obese, chest thrusts should be utilized.	**Mild obstruction:** Observe patient until obstruction is relieved. If obstruction persists, activate EMS. **Severe obstruction:** Utilize abdominal thrusts until obstruction is relieved or the child becomes unresponsive. If the child becomes unresponsive, begin steps of CPR starting with compressions.	**Mild obstruction:** Observe patient until obstruction is relieved. If obstruction persists, activate EMS. **Severe obstruction:** Deliver up to 5 back slaps and 5 chest thrusts until obstruction is relieved or the infant becomes unresponsive. If the infant becomes unresponsive, begin steps of CPR starting with compressions.

Emergency Contacts

Proper organization is necessary and to allow for the members of the dental team to work efficiently in managing a medical emergency should it occur. Emergency contact information should be posted next to telephones. This list should include the numbers for emergency medical services (EMS), fire, police/911, poison control, and the nearest hospital emergency center. If a number must be dialed for an outside line, this should be clearly indicated. Clear and simple directions on how to best access the facility should be posted next to the telephone so that the caller can provide this information to emergency personnel, in particular when the facility is located in a large multibuilding suite (Table 51-3).[7]

Action Plan

To prevent confusion in an emergency, each individual must know what his or her responsibilities are. To ensure effective action on the part of those members involved in managing an emergency, the dental team should review the emergency action plan periodically and complete a practice drill that simulates each member's role in the event of an actual emergency. The action plan should be reviewed with all new employees.

Action plans should be kept as simple as possible for ease of implementation. In most cases emergencies can be effectively managed by three to four members of the dental team. Team member 1, or the team leader, is generally the individual who encounters the emergency, and who then directs team members 2 and 3. Other members of the team remain available but clear of the emergency (Table 51-4 and Teamwork).[7,8]

Equipment

All dental offices should be equipped with a basic first aid kit, emergency drug kit, portable oxygen (size "E"/M-24 cylinder), and an AED. One individual should be designated to assess the equipment on a weekly basis to ensure that it is functioning and that items have not expired.

Oxygen, which is indicated in all emergency situations except hyperventilation, is the most useful drug in an emergency. A size "E"/M-24 cylinder provides oxygen for approximately 30 minutes and is recommended due to its portability. Smaller-sized cylinders do not contain an adequate amount of oxygen for proper management of an emergency, and larger cylinders lack the ease of portability. All members of the dental team

Table 51-3. Emergency Contact Information for Medical Assistance[7,8]

Facility information
- Complete address
- Phone number
- Location of office
- Basic directions (for example, intersecting streets and building number)

Emergency contacts (indicate if a number must be dialed for an outside line)
- EMS: 911
- Poison Control Centers: 1–800–222–1222
- Fire
- Police
- Ambulance
- Local emergency room

Reporting an emergency to EMS (911)
- EMS may request the following information:
  - Location of the emergency
  - The number you are calling from
  - Nature of the emergency (for example: chest pain, suspect possible heart attack)
  - Condition of the victim (age, consciousness, vitals)
  - Emergency treatment that is being administered
- Be prepared to follow instructions of dispatcher
- Stay on the line until instructed by the dispatcher to hang up

Table 51-4. Emergency Management Action Plan[7,8]

Team Member 1
- The individual who encounters the emergency
- Remains with the victim
- Directs team members 2 and 3
- Positions victim
- Monitors vitals
- Provides BLS as needed

Team Member 2
- Brings emergency equipment (first aid kit, emergency drug kit, O$_2$, AED)
- Prepares oxygen for delivery
- Prepares drugs for administration
- Prepares AED for use
- Assists with monitoring vitals
- Assists with BLS as needed

Team Member 3
- Activates EMS
- Records time of emergency
- Maintains documentation of emergency
- Meets rescue team at entrance and directs to emergency
- Assists as needed

Teamwork

Melissa, the office receptionist, has taken an emergency call from a patient's mother. A 16-year-old patient of the practice just got hit in the mouth by a baseball bat during an after-school game. The young gentleman arrives at the office and has evident trauma to his mouth. The dentist is with another patient. Mary Claire, the hygienist in the office, is currently making confirmation calls to patients scheduled for the next day. After learning that it would be another 15 minutes before Dr. Nichols could see the emergency patient, Mary Claire consults with Dr. Nichols to determine what type of radiographs need to be exposed on the young baseball player. Mary Claire reassures the patient, reviews the patient's medical history, obtains information about the emergency, and exposes the prescribed radiographs. When Dr. Nichols enters the operatory, he is presented with the information and radiographs needed to assist him in managing the dental emergency. Mary Claire displayed teamwork by offering help to Melissa by using her time wisely to make confirmation calls, ensuring a full schedule for the upcoming day. She also assisted Dr. Nichols with time management and supplied critical information needed to treat the emergency patient. ■

should be trained to distinguish oxygen, which is contained in a green cylinder, from other gases found in the dental setting, such as nitrous oxide, which is contained in a blue cylinder. Because emergencies rarely occur, instructions for the operation of the oxygen tank and administration recommendations should be laminated and attached to the tank (Table 51-5).[7,9]

First aid and emergency drug kits can be purchased as commercially prepackaged items; however, such kits may include items that the dental team is not adequately trained to use or administer. It is recommended to include only those items that the dental team is trained to administer and to seek professional training as needed. The American Dental Association's Council on Scientific Affairs offers the following suggestions in regard to emergency drug kits (Tables 51-6 and 51-7):

In designing an emergency drug kit, the Council suggests that the following drugs be included as a minimum: epinephrine 1:1000 (injectable), histamine-blocker (injectable), oxygen with positive-pressure administration capability, nitroglycerin (sublingual tablet or aerosol spray), bronchodilator (asthma inhaler), sugar and aspirin. Other drugs may be included as the doctor's training and needs mandate. It is particularly important that the dentist be knowledgeable about the indications, contraindications, dosages and methods of delivery for all items included in the emergency kit. Dentists

Table 51-5. Oxygen Delivery Systems[9,11]

Device	Indications	Flow Rate	Oxygen Concentration
Cannula	Patient is breathing and needs low levels of oxygen	2–6 L/min	25%–45%
Facemask	Patient is breathing and needs moderate levels of oxygen: • when cannula is not tolerated • when more oxygen is desired • when patient is in shock	8–15 L/min	40%–60%
Nonrebreather mask	Patient is breathing and needs high levels of oxygen: • when patient is in shock • when more oxygen is needed	10–15 L/min	60%–90%
Bag-valve mask	Patient has stopped breathing; used instead of mouth-to-mouth resuscitation	10–15 L/min	90%–100%

Table 51-6. Emergency Drugs[7,9,10]

Drug	Indication	Action	Administration
Aromatic ammonia	Syncope	Respiratory stimulant	Inhaled
Aspirin	Myocardial infarction	Antiplatelet	Chewed and swallowed
Bronchodilator (albuterol, Proventil)	Bronchospasm (asthma)	Beta$_2$-adrenergic agonist agent (bronchodilator)	Inhaled
Diphenhydramine	Mild allergic reaction	Antihistamine	Oral/intramuscular
Epinephrine	Severe allergic reaction or bronchospasm	Adrenergic agonist agent (bronchodilator)	Intramuscular
Glucose	Hypoglycemia	Antihypoglycemic agent	Ingested/intravenous
Nitroglycerin	Angina pectoris	**Vasodilator**	Sublingual
Oxygen	Respiratory distress	Increases blood oxygen	Inhaled

are also urged to perform continual emergency kit maintenance by replacing soon-to-be-outdated drugs before their expiration.

For offices in which emergency medical services, or EMS, personnel with defibrillation skills and equipment are not available within a reasonable time frame, the dentist may wish to consider an automated external defibrillator, or AED, consistent with AED training acquired in the BLS section of health care provider courses.[10]

Documentation

For all types of care, dental hygienists have a legal responsibility to maintain accurate records. It is important to record the treatment provided in an emergency situation. Because emergencies do not occur on a regular basis, it is best to keep an emergency treatment report form. This will ensure adequate and accurate documentation of the emergency. Forms should include the date

and time of the emergency, a description of the emergency, the time EMS was contacted and arrived, any treatment and drugs administered, the condition of the person when transported from the site, and any individuals present. A copy of the form should be kept in the patient's file and a copy should be given to the EMS (Table 51-8).[7]

MEDICAL AND DENTAL EMERGENCY MANAGEMENT

Even when the necessary measures have been taken to minimize the risk of occurrence of a medical or dental emergency, the potential for an emergency can never be completely eliminated (see Evidence-Based Practice). It is therefore critical that the dental hygienist be prepared to recognize and manage emergencies. Through careful observation, the hygienist can often

Table 51-7. *Emergency Equipment*[7,9,11]

- Portable oxygen tank (size "E"/M-24 cylinder)
- Nasal cannula/pocket ventilation mask/bag-valve mask (for adult, adolescent, and child)
- Automated external defibrillator
- Backboard
- Blanket
- Disposable syringes (2 mL with 18- through 21-gauge needles)
- Suction/aspirating tips (tonsil suction tips)
- Tourniquets
- Forceps
- Sterile bandages
- Saline solution
- Blood pressure cuff (large adult, adult, and child)
- Stethoscope
- Thermometer
- Instant cold packs
- **Ipecac syrup**
- Milk of magnesia

recognize the early signs and symptoms of an emergency, allowing for early intervention and reducing the risk of more serious complications. Tables 51-9 and 51-10 provide an overview of the medical and dental emergencies that may be encountered in the dental setting.

Evidence-Based Practice

Research has shown that an oral health-care provider will have to manage a medical emergency once every 1.4 years. In addition, research indicates that syncope is the most common medical emergency that occurs in the dental setting. Allergic reactions, diabetic emergencies, cardiac arrest, angina pectoris, myocardial infarction, asthma attacks, seizures, and postural hypotension, although less frequent, have also been reported. It is critical that oral health-care providers are fluent in prevention, preparedness, and management of medical emergencies that may transpire.[1,7,17] ■

Table 51-8. *Emergency Equipment*[7,9,11]

Emergency Treatment Report Form

Patient's Name: _____ Date: _____ Time: _____

Time EMS contacted: _____ Time EMS arrived: _____

Description of Emergency:

_____

_____

_____

Vitals:

Time	Pulse	Respiration	Blood pressure

Drugs Administered:

Time	Pulse	Respiration	Blood pressure

Description of Treatment Administered:

_____

_____

_____

Individuals providing treatment:

_____

_____

_____

Continued

Table 51-8. Emergency Equipment[7,9,11]—cont'd

Individuals present:

_____

_____

_____

Condition of patient when transported from site:

_____

_____

Recorded by: Print name: _____ Signature: _____

Table 51-9. Management of Medical Emergencies[7,11-23]

Medical Emergency	Signs and Symptoms	Management
Adrenal crisis (cortisol deficiency): a life-threatening condition that occurs when there is not enough cortisol, a hormone produced by the adrenal glands	Weakness Confusion Abdominal pain Anxious/stressed Rapid, weak pulse Low blood pressure Shock-like symptoms Loss of consciousness	Discontinue treatment, place patient in the supine position, activate EMS, open airway, monitor vital signs, and administer high-flow oxygen. If patient becomes unresponsive, initiate BLS.
Airway obstruction: physical blockage of the airway by an object	Inability to speak or cough forcefully Gagging Difficulty breathing Gasping **Cyanosis** of lips and fingernails	Discontinue treatment; position patient upright or as comfortable. Perform abdominal thrusts until the object is dislodged. If patient becomes unresponsive, position supine, activate EMS, and initiate BLS.
Allergic reaction: a reaction to an allergen that is generally mild to moderate and limited to localized areas of the body	**Delayed allergic reaction:** Erythema (rash) **Urticaria** (hives, itching) **Angioedema** (localized swelling of subcutaneous and/or submucosal tissues)	Discontinue treatment, administer antihistamine; epinephrine may be needed if patient experiences difficulty breathing.
Anaphylaxis: an immediate whole-body reaction to an allergen that results in the release of histamine and edema of the airways	**Immediate allergic reaction or anaphylaxis:** Urticaria Angioedema Respiratory distress Coughing, wheezing Low blood pressure Weak pulse Laryngeal edema with difficulty swallowing Dilation of pupils May progress to a sudden loss of consciousness and/or cardiac arrest	Discontinue treatment, administer epinephrine, administer oxygen, activate EMS, monitor vital signs, initiate BLS as needed.
Angina pectoris: chest pain that results from poor blood flow to the heart through the coronary arteries	Crushing chest pain or discomfort (tightness, squeezing, fullness, pressure) Pain may radiate to arms, neck, shoulder area, or back Nausea Fatigue Dizziness Anxiety Shortness of breath Sweating	Discontinue treatment, place patient in an upright position or as comfortable for breathing, activate EMS, administer oxygen by nasal cannula or facemask. Administer the patient's own nitroglycerin if available. Administer 1 0.4-mg tablet or metered spray sublingual. Repeat twice at 5-minute intervals for a total of three doses. Monitor vital signs. If symptoms persist, suspect a myocardial infarction.

Table 51-9. *Management of Medical Emergencies*[7,11-23] —cont'd

Medical Emergency	Signs and Symptoms	Management
Asthma attack: a sudden inflammation of the airways	Difficulty breathing Tightness in chest Coughing and wheezing Sweating Cold, pale, and clammy skin Faintness Nausea Rapid pulse	Discontinue treatment, position patient upright, and ensure airway is patent. Have patient self-administer his or her own bronchodilator if available or from emergency drug kit if needed. Provide supplemental oxygen and monitor vitals. If patient decompensates, activate EMS and administer epinephrine.
Burn (first degree): affects only the outer layer of skin **Burn (second degree):** affects the outer and under layers of skin	**First-degree:** Redness, swelling, and pain **Second-degree:** Intense redness Splotchy appearance Severe swelling and pain Blisters	**First- and second-degree:** Cool the burn under cool (not cold) running water until pain subsides, do not apply ice, butter, or ointments to the burn; do not break blisters. Cover the burn with a sterile gauze bandage.
Burn (third degree): affects the skin and underlying tissues	**Third-degree:** Charred, black or white Leathery in appearance Insensitive to touch	Discontinue treatment, activate EMS, observe for shock, raise burned body part above heart when possible, monitor vital signs, and initiate BLS as needed.
Chemical burn: damage to skin and/or underlying tissues due to chemical exposure	**Chemical burn:** Redness or discoloration present	Discontinue treatment; remove causative agent by rinsing off chemical with cool running water for 20–30 minutes (refer to Material Safety Data Sheet). Rewash burn area if burning continues after initial wash. Cover the burn with a sterile gauze bandage.
Cardiac arrest: a condition in which the heart suddenly and unexpectedly stops beating	Sudden loss of responsiveness/consciousness No breathing, pulse, or respiration	Activate EMS. Initiate BLS.
Diabetic coma (hyperglycemia, ketoacidosis): excessively high level of blood sugar	Confusion Lethargy Weakness Respiratory depression Weak, rapid pulse Low blood pressure Polyphagia (excessive hunger) Polydipsia (excessive thirst) Polyuria (excessive urination) Acetone breath odor Unconsciousness	Discontinue treatment, activate EMS, administer oxygen via nasal cannula, and monitor vital signs. If patient is conscious, have patient self-administer insulin if available. If patient becomes unresponsive, initiate BLS.
Fluoride (acute toxicity): administration of systemically toxic levels of fluoride	**Acute toxicity:** Abdominal pain Headache Diarrhea Nausea Weakness	Discontinue treatment, activate EMS. Induce vomiting using digital stimulation or ipecac syrup; administer fluoride-binding liquid such as milk, milk of magnesia, or lime water. Monitor vital signs.
Foreign body in eye: an object floating in the tears on the surface of the eye or embedded within the eye	Tearing Redness Pain Blinking	Discontinue treatment; wash hands. To examine the eye, pull the lower lid down and have the patient look up while holding the upper lid open. If the object is floating on the surface, flush with water or saline. If

Continued

Table 51-9. *Management of Medical Emergencies*[7,11-23] —cont'd

Medical Emergency	Signs and Symptoms	Management
		the object is embedded in the eye, do not attempt to remove and activate EMS.
Heart failure: a condition in which the heart cannot adequately pump blood throughout the body	Shortness of breath Persistent coughing or wheezing Edema (swelling) of the feet, ankles, legs, or abdomen Fatigue Increased heart rate	Activate EMS. Position patient upright and provide oxygen via nasal cannula or facemask. Monitor vital signs and initiate BLS as needed.
Hemorrhage: uncontrolled bleeding	**Of an extremity:** **Artery**—spurting blood **Vein**—oozing blood	Discontinue treatment; apply direct pressure to the site until bleeding stops; if possible, elevate the site that is bleeding above the heart. Position patient supine to decrease the occurrence of syncope; cover patient with a blanket to prevent loss of body heat. If bleeding does not stop, apply pressure to the supplying vessel.
	From tooth socket:	Pack area with sterile or hemostatic gauze and instruct patient to bite firmly. If bleeding continues, place a damp tea bag (tannic acid) in area of bleed and instruct patient to bite firmly and avoid rinsing. Position patient upright and have him or her lean forward; advise patient to breathe through mouth and pinch nose for 5–10 minutes.
Hyperventilation: overly rapid or deep breathing associated with anxiety	**Nosebleed:** Deep rapid breathing Shortness of breath Lightheadedness Tingling or numbness in fingers or feet Rapid heart rate Anxiety Tightness in chest	Discontinue treatment, position patient upright, and reassure patient. Instruct patient to take deep breaths, inhaling through the nose and exhaling slowly through pursed lips. Use of a paper bag is not recommended due to contraindications for patients with a history of asthma, chronic obstructive pulmonary disease, heart disease, stroke, or diabetes. Do not administer oxygen.
Insulin reaction (hypoglycemia, hyperinsulinism): level of blood sugar is too low	Irritation Confusion Hunger Sudden mood change Headache Feelings of dizziness Increased anxiety Bounding pulse Moist, cold, and pale skin Weakness Possible loss of consciousness	**Conscious patient:** Discontinue treatment; administer oral glucose. Observe patient for 1 hour before dismissal. **Unconscious patient:** Activate EMS, initiate BLS, monitor vital signs, and administer intramuscular glucagon or intravenous glucose.
Local anesthesia (hematoma): a bruise that results from small blood vessels breaking and leaking their contents into the soft tissue beneath the skin	**Hematoma:** Rapid swelling, redness postinjection	Discontinue treatment, position patient upright, apply pressure and ice to the affected area.

Table 51-9. *Management of Medical Emergencies*[7,11-23] —cont'd

Medical Emergency	Signs and Symptoms	Management
Local anesthesia (allergic reaction): see allergic reaction	**Allergic reaction:** Skin and mucous membrane reactions Allergic bronchial asthma attack	Discontinue treatment; administer antihistamine or bronchodilator. Epinephrine may be needed if patient experiences difficulty breathing. Monitor vital signs. See anaphylaxis.
Local anesthesia (anaphylaxis): See anaphylaxis	**Anaphylaxis:** See anaphylaxis	Discontinue treatment, monitor vital signs, and administer oxygen. If symptoms progress, activate EMS.
Local anesthesia (overdose): administration of systemically toxic levels of anesthetic	**Mild toxic overdose:** Anxiousness Restlessness Confusion Rapid pulse and respirations **Severe toxic overdose:** Drop in blood pressure Tremors Lethargy Shock-like symptoms Rapid, weak pulse Respiratory depression Unconsciousness	Discontinue treatment, activate EMS, open airway, monitor vital signs, administer oxygen, and initiate BLS as needed.
Myocardial infarction: damage or death of heart muscle due to blockage of blood flow through a coronary artery	Uncomfortable chest pain; may be mild to severe (pain not relieved by nitroglycerin) Pain may radiate to arms, neck, and shoulder area, or back Nausea Fatigue Dizziness Anxiety Shortness of breath Palpitations Sweating	Discontinue treatment, activate EMS, position patient upright or as comfortable, administer aspirin (if patient not allergic), monitor vital signs, administer oxygen, and initiate BLS as needed.
Respiratory failure: inability of the lungs to provide adequate oxygen	Rapid difficult breathing Cyanosis Confusion Loss of consciousness	Discontinue treatment; activate EMS. For conscious patient, position patient semisupine or upright; ensure airway is patent; provide supplemental oxygen via nasal cannula or facemask. Monitor vital signs. For unconscious patient, position supine; initiate BLS as needed.
Seizure (generalized): physical changes in behavior that occur after an episode of abnormal electrical activity in the brain	**Convulsive, generalized tonic-clonic seizure:** Aura Loss of consciousness Epileptic cry Involuntary tonic-clonic muscle contractions Altered breathing Involuntary urination and/or defecation	Discontinue treatment, position patient supine, do not move the patient from the dental chair, do not place anything in the patient's mouth, make treatment area safe by moving objects and equipment out of reach, and time the duration of the seizure. If the seizure lasts longer than 5 minutes or if multiple seizures occur, activate EMS, open airway, administer oxygen via nasal cannula or facemask, monitor vital signs, and initiate BLS as needed.

Continued

Table 51-9. *Management of Medical Emergencies*[7,11-23] —cont'd

Medical Emergency	Signs and Symptoms	Management
		Postseizure: allow patient to rest, arrange for transportation/patient support. Refer for medical follow-up.
Seizure (absence): a brief disturbance of brain function due to abnormal electrical activity in the brain	**Nonconvulsive absence seizure:** Sudden loss of consciousness, fixed posture, blank stare, muscle twitches	Discontinue treatment, monitor patient closely, make treatment area safe, and refer for medical follow-up.
Shock: inadequate blood supply to the body's organs, which may result in death	Cool and clammy skin Cyanosis Dilated pupils Weak rapid pulse Slow and shallow breathing or hyperventilation (rapid and deep) Nausea and vomiting Appears confused, weak, and anxious Condition leads to loss of consciousness without treatment	Discontinue treatment, activate EMS, position patient supine, maintain open airway, monitor vital signs, and keep patient warm and still; initiate BLS as needed.
Stroke (cerebrovascular accident): an interruption in blood supply to the brain	Sudden dizziness Loss of balance or coordination Impaired speech Confusion Paralysis on one side of the body or face Sudden severe headache Blurred vision	Discontinue treatment, activate EMS, position patient on paralyzed side, and keep head turned to side to prevent choking if vomiting occurs. Avoid giving patient food or drink. Monitor vital signs; administer oxygen; initiate BLS as needed.
Syncope: a brief loss of consciousness due to inadequate blood flow to the brain	Pale skin Dizziness Weakness Blurred vision Nausea Feeling of warmth Perception that the room is moving Trembling or shaking Shortness of breath Loss of consciousness	Discontinue treatment; position patient supine and elevate legs. Maintain airway; loosen tight clothing (necktie/belt); place a cool, damp cloth on forehead; wave aromatic ammonia below nose. Monitor vital signs and reassure patient upon regaining consciousness. If patient does not regain consciousness within 1 minute, differential diagnosis should include hypoglycemia, acute myocardial infarction, cerebrovascular accident, and cardiac arrest.

Table 51-10. *Management of Dental Emergencies*[24-27]

Dental Emergency	Signs and Symptoms	Management
Avulsed tooth: a tooth that has been knocked out of its socket	Tooth forcibly displaced from socket Bruising Swelling Trauma	Patient should be instructed to handle tooth by crown and avoid touching root. If able, reimplant tooth into socket. If unable to reimplant tooth into socket, transport tooth to oral health-care setting in Hanks balanced salt solution, milk, saline, saliva, or water (listed in order of preference).
Dislocated jaw: dislocation of the temporomandibular joint from its normal position	Deviation of normal movement Inability to close mouth Trismus	Position patient upright or as comfortable. Reassure patient and activate EMS. Closed reduction should be performed in the emergency room following the

Table 51-10. *Management of Dental Emergencies*[24-27]—cont'd

Dental Emergency	Signs and Symptoms	Management
		administration of a combination of sedatives and analgesics.
		Reduction technique: Place gloved thumbs wrapped with gauze on the patient's mandibular molars bilaterally, as far back as possible. Fingers are curved beneath the angle and body of the mandible. Apply downward and backward pressure on the mandible using thumbs while slightly opening the mouth. This helps disengage the condyle from the anterior eminence and reposition it back into the mandibular fossa.
		There is a risk of injury to the thumbs of the health-care provider as the mouth snaps closed with successful reduction. Therefore, it is recommended that the health-care provider wrap both thumbs with gauze.
Facial fracture: any break in the bones of the face	Pain Swelling Bruising Facial deformity	Position patient upright or as comfortable, reassure patient, and apply icepack to area to reduce pain and swelling. If bleeding is present, apply pressure to control the bleeding. Activate EMS.
Jaw fracture: a break in the mandible	Deviation of normal movement Inability to close mouth Pain Swelling Bruising Facial deformity	Position patient upright or as comfortable, reassure patient, and apply ice pack to area to reduce pain and swelling. Activate EMS.
Luxation: dislocation of a tooth in its socket	Tooth displaced in a labial, lingual, or lateral direction	Immediate reposition of tooth and splint placement is necessary. With primary dentition, extraction of tooth may be necessary.
Tooth fracture: any break in the tooth structure; may involve the anatomical crown and/or root	**Enamel:** **Enamel and dentin:** **Enamel, dentin, and pulp:** **Root fracture:**	Recontour or restore if indicated. Restore. Assess the need for endodontic therapy and restore accordingly. Assess the need for endodontic therapy and restore accordingly.

Case Study

Mr. Garcia is a 62-year-old male with a history of high cholesterol, elevated blood pressure, and angina pectoris. He is currently taking an antihyperlipidemic medication, a calcium channel blocker, and nitroglycerin as needed. Mr. Garcia states that he sees his doctor regularly and that his blood pressure and cholesterol levels are well controlled. Mr. Garcia shares with you that his son recently passed away earlier in the month. During treatment, Mr. Garcia complains of chest and arm pain. He is sweating and appears to be short of breath.

Vitals at the time of treatment:

Blood pressure: 162/84 mm Hg

Pulse: 68 beats per minute

Respirations: 14 breaths per minute

Case Study—cont'd

Case Study Exercises

1. Based on the information provided in the case, what emergency is Mr. Garcia most likely experiencing?
   A. Heart failure
   B. Myocardial infarction
   C. Cardiac arrest
   D. Angina pectoris
2. Management of the emergency that Mr. Garcia is experiencing would include all of the following EXCEPT which one?
   A. Administering nitroglycerin
   B. Placing in the supine position
   C. Administering oxygen
   D. Monitoring vital signs
3. If Mr. Garcia's symptoms persist, what emergency should be suspected?
   A. Heart failure
   B. Myocardial infarction
   C. Cardiac arrest
   D. Angina pectoris

4. Select all of the following that increase the risk of Mr. Garcia experiencing an emergency.
   A. History of high cholesterol
   B. History of hypertension
   C. The recent passing of his son
   D. Respirations at time of treatment
   E. Pulse at the time of treatment
   F. Blood pressure at time of treatment
5. The administration of nitroglycerin is indicated in the management of Mr. Garcia's emergency because it will allow for increased blood flow to the cardiac muscle.
   A. Both the statement and the reason are correct and related.
   B. Both the statement and the reason are correct but not related.
   C. The statement is correct but the reason is not.
   D. The statement is not correct, but the reason is correct.
   E. Neither the statement nor the reason is correct.

Review Questions

1. What is the recommended size for oxygen tanks in dental offices?
   A. A
   B. B
   C. C
   D. D
   E. E

2. In which of the following emergencies is the use of oxygen NOT indicated?
   A. Syncope
   B. Asthma
   C. Angina pectoris
   D. Hyperventilation

3. Immediately following the administration of a local anesthetic, the patient experiences edema of the tongue, pharyngeal tissue, and larynx. The patient is experiencing
   A. hyperventilation.
   B. asthmatic attack.
   C. anaphylactic reaction.
   D. shock.

4. Shortly after beginning the prophylaxis, the dental hygienist observes that the patient shows signs of angioedema and urticaria, then begins to cough and wheeze. Which of the following drugs is indicated for the management of this patient's condition?
   A. Nitroglycerin
   B. Epinephrine
   C. Albuterol
   D. Aspirin

5. The patient appears anxious and somewhat disengaged during the hygienist's review of the medical history. During treatment, the patient is tightly gripping the armrest. The patient suddenly sits up and exclaims that she is having difficulty breathing. What is the hygienist's assessment?
   A. Hyperventilation
   B. Anaphylaxis
   C. Asthma attack
   D. Hypoglycemia

Active Learning

1. With a peer, discuss the signs and symptoms of anaphylaxis. Discuss the emergency management of anaphylaxis.

2. Ask a peer to act out the signs and symptoms of an emergency. First identify the emergency, and then simulate the appropriate steps of handling the emergency that has been presented.

3. Locate the medical emergency equipment in a clinical setting. Identify the equipment and list emergencies that it may be used to treat.

4. Create a chart that depicts the steps of CPR. ■

REFERENCES

1. Malamed, SF. Knowing your patients. *JADA*, 2010;141: 3S-7S.

2. American Society of Anesthesiologists. ASA Physical Status Classification. 1995-2011. Available from: http:// asahq.org/resources/clinical-information/asa-physical-status-classification-system. Last approved October 15, 2014.

3. American Academy of Pediatrics. PACT: oral injury key points. 2011. Available from: http://www2.aap.org/ oralhealth/pact/ch10_key.cfm.

4. American Dental Association (ADA) Council on Access, Prevention, and Interprofessional Relations; ADA Council on Scientific Affairs. Using mouthguards to reduce the incidence and severity of sports-related oral injuries. *JADA*. 2006;137(12):1712-1720.

5. American Heart Association. (2011, March). *BLS for healthcare providers. Student manual.* South Deerfield, MA: Channing L. Bete Co., Inc.

6. American Heart Association. Part 5: adult basic life support. 2010. Available from: http://circ.ahajournals. org/content/122/18_suppl_3/S685.full.pdf+html.

7. Malamed SF. *Medical emergencies in the dental office.* 6th ed. St. Louis, MO: Mosby; 2007.

8. Haas DA. Preparing dental office staff members for emergencies, developing a basic action plan. *JADA.* 2010;141:8S-13S.

9. Rosenberg, M. Preparing for medical emergencies: the essential drugs and equipment for the dental office. *JADA.* 2010;141:14S-19S.

10. ADA Council on Scientific Affairs. Office emergencies and emergency kits. *JADA.* 2002;133:364-365.

11. Lexi-Comp, Inc. Dental office medical emergencies: oxygen delivery. 2010. Available from: http://www. crlonline.com/crlsql/servlet/crlonline.

12. Little JW, Falace DA, Miller CS, Rhodus NL. *Dental management of the medically compromised patient.* 8th ed. St. Louis, MO: Mosby; 2013.

13. American College of Emergency Physicians. What to do in a medical emergency: asthma and allergies. 2011. Available from: http://www.emergencycareforyou. org/Emergency-101/What-To-Do-In-A-Medical-Emergency/.

14. American College of Emergency Physicians. What to do in a medical emergency: fainting. 2011. Available from: http://www.emergencycareforyou.org/Emergency-101/ Emergencies-A-Z/Fainting/.

15. American College of Emergency Physicians. What to do in a medical emergency: shock. 2011. Available from: http://www.emergencycareforyou.org/Emergency-101/ Emergencies-A-Z/Shock/.

16. American Institute for Preventive Medicine. Emergency and first aid: shock. 2011. Available from: http:// www.healthy.net/scr/article.aspx?Id=1498.

17. Haas DA. Management of medical emergencies in the dental office: conditions in each country, the extent of treatment by the dentist. *Anesth Prog.* 2006;53:20-24.

18. Mayo Foundation for Clinical Education and Research. Burns: first aid. 1998-2011. Available from: http:// www.mayoclinic.org/first-aid/first-aid-burns/basics/ ART-20056649.

19. Mayo Foundation for Medical Education and Research. Chemical burns: first aid. 1998-2011. Available from: http://www.mayoclinic.org/first-aid/first-aid-chemical-burns/basics/art-20056667.

20. Mayo Foundation for Medical Education and Research. Heart attack: first aid. 1998-2011. Available from: http:// www.mayoclinic.org/first-aid/first-aid-heart-attack/ basics/art-20056679.

21. Mayo Foundation for Medical Education and Research. Nosebleeds: first aid. 1998-2011. Available from: http:// www.mayoclinic.org/first-aid/first-aid-nosebleeds/ basics/art-20056683.

22. Mayo Foundation for Medical Education and Research. Vasovagal syncope. 1998-2011. Available from: http:// www.mayoclinic.org/diseases-conditions/vasovagal-syncope/basics/symptoms/con-20026900.

23. WebMD LLC. Respiratory failure treatment and management. 1994-2011. Available from: http:// emedicine.medscape.com/article/167981-treatment.

24. Douglass AB, Douglass JM. Common dental emergencies. *Am Fam Phys.* 2003;67(3):511-517.

25. Flores MT, Andersson L, Andreasen JO, Bakland LK, Malmgren B, Barnett F. Guidelines for the management of traumatic dental injuries. *Dent Traumatol.* 2007; 23(3):130-136.

26. Prajer R., Grosso G. *DH note*s. Philadelphia, PA: F.A. Davis Company; 2011.

27. WebMD LLC. Mandible dislocation treatment and management. 1994-2011. Available from: http:// emedicine.medscape.com/article/823775-treatment# a1126.

Part XI

Future Vision

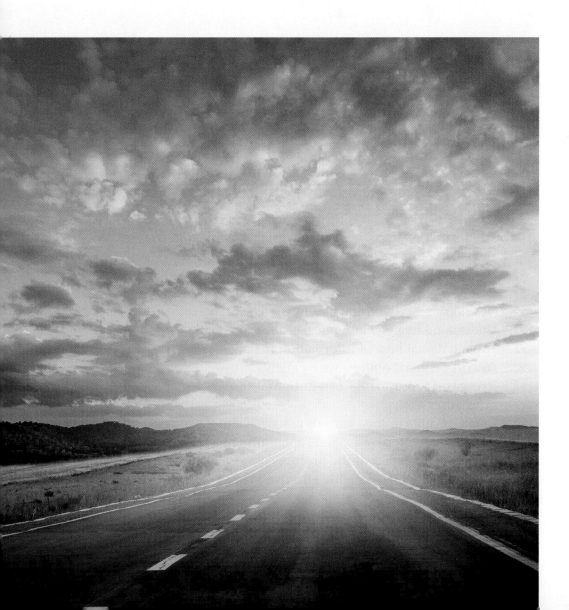

Chapter 52 | Practice Management

Ann-Marie C. DePalma, CDA, RDH, MEd, FADIA, FAADH

KEY TERMS

accounts receivable

Current Dental Terminology (CDT)

drama triangle

goal

huddle

mission statement

overhead

preferred provider organization (PPO)

SMART(ER) goals

Systemized Nomenclature of Dentistry (SNODENT)

usual, customary, and reasonable (UCR) fee plan

vision

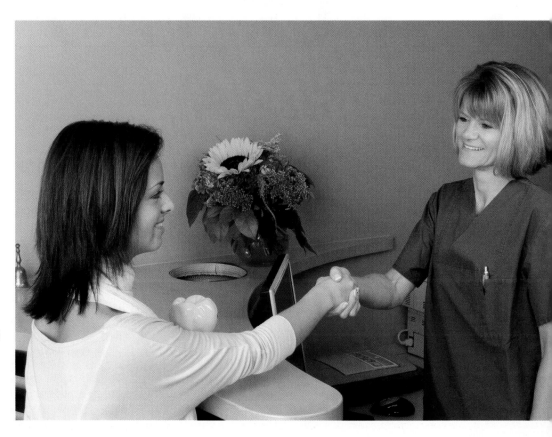

LEARNING OBJECTIVES

After reading this chapter, the student should be able to:

52.1 Define and discuss leadership in the dental practice.

52.2 Discuss components of communication.

52.3 Establish professional and personal goals.

52.4 Develop a practice vision and mission.

52.5 Understand hygiene and office production goals.

52.6 Explain dental benefit information to patients.

52.7 Discuss financial options with patients.

52.8 Recognize appropriate Current Dental Terminology codes for hygiene procedures.

52.9 Compare and contrast various practice team meetings.

52.10 Schedule an effective hygiene appointment as it relates to the practice management aspect of the practice.

52.11 Summarize habits of highly effective practices.

KEY CONCEPTS

- Leadership within the dental practice is not only the responsibility of the dentist/owner, but involves all team members.
- Communication is essential in all areas of the dental practice, between dentist and team members, between team members, and between patient and dentist/team members. Communication influences patient relationships and retention.
- The hygienist and all team members need to understand the vision, mission, and goals of the practice.
- The dental practice is a business that must be run efficiently to survive and prosper.

RELEVANCE TO CLINICAL PRACTICE

Dental hygienists devote most of their time to educating and motivating patients, and practicing their clinical skills. Despite its clinical focus, however, dentistry is a business, and hygienists need to develop leadership, communication, and problem-solving skills to be successful. Knowledge of and proficiency in using efficient business and clinical management systems are also necessary to contribute to the dental practice's success.

LEADERSHIP

For a business to grow and be effective, the leadership must be strong. Leadership stems not only from the owner but also from all members involved in the business. Leadership involves the position or function of a leader or the ability to lead by directing a group. What constitutes being an effective leader? A leader is one who has a clear sense of purpose and an orientation toward goal accomplishment, possesses a commitment to the service of others, has excellent communication skills, possesses an awareness of other's goals and the commitment to help others reach their goals, has the knowledge of what needs to be done and the desire to get things done, and possesses a sense of "ownership." All dental professionals, including hygienists, assistants, dentists, and business team members, possess three distinct leadership roles within a practice: leader of self, leader of teammates, and leader of patients. When each person assumes the responsibilities of each of these roles, the individual leaders and, ultimately, the practice will benefit.

As a leader of self, it is the hygienist's responsibility to maximize his or her talents to be an asset to the organization. The organization has a responsibility to provide a healthy environment, one that is conducive to growth and development. Asking the following questions can help hygienists clarify their role as leader of self:

- Are my personal and professional goals clear, and am I working toward these goals on a daily basis?
- Do I face challenges head on with the goal of resolving them?

- Do I know how to prioritize my time to make a difference in the organization/practice?
- Do I truly care about the organization/practice, teammates, and patients?

As a leader of teammates, an environment of mutual respect and heartfelt interest in helping others succeed is essential. Questions hygienists who are leaders of teammates should ask themselves include the following:

- Can my teammates count on me to support them or help them when needed?
- Do I communicate openly with team members, or do I keep things inside?
- Am I proud of our practice and my contributions to it?

All professionals in the practice have the responsibility and opportunity to lead patients to make decisions that are good for their oral and systemic health. Each patient has a defining moment when team members have the opportunity to influence whether or not the patient accepts treatment. As a leader of patients, dental hygienists can lead patients to better health by asking questions such as the following:

- Do I accept responsibility in helping patients make informed decisions regarding their health?
- Can the dentist and team count on me to communicate effectively with each patient about the value of the recommended treatment?
- Am I a good listener, taking the time to listen to the patient's desires or concerns, or am I only interested in my needs?

Although every team member has a responsibility to assume a leadership role within the practice, it is the hygienist who should empower others, from team members to patients, toward the common goal of optimum oral health. As a leader, the hygienist can use communication skills, knowledge, and commitment to influence others to achieve health goals. Education is the hallmark of the dental hygiene practice, and by educating others to achieve leadership roles, the hygienist not only expands her or his leadership skills but empowers other team members to become leaders.

Trust and the Drama Triangle

Trust is essential to leadership. Without the trust of an individual or group, the leader is ineffective. All relationships are based on trust. The first step in the trust relationship centers on keeping commitments. A leader allows individuals the opportunity to fulfill promises made or keep deadlines met. If either can't be achieved, the individual has the responsibility to inform the leader and seek alternatives. Trust is built when this occurs.

The leader does not allow gossip or faultfinding to destroy relationships, whether with team members or with patients. By following the principle of always praising in public and reprimanding in private, the leader builds a trusting relationship. The leader also avoids the **drama triangle**, a process defined in 1968 by Dr. Stephen Karpman,[1] which involves relationships and conflicts that occur in teams and groups. There are three interchangeable psychological components, or roles, involved in the drama triangle:

- Victim: The person who feels victimized, oppressed, helpless, hopeless, powerless, or ashamed in a situation; looks for a rescuer who will perpetuate his or her negative feelings; will not make decisions or solve problems; and often takes a dejected stance.
- Persecutor: The person who pressures, coerces, or persecutes the victim; sets strict limits unnecessarily; and blames, criticizes, or acts as the "critical parent."
- Rescuer: The person who intervenes, seemingly out of a desire to help the situation or the underdog; keeps victim dependent; and acts as a "marshmallow" parent.

The leader does not participate in or allow the drama triangle or gossip to control interactions within the team, especially if a member is not present. Leaders also allow individuals the opportunity, without becoming defensive, to voice issues that may be a concern. When team members understand that the team is a safe environment within which to discuss any issue, trust is built and shared. By avoiding gossip, encouraging team members to voice concerns, and providing frequent positive reinforcement, leaders empower their groups to achieve the highest level of performance. Steven M. R. Covey, in his book *Speed of Trust*, lists 13 behaviors that leaders and teams embody that influence the trust within an organization. These behaviors are:[2]

1. Talk Straight
2. Demonstrate Respect
3. Create Transparency
4. Right Wrongs
5. Show Loyalty
6. Deliver Results
7. Get Better
8. Confront Reality
9. Clarify Expectation
10. Practice Accountability
11. Listen First
12. Keep Commitments
13. Extend Trust

Using these behaviors, Covey believes that one is making a "deposit" into the trust account of another. To build this trust account, the behaviors need to be in balance; stressing one behavior over another places that behavior as a weakness rather than strength.

According to Covey,[2] decreasing trust decreases speed and increases costs, whereas increasing trust increases speed and decreases costs. Highly effective organizations/practices and leaders demonstrate these behaviors on a daily basis.

Additionally, there are numerous other professional leadership development strategies developed by psychologists, behavioral therapists, and military organizations. Depending on an individual and organization's focus, each stresses the importance of effective leaders demonstrating trust.

Vision, Mission, and Goals

Vision and goal setting are important components of leadership. In business, the **vision** is the stated aims and objectives of a business. For dentistry, the vision of the practice is a clear vision of what the practice should be, whether in the physical sense or in the types of patients to be treated. The dentist and team need to have a clear focus of what is wanted and needed for the practice to prosper. This focus centers on the physical properties of the office; the number, types, and responsibilities of all team members; and the type of patient population the practice will provide treatment for, along with any other attributes the leaders envision. To ensure success, all team members need to be involved in the development and implementation of the practice's vision, mission statement, and goals.

Vision

The vision for the practice is the ideal description of what the practice will look like in both the short- and long-term future. In defining a vision, questions that can be asked include the following:

- What is your ideal practice? How does it physically appear? What type of patients will be seen in the practice?

- What are the elements of excellent communication between doctor and team, between team members, between doctor/team and patients, and between doctor/team and referral sources?
- What are the practice's expectations for relationships with patients and others who work with the practice? Do patients understand the responsibilities, such as insurance balance payments, appointment cancellation policies, and radiographic protocols?
- What barriers, or obstacles, might be encountered? How can these barriers be overcome?
- What is being done to achieve the vision? What tools or education needs to be obtained to achieve the vision?

Mission Statement

The **mission statement** is created from the practice vision. The mission statement is the most important factor that stands as the foundation of success for the vision. All things related to the practice, the goals, the projects, and the plans should answer the question, "if we do this will we move closer to our ultimate mission?" The mission statement:

- states who you are,
- describes what you are about,
- contains highly emotional words that motivate the team to act, and
- is concise/brief.

Mission statements are written, posted declarations of the practice's main purpose and can change over time. The mission statement of a start-up practice may have a different appearance than one for a seasoned practice. It serves as the compass in assisting the practice in focusing on what is important and what is not, while keeping the practice vision in mind.

An example of a good mission statement would be: "Our mission at ABC Dental Center is to serve patients by providing the highest-quality dental care manifested by the promotion of long-term dental health."

Goals

A **goal** is an observable and measurable end result having one or more objectives to be achieved within a specific time frame. Goals help to keep team members focused and thus help the practice achieve the vision of the mission statement. Goals are categorized as high priority (must be done), medium priority (should be done), and low priority (would be nice to get done). Having clear practice goals establishes a strategic plan to help increase collections and production within the dental practice.

To accomplish a goal, one must write the goal, design a plan of action, list the steps to achieve the goal, determine the person(s) responsible for each task/step, activate each task/step at the correct time, and evaluate the process along the way. One way to achieve the goal is to use the **SMART** or **SMARTER** format. Use of the SMART format ensures that all relevant information is included in each goal. SMART represents:

- **S**pecific: with a clear end picture in mind
- **M**otivational: with rewarded steps along the way
- **A**ttainable: set a notch higher but achievable
- **R**elevant: in line with the mission
- **T**imely; time bound
- **E**valuate: change or update goals as necessary
- **R**eevaluate: allows for continuous improvement

SMART goals were first discussed in the November 1981 issue of *Management Review*.[3] Over the years, other goal-setting criteria have been discussed, including management by objectives, performance indicators, and strategic planning. A review of a business management text will provide information on the various types of goal-setting strategies that are available.

COMMUNICATION

Effective communication influences all aspects of a dental practice, including whether patients patronize the practice, accept treatment, pay for services, stay active in the practice, and refer others to the practice. Effective communication among team members and with patients is integral to successful practice. Patients are concerned about excellent care and treatment but also about the level of communication within the practice. Ineffective communication can result in a lack of commitment to treatment recommendations or failure to return to the practice.

Communication Barriers

Cultural, linguistic, biased-based, or assumption-based barriers influence effective communication. What may be appropriate for one culture, such as eye contact or a handshake, may be inappropriate for another. The same holds true for linguistic challenges—different areas of the country or different nationalities will use words differently, often with the same word having different meanings. Biased-based and assumption-based barriers reflect an individual history with a group or individual. An example would be assuming that someone who is shabbily dressed is homeless, when, in fact, the person may have substantial resources. Each barrier can affect communication between individuals.

Components of Communication

There are four components of communication: reading, writing, listening, and speaking. In dentistry, listening and speaking are more important than reading and writing. As discussed in Chapter 3, Communication Skills, listening is a key component of the collaborative process of motivational interviewing (MI). Listening is a master skill that involves a variety of tools, such as the following:

- Facing the patient when listening and maintaining eye contact (as culturally appropriate)

- Keeping an open mind to the subject matter and not becoming defensive
- Listening to the words spoken and picturing what the person is saying and how she or he is feeling
- Not interrupting or imposing one's own solutions while engaging in a trusting relationship in which one sincerely wants to help the other
- Asking open-ended questions to clarify or show understanding
- Providing feedback both as active and passive listening
- Taking notes as needed
- Paying attention to nonverbal signals such gestures, facial expressions, tone and volume of voice, and posture
- Repositioning oneself if the focus on the speaker is lost

Listening is a gift of time that helps build relationships, solves problems, ensures understanding, resolves conflicts, and improves accuracy. For dental hygienists, effective listening can increase patient acceptance and improve team communication and productivity. Refer to Chapter 3 for detailed information on using communication skills in the dental practice.

BUSINESS OF DENTISTRY AND DENTAL HYGIENE

The contemporary dental practice is a business. According to Merriam-Webster,[4] a business is a trade or profession involving the purchase or sale of goods or services. The dental professional, whether dentist, hygienist, assistant, or business team member, is the provider of a service and deserves to practice in the best manner to achieve maximum productivity and profitability. Dentists are the owners of the practice, but all team members are essential to the productivity and profitability of the practice. To contribute to the practice's success, hygienists need to understand the business of dental hygiene as it relates to the overall business of the practice.

Production and Collection Goals

As discussed earlier in this chapter, goals are established to achieve the practice's mission. Daily productivity goals for the dentist, hygienist, and practice are defined. These, along with the collection goals, determine the productivity of the practice. This does not mean that the practice is solely focused on numbers or dollars, but, as a business, the practice needs to collect a certain amount of revenue to pay its costs of doing business (the practice's **overhead**) and earn a profit. Major overhead expenses include salaries, payroll deductions, benefits, practice marketing and promotion, equipment, building/rent, and dental supplies. Minor overhead consists of office supplies, repair and maintenance of equipment and/or building, utilities, business insurance, postage, taxes, continuing education, dues/licenses, and professional fees such as accounting and legal services. Current general practice overhead averages around 70% to 75% of revenue, with the ideal being in the 55% to 65% range. Minor overhead should represent 10% to 15% of total overhead. These measurements are based on a percentage of collections. In dentistry, there are three main ways to reduce overhead: increase fees (collections), increase production, and/or decrease costs.

Collections represent money in the bank that can be used to pay the practice's bills, or overhead. Production figures do not necessarily take into account any adjustments the practice makes for insurance or other types of discounts such as senior/elder adjustments. The dentist/owner obtains practice overhead information from data collected either from the practice's accountant or from the office's accounting records. Such data should be recorded monthly and reviewed quarterly.

Production and collection goals are determined by taking the averages of each category over a period of time, usually a 3- to 6-month time frame. These figures are adjusted by a percentage of 5% to 20%, depending on the practice, to achieve a realistic goal that is attainable but not too easy to reach. Each dentist and each hygienist has an individual production goal, with all clinical team members participating in the daily office production goal. The daily production goals are multiplied either by the number of days the practice is open or by the number of days a practitioner works. For example, a team of three hygienists and one dentist might have a dentist production goal of $2,500/day, with each hygienist having a goal of $1,000/day production. If the dentist and two hygienists worked each day, the total office production for a day would be $4,500. Two hygienists work 2 days a week (total 8 days per month each), and the third hygienist works 4 days per week (16 days per month). Each hygienist would have the same daily production goal of $1,000, with the 8-day-a-month hygienist's monthly goal totaling $8,000 and the 16-day-a-month hygienist's goal totaling $16,000. The dentist works 4 days per week (16 days per month) with a goal of $40,000 per month. $40,000 plus $16,000 (8,000 x 2 hygienists) plus $16,000 equals $72,000 per month total office production (or 4,500 x 16 days = 72,000).

Practice management experts feel that a practice should be collecting 95% to 98% of monthly production. In this case, a 98% collection rate would be $70,560. Many practices have at least a 50% insurance-based practice. Insurance turnaround from submission to payment can vary depending on the insurance company and dental procedures. All dental practices that are submitting insurance claims should be filing electronically. Electronic claim submission is faster (payment is usually received with 3–7 days), is less expensive (no costs for paper and postage) and allows for easier claim follow-up. If a practice accepts assignment of insurance benefits (patients give permission for insurance company to pay the dental practice directly), there is a 30-day current insurance balance time frame. Any amount due is considered overdue on day 31, and payment should be required of the patient. Practices that do not enforce the 31-day rule may have high accounts receivable. **Accounts receivable** are the amounts due to the practice, whether private pay (to be paid by the patient) or insurance balances. To achieve the 95% to 98% collection percentages, a practice needs to actively engage in reduction of the accounts receivables (A/R) on a daily basis.

Many practices belong to a **preferred provider organization (PPO)**, a contract between a dental benefits provider (insurance company) and the provider of dental care (dentist and, in some states, public health dental hygienists) providing that, in return for the referral of dental patients, the dentist will provide procedures at a reduced rate. The dental practice benefits from a patient base and the insurance company benefits from reduced costs. Depending on the PPO contract, the dental practice may or may not be able to balance bill the patient (charge the patient for any difference between the fee paid by the insurance company and the practice's usual fee). For example, if the practice charges $100 for a service, but the agreed-upon fee that the insurance company pays is $75, the practice may be able to bill the patient for the balance of $25.

Dental practices must adjust their production numbers to reflect the fees established by insurance companies. The **usual, customary, and reasonable (UCR) fee plan** is used by PPOs and other insurance providers:

- **U**sual fee: The fee the dentist uses most often for a given dental procedure.
- **C**ustomary fee: The fee determined by the insurance benefit provider from actual submitted fees for specific procedures.
- **R**easonable fee: The fee determined by the insurance benefit provider for a particular procedure that requires a modification or special consideration by the insurance company or provider.

If a practice has a high PPO patient population, the amount of adjustments will be high. The practice therefore may not reach the 95% to 98% collection percentage. Hygienists need to be aware of this because although production may appear high, with the amount of adjustments the practice must take, the actual collection percentage is low. Practices rely on collections to pay their bills. If accounts receivables are high, collections will be low. Business collection experts have determined that the longer an account receivable remains unpaid, the less it is worth and the harder it is to collect. Each month a dollar stays on an account unpaid it decreases in value. The best way to achieve lower accounts receivables is to have firm, but flexible financial policies in place for all treatments, with discussions of policies at the time of service. Mailing information about patient accounts balances or making phone calls to patients assists in collecting unpaid balances, but neither of these strategies is as effective as in-person discussions.

Patient Financial Options

Many patients don't go to the dentist or decline treatment due to costs. Patients often will proceed with treatments once they understand their financial responsibilities and if the practice makes the treatments affordable for their budget. Using written financial agreements with all patients is an important component of this communication process. In this manner, patients understand the insurance and individual responsibilities and ways the office can assist in making the treatments affordable. Providing the patients with options for payments and treatments allows the patient a sense of control, yet, in actuality, the dental team controls these options. Offering patients various treatment options for their situation, and allowing them the option of accepting part of the treatment along with financial options that are beneficial for them and the practice, instills confidence and acceptance in patients. Using benefits, risks, alternatives to treatment, no treatment options (BRAN) provides patients the ability to determine their course of treatment and follows the legal requirements of informed consent (see Chapter 2 for further information on legal and ethical principles). Patients want the best treatment and look to dental professionals to provide that treatment, but in a manner that is fiscally responsible. On the other hand, the dental practice as a business in today's economy cannot survive with large accounts receivables. Offering a variety of payment options, such as the following, at the time of service benefits both patients and the practice:

- Offer an accounting reduction of 5–10% on all treatment if balance is paid in full before treatment.
- Offer payments by appointment, with the final payment due 1 week before the final appointment.
- Offer payment by credit card at time of service or by providing an authorization on the credit card for balances from insurance payments or insurance balances beyond 30 days, including use of health savings account credit cards. According to the Internal Revenue Service,[5] a health savings account is a tax-exempt trust or custodial account that is established to pay or reimburse certain medical expenses.
- Offer health-care financing options provided by outside third-party payers that pay the dental practice for services and collect monthly payments from patients, similar to credit card financing but only for health-care expenses). This may also include a cosigner on the account if the patient's credit is less than favorable. Examples of companies that offer health-care financing include Springstone Financing and Care Credit.

The Dental Hygienist's Role in Accounts Receivable

All dental team members—from business team, to assistant, to dentist, to hygienist—play important roles in maintaining low accounts receivables. A hygienist needs to understand the business/financial and clinical aspects of treatment acceptance. No treatment should be scheduled until the patient understands and completes all written financial agreements. The clinical team, however, should not be involved in the direct discussion of the financial options; that is the job of the business team. Clinical team members should focus on the aspects of treatment pertaining to clinical issues, allowing the "experts" of the practice in financial issues to communicate the intricacies of the financial arena of the practice. For example, often the clinical team may ask the patient, "will you be paying for that today," which requires a yes-or-no response, when the appropriate question by the business team would be, "Mrs. Patient, today's hygiene therapy appointment today was $100; how will you be taking care of that?" The business team member can then discuss the various options.

Current Dental Terminology and Periodontal Diseases

Current Dental Terminology (CDT) is a list of standardized terms and codes established by the American Dental Association (ADA) for the purpose of consistency in reporting dental services and procedures to dental benefit insurance plans.[6] CDT codes are revised approximately every 2 years with new codes or changes in the terminology of existing codes. A committee of members of the ADA, insurance company representatives, governmental representatives, and other interested parties (individuals, associations, or other groups) meet to evaluate and discuss current codes and advise alterations in the descriptors or the need for additional codes based on currently accepted treatment modalities.

Each category of dentistry is assigned a range of codes that begins with the letter D, signifying that the service is a designated dental service. The second number of the code represents the category, and the remaining digits represent the procedure or service. For example, in the CDT 2011–2012, common services are coded as follows:[6]

- preventive services—D0100–D0999—periodic oral evaluation = D0120
- preventive services—bitewing radiograph (4 films) = D0274
- preventive services—prophylaxis (adult) = D1110
- periodontal services—D4000–D4999—periodontal maintenance = D4910
- periodontal services— scaling and root planing 4 or more teeth in quadrant = D4341

Currently if the patient's periodontal status is known from the 1999 American Academy of Periodontology (AAP) Classification System,[7] it is not necessary to include it on insurance claims, unless required by the benefit provider or by procedure. It is, however, a good practice to begin to educate patients about the disease process and to inform them of their periodontal status. Just as electronic health records (EHRs) have changed the face of the medical practice, electronic dental records (EDRs) will change the face of the dental practice, allowing for more diagnosis-driven claims and procedure codes. With the advent of **Systemized Nomenclature of Dentistry (SNODENT)**, use of the classification system may be required in the future. SNODENT is a vocabulary designed for use in the electronic dental record environment.[8] Its purpose is to provide standardized terms for describing dental disease, capture clinical detail and patient characteristics, and permit analysis of patient care services and outcomes; it will be interoperable with EHRs and EDRs. EHRs/EDRs are components of the Health Information Technology for Economic and Clinical Health (HITECH) Act of 2009. The HITECH Act was part of the American Recovery and Reinvestment Act of 2009 (ARRA). ARRA contains incentives related to health-care information technology and creation of a national health-care infrastructure, and is designed to accelerate the adoption of EHR systems among providers by meaningful use of health information technology.

The hygienist uses communication skills to educate and encourage the patient to proceed with recommended treatments. The 1999 AAP Classification System does not include health; however, gingivitis or gingival diseases are considered.[7] With estimates by the ADA of 80% to 85% of the general population presenting with periodontal disease, hygienists need to educate patients on their specific periodontal situation, including gingival disease. Gingival diseases manifest as swollen, bleeding gingival tissues with no evidence of bone loss, either radiographically or clinically, and represent a reversible condition. Gingival diseases span a variety of conditions, and patients need to understand the importance of treatment (refer to Chapter 11, Periodontal Examination, for more in-depth information on periodontal diseases).

Other team members support and reinforce the dental hygienist's recommendations. Patients may agree with the hygienist to proceed with treatment, but decide not to proceed when confronted with treatment costs or to only proceed with treatment covered by their insurance plan. All team members need to understand and support the hygienist's treatment recommendations. Continuing to provide prophylactic care to patients who refuse recommended periodontal care creates a false sense of health in the patient and a loss of production for the practice. It also exposes the practice to potential liabilities. All documentation of the treatments and data recorded (including periodontal charting and radiographic findings) must correspond to claims submitted to the insurance benefit provider or fees charged to the patient. Many times, patients "only want what insurance covers," and business team members and practices try to accommodate the patient by alternating insurance codes for adult prophylaxis and periodontal maintenance procedures or other types of coding manipulation (dating treatment not on actual date of "cleaning" but on exact 6-month interval if patient was seen before 6-month date). Hygienists need to be aware that manipulation of insurance coding to obtain benefit is considered insurance fraud. Patients need to be educated about their disease or health status and treated accordingly. The hygienist needs to understand the implications of proceeding with situations such as these (please refer to Chapter 2 on ethical decision making).

Periodontal disease categories include chronic or aggressive periodontal disease, periodontitis as a manifestation of systemic diseases, necrotizing periodontal diseases, abscesses of the periodontium, periodontitis associated with endodontic lesions, and developmental or acquired deformities or conditions. All of these represent irreversible disease processes and are based on severity and extent of the disease. As with many other systemic diseases and disorders, early diagnosis and treatment of periodontal diseases/gingival diseases provide a better outcome. As hygienists in today's business-oriented dental practice, it is essential to educate and inform the patient of her or his periodontal disease or health status. How much disease does one allow before treating? Verbal skill training using learned communication techniques as a team is important to provide maximum benefit for patients and the practice.

Reaching Hygiene Goals
Periodontal Care

One way to achieve a daily or monthly hygiene goal is by treating active periodontal disease. The practice can develop protocols for gingival disease and periodontal disease based on evidence-based research that is current at the time, including treatment with the use of chemotherapeutics and power scalers. A series of appointments with intense patient education would be the hallmark of any program. Despite dental benefit providers' reluctance to cover additional treatment appointments, the verbal skills teams use to educate patients from initial contact through final appointment (including importance of regularly scheduled maintenance appointments) are crucial in patient's overall treatment acceptance and improvement of oral health. Use of third-party patient financing and credit card authorizations or other financing options will assist patients in receiving the treatments that are needed. Additionally, the hygienist can increase productivity by reviewing each day at the morning **huddle** (team meeting) any patients who require updated radiographs and/or periodontal charting. All periodontal charting should be done verbally so that the patient hears the numbers and sites of bleeding points. If available, an assistant or business team member can assist in the charting process, thereby reducing infection control issues. Making patients aware of their pocket depths and bleeding point numbers helps patients understand the disease progression. For example, "Mrs. Patient, we have found a number of bleeding points today, and because health is no bleeding points or pocketing, how do you feel about what we have diagnosed today?"

(See Chapter 3, Communication Skills, for information on motivational interviewing.) Dentist hygiene evaluations can be done at a natural break in the dentist's schedule rather than at the end of the hygiene appointment. This can reinforce the importance and urgency of the need for radiographs and other data collection information. Radiographs should be updated based on the ADA 2004 Guidelines for Prescribing Dental Radiographs.[9] Each practice should develop a radiographic protocol that allows full documentation of all needed diagnostic information and conforms to the current radiographic guidelines.

Fluoride Treatments

Many practices provide fluoride treatments for children and teenagers, but once the "insurance age" for fluoride occurs, the use of fluoride decreases. Many adults, however, would benefit from professional fluoride applications. Patients with xerostomia; patients with a high level of risk assessment for caries; those undergoing cancer therapy, including radiation and chemotherapy; or those who have frequent snacking, multiple restorations, orthodontics, or sensitivity issues can all benefit from professionally applied fluoride treatments, including fluoride varnish. Although this list is not exhaustive, these patients and others would also benefit from xylitol education and use as well. In-office tobacco cessation programs, dietary analysis, or adjunctive oral cancer screenings can also assist the hygienists and the team in achieving productivity goals and enhancing patient outcomes.

Increasing Perceived Value of Treatment

Use of an intraoral camera assists with patient education and treatment acceptance. Showing the patient the results of therapies, new areas of concern, or treatments that need to be completed enables the patient to understand and value the services provided. Seeing a gray area on a radiograph makes less of an impression than seeing a crack in a restoration in the mouth on a computer screen. Our role as dental hygienists is to help assist patients in valuing the needed dentistry. One way we do this is by using visual techniques and tools. The intraoral camera is one tool in the armamentarium to do that. Time should be scheduled into the hygiene appointment to allow sufficient time for data collection, including appropriate visualization of areas. Each hygienist should have access to available technology in the practice, and if the equipment is not readily available, discussions should ensue during the morning huddle to expedite the process. As with other data collection within dentistry, the hygienist should use the dentist's name in verbal communication to enhance the importance and value of recommendations. For example, "Mr. Patient, Dr. Jones, would like me to take photographs of these areas of concern. We want you to understand why we are concerned about your health."

Team Communication

Effective teams communicate daily on the needs of team members and patients. Efficient and effective daily meetings, or huddles, can reduce overall stress within the practice and increase productivity. To prepare the team for the day, huddles are usually held in the morning, but there are times that, due to other commitments, some team members cannot be in attendance. A problem-solving approach can be used to schedule the daily meeting at the best time for all team members.

At its most basic, the huddle can be a review of the day's schedule. Effective teams, however, plan for the day, eliminate bottlenecks in the schedule, and plan hygiene evaluations and emergency time. Each clinical team member evaluates her or his patient charts and discusses needs such as periodontal charting, radiographic updates, and restorative or hygiene treatments for patients and/or family. If there are multiple hygienists, they discuss the use of the intraoral camera and the best time for the dentist to do evaluations. If new patients will be seen that day, the business team informs the team of new patient information and needs. This information helps the team create a higher level of customer service for the patient and reinforces the value of the practice for the patient. If preset emergency time is not scheduled or has been filled, the team can identify appropriate times in the schedule that can be used for emergencies. Business and clinical team members also discuss patient financial concerns/issues and patient management issues. For patients who are up to date with all treatments and for whom no issues are present, the clinical team member need only state the patient's name and say "okay" or skip the patient altogether. Depending on the practice, some offices include information on business statistics such as the previous day's production and/or collection, the current day's scheduled production, and other important statistical information. The next available open appointments for the dentist and hygienists should also be noted. Noting next available appointments provides the clinical team information to discuss with the patient. For example, "Mrs. Patient, Dr. Jones's next appointment for a crown procedure is Tuesday at 10 a.m. Will this work for you?" Having the information readily available reinforces the need for and urgency of the treatment.

Routing Slips

Team members can make notes on printed copies of the daily schedules or, for practices that use digital charting, notes can be placed on individual patient routing slips. The routing slip can also be used as a communication tool between the clinical team and the business team. The hygienist can note further treatment needs; changes in the day's treatment (treatment not completed or additional treatment added); updates to patient information such as medical history, address, or insurance changes; and any other information the practice deems appropriate. Use of the routing slip decreases the need for members of the business team

to ask questions regarding what was done in the appointment, how much it was, and when the next treatment is, for example. Asking these questions conveys a sense of disorganization in the practice, in turn decreasing the value and trust the patient may have.

Other Meetings

Other types of team meetings should also be regularly scheduled to help implement goals and objectives, maintain open communication, strategize opportunities, or problem solve issues. These can include full team meetings scheduled every 4 to 6 weeks and departmental meetings if there are several hygienists, assistants, or business team members in each of the departments. The dentist(s) should attend each department's meeting to ensure that all team members share the same information and consistent protocols are used in the practice. Regularly scheduled meetings increase productivity and decrease stress.

Patient Scheduling

The practice's daily schedule affects productivity and can cause stress. Hygienists need an adequate amount of time to perform all clinical responsibilities and to provide patient education. Patient education drives the practice forward, because well-educated patients are more likely to accept treatments, refer patients, and remain with the practice. Hygiene appointments should be 60 minutes and include time for infection control procedures, clinical hygiene, and patient education.

The best way to determine exact times for procedures from regular prophylaxis to periodontal therapy appointments is to perform a procedural analysis. A procedural analysis breaks down each step of a procedure from start to finish and the actual time it takes to perform the procedure. Each hygienist in the practice should perform each procedure three to four times and then average their times. A timed procedure should include:

- Patient introductions from reception area
- Social graces in operatory
- Medical/dental history review
- Data collection, including intra-/extraoral evaluation, periodontal and restorative charting, and any other practice-specific data collection
- Dental hygiene procedures including radiographs
- Patient education
- Dentist evaluation
- Patient dismissal and transfer to business team
- Infection control procedures for breakdown/set up of operatory.

Each hygienist's individual procedural analysis average should then be discussed as a department and appropriate appointment lengths determined. The dentist uses the hygienists' recommendations to determine appointment lengths for the practice, which are relayed to the business team for implementation into the practice management software templates. There are numerous dental practice management software programs, such as Eaglesoft, Dentrix, and Practice-works, that allow practices to individualize schedules. Today's hygienist needs to be computer literate and comfortable using technology in the various aspects of clinical care. A hygienist may be required to schedule patients from the operatory and will be able to control her or his schedule based on individual patient needs and practice templates. Assistants and dentists can also perform procedural analysis for all major procedures in a similar fashion. These procedural analyses can assist the practice in seeing patients on time, and decrease stress levels in the practice.

The Appointment Book

The appointment book template can be incremented in 10-minute rather than 15-minute increments to allow for better time management. The following information should be included in the book for each appointment: patient name, phone, and address, and a description of the procedure with as much detail as possible. With this information, the clinical team can save time, focus on patient care, and decrease stress. The practice also should be aware of Health Insurance Portability and Accountability Act (HIPAA) considerations in posting the schedule, in paper or computer format, so as to be in compliance with current guidelines regarding protected patient information.

Scheduling

Reserving preblocked hygiene appointment times for procedures such as periodontal maintenance allows the hygienist to be efficient and productive. Preblocked hygiene appointments are appointments that represent a production amount equal to or greater than the fee for scaling and root planing (SCRP; CDT code D4341). Any procedure or group of procedures that equal the SCRP fee can be placed in these reserved appointments. By using the formula of providing half of the daily production goal from reserved appointments, the hygienist would perform a variety of procedures per day and achieve production goals. For example, the earlier example of hygiene production of $1,000 per day would result in reserved times equal to $500. This reserved amount would be divided by the fee for one quadrant of SCRP of $225 for this office or two reserved appointments per day per hygienist (500 divided by 225 = 2.2). Reserved appointments are scheduled daily to provide a variety of times for patients to chose from and to accommodate the hygienists' personal preferences. Other hygiene appointments are scheduled around the reserved appointments.

Reserved appointments are considered nonschedulable until 1 week before the appointment, when they can be released for other appointments. If scheduled times do not fit a particular patient's needs, the reserved time can be moved on a particular day to accommodate the patient, and still allow for provision of needed services. Depending on the practice, preblocked appointments

can be used for initial periodontal therapy, periodontal maintenance, new patient appointments, or combination appointments such as prophylaxis and radiographs. In this manner, both the practice and the patient achieve their goals. The practice gains production and the patients receive the treatment needed within a reasonable time frame.

Patients should be offered two appointment times for procedures, whether hygiene or restorative. Offering two options allows the patient to feel in control, and also allows the practice to create a schedule that maximizes productivity. A team member using good verbal skills might say, "Mr. Patient, Suzy, our hygienist, provides periodontal therapy on Mondays at 10 a.m. or Tuesdays at 4 p.m. Which would work for you?"

Communication to Avoid Cancellations and No-Shows

Even with appropriate scheduling, the practice and the hygienist may experience cancellations and no-show appointments. There is no way to completely eliminate these in any practice, but there are steps that can be implemented to reduce their occurrence. Communication is essential in helping to reduce cancelled appointments/no-shows. From the initial phone call, patients should understand the urgency and need for treatment. During the initial call, business team members should learn the patient's motivators and goals and use them throughout communications. An initial communication sheet detailing all patient information can be developed by the practice. This sheet can list pertinent patient demographic information and the patient's desires, needs, motivators, and challenges, which can be conveyed to the clinical team during the huddle on the day of the appointment. Questions that can be asked of the patient to determine her or his motivators include the following: What do you see as the goals for your teeth, your mouth, or your smile? How can we assist you to achieve these goals? See Chapter 3 for motivational interviewing questions.

The clinical team members can use this behavioral interviewing information to focus their communication with the patient. Before returning the patient to the business team, the clinical team reviews the day's treatment with the patient, explains the next treatment needed with benefits and risks, and discusses the time frame between appointments. First, the primary clinician, whether hygienist or dentist, raises the patient from a fully reclined position to a semireclined position, with the patient bib still in place. Placing the chair in the semi-upright position indicates the clinical portion is complete, but the appointment is not complete. Patient education can occur at this level (knee to knee, eye to eye), and the patient can be informed of the appropriate information. If the dentist is completing the hygiene evaluation, he or she asks if there are any questions and then leaves the operatory.

The hygienist reinforces any information the dentist presented and asks open-ended questions. When the discussion is complete, the hygienist removes the patient bib, sits the patient upright, and transfers the patient to the business team. The hygienist walks the patient to the business office, hands the business team the routing slip, and states the treatment rendered, future treatment needed, and time frame. This repetition reinforces patient education. When a patient hears something several times in varying formats, she or he is learning. When the patient hears information regarding the need and urgency of treatment from several sources, the patient will eventually understand the need and proceed. Patients may not immediately accept treatment recommendations, but with repetition and education, most will eventually proceed with needed treatments. The dental hygienist educates patients to make good choices for their dental health.

Hygiene/Dentist Discussion

Repetition is also a component of the hygiene evaluation by the dentist, which should occur after the hygienist collects all necessary data, and at a time that is convenient for the dentist. If the dentist waits to do the evaluation at the end of the hygiene appointment, the necessary time and transfer of information (education) may not occur. The hygienist may feel rushed to seat the next patient, the dentist may be rushed to complete his or her restorative patient or other hygiene patient evaluations, and the patient may want to be finished with the appointment. None of these is conducive to learning. During the hygiene evaluation, the hygienist can communicate a variety of information to the dentist:

• Personal patient information
• Medical/dental history updates as needed
• Oral cancer screening evaluation
• Periodontal and restorative evaluation, including bleeding points, probing depths, and caries evaluation
• Patient areas of concern
• Radiographs taken or that need to be taken
• Intraoral camera images taken
• Patient motivators and concerns

The dentist should read aloud any findings from radiographic evaluations. This helps educate the patient about his or her oral disease or health. Discussing findings in relationship to the patient's motivators and concerns adds a sense of need and urgency to treatment recommendations. The hygienist and dentist can discuss with the patient the importance of maintenance for the patient's particular situation. Additionally, the hygienist or dentist can ask the patient open-ended questions such as "What concerns you about treatment recommendations?" or "How can we make your visit more comfortable?" to elicit further information about the patient's motivators. Open-ended questions provide the dental professional with patient insights that are not gleaned from simple yes-or-no questions. The hygienist can also discuss any insurance or financial objections that the patient may have shared. This information can be shared with the dentist, and also

with the business team. Entire teams should develop verbal skills to answer commonly heard objections to treatments. No one verbal skill will work for every situation, but using feel, felt, found can help with patient objections. When hearing the discussion between the hygienist and dentist, the patient will hear the diagnosis and recommendations and begin to understand the importance and value of the hygiene appointment. During this discussion, the patient can be asked if there is anything that he or she would like to change about his or her mouth or smile, and if so, value-added dental services that the practice offers can be discussed. Patient education benefits both the patient and practice by creating healthy, educated patients and satisfied dental team members.

Hygiene Retention

Historically, the hygiene department was considered the "loss leader" of the practice—it brought patients in but did not produce profits for the practice. That has changed in today's technology-driven dental practice. Approximately 40% to 60% of the dentist's restorative treatments come from the hygiene department.[10] Without an effective system of monitoring the hygiene retention rate, the overall practice will suffer. Hygiene retention rates should be approximately 85% of the active patient family (an active patient is anyone who has been to the practice within 2 years). For example, an active patient family of 2,000 patients should have a hygiene retention rate of 1,700 patients. Does the practice have sufficient hygiene hours and appointments to maintain 85% retention and also include new patients or periodontal procedures?

Several methods can be used to determine whether the correct number of hygiene hours and appointments is available. Some practices hire a hygiene coordinator to maintain the hygiene schedule. Other practices have business team members who are responsible for both dentist and hygiene schedules. Either is acceptable as long as a dedicated system is in place. If a hygiene coordinator is implemented, this position has the following responsibilities:

• Determining that each hygienist is scheduled for daily production goals. Some practices also institute the use of a dedicated hygiene assistant to increase overall hygiene production. This dedicated hygiene assistant increases hygiene production by allowing the assistant to perform medical history review and other nonclinical or delegable assistant duties per state rules and regulations that allow the hygienist to concentrate on productive hygiene skills.
• Filling openings in the hygiene schedule as they occur, if possible.
• Confirming all hygiene appointments 2 days before appointment. If direct contact with the patient is not successful, a request for the patient to contact the office should be made. All patient contact information should be obtained at each appointment, including

the patient's preferred method of contact, whether home or cell phone, e-mail, or text messaging. The phrase "calling to confirm" should be avoided. The preferred phrasing is that the practice is "calling to remind you of your reservation with Dr. Jones or the hygienist, Sue." Appointments that are confirmed can be broken; reservations are made and not cancelled.

- Evaluating the restorative schedule 1 day in advance to determine whether there are any past-due hygiene patients and discussing such with a past-due patient at the restorative appointment.
- Having all hygiene appointments scheduled in the treatment room as appropriate before the end of an appointment, and sending reminder cards or letters 4 weeks before the next appointment. Patients may say they will call to schedule an appointment, but they often forget to make the call. Never let a patient leave without a scheduled appointment; to do so reduces productivity.
- Contacting hygiene patients who are overdue by 1 to 3 months by phone. If contact is not made and there is no response from the patient, send informational letters with patient-specific information.
- Contacting patients who are 4 months overdue in hygiene by phone and letter. If there is no response, place patients in the next year in the month that they were originally due.
- Sending a letter to patients who are over a year overdue that requests the patients to make a choice: Schedule an appointment and provide the best time to reach them; not schedule an appointment at this time, but contact them in the future; or be removed from the active patient list.

Calls and letters can be spaced throughout the month. For example, patients who are overdue by 1 to 3 months can be contacted in the first week of the month, those 4 months overdue in the second week, and so forth. Additionally, regular chart audits by the hygienists during the morning huddle can be critical to the success of the retention program. To determine the effectiveness of the retention program, the hygiene coordinator or business team member can divide the total number of unfilled appointments by the total number of available appointments for the month. This information can be discussed at monthly team meetings.

It is also important to note that the entire team is responsible for hygiene retention. Using communication skills and patient education, each team member stresses the need for and urgency of treatments based on the patient's individual motivators and desires. Any objections patients may voice can be addressed and overcome with appropriate verbal skills. Communication is essential to hygiene retention.

Professionalism and Appearance

Professionalism and the appearance of the team add to the perceived value of and trust in the practice. Members of the dental team should project professionalism in everything they say and do and in their appearance. Professional image websites, products, and consultants can assist the team in creating an image that displays professionalism and inspires trust in patients. Team members should also observe the office occasionally through the eyes of the patient—take time during a team meeting to do a "walk-through" of the practice. Team members should evaluate other areas of the practice from their normal area—for example, hygienists should review the business office and reception areas; business team members should review the clinical areas; and assistants and the dentist should review the sterilization/laboratory areas, bathrooms, and lunch area. Seeing the practice through the eyes of the patient allows the team to appreciate the appearance that the practice is portraying. An appearance that is inviting and professional helps increase the trust the patient will have and thus increase overall acceptance of recommendations.

Hygienists can also increase productivity by assuming the role of technology advisor in the practice. Strategic use of technology grows and protects practices. This includes using the latest products, such as digital radiography or other diagnostic tools, and social media. Contacting patients via texts or e-mails; being a voice in the social media world with blogs, Facebook, Twitter, or other accounts; and updating the practice's website regularly are as much a part of the hygienist's role in practice management as scaling and root planing. Depending on the individual practice and the hygienist's comfort, the hygienist is the ideal person to be the "face" of the practice in the technology world. Educating the patient about oral health and the practice with a mix of 80% education and 20% practice promotion in the digital arena will help increase the visibility of the practice as a leader in oral health for the community.

Habits of Effective Offices

Habits that every hygienist and team member should pursue to create the optimum practice include the following:

1. Teams should be open to change and focused on continuing education to promote lifelong learning.
2. Communication should be constant and provide clear messages sent and received for and between patients and team members.
3. Practice should focus on patient-centered care, not profit-focused care.
4. Phone skills and etiquette must be superb—you never know who is on the other end of the call.
5. Every team member should know, believe in, and uphold the practice philosophy and mission.
6. Every patient, every visit deserves the "red carpet treatment."
7. Every team member should give and receive respect and rewards every day—not just monetarily but verbally as well.

8. Community service should be a part of the practice philosophy and mission. The practice and its team are members of the larger community and need to be seen in the community as making a difference.

9. The practice should be noninsurance focused. Provide care and treatment based on the patient's need, not insurance coverage. Provide affordable payment options for patients to obtain the treatment they want and need.

The role of the hygienist in today's dental practice extends beyond cleaning patients' teeth. The hygienist needs to be aware of the intricacies of the business of dentistry and assist other team members in the overall development and management of the practice.

Case Study

Dental hygiene appointments in the practice regularly run behind schedule, and several patients have complained about the long wait when they arrive for their appointments.

Case Study Exercises

1. Dental hygienists need an adequate amount of time to perform all clinical responsibilities and to provide patient education. Dental hygiene appointments should be 30 minutes and include time for infection control procedures, clinical hygiene, and patient education.
   A. Both statements are true.
   B. Both statements are false.
   C. The first statement is true, but the second is false.
   D. The first statement is false, but the second is true.

2. All of the following strategies for addressing the dental hygiene scheduling delays are appropriate EXCEPT which one?
   A. Determine which dental hygienists are running behind schedule and advise them on how to speed up appointments.
   B. Change the schedule to 10-minute rather than 15-minute increments.
   C. Have each hygienist participate in a procedural analysis to determine appropriate appointment lengths.
   D. Reserve preblocked appointment times for procedures such as periodontal maintenance.

3. Creating a schedule with preblocked dental hygiene appointment times does which of the following?
   A. Allows the dental hygienist to make up time if earlier appointments run long
   B. Allows the dental hygienist to be efficient and productive
   C. Increases the dental hygienist's efficiency because all advanced procedures are performed at the beginning of the day

Review Questions

1. A leader is the
   A. employer.
   B. dentist.
   C. one with a commitment to others.
   D. one who decides the direction of the organization

2. All relationships are built on
   A. influence.
   B. trust.
   C. behaviors.
   D. selflessness.

3. A mission statement says who you are and what you are about, uses emotional words, and is short. A mission statement conveys why you are there and how many and what types of patients you see, uses logical words and is short.
   A. Both statements are correct.
   B. Neither statement is correct.

4. Goals should be written in _____ format.
   A. SMART
   B. MARST
   C. AMART
   D. START

5. Major overhead should represent which percentage of total overhead?
   A. 45–55%
   B. 55–65%
   C. 65–75%
   D. 75–85%
   E. 85–95%

Active Learning

1. Talk to family members and friends about what qualities make a good leader. Compare their responses to the leadership qualities discussed in the chapter and create a plan for developing two of the qualities.
2. Working in small groups, create a vision for a new dental practice. Use the questions related to vision in this chapter to guide you. Then write a mission statement for your practice. Share your work with the class. ▪

REFERENCES

1. Karpman SB. A Game Free Life. Drama Triangle Publications. San Francisco, CA. http://karpmandrama triangle.com/.
2. Covey MR. *Speed of trust.* New York, NY: Free Press; 2008.
3. Doran G, Miller A, Cunningham J. There's a S.M.A.R.T. way to write management's goals and objectives. *Management Review,* 1981;70(11):35-36.
4. Merriam-Webster business definition, http://www.merriam-webster.com/dictionary/business.
5. Department of the Treasury, Internal Revenue Service. Health Savings Accounts and Other Tax-Favored Health Plans Publication 969, Cat. No. 24216S. http://www.irs.gov/pub/irs-pdf/p969.pdf.
6. American Dental Association. *CDT, Current Dental Terminology, 2011-12 and 2013.* St. Louis, MO: Elsevier/Mosby; 2013.
7. Armitage GC. Development of a classification system for periodontal diseases and conditions. *Ann Periodontol.* 1999 Dec;4(1):1-6.
8. American Dental Association. SNODENT. Available from: http://www.ada.org/en/member-center/member-benefits/practice-resources/dental-informatics/snodent.
9. American Dental Association and U.S. Department of Health and Human Services. The Selection of Patients for Dental Radiographic Examinations. Revised 2004. http://www.ada.org/~/media/ADA/Science%20and%20 Research/Files/topics_radiography_examinations(1).ashx.
10. Jameson C. Patient retention in hygiene. *Dental Economics.* http://www.dentaleconomics.com/articles/print/volume-93/issue-9/departments/practice-elevation/patient-retention-in-hygiene.html.

RESOURCES

BOOKS:

American Dental Association. *CDT, Current Dental Terminology, 2011-12 and 2013.* St. Louis, MO: Elsevier/Mosby; 2013.

Covey MR. *Speed of trust.* New York, NY: Free Press; 2008.
Gaylor L. *Administrative dental assistant.* St. Louis, MO: Saunders Elsevier; 2007.
Iannucci J, Howerton L. *Dental radiology principles and techniques.* 3rd ed. St. Louis, MO: Saunders Elsevier; 2006.

ARTICLES:

DePalma AM. Nine habits of highly effective offices. *Dent Econ.* Oct 2007. http://www.dentaleconomics.com/articles/print/volume-97/issue-10/features/9-habits-of-highly-effective-offices.html
Hanneman A. principles for dental professionals to live by. *Dent Econ.* Oct 2007. http://www.dentaleconomics.com/articles/print/volume-97/issue-10/features/principles-for-dental-practices-to-practice-by.html.

INTERNET:

American Academy of Periodontology. Development of a classification system for periodontal diseases and conditions. Armitage GC. Development of a classification system for periodontal diseases and conditions. *Ann Periodontol.* 1999;4(1):1-6.
American Dental Association. SNODENT. Available from: http://www.ada.org/en/member-center/member-benefits/practice-resources/dental-informatics/snodent.
Carlos M. Effective listening skills. MC Solutions. Available from: http://www.slideshare.net/anscers/effective-listening-skills.
Conflict Resource Consortium, University of Colorado. International online training program on intractable conflict (I messages). Available from: http://www.colorado.edu/conflict/peace/treatment/istate.htm.
Free Management Library. Problem solving and decision making. Available from: http://managementhelp.org/personalproductivity/problem-solving.htm.
HITECH Act. Available from: http://www.healthit.gov.
Morningside Center. I messages and the Assertiveness Line. Available from: http://www.teachablemoment.org/elementary/imessages.html.
Myer P. Attitude is everything (SMART goals). Meyer Research Group. 2003. Available from: http://www.leadership-development-coaching.com/**drama-triangle**.html.
National Joint Committee for the Communicative Needs of Persons with Severe Disabilities. Communication definition. Available from http://www.asha.org/NJC/.

OTHER:

Jameson Management Systems

Chapter 53 | Career Development

Christine N. Nathe, RDH, MS

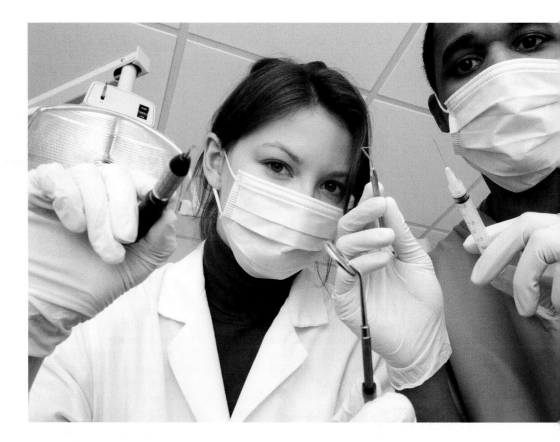

KEY TERMS

career development
career goal
curriculum vitae (CV)
resume

LEARNING OBJECTIVES

After reading this chapter, the student should be able to:

53.1 Describe employment opportunities for a dental hygienist.
53.2 Define the skills needed to find employment.
53.3 Prepare a resume for employment.
53.4 Describe interviewing skills.
53.5 Describe career development strategies.

KEY CONCEPTS

- Dental hygienists should carefully assess employment opportunities available to them.
- Specific skills are necessary to secure employment.
- For a lifetime of job satisfaction, dental hygienists should follow career development strategies.

RELEVANCE TO CLINICAL PRACTICE

Many dental hygienists have been and currently are employed by private dental practices, or, for those with advanced degrees, academic institutions. However, opportunities for employment in school-based clinics, medical practices, and other settings within comprehensive social and health systems networks are also becoming available to dental hygienists. This chapter discusses the skills and strategies needed to secure and maintain employment in a variety of settings.

EMPLOYMENT OPPORTUNITIES

Dental hygienists have a variety of career options upon graduation. Historically, private dental practices owned by one or two general dentists have employed most dental hygienists. Other private practices that employ dental hygienists include offices owned by periodontists, pediatric dentists, and sometimes orthodontists. Dental hygienists working in smaller private offices have an opportunity to become close to the few individuals they work with and be part of a unique dental family.

Larger practices, which may be owned by a corporation or insurance company, employ many dental hygienists and may include dental specialists such as orthodontists and general dentists. Dental hygienists interested in working with a diverse staff and in specialized areas of dentistry may be attracted to employment in a large practice. Employment in a large practice may also offer dental hygienists opportunities to pursue management positions.

School-based health clinics are now hiring dental hygienists. In some states, dental hygienists may also work in hospitals and nursing homes. Advanced degrees beyond a certificate or associate's degree may be required to pursue career options in clinics, hospitals, and nursing homes. For more information on the variety of opportunities available to dental hygienists, see Chapter 50, Alternative Practice Settings.

Other career options available to dental hygienists include working with the U.S. Public Health Service (USPHS), the National Health Service Corps (NHSC), Veteran's Affairs (VA) Dental Clinics, federal and state prisons, dental insurance companies, and the dental industry. The dental industry consists of companies that research, market, and sell products aimed at providing support to systems for the delivery of dental care. Positions with dental industry companies may be clinic based or involve health promotion activities, sales, marketing, research, or management/administration, and may require a bachelor's or master's degree.

The USPHS commissions dental hygienists as Health Services officers. USPHS dental hygienists treat patients in underserved and disadvantaged areas, respond to public health emergencies and natural disasters, educate communities about health, work in science or health administration, or concentrate on other areas within their specialty, such as promoting oral health initiatives or coordinating oral health projects (Table 53-1). As part of a multidisciplinary team of health professionals, USPHS dental hygienists enjoy excellent benefits and work/life balance, and are able to make a real difference in the nation's health. A bachelor's degree is required to become a Health Services officer.[1] (See Spotlight on Public Health and Teamwork.)

Through scholarship and loan repayment programs, the NHSC helps health professional shortage areas (HPSAs) in the United States obtain services from medical, dental, and mental health providers to meet their health-care needs. About half of all NHSC clinicians work in health centers supported by the Health Resources and Services Administration (HRSA), which provide preventive and primary care services to patients with low or no income.[2]

Spotlight on Public Health

Although students often enter dental hygiene school planning to practice in a private dental office, many dental hygienists find employment in public health settings. Dental public health focuses on oral health care and education of populations, with an emphasis on the utilization of dental hygiene sciences. The delivery of dental services for individuals and population-based dental public health at the national and local levels involves a variety of institutions, infrastructures, and activities.

Most dental public health practice follows steps similar to those taken by a dental hygienist in the private sector, but the focus is primarily on a population, including those who do not seek care, rather than just one patient in the chair.

Many dental hygienists choose to work in dental public health settings. Dental public health education is presented to dental hygiene students in all dental hygiene educational programs. Public health is embedded throughout the educator, researcher, administrator/manager, advocate, and clinician roles of a dental hygienist. ■

Table 53-1. Professional Roles of the Dental Hygienist

Role of the Dental Hygienist	Dental Public Health Responsibilities Embedded Throughout
Administrator/Manager	Develops and coordinates dental projects, clinics, or other related organization
Advocate	Provides dental health consultation to groups and lobbies to change laws to advance the practice of dental hygiene
Clinician	Provides clinical care to the population
Educator	Educates and promotes dental health education to patients and/or educates future dental hygienists
Researcher	Conducts research on dental hygiene

Teamwork

Dental hygienists working in public health routinely work with a variety of health and social service workers in a team paradigm. Collegial relationships are important to career satisfaction. Developing the ability to communicate with others professionally and respectfully fosters collegial relationships. Working well with others is paramount and can be accomplished if the dental hygienist strives to complement and collaborate within the team. ■

Dental hygienists who work in the dental clinic at a VA dental clinic, a military base, or a federal prison as a contract employee or as a U.S. civil service employee serve a specific population with a variety of providers.[3,4] Many state prisons employ dental hygienists as state employees, or more frequently as employees of a private health-care company that contracts with the specific prison.

Dental insurance companies frequently employ dental hygienists in a variety of consultant and administrative positions. Additionally, many dental companies that sell dental products, equipment, materials, and instruments hire dental hygienists to work in sales, research, marketing, education, and administration. Many dental hygienists have started their own companies that staff dental offices and clinics or write for dental hygiene periodicals. The opportunities for dental hygienists, particularly those with advanced degrees, are nearly endless.

Dental hygienists with advanced degrees are employed as instructors and professors in academic institutions that grant dental hygiene degrees, such as a master's degree in dental hygiene. These dental hygiene faculty members teach didactic and clinical courses and incorporate professional services into their careers by serving in leadership positions in professional and community organizations that focus on improving oral health in society. Dental hygiene professors in university settings conduct research and develop scholarly initiatives that develop and expand the scientific knowledge base of the dental hygiene discipline. All of these professionals play a critical role in advancing the profession by educating and mentoring future dental hygienists.

FINDING A POSITION

There are various ways to find a dental hygiene position. The American Dental Hygienists' Association (ADHA) provides job search information to help dental hygienists secure employment (Box 53-1).

Job search strategies include reading the classified ads in the newspaper and asking friends, family members, and acquaintances if they know of job openings. These methods are effective when looking for positions in private offices within the community. Scheduling an interview is the best way to find out whether the dental hygienist meets the employer's job requirements, and whether the practice meets the hygienist's expectations for employment.

Dental hygienists looking for employment outside a private office may find positions in VA dental clinics, the USPHS, federal prisons, and other federal and state entities by searching the specific government website or conducting a general search on the Internet for government dental hygiene positions. Most localities have agencies that place dental hygienists in temporary positions as needed. Some companies focus on helping dental hygienists find employment in other countries, which can be an interesting career option and lifetime adventure. In addition, more communities are employing dental hygienists in schools as part of a school-based health clinic or mobile health program that travels to various schools.

A personal interview is the best choice for gaining employment, but sending a cover letter and resume work well for times when a personal interview cannot be scheduled immediately. It is important to keep opportunities open, because a variety of changes could develop that would make some choices more appealing than others. For example, it may sometimes be necessary to work part time or full time or a different daily schedule, and during some periods of life it may be easier to relocate for job opportunities than during other times. Flexibility is helpful, as is the knowledge that dental hygiene practice continues to grow, including opportunities related to professional advancement.

Box 53-1. *Job Search Information*

Newspapers

Many dentists prefer not to use newspaper ads, and those who do often use a "blind ad" when looking for new employees, which requires that you respond to a post office box. This allows the dentist to remain anonymous, and puts the dental hygienist at a distinct disadvantage. You might find yourself applying for positions you don't want. If you are already employed, you may be sending a resume to someone whom you would rather didn't know your intentions. However, it is still a good idea to check newspapers on a daily basis. Classified ads from many of the nation's prominent newspapers are listed online with careerbuilder.com.

Because online employment resources are expanding rapidly, you may want to start by conducting a keyword search for employment resources on popular Internet search sites such as Infoseek, Lycos, AltaVista, Webcrawler, Yahoo, and Eblast. Indeed, some of these Internet portals maintain their own extensive employment listings.

Professional Publications

Professional journals, and other professional publications, contain a classifieds section in the back. These ads are often for positions in underserved, and sometimes exotic, locations. Check these publications if you are interested in relocating or are the adventurous type.

Unsolicited Cover Letters and Resumes

If you are in an area where the dental practice population makes it practical, you might consider sending a cover letter and resume to each practice. You might get lucky and have one land in an office with a new, unadvertised opening. Be sure to include a statement of flexibility, such as a willingness to work nontraditional hours or to substitute—it will make you more marketable—and ask that your resume be kept on file in case of future openings.

Local Professional Associations

Many local professional associations have an active job referral system. If you are new to an area, contact your state association, which can give you the name of the contact person for your local component.

Dental Auxiliary Placement Service

Most metropolitan areas have dental auxiliary placement services. Fee arrangements vary among agencies. Some charge the employer, some charge the employee, and some divide the placement fee between both parties. Most agencies are listed in the telephone directory, and many advertise in newspaper classified ads and in professional publications. If you decide to use one of these services, be sure you read and understand thoroughly any contracts into which you enter.

Temporary Placement Service

A temporary placement service is a company that provides employees to meet short-term need. "Temps" may be needed on short notice for short periods of time, to substitute for a dental hygienist who is ill, for example, or for planned, longer periods, such as for a maternity leave or vacation. Many temporary dental hygienists find ideal permanent situations this way. Before committing to a full-time position, both the dental hygienist and the employer are able to determine whether the hygienist's skills and strengths are best utilized in the position. Once again, it is important to understand the policies of the agency, especially the consequences of accepting a permanent position.

Dental Hygiene Schools

Dental hygiene programs usually have a job board or a faculty member who keeps track of open positions, both locally and around the state. Dentists consider programs to be good sources of potential applicants, and many call or write when a position is available.

Networking

An oral health-care community is much like a small town: Everybody knows everybody, and if they don't, they know someone who does. Call practicing dental hygienists in your community and let them know you are looking for a job. If a dentist you contact is not looking for a dental hygienist, ask him or her to pass on your resume to a colleague who may be. Dental supply representatives also are excellent resources. They visit offices on a routine basis and usually are knowledgeable about current employment situations. Dental supply representatives are concerned with creating and maintaining goodwill, and most are happy to help. ■

RESUME WRITING

A **resume** is a brief overview of the dental hygienist's educational credentials, employment history, accomplishments, professional organizational memberships, specific skills, and community activities. A potential employer will quickly peruse a resume, so the use of bullets and a short, condensed format is preferred.

There are several acceptable formats for resumes, and some include a vision or professional goal or objective. Chronological resumes list experience in reverse chronological order, and functional resumes emphasize individual skills and accomplishments. An organized resume is mandatory. The resume can be delivered personally to the practice or mailed with a cover letter and a page listing at least three references with current phone numbers and e-mail addresses if possible.[5] Always request permission from individuals who will be used as references in advance and keep them informed when applying for positions.

The resume should be factually correct and concise, and the cover letter should be written for the specific position that is being offered. The dental hygienist's goal should be congruent with that of the organization or office that has the available position. It is important to proofread the resume and cover letter in addition to running the spell-check feature in the word processing software to ensure that there are no spelling or grammatical errors.

Less frequently, a dental hygienist will be asked for a **curriculum vitae (CV)** instead of a resume. A CV is more descriptive than a resume, and typically is required for academic positions. Most entry-level dental hygiene positions do not require a CV. The information required on a CV is shown in Box 53-2.

INTERVIEWING

An interview is an opportunity for the dental hygienist to market his or her skills and accomplishments and discuss what he or she can do for a practice. Job applicants should be prepared to answer questions about what motivated them to pursue a career in dental hygiene and why they want the job they are applying for. They should also be prepared to explain how their skills and strengths will benefit the practice. Rehearsing responses to potential questions with a family member, friend, or fellow dental hygienist will build confidence. Sample interview questions developed by the ADHA are listed in Box 53-3.[5]

Schedule the interview at a time that works for the employer and the applicant, and be on time for the interview. Before interviewing, the applicant should determine a monthly or annual budget as a preparation for salary negotiations.

The interview is a two-way process; the potential employer learns about the dental hygienist, including his or her goals and skills, and the applicant learns about the potential employer's goals and the responsibilities of the position. Many employers may request a working interview, which would mean that the dental hygienist would work for 1 day with pay, to see if the employer felt comfortable with the potential employee and, vice versa, that the employee felt comfortable with the employer and staff. Effective communication is essential; be prepared to ask questions and clarify needs and expectations. Bringing a list of questions may be appropriate to help cover all potential needs. Some examples include questions related to who is responsible for scheduling, confirming, and filling last-minute openings; length of dental hygiene appointments; and/or flexibility in individualizing patient care appointments as needed. The ADHA provides recommendations for interviewees (Box 53-4). Within a few days of the interview, send a handwritten note to the interviewer thanking the interviewer for his or her time and briefly reiterating why your qualifications make you a good candidate for the position.

CAREER DEVELOPMENT

Career development can be defined as the creation of one's career. This begins during dental hygiene education and does not really end until retirement, or for some energetic and involved dental hygienists, long after retirement. All dental hygienists should take

---

Box 53-2. *Curriculum Vitae (CV) Essentials*

Date, Name, and Address
Licensure and certification
Educational history

Teaching
Employment history
Professional recognition
Professional membership
Extramural professional activities

Scholarly Achievements
Books
Chapters
Peer-reviewed articles
Editorial responsibilities
Invited lectures
Professional research presentations
Current grant and contract funding

Service
Patient care activities
Community service
University service

Box 53-3. *Sample Questions*

Tell me about yourself.

Tell me about your background.

Name some of your accomplishments.

Why did you go into dental hygiene?

Tell me about your strengths and your weaknesses.

What interests you about this position?

Do:

Arrive early.

Turn off your cell phone before the interview.

Be prepared to complete a formal job application.

Bring contact information for previous employers and a pen, and write neatly.

Be genuinely glad to meet your interviewer.

Greet the interviewer by his or her formal name (e.g., Dr. Atalay), stand up straight, and walk with energy.

Wait to be offered a chair before sitting down.

Be a good listener and communicator.

Be aware of nonverbal communication, especially eye contact.

Get a complete job description and explanation of expected duties.

Stress your achievements in a factual, sincere manner.

Show enthusiasm.

Bring multiple copies of your resume and reference pages.

Do Not:

Discuss marital status, age, race, religion, children, health, or political party membership.

Chew gum.

Answer questions with simple one-word answers; elaborate when possible.

Speak poorly of former employers or coworkers.

Speak of political or controversial issues. ■

Box 53-4. *Interviewing*

- Know the place and time of the interview and the correct pronunciation and name of the interviewer. Plan to arrive at the location early.
- Research the company or office. If possible, investigate present employees' length of employment and the turnover rate.
- Practice interviewing skills with a friend or family member.
- Prepare questions to ask during the interview.
- Dress in a conservative, professional manner.
- Greet the interviewer with direct eye contact, a firm handshake, and a smile. ■

time to carefully and thoughtfully decide their career goals. Questions to consider include the following:

- Why did you enter dental hygiene?
- What is your long-term goal?
- In what types of positions are you interested in gaining experience?
- What is your ideal position?

A **career goal** is a broad statement that reflects the final outcome that the dental hygienist wishes to accomplish. Career goals are written to accomplish a career milestone—for example, the dental hygienist expects to teach in a preclinical setting within the next 5 years. Strategies to reach this goal include applying to degree completion programs, taking education courses that include practical experience in clinical teaching, and then applying for an open clinical teaching position. By writing goals, the dental hygienist plans how to accomplish career aspirations.

Career planning is a lifelong process that involves much more than choosing a profession and obtaining a position. It focuses on reaching one's potential in the dental hygiene profession, determining success, assessing one's skills and interests, devising a professional career plan, and putting the career plan into action by advancing one's education.[6] The first step in career planning is setting short-term and long-term goals.

Career planning can continue to develop and change based on attainment of original career goals. Hovliaras-Delozier further describes options to enhance career satisfaction. She highlights the importance of evaluating career satisfaction and goals for the present and future. It is crucial for the dental hygienist to determine his or her level of skills and education, and explore career satisfaction, what other avenues he or she might pursue to gain more learning or certification, and the steps he or she can take to secure a high level of job satisfaction. Hovliaras-Delozier also describes the need to evaluate and make changes as necessary.[6] Some dental hygienists stay in the same position for many years, whereas others may decide to change positions. Regardless of which path the dental hygienist chooses, it is important that he or she fulfill basic obligations as a health-care provider (see Professionalism).

Professionalism

The traits associated with a health-care professional are all rooted in beneficence, the ethical principle that pertains to "doing good." Dental hygienists uphold the core value of beneficence by using their knowledge and skills to benefit the patient. Focusing on the patient's needs is satisfying as a provider and is the hallmark of professionalism. ■

SUMMARY

Although dental hygienists have historically practiced in private dental offices, new opportunities are available in other settings. Dental hygienists need specific skills to secure and maintain employment.

Mapping career goals, developing strategies to attain those goals, and crafting a well-written and organized resume and cover letter are all important to achieving success. Dental hygienists must be prepared and organized when scheduling interviews and must formulate their long-term goals and vision for a career.

Case Study

Irene Newman decided to follow her dream to become a dental hygienist. She had always liked her dental hygienist, and thought it seemed like an interesting career opportunity. After graduation, she practiced in a private dental practice owned by her cousin and enjoyed the patient interaction. However, after a few years, she decided she wanted to try something different. She was undecided as to whether she was interested in sales, teaching, or perhaps public health, so she met with one of her former professors. This sparked an interest in applying to a bachelor's degree completion program, and she was accepted. During the program, she was able to student teach in junior clinic and discovered that she enjoyed interacting with students. Upon graduation, she immediately applied to a graduate program in dental hygiene and was accepted. As part of her thesis project she worked to design an instrument that would detect subgingival calculus, which she felt would help her students and less experienced dental hygienists. While working with a dental instrument company as part of her thesis project, she met a few contacts and was hired as a research specialist for that company after graduation. Even better, the company let her continue practicing 1 day per week and teaching one-half day per week during the fall semester, because this was vital to instrument development. Although her initial goal was to practice in a private office, advancing her education allowed Irene to continue her career development and progress.

Note: Irene Newman was the first dental hygienist, and she was trained and hired by her cousin, Dr. Alfred C. Fones, the founder of dental hygiene.

Case Study Exercises

1. Describe your feelings about dental hygiene thus far in your educational career.
2. Describe your short- and long-term career goals.
3. Develop a career plan to attain these goals.
4. Develop a timeline that will assist in attainment of these goals.

Review Questions

1. School-based health clinics are now hiring dental hygienists. Many of these positions may require additional degrees.
   A. The first statement is true, but the second statement is false.
   B. The first statement is false, but the second statement is true.
   C. Both statements are true.
   D. Both statements are false.

2. One important aspect of career development is
   A. developing career goals.
   B. evaluating available dental hygiene positions.
   C. marketing oneself.
   D. attending additional clinical sessions.

3. Important guidelines to follow when interviewing for a potential position include which of the following?
   A. Arrive early.
   B. Organize your thoughts while waiting for the interview to begin.

   C. Discuss flexibility regarding child care with the potential employer.
   D. Discuss membership in local dental groups with the potential employer.

4. Resumes should include all of the following EXCEPT which one?
   A. Educational experience
   B. Employment experience
   C. Professional memberships
   D. Marital status

5. Cover letters should be sent to all potential employers. Cover letters should be sent regardless of whether an interview is scheduled or completed.
   A. The first statement is true, but the second statement is false.
   B. The first statement is false, but the second statement is true.
   C. Both statements are true.
   D. Both statements are false.

Active Learning

1. Construct a one-page resume. Ask your course instructor to provide feedback.
2. Develop a curriculum vitae. Ask your course instructor to provide feedback.
3. Write five interview questions. Working with a partner, take turns interviewing each other in class. At the end of the activity, give each other feedback and ask the course instructor for advice on interview skills. ▪

REFERENCES

1. U.S. Public Health Service. About us. Available from: http://www.usphs.gov/AboutUs/.
2. National Health Service Corps. The Corps experience. Available from: http://nhsc.hrsa.gov/corpsexperience/index.html.
3. Veterans Health Administration. VA dentistry. Available from: http://www.va.gov/dental/.
4. USAJOBS. Available from: https://www.usajobs.gov/.
5. American Dental Hygienists' Association. *Employment reference guide*. Chicago, IL: American Dental Hygienists' Association; 2010. https://www.adha.org/professional-benefits.
6. Hovliaras-Delozier CA. *Building a foundation for career success*. Chicago, IL: American Dental Hygienists' Association; 2011.
7. Hovliaras CR. Marketing yourself: embrace the challenge of enhancing your career in a tough economy. *RDH*. 2010;30(11). Available from: http://www.rdhmag.com/articles/print/volume-30/issue-11/features/marketing-yourself.html.

Chapter 54 | Lifelong Learning

Jonathan B. Owens, RDH, MS • Kris Johnson, RDHAP, BA

KEY TERMS

andragogy
continuing education
critical thinking
direct access
evidence-based practice
lifelong learning
pedagogy
PICO
self-directed learning

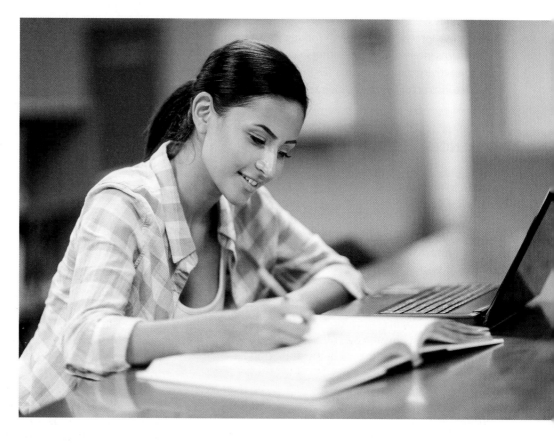

LEARNING OBJECTIVES

After reading this chapter, the student should be able to:

54.1 Define lifelong learning.
54.2 Describe the differences between andragogy and pedagogy.
54.3 Explain critical thinking.
54.4 Define evidence-based practice.
54.5 List various ways in which the Registered Dental Hygienist is able to obtain continuing education after graduation.
54.6 Explain why lifelong learning can be beneficial to both practitioner and patient.

KEY CONCEPTS

• Lifelong learning can help individuals remain current in their discipline.
• Professional responsibility requires the pursuit of continual learning.
• Multiple modalities exist to deliver advanced dental hygiene degrees and continuing education.
• Individual states determine the continuing education criteria for continued licensure.

RELEVANCE TO CLINICAL PRACTICE

The dental hygienist is an integral part of the health-care profession. The dental hygienist sees patients as often as every 3 to 6 months, giving the dental hygienist a unique opportunity to evaluate intraoral and extraoral tissues. Often, the dental hygienist is the first to identify lesions or abnormalities that are associated with systemic disease. As such, it is the dental hygienist's responsibility to stay abreast of new information and modalities in the dental hygiene field by making a commitment to lifelong learning. This chapter discusses the value and effects of lifelong learning for dental hygienists and outlines opportunities for continual study, such as advanced education, continuing education, and self-study.

WHAT IS LIFELONG LEARNING?

Lifelong learning can be described as self-directed, active learning that takes place over the course of a lifetime, beyond secondary, undergraduate, and graduate education. It includes formal education, self-study, and experiential learning.[1]

Lifelong learning includes, but is not limited to, the following aspects:

- Value—Value gaining continuous knowledge.
- Commitment—Commit to being a lifelong learner.
- Attitude—Embrace the right attitude toward lifelong learning.
- Plan—Develop the learning plan that best suits you professionally.
- Method—Combine the learning methods that work for you.
- Reading—Seek to read for an hour each day.
- Journaling—Reflect and write about personal growth and development.
- Library—Create your own library of references.
- Application— Regularly apply what you are learning.[2]

In earlier times, individuals completed their education, went to work, and relied on experience to maintain their professional integrity. Today, many professions require continuing education and to retain licensure. Most employers seek out individuals who are leaders and who are able to demonstrate high-level skills and knowledge. In fact, lifelong learning can be considered a primary strategy for maintaining employment.[3] The rapid pace with which new information is generated and delivered to the workforce requires consistent updating and integrating into daily routines. Gone are the days when a professional license made one the "expert." With access to information on the Internet, patients question and challenge care providers now more than ever.

Health-care professionals are accountable to the public when making treatment decisions, so it is imperative that the practitioner maintains up-to-date knowledge. When providers stay current in their discipline, they will be able to provide the highest-quality care to their patients, because, among other benefits, continued learning strengthens decision-making skills (Box 54-1).[4]

ADULT VERSUS CHILD LEARNERS

Malcolm Knowles, a scholar in adult education, brought the adult learning theory and the term *andragogy* to the United States in 1968. **Andragogy** applies to adult learners and is considered to be lifelong and life-wide learning.[5] It takes into consideration academic, purposeful learning, along with the unstructured experiential learning gained throughout life, such as through travel, accidents, and aging (Table 54-1). **Pedagogy,** on the other hand, describes how children learn, which tends to be a more teacher-centered process. Teachers are the experts; they tell students what and how to learn and are the evaluators of that learning. The way adults learn is vastly different from the way children learn. Adults have life experience and

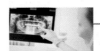

Advancing Technologies

It is estimated that there are 181,000 dental hygienists in the United States, and one must consider the body of knowledge held by members of the profession and the possibilities of communication among them. The ability of a hygienist on the East Coast to instantly communicate with a colleague 2,000 miles away highlights the ease with which a diverse group of professionals with similar interests or questions may contact each other. Different types of technology connect people almost constantly. Whether social networking via message boards, chat services, listservs, blogs, e-mail, phones, texting, Skype, Twitter, Facebook, Instagram, Pinterest, YouTube, or the as-yet-uncreated, ever-more-accessible new technology makes for limitless possibilities to share and discover information about oral health. ■

Box 54-1. *Key Points*

- Lifelong learning includes continuous reflection on current practice, and choosing to build on skills and to be the best dental hygienist you can be.
- Ask yourself: Where am I now in my profession? How is this working for my patients and myself? What can I do to raise my own professional bar?
- Incorporate technology into your practice to seek on-the-spot information references. It is impossible to have up-to-date knowledge on everything.
- Keep a portfolio of your educational accomplishments and to build on past knowledge and develop in the future.
- Participate in study clubs and/or discuss new learning with colleagues as a form of shared inquiry and new perspectives. ■

Table 54-1. *Principles and Applications of Adult Learning*

Principle	Application
Adults have an accumulation of life experience and knowledge	Life experiences and prior knowledge create new learning
Adults are self-directed	Shared inquiry, learning with others
Adults are goal oriented	Enjoy programs with clearly defined elements that lead to goal completion
Adults want to know that what they're learning applies and is relevant	Finding unexpected, yet beneficial relevance
Adult learners need to feel respected	Prior life experience can enhance the learning environment
Adult learners experience both intrinsic and extrinsic motivation for new information	The benefits of learning and appropriate challenge for growth
Adults learn best when they are active participants in their own learning	Shared inquiry, questions, activities, practice
There is no "one way" to adult learning	Consider various learning styles
Adults prefer timely and appropriate feedback	Feedback from instructor, peers, self
Adult learners do well in an informal, yet personal environment	Group interaction

are self-directed, goal oriented, and motivated, and they like to know that what they are learning will have application in their lives.[6] **Self-directed learning** is learning that is self-initiated, self-managed, and self-motivated, with independent goal setting and decision making as to what is worthwhile and applicable. In self-directed learning, teachers are more like coaches, or mentors, and peers are fellow collaborators.[7]

CRITICAL THINKING

An essential component of lifelong learning practice begins with acquiring critical thinking skills. **Critical thinking** is the process by which people analyze information, then clarify and evaluate it and derive newly constructed knowledge about that information. Courses in dental hygiene education programs emphasize critical thinking and problem solving as foundational knowledge for lifelong learning and evidence-based practice. According to the Foundation for Critical Thinking: "Critical thinking is self-guided, self-disciplined thinking which attempts to reason at the highest level of quality in a fair-minded way."[8]

Ideal critical thinking skills involve:

- Conceptualizing
- Analyzing
- Synthesizing
- Evaluating
- Observing
- Experiencing
- Reflecting
- Reasoning
- Communicating

To answer key questions in evidence-based patient care, a dental hygienist must be skilled in the ability to analyze research reports, determine their validity, and apply the information to practice. The act of engaging in the review of research builds a foundation for lifelong learning by providing recent knowledge to the dental hygienist, who can then look for additional training or education about current information trends. Critical thinking becomes essential when the dental hygienist seeks to integrate reliable research with clinical expertise and patient preferences and then design appropriate care plans for patients. The accelerating pace of change in the profession reinforces the need to prepare dental hygienists with the skills to cope with change, through learning, rather than simply to know treatment facts (see Application to Clinical Practice).[8]

EVIDENCE-BASED PRACTICE

Evidence-based practice (EBP) can be defined as the highest level of current available evidence teamed

Application to Clinical Practice

You are seeing a patient for the first time and notice on her health history that she takes a medication for anxiety known to cause dry mouth. Once you begin to work intraorally, you gain confirmation that this patient has signs of xerostomia. After questioning the patient about this, you realize she would most likely benefit from a new toothpaste for dry mouth. You suggest this to the patient, but when she learns the toothpaste has fluoride in it, she refuses, stating that she is strongly against the use of fluoride. Using your critical thinking skills, how would you address this situation? ▧

with the dental hygienist's own clinical competence. The dental hygiene diagnosis must employ EBP and to assure the best level of care for the patient. This requires reviewing current research that answers a specific question or series of questions by performing a systematic review.[9]

Key steps in the EBP process are the following:[10]

Step 1: Compose a well-defined question.

Step 2: Locate credible resources to help answer that question.

Step 3: Use critical thinking to determine the accuracy of evidence.

Step 4: Decide if evidence is relevant to application.

Step 5: Review efficacy of application and improve where necessary.

The acronym **PICO** can be used to remember how to form a well-defined question:

- Recognize the **patient's** condition.
- Consider the **intervention.**
- Utilize a **comparison intervention** if relevant.
- Acknowledge possible **outcome.**

For example:

Patient condition: Acute isolated periodontitis with 6-mm pockets #14 MF, #14 DL, and #15 ML

Intervention: Isolated scale root plane

Comparison intervention: Review oral hygiene thoroughly and have patient return in 3 weeks to reevaluate.

Outcome: Resolution of pocket depths?

Locate credible resources:

- Electronic database
- Current literature
- General resources
  - Offers background information on a subject
  - Refresh knowledge on a subject not often dealt with
  - Example: *Merck Manual*

- Filtered resources
  - High credibility
  - Clinical expert review
  - Example: Cochrane database
- Unfiltered resources
  - Less credible
  - Most recent information
  - Example: MEDLINE

Literature in health care is constantly evolving. The consummate dental hygienist spends time reading professional journals, investigating online resources, and participating in study groups or online discussions among colleagues and to stay abreast of new information (see Evidence-Based Practice).[10]

Evidence-Based Practice

Utilizing PICO, write a well-defined clinical question for the following case:

A 53-year-old woman presents with intraoral findings of white lines in a lacy network on the buccal mucosa, has a metallic taste in her mouth, and suffers from xerostomia. You suspect lichen planus, and need to decide what treatment, if any, she would benefit from.

Once you have written your question, list your top three resources to find the most current and credible information. ▧

Teamwork

The practice you work in has not had an up-to-date infection control system in place for a very long time. Recently, you started noticing sloppy cross-contamination occurring, and this bothers you. You've tried to mention it to other team members in a kind, but concerned way, yet nobody seems to care. You ask the doctor if he would mind appointing someone to be the Organization for Safety, Asepsis and Prevention (OSAP) charge for the office because you're concerned about the health and well-being of the patients. At the next team meeting, you are unanimously voted the charge for this task. After doing your research, you've learned that membership will cost the office an annual fee of $100, which will grant you access to the OSAP website.[32] Once you receive access to the OSAP website, you are amazed by how much you learn. The next month, at the team meeting, you are given time to update everyone on current and effective protocol for infection control. This information is well received and creates a newfound appreciation for sound procedures in this aspect of the practice. ▧

ADVANCED EDUCATION

Advanced education in dental hygiene includes courses of study beyond the level required for clinical practice known as an entry-level degree. Entry-level degrees include the certificate, associate, and bachelor's degrees specific to clinical dental hygiene. Various advanced education programs exist for the dental hygienist. The teaching methodology and location offerings in advanced educational programs range from traditional brick-and-mortar settings, to hybrid courses that combine on-campus classes with online coursework, to courses that are delivered completely online. Those seeking advanced education will be able to select a program that suits their lifestyle, learning style, and career goals from the variety of nationwide offerings.

Degree-Completion Programs

Since the mid-1980s, there has been discussion of making the entry level to practice clinical dental hygiene a baccalaureate degree, but the profession has had difficulty establishing this. The intent behind this movement is to advance the profession of dental hygiene.[11] The majority of the entry-level dental hygiene programs in the United States consist of schools that confer associate degrees or certificates to their graduates. Should graduates from an associate degree or certificate program desire a bachelor's degree, degree-completion programs exist throughout the country to meet their needs.[12] A candidate working toward a baccalaureate degree completion may select a major in dental hygiene or in a related field such as allied health or health sciences. However, choosing other programs such as business, nutrition, education, or gerontology will undoubtedly serve the practitioner well throughout his or her career in dental hygiene. After earning a baccalaureate degree, dental hygienists may hold positions in public health, education, administration, or corporate settings, in addition to traditional clinical settings. At this writing, the American Dental Hygienists' Association (ADHA) reports 335 entry-level dental hygiene programs and 57 degree-completion programs in the United States.[13]

The Importance of Accreditation

When selecting a college or university and before committing any money to a postsecondary educational institution, it is important to determine whether or not the institution is accredited. This is even more important when considering a nontraditional form of instruction—such as distance learning. With an accredited institution, a student has some assurance of receiving a quality education and gaining recognition by other colleges and by employers of the course credits and degrees earned. Accreditation is an affirmation that a college provides a level of quality in education that the general public has the right to expect and that the educational community recognizes.

Master's Degree Programs

Twenty-two dental hygiene programs currently offer a master's degree. Fourteen award a Master of Science in Dental Hygiene degree, and six confer a variety of degrees such as Master of Science, Master of Health Science, or Master of Community Oral Health.[13] A dental hygienist may undertake study in a discipline other than dental hygiene. Dental hygienists earning a master's degree in business, education, public health, administration, or other majors will bring a variety of knowledge and experience to their dental hygiene careers. Master's level coursework includes research methodology and the application of that methodology to a culminating thesis or project. Other topic areas that may be studied include leadership, educational theory, epidemiology, clinical practice, and basic sciences. Dental hygienists earning master's degrees are frequently employed in research settings, in the public health field, or in educational institutions as dental hygiene educators and administrators.[14]

Doctoral Degrees

Doctoral education meets the demand to increase a particular discipline's body of knowledge and the need to educate future researchers and advanced educators. At this time in the United States, dental hygienists who desire a doctoral degree must conduct their study and research in another discipline because no doctoral degrees currently exist in the field. The world's first PhD program in dental hygiene was opened in Namseoul University in South Korea in 2013. Doctoral degrees for the dental hygienist may include education, public health, biological sciences, public administration, or another field. The structure of doctoral education encompasses taking classes, leading seminars, formulating a dissertation proposal, conducting research, writing the dissertation, and defending the dissertation in front of a committee.

During the early 1990s, a Task Force Report on Dental Hygiene Education discussed the value of pursuing advanced degrees in dental hygiene. The report gave particular emphasis to setting goals for doctoral programs in dental hygiene that would expand research capability and generate new knowledge.[11] The document titled *Dental Hygiene: Focus on Advancing the Profession*, authored by the ADHA, reported that a research infrastructure is required to advance dental hygiene knowledge, and creating a doctoral-level pathway for dental hygienists would meet this need. The document further recommended curricular models for both a professional Doctor of Science in dental hygiene and an academic Doctor of Philosophy.[15]

Another document, the ADHA's National Research Agenda, includes a section with various topics listed that might guide research in the area of professional education and development.[16] Dental hygiene researchers are asked to investigate how other professions have established their entry level for practice at the master's or doctoral level.[15] Studies of this nature would provide information about the experiences of other professions that have pursued higher degrees for entry level into a profession. For nearly two decades, organized dental hygiene has discussed the idea of the doctoral degree in particular and advanced degrees in general.[11] Whether the profession moves in this direction or not depends on the course of decisions made by state boards, lawmakers, and professional leaders in education and clinical practice.

Direct Access

The entry-level degree for dental hygienists is required to gain additional credentials and/or education and to become a direct-access hygienist. **Direct access** means that a dental hygienist can initiate patient treatment without the authorization and supervision of a dentist and can establish a provider relationship with patients. Not all 50 states allow direct-access dental hygiene. Requirements as to the additional education and/or experience required to obtain this license or permit vary among the 35 states that do allow it.[17] The terminology used by states to label direct patient access are many and include titles such as *collaborative agreement* or *practice, affiliated practice agreement, registered dental hygienist in alternative practice, limited access permit, expanded practice dental hygienist, extended care permit, unsupervised practice, independent practice, remote* or *offsite supervision,* and *extended access endorsement.* Several states emphasize the public health aspect of direct-access dental hygiene by naming the position *public health dental hygienist, public health supervision,* or p*ublic health dental hygiene practitioner* (see Spotlight on Public Health).[18]

Alternative Practice Models

Over 50 other countries have a dental therapy practitioner (or similar) model. The traditional oral health-care delivery system is beyond the reach of many Americans due to lack of resources or minimal value relating to dental health; however, various new providers have been proposed. Needs for oral health education, prevention, and basic restoration procedures pervade a growing segment of the population who are unable to access services. The ADHA recommended one solution to the issue of limited access to dental care by proposing a new provider, the Advanced Dental Hygiene Practitioner (ADHP). This advanced practitioner was designed as a national license category for dental hygienists who would serve in community and public health settings as a solution for improving the oral health of underserved populations.[19] Currently, Metropolitan State University in the Minneapolis/St. Paul area of Minnesota offers a Master of Science in Advanced Dental Therapy (MSADT). Applicants to this program must be baccalaureate-prepared, licensed dental hygienists. An Advanced Dental Therapists (ADT) must practice in a collaborative arrangement with a dentist but without the dentist's supervision. In Alaska, Dental Health Aide Therapists (DHATs) have treated Alaskan Native tribes since 2004. Minnesota began training Dental Therapists (DTs) and ADTs in 2009 and graduated its first class in the summer of 2011. It is estimated that a single ADT will be able to provide care for 800 underserved people per year. Unfortunately, this licensure does not cross state lines.[20] See Chapter 50, Alternative Practice Settings, for more information.

The American Dental Association (ADA) proposed a Community Dental Health Coordinator (CDHC) who is recruited for training from the community in which the CDHC will work.

Each of these workforce models requires some type of specialized training. Although not all require a dental hygiene license, hygienists may be trained in these categories. The process of providing primary oral health care to people with low income, special needs, or minimal education or those who live in remote areas has been ineffective at best.[21] The goal of designing a workforce capable of providing care to those with the greatest need and fewest resources challenges all of the dental professions to join forces, learn together, and create solutions.

CONTINUING EDUCATION

Continuing education is training that occurs after formal education in a field of study and is designed to update the participant on new information and to reinforce previously learned concepts. Professional associations and licensing boards place a high value on continued learning, as evidenced by published standards and licensing requirements for continuing education. Nearly every state requires some form of ongoing, postlicensure study as one of the criteria for relicensure. The venue and type of continuing education delivery

Spotlight on Public Health

In California, a dental hygienist with a bachelor degree or its equivalent and 2,000 hours of practice in the 3 years immediately preceding may take coursework and apply for a license as a Registered Dental Hygienist in Alternative Practice (RDHAP). An RDHAP may practice without a dentist in dental shortage areas, persons' homes, schools, residential care facilities, and other institutions, thereby meeting the public health need to serve populations who lack access to care. Prophylaxis, periodontal treatment, fluoride varnish, sealant applications, and oral health instruction do not require a fully equipped dental operatory, thereby allowing for the delivery of less expensive care to patients in critical need of dental hygiene services. For detailed information on alternative practice settings, see Chapter 50. ■

may range from a short lecture format at a local component meeting to a multiple-day, hands-on course that includes lecture, role-play, and clinical skill practice.

Motivating factors for continued education vary among individuals. For some, the need for courses or units to meet licensure requirements provides the impetus to attend local or statewide meetings. Others choose subjects of interest as the criteria by which they select courses. Professionals might also determine topics with which they are unfamiliar or inexperienced and enroll in courses that will advance their professional knowledge and skill in that area. Continuing education programs not only educate health-care practitioners, they may also serve to infuse the participant with a renewed enthusiasm for practice and provide an opportunity to network with peers (see Teamwork).

The Standards for Clinical Dental Hygiene Care

Clinical Practice Standards, developed in 2008, help guide hygienists by clearly defining the practice of dental hygiene and discussing educational preparation, practice settings, and professional responsibilities.[22] This document points out the importance for the dental hygienist to continually learn, maintain competence, and be willing to evolve with the ever-changing health-care system.

State Requirements

After the first U.S. state established continuing education requirements for dental hygienists in 1969, 48 states and Washington, D.C., followed suit to mandate continuing education as a condition for license renewal. Each state has determined its own requirements for continuing education, with a wide variance of between 6 and 100 hours required per licensing period. Licensing periods vary between 1 and 5 years. State autonomy allowed for the creation of 49 different sets of requirements, but some similarities exist among them. Forty-four states require certification in cardiopulmonary resuscitation (CPR) as a condition of license renewal. To meet the postlicensure education mandate, self-study courses are allowed in 41 states. A variety of course subjects, such as medical emergencies, ethics, infection control, jurisprudence, or radiography, may be mandatory in one or more states. Consulting with a state's dental hygiene licensing and regulatory agency will assure that an applicant for licensure possesses the appropriate continuing education credentials.[23]

Professional Organizations

Professional organizations serve to set policy and guide the progress of the members they represent. Each of the organizations described here has evolved its own relationship with the dental hygiene profession. The individual missions have a different focus, but all of the organizations list lifelong learning as some component of their goals, and all endeavor to provide opportunities for educational enrichment.

American Dental Hygienists' Association

The ADHA has published many documents that underscore and expand upon the ADHA mission "to advance the art and science of dental hygiene and to promote the highest standards of education and practice in the profession."[24] The ADHA website, www.adha.org, is an unparalleled resource for the dental hygienist to learn about membership, education and careers, advocacy, current news and events, publications, state licensing requirements, leadership and governance, and links to other resources.

Because state licensing boards are being requested to include representation from the public in the regulation of professions, greater consumer representation will appear on professional boards. This action pushes state boards to change their focus from one of assessing entry-level competence to assuring continued professional competence. Dental hygienists will want to be active participants in developing the guidelines and the methods chosen for continued competence in their profession.

American Academy of Dental Hygiene

The American Academy of Dental Hygiene (AADH) is the organization that approves continuing education courses, based on the Academy of General Dentistry Pace Guidelines, for the dental hygiene professional. It is also responsible for developing the Standards for Continuing Education. It promotes lifelong learning by establishing adherence to a high standard of educational experience as a membership requirement. New members must show proof of attending 75 hours of AADH-approved continuing education in the 5 years preceding their application. Professional experience must include at least 750 hours per year for 5 of the last 8 years. To become a Fellow of the organization, an advanced degree and additional education in a field of specialty are required. Tenets of the AADH include fostering "the continuing pursuit of education and research in the art and science of dental hygiene" and recognizing excellence in practice and community service.[25]

The American Dental Education Association

The American Dental Education Association (ADEA), representing all facets of dental education, has published a list of competencies for entry into the profession of dental hygiene that emphasizes the value of lifelong learning. The Core Competencies outline behavior regarding adhering to the professional code of ethics, abiding by all state and federal laws, utilizing critical thinking and evidence-based decision making, accepting accountability, adapting self-assessment, integrating new scientific theories, recording accurate and complete records, communicating effectively, collaborating with other health-care professionals, and managing medical emergencies. The ability to base patient care on solid science requires consistent journal reading and attendance at courses or presentations that explain the research as it translates into practice.[26]

In 2006, the ADEA House of Delegates approved policy statements to serve as guidelines for dental education programs.[27] The guidelines underscored the expectation for all dental professionals to engage in lifelong learning. Under the Education heading, the policy states that students are to be encouraged during their educational programs to become lifelong learners and to study research concepts and apply them to their practices.

The International Federation of Dental Hygienists

The International Federation of Dental Hygienists (IFDH) was formed in 1986 in Oslo, Norway, as a global forum to unite dental hygiene associations in their missions to advance and represent the profession. The IFDH works with a variety of global partners as a worldwide promoter of access to oral health care. The IFDH promotes the exchange of knowledge among its members and member countries regarding the profession, its practice, and professional education programs. It also supports the development of research by dental hygienists who may be invited to present papers at the International Symposium on Dental Hygiene (ISDH).[28] The Symposium, held every 3 years, provides a source of lifelong learning for dental hygienists, who may learn from research paper presentations and network with hygienists from around the world.

Delivery of Continuing Education

As the complexity of the information required in dental hygiene practice increases, so do the opportunities to obtain the training and education necessary to maintain up-to-date knowledge. At one time, the only choice for education after graduation was through attendance at large state or national meetings. With the advent of state-mandated continuing education, demand for courses has increased and offerings have become more commonplace. The burgeoning technology sector has created a variety of delivery methods for oral health information and promises to continue innovating in ways that we can only imagine.

Professional Meetings

Professional meetings, whether local, state, or national in scope, offer educational courses for the attendees, and the larger the meeting, the greater the variety of courses that are available (see Professionalism). Advantages to attending courses in person are the potential for hands-on experience and other learning activities, the ability to experience different areas of the country or the world, and the opportunity to network with fellow professionals. Disadvantages include the cost of registration—which usually covers the costs for facilities, food, and presenters—and personal expenses for lodging and transportation. The time away from work and family may contribute to the overall personal cost of attending convention-type meetings.

Professionalism

The ADHA Bylaws and Code of Ethics contains a section titled "Standards of Professional Responsibility" in which categories of groups to whom hygienists have responsibility are listed. The importance of lifelong learning is underscored in the section on responsibility to ourselves as *individuals* who "continually strive for knowledge and personal growth." The section on responsibility to ourselves as *professionals* reminds dental hygienists to "enhance professional competencies through continuous learning and to practice according to high standards of care" and to "develop collaborative professional relationships and exchange knowledge to enhance our own lifelong professional development."[31] ■

Self-Study Opportunities

Mandated continuing education courses may be obtained through self-study, self-directed, or programmed learning courses. Self-study courses may be offered online through a college, university, or business website. Reading an article, paper, brochure, or book; completing a posttest on the content; and then sending the test to the provider is another type of self-directed learning. In a third category of self-study, a dental hygienist can purchase or rent a CD-ROM or DVD containing subject matter of relevance to the practitioner, and then watch or listen to the program. Once questions pertaining to the content of each course are answered, they are submitted to the provider, who issues a certificate of completion and awards continuing education units.

A variety of providers offer self-study opportunities for continuing education credit.

The ADHA presents opportunities for self-study of all three types. The ADHA website lists online courses worth 1 to 2 continuing education units each that are free or of minimal cost to members and provide information in a wide variety of subject areas.[29] Numerous dental product companies offer educational self-study courses covering topics of interest to dental hygienists, such as caries and dental decay prevention, the oral–systemic link, and the efficacy of toothpastes and mouthrinses, among many other subjects. Some companies and education providers broadcast webinars and podcasts that can be heard or watched from a computer screen or handheld media device. By checking the websites of dental product companies, a dental hygienist can peruse the self-study options available and select topics and delivery methods of interest. The convenience of self-study modalities that require little travel or cost and provide self-determined viewing times is likely to push this sector of education into considerable future growth (see Advancing Technologies).

Case Study

A colleague is frantic because he just realized that his license is almost due for renewal and he hasn't completed all of his continuing education needed for the licensing period. He says he should have paid closer attention to this, but he was distracted because his mother had been ill. He has been looking online for courses around the area, but hasn't found anything. Luckily, he has completed about two-thirds of his continuing education (CE) requirements.

Case Study Exercises

1. What would be a logical next step for the dental hygienist looking for quick CE units?
   A. Searching hard-copy and/or online journals for CE units
   B. Going to the local community center and taking a health-related course
   C. Asking a colleague for a course number and creating a forged completion certificate
   D. Searching the ADHA website for CE offerings
   E. Both a and d

2. Most states require dental hygienists to complete a set number of continuing education credits every _____ years.
   A. 3
   B. 1 to 5
   C. 4
   D. 2 to 5

3. How many states currently require cardiopulmonary resuscitation certification and to maintain licensure?
   A. 48
   B. 52
   C. 44
   D. 41

4. Consulting with a state's _____ and _____ agency will assure that an applicant for licensure possesses the appropriate continuing education credentials.
   A. board; licensing
   B. licensing; regulatory
   C. regulatory; dental
   D. legal; licensing

5. Each of the following may be mandatory in one or more states EXCEPT which one?
   A. Ethics
   B. Radiography
   C. Nutrition
   D. Jurisprudence
   E. Infection control
   F. Medical emergencies

6. The first U.S. state established continuing education requirements for dental hygienists in 1969. Forty-nine states and Washington, D.C., followed suit to mandate continuing education as a condition for license renewal.
   A. Both statements are true.
   B. Both statements are false.
   C. The first statement is true, but the second is false.

Review Questions

1. OSAP stands for which of the following?
   A. Occupational Safety and Protection
   B. Organization for Safety and Protocols
   C. Organic Students and Professors
   D. Organization for Safety, Asepsis and Prevention

2. Andragogy
   A. refers to the way in which children learn.
   B. is teacher-centered learning.
   C. is how adults learn.
   D. is lifelong.
   E. Both c and d

3. To become a Fellow of the AADH one must
   A. obtain an entry-level degree and be published in a professional journal.
   B. hold an advanced degree and additional education in a field of specialty.

   C. possess national speaker recognition and have been nominated as "mentor of the year."
   D. hold a teacher's credential and have at least 5 years of experience as an educator.

4. The acronym PICO stands for which of the following?
   A. Patient, intervention, critical, outcome
   B. Purpose, intent, compare, offer treatment
   C. Patient, intervention, comparison intervention, outcome
   D. Plan, infer, confirm resource, organize

5. The entry-level hygienist is a hygienist
   A. with a master's degree.
   B. who hasn't yet passed the state board.
   C. with less than 2 years of clinical practice.
   D. who has graduated from an associate, certificate, or dental-hygiene-specific baccalaureate program.

Active Learning

1. Use the Internet to find five different baccalaureate degree-completion programs for the dental hygienist.

2. Acquire and listen to a continuing education course through a product of your choice.

3. Take a walk with a fellow colleague and discuss where you intend to go in the profession of dental hygiene. Make sure it is a dialogue.

4. Research PubMed for information on current periodontal therapies.

5. Create a LinkedIn account on the Internet and reach out to a dental hygiene professional who intrigues you in terms of career direction. Ask the individual what path was taken to get where he or she is now.

6. Interview another hygienist, a mentor perhaps, who has gone on to further his or her education and find out if it has opened more career opportunities for the individual.

7. In 300 to 500 words, describe where you see yourself professionally in 5 years, and in 10 years. ■

REFERENCES

1. Oncology Nursing Society Position. Lifelong learning for professional oncology nurses. 2012. Available from: http://ons.metapress.com/content/2k7tw11401748747/fulltext.pdf.

2. Sarder R. *Learning. Steps to becoming a passionate lifelong learner.* New York, NY: Sarder Press; 2011.

3. Collins J. Lifelong learning in the 21st century and beyond. *RadioGraphics.* 2009;29:613-622. doi:10.1148/rg.292085179. Available from: http://radiographics.rsna.org/content/29/2/613.full.

4. McFadden JJ, Thiemann LJ. Evidence-based practice for lifelong learning. *AANA Journal.* 2009;77(6). Available from: http://www.aana.com/newsandjournal/Documents/educnews_1209_p423-426.pdf.

5. Reischmann J. 2004. Studies in pedagogy, andragogy, and gerontagogy. Available from: http://www.umsl.edu/~henschkej/henschke/more%20henschke_5_11_04/andragogy_A_banner_for_identity.pdf.

6. Collins J. Education techniques for lifelong learning. Principles of adult learning. *RadioGraphics.* 2004;24:1483-1489.

7. VanBriesen JM. Self-directed learning. 2011. Available from: http://www.nae.edu/File.aspx?id=37803.

8. Foundation for Critical Thinking. Defining critical thinking. 2013. Available from: http://www.criticalthinking.org/pages/defining-critical-thinking/766.

9. Journal of Dental Education. Introducing dental students to evidence-based decisions in dental care. 2008. Available from: http://www.jdentaled.org/content/72/1/87.full.pdf+html.

10. University of Minnesota Libraries. Evidence-based practice. An Interprofessional Tutorial.2013. Available from https://www.lib.umn.edu/apps/instruction/ebp/.

11. Henson H, Gurenlian J, Boyd L. The doctorate in dental hygiene: has its time come? *Access.* 2008:10-14.

12. American Dental Hygienists' Association. Degree completion dental hygiene programs. Available from: http://www.adha.org/resources-docs/71618_Degree_Completion_Programs.pdf.

13. American Dental Hygienists' Association. Number of dental hygiene education programs offered by state. August 14, 2015. Available from: http://www.adha.org/resources-docs/7525_Map_of_DH_Programs_Per_State.pdf.

14. American Dental Hygienists' Association. Dental Hygiene Education Curricula, Program, Enrollment and Graduate Information. October 21, 2014. Available from: http://www.adha.org/resources-docs/72611_Dental_Hygiene_Education_Fact_Sheet.pdf.

15. American Dental Hygienists' Association. Dental hygiene: focus on advancing the profession. 2005. Available from: http://www.adha.org/resources-docs/7263_Focus_on_Advancing_Profession.pdf.

16. American Dental Hygienists' Association. National dental hygiene research agenda. 2007. Available from: http://www.adha.org/resources-docs/7834_NDHRA_Statements.pdf.

17. American Dental Hygienists' Association. Direct Access 2014—37 states. Revised September 2015. Available from: http://www.adha.org/resources-docs/7524_Current_Direct_Access_Map.pdf.

18. American Dental Hygienists' Association. Direct access states. Revised September 2015. Available from: http://www.adha.org/resources-docs/7513_Direct_Access_to_Care_from_DH.pdf.

19. American Dental Hygienists' Association. Competencies for the Advanced Dental Hygiene Practitioner (ADHP). 2012. Available from: http://www.adha.org/resources-docs/72612_ADHP_Competencies.pdf.

20. Metropolitan State University. Master of Science in Advanced Dental Therapy (MSADT). 2013. Available from: http://www.metrostate.edu/msweb/explore/catalog/grad/index.cfm?lvl=G&section=1&page_name=master_science_advanced_dental_therapy.html.

21. American Dental Association. The Community Dental Health Coordinator. 2012. Available from http://www.ada.org/~/media/ADA/Advocacy/Files/ADA_Breaking_Down_Barriers-Community_Dental_Health_Coordinator.pdf.

22. American Dental Hygienists' Association. Standards for clinical hygiene practice. 2012. Available from: http://www.adha.org/resources-docs/7261_Standards_Clinical_Practice.pdf.

23. American Dental Hygienists' Association. States requiring continuing education for license renewal. (August 2015). Available from: https://www.adha.org/licensure.

24. American Dental Hygienists' Association. Mission and history. 2012. Available from: http://www.adha.org/mission-history.

25. American Academy of Dental Hygiene. Continuing education. 2015. Available from: http://www.aadh.org.

26. American Dental Education Association. Competencies for entry into the allied dental professions. 2011. Available from: http://www.adea.org/uploadedFiles/ADEA/Content_Conversion_Final/about_adea/governance/ADEA_Competencies_for_Entry_into_the_Allied_Dental_Professions.pdf.

27. American Dental Education Association. Policy statements 2011. 2011. Available from: http://www.adea.org/about_adea/governance/ACAEPToolkit/Documents/2009%20policy%20statements.pdf.

28. International Federation of Dental Hygienists. About the IFDH. 2013. Available from: http://www.ifdh.org/about.html.

29. American Dental Hygienists' Association. ADHA online CE courses. 2015. Available from: https://www.adha.org/ce-courses.

30. Bureau of Labor Statistics. Occupational outlook handbook: dental hygienists. 2012. Available from: http://www.bls.gov/ooh/healthcare/dental-hygienists.htm.

31. American Dental Hygienists' Association. Bylaws and code of ethics. 2012. Available from: http://www.adha.org/resources-docs/7611_Bylaws_and_Code_of_Ethics.pdf.

32. Organization for Safety, Asepsis and Prevention. OSAP member descriptions. 2013. Available from: http://www.osap.org/?page=JoinMembershipDescription

Glossary

A_{1C} Laboratory test that measures average blood glucose level over the last 2 to 3 months.

abrasion Removal of a surface by means of friction.

abrasives Toothpaste ingredients that aid in the removal of plaque/debris and staining.

absolute contraindication Circumstances under which a drug should absolutely not be administered.

abutment A tooth or an implant that provides support for a fixed bridge.

accounts receivable Amounts due to the practice, whether private pay (to be paid by the patient) or insurance balances.

achlorhydria The insufficient production of gastric acid in the stomach.

acid–base balance (pH) A solution's acidity or alkalinity (base) expressed as pH.

acid etching Process used to create a microscopic roughness on the tooth's enamel surface, which the sealant flows into; a mechanical bond is then created.

acidogenic bacteria Acid-producing microorganisms. Also called *cariogenic bacteria.*

acquired condition Condition that develops later in life.

acquired pellicle A thin film that coats the tooth immediately on exposure to saliva.

actinic cheilitis Severe sun damage to the lip.

active immunization Exposure of the body to an antigen to stimulate the body to produce its own antibodies.

active ingredients Ingredients that contribute to the therapeutic properties of the dentifrice.

activities of daily living (ADL) Tasks an individual performs involving self-care, such as eating, bathing, and dressing.

acute adrenal insufficiency A condition in which the adrenal glands do not produce adequate amounts of steroid hormones, primarily cortisol; but may also include impaired production of aldosterone (a mineralocorticoid), which regulates sodium conservation, potassium secretion, and water retention.

acute inflammation Inflammation that begins suddenly and is of short duration ($\leq$2 weeks).

acute respiratory infection Communicable disease (spread from one person to another) caused by bacteria, viruses, or fungi.

adaptation The manner in which the working end of an instrument is positioned against the tooth surface.

adaptive or acquired immune response Immunity acquired through contact with a disease-causing agent. Immunity can be acquired naturally through exposure to a disease or artificially through vaccination.

adaptive immune system Defense mechanism that recognizes specific antigens and produces the cells and processes required to eliminate the antigens. Also called *specific immune system.*

Addison disease Primary adrenal insufficiency in which the adrenal glands are damaged and cannot produce enough cortisol and, in many cases, not enough aldosterone.

Addisonian crisis Situation characterized by severe worsening of adrenal insufficiency symptoms, including sudden penetrating pain in the lower back, abdomen, or legs; severe vomiting or diarrhea; sudden drop in blood pressure; and/or loss of consciousness.

adjunctive screening techniques Technologies available to assist in the early screening or identification of precancerous or cancerous lesions within the oral cavity. These technologies enable practitioners to alert the patient to the need for a more definitive diagnosis and are considered screening tools only.

adolescence The period from puberty to adulthood.

adrenal insufficiency (AI) Hormonal disorder that occurs when the adrenal glands are not functioning properly to produce needed hormones.

Advanced Dental Hygiene Practitioner (ADHP) Midlevel oral health provider proposed by the American Dental Hygienists' Association to address access-to-care issues.

aerosols Invisible biologic contaminants less than 50 μm in diameter.

afferent nerve Sensory nerve that carries information from the periphery of the body to the central nervous system (CNS).

AIDS The late stage of HIV.

air polishing A technique performed using compressed air, water, and sodium bicarbonate powder.

akinesia Muscle rigidity.

ALARA Principle of radiation use As Low As Reasonably Achievable to minimize radiation exposure.

alternative practice setting A site other than a dental office where dental services are provided to patients.

alveolar bone proper A thin layer of bone that supports the root and gives attachment to the periodontal ligament; also called *lamina dura* or *cribriform plate.*

alveoli Bony sockets.

Alzheimer disease Irreversible, degenerative brain disease, affecting 1 in 10 adults older than 65 years.

ambivalence Having positive and negative feelings toward an action, person, or situation.

American Dental Hygienists' Association (ADHA) The largest professional organization representing dental hygienists in the United States. ADHA offers opportunities for professional development and leadership.

American Sign Language (ASL) A visual, gestural language that has its own vocabulary, grammar, and syntax and is recognized as a language different from English. Hand movements, body postures, and facial expression serve as words of the language.

amides Anesthetics that have nitrogen as part of their molecular makeup.

amplitude The distance the tip of an ultrasonic scaler moves or the length of the stroke.

amyotrophic lateral sclerosis (ALS) A serious neurological disease resulting in muscle weakness, disability, and eventually death; often called Lou Gehrig disease.

analgesia The absence of pain.

analog x-ray film Photographic film used to visualize objects exposed to x-rays; available in two types: nonscreen film used for intraoral radiographs and screen film used for extraoral radiographs.

anaphylaxis An immediate whole-body reaction to an allergen that results in the release of histamine and edema of the airways.

andragogy Lifelong and life-wide learning that includes academic, purposeful learning, as well as unstructured, life experiential learning such as travel, accidents, and aging.

anemia A condition that occurs when the body does not produce enough healthy red blood cells, resulting in the possible lack of oxygen to the organs.

anesthesia The absence of sensation to include all senses plus the attenuation of pain; process is required before surgery.

angina pectoris A condition caused by a lack of oxygen supply to the myocardium, generally due to constriction of the coronary arteries as a result of coronary artery disease, specifically atherosclerosis.

angioedema Localized swelling of subcutaneous or submucosal tissues, or both.

Angle classification of malocclusion System for classifying malocclusion based on the relationship of the maxillary first molar to the mandibular first molar and the relationship between the maxillary and mandibular canines, particularly when the first permanent molars are missing.

angular cheilitis Oral mucosa condition that occurs bilaterally at the commissures of the lips and appears as deep red cracks or inflamed ulcerated fissures with or without symptoms of discomfort.

angulation The angle between the bladed instrument working end and the surface of the tooth.

ankyloglossia Congenital condition that occurs when the lingual frenulum attaching the tongue to the floor of the mouth or lingual gingiva is too short, thick, or tight, and often results in the inability to properly raise or extend the tongue. Commonly referred to as *tongue-tied.*

anorexia nervosa An eating disorder in which the person sees herself as overweight no matter how dangerously underweight she becomes.

anteverted pelvis Tipping the pelvis forward to reduce muscle strain and decrease intervertebral disk pressure.

antibody Substance produced by plasma cells in response to specific antigens that bind with their antigen to form an immune complex, which identifies the antigen for destruction.

anticipatory guidance The process of providing information about upcoming developmental milestones to prepare patients and caregivers for future stages.

anticoagulant therapy A procedure that results in the prevention of coagulation (clotting) of blood.

antigen Substances that the immune system identifies as nonself.

antigen–antibody complexes The complex formed by the binding of antigen and antibody molecules.

antigingivitis agents Ingredients thought to reduce the pathogenicity of biofilm.

antimicrobial agents Ingredients that slow the growth of or kill microbes.

antitartar agents Ingredients that reduce crystal growth on tooth surfaces.

anxiolytic The ability to reduce or minimize anxiety and fear.

aphasia Speech or language deficits.

apoptosis Programmed cell death.

appliance Device designed to provide a function or therapeutic effect in the mouth.

aromatic ammonia Respiratory stimulant used in the management of syncope.

arrhythmias Irregular heart rhythms caused by a disturbance of the normal electrical conduction system of the heart or as a consequence of heart disease.

arthritis Chronic condition characterized by pain, swelling, and stiffness in the joints; can also compromise the immune system.

assessment The process of gathering information from the patient relative to general health and oral health status, medical history, medications, current needs, and concerns.

assessment instruments Instruments that help the dental hygienist collect data used to guide and determine treatment needs.

asthenia Varying degrees of weakness of voluntary muscles.

asthma A chronic lung disease characterized by inflammation and narrowing of the tracheobronchial tree.

atheroma Lipid deposits in subendothelial tissue.

atherosclerosis A buildup of fibrofatty deposit or plaque consisting of several lipids on the internal walls of medium and large arteries, which causes a narrowing of the lumen of the vessel.

atrial septal defect An opening between the left and the right atria.

attached gingiva Portion of the gingiva attached to the alveolar bone by collagen fibers.

attitudinal barrier Describes the difficulties or challenges experienced by a person with physical impairments as a result of another individual's misunderstanding, ignorance of the disability, dismissal of the individual as a "person" due to the disability, or unjust decisions about the individual's capabilities—for example, discrimination, pity, stereotypes, and fear of the impairment.

autistic spectrum disorders Pervasive developmental disorders that include conditions such as Asperger syndrome and Rhett disorder.

autoantibody Host tissue.

autoimmune disease Condition that occurs when the body identifies parts of an individual's own body (self) as antigens and mounts an immune response.

autoinoculation Spread of disease to other areas on the skin, eyes, and nostrils/nose.

automated external defibrillator (AED) Computer device that diagnoses cardiac rhythms and delivers electrical shocks to the heart.

autonomy The ethical principle and core value of self-determination.

autopolymerization The process by which sealants self-polymerize. Autopolymerizing sealants have two parts, a catalyst and base, which must be mixed uniformly and placed quickly because polymerization starts as the materials combine.

autosomal recessive Type of hereditary disease that results from an identical gene received from each parent.

avulsed tooth Tooth that has been knocked out of its socket.

bacteremia Bacteria migrating from the periodontal pocket to the bloodstream.

barrier-free design Universal design that allows accessibility for people with or without physical impairments.

basic life support (BLS) Emergency care that supports the ventilation and circulation of a victim experiencing a life-threatening illness or injury.

Bass brushing method Toothbrushing technique that targets the gingival margin.

battery Rendering an additional procedure, such as applying fluoride, without obtaining the patient's consent.

Bell palsy (BP) Weakness or paralysis of the facial muscles, usually on one side of the face, caused by unilateral inflammation of the seventh cranial nerve.

beneficence The ethical principle and core value that pertains to doing good.

benign migratory glossitis See **geographic tongue**.

best practice The use of scientific research as a guide to making sound patient care decisions and applying them to ensure the best possible health outcomes.

betel nut Fruit of the Areca catechu palm tree, which is native to southeast Asia; chewing betel nut products is strongly linked to oral cancer.

bias The tendency to introduce error into a measurement by favoring one answer, outcome, or value over others; types of bias include measurement bias, for example, of an instrument, and observational bias, for example, of a researcher.

binging Consuming large quantities of simple carbohydrates, which the body craves because it is being deprived of nutrients.

bioburden The number of viable organisms in or on an object or surface.

biofilm A colony of microorganisms within a protective polysaccharide slime layer that forms in dental tubing.

biohazard Something that poses a health risk for a practitioner.

biological age How a person's body ages physiologically. Medical assessments such as vital signs, bone density, basal metabolic rate, hearing, vision, balance, and flexibility are instruments used to measure a person's biological age.

biological marker A biochemical abnormality shared by all patients with a disease.

biomedical database Research resource database containing published literature on subjects of a biomedical nature.

biopsy Removal of a tissue for the purposes of obtaining a diagnosis.

bipolar disorder Condition characterized by extreme mood swings between euphoria and depression.

bipolar I disorder Condition diagnosed when a person experiences one or more manic episodes, without necessarily having experienced a subsequent depressive episode; also called *manic-depression*.

bipolar II disorder Condition diagnosed when a person suffers from less severe mania than bipolar I and at least one major depressive episode.

bisphenol A-glycidyl methacrylate (bis-GMA) A dimethacrylate monomer used to make dental sealants.

bisphosphonates The class of drugs most often prescribed for osteoporosis.

bisphosphonate-related osteonecrosis of the jaw (BRONJ) An area of bone in the jaw that has died and been exposed in the mouth for more than 8 weeks in a person taking any bisphosphonate.

bitewing radiograph An intraoral radiograph that shows the crowns of teeth of both the maxilla and the mandible on a single image.

bleeding on probing (BOP) Bleeding that occurs with gentle probing of the ulcerated soft tissue wall of an inflamed pocket/sulcus. Bleeding does not occur in health.

bleeding time Test that measures how long it takes a standardized skin incision to stop bleeding; normal readings range between 1 and 6 minutes.

blind Visual acuity of 20/200.

blinding A type of research control method. In a single-blinded study, the participant is unaware of what the intervention will be. A double-blinded study signifies that neither participant nor researcher is informed about the intervention. A nonblinded study, commonly known as open-label, means both the participant and the researcher are cognizant of the intervention.

blood pressure Pressure exerted on the walls of blood vessels. Measurement of blood pressure provides a means of screening general health and is recommended for all who present for oral care, including children.

body mass index (BMI) A measure of body fat calculated by a formula using an individual's height and weight.

bradycardia A sinus node dysfunction that results in less than 60 beats/min.

bradykinesia Slowness of motion.

Brännström hydrodynamic theory Widely accepted theory regarding the cause of dentin hypersensitivity. It hypothesizes that when physical stimuli such as cold or heat is applied to exposed dentin, fluids in the tubules are disturbed, producing an outward flow of tubular fluid through capillary actions. The fluid movement stimulates nerve receptors sensitive to pressure, which the patient perceives as sharp pain.

breach of contract Failure by the practitioner to render treatment in a reasonable time and within the standard of care.

bronchodilator Drug that dilates the bronchi and bronchioles of the lungs easing air flow to enhance breathing.

brush test See **exfoliative cytology**.

buffer To bring a low pH to normal level.

bulbar muscles Mouth and throat muscles responsible for eating and talking.

bulbar weakness Weakness of the facial muscles, difficulty chewing and swallowing, difficulty speaking, and weakness of the neck muscles; the affected nerves originate on the bulblike portion of the brainstem.

bulimia nervosa An eating disorder characterized by overeating, or binging, on large quantities of food.

calcium peroxide A whitening agent.

calculus Hard deposits in the oral cavity.

calculus ledges Subgingival, shelflike pieces of calculus that accumulate parallel to the cementoenamel junction (CEJ) of the tooth.

calculus rings Layer of calculus that encircles the buccal or lingual surface of the tooth, either subgingival or supragingival.

calculus spicules Small, needle-like or pointed pieces of calculus at the line angle that appears on the mesial and distal surfaces of the tooth.

calibration Process by which consistency among individuals collecting data is established to ensure accurate use of the data collection instrument.

cancer A general term that applies to a group of more than 100 diseases in which cells in a part of the body begin to grow out of control.

Candida albicans The most common fungus found in the mouth, often colonizes the irregular acrylic surfaces of the prosthesis and subsequently infects the underlying oral mucosa.

carbamide peroxide A whitening agent.

cardiovascular surgery Surgery on the heart or large vessels that bring blood to and from the heart.

career development Creation of one's career.

career goal Broad statement that reflects the final outcome that the dental hygienist wishes to accomplish.

caries A transmissible bacterial infectious disease process of the mineralized oral structures. The disease occurs on a continuum, resulting from repeated cycles of demineralization and remineralization over an extended period.

caries management by risk assessment (CAMBRA) An evidence-based disease-management protocol designed for clinical practice.

cariogenesis The development of caries.

cariogenic Likely to promote dental caries.

cariogenic bacteria Acid-producing microorganisms. Also called *acidogenic bacteria*.

cariology The study of dental caries.

cariostatic A substance that inhibits the formation of dental caries.

carious lesion Also known as tooth decay. A breakdown of teeth, either the crown or the root. A carious lesion is a sum of several factors, such as bacteria interacting with sugars, and production of acids that break down tooth structure. It is a detectable change in the tooth structure that results from the biofilm-tooth interactions occurring due to the disease caries.

carrier A person who may transmit an infectious agent to others regardless of whether there are signs or symptoms of disease.

case—control study Studies in which participants are selected based on their disease and compared with people who do not have the disease. Researchers look back in time to identify factors or exposures that might be associated with illness.

case report A report on the treatment of one single patient.

case series A collection of reports on the treatment of individual patients.

cataract A cloud that develops over the lens of the eye and prevents light from passing through.

cavitation Rapid movement of air bubbles from the tip of an ultrasonic scaler insert.

cavity The end result of a localized chemical dissolution of the tooth structure caused by metabolic events taking place in the biofilms that cover the affected tooth surface(s) and denote a hole in the tooth. Also called *dental decay* or *cavitation*.

celiac sprue A red blood disorder associated with the body's inability to properly metabolize gluten.

cell-mediated immunity Immune responses mediated by cells as opposed to soluble molecules like antibodies.

cementoenamel junction Point where the cementum of the tooth root and the enamel of the tooth crown meet; 60% of the time the cementum overlaps enamel, 30% of the time the cementum and enamel meet, and 10% of the time the cementum fails to meet the enamel, creating a small gap.

centric occlusion The voluntary position of the dentition that allows the maximum contact when the teeth occlude.

cerebral palsy (CP) A nonprogressive neuromuscular disorder caused by brain abnormalities or damage. Impairments may be characterized as sensory, motor, and emotional disturbances, and include seizure disorders and cognitive disorders.

chemokines A large group of small proteins that guide white blood cells to sites where they are needed.

chemotherapy A systemic drug regimen designed to specifically kill rapidly dividing cells.

chief complaint The patient's reason for seeking dental care.

cholinergic crisis Condition that typically results from overmedication. Signs and symptoms include excess salivation, abdominal pain, vomiting, diarrhea, and respiratory distress.

chorea Quick, dancelike, uncontrollable movements of the limbs.

chronic inflammation A longer-lived inflammatory response that continues for more than a few weeks because the body is unable to resolve the infection.

chronic obstructive pulmonary disease (COPD) Progressive lung disease that obstructs airflow from the lungs, affecting approximately 6% of the population.

chronological age The number of years a person has lived; usually categorized into the following age brackets: younger old (aged 65–75 years), older-old (aged 75–85 years), and oldest old (aged 85+ years).

circadian rhythms Physical, mental, and behavioral changes that follow a roughly 24-hour cycle, responding primarily to light and darkness in an organism's environment.

civil law Pertains to a wrongful act against a person that violates his or her person (body), privacy, or property or contractual rights. Civil law is made up of two categories: tort law and contract law.

clinical attachment level (CAL) Measurement of the distance of the junctional epithelium from a fixed reference point, the cementoenamel junction. Best single measurement of tooth support.

closed-ended questions Questions that elicit a "yes" or "no" answer.

cochlear implant An electronic device consisting of an external portion behind the ear surgically attached to a second part under the skin that gives a representation of sound through a microphone and speech processor via signals sent directly to the auditory nerve of the brain.

coinfection Simultaneous development of infections.

col A concave-shaped depression in the papilla.

collagen A tough, flexible, white material that provides strength and resilience, and is a major component of all connective tissue; the most abundant protein in the body.

collimation Shaping the x-ray beam to the area that is to be imaged.

comorbidities Multiple chronic diseases.

complement A set of soluble molecules that can bind to certain molecules that are common among microbial cells.

complement cascade A process triggered when the first complement molecule, C1, encounters an antigen–antibody complex. Each of the complement proteins performs its specialized work, acting, sequentially, on the molecule next in line. The end product is a cylinder that punctures the cell membrane and, by allowing fluids and molecules to flow in and out, kills the target cell.

complement system A series of approximately 25 proteins that work to assist the work of antibodies in destroying bacteria.

complete blood cell count (CBC) Blood test to determine the number of red blood cells, white blood cells, and platelets in the body.

complete denture A removable prostheses fabricated to replace all of the teeth in a single arch or the entire dentition, as well as the adjacent tissues.

complete mouth radiographic series (CMS) A combination of periapical and bitewing radiographs, typically 18 to 20 radiographs, showing all the teeth in the oral cavity; also called a *full-mouth series* (sometimes abbreviated FMX).

composite veneer A mixture of glass filler particles and polymerizable (either self- or light-activated) resin used to correct misalignment or discoloration of teeth, and to perfect the look of teeth; also called a *direct veneer*.

computed radiography (CR) A digital imaging system that uses photostimulable phosphor (PSP) plates to capture an image that is viewed on a computer after the PSP plate is scanned.

computer-aided design/computer-aided manufacturing (CAD/CAM) Computer software that is used to both design and manufacture products.

confidentiality The ethical principle and core value that in health-care deals with nondisclosure of personal information about the patient, which could potentially cause harm.

confounders A situation in which the effect or association between an exposure and outcome is distorted by the presence of another variable. *Positive* confounding (when the observed association is biased away from the null) and *negative* confounding (when the observed association is biased toward the null) both occur.

congenital condition Present from birth.

congenital heart disease (CHD) An abnormality of the heart structure or function, or both, caused by abnormal heart development before birth.

conscious sedation Central nervous system depression such that mental and physical functions are diminished while maintaining consciousness; typically accomplished by a drug.

continuing education Training that occurs after formal education in a field of study and is designed to update the participant on new information and to reinforce previously learned concepts.

contrast The difference between two neighboring areas on the radiograph.

convalescent stage Period when the body begins to restore itself.

coronal caries A cavity, or decay, on the crown of the tooth.

coronary heart disease A narrowing of the small blood vessels that supply blood and oxygen to the heart.

C-reactive protein One of the acute-phase proteins that increase during systemic inflammation.

criminal law Pertains to crimes against society as outlined by statutory law for which the state (government) may institute criminal proceedings in a court of law.

critical thinking The process by which people analyze information, then clarify and evaluate it, and derive newly constructed knowledge about that information.

cross-contamination Indirect passage of harmful substances between patients through unsterile equipment, procedures, or products.

crown A restoration made to completely cover a tooth and improve the function and esthetics of the tooth; sometimes referred to as a cap.

curettage The removal of the soft tissue in the periodontal pocket.

Current Dental Terminology (CDT) Standardized terms and codes established by the American Dental Association for the purpose of consistency in reporting dental services and procedures to dental benefit insurance plans.

curriculum vitae (CV) Overview of the dental hygienist's education, employment history, accomplishments, professional organization memberships, skills, and community activities that is more descriptive than a résumé and is typically required for academic positions.

curve of Spee An anatomic curvature of the occlusal alignment of the teeth, beginning at the cusp tip of the mandibular canine, following the buccal cusps of the premolars and molars, and continuing to the anterior border of the ramus.

cyanosis Dark blue to purple discoloration of the skin or mucous membranes caused by inadequate oxygen in the blood.

cyclothymic disorder Condition diagnosed when a person experiences mood swings similar to but not as intense as bipolar disorder.

cystic fibrosis (CF) An inherited, lifelong disease that affects multiple organs, including the lungs, pancreas, and liver, resulting in a shortened life expectancy.

cytokines Varied and powerful chemical messengers that are secreted by the cells of the immune system and mediate the inflammatory response.

cytologic smear Technique in which tissues are wiped with a spatula and the harvested cells are smeared on a glass slide. The slide is sprayed with a fixative, then stained and examined under the microscope.

data Qualitative and quantitative information collected as a result of research.

deaf Having partial or complete lack of the sense of hearing.

definitive diagnosis Final diagnosis based on test results, such as blood tests and biopsies; a condition or patient problem that is readily identifiable.

dementia Brain disorder that results in deterioration of memory, concentration, and judgment, and may cause emotional disturbance and personality changes.

demineralization The loss of calcium and phosphate from the enamel surfaces of teeth that occurs when acid-producing *Mutans streptococci* (MS) and other cariogenic bacteria metabolize dietary fermentable carbohydrates.

demyelination Destruction of the myelin sheath.

density A property of the image receptor to block visible light. A radiograph with increased density appears blacker or darker; a radiograph with decreased density appears whiter or lighter.

dental anxiety A nonspecific ambiguous feeling of unease. It is anticipatory in nature, because there is no immediate threat and the source of the future threat is unknown.

dental decay Derived from the Latin words meaning "rottenness or decay" and is commonly used interchangeably with the terms *cavity* and *cavitation*.

dental erosion A loss of tooth structure caused by acid exposure from foods and beverages (exogenous sources) and/or gastric contents (endogenous sources).

dental fear A mental, emotional, or physical reaction to a known danger, stimulus, or an immediate threat.

dental floss Cord of thin filaments used to remove food from between teeth and dental plaque biofilm from the sides of the teeth.

dental hygiene process of care The framework to identify the causes of a condition that can be treated or prevented by the dental hygienist. It includes six steps: assessment, diagnosis, planning, implementation, evaluation, and documentation.

dental hygiene treatment plan The dental hygienist's recommended treatment and outcomes related to the established assessments and diagnosis.

dental hygienist A licensed, preventative oral health professional who provides a variety of oral health services to patients.

dental phobia Significant fear, to the degree of being excessive, irrational, and persistent in response to either the presence of the threat or stimulus or the anticipation of that threat.

dentin tubules Small channels that make up dentin and contain odontoblastic processes bathed by tissue fluids and minerals.

denture Oral prosthesis that replaces all the teeth in the dentition.

denture-induced fibrous hyperplasia See **epulis fissuratum**.

denture stomatitis Inflammation of the underlying soft tissues that occurs as a result of mechanical, chemical, thermal, bacterial, viral, and allergic stimuli.

depolarize To cause the channels in nerve cell membranes to change shape in response to a stimuli and allow the influx of sodium ions.

desensitization Gradually introducing objects or procedures to an individual so that he or she will become accustomed to them and begin to accept them.

determinants Various factors that, combined together, affect the health of individuals and communities. The determinants of health include: the social and economic environment; the physical environment; and the person's individual characteristics and behaviors.

deterministic effects Dose-dependent effects.

developmental disability Cognitive impairment, acquired or congenital. Also called *intellectual disability*.

diabetes mellitus Chronic metabolic disease caused either by the body's insufficient production of insulin or the body's inability to respond to the insulin produced.

diabetic retinopathy Damage to the blood vessels in the retina.

diastolic blood pressure Arterial pressure between heartbeats when the heart rests; normal diastolic blood pressure is less than 80 mm Hg.

dichotomous scale A scale that measures a factor that has only two variables when the variable of interest is either present or absent.

dietary adequacy Number of servings of each food group consumed.

dietary assessment Screening to determine dietary adequacy, usual eating habits, and patterns of consuming cariogenic foods and beverages.

Dietary Guidelines for Americans, 2010 Recommendations for healthy Americans and those at increased risk for chronic disease (aged ≥2 years) that emphasize daily energy balance, physical activity, a healthy body weight, nutrient-dense foods, food safety, and healthy eating patterns that meet the nutritional needs for general and specific population groups.

differential diagnosis Process of distinguishing a disease from other diseases with similar signs and symptoms.

differential gene expression Gene expression that responds to signals or triggers; a means of gene regulation.

digital impression A computer-generated image of a tooth prepared for a restoration, such as a crown, onlay, or inlay; used in CAD/CAM technology.

digital motion activation Moving the periodontal instrument by flexing three fingers: thumb, index, and middle finger.

digital radiography (DR) A digital imaging system that uses sensors and flat-panel detectors to capture images that are directly connected to a computer, providing a near-instantaneous image.

diphenhydramine Antihistamine used to treat the symptoms of allergies/allergic reactions.

diplopia Double vision.

direct access Policies that allow dental hygienists to initiate patient care, treat patients, and maintain provider–patient relationships without the authorization or supervision of a dentist.

direct restoration A soft, malleable filling material placed directly on a tooth.

direct supervision Requirement by most states for a dentist to be present when a dental hygienist is performing certain procedures. The dentist must order, control, and assume full professional responsibility for the procedure. Such procedures must be checked and approved by the supervising dentist before dismissal of the patient from the office of said dentist.

disinfectants Agents used to destroy or inhibit the growth of microorganisms.

drama triangle Group conflict involving a victim, persecutor, and rescuer.

dynamic sitting Alternating between sitting and half standing.

dysarthria Difficulty speaking.

dysgeusia Impaired sense of taste.

dysphagia Difficulty swallowing.

dysphonia Speaking or voice impairments.

dysplasia Precancerous lesion.

dyspnea Difficulty breathing.

dysthymic disorder Chronic, less intense bouts of depression.

dystonia Constant writhing, twisting, uncontrollable movement.

early childhood caries (ECC) In children younger than 6 years, the presence of one or more decayed, missing, or restored primary teeth. Also called *baby bottle decay*.

efferent nerve Motor nerve that carries information away from the central nervous system to the periphery of the body.

empirical evidence Knowledge acquired through experimentation and observation.

endocrine system A system of glands and cells that work with the nervous system (neuroendocrinology) producing hormones that are released directly into the bloodstream.

engineering controls (EC) Measures to isolate or remove bloodborne pathogen hazards from the workplace; for example, sharps container, instrument cassette, needle recapping device.

epithelial dysplasia Oral precancer.

epulis fissuratum Lesion caused by chronic trauma, most commonly from an ill-fitting denture; commonly occurs in the vestibular mucosa and clinically appears as folds of fibrous connective tissue. Also called *inflammatory fibrous hyperplasia* or *denture-induced fibrous hyperplasia*.

epulis gravidarum Single, tumor-like growths of gingival tissue that occur most frequently in an area of inflammatory gingivitis or other areas of recurrent irritation, or from trauma or any source of irritation. Also called *pregnancy granuloma*.

ergonomics the scientific study of equipment design and workspaces focused on maximizing productivity by minimizing operator fatigue and discomfort.

erythema migrans See **geographic tongue**.

erythema multiforme (EM) Skin disorder that occurs primarily in children and young adults and presents as multiple types of skin lesions. EM occurs as an allergic reaction or as a reaction to infection.

erythroplakia Term used by some clinicians to describe a suspicious red oral area that may be at increased risk for oral cancer.

ester Anesthetic that has oxygen in its molecular makeup.

ethical decision-making A method to resolve ethical dilemmas. Steps include identifying the ethical dilemma, gathering the facts, listing the options, applying ethical principles to the options, choosing the best option and implementing the decision, and evaluating the decision.

evaluation The measurement of the outcomes of dental hygiene treatment.

evidence-based care (EBC) A patient-centered approach to care that merges the best available research with clinical expertise and patient preferences.

evidence-based decision-making (EBDM) The process of locating, interpreting, and appropriately applying scientific evidence to support patient care decision-making; however, evidence alone does not replace sound clinical judgment.

evidence-based dental hygiene practice The combined use of current, relevant, scientifically sound evidence and professional clinical judgment to evaluate information to determine and provide optimal patient-centric, comprehensive oral care, with consideration for the patient's point of view.

evidence-based practice A way of providing health care that is guided by a thoughtful integration of the best available scientific knowledge with clinical expertise and patient beliefs. This type of practice reflects the interests, values, needs, and choices of the individuals served.

excisional biopsy Complete removal of the lesion for diagnosis.

exfoliative cytology Screening technique in which cells are harvested with a small brush that can penetrate to the basal cells of the epithelium, where dysplasia first develops. The slide is screened by a special computer system that is calibrated to pick up abnormal cells; then a pathologist examines the slide.

exostosis Bony outgrowth on the maxillary or mandibular alveolar ridges, which is usually asymptomatic.

explorer A flexible, thin assessment instrument using the clinician's tactile sense to evaluate tooth surfaces.

expressed consent Oral or written agreement to treatment.

external locus of control The belief that control of future outcomes resides primarily outside oneself, either with more powerful others or because of fate or chance.

external whitening Products such as whitening strips, rinses, and toothpastes that are applied to the exterior of the teeth.

extrinsic stain A stain that forms on the outer surface of enamel within biofilm and is caused by external factors; can be removed with hand instruments, ultrasonic instruments, or polishing.

exudate A collection of dead white blood cells (neutrophils) that is indicative of infection. It may be a pearly white to a pale yellow. Also called *suppuration*.

familial Passed from parent to child.

feldspar A cleaning agent that is low in abrasives and available in powder form; can be mixed with water or sodium fluoride to polish the teeth.

festination Walking with short, shuffling steps; also known as *propulsive gait*.

fibrin Substance produced during the coagulation process that helps platelets adhere to each other and the walls of the injured blood vessel.

fibroma Reactive hyperplasia of fibrous connective tissue in response to local irritation or trauma. Also called *irritation or traumatic fibroma* or *focal fibrous hyperplasia*.

fibromyalgia (FM) Disorder that causes muscle pain and fatigue. Patients typically have "tender points" that experience pain when pressure is applied to these areas. Typical tender points are the neck, shoulders, back, hips, arms, and legs.

fibrosis Thickening and hardening of the skin of the hands and face.

fiduciary A relationship between persons in which one person acts for another in a position of trust.

field cancerization A concept encompassing four general ideas: (a) abnormal tissue surrounds the tumor that may not be apparent clinically, (b) potentially cancerous cells can arise at multiple locations simultaneously, (c) oral cancer can consist of several independent lesions that can coalesce into one tumor, and (d) the incomplete removal of abnormal tissue borders after surgery may explain recurrences. Also called *cancer fields*.

file Instrument with numerous cutting edges that is used primarily to remove and break large, solid parts of calculus into smaller pieces.

filled sealants Sealants with silica and quartz particles added to increase strength and hardness.

finger spelling (American Manual Alphabet) The manual reproduction of English using the hands and fingers; often combined with sign language.

fissured tongue Fairly common condition of unknown cause that affects the dorsum of the tongue in which multiple deep fissures or grooves are present.

fixed bridge A partial denture used to replace one or multiple teeth.

flat panel detector Digital imaging sensor used for extraoral radiographs.

flavoring agents Ingredients that add flavors preferred by consumers to dentifrices.

focal fibrous hyperplasia See **fibroma**.

food debris Food that remains in the mouth after eating.

Fordyce granules Ectopic sebaceous glands that commonly occur on the labial and buccal mucosa, retromolar area, and anterior tonsillar pillar. Present in 80% of the population, they present as multiple yellowish white papules and are usually asymptomatic.

formative evaluation Ongoing process accomplished by reviewing the patient's history at each appointment during the treatment series and assessing any changes.

free gingiva Portion of the gingiva that is not attached to the tooth by gingival fibers, and forms the soft tissue wall of the gingival sulcus. Also called *unattached gingiva*.

fremitus Palpable or visual movement of a tooth when in function because of hyper or traumatic occlusion.

frequency The number of times an ultrasonic instrument tip vibrates or cycles per second (cps).

fulcrum A finger used to stabilize the hygienist's hand when performing instrumentation and assessment.

functional age How a person interacts mentally and physically with his or her surroundings; measured by the ability to perform certain activities of daily living (ADLs).

functional capacity The ability of an individual to perform basic daily activities. Adequate functional capacity is defined as the individual being able to perform activities that meet a 4 metabolic level of endurance, also known as 4 metabolic equivalents (METs).

furcation Area where the roots of a tooth separate, putting the tooth at greater risk for attachment loss and a poorer prognosis after periodontal therapy than teeth without furcation involvement.

furcation probe A type of periodontal probe used to evaluate the bone in areas of furcation on multi-rooted teeth.

gender Socially defined differences between men and women.

general supervision Procedures provided by a dental hygienist that are based on instructions given by a licensed dentist but do not require the physical presence of the supervising dentist during the performance of those procedures.

geographic tongue Benign inflammatory condition with an unknown cause, but nutritional deficiency, stress, and heredity may play a role. Most commonly involves the dorsal and lateral portions of the tongue and presents as single or multiple pink to red denuded areas of filiform papillae that are bordered by a white or yellowish rim. Also called *benign migratory glossitis, erythema migrans,* or *wandering rash of the tongue.*

germicide An agent that destroys microorganisms.

gingival crevicular fluid An inflammatory exudate that results from the increased vascular permeability of inflamed gingival tissue.

gingival embrasure The area between the teeth.

gingival epulis (pl., epulides) Generic clinical descriptive term for a focal noninfectious enlargement or lump of the gingiva.

gingival fibromatosis Uncommon diffuse enlargement of the gingiva that is not caused by local inflammation or infection. Also called *gingival hyperplasia* or *gingival overgrowth.*

gingival recession Reduction of the gingival margin to a position apical to the cementoenamel junction, exposing the root surface.

gingival sulcus The space between the free gingiva and the tooth surface into which an instrument such as a periodontal probe or curette can be inserted.

gingivitis Inflammation localized to the gingival tissue with no apical migration of the junction epithelium.

glaucoma No peripheral vision, from conditions that cause damage to the optic nerve.

glucagon Hormone secreted in response to low concentration of glucose in the blood.

glucometer A glucose meter or medical device for determining the approximate concentration of glucose in the blood.

glycocalyx Sticky extracellular matrix produced by biofilm microorganisms, which help maintain the overall integrity of the biofilm.

goal Observable and measurable end result having one or more objectives to be achieved within a specific time frame.

grading A measure of the changes in cells affected by cancer compared with similar healthy cells.

grit Particles that are found in abrasive agents; the abrasiveness of prophy pastes depends on the particle size.

guide dog A dog trained to assist a person who has a disability.

G.V. Black classification of caries Charting system that classifies caries by tooth type and location or surface with caries; also used to classify restorations and lesions.

hairy tongue Occurs when the filiform papillae become abnormally elongated and give the dorsum of the tongue a hairlike appearance.

halitosis An oral condition characterized by a noticeable malodorous smell that is emitted during breathing or speaking.

handle rolling Turning the handle of the instrument between the thumb and index finger to readapt the instrument to the surface of the next tooth.

health Defined by the World Health Organization as "a state of complete physical, mental, and social well-being and not merely the absence of disease or infirmity."

health disparities Population-specific differences in the presence of disease, health outcomes, quality of health care, and access to health-care services that exist across racial and ethnic groups.

health education Providing learning experiences designed to foster behavior conducive to health.

health promotion Defined by the World Health Organization as "the process of enabling people to increase control over their health and its determinants, and thereby improve their health."

hearing aid A device that amplifies sounds, making the sound louder so that the person can hear better.

hearing dog A dog trained to alert the profoundly deaf person to sounds such as the doorbell, telephone, or smoke alarm, leading the person to the sound source.

heart block Type of arrhythmia that is caused by the malfunction of the heart's electrical system.

heart failure A condition where the heart cannot pump enough blood to meet the body's needs under normal physiological conditions.

hemianopsia Loss of half of visual field.

hemophilia A group of inherited bleeding disorders in which the body is unable to form clotting factors, which results in spontaneous bleeding and the inability to produce clots quickly enough to stop bleeding.

hemostasis Termination of bleeding.

hepatitis Inflammation of the liver caused by a virus or nonviral means such as excessive alcohol consumption.

hertz (Hz) Unit of energy that measures cycles per second (cps).

HIV Virus that attacks CD4$^+$ helper T cells, resulting in impaired immune function.

Hodgkin disease A white blood cell disorder in which there is uncontrolled growth (neoplasm) of B lymphocytes.

hoe A large appliance with a single cutting edge created by the connection of the beveled toe and face of the razor blade.

holistic Concept that holds that all aspects of people's needs including psychological, physical, and social should be taken into account and seen as a whole.

huddle Team meeting.

human herpesvirus Eight herpes viruses for which there is no cure.

human papillomavirus (HPV) Family of more than 100 viruses, of which a few sexually transmitted types (types 16, 18, and others) have been linked to pharyngeal, tonsillar, and some oral cancers, as well as cervical and rectal cancers.

humectants Ingredients that prevent water loss from a preparation to prevent dehydration of the formulation.

humoral immunity Immune response mediated by soluble molecules such as complement and antibodies.

Huntington disease (HD) An inherited brain disorder characterized by progressive physical, cognitive, and psychological deterioration.

hydrocephalous Abnormal accumulation of cerebrospinal fluid in the ventricles of the brain that may cause enlargement of the skull and may affect as many as 90% of children with myelomeningocele.

hydrogen peroxide A whitening agent.

hydroxyapatite Also called hydroxyapatite (HA). A naturally occurring mineral form of calcium apatite with the formula $Ca5(PO4)3(OH)$, but is usually written $Ca10(PO4)6(OH)2$ to denote that the crystal unit cell comprises two entities.

hyperacusis Sensitivity to sound.

hyperinsulinism Too low a level of blood sugar.

hypertension An abnormally elevated blood pressure; systolic blood pressure of 140 mm Hg or higher and diastolic blood pressure of 90 mm Hg or higher.

hypertonic Overactive muscles, contracting when they should be at rest.

hyperventilation Deep, rapid, irregular breathing.

hypotension Abnormally low blood pressure; may be associated with fasting, rest, syncope, shock, hemorrhage, medications such as antidepressants, and systemic diseases such as Addison's disease, hypothyroidism, anemia, and heart failure.

hypotonic Decreased muscle tone.

iatrosedation A relaxed state induced by actions rather than drugs; a method of anxiety reduction that is psychologically based.

illumination Using the mirror to reflect light onto intraoral surfaces that may otherwise be dark and difficult to see.

immune complex Substance formed when an antibody binds to an antigen to target the antigen for destruction.

immunodeficiency State of missing or dysfunctional components of the immune system that leads to increased susceptibility to infection.

immunoglobulin A large, Y-shape protein produced by plasma cells that is used by the immune system to identify and neutralize pathogens such as bacteria and viruses.

immunological memory The body's ability to remember previous encounters with antigens, which enables the immune system to respond very quickly to a subsequent infection.

implant Support for a fixed bridge.

implant maintenance A protocol or a set of guidelines, designed to assist clinicians in maintaining dental implants for long term success.

implied consent Agreement to treatment communicated by the patient's actions; for example, arriving for an appointment and allowing treatment to proceed.

inactive ingredients Ingredients that help maintain the toothpaste's consistency to make it more palatable to the consumer.

incidence The number of new cases of a disease or condition over a specified period.

incisional biopsy Removal of a representative portion of the lesion for diagnosis.

index Scoring system for clinical disease; an indicator or measuring device.

indirect restoration A crown, inlay, onlay, or veneer that is customized for a precise fit in the patient's mouth and usually fabricated at a dental laboratory.

indirect vision Using a dental mirror to view an intraoral structure that cannot be seen directly.

induration Hardening of normally soft tissue caused by an invading tumor.

infective endocarditis An infection caused by bacteria that enter the bloodstream and settle in the heart lining, a heart valve, or a blood vessel.

infiltration Injection of anesthesia that affects an area close to the nerve endings.

inflammation Redness, heat, edema, and pain caused by the body's response to injury.

inflammatory fibrous hyperplasia See **epulis fissuratum**.

inflammatory papillary hyperplasia Common hyperplastic response to reactive tissue growth on the hard palate beneath the denture that may be caused by an ill-fitting denture, poor oral hygiene, and wearing a denture 24 hours a day. Also called *papillary hyperplasia of the palate* or *palatal papillomatosis*.

informed consent The patient agrees to treatment after having been informed by the practitioner of his or her health status, the risks and benefits of the treatment options available, the consequences of not receiving treatment, and all financial implications.

informed refusal The patient's decision to refuse recommended treatment or referrals; should be signed and dated, and kept in the patient's record.

inlay An indirect restoration that is precisely fitted to a cavity in a tooth and permanently cemented into place, restoring the occlusal surface without including the cusp of a posterior tooth.

innate immune response The body's immediate protection against an invading pathogen, or nonspecific immunity, the natural resistances with which a person is born.

innate immune system Defense mechanisms that people have from birth, including mechanical barriers such as skin and mucous membranes, as well as some leukocytes. Also called *nonspecific immune system.*

innate susceptibility Immune responses that are present from birth and not learned, adapted, or permanently heightened as a result of exposure to microorganisms, in contrast to the responses of T and B lymphocytes in the adaptive immune system.

in situ Cancer that has not metastasized.

insulin Hormone secreted in response to high concentrations of glucose in the blood.

intellectual disability Cognitive impairment, acquired or congenital. Also called *developmental disability.*

intention tremors Trembling during voluntary movement.

interconceptual Between pregnancies.

interdental brushes Specially designed brushes with small nylon filaments twisted onto a stainless-steel wire that are used to access and clean the col area.

interleukin Any of several lymphokines that promote macrophages and killer T cells and B cells and other components of the immune system.

internal locus of control The belief that control of future outcomes resides primarily within oneself.

internal whitening Placement of a whitening agent inside a tooth.

International Federation of Dental Hygienists (IFDH) A professional organization that serves to unite dental hygiene associations from around the world with the common cause of promoting dental health.

International Normalized Ratio (INR) Test that measures the body's ability to clot and compares it with an average. The higher the INR, the longer it takes blood to clot.

International Standards Organization (ISO) designation system System that uses a two-digit code to label the teeth. The first number in the two-digit code indicates the quadrant, and the second indicates the specific tooth in the quadrant. The digits 1 through 4 depict the four permanent quadrants starting with the maxillary right, then maxillary left, mandibular left, and mandibular right. A second digit is used to identify the tooth number beginning at the midline and sequentially numbering the teeth with number 1 for the central incisor to number 8 for the third molar. The numbers 5, 6, 7, and 8 depict the four primary quadrants.

intervention A treatment that at least one group of participants in a research study receives, whereas another group receives a placebo, or standard of care.

intrinsic endogenous stain Staining that occurs during tooth development and is incorporated into the structure of the tooth.

intrinsic exogenous stain Staining that occurs within the tooth because of changes from outside sources, including smoking and use of smokeless tobacco products, such as chewing tobacco, dissolvable tobacco, and snuff.

intrinsic stain Discoloration of teeth from within; a stain that forms on the inner surface of enamel and cannot be removed with hand instruments, ultrasonic instruments, or polishing.

in vitro **research** An experimental study conducted without human participants; used primarily to evaluate safety, toxicity, and potential therapeutic effects.

ionizing radiation Electromagnetic radiation that produces ions as it travels through matter; x-ray.

iontophoresis A physical process in which ions flow diffusively in a medium driven by an applied electric field.

ipecac syrup Agent that induces vomiting.

irreversible index An index that measures factors that cannot be changed; for example, a dental caries index called DMFT or DMFS.

irritation fibroma See **fibroma**.

ischemia Local loss of blood supply.

ischemic heart disease Insufficient blood flow to the heart.

isotonic Having the same osmotic pressure as another solution.

junctional epithelium Tissue attachment that lies at the base of the gingival sulcus.

justice The fair treatment of individuals; equitable allocation of health-care dollars and resources.

justification Principle of prescribing radiographs based on clinical findings, not on the basis of routine or a predetermined time interval.

laser An instrument that produces a very narrow, intense beam of light energy. When laser light comes in contact with tissue, it causes a reaction. Lasers are used in dentistry to perform a variety of soft and hard tissue procedures. There are different lasers for different procedures, some used for surgery, some to cure restorative materials and enhance tooth bleaching, and others to remove tooth structure for elimination of disease and restoration.

latent image An image that is created on either analog x-ray film or digital imaging (PSP plates and sensors) that is not visible to the naked eye until it is processed either via chemical (analog x-ray film) or by a computer (PSP plates and sensors).

latent period The time from when the infectious agent enters the body until the first symptoms emerge; incubation stage.

lateral cephalometric skull radiograph Radiograph that shows the anterior portion of the patient's head from a lateral view; frequently made in orthodontics to evaluate the position of the jaws in relation to each other and the skull base.

lavage Feature on an ultrasonic scaler used to adjust the flow of water from the tip.

lead apron A flexible shield placed over the thorax and pelvis of a patient with lead or lead equivalent thickness to block x-rays from exposing this area of the patient.

leeway space The spacing that dentists preserve during the mixed dentition period to allow for adequate space for the permanent dentition to erupt.

legal blindness Visual acuity of 20/200.

leukemia Cancer of the white blood cells in bone marrow and the circulating blood.

leukoedema Asymptomatic condition that is caused by a harmless accumulation of glycogen in the surface cells and affects non-whites, particularly African Americans, more often than other populations. Clinically appears bilaterally on the buccal mucosa as a grayish white opalescence that disappears when stretched.

leukoplakia Term used by some clinicians to describe a suspicious white oral area that may be at increased risk for oral cancer.

levels of evidence A means of evaluating the quality of a research study. Levels of evidence range from 1 to 6, with level 1 being the highest level of evidence.

lichen planus (LP) Condition that presents as a rash on the skin or painful oral lesions; it typically affects middle-aged adults.

lifelong learning Self-directed, active learning that takes place over the course of a lifetime, beyond secondary, undergraduate, and graduate education. It includes formal education, self-study, and experiential learning.

linea alba Condition commonly found bilaterally on the buccal mucosa along the line of occlusion. Clinically appears as a thickened white line in response to friction.

lipopolysaccharide (LPS) Large molecule consisting of a lipid and a polysaccharide joined by a covalent bond; it is found in the outer membrane of Gram-negative bacteria, acts as an endotoxin, and elicits strong immune responses in animals.

lipoxins Lipids that encourage the resolution of inflammation by limiting the migration of additional polymorphonuclear leucocytes (PMNs) into the site of inflammation, activating noninflammatory monocytes, and stimulating the removal of dead PMNs by macrophages.

lip reading Recognizing spoken words by watching a person's lips, face, and gestures.

literature review A comprehensive, preliminary investigation into existing scientific literature to determine the course of research on a topic, or whether further research is actually required.

local anesthesia Absence of sensation in a small area of the body.

locus of control An individual's beliefs about what factors determine his or her rewards or outcomes in life.

lower motor neurons Spinal nerves that branch out from the spinal cord to the other parts of the body.

lumen An opening or hollow space.

luxation Dislocation of a tooth in its socket.

macular degeneration Condition that affects the center of visual field.

magnetostrictive ultrasonic scaler Type of scaler that has an elliptical, or figure-eight, motion.

magnification loupes Lenses used to improve visual perception.

maintenance Ongoing treatment that occurs either after active therapy or as a routine prophylaxis.

major depressive disorder An acute occurrence of depression in which sufferers exhibit symptoms severe enough to limit everyday normal functioning.

major histocompatibility complex (MHC) Nucleated cell markers that signal "self," communicating that certain cells are part of the body.

malar Red butterfly rash commonly found on the face of patients with systemic lupus erythematosus.

malocclusion A misalignment problem that may lead to serious oral health complications.

mandibular torus (pl., tori) See **torus mandibularis**.

manual polishing A technique performed by using a porte polisher, which uses an orangewood tip attached to a contra-angle.

manual toothbrush The oral self-care device used by most people to remove plaque biofilm.

materia alba A loosely attached accumulation of bacteria that can be easily removed by mechanical actions such as vigorous rinsing or a strong spray of water. The color is generally white to yellow, and it is thick and cottage cheese–like in texture.

matrix metalloproteinases (MMPs) Substances secreted during the inflammatory process that increase collagen breakdown, and activate cytokines and chemokines.

mean score A statistic used for descriptively analyzing data that are at least interval scaled; computed by adding each score in the distribution and dividing by the number of scores.

measurable outcomes Results of dental hygiene care that can be quantified—for example, probing, plaque control, bleeding points, and retention of sealants.

medical model Approach to care that supports prevention of dental diseases and, if present, early and minimally invasive treatment.

meninges The tissues covering the spinal cord.

menopause The stage when menstruation ceases, typically between ages 45 and 55 years.

mental disorder A clinically significant behavioral or psychological syndrome or pattern that occurs in an individual and is associated with present distress or disability or with a significantly increased risk for suffering death, pain, disability, or an important loss of freedom.

meta-analyses Analyses to determine whether the volume of evidence supports an association between diseases.

metabolic equivalents A unit of measurement that represents the amount of oxygen consumption needed for physical activity; used to evaluate physical status.

metabolic syndrome Cluster of conditions that includes high blood pressure and blood sugar levels, abnormal cholesterol levels, and excess body fat around the waist; it is an early indicator of increased diabetes risk.

metastasis A distinct form of cancerous spread that occurs when malignant cells enter blood or lymphatic vessels and travel to distant sites.

microorganism An organism too small to be viewed by the unaided eye, as bacteria, protozoa, and some fungi and algae.

microstomia Abnormal smallness of the mouth.

mission statement Written declaration of the practice's main purpose.

mobile dental clinic A self-contained dental operatory with all equipment necessary for delivery of dental treatment.

modifiable risk factor Behavior that can be changed.

modified Widman flap A type of periodontal surgery used to gain access to the deeper periodontal structures using a flap reflected from the root and alveolar surfaces. It is indicated in active pockets over 4mm deep that are not responding to initial treatment; pockets beyond the muco-gingival line with bone loss; or pockets with marginal deformity.

Mohs scale of hardness A scale comparing the hardness value of ingredients found in prophy pastes and air-polishing powders compared with enamel, dentin, and cementum.

mood disorder Disturbance in a person's mood or emotional state beyond what is considered normal, everyday variation.

motion activation Movements of the instrument to create a stroke on the surface of the tooth.

motivational interviewing "A collaborative, person-centered form of guiding to elicit and strengthen motivation for change."

motor neurons Nerve cells that control the muscles.

mucogingival junction Junction of attached gingiva and alveolar mucosa, delineated by a distinct color change.

mucositis Inflammation of the mucous membrane lining the digestive tract from the mouth to the anus.

multidisciplinary team (MDT) A group of professionals from different health-care disciplines working together to direct and coordinate a cancer patient's care.

multiple sclerosis (MS) A chronic, inflammatory, autoimmune disease that results in demyelination in the central nervous system.

muscular dystrophies (MD) Group of more than 30 genetic diseases characterized by progressive weakness and degeneration of the skeletal muscles that control movement.

musculoskeletal disorders (MSD) Conditions that develop over time from the chronic use of repetitive, forceful, and awkward movements or postures at work or at home.

myasthenia gravis (MG) Autoimmune disorder of neuromuscular transmission characterized by varying degrees of weakness of voluntary muscles that is usually progressive.

myasthenic crisis The need for respiratory assistance because of muscle weakness. Signs include the inability to swallow, speak, or maintain an open airway, double vision, tachycardia, and profound muscle weakness.

myelinated A-delta fibers Sensory nerve fibers that are found on the pulpal side of the dentin tubules and elicit a well-localized, sharp pain considered responsible for dentin hypersensitivity.

myelomeningocele See spina bifida.

myocardial infarction A condition caused by lack of adequate blood flow to the cardiac tissue leading to cell and tissue death of the affected areas of the heart muscle; commonly referred to as a heart attack.

nadir The lowest point. When used in reference to chemotherapy, it describes the point when blood cell counts are at their lowest after a chemotherapy treatment.

National Dental Hygienists' Association (NDHA) A professional organization dedicated to increasing the number of minority dental hygienists, assisting in the access to oral care for underserved communities, and promoting the highest educational and ethical standards for dental hygienists.

negative aspiration After creating negative pressure within the cartridge, no blood is drawn into the cartridge.

nerve block Anesthetic injection that is deposited near a nerve trunk or nerve plexus.

neurological impairments Disorders of the nervous system.

nonionizing radiation Radiation that does not cause ionization of cells.

nonmaleficence Do no harm.

nonmodifiable risk factor Personal attributes or genetics that cannot be changed.

non-nutritive habits Behaviors such as thumb/digit sucking, use of pacifiers, tongue thrusting, bruxism, fingernail biting, and intraoral/perioral piercings that can affect the positioning of the primary and permanent dentition.

nonverbal communication The body language of the speaker, including facial expressions, posture, use of hand gestures, body movements, and even the type of handshake given.

nosocomial pneumonia Pneumonia acquired in a hospital or other health-care setting such as a nursing home. Also known as hospital-acquired pneumonia or health-care–associated pneumonia.

nutrient imbalance Disproportion in the amount of energy and nutrients an individual obtains from his or her diet.

nutritional counseling The process of providing education regarding diet and oral health, assisting individuals in assessing dietary and oral health risks, and collaborating with the individuals to facilitate positive change.

occlusal radiograph An intraoral radiograph that shows an entire tooth similar to a periapical radiograph but with different angles, giving a distorted image of the tooth.

odds ratio The odds of a person having a disease if they are exposed to a risk factor compared with having the disease if they are not exposed to that same factor.

onlay An indirect restoration that is precisely fitted to a cavity in a tooth, covers a cusp(s), and is permanently cemented into place.

open-ended dialogue Questions designed to encourage individuals to give a thoughtful response sharing information and feelings.

open flap debridement A periodontal procedure in which the supporting alveolar bone and root surfaces of teeth are exposed by cutting the gingiva to provide increased access for scaling and root planing.

opportunistic infections Infections caused by microorganisms that are only capable of producing disease because of the impairment of the immune system.

optimization Principle that seeks to maximize diagnostic yield and minimize patient exposure. The decision to use ionizing radiation for diagnostic purposes is made only after careful consideration of the patient's dental and general health needs as revealed by medical and dental histories and a clinical examination.

oral and maxillofacial pathology The specialty of dentistry that deals with the cause, pathogenesis, identification, and management of diseases that affect the oral and maxillofacial regions.

oral irrigator Interdental cleaning aid that uses pulsating lavage and a variable pressure setting to clean the interproximal area.

oral squamous cell carcinoma (OSCC) Squamous cell carcinoma is a histologically distinct form of cancer deriving from epithelium. It arises from mutated ectodermal or endodermal cells lining body cavities. OSCC occurs in the squamous cell epithelium that covers the oral cavity, lips, and throat. It originates from the oral keratinocytes where DNA mutations can be spontaneous, and carcinogens from tobacco and alcohol increase the mutation rate.

ordinal scale A scale characterized by rank ordering.

orthopnea Difficulty breathing in a supine position.

orthostatic hypotension A form of low blood pressure that occurs when there is a sudden change from the horizontal position to the upright position or by prolonged standing, resulting in syncope.

osseointegration The direct biological attachment of living bone to a titanium implant surface without any intervening soft tissue.

osteonecrosis Bone tissue death.

osteopenia Bone density that is lower than normal peak density but not low enough to be classified as osteoporosis.

osteoplasty Removal of nonsupporting bone to improve bone morphology.

osteoporosis Disease characterized by a thinning and weakening of the bones resulting in bone fractures of the hip, wrist, and spine.

osteoradionecrosis (ORN) Nonhealing, dead bone that is a complication of radiation therapy and results from functional and structural bony changes that may not be expressed for months or even years.

osteotomy Removal of supporting bone.

overdenture A type of complete denture that is supported by retained natural roots or dental implants rather than the alveolar ridge.

overhead Costs of doing business including salaries, payroll deductions and benefits, practice marketing and promotion, equipment, building/rent, dental supplies, office supplies, repair and maintenance of equipment and/or building, utilities, business insurance, postage, taxes, continuing education, dues/licenses, and professional fees such as accounting and legal services.

over-the-counter (OTC) whitening Products such as toothpastes and whitening strips that can be purchased to whiten the teeth without a prescription; their main ingredient is hydrogen peroxide in a weakened concentration.

palatal torus (pl., tori) See **torus palatinus**.

palliative Care that provides relief without curing.

Palmer notation A system in which a right-angle symbol (⌋) designates each quadrant. The permanent teeth are then numbered sequentially starting at the midline with #1 and moving posterior to #8. The tooth number is placed in the right-angle symbol. Letters beginning with A are used in the symbol to identify primary teeth.

pantomograph Extraoral radiograph made with the source of radiation and image receptor moving around the patient's head creating a focal trough around the jaws, and showing the entire maxilla and mandible and surrounding structures superiorly to the orbits and inferiorly to the hyoid.

papilla The portion of the gingival tissue that fills the interproximal space between the adjacent teeth. Also called *interdental gingiva*.

parafunctional habits Behaviors exhibited by a patient that include bruxism, nail biting, ice chewing, and excessive picking at restorations.

paralysis No sensation and no voluntary movement.

paraplegia Paralysis of the lower limbs.

paresis Partial or slight paralysis.

paresthesia Sensation of numbness, tingling, or sharp, prickling pain that can signal compression of a nerve.

Parkinson disease (PD) Progressive neurological disorder caused by a reduction in the brain cells that produce the chemical dopamine, which plays a major role in muscle control; characterized by involuntary muscle movements and tremors of the head, arms, and legs, which cause fine motor skill, balance, and gait problems.

paroxysmal pain syndromes Short-duration, intense, electric, or shocklike pains that occur at a high frequency.

partial participation A technique that nurtures the desire of children aged 2 to 5 years to assert control over a situation by involving them as helpers during the dental hygiene appointment.

partial thromboplastin time (PTT) Test that measures the body's ability to clot; involves adding a reagent to the patient's skin at the time of testing. Normal range is 25 to 40 seconds; severe bleeding problems are indicated when readings are more than 50 seconds.

passive immunity Acquired through transfer of antibodies or activated T cells from an immune host; is transient, lasting only a few months.

passive immunization Temporary immunity passed from mother to child through the placenta or by delivering antibodies to the body through an injection.

patent ductus arteriosus A congenital heart defect in which the ductus arteriosus blood vessel, which connects the pulmonary artery to the descending aorta, does not close after birth.

paternalism Telling a person what to do like a father manages a child.

pathogenic Disease producing.

pathophysiology The study of the functional changes associated with diseases.

patient advocacy Any activity that ultimately benefits a patient. Using that definition, it can apply to caregiving for an individual patient, to groups that develop policies and advice that help patients, or to government groups that develop legislation to improve systems or processes for patients.

pedagogy Teacher-centered learning. Teachers are the experts; they tell students what and how to learn, and are the evaluators of that learning.

pellicle formation The preconditioning stage that defines reversible–irreversible attachment of the colonizing bacteria on the tooth surface.

people-first language Describing a person with a health impairment or disability first as a person followed by the diagnosis; for example, person with a hearing impairment.

periapical radiograph An intraoral radiograph that shows an entire tooth on a single image.

peri-implantitis An inflammatory reaction of the soft and hard tissues with subsequent loss of supporting bone surrounding an implant.

peri-implant mucositis The reversible, inflammatory reaction in the soft tissues surrounding an implant.

periodontal debridement Removal of plaque biofilm and calculus that have accumulated on the teeth to maintain oral health.

periodontal disease A group of diseases characterized by bacterial infection of the periodontium including the gingiva, periodontal ligament, bone, and cementum.

periodontal healing After nonsurgical periodontal therapy, healing occurs as repair of existing tissues rather than regeneration of tissues lost in the disease process.

periodontal maintenance (PM) Treatment that includes site-specific scaling and root planing in areas that have shown disease progression, signs of inflammation, or both.

periodontal medicine Refers to the role of systemic factors on periodontal disease (PD), and the association of PD with chronic diseases of aging such as diabetes and cardiovascular disease (CVD).

periodontal probe An assessment instrument calibrated with millimeter markings used to evaluate the health of the periodontium.

periodontal risk assessment The process of identifying factors that may increase the onset, severity, and/or progression of periodontal disease.

Periodontal Screening and Recording (PSR) Tool used to identify the need for a comprehensive periodontal assessment.

periodontal surgery Surgical treatments that aim to reduce pocket depth and/or restore gingival contour to a state that can be maintained free of inflammation by the patient.

periodontitis Inflammation of the structures of the periodontium marked by apical migration of the junctional epithelium.

periodontium The functional system of hard and soft tissues comprised of the gingiva, cementum, periodontal ligament, and alveolar bone that surround and attach teeth to the bone and provide support, protection, and nourishment to the teeth.

perioscopy A nonsurgical procedure performed with a fiberoptic endoscope connected to a color high-definition monitor to diagnose and treat dental and periodontal diseases.

peripheral giant cell granuloma Uncommon, but not rare, cause of focal gingival enlargement. The cause is unknown, but it may represent a reaction to irritants trapped within the sulcus. Lesions are purple dome-shaped nodules on the gingiva, usually anterior to the molars, and are usually less than 1 cm in size.

peripheral ossifying fibroma (POF) Uncommon, but not rare, cause of focal gingival enlargement that occurs only on the gingiva. The cause is unknown, but it may represent a reaction to irritants trapped within the sulcus. The POF is most common in the anterior maxillary arch and colors range from red to pink, or ulcerated from trauma.

permucosal seal The soft tissue interface formed with the implant fixture and abutment; also called the *biologic.*

personal protective equipment (PPE) Attire worn to prevent disease transmission; consists of protective clothing, protective eyewear, mask, and appropriate gloves for the procedure being performed. Face shields, bouffant surgical caps, and surgical shoe covers are optional.

pH A numeric scale used to specify the acidity or alkalinity of an aqueous solution.

phagocytes Cells that protect the body by ingesting (phagocytosing) harmful foreign particles, bacteria, and dead or dying cells.

pharmacokinetics A drug's action as it moves through the body.

photophobia Sensitivity to light.

photopolymerization The process by which sealants are polymerized by visible light. A curing light is used to harden the sealant once it has been placed into pits and fissures.

photostimulable phosphor (PSP) plate Plate made of "europium-doped" barium fluorohalide, which absorbs and stores energy when exposed by x-rays, creating a latent image.

physical disability Any impairment to physical activity.

PICO Acronym used to remember how to form a well-defined question: Recognize the **P**atient's condition, consider the **I**ntervention, use a **C**omparison intervention if relevant, acknowledge possible **O**utcome.

piezoelectric ultrasonic scaler Type of scaler that generates a linear motion.

pivoting A joint swinging movement of the arm and hand conducted by balancing on the fulcrum finger.

plasmapheresis A method of treating the blood plasma to remove the acetylcholine receptor antibodies from the plasma to decrease the autoimmune response.

pleurisy Inflammation of the pleura, characterized by a dry cough and pain on the affected side.

polishing A technique used to remove extrinsic stains that cannot be removed with hand or ultrasonic instruments from enamel surfaces or before sealant placement.

polymerization A chemical reaction in which monomers are linked to create a polymer. Refers to hardening of dental sealants.

polymorphonuclear neutrophil (PNM) Granular leukocyte (or white blood cell) that moves to a cell, adheres to immune complexes, and engulfs microorganisms, and so on, with phagocytes. These, in turn, eat the microorganisms, along with other foreign particles.

pontic An oral prosthesis designed to replace a single missing tooth.

porcelain veneer Thin pieces of porcelain used to recreate the natural look of teeth while also providing strength and resilience comparable with natural tooth enamel; also called an *indirect veneer*.

portable unit A lightweight, self-contained system with a compressor for providing dental care that requires little space and can be configured to fit most spaces.

positive aspiration After creating negative pressure within the cartridge, blood is drawn into the cartridge.

post–cardiovascular surgery The interim following surgery on the heart or large vessels that bring blood to and from the heart.

power polishing A technique performed by using a slow-speed handpiece, disposable prophy angle or prophy brush, and prophy paste.

power toothbrush Battery-operated toothbrush available with a variety of brush heads and bristle designs, and oscillating and high-velocity sonic brushing action to simplify the brushing process.

preconceptual Before pregnancy.

preferred provider organization (PPO) Contract between a dental benefits provider (insurance company) and the provider of dental care (dentist and, in some states, public health dental hygienists) that in return for the referral of dental patients, the dentist will provide procedures at a reduced rate.

pregnancy tumor Cases of pyogenic granuloma that appear to be influenced by high hormone levels such as at puberty or during pregnancy. See **pyogenic granuloma**.

presbycusis Age-related hearing loss, progresses over many years and usually affects hearing high-frequency sounds.

presbyopia A condition that makes it difficult to see things at close range.

preservatives Ingredients that preserve the dentifrice and prevent bacterial growth.

prevalence The number of cases of a disease or condition per population at risk at a particular point in time.

primary prevention Disease prevention measures such as vaccinations that aim to stop diseases from occurring.

primary research Studies related to human beings that may be observational or involve trials to evaluate the efficacy of a particular intervention. Also known as clinical or basic research.

primate spacing Spacing between the maxillary lateral and canine and the mandibular canine and first molar that is essential to allow the larger permanent teeth to erupt without difficulty.

probe depth Depth of the gingival sulcus determined by the distance from the edge of the free gingival margin to the junctional epithelium using a calibrated periodontal probe.

prodromal stage The period when general symptoms such as fever, nausea, and headache occur. This stage is communicable.

professional whitening Methods that contain a higher concentration of whitening agents than over-the-counter products and are available only with a prescription.

prognosis A prediction for whether the patient's disease will heal.

prophylaxis Preventive care, including removal of plaque, stain, and calculus to prevent irritation of the tissues and prevent the initiation of periodontal disease.

prophy paste Abrasive paste that is used during manual or power polishing to remove extrinsic stain from the enamel surface.

prosthesis Artificial replacement of a missing body part.

protective oral appliance Device worn to reduce/prevent injury to the oral cavity.

protective stabilization The restriction of a patient's movements to decrease the risk for injury to the patient and dental hygienist, and allow for safe completion of treatment.

prothrombin time (PT) Test that measures the body's ability to clot. Normal range for clotting to occur using this test is between 11 and 16 seconds.

proxemics The study of set measurable distances between people as they interact.

psychosocial disability Inappropriate behaviors with social interrelations.

ptosis Drooping eyelids.

puberty Developmental stage when an individual is capable of reproduction, typically between ages 11 and 14 years in girls and 13 and 16 years in boys.

public health The science of protecting and improving the health of families and communities through promotion of healthy lifestyles, research for disease and injury prevention, and detection and control of infectious diseases.

pulse The rate at which the heart beats.

pyogenic granuloma Uncommon, but not rare, blood vessel proliferation in response to local irritation, trauma, or poor oral hygiene. See **pregnancy tumor**.

quadriplegia Paralysis of all four limbs.

quality assurance Systematic monitoring of services provided to ensure that standards of care are being met.

radiation caries Tooth decay of the cervical regions, incisal edges, and cusp tips secondary to xerostomia induced by radiation therapy to the head and neck.

radiograph The resultant image after a patient or object is exposed to x-rays.

radiolucent Areas that appear dark or black on the radiograph; also used to describe any part of the patient that allows the transmission of x-rays to the image receptor.

radiopaque Areas that appear light or white on the radiograph; also used to describe any part of the patient that blocks the transmission of x-rays.

randomization A study control method by which researchers assign participants in a trial to either an experimental or a control group by chance. Randomization is not a haphazard assignment; it is performed using a carefully planned strategy.

randomized controlled trial A carefully planned study in which at least one group of participants receives some sort of intervention, or treatment, while the other group receives a placebo, or standard of care.

Raynaud phenomenon An intensified reaction to cold or anxiety that elicits discoloration and numbness in the fingers, toes, ears, and nose. Fingers will characteristically become white and then blue, because of spasm of the vasculature and the resulting diminished blood supply.

reactive conditions Conditions that result from the reaction of tissues to mechanical trauma, heat, medications, or other environmental factors.

recrudescence Becoming reactivated after a period of inactivity.

recurrent caries Decay at a site where caries has previously occurred. It may be due to numerous factors, which may include inadequate removal of the initial decay, usually beneath a restoration, poor oral hygiene, or other factors.

reference citation A numbered or annotated section of text within a manuscript that refers to, or cites, the source of information and corresponds to the author(s) published (or unpublished) work listed in the references.

referral Recommendation of a patient to another health-care provider for treatment.

reflective listening A two-way feedback loop of communication wherein the listener restates what the speaker has communicated.

refractory Indicates disease that is relatively nonresponsive to repeated conventional treatment.

regenerative techniques Incorporate surgical technique, biological concepts, and biomaterial enhancement to promote regeneration of periodontal tissues.

registered dental hygienist The credential earned by graduates of accredited dental hygiene education programs in colleges and universities.

Registered Dental Hygienist in Alternative Practice (RDHAP) License category created by the California state legislature to deliver dental hygiene care in settings outside a dental office such as residential facilities, schools, and areas where there is a shortage of dental care providers.

regurgitation The incomplete closure of the valve leading to backflow of blood through the valve.

relative contraindication Drug may be administered after weighing the risks.

relative risk The probability of developing a disease if the person is exposed to the risk factor compared with a person who is not exposed to that same risk factor.

relaxation response Process by which the heart and respiratory rates decrease, blood pressure is lowered, and muscle tension decreases following the stress response.

reliability The extent to which a method or a measurement repeatedly and consistently produces the same outcome or results, performed under identical conditions.

remineralization The natural repair process where calcium and phosphate ions use fluoride as a catalyst to rebuild the crystalline structure histologically in the subsurface lesion.

removable partial denture An oral prosthesis that replaces multiple, but not all, teeth in an arch.

rescue breathing Breaths provided by a rescuer in an emergency situation when respirations are absent or inadequate.

resolvins Anti-inflammatory lipids.

respiration Inhalation and exhalation of air.

résumé Brief overview of the dental hygienist's educational credentials, employment history, accomplishments, professional organization memberships, skills, and community activities.

retraction Using the head of the mirror to hold the patient's cheek, lip, or tongue out of the working area or field of vision.

reversible index An index that measures damage or factors that can be reversed or changed; for example, plaque, gingivitis, and bleeding.

rheumatic heart disease A systemic inflammatory condition that demonstrates cardiac manifestations and is caused by group A β-hemolytic streptococci.

rheumatoid arthritis (RA) An autoimmune disease that results in pain, swelling, and loss of function in the joints.

risk The probability that loss, harm, or injury will occur if nothing is changed.

risk assessment The evaluation of the qualitative and quantitative information gained during the assessment and screening process.

risk factor A behavior or attribute that has a direct causal effect on the onset and/or progression of the disease.

risk indicator Similar to a risk factor except it does not meet the criteria of evidence; it is biologically plausible, but research has shown only an association with the disease.

risk marker A factor that has not demonstrated a causal or biological relationship with oral disease through research but has been associated with the disease when looking at populations or data over a long period.

root caries Refers to decay of the root surface of a tooth.

Russell periodontal index is a measure of the extent of periodontal disease in an individual that considers the amount of bone loss around the teeth and the degree of gingival inflammation. It is used frequently in the epidemiologic investigation of periodontal disease.

saliva Fluid that is produced by the parotid, submandibular, and sublingual glands, and is an important factor in the caries process.

salivary diagnostics The use of saliva to look for indicators of health conditions or diseases.

scaling and root planing (SRP) Instrumentation of the crown and root surfaces of the teeth with hand, sonic, or ultrasonic instrumentation to remove plaque biofilm, calculus, and stains.

schizophrenia A group of disorders characterized by disturbed or distorted perceptions of reality, odd physical behaviors or speech, and random, illogical thinking. Frequently those suffering from schizophrenic disorders are delusional or have hallucinations.

scleroderma (SC) A debilitating disease of the connective tissue with no known cause, although it is suspected to be autoimmune in nature. In patients with SC, excessive amounts of collagen are produced and deposited into the connective tissue, producing a hard appearance of the skin.

scoliosis Abnormal curvature of the spine.

scope of practice Rules and regulations defining what services dental hygienists can provide.

sealant A resin material that is placed into the pits and fissures of teeth at risk for caries.

secondary caries Also known as recurrent caries. Decayed areas that appear at a location with a previous history of caries.

secondary prevention Measures such as clinical screening and self-examinations done to facilitate early detection and treatment of diseases to prevent further progression.

secondary research Literature reviews and meta-analyses.

selective polishing Polishing of specific teeth that present with only extrinsic stains; used to reduce damage to the enamel, cementum, and dentin.

self-care disability Inability to care for self independently.

self-directed learning Self-initiated, self-managed, self-motivated learning, with independent goal-setting and decision-making as to what is worthwhile and applicable. Teachers are more like coaches, or mentors, and peers are fellow collaborators.

self-efficacy The ability to take charge and make decisions.

self-etching Any sealant that eliminates the steps of phosphoric acid etching and rinsing.

senescence The aging process.

sensitivity The ability of the index or test to correctly identify those patients with the disease.

sensor Component of digital imaging system made of silicon crystals; the crystal bonds are broken when exposed to x-rays, creating a latent image on the sensor.

sensory disability Any disability relating to a sensory organ such as sight and sound.

seroconversion The development of antibodies.

service animal Any animal trained to assist a person who has a disability.

sex Biological differences between male and female individuals.

sickle cell anemia An inherited disorder in which the body makes red blood cells that are crescent shaped rather than the normal disc shape; found mostly in black individuals and those of Mediterranean origin.

Sievert SI unit that refers to dose equivalent.

simplified portable unit A system that uses available resources and an ultrasonic scaler along with a cordless handpiece and basic dental hygiene instrument setup to deliver care to patients who cannot travel to the dental office.

sinus bradycardia A slow heart rate of less than 60 beats/min.

Sjögren syndrome (SS) Autoimmune disease that affects the salivary and lacrimal glands. Immune cells (primarily T cells) attack the glands, causing tissue destruction, which impairs the patient's ability to produce saliva and tears.

SMART(ER) goals Acronym for goals that are Specific, Motivational, Attainable, Relevant, Timely, Evaluate, Reevaluate.

smear layer A thin layer of organic debris that develops on the tooth surface after procedures such as root planing or cutting with a dental bur, covers the tubules, and provides relief from dentin sensitivity.

societal trust The shared expectation that people will manifest sensible and reciprocally beneficial behavior in their interactions with others.

sodium perborate A whitening agent.

somnolence Severe drowsiness.

sonic scaler Device that is connected to the dental unit's compressed air valve and activated by the unit's foot control.

spasticity Feelings of stiffness and a wide range of involuntary muscle spasms (sustained muscle contractions or sudden movements). One of the more common symptoms of conditions such as multiple sclerosis (MS).

spatter Biologic contaminants that are greater than 50 μm in diameter and may be visible.

special needs A term used in clinical diagnostic and functional development to describe individuals who require assistance for disabilities that may be medical, mental, or psychological. The *Diagnostic and Statistical Manual of Mental Disorders* and the *International Classification of Diseases* 9th edition both give guidelines for clinical diagnosis.

speckled leukoplakia Mixture of red and white areas in leukoplakia.

spina bifida (SB) Birth defect in which the backbone and spinal canal do not close before birth. It is a neural tube defect in which the bones of the spine do not completely form, resulting in an incomplete spinal canal. This causes the spinal cord and meninges, the tissues covering the spinal cord, to stick out of the child's back. Also called *myelomeningocele*.

spinal cord injury (SCI) Damage that usually begins with a sudden, traumatic blow to the spine that fractures or dislocates vertebrae.

spinal muscular atrophy (SMA) Hereditary disease characterized by progressive hypotonia and muscular weakness.

squamous cell carcinoma Oral cancer.

staging Procedure that determines how large a cancer is and whether it has spread to other parts of the body.

standard precautions Steps introduced in 1996 by the Centers for Disease Control and Prevention to protect workers and patients; include pathogens that can spread by blood or any other body fluid, excretion, or secretion. Standard precautions apply to: (a) contact with blood; (b) all body fluids, secretions, and excretions excluding sweat; (c) nonintact skin; and (d) mucous membranes.

statistical significance The level of probability that an association between two or more variables occurred by chance alone; expressed as *p* value, which refers to the level of significance.

stenosis The incomplete opening of the valve.

sterilization The destruction or removal of all forms of life, specifically microorganisms, from materials or objects. Methods of sterilization used in dental offices are moist heat (steam under pressure), dry heat, and chemical vapor.

stochastic effects All-or-nothing effects, for example, radiation-induced damage, such as cancer, either will or will not occur because of ionizing radiation exposure.

stress response The physical, emotional, psychological, and behavioral response to a particular situation or stressor.

stroke A cerebrovascular disorder resulting from disruption of the blood supply to the brain leading to neurological impairments of the central nervous system.

subgingival biofilm Biofilm located within the periodontal pocket or sulcus.

subgingival (serumal) calculus Calculus that forms apical to the gingival margin. It is usually dark to black, because of the blood pigment, hemosiderin. It is not visible through an oral examination but is often seen with a radiographic examination.

substantivity The ability to remain on the skin after rinsing and drying to inhibit the growth of bacteria.

summative evaluation Results process made by comparing initial assessments with assessments taken at the evaluation appointment.

superinfection An infection that develops when another infection is present; for example, hepatitis D can only replicate itself if hepatitis B is present.

supervised neglect Regularly examining a patient who shows signs of disease but not informing the patient of the disease's presence or progress.

suppuration A collection of dead white blood cells (neutrophils) that is indicative of infection. It may be a pearly white to a pale yellow. Also called *exudate*.

supragingival biofilm Biofilm that accumulates on the clinical crown.

supragingival (salivary) calculus Calculus located above the gingival margin. It appears creamy white to yellow and changes color as it is exposed to foods and tobacco products.

surfactants Surface-active agents that add foaming characteristics, reduce surface tension, and suspend plaque and debris in an emulsion for easier removal during mechanical cleaning.

surgical model Treatment that ends when teeth are restored.

systematic search A strategized tactic for locating answers to clinical and other questions by mining scientific and biomedical databases.

systemic lupus erythematosus (SLE) Autoimmune disease in which there is inflammation and damage to various tissues in the body.

Systemized Nomenclature of Dentistry (SNODENT) Vocabulary designed for use in the electronic dental record environment to provide standardized terms for describing dental disease, to capture clinical detail and patient characteristics, to permit analysis of patient care services and outcomes, and will be interoperable with electronic health records and electronic dental records.

systolic blood pressure Arterial pressure when the heart muscle contracts and forces blood into the circulation; normal systolic blood pressure is less than 120 mm Hg.

tachyarrhythmia A fast, irregular pulse rate caused by a cardiovascular instability.

tachycardia An unusually rapid heart rate, more than 100 beats/min in adults.

tachypnea Rapid breathing.

tactile finger spelling Tactile sign language combined with American Sign Language.

tactile sign language (TSL) Using a method called *print on palm*, the person communicating with the deaf-blind person prints large block letters on the deaf-blind person's palm. Each letter is written in the same location on the palm.

telecommunications device for the deaf (TDD) Device that provides relay services with a three-way call to an operator who serves as the communicator to the deaf person.

teletypewriter (TTY) Device that sends text messages by telephone using a keyboard and visual display and/or printer.

tendency Occurs when the mesial cusp of the maxillary first molar is either mesial or distal to the central groove of the mandibular molar by less than the width of a premolar.

tertiary prevention Measures taken with chronic diseases or after advanced disease states in which rehabilitation is necessary to regain optimal health.

therapeutic polishing Polishing done with a prophy paste that includes ingredients added for remineralization and to reduce hypersensitivity.

thickening agents Ingredients that stabilize dentifrice formulations and prevent separation of liquid and solid phases.

thrombocytopenia Platelet count less than 150,000 cells/mm.

thrombogenic Causing or resulting in coagulation of the blood.

thrombus Final product of the blood coagulation step.

thymectomy Surgical removal of the thymus.

thyroid collar A flexible shield with lead or lead equivalency that covers the neck, specifically the thyroid, blocking x-rays from exposing this area.

tidal volume The amount or volume of air/gas in the lungs obtained from normal inspiration and released on normal expiration.

tinnitus The perception of sound or ringing in the ears or head when no external source is present. The sound may be continuous or intermittent, vary in pitch, and occur in one ear or both.

tissue autofluorescence Technology that makes abnormal tissues appear black in contrast with the green-tinged fluorescence of normal tissues under that particular wavelength of light.

tissue reflectance Technology that causes abnormal tissues to reflect extra light so that they appear more intensely white.

titanium Elementary substance combined with traces of aluminum and vanadium to form an alloy that is compatible with human tissues and used in dental implants.

titer The concentration of a substance in a solution.

titration The act of administering a drug in increments over time until the desired endpoint is reached.

toluidine blue dye Dye that has an affinity for nucleic acids, which are more plentiful in actively dividing cells, including dysplastic and cancerous cells.

Tomes fiber Odontoblastic process in the dentin tubules.

tooth mobility Movement of a tooth that is greater than normal physiologic movement.

torus mandibularis (pl. tori) Common bony outgrowth found bilaterally on the lingual aspect of the mandibular alveolar bone, most often in the premolar area.

torus palatinus (pl. tori) Bony nodular growth present on the midline of hard palate.

transillumination Directing light off the mirror and through the anterior teeth to create light passing through the tooth. Used to view calculus deposits, decay, and restorations on anterior teeth.

traumatic brain injury (TBI) A form of acquired brain injury that occurs when a sudden trauma causes damage to the brain.

traumatic fibroma See **fibroma**.

treatment plan Delineates the treatment interventions that the dental hygienist and the patient will implement.

trigger points Hyperirritable spots in the fascia surrounding skeletal muscle. Trigger points are discrete, focal, hyperirritable spots located in a taut band of skeletal muscle. They produce pain locally and in a referred pattern and often accompany chronic musculoskeletal disorders.

trismus A prolonged spasm of the muscles of the jaw.

tuberculosis (TB) Primarily an infection of the lungs caused by *Mycobacterium tuberculosis*; can also infect the oral cavity, lymph nodes, kidneys, and bone; may be contracted when a person inhales contaminated droplets from an infected person who coughs, sneezes, breathes heavily, or sings.

tumor A mass of tissue formed by abnormal cells.

tumor board Multidisciplinary group of health-care providers that collaborates to determine patient care; can include oral and general surgeons, radiologists, dentists, oral and general pathologists, speech pathologists, pharmacologists, social workers, and others.

two-way communication The verbal and nonverbal exchange of thoughts and information between individuals; the primary mode of communication for dental hygienists in the professional setting.

ultrasonic cleaner A device that transmits high-energy and high-frequency vibrations to a fluid-filled container to dislodge particles from immersed objects.

ultrasonic scaler Device that has its own electronic generator and a foot pedal attached to the unit.

unfilled sealants Sealants that have less strength and hardness but usually do not require occlusal adjustment because occlusal forces will wear away any areas of the sealant that are high.

universal instruments Instruments, often with complex shanks, that are used in all areas of the mouth.

universal numbering system Uses the numbers 1 to 16 for the maxillary arch beginning with the maxillary right third molar and ending with the maxillary left third molar. Continues with the mandibular left third molar, #17, and ends with the mandibular right third molar, #32. The primary dentition is identified using letters of the alphabet. An A is assigned to the maxillary right second molar and lettering continues sequentially around the upper arch to J, the second molar of the maxillary left quadrant. The letter K is the second molar of the mandibular left quadrant, and lettering continues sequentially around the lower arch to T, the second molar of the mandibular right quadrant.

universal precautions Steps taken by health-care workers to protect workers and patients based on the concept that all blood and body fluids are contagious.

upper motor neurons Nerves that lie within the spinal cord.

urticaria Outbreak of red, itchy patches on the skin, commonly referred to as hives.

usual, customary, and reasonable (UCR) fee plan System used by preferred provider organizations and other insurance companies to determine fees based on the fee the dentist most often charges for a given procedure, the fee determined by the insurance provider from actual submitted fees for specific procedures, and the fee determined by the insurance benefit provider for a particular procedure that requires a modification or special consideration by the insurance company or provider.

vaccination The administration of antigenic material (a vaccine) to stimulate an individual's immune system to develop adaptive immunity to a pathogen.

validity The extent to which a study or index measures what it is intended to measure.

vasoconstrictor A nerve or drug that causes a decrease in the diameter of the lumen of a blood vessel.

vasodilator Agent that causes dilation of the blood vessels.

ventricular fibrillation Uncoordinated contraction of the ventricle cardiac muscle.

ventricular septal defect An opening in the septum between the ventricles that allows oxygenated blood to flow from the left ventricle into the right ventricle.

ventricular tachycardia Three or more consecutive depolarizations occurring greater than 100 beats per minute.

ventriculoatrial shunt Port placed in patients with hydrocephalus to allow cerebrospinal fluid to flow from the cerebral ventricular system to the cardiac atrium.

ventriculoperitoneal shunt Port placed in patients with hydrocephalus to remove excess cerebrospinal fluid from the brain's ventricles into the peritoneal cavity of the abdomen.

veracity The ethical principle and core value related to honesty.

verbal communication Written and oral communication between individuals.

vertebra Rings of bone that surround the spinal cord.

vision Stated aims and goals of a business.

vital tissue staining technology Uses toluidine blue dye to visualize proliferating cells; does not distinguish between cells that are proliferating because of normal healing responses and those that are precancerous or cancerous.

von Willebrand disease The most common inherited bleeding disorder caused by a lack of glycoprotein Ib, which reduces the body's ability to clot.

wandering rash of the tongue See **geographic tongue**.

warfarin A prescription drug with anticoagulating properties.

wellness Defined by the National Wellness Institute as "an active process through which people become aware of and make choices toward a more successful existence."

wellness model Health-care strategy focused on guiding patients toward risk reduction and disease prevention.

Wickham striae Lesions characterized by a network of lines, which are lacy in appearance.

woodstick A triangular-shaped device traditionally made of soft wood such as balsa, bass, or birch used for interdental cleaning.

work practice controls (WPC) Measures to reduce the risk for exposure by changing the way that a task is performed; for example, recapping a needle using the one-handed scoop technique.

wrist motion activation The rotating movement of the hand and wrist as one unit that allows the hygienist to apply additional power for the instrumentation stroke.

xerophthalmia Dry eyes.

xerostomia Dryness of the mouth.

x-ray Electromagnetic radiation that produces ions as it travels through matter; referred to ionizing radiation.

REFERENCES

1. Welch MR, Rivera RE, Conway BP, Yonkoski J, Lupon PM, Glancola, R. Determinants and consequences of social trust. *Social Inquiry*. 2005;75(4):453-473.
2. Rollnick S, Miller W, Butler C. *Motivational Interviewing in Health Care: Helping Patients Change Behavior*. New York: The Guilford Press; 2008:210.
3. Hall ET. *The Hidden Dimension*. Garden City, NY: Doubleday; 1966.

Photo and Illustration Credits for Part Openers and Chapter Openers

Chapter 2: © iStock / Thinkstock
Chapter 3: © Stockbyte / Thinkstock
Chapter 4: © Bratila Andrei / iStock / Thinkstock
Chapter 5: © Bota Finna Zsolti / iStock / Thinkstock
Chapter 6: © kasto80 / iStock / Thinkstock
Part III: © DTKUTOO / iStock / Thinkstock
Chapter 12: © Chalabala / iStock / Thinkstock
Chapter 13: © Lighthaunter / iStock / Thinkstock
Chapter 14: © Creatas Images / Creatas / Thinkstock
Chapter 16: © Glayan / iStock / Thinkstock
Chapter 17: © Katarzyna Bialasiewicz / iStock / Thinkstock
Chapter 18: © Creatas Images / Creatas / Thinkstock
Chapter 20: © Chalabala / iStock / Thinkstock
Chapter 21: © Ade Hughes / Hemera / Thinkstock
Chapter 23: © bgbs / iStock / Thinkstock
Chapter 28: © Jan Mika / iStock / Thinkstock
Chapter 29: © Ocskaymark / iStock / Thinkstock
Chapter 31: © goce / iStock / Thinkstock
Part VIII: © Creatas Images / Creatas / Thinkstock
Chapter 34: © Creatas Images / Creatas / Thinkstock

Chapter 35: © Ryan McVay / DigitalVision / Thinkstock
Part IX: © andresrimaging / iStock / Thinkstock
Chapter 36: © DenKuvaiev / iStock / Thinkstock
Chapter 37: © Sergey Nivens / iStock / Thinkstock
Chapter 38: © Sebastian Kaulitzki / Hemera / Thinkstock
Chapter 39: © humonia / iStock / Thinkstock
Chapter 40: © melnichuk_ira / iStock / Thinkstock
Chapter 41: © stockdevil / iStock / Thinkstock
Chapter 42: © MEHMETTAYLAN / iStock / Thinkstock
Chapter 43: © mtmphoto / iStock / Thinkstock
Chapter 44: © Ingram Publishing / Thinkstock
Chapter 45: © prudkov / iStock / Thinkstock
Chapter 47: © Fotovika / iStock / Thinkstock
Chapter 48: © Catherine Yeulet / iStock / Thinkstock
Chapter 50: © Olaf Bender / iStock / Thinkstock
Part X: © Braden Gunem / iStock / Thinkstock
Part XI: © shansekala / iStock / Thinkstock
Chapter 52: © Hightower_NRW / iStock / Thinkstock
Chapter 53: © Creatas Images / Creatas / Thinkstock
Chapter 54: © Michael Jung / iStock / Thinkstock

Index

A

A-beta fibers, 449–450
A-delta fibers, 449–450
Abdominal exercises, 400
Abfraction, 223, 223f
Abrasion, 223, 223f, 461
Abrasive agents, for polishing, 461–462
Absence seizure, 814t
Absolute contraindication, 542
Absorption, of local anesthetics, 530–531
Abutments
    biofilm retention on, 380
    dental implant, 385
    fixed bridge, 379
    for overdentures, 386
Accounts receivable, 825–826
Accreditation, 587, 846
Acetylcholine receptors, 676
Acetylsalicylic acid. See Aspirin
Achieving a Better Life Experience (ABLE)
        Act, 774t
Achlorhydria, 755
Acid etch, 366, 369
Acid–base balance, 531
Acidogenic bacteria, 346
Acidulated phosphate fluoride (APF), 479
Acquired immunity, 56, 56f
Acquired pellicle, 231
Acromegaly, 667–668
Actinic cheilitis, 173, 173f
Actinomyces viscosus, 231
Action plan, for emergencies, 806, 807t
Active immunity, 56
Active immunization, 87
Active ingredients
    in dentifrices, 335–336, 339t–340t
    in mouthrinses, 337, 339t–340t
Activities of daily living (ADL), 751
Acute adrenal insufficiency, 682
Acute inflammation, 58–59, 198, 198f
Acute myocardial infarction, 602
Adaptive/acquired immune response, 56
Adaptive immune system, 674
Addison disease, 681–682
Addisonian crisis, 682
Adenoids, 55, 56f
Adenoma, 667
Adhesives, 456
Administrators, dental hygienists as, 5
Adolescence, 726t, 738
Adolescents. See also Children
    dental trauma risks in, 739
    health promotion and prevention in, 47–48
    peer pressure on, 48
    smoking in, 49, 293
    tobacco use by, 739
Adrenal cortex, 664–665
Adrenal crisis, 810t
Adrenal gland
    anatomy of, 664–665
    diseases of, 669
Adrenal insufficiency (AI), 681–682
Adrenal medulla, 665
Adrenocortical insufficiency, 667
Adrenocorticotropic hormone (ACTH), 665,
        667, 669

Adrenocorticotropin, 669, 682
Advanced dental hygiene practitioner
        (ADHP), 791
Advanced dental therapist (ADT), 16, 847
Advanced education, 846–847
Advanced glycation end products, 62
Advocacy, 549, 796
Advocates, dental hygienists as, 5, 796
Aerosols, 85, 612
Affordable Care Act, 42, 775
Age
    biological, 753–754
    chronological, 753
    dentin hypersensitivity and, 451
    functional, 754
    periodontal disease risks based on, 297
Age-related macular degeneration, 623t
Agencies
    infection control, 93–94
    rulemaking authority of, 10
Aggregatibacter actinomycetemcomitans, 61
Aggrenox, 697t
Aging. See also Elderly
    brain changes, 755
    cardiovascular system changes, 754
    chronic conditions secondary to, 751
    definition of, 753–754
    endocrine system changes, 755
    gastrointestinal system changes, 755
    hearing declines secondary to, 756
    immune system changes, 755–756
    integumentary system changes, 756–757
    musculoskeletal system changes, 756
    nervous system changes, 755
    normal changes associated with, 758t
    physical disabilities secondary to, 751
    physiological, 754–757
    respiratory system changes, 754–755
    sensory system changes, 756
    taste sensation affected by, 765
AIDS. See also HIV
    description of, 86
    Kaposi sarcoma associated with,
        90, 683f
    occupational exposure to, 703
Air polishing, 468f, 468t, 468–471, 573
Airway
    assessment of, 805t
    obstruction of, 806t, 810t
Akinesia, 655
ALARA principle, 182, 255
Alcohol
    abuse of, 639t, 639–640, 641t
    anticoagulants and, 657
    cancer risks, 709b
    in mouthrinses, 337, 479, 639
    oral squamous cell carcinoma risks,
        172, 297
Aldosterone, 665, 682
Alkaline peroxide, 381t
All-ceramic crown, 476
Allergic reactions
    to local anesthetics, 542, 813t
    management of, 810t
Alpha-blockers, 744
5-Alpha-reductase inhibitors, 744

Alternative current impedance
        spectroscopy, 353
Alternative practice
    allowable duties in, 798
    backpack, 794
    case study of, 792–793
    definition of, 791
    dental charting in, 798
    dental practice acts applicability in, 799
    description of, 847
    flying hygienists, 794–795
    freestanding building, 793–794
    hospitals, 796–797
    institutions, 798
    intermediate care facilities, 795
    mobile dental clinics, 791–792
    portable units, 792
    prisons, 798
    private homes, 797
    schools, 797
    simplified portable units, 792
    skilled nursing facilities, 795
    street outreach, 797–798
    workplace, 798
Aluminum trihydroxide, 469
Alveolar bone
    anatomical abnormalities of, 451b
    anatomy of, 191f, 193–194
    osteoporosis effects on loss of, 295
    resorption of, 202
    stimulation of, 390
Alveolar bone proper, 193
Alveolar crest fibers, 194t
Alveolar process, 184t
Alveolar ridge
    chronic inflammation of, 379
    palpation of, 182, 182f
Alveoli, 193, 611, 612f, 754
Alveologingival fibers, 192t
Alzheimer disease
    definition of, 757
    description of, 751
    early/mild stage of, 758–759, 759t
    epidemiology of, 757
    etiology of, 757
    genetic factors, 757
    incidence of, 757
    late/severe stage of, 758, 759t, 760
    middle/moderate stage of, 758–760, 759t
    patient education about, 761t
    prevalence of, 757
    risk factors for, 757
    signs and symptoms of, 758–759
    stages of, 758–760, 759t
Amalgam
    dental charting symbols for, 219t, 221
    intrinsic stains caused by, 235
Ambivalence, 31–32
American Academy of Dental Hygiene
        (AADH), 848
American Academy of Pediatric Dentistry
        (AAPD)
    anticipatory guidance as defined by, 724
    dental home concept of, 47, 724
    early childhood caries as defined by, 351
    perinatal oral health guidelines, 742

American Academy of Periodontology
(AAP), 59, 296, 440, 557, 573, 826
American Conference of Governmental
Industrial Hygienists (ACGIH), 521
American Dental Association (ADA)
caries risk assessment questionnaires,
249–250, 296
contact information for, 94t
Council on Scientific Affairs, 807
electronic databases of, 75t
function of, 94
Give Kids A Smile program, 723
health history form of, 123
oral health during pregnancy, 741
pediatric dentistry as defined by, 723
radiograph prescription guidelines,
264, 265t
Seal of Acceptance program, 339
tuberculosis recommendations of, 91
American Dental Education Association
(ADEA), 59, 848–849
American Dental Hygienists' Association
(ADHA)
*Applied Standards of Clinical Dental Hygiene
Practice*, 305
code of ethics of, 13b, 14t, 16, 233, 849
continuing education
recommendations, 848
Governmental Affairs section of, 11
history of, 5
job interview recommendations from,
838, 839b
job search resources, 836, 837t
National Research Agenda, 846
oral health practitioner as defined by, 235
Public Health and Advocacy Forums, 708
self-study opportunities, 849
Standards for Clinical Dental Hygiene Practice,
4, 11, 123, 298, 305, 308, 549,
554, 848
tobacco cessation promotion by, 139
American Diabetes Association, 63
American Heart Association (AHA), 148
American Lung Association (ALA), 612
American National Standards Institute
(ANSI)
analog film physical sizes, 260, 262t
contact information for, 94t
description of, 93
protective eyewear standards of, 95
American Recovery and Reinvestment Act
(ARRA), 826
American Sign Language (ASL),
628–629, 629
American Society of Anesthesiologists (ASA)
physical status classification system,
804, 804t
risk classification system of, 123, 148, 149t
Americans with Disabilities Act, 10, 582, 584,
621–622, 625, 629–630, 774t, 775
Amides, 527, 530, 530t, 542
Amifostine, 711t
Amorphous calcium phosphate (ACP),
349–350, 456, 574
Ampicillin, 601t
Amyotrophic lateral sclerosis (ALS),
649–650
Analgesia, 514
Analog x-ray film, 259, 261t–262t,
261–262, 262f

Anaphylaxis, 810t, 813t
Andragogy, 843
Androgens, 665
Anemia
aplastic, 700
definition of, 698
iron-deficiency, 699
pernicious, 699
sickle cell, 700
Anesthesia
infiltration, 527, 527f
local. *See* Local anesthesia
nerve block. *See* Nerve block anesthesia
topical, 533t, 533–534, 573
Angina pectoris, 132t–133t, 601–602, 602t,
760t, 810t
Angioedema, 810t
Angiotensin-converting enzyme
inhibitors, 603t
Angiotensin receptor blockers, 603t
Angle classification, of malocclusion, 224
Angular cheilitis, 272t, 699, 765
Angulation, 421
Ankyloglossia, 168–169
Anorexia nervosa, 638–639, 639t
Anterior crossbite, 225, 225f
Anterior crowding, 219t
Anterior midline, 179, 179f, 183t
Anterior sickle scalers, 423, 423f
Anterior superior alveolar nerve (ASA)
anatomy of, 528–529
anesthetic block of, 538–539, 543t
Anterior teeth
complex shanks for, 418
universal curets for, 425, 425b
Anterior version pelvic position, 396–397
Anteverted pelvis, 398
Antiarrhythmic agents, 596t
Antibiotics
in myasthenia gravis, 677t
prophylactic use of
for cardiac conditions, 148, 600, 605b
guidelines for, 686, 695
indications for, 745t
Plavix and, 694
systemic, for periodontal infections,
437, 439
vitamin K production affected by, 696
Anticholinergics, 786t
Anticipatory guidance
in adults, 740
in children, 724, 730t–731t
Anticoagulants, 605, 656. *See also* Blood-
thinning drugs
Antigen
definition of, 56, 673
hepatitis B surface antigen, 88
Antigen-presenting cells, 674
Antigen–antibody complexes, 56
Antigingivitis agents, 336–337, 340t
Antihypertensive medications, 599t
Antileukotrienes, 615t
Antimicrobial agents, 336–337, 434–435,
574, 574t
Antirejection medications, for organ
transplantation, 686
Antiseizure medications, 786t
Antitartar agents, 336, 339t
Anxiety. *See* Dental anxiety
Anxiolytic, 514

Aphasia, 656
Aplastic anemia, 700
Apoptosis, 675
Appendix, 55, 56f
Appointment(s). *See also* Maintenance
appointment; Scheduling of patients
for children, 729–733
confirming of, 831
for elderly, 752
for infants, 47
in physically impaired patients, 777,
778t–780t, 780–782
reserved, 829
value of, communication used to create,
32–33
Area-specific explorer, 160t
Arestin, 435, 435t, 574t
Aripiprazole, 642t
Arrhythmias, 133t, 596, 596t
Arthritis, 132t, 751, 760t
Articaine, 532t
Artificial joints, 132t
Artificially acquired immunity, 56
Aspartate aminotransferase, 205
Aspiration pneumonia, 63, 759
Aspirin, 693–694
Assessment
definition of, 155
dental anxiety, 495–496, 498
dental fear, 495–496, 498
in dental hygiene process of care, 4, 46–47
evaluation of data from, 554–555
risk-based. *See* Risk assessment
technological advances in, 162
Assessment, Diagnosis, Planning,
Implementation, Evaluation, and
Documentation (ADPIED), 549,
550t–553t, 561
Assessment instruments
community setting use of, 158
definition of, 155
explorer, 157–158, 158f, 159t–160t, 160f
furcation probe, 160–163, 161f–162f, 163t
mouth mirror, 155f–157f, 155–157
periodontal probe, 160–162, 161f
summary of, 163
Assessment stroke, 421, 422t
Assessment surveys, 496
Asthenia, 653
Asthma, 133t, 614, 614f, 614t–615t, 616b
Asthma attack, 615–616, 811t
Asymmetric tonic neck reflex, 779t
Ataxic palsy, 651–652
Atherogenesis, 595
Atheroma, 63, 595
Atherosclerosis, 597–598, 602
Atherosclerotic cardiovascular diseases
(ACVD), 60
Athetoid palsy, 651–652
Atorvastatin, 598t
Atria, 593, 593f
Atrial fibrillation, 596t, 596–597
Atrial septal defect, 603, 604f
Atridox, 435, 435t, 574t
Attached gingiva, 193, 203, 203f
Attachment loss
calculus as risk factor for progression
of, 570
peri-implantitis as, 573
smoking as cause of, 292–293

Attitudinal barrier, 775
Attrition, 223, 223f
Auditory system, 627
Auricular regions, 178, 178f, 183t
Autism spectrum disorders (ASD), 635–636, 637t, 641t–643t
Autoantibodies, 755
Autoclave, 105f
Autoclaving
    description of, 105, 105f
    of mouth mirrors, 156–157
    of power scaling instruments, 413
Autofluorescence, 183t, 184
Autoimmune diseases, 674, 755–756
Autoinoculation, 109
Automated external defibrillator (AED), 805, 806t
Automated instruments, 401
Autonomy
    definition of, 12, 42
    example of, 14t
    by health-care provider, 13
    informed consent and, 12
    in motivational interviewing, 31, 31f
    treatment refusal as form of, 13
Autopolymerized sealants, 365
Autosomal recessive hereditary disease, 785
Avulsed tooth, 814t
Azithromycin, 601t

B

B cells
    development of, 674
    in periodontitis, 60
Baby boomers, 751
Baby bottle decay, 726–727
Baccalaureate degree, 846
Background radiation dose, 263
Backpack, 794
Bacteremia, 61, 148, 594
Bacteria
    acidogenic, 346
    caries caused by, 346
    cariogenic, 346–347, 351
    in oral cavity, 593
    oral disease risks and, 294
Bacterial endocarditis, subacute, 594
Bacterial meningitis, 92t
Barrett's esophagus, 739
Barrier film, 101
Barrier-free design, 775
Basal lamina, 191
Basic erosive wear examination (BEWE), 452
Basic life support, for emergencies, 805, 805t–806t
Basic research, 74–75
Bass brushing method, 322, 322f, 323t
Battery, 313
Beaver tail tips, for power scaling devices, 412, 412f
Behavior modification, 569
Behavioral change models
    learning ladder, 44, 44f
    locus of control, 44–45
    Maslow's hierarchy of needs, 44, 44f
    social cognitive theory, 45
    social learning theory, 45
    theory of reasoned action/planned behavior, 45

Behavioral management, of special-needs patients, 586
Bell palsy, 650–651
Beneficence
    definition of, 14t
    example of, 14t
    nonmaleficence versus, 15
Benign migratory glossitis, 169
Benign prostatic hyperplasia (BPH), 744
Benson, Herbert, 501
Benzocaine, 533t
Benzoyl-DL-arginine-naphthylamide (BANA), 205
Benzydamine hydrochloride, 711t
Best practice, 71
Beta blockers, 531, 531t, 601, 603t
Betel nut products, 172, 236, 236t
Beyond a reasonable doubt standard, 11
Bezafibrate, 598t
Bias, 74
Bidigital palpation, 177, 177f, 181
Bilateral palpation, 177, 177f
Bimanual palpation, 177, 177f, 180
Binging, 638
Bioburden, 104
Biofeedback, 505
Biofilm
    on abutment teeth, 380
    bacteria that cause, 231, 434
    body's response to, 235
    cellular communication of, 232
    characteristics of, 434
    control of, 231
    definition of, 231, 409
    description of, 102
    formation of, 231–232, 434, 434f
    gingivitis and, 232
    glycocalyx in, 232
    ideal areas for, 294
    inflammation secondary to, 235
    microbiology of, 232
    oral disease risks and, 294
    plaque, 57
    power scaling for removal of, 377, 378f
    in special-needs patients, 585
    subgingival, 231f, 232, 434, 595
    supragingival, 231f, 232
    ultrasonic scaling for removal of, 377, 378f
Biographical data, in health history, 127, 129
Biohazard, 521
Biological age, 753–754
Biological indicators, for sterilization monitoring, 105, 105f
Biological marker, 649
Biological seal, 203
Biological sex, 737
Biomedical database, 75, 75t
Biopsy
    definition of, 169
    excisional, 169, 185–186, 186f
    incisional, 185, 555
    pathology report from, 187
    punch, 186
    sample preservation, 186, 186f
    specimen examination, 187
    submitting of, 186–187
    types of, 185–186
Biotransformation, 530
Bipolar disorder, 636–637, 642t–643t
Bisphenol A, 371

Bisphenol A-glycidyl methacrylate, 365
Bisphosphonate-related osteonecrosis of the jaw (BRONJ), 295, 716–717, 742–743, 761t, 763
Bitewing radiographs, 256–257, 257f, 352, 357t–358t, 568
Black line stain, 236t
Bladed tips, for power scaling devices, 411
Bleeding
    evaluation of, 558
    flossing to reduce, 324
    oral disease risks and, 294
    on probing, 196t, 200, 200f, 209t, 390, 570, 570f
Bleeding disorders, 136t, 697–698
Bleeding index, 247
Bleeding time, 692, 692t
Bleomycin sulfate, 514
Blinding, 74
Blindness, 621–622
Blood
    disposal of, 108
    oxygen levels in, 613, 613f
Blood clot, 691, 692f
Blood pressure
    classification of, 599, 599t
    definition of, 144
    diastolic, 144
    measurement of, 144–147, 599–600, 667
    systolic, 144
Blood pressure cuff, 145–147
Blood-thinning drugs
    antibiotics effect on, 696
    aspirin, 693–694
    description of, 693
    herbal medications interfering with, 697
    miscellaneous types of, 697t
    Plavix, 694, 697t
    statins effect on, 696–697
    warfarin, 695–696
Blood transfusion, 136t
Blood vessels
    anatomy of, 594f, 598f
    atherosclerosis of, 597–598, 598t
    as lymphoid organ, 55, 56f
Bloodborne pathogens
    engineering controls for, 94–95
    exposure control plan for, 112
    work practice controls for, 94–95
Body fluids, 108
Body language, 26
Body mass index (BMI), 140, 141t
Body temperature, 142
Bone
    alveolar. See Alveolar bone
    dental implant and, interface between, 386–387
    postmenopausal loss of, 742–743
Bone grafting, 387
Bone marrow
    as lymphoid organ, 55, 56f
    platelet formation in, 691
Brachial artery, for pulse assessment, 146
Bradycardia, 596
Bradykinesia, 655
Braille, 622, 627, 631
Brain, 755
Brånemark, Per-Ingvar, 384
Brännström hydrodynamic theory, 450, 450f, 482
Breach of contract, 313

Breastfeeding, 741–742
Bright Futures, 47
Bronchitis, chronic, 616b
Bronchodilators, 614t, 616
Brown stain, 236t
Brush
    interdental, 325–326, 327f
    toothbrush. See Toothbrushes
Brushing
    of teeth. See Toothbrushes
    of tongue, 322, 323f
Bruxism, 778t
Buccal mucosa
    bimanual palpation of, 177, 177f, 180
    inspection of, 180, 180f
    palpation of, 177, 177f, 180, 180f, 184t
Buccal nerve
    anatomy of, 529
    anesthetic block of, 541, 541f, 544t
Buccoversion, 227
Buffer, 347
Bulbar muscles, 654
Bulbar weakness, 676
Bulimia nervosa, 638–639, 639t
Bulla, 176t
Bupivacaine, 532t
Burns, 811t

C
C1, 56
C-fibers, 449
C-reactive protein (CRP), 57, 61–62, 595
Calcitonin, 664
Calcium carbonate, 469
Calcium channel blockers, 601
Calcium peroxide, 481
Calcium phosphate, 357t–358t
Calcium phosphate rinse, 711t
Calcium phosphate technology, for dentin
        hypersensitivity, 453t, 454
Calcium phosphosilicate, 469
Calcium sodium phosphosilicate (CSP), 350
Calculus
    attachment loss progression and, 570
    body's response to, 235
    definition of, 233
    on dental implants, 388, 388f
    dentifrice and mouthrinse active
        ingredients for reduction in, 339t
    detection of, 233–234
    formation of, 233
    forms of, 233
    indices of, 204, 246–247, 247t
    location of, 233
    periodontal disease risks, 233
    as plaque biofilm, 204, 231
    radiographic appearance of, 259t
    removal of
        description of, 235
        instrument angulation for, 421
        instrumentation strokes for,
            422–423, 423f
        sickle scalers, 422–423, 423f
        universal curets, 424, 424b
    subgingival, 231f, 232–233
    supragingival, 231f, 232–233, 338, 388,
        568f, 570
    Volpe-Manhold Index of, 241, 244t, 246
Calculus ledges, 233, 233t
Calculus rings, 233, 233t

Calculus spicules, 233, 233t
Calibration, 241
California Dental Association, 64
California Dental Hygienists'
        Association, 649
Calorie needs, 279, 279t–280t
Canadian Dental Hygienists' Association,
        13b, 14t, 16
Canadian Oral Health Strategy, 15
Cancellations, 829–830
Cancellous bone
    description of, 194
    radiographic appearance of, 259t
Cancer. See also Oral cancer; Oral squamous
        cell carcinoma (OSCC)
    in African Americans, 708
    chemotherapy-associated complications
        description of, 701, 709–710
        infections, 711–712
        oral mucositis, 710t–712t, 710–711, 711
        prevalence of, 709
    definition of, 707
    incidence of, 708
    information resources for survivors
        of, 716b
    multidisciplinary team approach to,
        707, 718
    prostate, 744
    race and, 708
    risk factors for, 708, 709b
    skin, 756
    smoking as risk factor for, 709b, 715
    staging of, 707, 708t
    thyroid, 668
    TNM staging of, 708t
    tongue, 713, 713f
    treatment of
        chemotherapy, 709–712
        cytoreductive therapy, 710
        oral care before, 745
        oral complications of, 701, 709–710,
            716–718
        oral evaluation before, 712, 712b
        planning strategies for, 718
        radiation therapy, 709, 716–718
Candida albicans, 171, 383, 711–712, 765
Candidiasis, oral, 615, 711–712, 765
Canines, 726t–727t
Cannabis abuse, 639t, 640
Carbamazepine, 642t
Carbamide peroxide, 481, 484
Carbohydrates
    fermentable, 273, 346, 348
    refined, 347
Cardiac arrest, 811t
Cardiac glycosides, 603t
Cardiogenic shock, 597
Cardiologist, 560t
Cardiopulmonary resuscitation (CPR), 805,
        805t–806t
Cardiovascular disease (CVD)
    angina pectoris, 601–602, 602t
    anticoagulant therapy, 605
    arrhythmias, 596, 596t
    atherosclerosis, 597–598, 602
    atrial fibrillation, 596t, 596–597
    atrial septal defect, 603, 604f
    bradycardia, 596
    congenital heart disease, 603–604
    deaths caused by, 592–593
    definition of, 592

description of, 55
    in elderly, 760t–761t, 763
    environmental factors, 595
    exacerbation of, 595
    heart, 592–593, 593f
    heart block, 597
    heart failure, 603, 603t
    hypertension. See Hypertension
    infective endocarditis, 148, 600
    inflammatory mediators and, 61
    inflammatory products in, 594, 595f
    ischemic heart disease, 601–602
    myocardial infarction, 602
    overview of, 591–592
    patent ductus arteriosus, 603–604, 604f
    periodontal disease and, 60–61, 594–595
    premature ventricular contractions, 597
    prevalence of, 592
    rheumatic heart disease, 600–601
    risk assessment of, 122
    risk factors for, 592, 592f
    sudden cardiac death, 602
    tachycardia, 596, 596t
    valvular heart disease, 604–605
    ventricular fibrillation, 596t, 597
    ventricular septal defect, 603, 604f
    ventricular tachycardia, 596t, 597
Cardiovascular surgery, 591, 605–606
Cardiovascular system
    age-related changes of, 754
    health history review of, 132t–133t
Cardiovascular training, 401
Career development, 838–839. See also
        Employment
Career planning, 839
Caregiver, 583t, 584, 586
Caries
    alternative current impedance
        spectroscopy for, 353
    bacteria that cause, 346
    Caries-Risk Assessment Tool, 249
    case study of, 359
    causes of, 346–348, 556f, 746
    cavity caused by, 345
    in children, 297
    classification of, 350–352
    coronal, 350–351
    definition of, 345, 726
    demineralization caused by, 346–348, 350
    dental charting symbols for, 219t
    detection of, 227–228, 352–353
    determinants–confounders model of,
        346, 347f
    dietary counseling for individuals at risk
        for, 348
    dietary factors involved in, 273, 283, 285b
    digital fiber-optic transillumination of, 353
    early childhood, 350–352, 726–727
    in elderly, 767
    electrical monitor for, 353
    explorers for detection of, 158
    fermentable carbohydrates and, 273,
        346, 348
    flossing to reduce risk of, 324
    foods that protect against, 273
    genetic factors, 745–746
    G.V. Black's classification of, 221,
        221t–223t, 350
    host factors associated with, 347
    incipient, 220t, 371–372
    indices of, 243–244

interproximal, 257
laser fluorescence of, 353
light-emitting diodes for detection of, 353
management of
  dental hygienist's role in, 353–354
  "minimally invasive" approach to, 353
in physically impaired patients, 778t
pit and fissure, 365
polysaccharides associated with, 231, 346
prevalence of, 365
prevention of
  calcium sodium phosphosilicate, 350
  Caries Management by Risk Assessment
    protocol for, 349, 354–355, 355t–358t
  casein phosphopeptide-amorphous
    calcium phosphate, 349–350
  chewing gum for, 349–350
  chlorhexidine mouthrinses and varnish
    for, 349, 357t–358t
  dentifrices for, 336, 339t
  fluoride for, 348–349, 349f, 357t–358t,
    365, 635, 717
  fluoride-releasing dental materials, 350
  mouthrinses for, 337, 339t, 349
  saliva's role in, 347, 348b
  sealants for, 357t–358t
  tricalcium phosphate, 350
  xylitol, 350, 357t
quantitative light-induced fluorescence
  of, 353
radiation, 717
radiographic detection of, 352, 357t
recurrent, 351
refined carbohydrates and, 347
remineralization process, 348
reversibility of, 346
risk assessment for
  in children, 727, 730t
  description of, 250, 354–355,
    355t–358t, 366
  in special-needs patients, 585
risk factors for, 231, 355, 366, 574, 717
root, 349, 351
secondary, 351
sex differences in, 745–746
staining caused by, 235
tactile detection of, 352
visual detection of, 227, 352
in women of childbearing age, 739
xerostomia as risk factor for, 296, 355, 717
Caries Management by Risk Assessment
  (CAMBRA), 250, 349, 354–355,
  355t–358t, 555, 587, 650, 654
Caries-Risk Assessment Tool (CAT), 249
Cariogenesis, 345
Cariogenic bacteria
  demineralization caused by, 347
  description of, 346
  vertical transmission of, in children, 351
Cariogenic foods, 273
Cariology, 345
Cariostatic foods, 273
Carious lesions
  classification of, 350–352
  definition of, 345
  multifactorial process involved in, 346f,
    346–347
  tactile detection of, 352
Carpal tunnel syndrome, 395
Carrier, 85
Case presentation, 312–313

Case report, 74
Case–control study, 74
Casein phosphopeptide-amorphous calcium
  phosphate (CPP-ACP), 349–350, 456,
  635, 717
Cataracts, 622, 624f
Cavitation, 410
Cavity, 345
CD8+ cells, 674
Cefazolin, 601t
Ceftriaxone, 601t
Celiac sprue, 700
Cementoenamel junction (CEJ)
  dentin hypersensitivity and, 451b
  description of, 192
  free gingival level at, 200
  mucogingival line to, 203f
Cementum
  anatomy of, 191f, 193
  radiographic appearance of, 259t
Centers for Disease Control (CDC), 93, 94t
Centric occlusion, 227
Cephalexin, 601t
Cerebral palsy (CP), 651–652
Cerebrovascular accident. See Stroke
Cervical lymph nodes, 179, 179f
Cervical vertebrae, 787
Cetacaine, 533t
Change
  in behavior, 31, 46
  readiness for, 46
Charge-coupled device (CCD), 263
Charters tooth-brushing method, 323t
Charting. See Dental charting
Charts. See Dental charts
Chemical burn, 811t
Chemical disinfectants, 106–108
Chemical indicators, for sterilization
  monitoring, 104–105, 105f
Chemical sterilization, 106–108
Chemical vapor sterilization, 106
Chemokines, 674
Chemotherapy
  bisphosphonates used with, 743
  oral complications caused by, 701,
    709–710
  in physically impaired patients, 786t
Chewing, 274
Chewing gum, 349–350, 742
Chickenpox, 89–90, 92t, 109t
Chief complaint, 129–130, 307
Children. See also Adolescents
  age-based characteristics of, 724t–725t
  anticipatory guidance in, 724, 730t–731t
  behavior guidance techniques for, 728–729
  body temperature ranges in, 142
  caries in
    description of, 297, 324
    early childhood, 350–352, 726–727
    risk assessment for, 355t–356t, 730t
  communication with, 728–729
  dental appointment procedures for,
    729–733
  dental fear and anxiety in
    desensitization techniques for, 728
    management of, 506
    modeling techniques for, 501
  dentition in, 725–726, 726t–727t
  desensitization approach for, 728
  diabetes mellitus in, 295

distraction techniques for, 500–501,
    728–729
Erikson's psychosocial stages,
    725t–726t, 729
fluoride for, 730t, 731–732
greeting of, 730, 730f
health promotion and prevention in, 47
hearing loss in, 621
hepatitis A in, 87
hepatitis E in, 89
hypertension in, 146
injury prevention discussions with, 731t
nutrition discussions with, 731t
obesity in, 140
oral health of
  caries. See Children, caries in
  dental trauma, 727–728
  Healthy People 2020 objectives for, 43
  malocclusion, 727, 727f–728f
  non-nutritive habits, 727
  public health rationale for, 723
oral hygiene in, 730t
physical techniques used with, 729, 729f
piercings by, 727
primary dentition in, 725–726, 726t
vision impairment in, 622, 624
Chlorhexidine
  caries prevention using, 349, 357t–358t
  in chronic obstructive pulmonary disease
    patients, 617
  description of, 110
  local delivery of, 574t
  mouthrinses with, 349, 357t–358t
  oral irrigator use of, 330, 330t
  oral mucositis prevention using, 711
  plaque removal using, around dental
    implants, 389
  varnish with, 349
Chloroxylenol PCMX, 110–111
Chlorpromazine, 642t
Choking, 806t
Cholesterol, 696–697
Cholestyramine, 598t
Cholinergic crisis, 677
Cholinesterase inhibitors, 676
Chorea, 652–653
Chronic bronchitis, 616b
Chronic Epstein-Barr virus infection, 90
Chronic inflammation, 59, 198, 198f, 594
Chronic ischemic heart disease (CIHD), 602
Chronic obstructive pulmonary disease
    (COPD), 133t–134t, 514, 615–617,
    760t, 762
Chronic periodontitis, 198f, 206
Chronological age, 753
Chronological resume, 838
Cigarette smoking
  cessation of, 48–50, 49b
  periodontal disease risks, 58
CINAHL, 75t
Circadian rhythms, 664
Circular fibers, 192t
Citalopram, 642t
Civil law, 11–12
Civil offense, 11
Class I malocclusion, 224, 225f
Class II malocclusion, 224–225, 225f
Class III malocclusion, 225, 225f
Cleaning
  of instruments, 104
  of patient care area, 100

Client self-care commitment model, 3
Clindamycin, 601t
Clinical attachment level (CAL), 196t, 200–201, 201f, 441, 558
Clinical contact surfaces, 100, 100t
Clinical examination
    evaluation of, 554–555
    gloves used in, 96–97
Clinical indices. See Indices
Clinical question
    PICO question, 72–73, 73f
    studies used to answer, 75t
Clinician
    cultural competence of, 557
    dental hygienists as, 4
Clofibrate, 598t
Clomipramine, 641t
Closed-ended questions, 29t, 29–30
Clot formation, 691, 692f
Clotting determination, 692t, 692–693
Clozapine, 642t
Cocaine abuse, 639t, 640
Cochlear hearing loss, 627t
Cochlear implant, 628
Cochrane Library, 75t
Code of ethics, 10, 13b, 14t, 16, 233, 849
Cognitive disabilities, 751
Cognitive impairment, 583t, 584, 755
Cognitive Vulnerability Model, 493–494, 494f
Cogwheeling, 655
Cohort study, 74
Coinfection, 88
Col, 323f, 323–324
Colestipol, 598t
Colitis, 134t
Collaboration
    in dental hygiene practice, 47, 140, 309, 462
    in dental implant therapy, 387
    in motivational interviewing, 31, 31f
Collagen, 192
Collagenase, 57
College of Registered Dental Hygienists of Alberta (CRDHA)
    description of, 123, 130
    health history used by, 140
Collimation, 264, 264f
Colony-forming units, 102
Communication
    ambivalence during, 31–32
    audience considerations during, 27–28
    in autism spectrum disorder patients, 636
    barriers to, 823
    breakdowns in, 27–28
    cancellation avoidance through, 829–830
    case study of, 36
    with children, 728–729
    components of, 823–824
    definition of, 25
    dental fear and anxiety managed with, 499–500
    dental hygiene appointment value created through, 32–33
    in dental practice, 823–824, 828
    between dentist and dental hygienist, 830
    dialogue as form of, 28–30, 29t
    eye contact as form of, 729
    generational differences, 28, 29t
    with hearing-impaired patients. See Hearing loss, communication methods for

KISS principle for, 27
message in, 27, 28t–29t
in motivational interviewing, 823
no-show avoidance through, 829–830
nonverbal, 26–27
in nutritional counseling, 275–276, 276f
in patient interview, 554
with physically impaired patients, 776–777, 777t
positive, 499–500
proxemics in, 26f–27f, 26–27
two-way, 25, 26t, 497
types of, 25–27
verbal, 25–26
with vision-impaired patients, 624–625
withholding of information by patient during, 29
written, 25–26
Community Alternative Programs/Department of Developmental Disabilities (CAP/MRDD), 651
Community dental health coordinator (CDHC), 847
Community Periodontal Index of Treatment Needs (CPITN), 195, 248–249
Comorbidities, 584
Complement, 674
Complement system, 56
Complementary metal oxide semiconductors (CMOS), 263
Complete blood cell count (CBC), 692
Complete denture, 380, 380f
Complete mouth radiographic series (CMS), 257
Composite restorations, 478
Composite veneer, 477–478
Computed radiography, 259–260, 261t, 262, 262f
Computer-aided design/computer-aided manufacturing (CAD/CAM), 477, 477f
Computer-assisted tomography, 478
Computer-based dental charts, 555, 570f
Computer-based dental practice management software, 555
Computerized patient records, 314
Conceptual models, 3
Conductive hearing loss, 627t
Cone beam computed tomography, 263
Confidentiality, 14t, 16
Conflicts of interest, scientific paper disclosure of, 76–77
Congenital, 168
Congenital deafness, 627
Congenital heart disease (CHD), 603–604
Congestive heart failure. See Heart failure
Conjunctivitis, 92t
Conscious sedation, 513
Consent
    expressed, 313
    implied, 313
    informed. See Informed consent
Constipation, 755
Contact dermatitis, 97
Continuing care, 574–575
Continuing education
    American Academy of Dental Hygiene approval of courses for, 848
    American Dental Hygienists' Association support for, 848

Clinical Practice Standards, 848
definition of, 847
delivery of, 849
in laser technology, 438
professional meetings for, 849
self-study opportunities, 849
state requirements for, 848
Continuous quality improvement, 561
Contract law, 11–12
Contrast, of radiographs, 258, 258f
Convalescent stage, 85
Corah's Dental Anxiety Scale-Revised, 496, 497f
Core values
    autonomy, 12–13, 14t
    beneficence, 14t, 15
    confidentiality, 16–18, 17t
    definition of, 12
    description of, 12
    justice, 14t, 15–16
    list of, 14t
    nonmaleficence, 10, 14t, 15
    social trust, 18
    veracity, 14t, 16
Coronal caries, 350–351
Coronary arteries, 593
Coronary artery disease (CAD), 601
Coronary heart disease, 595
Corporations, dental hygienists in, 4–5
Cortical bone
    description of, 193–194
    radiographic appearance of, 259t
Corticosteroids
    multiple sclerosis treated with, 679
    in physically impaired patients, 786t
    respiratory diseases treated with, 614t–615t, 667
    systemic lupus erythematosus treated with, 681
Cortisol, 665, 667, 682, 810t
Cosmetic whitening. See Esthetic dentistry; Tooth whitening
Covered entities, 16, 18
Cribriform plate, 193
Criminal law, 11
Critical instruments and equipment, 107, 107t
Critical pH, 347
Critical thinking, 844
Critical-thinking process, 658
Cross-contamination, 103
Cross-sectional studies, 292
Crossbite, 225, 226f, 727f
Crown (anatomic), 450f
Crown (restoration)
    all-ceramic, 476
    computer-aided design/computer-aided manufacturing of, 477, 477f
    crowning process for, 476–477
    definition of, 476
    indications for, 476
    materials for, 476
    porcelain-fused-to-metal, 476
    temporary, 476
Cryotherapy, 711t
Crystal HD mirror, 157
Culture
    dimensions of, 33–35, 34t–35t
    individualism in, 33, 34t
    long-term orientation in, 35, 35t
    masculinity in, 34t, 35

personal space differences based on, 27
power/distance in, 33, 34t
uncertainty/avoidance index in, 34t–35t, 35
Curets
  Gracey
    description of, 419, 420f, 425–426
    design of, 426
    sharpening of, 428–429
    technique for, 427b, 427f
    working end of, 420, 420f, 426
  universal
    for anterior teeth, 425, 425b
    calculus removal stroke, 424, 424b
    for posterior teeth, 425, 426b
    sharpening of, 429
Curettage, 421
Current Dental Terminology (CDT), 826–827
Curriculum vitae (CV), 838, 838b
Curve of Spee, 227
Curved explorer, 159t, 233
Cushing syndrome, 667, 669
Cutting edges
  definition of, 419
  dullness of, 428
  of files, 426
  illustration of, 420f
  sharpening of, 428
Cyanosis, 810t
Cyclothymic disorder, 637
Cystic fibrosis, 617, 776t, 784–785
Cytokines, 56–57, 61, 594, 674
Cytological smear, 184–185
Cytomegalovirus (CMV), 90, 92t
Cytoreductive therapy, 710
Cytotoxic T cells, 674

D
Dairy foods, 281t–282t
Dangerousness, 493, 494f
Darkroom, 100–101
Data collection, 242
Databases, 75, 75t
Daylight loader, 101
DDAVP. See Desmopressin acetate
Deaf, 627
Deaf-blind patients, 630–631
Debridement
  definition of, 434
  endoscopic, 439
  maintenance appointment, 572–573
  nonsurgical, 439
Decalcification, 223, 224f
Decision making
  autonomy in, 12–13
  ethical model of, 18–20, 19b
  evidence-based, 71, 554
  health history used in, 147–148
  informed consent and, 13, 15
  shared, 13
Decontamination of instruments, 104
Deep cervical lymph nodes, 179, 179f
Defibrillators, 597
Definitive diagnosis, 307
Degloving, 97, 98f
Degree-completion programs, 846
Dehydration, 755, 765
Deinstitutionalization, 773
Dementia, 751, 754, 761t

Demineralization
  definition of, 483
  dental fluorosis as cause of, 483
  description of, 346–348, 350
  tooth whitening as cause of, 482
Demyelination, 679
Density, of radiographs, 258, 259f
Dental anxiety
  assessment of, 495–496
  case study of, 507–508
  in children
    management of, 506
    modeling techniques for, 501
  definition of, 491
  effects of, 492–494
  etiology of, 492–493
  learning of, 493
  management of
    assessment, 495–496, 498
    biofeedback, 505
    cognitive and behavioral strategies, 499–501
    communication as part of, 499–500
    comprehensive program for, 499
    dental environment considerations, 499
    distraction, 500–501, 728–729
    expectation setting and, 500
    focused attention, 503–504
    focused breathing, 502, 502b
    guided relaxation, 503, 504b
    hypnosis, 504–505
    interview, 496–498
    modeling, 501
    pain control management as part of, 505–506
    pharmacological agents for, 505
    progressive muscle relaxation, 502, 503b
    rapport building for, 500
    relaxation techniques, 501–505
    staff considerations, 499
    systemic desensitization, 505, 506b
    Tell–Show–Do, 501
  onset of, 492–493
  personality traits associated with, 493
  signs of, 495b
  systemic stress caused by, 514
Dental auxiliary placement service, 837t
Dental Beliefs Survey, 496
Dental care
  access to, 42, 139, 351, 791
  barriers to, 5, 42, 773, 775, 791
  disparities in, 42
  evidence-based, 71
  financial barriers to, 773, 775
  socioeconomic conditions' effect on, 42
Dental caries. See Caries
Dental charting
  in alternative practice settings, 798
  description of, 217
  evaluation data documented by, 554
  by hand, 219
  symbols used in, 219t–221t
Dental charts. See also Periodontal chart
  computer-based, 555, 570f
  description of, 217
  tooth numbering system used in, 217, 217f–218f
  updating of, at maintenance visit, 568
Dental decay, 345, 745–746
Dental emergencies, 814t–815t

Dental endoscopy, 438
Dental erosion
  basic erosive wear examination for, 452
  description of, 273
Dental fear
  assessment of, 495–496
  case study of, 507–508
  dangerousness and, 493, 494f
  definition of, 491
  dental phobia versus, 492
  disgustingness and, 494
  embarrassment and, 494
  etiology of, 492–493
  fear of pain as cause of, 493
  learning of, 493
  management of
    assessment, 495–496, 498
    biofeedback, 505
    cognitive and behavioral strategies, 499–501
    communication as part of, 499–500
    comprehensive program for, 499
    dental environment considerations, 499
    distraction, 500–501, 728–729
    expectation setting and, 500
    focused attention, 503–504
    focused breathing, 502, 502b
    guided imagery, 503, 504b
    guided relaxation, 503, 504b
    hypnosis, 504–505
    interview, 496–498
    modeling, 501
    pain control management as part of, 505–506
    pharmacological agents for, 505
    progressive muscle relaxation, 502, 503b
    rapport building for, 500
    relaxation techniques, 501–505
    staff considerations, 499
    systemic desensitization, 505, 506b
    Tell–Show–Do, 501
  onset of, 492–493
  past traumatic experience as cause of, 493
  perception and, 493–494
  personality traits associated with, 493
  prevalence of, 491
  professionalism and, 492
  signs of, 495b
  systemic stress caused by, 514
  uncontrollability and, 493, 494f
  unpredictability and, 493, 494f
  vicious cycle of, 492, 492f
Dental Fear Survey (DFS), 496
Dental floss, 324–326, 325f
Dental floss holder, 325t, 327, 327f
Dental follicle, 259, 260f
Dental health-care personnel (DHCP)
  fingernail care in, 110
  hair in, 109–110
  hand care by, 110
  hand hygiene in, 110–112, 111f
  health maintenance by, 109
  infection control by, 109–112
  jewelry worn by, 110
  nail care in, 110
  personal protective equipment worn by. See Personal protective equipment (PPE)
  skin care in, 110
  standard precautions used by, 85

universal precautions used by, 85, 702
vaccination recommendations for, 109t
Dental history
  evaluation of, 554
  questions for, 496b
  review of, 109
  updating of, 567–568
Dental home, 47, 724
Dental hygiene
  conceptual models for, 3
  definition of, 4
  for dental implants, 387–389, 388b
  direct-access, 847
  as discipline, 3
  esthetic restorations, 479
  evidence-based, 71
  for fixed bridges, 379
  future of, 5
  goals of, 775
  growth of, 654
  history of, 4
  for oral appliances, 376–378
  for prostheses, 376–378
  tooth whitening and, 482
  treatment plans for. *See* Treatment plans
Dental Hygiene Committee of
    California, 649
Dental hygiene diagnosis (DHDx)
  assessment data used in, 307, 310
  case examples of, 307
  definition of, 305–306, 571
  definitive diagnosis, 307
  differential diagnosis, 307
  formulating of, 307–308
  historical perspective on, 305
  overview of, 305
  purpose of, 306
  Standards for Clinical Dental Hygiene Practice
    used in, 305–306
  terminology associated with, 306–307, 307t
Dental hygiene process of care
  Assessment, Diagnosis, Planning,
    Implementation, Evaluation, and
    Documentation, 549, 550t–553t
  description of, 4, 46–47, 298, 306f
  self-care devices and, 320t
Dental hygiene schools, 837t
Dental hygienists
  administrative roles of, 5
  as advocates, 5, 796
  caries management role of, 353–354
  as clinician, 4
  collaboration with other health-care
    professionals, 47, 309, 462
  in corporations, 4–5
  definition of, 3
  dentist and, communication between, 830
  education of, 3, 5
  as educators, 5
  functions of, 795
  licensure requirements for, 3
  local anesthesia administration by, 533
  nutritional counseling role of, 274, 353
  in pediatric dentistry, 724–725
  practice settings for, 3
  professional appearance of, 499, 831
  in public health settings, 5
  reimbursement for, 5
  as researcher, 5
  roles of, 4f, 4–5, 836t
  scope of practice, 4–5

Dental imaging systems
  analog x-ray film, 259, 261t–262t,
    261–262, 262f
  computed radiography, 259–260, 261t,
    262, 262f
  digital, 259–263, 262f–263f
  digital radiography, 228, 259–260, 261t,
    262–263, 263f
  photostimulable phosphor plates used in,
    259–260, 262, 262f
  types of, 259–260
Dental implants. *See* Implant(s)
Dental insurance, 569
Dental laboratory, 102–103
Dental phobia
  definition of, 491
  dental fear versus, 492
Dental practice
  accounts receivable, 825–826
  appointment book used in, 829
  collection goals for, 824–825
  communication in, 823–824
  Current Dental Terminology, 826–827
  effective, habits of, 831–832
  fluoride treatments, 827
  goals of, 823–825
  hygiene goals, 827–828
  hygiene retention, 830–831
  insurance claims, 824
  leadership in, 821–823
  meetings in, 828
  mission statement of, 823
  overhead costs of, 824
  patient financial options, 825–826
  perceived value of treatment, 827, 831
  preferred provider organization, 825
  production goals for, 824–825
  professionalism in, 831
  routing slips used in, 828
  scheduling of patients, 828–829
  team communication in, 828
  technology use in, 831
  trust in, 822
  usual, customary, and reasonable fee
    plan, 825
  vision in, 822–823
Dental practice acts
  access to, 11
  in alternative practice settings, 799
  local anesthesia requirements under, 530
  state regulation of, 10
  as statutory law, 10
Dental radiograph equipment,
    100–101, 101f
Dental R.A.T., 162
Dental trauma, 727–728, 739, 805
Dental unit water lines, 102, 102f
Dentifrices
  abrasives in, 336
  active ingredients in, 335–336, 339t–340t
  adverse reactions to, 338–339
  flavoring agents in, 336
  fluoride in, 336, 339, 349
  humectants in, 336
  inactive ingredients in, 335–336
  indications for, 335–336
  potassium-containing, 455
  prescription-strength, 338
  preservatives in, 336
  regulation of, 335
  surfactants in, 336

thickening agents in, 336
tooth sensitivity reduction using,
    336, 340t
Dentin
  anatomy of, 449–450, 450f
  exposed, 451b
  radiographic appearance of, 258, 260f
Dentin hypersensitivity
  age of patient and, 451
  anatomy of, 449–450, 450f
  Brännström hydrodynamic theory of,
    450, 450f, 482
  case study of, 457
  causative factors, 450, 450f
  definition of, 449–450
  diagnosis of, 452, 453b
  gender predilection for, 451
  hydrodynamic theory of, 450, 450f, 482
  overview of, 449
  patient education plan for, 454b, 454–455
  phases of, 452
  predisposing factors, 450, 451b
  prevalence of, 450–452
  prevention of, 454, 454b
  screening for, 453b
  sites of, 452
  smear layer and, 450
  teeth commonly affected by, 451
  after tooth bleaching/whitening, 452, 482
  transient, 452
  treatment of
    adhesives, 456
    blocking agents, 453t, 453–454
    calcium compounds, 456
    calcium phosphate technology, 453t, 454
    delivery modes for, 454–457
    dental fear and anxiety reduced
      through, 506
    desensitizing agents, 452–455, 453t
    fluorides, 456–457
    home-applied options for, 455, 457
    iontophoresis, 456
    lasers, 456–457
    periodontal plastic procedures, 457
    plan for, 454b, 454–455
    potassium nitrate, 456
    potassium oxalates, 456
    professional options for, 456–457
    protein precipitants, 453t, 454
    resins, 456
    restorative procedures, 457
Dentin tubules
  anatomy of, 449
  blocking/obtundation agents for, 453t,
    453–454
  exposure of, 450, 451b
  sensory nerve fibers in, 449–450
Dentistry
  goals of, 375, 723
  minimally invasive, 353
  pediatric. *See* Pediatric dentistry
Dentition. *See also* Teeth
  in children, 725–726, 726t–727t
  in elderly, 767
Dentogingival fibers, 192t
Denture(s)
  complete, 380, 380f
  fixed partial, 379, 379f
  function of, 376t
  history of, 378
  implants versus, 390

occlusal force reductions caused by, 390
oral mucositis in patients with, 710
patient education about, 384
removable partial, 220t, 380–383
Denture-induced fibrous hyperplasia, 170
Denture stomatitis, 383
Depolarization, 530
Dermis, 757
Desensitizing agents
 dentin hypersensitivity managed with,
   452–455, 453t
 at maintenance appointment, 573
 manual polishing used to apply,
   463–465
 Porte polisher used to apply, 463–465
 tooth whitening and, 483
Desipramine, 641t
Desmopressin acetate, 698
Determinants–confounders model, of caries,
   346, 347f
Deterministic effects, of ionizing
   radiation, 263
Developmental Disabilities Assistance and
   Bill of Rights Act Amendments of
   2000, 774t
Diabetes mellitus
 in children, 295
 complications of, 666
 definition of, 665–666
 dental hygiene considerations for,
   666–667
 in elderly, 760t
 glycemic control of, 295
 health history considerations for, 135t
 hypertension risks, 666
 maintenance visit assessment of, 569
 oral problems caused by, 666
 periodontal disease risks, 62–63,
   294–295, 569
 periodontitis and, 61
 prevalence of, 61, 62f, 663
 risk factors for, 63
 screening guidelines for, 63
 sleep apnea and, 666
 symptoms of, 762
 treatment of, 569
 type 1, 666, 674
 type 2, 666
 xerostomia risks, 295
Diabetic coma, 811t
Diabetic ketoacidosis, 667, 811t
Diabetic retinopathy, 622, 623t
DIAGNOdent, 228
Diagnosis
 definition of, 305
 definitive, 307
 dental hygiene. *See* Dental hygiene
   diagnosis (DHDx)
 in dental hygiene process of care, 4, 47
 evaluation of, 555
 periodontal, 555
*Diagnostic and Statistical Manual of Mental
   Disorders* (DSM), 635
Dialogue with patient
 closed-ended questions in, 29t, 29–30
 open-ended, 28, 29t
Diamond-coated tips, for power scaling
   devices, 411
Diastolic blood pressure (DBP), 144, 666
Diazepam, 586
Dichotomous scale, for indices, 242

Diet
 analysis form for, 284t
 caries risks affected by, 273, 283, 285b
 dental health effects on, 273–274
 oral conditions that affect, 273–274, 274f
 oral health affected by, 271–273
Diet record, 277
Dietary adequacy, 275, 283
Dietary assessment
 calorie needs, 279, 279t–280t
 case study of, 286
 computer-assisted, 277
 diet adequacy, 283
 dietary modifications, 283
 documentation, 283
 food group recommendations, 279,
   281t–282t, 283
 food record, 275, 277–278, 278b
 indications for, 274
 lifestyle modifications, 283
 nutrition education, 279, 279f
 patient history review, 278–279
 progress monitoring, 283
 steps involved in, 277–283
 24-hour recall, 275, 275t
Dietary Guidelines for Americans, 2010,
   274, 275b
Differential diagnosis, 170, 307
Differential gene expression, 57
Diffusion hypoxia, 515
Digital fiber-optic transillumination
   (DIFOTI), 353
Digital imaging systems, 259–263, 262f–263f
Digital motion activation, of instruments, 421
Digital periodontal chart, 208, 211f
Digital radiography, 228, 259–260, 261t,
   262–263, 263f, 478
Diplopia, 654
Dipyridamole, 697t
Direct access, 847
Direct supervision, 799
Direct transmission, of infections, 85
Disabilities. *See also* Special-needs patients
 categories of, 582t
 physical. *See* Physical impairment
Disease-modifying antirheumatic drugs
   (DMARDs), 680–681
Disinfectants
 chemical, 106–108
 description of, 94, 100
 germicidal activity for, 107, 107t
 high-level, 107
 hospital, 108
 household products as, 381t
 intermediate, 108
 low-level, 108
 shelf life of, 108
Disinfection
 ecofriendly practices in, 103
 of nitrous oxide/oxygen sedation
   equipment, 521
 of oral appliances, 381t
 of patient care area, 100
 of prostheses, 381t
Dislocation of jaw, 814t–815t
Disposable mirrors, 156–158
Distraction techniques, for dental fear and
   anxiety, 500–501, 728–729
Diuretics, 599t, 603t
DMFS index, 243
DMFT index, 243

Docetaxel, 744
Doctoral education, 846–847
Documentation
 definition of, 4
 in dental hygiene process of care, 4, 47
 of dietary assessment, 283
 of emergencies, 808
 of evaluation, 553t
 of extraoral examination, 176
 of infection control, 112–113
 of intraoral examination, 176
 local anesthesia, 537
 of maintenance appointment, 575
 of referral, 561
 risk management through, 12
 standards for, 313–314
Domestic violence, 744
Dorsum of tongue, 181, 181f
Double-blind study, 74
Double-ended explorer, 158, 158f
Down syndrome, 581
Drama triangle, 822
Dressings, 442, 444
Drooling, 780t
Drug-induced asthma, 614
Drug kits, for emergencies, 807, 808t–809t
Drugs. *See* Medications
Dry-heat sterilization, 106
Dry mouth. *See* Xerostomia
Duchenne muscular dystrophy, 784
Dynamic sitting, 398, 398f–399f
Dysarthria, 650, 779t
Dysgeusia, 680, 712
Dyskinetic palsy, 651–652
Dysphagia, 653, 657, 678
Dysphonia, 654
Dysplasia
 definition of, 172
 grading of, 175
 oral squamous cell carcinoma versus, 175
 prognosis for, 175
 treatment of, 175
Dyspnea, 144
Dysthymic disorder, 637
Dystonia, 653

E

Ear thermometer, 142
Ear to chest exercise, 102
Early childhood caries (ECC), 350–352,
   726–727
Early childhood stage, 725t
Ears
 examination of, 178
 health history review of, 131t
Eastman Interdental Bleeding Index, 247
Eating patterns, 139
Edge-to-edge bite, 225, 226f
Education
 advanced, 846–847
 continuing. *See* Continuing education
 description of, 3, 5
Education of All Handicapped Children
   Act, 774t
Educators, dental hygienists as, 5
Elderly. *See also* Aging
 angular cheilitis in, 765
 appointment scheduling for, 752
 autoimmune diseases in, 755–756
 caries in, 767

caries risk assessment in, 355t–356t
chronic conditions in, 751
chronic ischemic heart disease in, 602
cognitive impairment in, 755
comprehensive dental care for, 752
constipation in, 755
dehydration in, 755
demographic changes in, 751
dentition in, 767
denture stomatitis in, 383
diseases and conditions that affect
  Alzheimer disease. *See* Alzheimer
    disease
  arthritis, 751, 760t
  cardiovascular disease, 760t–761t, 763
  chronic obstructive pulmonary disease,
    760t, 762
  dementia, 751, 754, 761t
  diabetes mellitus, 760t, 762–763
  osteoporosis, 761t, 763
  Parkinson disease, 761t, 763
  stroke, 761t, 763–764
  types of, 760t–761t
gingivitis in, 767
health promotion and prevention in, 48
hearing impairment in, 621, 756
hearing loss in, 756
heat stroke in, 757
homebound, 751–753
hypotension in, 754
immobilized, 752
institutionalized, 751–753
in long-term care facilities, 751
oral cancer in, 766–767
oral candidiasis in, 765
oral changes in, 764–765
oral conditions in, 765–767
oral mucosa in, 765
periodontal disease in, 767
periodontal structures in, 767
periodontitis in, 767
plaque removal in, 766
population growth of, 751–752
skin infections in, 757
stereotypes associated with, 752
tongue in, 765
transportation for, 752–753
vision impairment in, 621, 756
xerostomia in, 761t, 765
Electrical caries monitor, 353
Electromagnetic radiation, 255
Electronic dental records (EDR), 122
Electronic health records, 314, 826
Electronic patient records, 314
Electronic thermometer, 142
Emergencies
  action plan for, 806, 807t
  basic life support for, 805, 805t–806t
  cardiopulmonary resuscitation for, 805,
    805t–806t
  dental, 814t–815t
  documentation of, 808
  drug kits for, 807, 808t–809t
  emergency contacts for, 806, 807t
  equipment for, 809t–810t
  first aid kit for, 806–807
  management of, 808–809, 810t–815t
  medical, 810t–814t
  medical consultation to prevent, 804
  medical history assessment to
    prevent, 803

  oxygen delivery systems for, 806–807, 808t
  preparedness for, 803, 805–808
  prevention of, 803–805
  psychological assessment to prevent, 804
Emergency contacts, 806, 807t
Emphysema, 616b
Employees
  exposure control plans for, 112
  training of, 112
Employment
  as faculty members, 836
  how to find, 836, 837b
  in insurance companies, 836
  interview for, 836, 838
  job search, 836, 837t
  opportunities for, 835
  resume writing for, 838
Emulsion, 261
Enamel
  anatomy of, 449, 450f
  dysplasia of, 630
  hypoplasia of, 726
  loss of, 451b
  radiographic appearance of, 260f
End-stage renal disease, 134t–135t
End-to-end bite, 225, 226f
Endocrine system
  adrenal gland, 664–665
  age-related changes in, 755
  anatomy of, 663f–664f, 663–665
  gonads, 665
  health history review of, 135t
  hypothalamus, 663f–664f, 663–664
  ovaries, 665
  pancreas, 665
  parathyroid glands, 664
  pineal gland, 663f–664f, 663–664
  pituitary gland, 663f–664f, 663–664
  testes, 665
  thyroid gland, 664
Endocrinologist, 560t
Endodontic restorations, 221
Endodontist referral, 559t
Endoscope explorer, 438, 438f
Endosteal implants, 385, 385t, 386f
Energy Star, 103
Engineering controls, 94–95
Environmental protection, 103
Environmental Protection Agency (EPA),
  93, 94t
Epinephrine, 531
Epithelial cells, 675
Epithelial desquamation, 545
Epstein-Barr virus, 90
Epulis fissuratum, 170
Epulis gravidarum, 741
Equipment
  for emergencies, 809t–810t
  Spaulding classification scheme for, 106
Ergonomics
  case study of, 405
  definition of, 395–396
  exercises. *See* Exercise(s)
  operator stool, 397–399
  standing, 399
ERIC, 75t
Erikson's psychosocial stages, 725t–726t, 729
Erosion, 224, 224f
Eruption patterns, for dentition, 726t–727t
Er:YAG laser, 437
Erythema migrans, 169

Erythema multiforme (EM), 685f–686f,
  685–686
Erythroplakia, 173–174
Essential hypertension, 598
Esters, 527, 530, 530t
Esthetic dentistry
  case study of, 485
  professionalism and, 484–485
  restorations. *See* Esthetic restorations
  tooth whitening. *See* Tooth whitening
  treatment plan for, 484–485
Esthetic restorations
  dental hygiene considerations for, 479
  direct
    composites, 478
    definition of, 475
    glass ionomer, 478–479
    indirect restorations versus, 475
  indirect
    crown. *See* Crown (restoration)
    definition of, 475
    direct restorations versus, 475
    inlay, 476
    onlay, 476
    porcelain veneer, 476–478
  patient education about, 479–480
  polishing of, 479
Estrogen, 665, 738
Ethical decision-making model, 18–20, 19b
Ethical dilemmas, 20
Ethical principles
  autonomy, 12–13, 14t
  beneficence, 14t, 15
  confidentiality, 16–18, 17t
  justice, 14t, 15–16
  list of, 14t
  nonmaleficence, 10, 14t, 15
  social trust, 18
  understanding of, 12
  veracity, 14t, 16
Ethics
  definition of, 9
  laws versus, 9–10
  moral values as source of, 9
  of nitrous oxide/oxygen sedation, 519, 522
Evacuation systems, 102
Evaluation
  of assessment data, 554
  of care, 556–557, 575
  case study of, 562
  of clinical examination, 554–555
  cultural competence during, 557
  definition of, 549
  in dental hygiene process of care, 4, 47
  of diagnosis, 555
  documentation of, 553t
  formative, 550t–553t, 554, 557
  of implementation, 556
  at maintenance appointment, 575
  of patient history, 554
  of plan, 556
  qualitative, 557
  quantitative, 557–558
  of radiographs, 555
  reevaluation, 557–558
  referrals, 558–561, 559t–560t
  summative, 550t–553t, 554, 557
  taxonomy of, 549, 550t
  threefold process of, 549
  tools for, 549, 554
  of vital signs, 554

Evidence
 application of, 76
 case report, 74
 case series, 74
 case–control study, 74
 clinical recommendations based on, 76
 cohort study, 74
 evaluation of, 75–76
 in vitro studies, 74
 levels of, 73–74
 literature review, 74
 meta-analyses, 73
 randomized controlled trial, 74
 reliability of, 76
 search for, 74, 75t
 systematic reviews, 73–74
 validity of, 76
Evidence-based care (EBC)
 definition of, 71–72
 instrumentation as defined by, 417
 levels of evidence, 73–74
Evidence-based decision making, 71, 554
Evidence-based dental hygiene care
 description of, 71
 PICO question, 72–73, 73f
Evidence-based medicine, 243
Evidence-based practice (EBP), 308, 844–845
Evidence-based process
 literature search. *See* Literature search
 outcome evaluation, 76
 PICO question, 72f, 72–73
 steps in, 72, 72f, 72t
 tenets of, 72f
Evocation of change, 31
Examination gloves, 96–97, 101f
Excisional biopsy, 169, 185–186, 186f
Exercise(s)
 hand, 401–402, 679t
 leg, 404, 404f
 neck stretches, 402
 shoulder stretches, 402–403, 403f
 upper body stretches, 403f–404f, 403–404
 wrist extensor, 402
 wrist flexor, 402
Exercise-induced asthma, 614
Exfoliative cytology, 183t, 185
Exocrine glands, 663
Exostosis/exostoses, 169
Explorer
 calculus detection using, 233–234
 description of, 157–158, 158f, 159t–160t, 160f
 endoscope, 438, 438f
Exposure control plans, 112
Exposure incident report, 112, 113t
Expressed consent, 313
Expressed contract, 12
External chemical indicators, for sterilization monitoring, 104, 105f
External locus of control, 45
Extracellular polysaccharides, 346
Extraoral examination
 diagnostic aids for, 182–185
 documentation of, 176
 ears, 178
 face, 177, 177f
 lymph nodes, 177, 177f
 at maintenance visit, 568
 nose, 178
 objectives of, 168
 palpation, 177, 177f

 principles of, 176–177
 procedure for, 177f–182f, 177–182
 skin, 177–178
 steps involved in, 183t–184t
 warning signs during, 176
Extraoral radiographs, 256–258, 258f
Extrinsic asthma, 614
Extrinsic stains
 air polishing of, 464t
 description of, 236, 338, 461
 manual polishing of, 463–464
Exudate, 197t, 202, 209t
Eye(s)
 examination of, 178
 foreign bodies in, 811t–812t
 health history review of, 131t
 protrusion of, 178
Eye contact, 729
Eyewear, protective, 95f–96f, 95–96
Ezetimibe, 598t

F

Face, of working end, 419, 419f
Face shields, 96, 97f
Facial examination, 177, 177f, 183t
Facial fracture, 815t
Facioscapulohumeral muscular dystrophy, 784
Factor replacement treatments, 698
Fair Housing Amendments Act, 774t
Fear. *See* Dental fear
Feldspar, 462
Fenofibrate, 598t
Fermentable carbohydrates, 273, 346, 348
Festination, 655
Fibrin, 691, 692f, 693, 695
Fibroblasts, 57
Fibroma
 description of, 170
 excisional biopsy of, 186f
 illustration of, 170f–171f
 peripheral ossifying, 170–172, 171f
Fibromyalgia (FM), 682
Fibrosis, 677–678
Fiduciary relationship, 16
Field cancerization, 714
Fight-or-flight syndrome, 491, 494–495
Files, 426, 428, 428b
Filiform papillae, 169
Film speed, 261
Finger spelling, 629, 631
Fingernails, 110
Finishing strips, 462
First aid kit, 806–807
First-degree burn, 811t
First-degree heart block, 597
Fissured tongue, 169
Fitness, 401
Fixed bridge, 379, 379f
Fixed orthodontic appliances, 376–377, 377f–378f
Fixed partial denture, 379, 379f
Flap procedures, 441–442
Flavoring agents
 in dentifrices, 336
 in mouthrinses, 336
Floor of mouth, 181–182, 182f, 184t
Florida Probe, 59, 162
Floss, 324–326, 325f
Floss holder, 325t, 327, 327f

Flossing
 dental floss for, 324–326, 325f
 of dental implants, 389, 389f
 of fixed bridge, 380f
 oral irrigator for, 327f, 329f
Flowmeter, 516–517, 517f, 520
Fluid imbalance, xerostomia secondary to, 275
Fluorescence, quantitative light-induced, 353
Fluoride
 acidulated phosphate, 479
 in adults, 827
 anticipatory guidance for, 730t
 application methods for, 349f
 caries prevention using, 348–349, 349f, 357t–358t, 365, 635, 717
 case study of, 340
 in children, 730t
 dentin hypersensitivity treated with, 456–457
 in dentifrices, 336, 339, 349
 emergencies associated with, 811t
 in mouthrinses, 337, 339
 sealants that release, 366
 in water, 339
Fluoride varnish, 479
Fluorohydroxyapatite, 348
Fluorosis, 338, 349, 461, 483
Fluoxetine, 641t
Fluvoxamine, 642t
Flying hygienists, 794–795
Focal fibrous hyperplasia, 170
Focused attention, 503–504
Focused breathing, 502, 502b
Fogging, of mouth mirror, 157
Food
 cariogenic, 273
 cariostatic, 273
 consistency of, 273
 portion sizes for, 278, 279b
Food debris, 232
Food diary, 558
Food groups, 279, 281t–282t
Food record, 275, 277–278, 278b
Foot-controlled sink, 111f
Forced-air dry-heat sterilizer, 106
Forced expiratory volume in 1 second (FEV1), 612, 614
Fordyce granules, 169
Foreign bodies, 811t–812t
Formative evaluation, 550t–553t, 554, 557
Four-unit bridge, 379
Fractured tooth, 220t, 221
Fractures, 815t
Frail older adult, 754
Free gingiva
 anatomy of, 192, 193f
 level of, 200, 201f
 margin of, 196t, 210t
Free gingival groove, 193f
Freestanding building, 793–794
Fremitus, 197t, 202–203, 203f, 211t
Frenum pull, 210t
Frequency, 255, 409
Fruits, 281t–282t
Fulcrum, 420, 420f
Functional age, 754
Functional capacity, 150
Functional shank, 419, 419f
Functionally dependent older adult, 754
Functionally independent older adult, 754

Functioning tumors, 667
Fungal infections
    opportunistic, 380
    treatment of, 171
Fungiform papillae, 169
Furcation
    definition of, 201
    evaluation of, 558
    Glickman classification system, 196t,
        201f–202f
Furcation involvement, 196t, 201, 209t
Furcation probe, 160–163, 161f–162f, 163t,
    201, 201f

G

Gag reflex, 778t
Gastroesophageal reflux disease (GERD),
    134t, 739
Gastrointestinal system
    age-related changes of, 755
    health history review of, 134t
Gemfibrozil, 598t
Gender
    calorie needs based on, 279t–280t
    periodontal disease risks based on, 297
    sex versus, 737–738
Gender differences, 738
General anesthesia, hospital dentistry with,
    583t, 585
General anesthetics, 513
General supervision, 799
Generalized tonic-clonic seizure, 813t–814t
Generational differences, in communication,
    28, 29t
Genetic tests, 206
Genetics, periodontal disease risks and,
    297–298
Genital herpes, 92t
Genitourinary system, health history review
    of, 134t–135t
Geographic tongue, 169, 169f
German measles. *See* Rubella
Germicide, 100
Gingiva
    anatomy of, 191f–193f, 191–193
    attached, 193, 203, 203f
    color of, 196t, 694
    dentifrice-related irritation of, 338
    enlargement of, from antihypertensive
        drugs, 600
    fiber groups of, 192f, 192t
    fibromatosis of, 170, 171f
    free, 192, 193f
    healthy, 694
    indices for assessing, 247–249, 248t
    inflammation of, 196t, 198, 198f
    inspection of, 181, 181f, 184t
    recession of, 193, 201f, 203, 293f, 451
    surface texture of, 199
    tooth whitening-induced irritation of,
        482–483
    wound healing in, 557
Gingival crevicular fluid
    biochemical assays of, 205
    menstruation-related hormonal changes
        effect on, 739
Gingival description, 196t, 198–199,
    199t, 208t
Gingival embrasure, 323, 323f
Gingival epulis, 170, 171f

Gingival Index (GI), 247, 248t
Gingival margin
    contour of, 198
    free, 196t
    height of, 210t
Gingival mucosa, 272t
Gingival pocket, 200
Gingival sulcus
    around implants, 390
    bacteria accumulation in, 232
    depth of, 196t, 199, 200f
    description of, 192–193
Gingivectomy, 441
Gingivitis
    biofilm and, 232
    definition of, 206
    description of, 232
    diabetes mellitus as risk factor for, 295
    in elderly, 767
    enzymes associated with, 205
    immune response genes in, 57
    in pregnancy, 740
    sex-based differences in, 738
    T cells in, 60
Give Kids A Smile (GKAS), 723
Glass-ionomer cements,
        fluoride-releasing, 350
Glass-ionomer restorations, 478–479
Glatiramer acetate, 680
Glaucoma, 622, 623t
Glazed porcelain, 479
Glickman index, 196t, 201f–202f
Glossitis, 272t
Glossodynia, 272t
Gloves, 96–99, 98f, 101f
Glucagon, 665
Glucocorticoids, 665
Glucometer, 63
Gluten, 700
Glycine, 468
Glycocalyx, 102, 232
Goals
    career, 839
    dental practice, 823–825
Gonadocorticoids, 665
Gonads, 665
Google Scholar, 75t
Gow-Gates block, 529, 541
Gowns, 95, 95f
Gracey curets
    description of, 419, 420f, 425–426
    design of, 426
    sharpening of, 428–429
    technique for, 427b, 427f
    working end of, 420, 420f, 426
Grading, 175
Grains, 281t–282t
Granulocytes, 674
Granuloma
    peripheral giant cell, 171
    pyogenic, 172
Grasp
    for explorer, 158, 160f
    for mouth mirror, 157f
    for probes, 161
Gravity displacement sterilizer, 106
Greater palatine nerve
    anatomy of, 528
    anesthetic block of, 539f, 539–540, 543t
Group A ß-hemolytic streptococci, 600
Growth factors, 691

Growth hormone, 667
GTR. *See* Guided tissue regeneration
Guide dog, 625
Guided imagery, 503, 504b
Guided relaxation, 503, 504b
Guided tissue regeneration, 442–443
G.V. Black's caries classification system, 221,
    221t–223t, 350

H

Hader bar and clips, 386
Hair, 109–110
Hairy tongue, 169
Halitosis, 232, 337
Haloperidol, 641t
Hand care, 110
Hand exercises, 401–402, 679t
Hand hygiene, 110–112, 111f
Hand instruments
    description of, 400–401
    periodontal debridement using, 434
    stain removal using, 461
Hand lotions, 110
Hand-scrubbing, of instruments, 104
Hand wash, 111
Handle
    definition of, 418
    rolling of, 421
Handpieces, 401, 465f–466f
Hard palate, 182, 182f, 184t
Hard tissue examination
    caries classification, 221, 221t–223t
    dental charts, 217, 219t–221t
    noncarious lesions, 223–224
    occlusion analysis, 224–225, 225f
    overbite, 226f–227f, 226–227
    overjet, 227, 227f
    pulp testing, 227
    teeth malrelations, 225f–227f, 225–227
Hawley retainer, 377f
Hazard communication program, 113
Hazard Communication Standard, 113
Head and neck cancers, 168, 712–715, 760t.
        See also Oral cancer; Oral squamous
        cell carcinoma (OSCC)
Headlights, 400
Health
    definition of, 41
    factors that affect, 42
    optimal, 42
    patient's responsibility for, 41
    wellness versus, 41
Health belief model, 45–46, 46f
Health-care providers
    autonomy by, 13
    dental hygienist's collaboration
        with, 47
    hepatitis C prevalence in, 88
    with infectious diseases, work restrictions
        for, 93t
    patient and, relationship between,
        16, 18
Health care system, 42
Health disparities, 42
Health education, 42
Health history
    American Dental Association, 123
    conducting of, 123
    decision-making based on, 147–148
    disease-oriented focus of, 123

elements of
  biographical data, 127, 129
  chief complaint, 129–130, 307
  family history, 130
  general health questions, 130
  medication history, 139–140, 140b
  occupation history, 139
  oral history, 130, 137t–138t
  personal psychosocial history, 138–139
  vital signs. *See* Vital signs
focus of, 123
forms of, 122
medical conditions reviewed in, 131t–137t
preparation of, 122–123
purpose of, 122
questionnaire for, 124f–127f
review-of-systems approach, 127,
    128f–129f, 131t–137t
samples of, 123, 124f–127f
signing of, 150
of special-needs patients, 584
updating of, 150
Health Insurance Portability and
    Accountability Act (HIPAA)
  covered entities under, 16
  description of, 129
  patient record protections under, 314
  Privacy Rule of, 16, 17t
  protected health information access under,
    16–18, 17t
  Security Rule, 18
Health professional shortage areas, 835
Health promotion
  in adolescents, 47–48
  in children, 47
  definition of, 42
  in elderly, 48
  Healthy People 2020 for, 42–43
  in infants, 47
  models for, 45–46
Health savings account, 825
"HealthPartners Dental Group and Clinics
    Periodontal Risk Assessment
    Guideline," 59
Healthy People 2020, 42–43
Hearing aid, 628
Hearing impairment
  in children, 621
  communication options for, 621
  definition of, 627
  in elderly, 621, 756
Hearing loss
  caries prevention in patients with, 630
  causes of, 627–628
  in children, 621
  communication methods for
    American Sign Language, 628–629, 629f
    electronic aids, 629–630
    finger spelling, 629, 631
    hearing dogs, 630
    interpreters, 629
    lipreading, 628
    traditional, 630
  deaf-blind patients, 630–631
  dental hygiene considerations for, 630
  in elderly, 756
  noise-induced, 627, 628f
  oral health and, 630
  patient factors associated with, 628
  self-care considerations, 630
  types of, 627, 627t

Heart, 592–593, 593f
Heart block, 597
Heart failure, 133t, 603, 603t, 812t
Heart transplantation, 606
Heat stroke, 757
Heavy-duty utility gloves, 97, 103–104
Height, 140, 141t
Helper T cells, 60, 674, 683
Hematocrit, 692t
Hematologic system, health history review
    of, 136t
Hematological system
  clot formation, 691, 692f
  description of, 691
Hematoma, 542, 812t
Hemianopsia, 656
Hemoglobin, 692t, 699–700
Hemoglobin A1c, 62, 569, 666
Hemophilia A, 698
Hemophilia B, 698
Hemorrhage, 812t
Hemorrhagic stroke, 656–657
Hemostasis, 595f, 691
Heparin, 605
Hepatitis
  definition of, 86, 702
  non-ABCDE, 702
  occupational exposure to, 702–703
  symptoms of, 86–87
  transmission of, 86
Hepatitis A virus (HAV), 87–88, 92t
Hepatitis B surface antigen (HBsAg), 88
Hepatitis B virus (HBV)
  description of, 88, 92t, 702
  exposure to, 113t
  vaccination for, 109t
Hepatitis C virus (HCV), 88, 92t, 113t, 702
Hepatitis D virus (HDV), 88, 702
Hepatitis E virus (HEV), 88–89
Hepatitis TT, 702
Herbal medications, 697
Herbal supplements, 657
Herpes labialis, 92t
Herpes simplex virus, 89, 92t
Herpes zoster, 92t. *See also* Shingles
Herpetic gingivostomatitis, 89
Herpetic whitlow, 92t
Hertz, 409
Hexachlorophene, 110–111
Hierarchy of needs, 44, 44f
High-density lipoprotein (HDL), 598
High-level disinfectants, 107
Highly active antiretroviral therapy
    (HAART), 296, 683
Hippocratic Oath, 12, 13b, 15
History. *See* Dental history; Health history;
    Medical history
HIV. *See also* AIDS
  definition of, 683
  dental hygiene considerations for, 683
  description of, 86
  exposure incident report for, 113t
  highly active antiretroviral therapy
    for, 296
  necrotizing ulcerative gingivitis associated
    with, 296, 296f
  occupational exposure to, 703
  pathogenesis of, 683
  postexposure prophylaxis for, 86,
    87t, 113t
  treatment of, 683

Hodgkin disease, 701–702
Hoes, 426, 427b
Holistic care, 41
Home care, 571
  for amyotrophic lateral sclerosis patients, 649
  for cerebral palsy, 652
  for Huntington disease, 653
  for Parkinson disease patients, 655–656
  for stroke patients, 658
Homebound elderly, 751–753
Homeless patients, 798
Honesty, 16
Horizontal bitewing radiographs, 256–257
Hormone(s)
  adrenal cortex, 665
  adrenal medulla, 665
  definition of, 664
  negative feedback mechanism of, 664
  positive feedback mechanism of, 664
  tropic, 664
Hormone replacement therapy, 739, 742
Hospital dentistry with general anesthesia,
    583t, 585
Hospital disinfectants, 108
Housekeeping surfaces, 100, 100t
Huddle, 827–828
Human herpesviruses, 89–90
Human Needs Conceptual Model, 557
Human needs model, 3
Human papillomavirus (HPV), 172–173,
    714t, 714–715
Humectants, 336
Humoral immunity, 674
Huntington disease (HD), 652–653
Hydrocephalus, 785
Hydrodynamic theory, of dentin
    hypersensitivity, 450, 450f, 482
Hydrogen peroxide, 481
Hydroxyapatite, 347
Hygiene retention, 830–831
Hyperactive gag reflex, in physically
    impaired patients, 778t
Hyperacusis, 650
Hyperbaric oxygen therapy, for
    osteoradionecrosis, 716
Hyperglycemia, 61
Hyperinsulinism, 812t
Hypertension
  antihypertensive medications for, 599t
  in children, 146
  classification of, 146, 147t
  definition of, 146, 598
  diabetes mellitus as risk factor for, 666
  in elderly, 761t
  essential, 598
  health history review of, 132t
  prevalence of, 598
  risk factors for, 599
  treatment of, 599
Hyperthyroidism, 668
Hypertonic, 650, 775
Hyperventilation, 144, 812t
Hypnosis, 504–505
Hypocalcification, 224, 224f, 483–484
Hypogeusia, 272t
Hypoglycemia, 812t
Hypoparathyroidism, 668
Hypoplasia, 224, 224f
Hypotension, 146, 754
Hypothalamus, 663f–664f, 663–664
Hypotonic, 775

I

Iatrosedation, 499
"Ill-E-O-So-As" stretch, 404, 404f
Illicit substances, 139
Illuminated tips, for power scaling
    devices, 411
Illumination, mouth mirrors for,
    155–156, 156f
Immobilized elderly, 752
Immune complex, 674
Immune diseases and disorders
    adrenal insufficiency, 681–682
    erythema multiforme, 685f–686f, 685–686
    fibromyalgia, 682
    HIV/AIDS. See AIDS; HIV
    lichen planus, 684f, 684–685
    multiple sclerosis, 679–680
    myasthenia gravis, 676–677, 677t
    rheumatoid arthritis, 680–681
    scleroderma, 677–679, 679t
    Sjögren syndrome, 675f, 675–676
    systemic lupus erythematosus, 675, 681
Immune response
    adaptive/acquired, 56
    cells of, 674
    innate, 56
    pathogens that elicit, 594f
Immune system
    acquired immunity, 56
    age-related changes in, 755–756
    complement cascade, 56–57
    function of, 673
    innate immunity, 56, 56f
    lymphoid organs, 55–56, 56f
    purpose of, 55
    research on, 57
Immunity
    acquired, 56, 56f
    active, 56
    humoral, 674
    innate, 56, 56f
    passive, 56
Immunization, 87
Immunodeficiency diseases, 674–675
Immunoglobulins, 674
Immunological memory, 673
Implant(s)
    abutment of, 385
    bone interface with, 386–387
    calculus formation on, 388, 388f
    collaborative approach to, 387
    continuing care intervals for, 388
    continuing education programs on, 390
    debridement of, 389
    dental charting symbols for, 220t
    dental hygiene considerations for,
        387–389, 388b
    dentures versus, 390
    endosteal, 385, 385t, 386f
    failure of, 204, 204f, 387f, 573
    flossing of, 389, 389f
    gingival sulcus depth around, 390
    history of, 384
    instruments used in cleaning of,
        388–389, 389f
    maintenance care of, 573–574
    mobility assessments, 388
    osseointegration of, 384–386, 387f, 573
    patient education about, 389
    peri-implant assessment, 203–204, 204f

peri-implant disease, 387, 573
    periodontal probing of, 390
    probing of, 390
    prostheses supported with, 386, 386f,
        388–389
    radiographic assessment of, 388, 573
    retention of, 386
    self-care of, 389
    soft tissue interface with, 386–387
    subperiosteal, 385, 385t
    technological advances in, 384–385
    titanium, 384
    transosteal, 385, 385t
    types of, 385, 385t
Implant probe, 161f
Implant-supported lingual bar, 380
Implant tips, for power scaling devices,
    411, 411f
Implantable pacemakers, 597
Implantologist referral, 560t
Implementation
    in dental hygiene process of care, 4, 47
    evaluation of, 556
Implied consent, 313
Implied contract, 12
In-office tooth whitening, 481, 481f
In vitro studies, 74
Inactive ingredients
    in dentifrices, 335–336
    in mouthrinses, 336–337
Incidence, 292
Incipient caries, 220t, 371–372
Incisional biopsy, 185, 555
Incisive nerve
    anatomy of, 529
    anesthetic block of, 541–542, 542f, 544t
Incisors, 726t–727t
Independent practice hygienist, 792–793
Indices
    calculus, 204, 246–247, 247t
    calibration, 241
    characteristics of, 241–242
    Community Periodontal Index of
        Treatment Needs, 248–249
    definition of, 241
    dichotomous scale for, 242
    DMFS, 243
    DMFT, 243
    Gingival Index, 247, 248t
    gingival status, 247–249, 248t
    irreversible, 243
    Modified Gingival Index, 247–248, 248t
    for oral disease risk assessment, 249–250
    for oral hygiene measurement, 244t,
        244–246
    ordinal scale for, 243
    periodontal, 249
    periodontal disease, 248
    periodontal scoring and recording
        index, 249
    periodontal status, 247–249
    plaque, 244t, 244–246, 554
    plaque biofilm, 197t, 204
    plaque control record, 197t, 204, 244t,
        244–245, 245f
    Quigley-Hein Plaque Index, 244t, 246
    reliability of examiner, 241–242
    reversible, 243
    Russell periodontal index, 248
    Rustogi modification of the Navy Plaque
        Index, 244t, 245f

significant caries, 243
    Silness Löe Plaque Index, 244t, 245–246
    types of, 242–250
    Volpe-Manhold Index, 241, 244t
Indirect transmission, of infections, 85
Indirect vision, 155, 155f
Individualism, as cultural dimension, 33, 34t
Individuals With Disabilities Act (IDEA), 774t
Induration, 174
Infancy stage, 725t
Infants
    characteristics of, 724t
    dental hygiene appointment in, 731
    health promotion and prevention in, 47
Infection
    chemotherapy-associated, 711–712
    maternal, fetal exposure to, 740
    opportunistic, 86
    process of, 85, 86f
Infection control
    agencies involved in, 93–94
    clinical contact surfaces, 100, 100t
    dental laboratory, 102–103
    dental radiograph equipment,
        100–101, 101f
    dental unit water lines, 102, 102f
    documentation of, 112–113
    ecofriendly challenges for, 103
    engineering controls for, 94–95
    evacuation systems, 102
    housekeeping surfaces, 100, 100t
    in patient care area, 99t, 99–103
    personal protective equipment for. See
        Personal protective equipment (PPE)
    record-keeping, 112–113
    resources and references for, 93–94, 94t
    surface barriers, 100, 100f
    work practice controls for, 94–95
Infectious asthma, 614
Infectious diseases
    AIDS, 86, 90
    carrier of, 85
    convalescent stage of, 85
    hepatitis. See Hepatitis
    HIV, 86
    human herpesviruses, 89f, 89–90
    latent period of, 85
    prevention of, 85–86
    prodromal stage of, 85
    reservoirs for, 85, 86f
    stages of, 85
    standard precautions against, 85–86
    summary of, 92t
    transmissible, 85–86
    transmission mode for, 85
    tuberculosis, 90–91, 91t–92t
    universal precautions against, 85, 702
    work restrictions for health-care providers
        infected with, 93t
Infectious mononucleosis, 90
Infective endocarditis, 148, 600, 601t
Inferior alveolar nerve (IAN)
    anatomy of, 529
    anesthetic block of, 540f, 540–541, 544t
Infiltration anesthesia, 527, 527f
Inflammation
    acute, 58–59, 198, 198f
    biofilm as cause of, 235
    chronic, 59, 198, 198f, 594
    destructive effects of, 58
    gingival, 196t, 198, 198f

under pontic, 379
reduction of, 64
resolution pathways for, 58–59
signs of, 196t, 198, 198f
in type 2 diabetes, 61
Inflammatory fibrous hyperplasia, 170
Inflammatory papillary hyperplasia,
170–171
Inflammatory response, 594
Influenza vaccination, 109t
Informed consent
definition of, 313
description of, 12–13, 15, 42
elements of, 15b
for nitrous oxide/oxygen sedation,
519, 522
PARQ used to obtain, 556
for protective stabilization, 729
for tooth whitening, 484
for treatment plan, 313, 571–572
Informed refusal, 42, 313, 378, 572
Infraorbital nerve block, 539, 539f, 543t
Infrared spectrophotometry, 521
Infraversion, 227
Inhalers, for asthma, 615
Inlay, 476
Innate immune response, 56
Innate immune system, 674
Innate immunity, 56, 56f
Innate susceptibility, 57
Inspection
of buccal mucosa, 180, 180f
of gingiva, 181, 181f, 184t
of palate, 182, 182f, 184t
of tongue, 181, 181f
Institutionalized elderly, 751–753
Institutions, 798
Instrument(s)
activation of
adaptation, 420–421
angulation, 421
digital motion, 421
handle rolling, 421
pivoting, 421
strokes, 421–423, 422t
wrist motion, 421
automated, 401
case study of, 429
classification of, 107t
double-ended, 418, 418f
files, 426, 428, 428b
Gracey curets
description of, 419, 420f, 425–426
design of, 426
sharpening of, 428–429
technique for, 427b, 427f
working end of, 420, 420f, 426
grasp of, 420, 420f
hand, 400–401
handle of, 418
hoes, 426, 427b
identification of, 419–420
for implants
dental hygiene, 388–389, 389f
maintenance care, 573
microultrasonic, 413–414
modified pen grasp of, 420, 420f
selecting of, 400–401
shank of, 418f, 418–419
sharpening of, 428–429
Spaulding classification scheme for, 106

strokes, 421–423, 422t
universal, 418
working ends of
design of, 418f–419f, 418–419
identification of, 420, 420f
Instrument processing
area for, 103
cleaning, 104
decontamination, 104
ecofriendly practices in, 103
packaging, 104
steam sterilization, 103
sterilization monitoring, 104–105, 105f
transportation, 103
Insulin, 665
Insulin reaction, 812t
Insulin resistance, 62
Insurance
dental, 569
liability, 12
Insurance claims, 824
Integumentary system. *See also* Skin
age-related changes in, 756–757
health history review of, 131t
Intellectual disability, 582t
Intention tremors, 651
Intentional torts, 11
Intercircular fibers, 192t
Interconceptual counseling, 739–740
Interdental area
anatomy of, 322–324, 323f
cleaning of. *See* Interdental cleaning
Interdental brush, 325–326, 327f
Interdental cleaning
aids for, 324f–327f, 324–327
dental floss, 324–326, 325f
dental floss holder, 325t, 327, 327f
interdental anatomy, 322–324, 323f
interdental brush, 325–326, 327f
patient education about, 330, 479
toothpicks for, 327
wood sticks for, 326, 327f
Interdental gingiva. *See* Papilla
Interdental papillae, 199
Interdisciplinary care, 283, 285t
Interexaminer reliability, 242
Intergingival fibers, 192t
Interleukins
-1, 206, 297
-6, 738–739
description of, 56
Intermediate care facilities, 795
Intermediate disinfectants, 108
Intermediate-pulpal anesthesia, 531
Internal chemical indicators, for sterilization
monitoring, 104, 105f
Internal locus of control, 45
Internal whitening, 481–482
International Caries Detection and
Assessment System (ICDAS II), 352
International Congress of Oral
Implantologists (ICOI), 390
International Ergonomics Association, 396
International Federation of Dental
Hygienists (IFDH)
code of ethics of, 13b, 14t, 16
description of, 5, 849
International Normalized Ratio (INR),
604–605, 605b, 657, 692, 692t, 696
International Standards Organization (ISO)
designation system, 219, 271

Interpapillary fibers, 192t
Interpreters, 629
Intersex, 737
Intervention, 74
Interview
employment, 836
patient, 123–124
questions for, 496b
Intimate distance, 26f, 26–27
Intimate partner violence, 744
Intracellular polysaccharides, 346
Intraexaminer reliability, 242
Intraoral examination
diagnostic aids for, 182–185
documentation of, 176
gingiva, 181, 181f
at maintenance visit, 568
objectives of, 168
oral cavity, 180
principles of, 176–177
procedure for, 177f–182f, 177–182
steps involved in, 183t–184t
tongue, 181, 181f
warning signs during, 176
Intraoral radiographs, 256f–257f, 256–257
Intrinsic asthma, 614
Intrinsic factor, 699
Intrinsic stains, 235–236, 461
Iodine, 110–111, 668
Iodine-deficiency goiter, 668
Iodophor, 110–111
Ionizing radiation
background dose of, 263
biological matter effects of, 263
collimation of, 264, 264f
definition of, 255, 263
deterministic effects of, 263
operator exposure to, 264
protection guidelines for, 263–266
quality-assurance program for, 266
safety considerations for, 266
stochastic effects of, 263
Iontophoresis, for dentin
hypersensitivity, 456
Iron-deficiency anemia, 699
Irreversible index, 243
Irritation fibroma, 170
Ischemic heart disease (IHD), 601–602, 760t
Ischemic stroke, 656
Islets of Langerhans, 665, 674
Isoniazid, 91, 617
Isotonic solution, 535
Isthmus, 664

J

Jaw
bisphosphonate-related osteonecrosis
of the, 295, 716–717, 742–743,
761t, 763
dislocation of, 814t–815t
fracture of, 815t
Jewelry, 110
Job interview, 838, 839b
Job search, 836, 837t
Junctional epithelium, 435
Justice
definition of, 14t, 15
in dentistry, 15
example of, 14t
Justification principle, 255

K

Kaposi sarcoma, 90, 296, 683f
Kelvin, Lord, 241
Keratins, 191
Ketoacidosis, diabetic, 667
KISS principle, 27
Knee-to-knee position, 731–732, 732f

L

Labial mucosa, 180, 184t
Labioversion, 227
Laboratory, dental, 102–103
Lactobacillus, 346
Lamina dura, 259, 260f
Lamina propria, 192
Lamotrigine, 643t
Large intestine, age-related changes in, 755
Laser(s)
    dentin hypersensitivity treated with, 456–457
    periodontal therapy use of, 437–438
Laser fluorescence, for caries detection, 353
Latent image, 259
Latent period, 85
Latent tuberculosis, 91, 91t, 617
Lateral cephalometric skull radiograph, 258, 258f
Lateral rotation, 403, 404f
Lateral surface, of working end, 419, 419f
Lateral trunk stretch, 403, 403f
Latex allergy, 97, 99
Lavage, 410
Law, 9-12
Lead apron, 263–264
Leadership, 821–823
Learners, 843–844
Learning ladder, 44, 44f
Leeway space, 227
Leg exercises, 404, 404f
Legal blindness, 622
Legal guardian, 583t, 584
Lesions, intraoral, 176, 176t
Leukemia, 136t, 701
Leukoedema, 169
Leukoplakia, 173, 173f–174f, 293, 293f
Levetiracetam, 643t
Levonordefrin, 531
Liability insurance, 12
Libman-Sacks endocarditis, 681
Licensure
    in Canada, 11
    description of, 3
    purpose of, 10
    state regulation of, 10
Lichen planus (LP), 684f, 684–685
Lidocaine, 532t–533t, 533
Life cycles, 738
Lifelong learning
    adult learners, 843–844, 844t
    advanced education, 846–847
    aspects of, 843
    child learners, 843–844
    continuing education, 847–849
    critical thinking, 844
    definition of, 843
    description of, 127
    evidence-based practice, 844–845
Light-emitting diode whitening machine, 481f
Light-emitting diodes, for caries detection, 353

Linea alba, 169–170
Lingual nerve, 529
Lingual retainers, 294, 295f
Linguoversion, 227
Lip(s)
    in elderly, 765
    palpation of, 180, 180f, 184t
Lipid-lowering medications, 598t
Lipopolysaccharides (LPS), 57, 61, 434
Lipoxins, 58
Lipreading, 628
Listening
    benefits of, 824
    reflective, 31–32, 32b
Literature search
    databases used in, 75, 75t
    description of, 74–75
    evaluation of evidence from, 75–76
    resources used in, 75
    systematic, 71
Lithium, 642t
Liver diseases, 134t
Lobene stain index, 244t
Local anesthesia
    adverse local reactions to
        epithelial desquamation, 545
        hematoma, 542, 812t
        needle breakage, 545
        paresthesia, 542, 544
        postinjection lesions, 545
        trismus, 544
    anterior superior alveolar nerve block, 538–539, 543t
    application of, 535–537
    buccal nerve block, 541, 541f, 544t
    case study of, 545
    definition of, 527
    documentation of, 537
    elevated levels of, 544t
    Gow-Gates block, 529, 541, 544t
    greater palatine nerve block, 539f, 539–540, 543t
    incisive nerve block, 541–542, 542f, 544t
    inferior alveolar nerve block, 540f, 540–541, 544t
    infiltration anesthesia, 527, 527f
    infraorbital nerve block, 539, 539f, 543t
    malignant hyperthermia caused by, 542
    mandibular injection sites for, 544t
    maxillary injection sites for, 543t
    medical conditions secondary to, 542
    mental nerve block, 541–542, 542f, 544t
    methemoglobinemia caused by, 542
    middle superior alveolar nerve block, 538–539, 543t
    nasopalatine nerve block, 540, 540f, 543t
    pain management uses of, 529–530
    patient positioning for, 536
    posterior superior alveolar nerve block, 538f, 538–539, 543t
    in special-needs patients, 585
    syringe for application of, 535–536
    systemic reactions to, 542
    treatment entry for, 537
    trigeminal nerve, 527–530, 528f–529f
Local anesthetics
    absorption of, 530–531
    allergic reactions to, 542, 813t
    amides, 527, 530, 530t, 542
    asthma contraindications for, 615
    biotransformation of, 530

    cardiac considerations for, 531
    distribution of, 530
    dosage of, 531, 533
    duration of action, 531
    esters, 527, 530, 530t
    excretion of, 530
    goal of, 529–530
    injectable types of, 527
    maximum recommended dose for, 531
    metabolism of, 530
    in myasthenia gravis, 677t
    overdose of, 813t
    pain management using, 529–530
    pharmacokinetics of, 530–531
    types of, 532t
    vasoconstrictors, 531, 531t–532t, 544t
    in vision-impaired patients, 626
Local drug delivery, 435t, 435–437, 574, 574t
Local professional associations, 837t
Locus of control, 44–45
Long-pulpal anesthesia, 531
Long-term care facilities, 751
Long-term oral health, 32
Long-term orientation (LTO), 35, 35t
Longitudinal studies, 292
Lorazepam, 586
Lou Gehrig disease. *See* Amyotrophic lateral sclerosis (ALS)
Loupes, 400, 400b
Lovastatin, 598t
Low-back pain, 396
Low-level disinfectants, 108
Low vision, 622
Lower motor neurons (LMNs), 787
Lumen, 531
Lung(s), 611, 612f
Lung capacity
    age-related declines in, 754
    description of, 515, 612, 613b
Luxation, 815t
Lymph nodes
    anatomy of, 55, 56f
    cervical, 179, 179f
    palpation of, 177, 177f, 179, 179f
    supraclavicular, 179, 180f, 184t
Lymphatic system, 136t
Lymphatic vessels, 56, 56f
Lymphoid organs, 55–56, 56f

M

Macrophages, 674
Macular degeneration, 622, 623t
Magnetostrictive power scaling devices, 409, 409f–410f
Magnification loupes, 400, 400b
Maintenance appointment
    assessments included in, 567–571
    calculus evaluations, 570
    care plan for, 567
    compliance with schedule for, 568
    continuing care intervals, 574–575
    debridement, 572–573
    definition of, 567
    dental chart updating at, 568
    dental hygiene treatment plan, 571–575
    diabetes management at, 569
    documentation of, 575
    evaluation of care at, 575
    extraoral examination during, 568

homecare assessments, 571
implant care at, 573–574
intraoral examination during, 568
medical history review, 567–568
oral risk assessments, 568–569
periodontal charting at, 570, 570f
plaque evaluations at, 570
polishing at, 573
radiographs at, 568
smoking cessation promotion at, 569
Maintenance therapies, 572
Major depressive disorder (MDD), 637,
  641t–642t
Major histocompatibility complex (MHC), 673
Malar rash, 681
Malignant hyperthermia, 542
Malnutrition
  definition of, 271
  nutrient imbalance associated with, 271
  oral conditions associated with,
    273–274, 274f
  oral signs associated with, 272t
  oral tissue development affected by, 272
  periodontitis and, 272
  prevalence of, 271
Malocclusion
  Angle classification of, 224
  in children, 727, 727f–728f
  Class I, 224, 225f
  Class II, 224–225, 225f
  definition of, 727
  in physically impaired patients, 778t
Malodor, oral, 232, 337
Malpractice, 11–12
Mandibular nerve, 529, 529f
Mandibular teeth, 726t
Mandibular torus, 170
Mantoux tuberculin skin test, 91
Manual polishing, 463t, 463–464
Manual toothbrushes, 319, 320f
Masculinity, 34t, 35
Masks, 96, 96f
Maslow's hierarchy of needs, 44, 44f
Master's degree programs, 846
Materia alba, 232
Material safety data sheets (MSDS), 113
Maternal periodontitis, 64, 740–741
Matrix metalloproteinases (MMPs), 57–58
Maxillary nerve, 528f, 528–529
Maxillary teeth, 726t
Maximum recommended dose (MRD), 531
Measles, mumps, and rubella
    vaccination, 109t
Measurable outcomes, 549
Medicaid, 775
Medical emergencies, 810t–814t. See also
    Emergencies
Medical history
  assessment of, for emergency
    prevention, 803
  evaluation of, 554
  in periodontium evaluation, 204
  review of, 109, 567–568
  updating of, 150, 567–568
Medical model, 723, 723t
Medical waste, 108, 112
Medicare, 775
Medication history, 139–140, 140b
Medications. See also specific medication
  asthma induced by, 614
  caries risks, 355

gingival fibromatosis caused by, 170, 171f
  local delivery of, 435t, 435–437
  need-specific, 657
  oral disease risks, 296
  in physically impaired patients, 786t
  during pregnancy, 741–742, 742t
  premedication, 148, 150
  special-needs patient's use of, 583t,
    584, 586
  xerostomia caused by, 296, 366, 585, 600,
    655, 751, 766
MedlinePlus, 75t
Melanin, 756
Memory
  age-related declines in, 755
  immunological, 673
Memory cells, 674
Men
  prostate disease in, 744–745
  puberty in, 738
Meninges, 785
Meningitis, bacterial, 92t
Meningococcal vaccination, 109t
Menopause, 742–743
Menstruation, 739
Mental disorders
  anorexia nervosa, 638–639, 639t
  autism spectrum disorders, 635–636, 637t,
    641t–643t
  bipolar disorder, 636–637, 642t–643t
  bulimia nervosa, 638–639, 639t
  categories of, 635
  definition of, 635
  eating disorders, 638–639, 639t
  medications for, 641t–643t
  mood disorders, 636–637
  pervasive developmental disorders, 635–636
  prevalence of, 635
  schizophrenia, 637–638, 642t
  substance dependence and abuse. See
    Substance dependence and abuse
Mental impairment, 779t
Mental nerve
  anatomy of, 529
  anesthetic block of, 541–542, 542f, 544t
Mepivacaine, 532t
Meta-analyses, 61, 73
Metabolic equivalents (METs), 150
Metabolic syndrome, 62, 666
Metastasis, 175, 707
Metastatic tumors, 707
Methamphetamine abuse, 639t, 640, 641t
Methemoglobinemia, 542
Methicillin-resistant Staphylococcus aureus, 785
Methylphenidate hydrochloride, 641t
Microabrasion, 484
Microbiological testing, 205
Microorganisms, 346
Microstomia, 678
Microultrasonic instruments, 413–414
Middle superior alveolar nerve (MSA)
  anatomy of, 528–529
  anesthetic block of, 538–539, 543t
Midwest Daries I.D. detection handpiece, 228
Milgrom, Peter, 500–501, 503
Mineralocorticoids, 665
Minimally invasive dentistry, 353
Minocycline hydrochloride, 436–437,
    483, 574t
Minute volume, 515, 520
Mirror, mouth, 155f–157f, 155–157, 549

Missing teeth
  charting of, 219, 220t
  replacement of, 378
Mission statement, 823
Mitral valve prolapse, 604
Mixed dentition, 726, 726t
Mixed hearing loss, 627t
Mixed palsy, 651
Mobile dental clinics, 791–792
Modeling, for dental fear and anxiety
    management, 501
Modified Dental Anxiety Scale, 496, 498f
Modified Gingival Index (MGI),
    247–248, 248t
Modified pen grasp
  for explorer, 158, 160f
  illustration of, 420f
  for mouth mirror, 157f
  for probes, 161
Modified Stillman tooth-brushing
    method, 323t
Modified Widman flap, 441–442
Mohs hardness value, 462, 462t, 468
Mohs scale of hardness, 462
Moist heat: steam under pressure
    sterilization, 105–106
Molars, 726t–727t
Mononuclear phagocytes, 674
Mood disorders, 636–637
Motivation, for behavior change, 46
Motivational Interviewing in Healthcare
    (Rollnick), 30
Motivational interviewing (MI)
  autonomy in, 31, 31f
  clinical practice applications of, 29
  collaboration in, 31, 31f
  communication in, 823
  definition of, 30
  evocation of change, 31
  health promotion through, 46
  open-ended questions used in, 30–31
  pillars of, 31–32
  public health applications of, 31
  reflective listening in, 31–32, 32b
  smoking cessation through, 48
Motor nerves, 648f
Motor neurons, 785, 787
Mouth
  floor of, 181–182, 182f, 184t
  health history review of, 131t
Mouth mirror, 155f–157f, 155–157, 549
Mouth prop, 587, 680
Mouthrinses
  active ingredients in, 337, 339t–340t
  adverse reactions to, 338–339
  alcohol in, 337, 479, 639
  as antigingivitis agents, 337
  caries prevention using, 337, 339t, 349
  chemical burning caused by, 338
  chlorhexidine, 349
  compounded, 338
  description of, 109
  fluoride in, 337, 339
  inactive ingredients in, 336–337
  indications for, 336–337
  prescription-strength, 337
  regulation of, 335
  staining caused by, 479
  topical pain relief using, 338
Mucogingival defects, 197t, 203
Mucogingival junction, 193, 193f, 210t

Mucogingival surgery, 442
Mucositis, oral, 701, 710t–712t, 710–711, 711
MuGard, 712t
Multidisciplinary team approach, 707, 718
Multiple sclerosis (MS), 679–680
Mumps, 92t
Muscle mass, 756
Muscular dystrophy, 776t, 784, 784t
Musculoskeletal disorders
    description of, 395
    operator stool and, 397
    prevention of, 396–397, 399
    stretching exercises for, 401
    types of, 395–396
Musculoskeletal system
    age-related changes in, 756
    health history review of, 132t
Mutans streptococci, 346, 727
Myasthenia gravis (MG), 653–654,
    676–677, 677t
Myasthenic crisis, 677
Mycobacterium tuberculosis, 90–91, 617
Myelinated A-delta fibers, 450
Myelomeningocele, 785
Myocardial infarction (MI), 132t, 602,
    760t, 813t
Myofascial pain syndrome, 395–396
Myotonic muscular dystrophy, 784
MyPerioID PST, 59, 250
MyPerioPath test, 250
MyPlate, 279, 279f

N

Nabers probe, 196t, 201f
Nail care, 110
Nasopalatine nerve
    anatomy of, 528, 528f
    anesthetic block of, 540, 540f, 543t
National Board Dental Hygiene
    Examination, 10
National Call to Action, 15
National Dental Association, 4
National Dental Hygienists' Association
    (NDHA), 5
National Diabetes Education Program, 663
National Health and Nutrition Examination
    Survey (NHANES), 243–244, 249, 351
National Health Service Corps (NHSC), 835
National Institute for Dental Research
    (NIDR), 246
National Institute for Occupational Safety
    and Health (NIOSH), 93, 94t
National Museum of Dentistry, 636
National Voter Registration Act of 1993, 774t
National Wellness Institute, 41
Natural killer cells, 674
Navel in and up exercise, 401
Nd:YAG laser, 437
Neck stretches, 402
Necrotizing ulcerative gingivitis, 296, 296f
Needle
    breakage of, 545
    recapping of, 536–537
Negative aspiration, 536
Negative feedback mechanism, 664
Negligence, 11
Nerve block anesthesia
    anterior superior alveolar nerve,
        538–539, 543t
    description of, 527, 528f

greater palatine nerve, 539f, 539–540, 543t
incisive nerve, 541–542, 542f, 544t
inferior alveolar nerve, 540f, 540–541, 544t
infraorbital nerve, 539, 543t
mental nerve, 541–542, 542f, 544t
middle superior alveolar nerve,
    538–539, 543t
nasopalatine nerve, 540, 540f, 543t
posterior superior alveolar nerve, 538f,
    538–539, 543t
Nervous system, 755
Networking, 837t
Neurofibrillary tangles, 757
Neurological impairments
    amyotrophic lateral sclerosis, 649–650
    Bell palsy, 650–651
    categories of, 647, 648f
    cerebral palsy, 651–652
    definition of, 647
    future increases in, 647
    Huntington disease, 652–653
    myasthenia gravis, 653–654
    Parkinson disease, 654–656
    prevalence of, 647
    stroke, 656–658
Neurological system, health history review
    of, 136t
Neuromuscular junction (NMJ), 676
Neutral pelvic position, 398
New Freedom Initiative, 774t
Niacin, 598t
Nicotinic acetylcholine receptors, 676
Nightguard, 376t, 377f
Nitrates, 601, 602t
Nitroglycerin, 810t
Nitrous oxide
    properties of, 515
    sedation using. See Nitrous oxide/oxygen
        sedation
    trace, 521
Nitrous oxide/oxygen sedation
    administration of, 520–521
    armamentarium for
        disinfection of, 521
        flowmeter, 516–517, 517f, 520
        portable unit, 516, 516f
        reservoir bag, 517, 517f
        scavenging nasal hood, 517, 517f
        sterilization of, 521
    in asthmatic patients, 615
    best practices for, 522
    biohazard risks, 521
    case study of, 522–523
    chronic obstructive pulmonary disease as
        contraindication for, 514
    contraindications for, 514–515
    ethical responsibilities, 519, 522
    expectations of, 518–519
    gas properties, 515
    goal of, 518
    hospital use of, 514
    indications for, 514
    informed consent for, 519, 522
    legal responsibilities, 519
    overview of, 513
    patient monitoring during, 520
    pregnancy contraindications for, 514
    preoperative assessment, 519, 519f
    risk assessment, 519
    signs and symptoms of, 518–519
    in special-needs patients, 586

standards of care for, 522
titration of, 518, 520, 522
trace gas minimization, 521–522
vomiting concerns, 518
NK cells. See Natural killer cells
No-shows, 829–830
Nocebo effect, 504, 505b
Nodule, 176t
Noise-induced hearing loss, 627, 628f
Non-nutritive habits, 727, 730t
Nonblinded study, 74
Noncarious lesions, 223–224
Noncritical instruments and
    equipment, 107t
Nonionizing radiation, 263
Nonmaleficence
    beneficence versus, 15
    definition of, 14t
    description of, 10, 15
    example of, 14t
Nonscreen analog x-ray film, 259, 261–262
Nonsteroidal anti-inflammatory drugs, 762
Nonsurgical periodontal therapy
    bacteria after, 435
    definition of, 417
    goal of, 433–434
    lasers, 437–438
    local drug delivery, 435t, 435–437
    multi-appointment sequence for, 556
    periodontal healing after, 434–435
    periodontal health benefits of, 417
    perioscopy, 438f, 438–440
    systemic antibiotics, 437, 439
Nonverbal communication, 26–27
Nose
    examination of, 178
    health history review of, 131t
Nosocomial infections, 613
Nosocomial pneumonia, 63–64, 613
Nutrient imbalance
    conditions associated with, 285t
    malnutrition and, 271. See also
        Malnutrition
    oral manifestations associated with,
        271–272
Nutrition status assessment, 138
Nutritional counseling
    for caries-prone individuals, 348
    in children, 731t
    communication skills used in,
        275–276, 276f
    dental hygienist's role in, 274, 353
    dietary improvements with, 274
    goals of, 558
    objectives of, 278b
    Oral Health Evaluation form used in,
        276t–277t

O

Obesity
    in children, 140
    oral disease risks, 296
    prevalence of, 140
Obturator, 376t
Occlusal force, 390
Occlusal radiographs, 257, 257f
Occlusion, 727f. See also Malocclusion
    alveolar bone resorption caused by trauma
        to, 202
    analysis of, 224–225, 225f

centric, 227
considerations for, 227
examination of, 184t
Occupation history, 139
Occupational exposures
    to hepatitis, 702–703
    to HIV/AIDS, 703
Occupational Safety and Health
        Administration (OSHA)
    Bloodborne Pathogens standard, 112
    description of, 93, 94t
    Hazard Communication Standard, 113
    hepatitis B vaccination
        recommendations, 702
    record-keeping requirements of, 112
Odds ratio, 292
Odontoblasts, 449
Odontogram, 554
Office waste management plan, 108
Oils, 281t–282t
Olanzapine, 642t
Older adults. *See* Elderly
O'Leary Plaque Record, 554, 556–557
Olmstead v. L.C., 582, 774t
Onlay, 476
Opaque sealants, 365
Open bite, 226, 226f, 728f
Open-ended dialogue/questions
    description of, 28, 829
    example of, 29t
    in motivational interviewing, 30–31
Open flap therapy, 441–442
Open-label study, 74
Operator stool, 397–399
Operatory, exercises in, 401–404, 402f–404f
Ophthalmic nerve, 527–528, 528
Opportunistic infections, 86, 380
Opportunistic pathogens, 58
Optimization principle, 255
Oral and maxillofacial pathologist
        referral, 559t
Oral and maxillofacial pathology. *See also*
        specific pathology
    acquired, 168
    congenital, 168
    definition of, 168
    developmental, 168–170, 169f
    reactive lesions, 170f–171f, 170–172
Oral and maxillofacial radiologist
        referral, 559t
Oral and maxillofacial surgeon referral, 559t
Oral appliances
    complications associated with, 383–384
    definition of, 375
    dental hygiene considerations for,
        376–378
    disinfection of, 381t
    patient education about, 378
    plaque biofilm formation on, 375
    professional cleaning of, 380–383
    removable, 375
    self-care of, 378
    types of, 376t
Oral cancer. *See also* Cancer
    age of patient and, 297
    demographics of, 714–715
    description of, 712–713
    in elderly, 766–767
    human papillomavirus and, 714t, 714–715
    incidence of, 168, 172–176, 766
    information resources for survivors of, 716b

metastasis of, 713
morbidity and mortality associated
        with, 715
multidisciplinary team approach to,
        707, 718
prevalence of, 297b
risk factors for, 766
screening for, 183t, 685, 713
self-examination for, 714b
signs and symptoms of, 714b
squamous cell carcinoma. *See* Oral
        squamous cell carcinoma (OSCC)
survival rates for, 713
treatment
    of oral complications caused by, 716–718
    overview of, 715–716
    planning strategies for, 718
    vital dye staining for, 183t, 184
Oral candidiasis, 615
Oral cavity
    bacteria in, 593, 611
    hard deposits in, 233–235. *See also*
        Calculus
    malodor from, 232, 337
    pH of, 347
    respiratory pathogens in, 611, 613
    soft deposits in
        acquired pellicle, 231
        biofilm, 231–232
        food debris, 232
        materia alba, 232
    visual inspection of, 180, 180f
Oral contraceptives, 739
Oral diseases
    cardiovascular diseases and, 60–61
    diabetes mellitus and, 61–63
    local contributing factors, 294, 294f
    malignancies as cause of, 375
    respiratory diseases and, 611–612
    risk assessment indices for, 249–250
    risk factors for
        bacteria, 294, 294b
        biofilm, 294
        bleeding, 293–294
        diabetes mellitus, 294–295
        immunosuppression, 296, 296f
        local contributing factors, 294, 294f
        medications, 296
        modifiable, 291–296
        obesity, 296
        oral health status, 293–294
        osteoporosis, 295
        smoking, 292f–293f, 292–293
        tobacco use, 292f–293f, 292–293
    systemic diseases and, connection
        between, 60–64, 560
Oral health
    alcohol effects on, 639
    benefits of, 737
    definition of, 567
    dietary risk factors that affect, 271–273
    in elderly, 48
    Healthy People 2020 objectives for, 43
    hearing loss and, 630
    long-term, 32
    oral disease risks and, correlation
        between, 293–294
    physician's participation in, 352
    risk assessment benefits for, 298
    socioeconomic status and, 235
    systemic diseases and, 60–64, 296, 555f

systemic health and, 567, 593–595
traditional education approaches to, 30–31
Oral health care
    access to, 42, 139, 351, 791
    barriers to, 773, 775, 791
    direct access to, 791
    financial barriers to, 773, 775
    interdisciplinary collaboration in, 59
    public health/safety net arena delivery
        of, 16
    teamwork in, 59
Oral Health Evaluation, 276t–277t
Oral Health Information Suite, 194
Oral health-related quality of life model, 3
Oral history, 130, 137t–138t
Oral hygiene
    assessment of, 197t, 204
    in children, 730t
    extrinsic stains caused by lack of, 236
    indices that measure, 244t, 244–246
    nosocomial pneumonia risk reductions
        with, 63
Oral hygiene index, 244, 244t–245t
Oral mucosa, 765
Oral mucositis, 701, 710t–712t, 710–711, 711
Oral pathology, 555
Oral prostheses. *See* Prostheses
Oral sedation, in special-needs patients,
        585–587
Oral squamous cell carcinoma (OSCC)
    alcohol use and, 172, 297
    appearance of, 173f–174f, 173–174
    demographics of, 172
    diagnosis of, 174–175, 175f
    dysplasia versus, 175
    grading of, 175
    histologic appearance of, 175f
    human papillomavirus and, 172–173
    illustration of, 172f
    in situ, 175
    metastasis of, 175
    prognosis for, 175–176
    risk factors for, 172–173, 297b, 568
    sites of, 713
    staging of, 175, 176b
    TNM staging of, 175, 176b
    in tongue, 713, 713f
Oral thermometer, 142
Orange stain, 236t
Oraqix, 533–534
Ordinal scale, for indices, 243
Organ transplantation, 686
Organization for Safety and Asepsis Protocol
        (OSAP), 94, 94t, 100
Organizations, professional, 5
Oropharyngeal cancer, 168
Orthodontic aligner, 376t, 377f
Orthodontic appliances
    air polishing of, 468t
    oral disease risks, 294, 295f
Orthodontist referral, 559t
Orthopnea, 144
Orthostatic hypotension, 146
Osseointegration, 384–386, 387f, 573
Ossicles, 756
Osteoblasts, 756, 763
Osteoclasts, 756, 763
Osteonecrosis of the jaw, bisphosphonate-
        related, 295, 716–717, 742–743,
        761t, 763
Osteopenia, 742

Osteoplasty, 442
Osteoporosis, 132t, 295, 742–743, 761t, 763
Osteoradionecrosis, 716–717, 743–744
Osteotomy, 442
Outcome evaluation, 76
Ovaries, 665
Over-the-counter whitening products, 480
Overbite, 226f–227f, 226–227
Overdentures
    abutment systems for, 386
    definition of, 386
    implant-supported lingual bar for, 380
Overgloves, 97
Overjet, 227, 227f
Oxcarbazepine, 643t
Oxygen. *See also* Nitrous oxide/oxygen
        sedation
    delivery systems for, 806–807, 808t
    properties of, 515
Oxytocin, 664

P

p value, 75
Pacemakers, 597
Packaging, of instruments, 104
Pain
    fear of, 493
    low back, 396
    paroxysmal, 680
Pain management
    in dental fear and anxiety management,
        505–506
    hypnosis for, 505
    local anesthetics for, 529–530
    in oral mucositis, 711t
Palatal papillomatosis, 170–171
Palatal torus, 170
Palate, 182, 182f, 184t
Palliative, 675
Palmer notation, 217
Palpation
    of alveolar process, 184t
    of alveolar ridge, 182, 182f
    of anterior midline, 179, 179f, 183t
    of auricular regions, 178, 178f, 183t
    of buccal mucosa, 177, 177f, 180,
        180f, 184t
    extraoral, 177, 177f
    of floor of mouth, 181–182, 182f, 184t
    of lips, 180, 180f, 184t
    of parotid gland, 178, 178f, 183t
    of pharynx, 184t
    of posterior triangles, 179, 180f
    of sternocleidomastoid muscle, 179,
        179f, 184t
    of submandibular triangle, 178–179,
        179f, 183t
    of submental triangle, 179, 179f, 183t
    of temporomandibular joint, 178,
        178f, 183t
    of thyroid cartilage, 179, 179f
    of tongue, 181, 181f
    of tonsils, 182, 184t
Pancreas, 665
Panoramic radiographs, 568
Pantomographs, 257–258, 258f
Papilla, 193, 193f
Papillary hyperplasia of the palate, 170
Papoose boards, 587
Papule, 176t

Parafunctional oral habits, 450, 451b
Paralysis, 787
Paraplegia, 787
Parasympathetic nervous system, 494–495
Parathormone, 664
Parathyroid glands, 664
Parathyroid hormone, 668
Paresis, 785
Paresthesia, 174, 542, 544
Parkinson disease (PD), 654–656, 761t, 763
Parotid gland
    palpation of, 178, 178f, 183t
    swelling of, in Sjögren syndrome, 675, 675f
Paroxetine, 642t
Paroxysmal pain syndromes, 680
Partial participation, 729
Partial thromboplastin time (PTT), 692–693
Particulate radiation, 255
Particulate respirator mask (PRM), 96
Passive immunity, 56
Passive immunization, 87
Patent ductus arteriosus, 603–604, 604f
Paternalism, 42
Paternalistic care, 13
Pathology report, 187
Patient
    advocacy for, 549
    eyewear for, 96, 96f
    health-care provider and, relationship
        between, 16, 18
    withholding of information by, 29
Patient care area
    cleaning of, 100
    clinical contact surfaces in, 100, 100t
    dental radiograph equipment,
        100–101, 101f
    disinfection of, 100
    housekeeping surfaces in, 100, 100t
    infection control in, 99t, 99–103
    surface barriers in, 100, 100f
Patient compliance
    dental insurance effects on, 569
    with maintenance schedule, 568
    with treatment, 556
Patient education
    dentures, 384
    esthetic restorations, 479–480
    interdental cleaning, 330, 479
    oral appliances, 378
    periodontal disease, 58
    plan, for dentin hypersensitivity, 454b,
        454–455
    prostheses, 378, 384
    tooth whitening, 482, 484
Patient history. *See also* Dental history;
        Health history; Medical history
    evaluation of, 554
    importance of, 123–127
    role of, 123–127
Patient interview
    communication in, 554
    dental anxiety and fear assessments,
        496–498
    description of, 123–124
Patient records, 314
Pedagogy, 843
Pediatric dentistry. *See also* Children;
        Infant(s)
    anticipatory guidance benefits of, 724,
        730t–731t
    aspects of, 723–725

dental hygienist's role in, 724–725
    evolution of, 723
    goals of, 723
    surgical model versus medical model of,
        723, 723t
Pedodontist referral, 559t
Peer pressure, 48
Peer review, 561
Pellicle formation, 231
People-first language, 581, 776, 777t
Perceived severity, 45–46
Perceived susceptibility, 45–46
Perceived value of treatment, 827, 831
Peri-implant assessment, 203–204, 204f
Peri-implant disease, 387
Peri-implant mucositis, 387, 389
Peri-implantitis, 197t, 203, 387, 573
Periapical radiographs, 255–256, 256f
PerioChip, 435, 435t, 574t
Periodontal care, 827
Periodontal chart. *See also* Dental charting;
        Dental charts
    definition of, 208
    digital, 208, 211f
    illustration of, 570f
    maintenance appointment assessment of,
        570, 570f
    periodontal examination findings charted
        on, 208, 208t–211t
Periodontal debridement
    definition of, 417–418, 433
    instrumentation used in, 439
    periodontal health benefits of, 417
Periodontal defects, 440
Periodontal diagnosis, 555
Periodontal disease index (PDI), 248
Periodontal disease (PD). *See also* Gingivitis;
        Periodontitis
    bacteria associated with, 232, 294, 294b
    cardiovascular diseases and, 60–61,
        594–595
    characteristics of, 206
    classification of, 206t–207t, 206–208
    definition of, 197t
    description of, 55
    in diabetes mellitus patients, 62–63,
        294–295
    dietary recommendations for, 272
    in elderly, 767
    features of, 57
    innate susceptibility to, 57
    maternal, 64
    pathogenesis of, 57–60
    patient adherence as risk factor for, 58
    patient education about, 58
    peri-implantitis, 197t, 203
    in physically impaired patients, 778t
    in pregnancy, 64, 297, 740
    preterm low birth weight associated
        with, 64
    refractory, 207
    risk assessment tools for, 59
    risk factors for
        age, 297
        description of, 57–58, 592f
        diabetes mellitus, 62–63, 294–295, 569
        genetics, 297–298
        history of disease as, 298
        list of, 572b
        nonmodifiable, 297–298, 569
        obesity, 296

osteoporosis, 295–296, 742
plaque, 570
race, 297
sex, 297
smoking, 58, 292f, 292–293, 558, 569
stress and, 139
systemic diseases and, 55, 60–64, 296, 433
treatment of
nonsurgical. *See* Nonsurgical periodontal therapy
overview of, 433
surgical. *See* Periodontal surgery
types of, 433, 827
in women of childbearing age, 739
Periodontal examination
adjunctive techniques, 205–206
case study of, 212
charting of findings of, 208, 208t–211t
comprehensive
bleeding on probing, 196t, 200, 200f, 209t
clinical attachment level, 196t, 200–201, 201f
contributing factors, 197t, 198t, 204
elements of, 195–196
free gingival margin level, 196t, 200, 201f, 210t
fremitus, 197t, 202–203, 203f, 211t
frenum pull, 210t
furcation involvement, 196t, 201, 209t
gingival description, 196t, 198–199, 199t, 208t
instruments and materials for, 196
mucogingival defects, 197t, 203
mucogingival junction, 193, 193f, 210t
oral hygiene assessment, 197t, 204
overview of, 195–196
peri-implantitis, 197t, 203
probing depths, 196t, 199–200, 200f, 208t
procedure for, 196, 196t–197t, 198–204
radiographs, 197t
suppuration, 197t, 202, 209t
tooth mobility, 197t, 202f, 202–203, 210t
description of, 194
genetic tests, 206
gingival crevicular fluid biochemical assays, 205
medical history used in, 204
microbiological testing, 205
periodontal risk assessment, 194–195
periodontal screening and recording, 195, 195t
radiographs, 204–205
subgingival temperature, 205–206
summary of, 208
Periodontal healing, 440
Periodontal index, 249
Periodontal ligament
anatomy of, 191f, 193, 193f
fiber groups of, 194t
Periodontal ligament space, 259, 260f, 678
Periodontal maintenance, 445, 573
Periodontal medicine, 55
Periodontal probe
description of, 160–162, 161f
junctional epithelium puncture by, 200
Periodontal prognosis, 557
Periodontal regeneration, 440
Periodontal risk assessment
description of, 194–195
in special-needs patients, 585–586

Periodontal scoring and recording (PSR) index, 249
Periodontal screening and recording (PSR), 195, 195t
Periodontal screening examination, 248
Periodontal surgery
complications of, 442
dental hygiene considerations, 444–445
dressings used in, 442, 444
flap procedures, 441–442
gingivectomy, 441
goals of, 440–441
guided tissue regeneration, 442–443
modified Widman flap, 441–442
open flap, 441–442
regenerative, 442
repositioned flap, 442
surgical pack, 442, 443f–444f
sutures, 442, 444
Periodontal therapy
goal of, 433
hemoglobin A1c reductions after, 62
maintenance visits, 445
nonsurgical. *See* Nonsurgical periodontal therapy
nosocomial pneumonia risk reductions with, 63
in pregnancy, 64
surgical. *See* Periodontal surgery
Periodontal tips, for power scaling devices, 411, 411f
Periodontist referral, 559t, 572b
Periodontitis
atherosclerotic cardiovascular diseases risks, 61
B cells in, 60
chronic, 198f, 206
definition of, 206
diabetes mellitus and, 61, 295
in elderly, 767
enzymes associated with, 205
immune response genes in, 57
malnutrition and, 272
maternal, 64, 740–741
metabolic syndrome associated with, 62
pathogenesis of, 57
plasma cells in, 60
in pregnancy, 740–741
risk factors for, 58
Periodontium
alveolar bone, 191f, 193–194
anatomy of, 191f–193f, 191–194
cementum, 191f, 193
description of, 191
gingiva. *See* Gingiva
indices for assessing, 247–249
landmarks of, 193f
malnutrition signs on, 272t
periodontal ligament, 191f, 193, 193f, 194t
radiographic evaluation of, 204–205
sex hormones effect on, 738
Periodontology, 440–441
PerioPredict Genetic Test, 59
Perioscopy, 438f, 438–440
Periosteum, 194
Periostogingival fibers, 192t
Peripheral giant cell granuloma, 171
Peripheral ossifying fibroma, 170–172, 171f
Peristalsis, 755

Permanent teeth
description of, 726, 727t
numbering systems for, 217, 218f
Permucosal seal, 387
Pernicious anemia, 699
Personal distance, 26f, 26–27
Personal protective equipment (PPE)
clothing, 95, 95f
description of, 93
eyewear, 95f–96f, 95–96
face shields, 96, 97f
gloves, 96–99, 98f
gowns, 95, 95f
illustration of, 95f–98f
instrument transportation using, 103
masks, 96, 96f
Personal psychosocial history, 138–139
Personal space
cultural differences in, 27
levels of, 26f–27f, 26–27
Pervasive developmental disorders, 635–636
Petechiae, 697
Peyer patches, 56, 56f
pH, 531
Phagocytes, 674
Pharmacokinetics, 530–531
Pharynx
inspection of, 181f
palpation of, 184t
squamous cell carcinoma of, 172
Phentolamine mesylate, 585
Photophobia, 650
Photopolymerized sealants, 365
Photostimulable phosphor plates, 259–260, 262, 262f
Physical disability, 582t
Physical impairments
barrier-free architectural designs, 775
caregiver teaching, 781–782
classification of, 776
communication considerations, 776–777, 777t
definition of, 773
dental hygiene appointment, 777, 778t–780t, 780–782
in elderly, 751
etiology of
congenital conditions, 785
cystic fibrosis, 776, 776t, 784–785
developmental conditions, 785
muscular dystrophy, 776, 776t, 784, 784t
spina bifida, 785
spinal cord injury, 787
spinal muscular atrophy, 785
traumatic brain injury, 786–787
etiquette considerations for, 776–777
health-care access barriers, 773, 774–775
historical perspective on, 773, 774t
medications commonly used in patients with, 786t
oral characteristics of patients with, 778t
oral hygiene care in, 780
physical contact for, 777
prevalence of, 773
primitive reflexes in patients with, 779t
teaching of patients, 780
toothbrush modifications in patients, 781, 781f
wheelchair
etiquette for, 777
transfer from, 779t, 782–784

Physician
in pediatric oral health, 352
referral to, 560t
of special-needs patients, 584
Physiological aging, 754–757
PICO format, 72–73, 73f, 845
Piercings, 727
Piezoelectric power scaling devices, 409, 409f
Pigtail explorer, 160t, 233
Pineal gland, 663f–664f, 663–664
Pits and fissures
caries in, 365
sealant placement in, 366–367, 367f
Pituitary gland
anatomy of, 663f–664f, 663–664
diseases of, 667–669
Pituitary tumors, 667
Pivoting, 421
Placebo effect, 500
Plagiarism, 78, 78t
Planning, in dental hygiene process of
care, 4, 47
Plaque
indices of, 244t, 244–246, 554, 557
maintenance appointment evaluation
of, 570
in vision-impaired patients, 626
Plaque Assessment Scoring System (PASS),
554, 557
Plaque biofilm
calculus as, 204
description of, 57
on oral appliances, 375
Plaque biofilm index, 197t, 204
Plaque (brain), 757
Plaque control record, 197t, 204, 244t,
244–245, 245f, 570
Plaque Index, 197t, 204
Plaque (skin lesion), 176t
Plasma cells, 60, 674
Plasmapheresis, 676
Platelet count, 692t
Platelets
bone marrow formation of, 691
in clotting, 692f
Plavix, 694, 697t
Pleurisy, 680
Pneumonia
aspiration, 63, 759
nosocomial, 63–64, 613
Pocket depth, 199, 200f, 250, 328t, 441, 827
Polishing
abrasive agents used in, 461–462, 462t
air, 468f, 468t, 468–471, 573
case study of, 470
esthetic restorations, 479
finishing strips used in, 462
at maintenance appointment, 573
manual, 463t, 463–464
Porte polisher, 463–465
power, 465–468, 466t
purpose of, 461
restorations, 463
selective, 461
stains treated with, 461
therapeutic, 462
Polycarbonate lenses, 96
Polycythemia, 701
Polymerization, 365
Polymorphonuclear neutrophils
(PMNs), 58–59

Polypharmacy, 657
Polysaccharides, 231, 346
Pontic, 379
Porcelain
description of, 463
glazed, 479
Porcelain-fused-to-metal crown, 476
Porcelain veneer, 476–478
Porphyromonas gingivalis, 595
Portable units, 792
Porte polisher, 463–465
Positive aspiration, 536
Positive feedback mechanism, 664
Positive reinforcement, 728
Post-cardiovascular surgery, 605–606
Posterior crossbite, 225, 226f
Posterior pharyngeal wall, 182
Posterior sickle scalers, 423, 424f
Posterior superior alveolar nerve (PSA)
anatomy of, 528
anesthetic block of, 538f, 538–539, 543t
hematoma at injection site for, 542
Posterior teeth
complex shanks for, 418
universal curets for, 425, 426b
Posterior triangles, 179, 180f
Postexposure prophylaxis, for HIV exposure,
86, 87t
Postherpetic neuralgia, 90
Postpartum care, 742
Posture
anteverted pelvis and, 398
tips for improving, 399–400
unhealthy types of, 396, 397t
Potassium-containing dentifrices, 455
Potassium nitrate, 456
Potassium oxalates, 456
Povidone-iodine, 668
Power/distance, as cultural dimension,
33, 34t
*Power of Habit: Why We Do What We Do in Life
and Business, The* (Duhigg), 49
Power polishing, 465–468, 466t
Power scaling
biofilm removal using, 377, 378f
procedure for, 412–413
Power scaling devices
advantages for, 410
amplitude of, 410
care and maintenance of, 413
contraindications for, 410–411
definition of, 409
disadvantages for, 410
indications for, 410
lavage control feature of, 410
magnetostrictive, 409, 409f–410f
mechanism of action, 409
microultrasonic instruments, 413–414
piezoelectric, 409, 409f
sonic scalers, 409
tips used by, 410f–411f, 410–412
types of, 409–413
ultrasonic scalers, 409f, 409–411
Power toothbrushes, 319–321, 321f,
597, 766
Pradaxa, 697t
Pravastatin, 598t
Prayer, 504
Preconception counseling, 739–740
Preferred provider organization
(PPO), 825

Pregnancy, 64–65
adverse outcomes of, 740
cytomegalovirus exposure prevention
during, 90
dental hygiene during, 741
epulis gravidarum during, 741
gastroesophageal reflux disease during, 739
gingivitis during, 740
health history review, 135t
medications during, 741–742, 742t
nitrous oxide/oxygen sedation
contraindications in, 514
oral care during, 741
periodontal disease during, 64, 297, 740
periodontitis in, 740–741
postpartum care, 742
radiation safety during, 266
radiographs during, 741
supine hypotensive syndrome in, 741
Pregnancy tumor, 172
Premature ventricular contractions (PVCs), 597
Premedication, 148, 150, 584, 601t, 605
Premolars, 727t
Presbycusis, 756
Presbyopia, 756
Preschool stage, 725t
Prescription-strength dentifrices and
mouthrinses, 338
Preservatives, in dentifrices, 336
Prevacuum steam sterilizers, 106
Prevalence, 292
Preventive services
caries. *See* Caries, prevention of
Healthy People 2020 objectives for, 43
PreViser analytic software, 59
Prevotella intermedia, 740
Prilocaine, 532t
Primary biliary cirrhosis, 737
Primary dentition, 725–726, 726t
Primary hemostasis, 595f
Primary prevention, 86
Primary progressive multiple sclerosis, 679
Primary research, 74–75
Primary sclerosing cholangitis, 737
Primary teeth, numbering systems for,
217, 218f
Primate spacing, 227
Primitive reflexes, 779t
Print on palm, 631
Prisons, 798
Privacy Rule, of HIPAA, 16, 17t
Private homes, 797
Probe
furcation, 160–163, 161f–162f, 163t,
201, 201f
periodontal, 160–162, 161f
Probing
around implants, 390
bleeding on, 196t, 200, 200f, 209t, 390,
570, 570f
depths in, 196t, 199–200, 200f, 208t, 573
Procedural analysis, 828
Process of care. *See* Dental hygiene process
of care
Prodromal stage, 85
Professional
discipline, 3
liability insurance, 12
negligence, 11
organizations, 5, 847–848
publications, 837t

Professionalism
  benefits of, 831
  in dental fear patients, 492
  esthetic dentistry and, 484–485
  evaluation and, 561
  lifelong learning as part of, 127
Progesterone, 665, 738–739
Prognosis, 556–557
Progressive muscle relaxation, 502, 503b
Progressive relapsing multiple
    sclerosis, 679
Prophy angle, 465, 465f
Prophy pastes, 461, 462t, 465f, 466–467, 478
Prophylaxis, 573
Prospective cohort study, 74
Prostate cancer, 744
Prostate diseases, 744–745
Prostate-specific antigen, 744
Prostheses
  complications associated with, 383–384
  daily care of, 384
  definition of, 375
  dental hygiene considerations for, 376–378
  disinfection of, 381t
  fixed, 376, 377f
  fixed partial denture, 379, 379f
  implant-supported, 386, 386f, 388
  patient education about, 378, 384
  professional cleaning of, 380–383
  removable, 375, 377, 380–383
  removable partial denture, 380
  self-care of, 378–379
  types of, 375, 376t
Prosthetic heart valves, 133t, 604
Prosthodontist referral, 560t
Protease, 683
Protected health information (PHI)
  description of, 16
  disclosure of, 18
  identifiers for, 16, 17t
  patient access to, 16, 18
  Security Rule provisions for, 18
Protective stabilization, 729
Protein foods, 281t–282t
Protein precipitants, 453t, 454
Prothrombin time (PT), 604–605, 692–693
Protrusion, 728f
Proxemics
  description of, 26f–27f, 26–27
  in nonverbal communication, 26, 27f
  in verbal communication, 25
Pseudomonas aeruginosa, 784–785
Pseudopocket, 200
PSR probe, 161f
Psychiatric conditions, 137t
Psychosocial disability, 582t
Psychosocial history, 138–139
Ptosis, 654
Puberty, 738
Public distance, 26f, 27
Public health settings, 5
Pulp cavity, 450f
Pulp testing, 227
Pulsating oral irrigator, 327f–329f, 327–330
Pulse assessment, 143–144
Pulse oximeter, 613, 613f, 615
Punch biopsy, 186
Pupil dilation, 178
Purified protein derivative, 617–618
Purkinje fibers, 593, 593f
Pustule, 176t

Pyogenic granuloma, 172
Pyridostigmine, 676

Q

Quadriceps stretch, 404, 404f
Quadriplegia, 787
Qualitative evaluation, 557
Quality assurance, 561
Quantitative evaluation, 557–558
Quantitative light-induced fluorescence, 353
Quaternary ammonium, 110–111
Questions
  closed-ended, 29t, 29–30
  open-ended, 28, 29t
Quetiapine, 642t
Quigley-Hein Plaque Index (QHPI), 244t, 246
Quitlines, for smoking cessation, 708
QunatiFERON-TB Gold test, 91

R

Race, periodontal disease risks based on, 297
Radial artery, for pulse assessment, 143
Radiation
  ionizing. *See* Ionizing radiation
  nonionizing, 263
  operator exposure to, 264
  quality-assurance program for, 266
  safety considerations for, 266
  types of, 255
Radiation therapy-associated complications
  candidiasis, 711–712
  caries, 717
  description of, 701
  dysgeusia, 712
  osteoradionecrosis, 716–717, 743–744
  temporomandibular joint dysfunction,
    717–718
  tissue necrosis, 717
Radiographs
  ALARA principle for, 182, 255
  bitewing, 256–257, 257f, 352,
    357t–358t, 568
  calculus on, 259t
  cancellous bone on, 259t
  caries detection using, 352, 357t
  case study of, 266–267
  cementum on, 259t
  complete mouth radiographic series, 257
  contrast of, 258, 258f
  cortical bone on, 259t
  definition of, 255
  density of, 258, 259f
  dental follicle on, 259, 260f
  dental implant assessments, 388
  dentin on, 258, 260f
  enamel on, 260f
  evaluation of, 555
  extraoral, 256–258, 258f
  history of, 256
  of implants, 388, 573
  indications for, 265t
  intraoral, 256f–257f, 256–257
  justification principle for, 255
  lateral cephalometric skull, 258, 258f
  at maintenance visit, 568
  normal appearances on, 258–259, 260f
  occlusal, 257, 257f
  operator exposure to, 264
  optimization principle for, 255

  panoramic, 568
  pantomographs, 257–258, 258f
  periapical, 255–256, 256f
  in periodontal examination, 197t
  of periodontium, 204–205
  in pregnancy, 741
  prescription of, 264–266, 265t
  radiolucencies on, 258, 259t
  radiopacities on, 258, 259t
  root formation on, 259, 261f
  screening uses of, 182
  terminology associated with, 256–259
Radiography
  computed, 259–260, 261t, 262, 262f
  digital, 228, 259–260, 261t, 262–263, 263f
Radiolucencies, 258, 259t
Radiopacities, 258, 259t
Radiopaque, 258
"Ramfjord teeth," 246
Randomization, 74
Randomized controlled trial, 74
Rapport, 500, 557, 561
Raynaud phenomenon, 677–679
Reactive lesions, 170f–171f, 170–172
Record keeping, 112
Recrudescence, 89
Recurrent caries, 351
Red blood cell disorders
  anemia. *See* Anemia
  celiac sprue, 700
  polycythemia, 701
Red stain, 236t
Reevaluation, 557–558
Reference citation, 77, 77t
Referrals, 558–561, 559t–560t, 572, 572b
Refined carbohydrates, 347
Reflective listening, 31–32, 32b
Refractory, 207
Refusal of treatment
  by children, 728f
  description of, 13, 42, 313
  informed refusal, 42, 313, 378, 572
Regenerative periodontal surgery, 442
Registered dental hygienist (RDH), 3
Registered Dental Hygienists in Alternative
    Practice (RDHAP), 462, 791–792,
    797, 847
Registered dietitian, 560t
Regulated medical waste, 108, 112
Regulatory T cells, 60
Regurgitation, 604
Rehabilitation Act of 1973, 774t
Relapsing/remitting multiple sclerosis, 679
Relative contraindication, 542
Relative risk, 292
Relaxation response, 501
Relaxation techniques
  focused attention, 503–504
  guided imagery, 503, 504b
  guided relaxation, 503, 504b
  overview of, 501–502
  patient preparation for, 502, 502b
Reliability, 76, 241–242
Remineralization, 348, 462
Removable partial denture
  cleaning of, 381–383
  dental charting symbols for, 220t
  description of, 380
  patient education about, 384
Renin-angiotensin-aldosterone system, 599t
Repositioned flap, 442

Rescue breathing, 805, 805t
Research
    amount of, 71
    basic, 74–75
    immune system, 57
    primary, 74–75
    secondary, 75
Research databases, 75, 75t
Researchers, dental hygienists as, 5
Reservoir bag, for nitrous oxide/oxygen
        sedation, 517, 517f
Residual, 110
Resins, for dentin hypersensitivity, 456
Resolvins, 58
Respiration, 144
Respiration rate, 144
Respiratory diseases
    acute, 612
    asthma, 614, 614f, 614t–615t, 616b
    chronic, 612
    chronic obstructive pulmonary disease,
        615–617
    cystic fibrosis, 617
    description of, 612–613
    oral diseases and, 611–612
    prevention of, 611
    stress effects on, 612
    symptoms of, 612b
    tuberculosis. See Tuberculosis
Respiratory failure, 813t
Respiratory infections
    acute, 613, 613b
    in dental hygienists, 613
    description of, 63–64
Respiratory system
    age-related changes of, 754–755
    anatomy of, 611, 611f
    health history review of, 133t–134t
    lower, 611
    physiology of, 515
    upper, 611
Respondeat superior, 12
Restorations
    after caries treatment, 345
    composite, 478
    by dental hygienists, 799
    endodontic, 221
    glass-ionomer, 478–479
    implant-supported, 386, 386f, 389
    oral disease risks, 294, 294f
    polishing of, 463
    tooth whitening effects on, 483
Restorative materials
    dentin hypersensitivity treated with, 457
    fluoride-releasing, 350
    glass ionomer, 457
    porcelain, 463
    radiographic imaging of, 257
Restriction devices, for special-needs
        patients, 587
Resume writing, 838
Retaining appliance, 376t, 377f
Retraction, mouth mirrors for, 155, 156f, 157
Retroauricular palpation, 178f
Retrospective cohort study, 74
Reversible indices, 243
Review-of-systems approach, to health
        history, 127, 128f–129f, 131t–137t
Rheostat, 465, 465f
Rheumatic heart disease (RHD), 600–601
Rheumatism, 132t

Rheumatoid arthritis (RA), 675, 680–681
Rhodium, 157
Right angle design explorer, 160t
Rinses, mouth, 109
Risk, 194, 291
Risk assessment
    cardiovascular diseases, 122
    caries
        in children, 727
        description of, 250, 354–355,
            355t–358t, 366
        in special-needs patients, 585
    case study of, 299–300
    definition of, 291
    health history used in. See Health history
    at maintenance visit, 568
    nitrous oxide/oxygen sedation, 519
    oral disease, 249–250, 568
    oral health improvements through, 298
    periodontal
        description of, 194–195
        in special-needs patients, 585–586
    periodontal disease, 59
    before sealant placement, 366
    system for, 149t–150t
    systematic approach to, 298, 299t
    teamwork involved in, 298
    technological advances in, 298
Risk factors
    for atherosclerosis, 598
    for cancer, 708, 709b
    for cardiovascular disease, 592, 592f
    care plan based on, 567
    for caries, 231, 355, 366, 574
    definition of, 55, 291
    for diabetes mellitus, 63, 294–295
    evaluation of, 557
    for hypertension, 599
    modifiable
        bacteria, 294, 294b
        biofilm, 294
        bleeding, 293–294
        definition of, 291–292
        diabetes mellitus, 294–295
        immunosuppression, 296, 296f
        local contributing factors, 294, 294f
        medications, 296
        modifiable, 291–296
        obesity, 296
        oral health status, 293–294
        osteoporosis, 295
        smoking, 292f–293f, 292–293
        tobacco use, 292f–293f, 292–293
    nonmodifiable, 292, 297–298, 569, 656
    for periodontal disease. See Periodontal
        disease, risk factors for
    types of, 55
Risk indicator, 292, 347
Risk management, 12
Risk marker, 292
RiskCalculator, 194
Risperidone, 642t
Rolling stroke tooth-brushing method, 323t
Rollnick, Steven, 30
Röntgen, Wilhelm, 256
Root
    anatomy of, 450f
    exposure of, 457
    radiographic imaging of, 259, 261f
Root canal, 450f
Root caries, 349, 351

Root planing
    definition of, 417
    stroke for, 421, 422t
Root surface, 440
Roseola, 90
Rotator cuff disorders, 395
Routing slips, 828
Rubella, 92t
Rule, 10
Rulemaking, 10
Russell periodontal index, 248
Rustogi modification of the Navy Plaque
        Index (RMNPI), 244t, 245f

S
Safety syringes, 530
Saliva
    in caries prevention, 347, 357t
    composition of, 275
    fluid intake to maintain, 275
    sealant failure caused by contamination
        from, 367
Saliva substitutes, 683, 766
Salivary diagnostics, 713
Salivary flow
    rate of, 347, 348b
    testing of, 357t–358t
Salivary glands
    in elderly, 765
    swelling of, 675, 675f
Scaling, 417
Scaling and root planing (SRP)
    bacteria disruption caused by, 611
    clinical attachment levels affected
        by, 441
    definition of, 433
    goal of, 434
    indications for, 441
    instrumentation used in, 434
    lasers and, 437–438
Scaling stroke, 421, 422t
Scavenging nasal hood, 517, 517f
Scheduling of patients
    description of, 828–829
    elderly, 752
Schizophrenia, 637–638, 642t
School-age stage, 726t
School-based health clinics, 835
School nurses, 797
Schools, 797
Schwartz, Gary, 25
Scientific paper
    abstract portion of, 76
    acknowledgments section of, 77
    conflicts of interest disclosures in, 76–77
    discussion/conclusion section of, 76
    introduction section of, 76
    materials and methods section of, 76
    parts of, 76–77
    plagiarism in, 78, 78t
    references section of, 77, 77t
    results section of, 76
    title of, 76
    writing of, 77–78
Scleroderma (SC), 675, 677–679, 679t
Scoliosis, 651
Scopus, 75t
Screening
    domestic abuse, 744
    oral cancer, 183t, 685, 713

periodontal examination, 248
radiographs for, 182
Sealants
    air polishing of, 468
    autopolymerized, 365
    caries prevention using, 357t–358t
    classification of, 365t
    composition of, 365–366
    contraindications for, 366–367
    definition of, 365
    dental charting symbols for, 220t
    fillers added to, 365
    fluoride-releasing, 366
    four-handed delivery of, 367
    incipient caries and, 371–372
    indications for, 366–367
    mechanism of action, 366
    opaque, 365
    photopolymerized, 365
    pit and fissure, 366–367, 367f
    placement of, 367–371, 368f–370f
    replacement of, 371
    retention of, 371
    risk assessment before using, 366
    self-etching, 366
    tinted, 365
    tooth anatomy considerations for, 366, 367f
    tooth isolation for, 369, 371
    types of, 365t
    unfilled, 365
Second-degree burn, 811t
Second-degree heart block, 597
Secondary caries, 351
Secondary hemostasis, 595f
Secondary prevention, 86
Secondary progressive multiple sclerosis, 679
Secondary research, 75
Security Rule, of HIPAA, 18
Sedation. See Nitrous oxide/oxygen sedation
Seizure disorders, 136t, 813t–814t
Selective polishing, 461
Self-assessment, 561
Self-care
    devices for
        dental floss, 324–326, 325f
        dental floss holder, 325t, 327, 327f
        dental hygiene process of care and, 320t
        health-care claims on, 321
        interdental brush, 325–326, 327f
        interdental cleaning, 322–327, 323f–327f
        oral irrigator, 327f–329f, 327–330
        overview of, 319
        patient education about, 330–331
        technological advances in, 319
        toothbrushes. See Toothbrushes
        toothpicks, 327
        wood sticks, 326, 327f
    in hearing-loss patients, 630
    implants, 389
    oral appliances, 378
    prostheses, 378–379
Self-care disability, 582t
Self-determination, 12, 14t
Self-efficacy, 45–46, 568–569
Self-etching sealants, 366
Semicritical instruments and equipment, 107, 107t
Senescence, 754
Sensorineural hearing loss, 627t
Sensors, for digital radiography, 260, 262–263, 263f

Sensory disabilities
    Americans with Disabilities Act provisions for, 622
    description of, 582t, 621
    hearing loss. See Hearing loss
    vision impairment. See Vision impairment
Sensory nerves, 648f
Seroconversion, 88
Service animal, 625
Sex, gender versus, 737–738
Sex differences
    definition of, 737
    in dental decay, 745–746
Sex hormones, 665, 738–739
Sexually transmitted infections/diseases, 135t
Shade matching, 478
Shank
    description of, 418f, 418–419
    of files, 426, 428
Shared decision-making, 13
Sharpening, of instruments, 428–429
Sharpey's fibers, 193, 194t
Sharps disposal, 108
Shepherd hook explorer, 159t
Shingles, 89–90, 92t
Shock, 814t
Short-pulpal anesthesia, 531
Shoulder stretches, 402–403, 403f
Sicca syndrome, 675
Sickle(s)
    anterior, 423, 423f
    calculus removal stroke with, 422–423, 423f
    posterior, 423, 424f
    shank of, 419
    sharpening of, 429
Sickle cell anemia, 700
Sievert, 263
Sign language, 628–629, 631
Significant caries index, 243
Silness Löe Plaque Index, 244t, 245–246
Simple goiter, 668
Simplified portable units, 792
Simvastatin, 598t
Single-blind study, 74
Single-ended explorer, 158, 158f
Sinoatrial node, 593
Sinus bradycardia, 143
Sitting, 396, 398, 398f–399f
Sjögren syndrome, 622, 675f, 675–676
Skilled nursing facilities, 795
Skin. See also Integumentary system
    anatomy of, 757
    examination of, 177–178
    infections of, in elderly, 757
    lichen planus-related lesions of, 684, 684f
    petechiae of, 697
Skin cancer, 756
Skin care, 110
Sleep apnea, 666
Sliding board, 783
SMART format, 823
Smear layer, 450
Smokeless tobacco, 293, 451b
Smoking
    attachment loss secondary to, 292–293
    cancer risks, 709b, 715
    cessation of, 48–51, 49b, 569, 708
    chronic obstructive pulmonary disease secondary to, 615
    clinical findings associated with, 292b
    extrinsic stains caused by, 236

oral disease risks, 292f–293f, 292–293
oral squamous cell carcinoma risks, 172, 709b
periodontal disease risks, 58, 292f, 292–293, 558, 569
Snore guard, 376t, 377f
Social cognitive theory, 45
Social distance, 26, 26f
Social learning theory, 45
Social reinforcers, 728
Social trust, 14t, 18
Socioeconomic status, 235
Sodium fluoride varnish, 456, 479
Sodium hyaluronate, 711t
Sodium hypochlorite, 381t
Sodium perborate, 481
Soft drinks, 273
Soft palate, 182, 182f, 184t
Soft tissue–dental implant interface, 386–387
Somnolence, 649
Sonic scalers, 409
Sonography, 205
Spastic palsy, 651
Spasticity, 679
Spatter, 85
Spaulding classification scheme, 106
Special-needs patients. See also Disabilities
    behavioral management of, 586
    best practices in, 586–588
    biofilm in, 585
    caregiver involvement with, 583t, 584, 586
    caries risk assessment in, 585
    categories of, 582–583
    cognitive ability of, 583t, 584
    comorbidities in, 584–585
    cooperation level of, 583t, 584
    definition of, 581
    dental hygiene considerations for, 583t
    dental hygienist experience with, 583t, 585
    dental management of, 587–588
    desensitization of, 586
    health history of, 584
    health stability of, 583t, 584
    historical legislation for, 582
    hospital dentistry with general anesthesia for, 583t, 585
    immobilization of, 587
    last visit by, 583t, 585
    legal guardian for, 583t, 584
    local anesthesia for, 585
    management of, 583t, 583–586
    medical management of, 586–587
    medication use by, 583t, 584, 586
    mouth prop for, 587
    nitrous oxide in, 586
    office setting considerations for, 583t, 584–585
    office treatment decisions for, 583t
    oral sedation in, 585–587
    papoose boards for, 587
    periodontal risk assessment in, 585–586
    physician of, 584
    premedication for, 584
    preventative and disease management programs in, 587
    restriction devices for, 587
    stabilization of, 587
    statistics regarding, 581, 582f
    support staff experience with, 583t, 585
    terminology changes for, 581
    time management of appointment for, 586

treatment plan for, 587–588

visualization by, 586

Sphygmomanometer, 145145

Spina bifida (SB), 785

Spinal cord injury (SCI), 787

Spinal muscular atrophy, 776t, 785

Spinal rotation, 403, 404f

Spleen, 56, 56f

Splint, 376t

Spore tests, 105, 105f

Sports guard, 376t

Squamous cell carcinoma

oral. *See* Oral squamous cell carcinoma (OSCC)

pharyngeal, 172

Stable angina, 601

Staff

in dental anxiety and fear management, 499

experience of, with special-needs patients, 583t, 585

Stages of change model, 46

Staging of cancer, 707, 708t

Stain(s)

extrinsic

description of, 236, 338, 461

manual polishing removal of, 463–464

tooth whitening for, 483

intrinsic, 235–236, 461, 726

Staining, toluidine blue dye for, 183t, 184, 185t

Standard of care

definition of, 11

determination of, 11

legal obligation to adhere to, 306, 649, 803

nitrous oxide/oxygen sedation, 522

refusal of treatment that doesn't match, 13

Standard of practice, 11

Standard precautions, 85–86

Standards for Clinical Dental Hygiene Practice, 4, 11, 123, 298, 305, 308, 549, 554, 848

Standing, 399

Stannous fluoride, 349

Staphylococcus aureus, 92t

Startle reflex, 779t

State(s)

dental hygiene practice acts regulated by, 10

legislative processes of, 11

licensure regulation by, 10

State dental boards

functions of, 10, 11b

rulemaking authority of, 10

State licensing boards, 848

Static-air sterilizer, 106

Static sitting, 396

Statins, 696–697

Statistical significance, 75

Statutory law

civil law, 11–12

criminal law, 11

dental hygiene practice acts as, 10

Steam sterilization, 103, 105–106

Stem cells, 764

Stenosis, 604

Stensen duct, 180

Stent, 376t

Stephan curve, 347, 347f

Sterile surgeon gloves, 97

Sterilization

autoclaving, 105, 105f

biological indicators for, 105, 105f

chemical, 106–108

chemical indicators for, 104–105, 105f

chemical vapor, 106

definition of, 100

dry-heat, 106

moist heat: steam under pressure, 105–106

monitoring of, 104–105, 105f

of nitrous oxide/oxygen sedation equipment, 521

steam, 103, 105–106

Sterilization log, 112

Sternocleidomastoid muscle, 179, 179f, 184t

Stethoscope, 145

Stevens-Johnson syndrome, 685, 685f

Stillman tooth-brushing method, 323t

Stochastic effects, of ionizing radiation, 263

Stomatitis, denture, 383

Straight explorer, 159t

Street outreach, 797–798

Streptococcal Group A infection, 92t

Streptococcal pharyngitis, 600

Streptococcus mutans, 61, 231–232, 346

Streptococcus sanguinis, 231–232, 595

Streptococcus sobrinus, 346

Stress

cortisol release caused by, 667

periodontal disease associated with, 139

respiratory conditions affected by, 612

Stress response, 494–495

Stretches, 402–403, 403f

Stroke (cerebrovascular), 136t, 656–658, 691, 761t, 763–764, 814t

Strokes (instruments), 421–423, 422t

Subacute bacterial endocarditis, 594

Subacute infective endocarditis, 600

Subgingival calculus

biofilm caused by, 434, 595

description of, 231f, 232–233

removal of, 421

Subgingival temperature, 205–206

Submandibular triangle, 178–179, 179f, 183t

Submental triangle, 179, 179f, 183t

Subperiosteal implants, 385, 385t

Substance dependence and abuse

alcohol, 639t, 639–640, 641t

cannabis, 639t, 640, 641t

cocaine, 639t, 640, 641t

methamphetamines, 639t, 640, 641t

Sucrose, 346

Sudden cardiac death, 602

Sulcular tooth-brushing method, 323t

Sulcus depth, 199, 200f

Summative evaluation, 550t–553t, 554, 557

Superinfection, 88

Supervised neglect, 558

Supine hypotensive syndrome, 741

Suppuration, 197t, 202, 209t

Supraclavicular lymph nodes, 179, 180f, 184t

Supragingival calculus, 231f, 232–233, 338, 388, 568f, 570

Suprarenal gland. *See* Adrenal gland

Supraventricular tachycardia, 596t, 597

Supraversion, 227

Surface barriers, 100, 100f

Surfactants

in dentifrices, 336

description of, 100

in mouthrinses, 337

Surgical model, 723, 723t

Surgical pack, 442, 443f–444f

Sutures, 442, 444

Swivel tips, for power scaling devices, 411, 411f

Symbols, for dental charting, 219t–221t

Sympathetic nervous system, 494–495

Sympatholytics, 599t

Syncope, 809, 814t

Systemic desensitization, 505, 506b

Systemic diseases

cardiovascular diseases, 60–61

diabetes mellitus, 61–63

oral diseases and, connection between, 60–64, 555f, 560

periodontal diseases and, 55, 60–64, 296, 433

respiratory infections, 63–64

Systemic health, 567, 593–595

Systemic lupus erythematosus (SLE), 675, 681

Systemized Nomenclature of Dentistry (SNODENT), 826

Systolic blood pressure (SBP), 144, 666

T

T cells

cytotoxic, 674

description of, 56–57

development of, 674

in gingivitis, 60

helper, 60, 674, 683

regulatory, 60

Tachyarrhythmias, 143

Tachycardia, 143, 596, 596t, 653

Tachypnea, 144

Tactile finger spelling (TFS), 631

Tactile sign language (TSL), 631

Teeth. *See also* Dentition; *specific tooth entries*

anatomy of

description of, 449–450, 450f

sealant placement considerations for, 366, 367f

surfaces, 219f

avulsed, 814t

bleaching of, 452. *See also* Tooth whitening

cosmetic whitening of. *See* Tooth whitening

discoloration of, 482

in elderly, 767

eruption patterns for, 726t–727t

fracture of, 815t

malnutrition signs on, 272t

malposition of, 227

malrelations of, 225f–227f, 225–227

mandibular, 726t

maxillary, 726t

missing

charting of, 219, 220t

replacement of, 378

mixed, 726, 726t

mobility of, 197t, 202f, 202–203, 210t, 558

numbering systems for, 217, 217f–218f

permanent, 726, 727t

primary, 725–726, 726t

sensitivity reduction in, using dentifrices, 336, 340t

surfaces of, 219f

trauma to, 727–728

Telecommunications Act, 774t
Telecommunications device for the deaf (TDD), 629
Teletypewriter (TTY), 622, 629
Tell–Show–Do, 501, 728, 780
Temporary placement service, 837t
Temporomandibular disorders (TMDs), 739
Temporomandibular joint
  dysfunction of, 717–718
  palpation of, 178, 178f, 183t
Terminal shank, 419, 419f
Tertiary prevention, 86
Testes, 665
Testosterone, 665
Tetanus, diphtheria, pertussis vaccination, 109t
Tetracycline-related intrinsic stains, 235, 461, 483, 726
Theory of reasoned action/planned behavior, 45
Therapeutic polishing, 462
Thermometers
  body temperature measurement using, 142
  subgingival temperature measurement using, 205
Thickening agents, in dentifrices, 336
Thioridazine, 642t
Third-degree heart block, 597
Thoracic outlet syndrome, 395
Thoracic vertebrae, 787
Three-unit bridge, 379
Throat, health history review of, 131t
Thrombi, 696
Thrombocytopenia, 692–693, 702
Thrombogenic, 604
Thromboxane, 693
Thrombus, 595, 595f
Thymectomy, 676
Thymoma, 676
Thymus, 56, 56f
Thyroid cartilage, 179, 179f
Thyroid collar, 263–264
Thyroid disease, 135t
Thyroid disorders, 663, 668
Thyroid gland
  anatomy of, 663f, 664
  cancer of, 668
  palpation of, 179, 668
Thyroxine, 664
Tidal volume, 515
Tinnitus, 627–628, 756
Tinted sealants, 365
Tips, for power scaling devices
  care and maintenance of, 413
  types of, 410f–411f, 410–412
Tissue autofluorescence, 183t, 184
Tissue engineering, 387, 764
Tissue reflectance, 183t, 184, 185f
Titanium implants, 384
Titer, 88
Titration, 518, 520, 522
TNM staging, 175, 176b, 708t
Tobacco use
  in adolescents, 293, 739
  alcohol use and, 639
  attachment loss secondary to, 292–293
  cancer risks, 709b, 713f
  cessation of, 48–51, 49b, 139, 569, 708
  extrinsic stains caused by, 236, 483
  oral disease risks, 292f–293f, 292–293
  oral squamous cell carcinoma risks, 172

periodontal disease risks, 58, 292f, 292–293, 558, 567, 569, 595
  smokeless, 293
  tongue cancer caused by, 713f
  tooth whitening for stains caused by, 483
Toluidine blue dye, 183t, 184, 185t
Tomes fibers, 449
Tongue
  cancer of, 713, 713f
  dorsum of, 181, 181f
  in elderly, 765
  fissured, 169
  geographic, 169, 169f
  inspection of, 181, 181f, 184t
  malnutrition signs on, 272t
  palpation of, 181, 181f
  ventral surface of, 181–182
Tongue brushing, 322, 323f
"Tongue-tied." See Ankyloglossia
Tonic labyrinthine reflex, 779t
Tonsils
  anatomy of, 56, 56f
  inspection of, 182
  palpation of, 182, 184t
Tooth erosion
  basic erosive wear examination for, 452
  description of, 273
Tooth loss
  extractions as cause of, 767
  prevalence of, 375
  replacement options for, 378
  sex differences in, 745
Tooth mobility, 197t, 202f, 202–203, 210t, 558
Tooth numbering systems, 217, 217f–218f
Tooth whitening
  case study of, 485
  contraindications for, 482, 482b
  dental hygiene considerations for, 482
  description of, 336–337, 339t
  desensitizing agents used with, 483
  external methods of, 480–481
  fluorosis treated with, 483
  gingival irritation caused by, 482–483
  hypocalcification treated with, 483–484
  in-office methods of, 481, 481f
  indications for, 482
  informed consent for, 484
  internal, 481–482
  maintenance of, 482
  microabrasion and, 484
  oral examination before, 480
  over-the-counter products for, 480
  patient education about, 482, 484
  restorations affected by, 483
  side effects of, 482–483
  take-house methods of, 480f, 480–481
  tetracycline stains treated with, 483
  tobacco stains treated with, 483
  tooth sensitivity caused by, 482
  Van Haywood's approach to, 485
  Vita shade guide, 480, 480f
  whitening strips and gels for, 480f, 480–481
Toothbrushes
  Bass brushing method, 322, 322f, 323t
  bicycle handlebar grip for, 781, 781f
  brush selection, 321–322
  brushing methods and techniques, 322, 322f, 323t
  history of, 319
  industry standard for, 321–322
  manual, 319, 320f

modifications to, for physically impaired patients, 781, 781f
  power, 319–321, 321f, 597, 766
  scientific evidence about, 320–321
  sign language for, 629f
  usage of, 321–322, 322f
Toothpaste. See Dentifrices
Toothpicks, 327
Topical anesthesia, 533t, 533–534, 573
Topiramate, 643t
Torsoversion, 227
Tort law, 11–12
Torus mandibularis, 170
Torus palatinus, 170
Tracheobronchial tree, 614f
Trans-septal fibers, 192t
Transcription, 683
Transfer board, 651, 652f
Transgingival fibers, 192t
Transient ischemic attack (TIA), 136t
Transillumination, 156
Transmissible diseases, 85–86
Transosteal implants, 385, 385t
Transplantation, 686
Transportation, for elderly, 752–753
Transtheoretical model, 46
Trauma
  dental, 727–728
  occlusal, 202
  in physically impaired patients, 778t
  prevention of, 805
Traumatic brain injury (TBI), 786–787
Traumatic fibroma, 170
Treatment
  algorithm for, 571f
  costs of, 310
  nonsurgical. See Nonsurgical periodontal therapy
  patient compliance with, 556
  refusal of, 13, 42, 313, 728f
  self-care devices for. See Self-care, devices for
  surgical. See Periodontal surgery
Treatment outcomes, 557–558
Treatment plans
  case examples of, 310–312
  description of, 4, 305
  determinants of, 308
  esthetic dentistry, 484–485
  as expressed contracts, 12
  financial implications section of, 310
  format of, 309–310
  four-prong approach to, 310, 310t–311t
  individualized, 309
  informed consent for, 313, 571–572
  for special-needs patients, 587–588
  Standards for Clinical Dental Hygiene Practice requirements for, 308
  three-prong approach to, 310
  treatment options included in, 310
  treatment risks and benefits included in, 310
Tremors, 655, 779t
Tricalcium phosphate, 350
Triclosan, 110–111, 336
Tricyclic antidepressants, 531
Trigeminal nerve
  local anesthesia of, 527–530, 528f–529f
  mandibular branch of, 529, 529f
  maxillary branch of, 528f, 528–529
  ophthalmic branch of, 527–528, 528f

Trigger points, 396
Triiodothyronine, 664, 668
Triple-bend tips, for power scaling devices, 412, 412f
Trismus, 544
Tropic hormones, 664
Trust, 18, 822
Tubercle bacillus, 90
Tuberculin skin test (TST), 91
Tuberculosis, 134t
   definition of, 617
   description of, 90–91, 91t–92t
   infection-control plan for, 112
   latent, 617
   purified protein derivative test for, 617–618
   screening for, 617–618
   symptoms of, 617
   transmission of, 617
Tumor
   benign, 707
   grading of, 707–708
   malignant, 707
   metastatic, 707
   pituitary, 667
Tumor necrosis factor alpha
   description of, 57–58
   insulin resistance and, 62
Turesky Modification of Quigley-Hein Plaque Index (TMQHPI), 246
24-hour recall, 275, 275t
Twinrix, 87
Two-way communication, 25, 26t, 497

U
Ulcers, 134t
Ultrasonic cleaners
   description of, 104
   oral appliance cleaning using, 381
   prosthesis cleaning using, 381
Ultrasonic instruments
   aerosols caused by, 612
   chronic obstructive pulmonary disease as contraindication for use of, 617
   diamond-coated, 439
   periodontal endoscope, 439
   scaling and root planing using, 434
Ultrasonic scalers, 409f, 409–411, 597
Ultrasonic scaling, for biofilm removal, 377, 378f
Uncertainty/avoidance index (UAI), 34t–35t, 35
Uncontrollability, 493, 494f
Underjet, 226, 226f
Unfilled sealants, 365
Unintentional torts, 11
Universal curets
   for anterior teeth, 425, 425b
   calculus removal stroke, 424, 424b
   for posterior teeth, 425, 426b
   sharpening of, 429
Universal instruments, 418
Universal numbering system, 217, 217f
Universal precautions, 85, 702
Unpredictability, 493, 494f
Unstable angina, 601
Upper body stretches, 403f–404f, 403–404
Upper motor neurons (UMNs), 787
Upper trunk extension, 403
Urinary system, age-related changes in, 755
Urticaria, 810t

U.S. Food and Drug Administration, 94, 94t
U.S. Public Health Service (USPHS), 835
Usher syndrome, 630
Usual, customary, and reasonable (UCR) fee plan, 825
Utility gloves, 97

V
Vaccinations
   chickenpox, 90, 109t
   definition of, 56
   for dental health-care personnel, 109t
   hepatitis A, 87–88
   shingles, 90
Validity, 76, 249
Valproic acid, 642t
Values
   core. See Core values
   definition of, 12
Valvular heart disease, 604–605
Varicella zoster virus (VZV)
   description of, 89–90, 92t
   vaccination for, 109t
Varnish
   chlorhexidine, 349
   fluoride, 479, 731–732
   sodium fluoride, 456
Vasoconstrictors, 531, 531t–532t, 544t
Vegetables, 281t–282t
VELscope Vx, 685
Veneer
   composite, 477–478
   porcelain, 476–478
Venlafaxine, 642t
Ventricles, of heart, 593, 593f
Ventricular fibrillation, 596t, 597
Ventricular septal defect, 603, 604f
Ventricular tachycardia, 596t, 597
Ventriculoatrial shunt, 785
Ventriculoperitoneal shunt, 785
Veracity
   definition of, 14t
   description of, 16
   example of, 14t
Verbal communication, 25–26
Vertebra, 787
Vertical bitewing radiographs, 257, 568
Vertical releasing incisions, 442
Vertical transmission, 351
Vesicle, 176t
Viral hepatitis. See Hepatitis
Viridans streptococci, 600
Virtual dentistry, 653
Vision (dental practice), 822–823
Vision impairment
   causes of, 622, 623t–624t
   in children, 622, 624
   communication methods for, 624–625
   deaf-blind patients, 630–631
   dental hygiene considerations for, 626, 627b
   dental office access provisions, 625b
   in elderly, 621, 756
   guiding and seating patients with, 625, 626b
   large-print materials for, 625
   local anesthetic administration considerations, 626
   oral clinical findings in, 622
   oral self-care instruction for, 626–627

   patient factors associated with, 622, 624
   prevalence of, 621
VITA Easyshade Advance shade matching, 478
Vita shade guide, 480, 480f
Vital signs
   blood pressure, 144–147
   body mass index, 140, 141t
   body temperature, 142
   height, 140, 141t
   pulse, 143–144
   respiration, 144
   weight, 140, 141t
Vital tissue staining, 183t, 184–185
Vitamin B12 deficiency, 699, 755
Vitamin K, 695–696
Voice, 177–178
Volpe-Manhold Index (VMI), 241, 244t, 246
von Willebrand disease, 697–698

W
"Walking bleach" technique, 481
Wand, 530
Wand anesthesia, 478
Wandering rash of the tongue, 169
Warfarin, 605, 657, 695–696, 763
Waste
   disposal of, 108
   laboratory, 102
   medical, 108, 112
   office management plan for, 108
Water flosser, 327, 328f–329f, 329
Water lines, dental unit, 102
Wavelength, 255
Weight, 140, 141t
Wellness
   definition of, 41
   functional ability and, 41
   health versus, 41
   optimal, 42
   patient's responsibility for, 41
Wellness mode, 791
Wheelchair
   etiquette for, 777
   oral hygiene considerations for patients in, 781, 782f
   transfer from, 779t, 782–784
White blood cell disorders, 701–702
"White clots," 691
White-coat syndrome, 500b
Whitening, tooth
   case study of, 485
   contraindications for, 482, 482b
   dental hygiene considerations for, 482
   description of, 336–337, 339t
   desensitizing agents used with, 483
   external methods of, 480–481
   fluorosis treated with, 483
   gingival irritation caused by, 482–483
   hypocalcification treated with, 483–484
   in-office methods of, 481, 481f
   indications for, 482
   informed consent for, 484
   internal, 481–482
   maintenance of, 482
   microabrasion and, 484
   oral examination before, 480
   over-the-counter products for, 480
   patient education about, 482, 484
   restorations affected by, 483

side effects of, 482–483
take-house methods of, 480f, 480–481
tetracycline stains treated with, 483
tobacco stains treated with, 483
tooth sensitivity caused by, 482
Van Haywood's approach to, 485
Vita shade guide, 480, 480f
whitening strips and gels for, 480f, 480–481
Wickham striae, 684, 684f
Williams probe, 161f
Wisdom teeth, 726, 727t
Women
bone loss in, 742–743
dental decay in, 745–746
domestic violence in, 744
gastroesophageal reflux disease in, 739
gingivitis in, 738
interconceptual counseling for, 739–740
life cycles of, 738
menopause in, 742–743
menstruation in, 739
osteoporosis in, 742–743
preconception counseling for, 739–740
pregnancy. *See* Pregnancy

puberty in, 738
tooth loss in, 745
Wood sticks, 326, 327f
Work practice controls, 94–95
Working ends, of instruments
cutting edge of, 419f, 420
design of, 418f–419f, 418–419
Gracey curets, 420, 420f, 426
identification of, 420, 420f
Workplace, 798
World Health Organization (WHO)
global health-care systems ranking by, 42
health as defined by, 41
health promotion as defined by, 42
significant caries index, 243
Wrist extensor exercise, 402, 402f
Wrist flexor exercises, 402, 402f
Wrist motion activation, of instruments, 421
Written communication, 25–26

X

X-rays, 255–256. *See also* Radiographs
Xerophthalmia, 675

Xerostomia
antihypertensive drugs as cause of, 600
caries risk associated with, 296, 355, 717
diabetes mellitus and, 295
diet affected by, 273
in elderly, 761t, 765
fluid imbalance and, 275
fluoride treatments in patients with, 827
in HIV/AIDS patients, 683
medication-induced, 296, 366, 585, 600, 655, 751, 766
mouthrinses for, 337
radiation therapy as cause of, 701
saliva substitutes for, 683, 717, 766
in Sjögren syndrome, 675f
Xylitol, 350, 357t, 675–676, 681, 742

Y

Yellow stain, 236t

Z

Ziprasidone, 642t